Kellie May
40702 County Road 26
Scottsbluff, NE 69361-6912

EXCLUSIVE ADA STUDENT MEMBERSHIP

JOIN THE ADA AT THE STUDENT RATE OF ONLY $43 ANNUALLY AND RECEIVE A FREE COPY OF *THE HEALTH PROFESSIONAL'S GUIDE TO POPULAR DIETARY SUPPLEMENTS*

Informational card must be returned to be eligible for this special ADA offer

BEGIN YOUR FUTURE IN

GET CONNECTED AND STAY INFORMED

Information

Scientific and practical information you need for career success

- *Journal of the American Dietetic Association*
  Learn about new research, practice information, and industry and association news in this monthly peer-reviewed scientific journal.

- *Scientific Summaries*
  Access through the member-only Web site to ADA's Scientific Summaries addressing the "hot" research studies in the five priority emerging areas including Obesity, Complementary Care and Dietary Supplements, Retail Food, and Human Genome and Biotechnology.

- *Dietetics in Practice*
  Enhance your knowledge and skills in a variety of practice areas with this easy-to-use quarterly newsletter. Features include Industry News and Washington Wire, short summaries of current research, and cutting edge references and other sources of hard-to-find information.

- *Member-Only Pricing*
  Member-only pricing discounts on books, client and consumer education publications; registration for the Food & Nutrition Conference & Exhibition; and other ADA products and services.

- *ADA's Member-Only Web Site: www.eatright.org*
  Features include the online version of the *Journal of the American Dietetic Association*, and news about the association's strategic actions. The general Web site offers a variety of other valuable resources including links to affiliate dietetic associations.

- *Access to PubMed*
  A service of the National Library of Medicine, PubMed provides access to more than 11 million citations from Med-Line and additional life science journals.

- *Member Service Center*
  The ADA Member Service Center provides streamlined communications with ADA, via a live voice answering the ADA telephones, for your routine questions, dues payments, or to place catalog orders.

- *ADA's Student Services*
  Student Center Web site provides student members with a comprehensive and up-to-date list of resources to assist them in learning about the profession as well as planning and building their careers. The member-only Web site offers an e-group, which is a threaded chat for students to share ideas and thoughts as well as ask practitioners questions. *Student News*, an online newsletter, keeps students informed of current trends and professional issues. Ongoing communications with national Student Dietetics Clubs regarding ADA activities and practice updates. FNCE Student Track designed specifically for dietetics students to network with each other and educators, to learn about career options and plan for their future in dietetics.

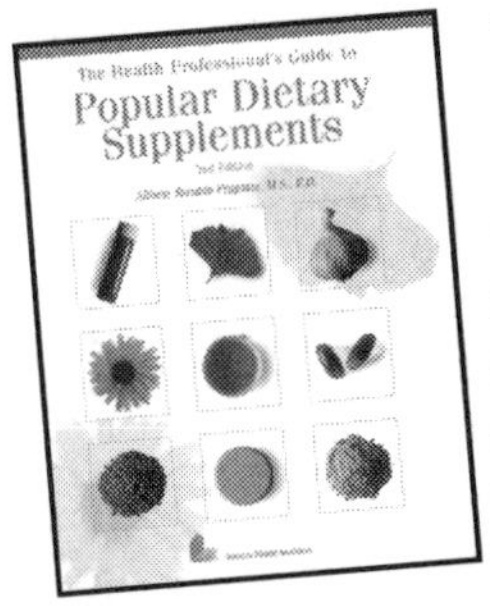

Yours Free with Membership

The Health Professional's Guide to Popular Dietary Supplements

More than 70 vitamins, minerals, amino acids, ergogenics, herbals, enzymes, and other supplements are covered in this new guide.

☐ **Yes! I would like to become an ADA Student Member and receive my complimentary copy of *The Health Professional's Guide to Popular Dietary Supplements***

P9-BZO-992

Name: ______________________

Address: ______________________

College/University : ______________________

City: ______________________

State: __________ Zip Code: __________

Phone: ______________________

Email: ______________________

AMERICAN DIETETIC ASSOCIATION

Tracking # HADA09107

EXCLUSIVE ADA STUDENT MEMBERSHIP

JOIN THE ADA AT THE STUDENT RATE OF ONLY $43 ANNUALLY AND RECEIVE A FREE COPY OF *THE HEALTH PROFESSIONAL'S GUIDE TO POPULAR DIETARY SUPPLEMENTS*

Informational card must be returned to be eligible for this special ADA offer

Education

Learn valuable information through conferences, workshops, journal articles, and the online education center

- *Annual Food & Nutrition Conference and Exhibition*
  Broaden your knowledge and skills while connecting with your peers at this conference, which offers more than 100 cutting-edge education programs and networking functions. Receive member rates for conference registration as well as special member prices at the ADA Bookstore.

- *Scholarships*
  See your profession continue to grow through the American Dietetic Association Foundation scholarship program that encourages eligible students to enter the field and helps dietetics professionals enhance their career.

- *ADA's Education Opportunities*
  ADA offers many education opportunities via the annual Food and Nutrition Conference, educational articles in the *Journal of the American Dietetic Association* and through the many publications listed in the Products and Services Catalog. These opportunities allow dietetics students and professionals to be on the cutting edge of their profession and to be ready for their next career opportunity.

- *ADA's Book & Publication Catalog*
  Turn to this resource for the latest in peer-reviewed and practice-related professional materials as well as a vast array of client and consumer education publications. Receive member-preferred pricing on publications and other ADA products and services.

- *Virtual Reality Bookstore*
  Choose from 75,000 book and software titles as well as expert reviews on the member-only Web site. Access more than 15,000 book reviews based on your member profile on the member-only Web site.

Networking

An active community of professionals sharing knowledge, skills and ideas.

- *Affiliate Dietetic Associations*
  Build partnerships and network with your colleagues at the state and district level. All ADA members receive automatic membership in an affiliate (state) association of their choice.

- *Dietetic Practice Groups*
  Gain insight into specialized areas of food and nutrition, and network with your colleagues. Enroll in one or more of these 28 different practice groups.

  - Clinical Nutrition Management
  - Consultant Dietitians in Health Care Facilities
  - Diabetes Care and Education
  - Dietetic Educators of Practitioners
  - Dietetic Technicians in Practice
  - Dietetics in Developmental and Psychiatric Disorders
  - Dietetics in Physical Medicine and Rehabilitation
  - Dietitians in Business and Communication
  - Dietitians in General Clinical Practice
  - Dietitians in Nutrition Support
  - Food and Culinary Professionals
  - Gerontological Nutritionists
  - HIV/AIDS
  - Hunger and Environmental Nutrition
  - Management in Food and Nutrition Systems
  - Nutrition Education for the Public
  - Nutrition Educators of Health Professionals
  - Nutrition Entrepreneurs
  - Nutrition in Complementary Care
  - Oncology Nutrition
  - Pediatric Nutrition
  - Public Health/Community Nutrition
  - Renal Dietitians
  - Research
  - School Nutrition Services
  - Sports, Cardiovascular, and Wellness Nutrition
  - Vegetarian Nutrition
  - Women and Reproductive Nutrition

- *Leadership Opportunities*
  Leadership opportunities are also available to members who choose to become involved. Progression responsibilities as a volunteer can also positively support a professional in their work roles.

* *Exclusive ADA Student Membership price is valid until December 2005. Payment to be made in US Dollars*

** *In order to be eligible for this promotional offer, you must become an ADA Student Member.*

Discovering **Nutrition**

NO POSTAGE NECESSARY IF MAILED IN THE UNITED STATES

BUSINESS REPLY MAIL
FIRST-CLASS MAIL PERMIT NO 40 SUDBURY MA

POSTAGE WILL BE PAID BY ADDRESSEE

ATTN: MARKETING DEPARTMENT
JONES AND BARTLETT PUBLISHERS
40 TALL PINE DRIVE
SUDBURY MA 01776-9849

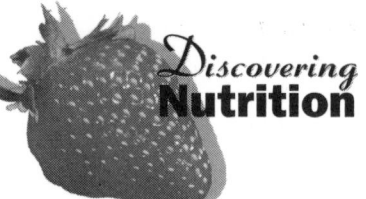

Life stage group	Choline (mg/d)	Calcium (mg/d)	Phosphorus (mg/d)	Magnesium (mg/d)	Iron (mg/d)	Zinc (mg/d)	Selenium (μg/d)	Iodine (μg/d)	Copper (μg/d)	Manganese (mg/d)	Fluoride (mg/d)	Chromium (μg/d)	Molybdenum (μg/d)
Infants													
0-6 mo	125*	210*	100*	30*	0.27*	2*	15*	110*	200*	0.003*	0.01*	0.2*	2*
7-12 mo	150*	270*	275*	75*	11	3	20*	130*	220*	0.6*	0.5*	5.5*	3*
Children													
1-3 y	200*	500*	460	80	7	3	20	90	340	1.2*	0.7*	11*	17
4-8 y	250*	800*	500	130	10	5	30	90	440	1.5*	1*	15*	22
Males													
9-13 y	375*	1,300*	1,250	240	8	8	40	120	700	1.9*	2*	25*	34
14-18 y	550*	1,300*	1,250	410	11	11	55	150	890	2.2*	3*	35*	43
19-30 y	550*	1,000*	700	400	8	11	55	150	900	2.3*	4*	35*	45
31-50 y	550*	1,000*	700	420	8	11	55	150	900	2.3*	4*	35*	45
51-70 y	550*	1,200*	700	420	8	11	55	150	900	2.3*	4*	30*	45
>70 y	550*	1,200*	700	420	8	11	55	150	900	2.3*	4*	30*	45
Females													
9-13 y	375*	1,300*	1,250	240	8	8	40	120	700	1.6*	2*	21*	34
14-18 y	400*	1,300*	1,250	360	15	9	55	150	890	1.6*	3*	24*	43
19-30 y	425*	1,000*	700	310	18	8	55	150	900	1.8*	3*	25*	45
31-50 y	425*	1,000*	700	320	18	8	55	150	900	1.8*	3*	25*	45
51-70 y	425*	1,200*	700	320	8	8	55	150	900	1.8*	3*	20*	45
>70 y	425*	1,200*	700	320	8	8	55	150	900	1.8*	3*	20*	45
Pregnancy													
≤18 y	450*	1,300*	1,250	400	27	13	60	220	1,000	2.0*	3*	29*	50
19-30 y	450*	1,000*	700	350	27	11	60	220	1,000	2.0*	3*	30*	50
31-50 y	450*	1,000*	700	360	27	11	60	220	1,000	2.0*	3*	30*	50
Lactation													
≤18 y	550*	1,300*	1,250	360	10	14	70	290	1,300	2.6*	3*	44*	50
19-30 y	550*	1,000*	700	310	9	12	70	290	1,300	2.6*	3*	45*	50
31-50 y	550*	1,000*	700	320	9	12	70	290	1,300	2.6*	3*	45*	50

Sources: Data compiled from *Dietary Reference Intakes for Calcium, Phosphorus, Magnesium, Vitamin D, and Fluoride.* Washington, DC: National Academy Press; 1997. *Dietary Reference Intakes for Thiamin, Riboflavin, Niacin, Vitamin B_6, Folate, Vitamin B_{12}, Pantothenic Acid, Biotin, and Choline.* Washington, DC: National Academy Press; 1998. *Dietary Reference Intakes for Vitamin C, Vitamin E, Selenium, and Carotenoids.* Washington, DC: National Academy Press; 2000. *Dietary Reference Intakes for Vitamin A, Vitamin K, Arsenic, Boron, Chromium, Copper, Iron, Manganese, Molybdenum, Nickel, Silicon, Vanadium, and Zinc.* Washington, DC: National Academy Press; 2001. These reports may be accessed via http://nap.edu.

Discovering Nutrition

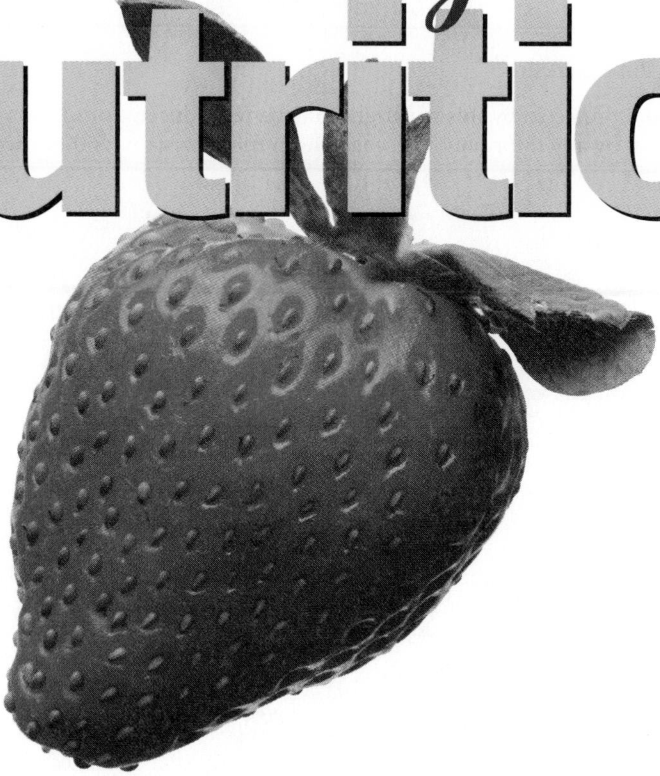

Paul Insel
Stanford University

R. Elaine Turner
University of Florida

Don Ross
California Institute of Human Nutrition

AMERICAN DIETETIC ASSOCIATION

JONES AND BARTLETT PUBLISHERS
Sudbury, Massachusetts
BOSTON TORONTO LONDON SINGAPORE

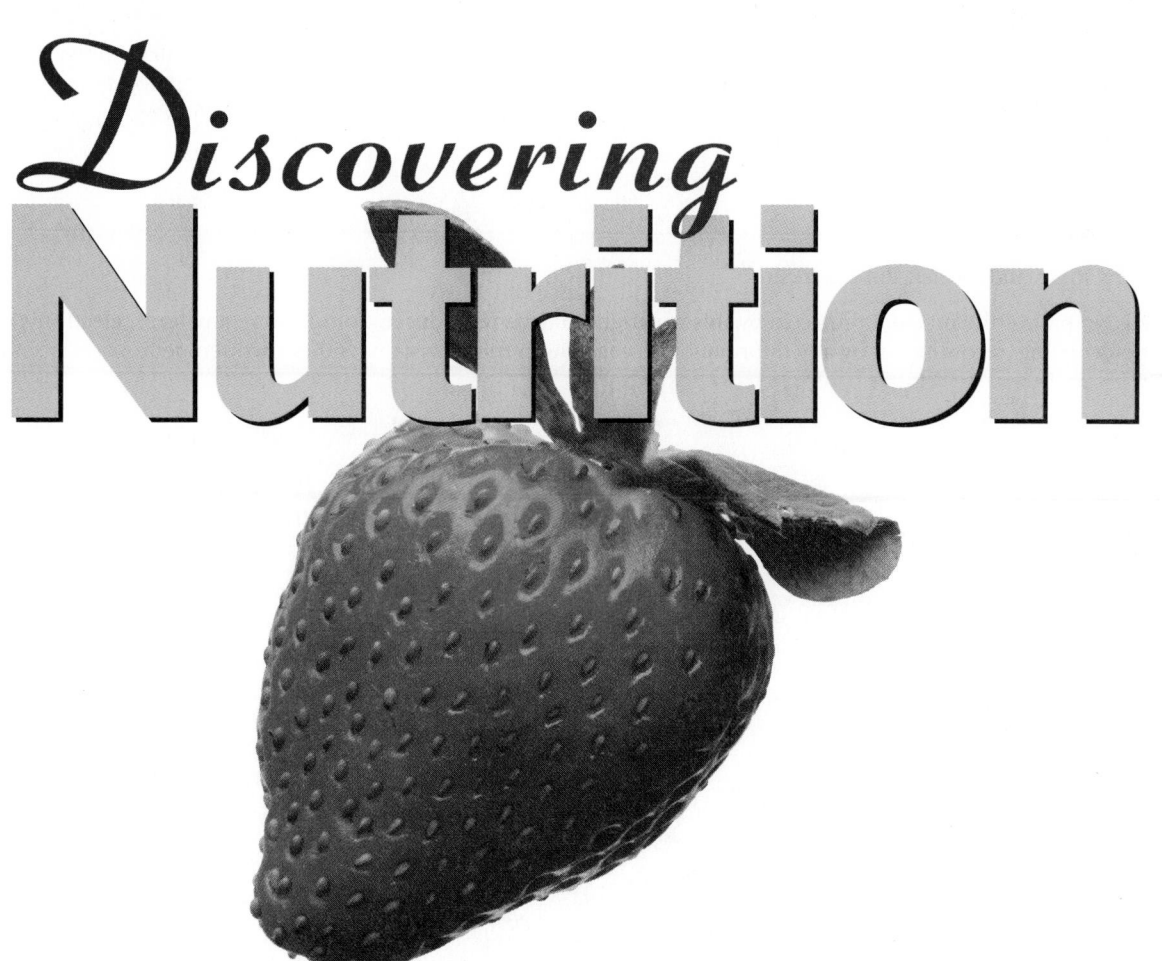

World Headquarters
Jones and Bartlett Publishers
40 Tall Pine Drive
Sudbury, MA 01776
978-443-5000
info@jbpub.com
http://health.jbpub.com

Jones and Bartlett Publishers Canada
2406 Nikanna Road
Mississauga, ON L5C 2W6
CANADA

Jones and Bartlett Publishers International
Barb House, Barb Mews
London W6 7PA
UK

Production Credits

Chief Executive Officer: Clayton Jones
Chief Operating Officer: Don W. Jones, Jr.
Executive V.P. & Publisher: Robert W. Holland, Jr.
V.P., Design and Production: Anne Spencer
V.P., Manufacturing and Inventory Control: Therese Bräuer
Director, Sales and Marketing: William Kane
Editor-in-Chief: J. Michael Stranz
Acquisitions Editor: Kristin L. Ellis
Production Editor: Julie C. Bolduc
Editorial Assistant: Corinne G. Hudson
Senior Marketing Manager: Nathan J. Schultz
Director of Interactive Technology: Adam Alboyadjian
Web Site Designer: Kristin E. Ohlin
Interactive Technology Associate: Dawn Mahon-Priest
Text Design: Studio Montage
Illustration: Imagineering Scientific and Technical Artwork, Studio Montage, and Nesbitt Graphics
Composition: Nesbitt Graphics, Inc.
Copyediting: Cindy Kogut, Editorial Ink
Cover Design: Anne Spencer
Cover Photo: © Betty Sederquist
Printing and Binding: Courier Companies
Cover Printing: Lehigh Press

Dedication

To Philip and Claire with love and toyfuls.

To Allen, Mitchell, and Teddy for their love, patience, and understanding.

To Donna and Mackinnon, the true stars who nourish my spirit.

Library of Congress Cataloging-in-Publication Data

Insel, Paul M.
Discovering nutrition / Paul Insel, R. Elaine Turner, Don Ross; technical review by the American Dietetic Association.
p. ; cm.
Includes bibliographical references and index.
ISBN 0-7637-0910-7 (pbk. : alk. paper)
1. Nutrition.
[DNLM: 1. Nutrition. 2. Diet. QU 145 I5955d 2003] I. Turner, R. Elaine. II. Ross, Don, 1952- III. American Dietetic Association. IV. Title.
QP141 .I628 2003
613.2—dc21

2002009854

Printed in the United States of America
06 05 04 03 02   10 9 8 7 6 5 4 3 2 1

The material in this book has been technically reviewed by the American Dietetic Association.

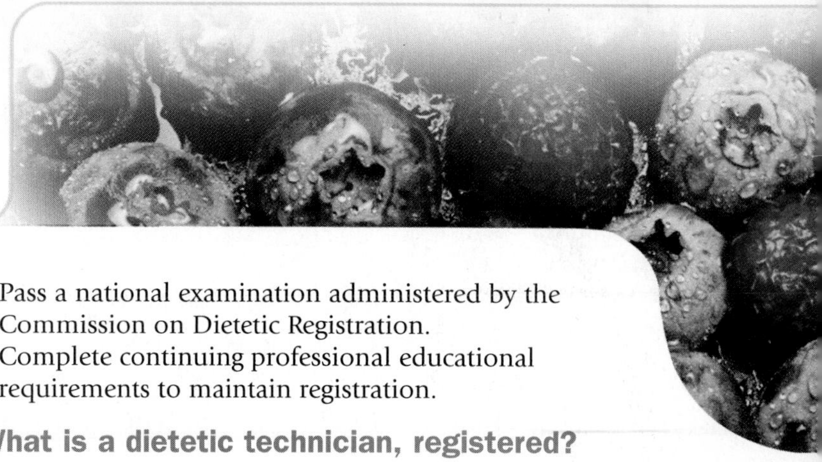

American Dietetic Association
216 W. Jackson Blvd.
Chicago, IL 60606
(800) 877-1600

www.eatright.org

With nearly 70,000 members, the American Dietetic Association is the nation's largest organization of food and nutrition professionals.

ADA was founded in Cleveland, Ohio, in 1917 by a visionary group of women, led by ADA's first president, Lulu C. Graves, and co-founder Lenna F. Cooper, who were dedicated to helping the government conserve food and improve the American public's health and nutrition during World War I.

Members

Approximately 75 percent of ADA's members are registered dietitians (RDs) and four percent are dietetic technicians, registered (DTRs). Other ADA members include clinical and community dietetics professionals, consultants, foodservice managers, educators, researchers, dietetic technicians, and students.

ADA members represent a wide range of practice areas and special interests, including public health; sports nutrition; medical nutrition therapy; nutrition counseling for weight control, cholesterol reduction, diabetes, heart and kidney disease, and many other health concerns; foodservice management in business, hospitals, restaurants, long-term care facilities, and education systems; education of other health-care professionals; and scientific research. Members can also join 28 special interest or dietetic practice groups.

What is a registered dietitian?

A registered dietitian is a food and nutrition expert who has met the minimum academic and professional requirements to qualify for the credential "RD." In addition to RD credentialing, many states have laws that regulate the licensure or credentialing of dietitians and nutrition practitioners. Frequently these state requirements are met through the same education and training required to become an RD.

Registered dietitians must:

- Complete at least a bachelor's degree and course work approved by ADA's Commission on Accreditation for Dietetics Education.
- Complete an accredited and supervised experiential practice program at a health-care facility, community agency, or foodservice corporation.
- Pass a national examination administered by the Commission on Dietetic Registration.
- Complete continuing professional educational requirements to maintain registration.

What is a dietetic technician, registered?

Dietetic technicians, registered (DTRs), often working in partnership with registered dietitians, screen, evaluate and educate patients; provide guidance in prevention of diseases such as diabetes and obesity; and monitor the progress of a patient or client. DTRs provide expert assistance in hospices, home health-care programs, day-care centers, foodservice operations, government, and community programs such as Meals on Wheels.

Dietetic technicians, registered must:

- Complete at least a two-year associate's degree in an approved dietetics technology program from an accredited U.S. college or university.
- Complete a minimum of 450 hours of supervised practice experience in community programs, health care, and foodservice facilities.
- Pass a nationwide examination and continuing education courses throughout their careers.

Commission on Dietetic Registration

The Commission on Dietetic Registration, the credentialing agency for ADA, awards credentials at entry, fellow, and specialty levels to individuals who have met its standards for competency to practice in the profession, including successful completion of its national certification examination and recertification by continuing professional education and/or examination.

Start thinking now about a career in dietetics

Within the field of dietetics, you can choose to be either a registered dietician (RD) or a dietetic technician, registered (DTR). Whichever option you choose, you'll share your knowledge of food and nutrition to help people make healthful food choices.

Scholarship information

The American Dietetic Association Foundation (ADAF) offers scholarships to encourage eligible students to enter the field of dietetics. Once you are enrolled in a college dietetics program accredited by the Commission on Accreditation for Dietetics Education you may be eligible for an ADAF scholarship.

Brief Contents

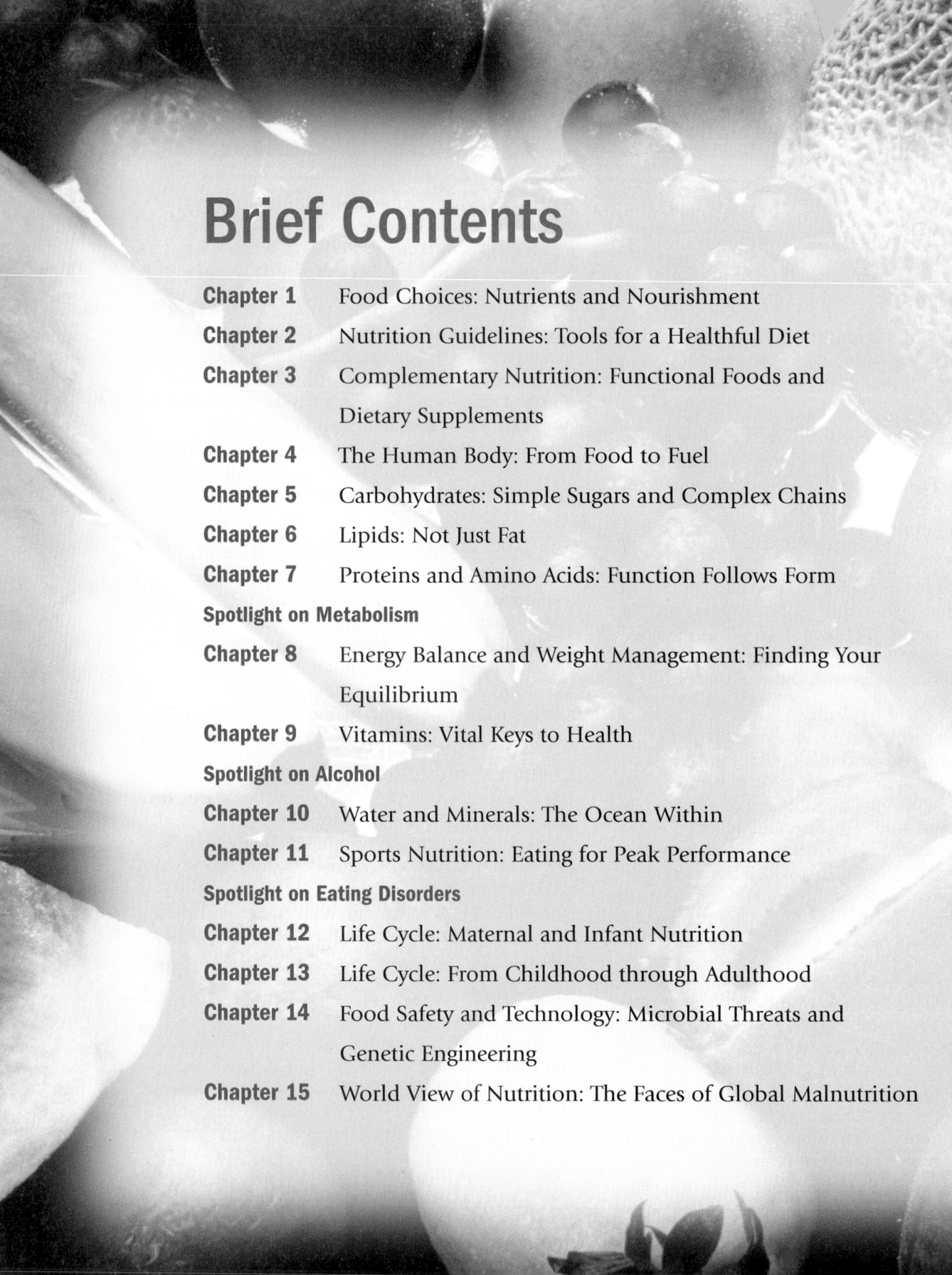

Table of Contents

Preface

Learning nutrition can be exciting and understandable. Our new book, *Discovering Nutrition,* takes students on a fascinating journey beginning, perhaps, with curiosity and ending, we hope, with a solid knowledge base and a healthy dose of skepticism for the endless ads and infomercials promoting "new" diets and food products. We want students to learn enough about their nutritional and health status to use this new knowledge in their everyday lives. Our mission is to give students the tools to interpret more logically the nutrition information provided by the evening news, on food labels, in popular magazines, and by government agencies. Our goal is to help them become sophisticated consumers of both nutrients and nutrition information. Hopefully, students will come to understand that knowledge of nutrition allows them to personalize information, rather than follow every guideline issued for an entire population.

Discovering Nutrition is unique in its behavioral approach. It challenges students to act, not just memorize the material. Familiar experiences and choices draw students into each chapter and analogies illuminate difficult concepts.

In addition, we address important questions that students often raise concerning such issues as ethnic diets, functional foods, nutrient supplements, phytochemicals, vegetarianism, diets for athletes, food safety, and fad diets. We focus attention on alcohol, eating disorders, and complementary nutrition. Some instructors may wish to cover metabolism so we included a Spotlight on Metabolism to provide a friendly tour of the metabolic pathways. Throughout the book, the relationship of diet and health is incorporated into appropriate chapters (e.g., lipids and cardiovascular disease, carbohydrates and diabetes).

Nutrition research shows that people often respond idiosyncratically to food. Some of us, for example, find that we can liberally salt our food with no effect on our blood pressure. Others who are salt sensitive find that even a small amount of salt sends their systolic blood pressure soaring. *Discovering Nutrition* brings up-to-date nutritional research into your class. It features the latest standards, such as the recent releases of Dietary Reference Intakes, guidelines from the National Cholesterol Education Program, and the *HealthierUS* initiative. *Discovering Nutrition* provides students with tools, such as the ancillary diet analysis software, to track and analyze their personal nutrient intakes. In addition, the book's web site, http://nutrition.jbpub.com/discovering, offers access to the constantly emerging developments in nutrition.

Presidential 2002 *HealthierUS* Initiative

Increasing personal fitness and becoming healthier is critical to achieving a better and longer life. Extensive research has shown that improving overall health, and thus preventing disease and premature death, is as easy as making small adjustments and improvements in the activities of daily life. The Presidential *HealthierUS* initiative uses the resources of the federal government to alert Americans to the vital health benefits of simple and modest improvements in physical activity, nutrition, and behavior. To achieve optimal health and nutrition, *Discovering Nutrition* delivers the tools for students to follow the *HealthierUS* initiative and incorporate positive behavior changes in their everyday lives.

Accessible Science

Discovering Nutrition makes use of the latest in learning theory and balances the behavioral aspects of nutrition with an accessible approach to scientific concepts. You will find the book to be a comprehensive resource that communicates nutrition both graphically and personally.

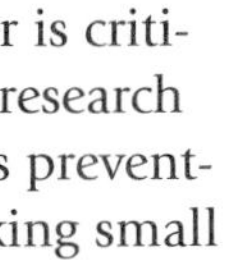

We present technical concepts in an engaging, non-intimidating way with an appealing, stepwise, parallel development of text and annotated illustrations. Illustrations in all chapters use consistent representations. Each type of nutrient, for example, has a distinct color and shape. Icons of

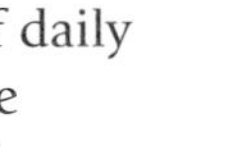

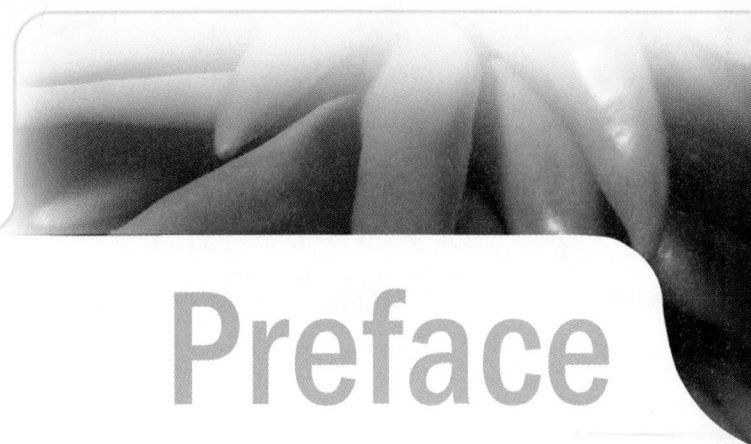

an amino acid, a protein, a triglyceride, and a glucose molecule represent "characters" in the nutrition story and are instantly recognizable as they appear throughout the book.

This textbook is unique in the field of nutrition and leads the way in depicting important biological and physiological phenomena, such as emulsification, glucose regulation, digestion and absorption, and fetal development. Extensive graphic presentations make nutrition and physiological principles come alive. The illustrations use pictures to teach and are part of a multimedia package that coordinates the text with illustrations and software. The EatRight Analysis and the Be Healthy Version 4.0 software programs are fully integrated ancillaries designed to help students track their diets, make choices, and hone their nutritional skills.

In addition to these strengths, the contents of this book have been technically reviewed by the American Dietetic Association, the nation's largest organization of food and nutrition professionals with more than 70,000 members.

The Pedagogy

Discovering Nutrition focuses on teaching behavioral change, personal decision making, and up-to-date scientific concepts in a number of novel ways. The interactive approach that addresses different learning styles makes it the ideal text to ensure a high likelihood of success by students. Beginning with Chapter 1, the material engages students in considering their own behavior in light of the knowledge they are gaining. The pedagogical aids that appear in most chapters include:

Think About It questions at the beginning of each chapter present realistic nutrition-related situations and ask the students to consider how they would behave in such circumstances.

The **Key to Illustrations** at the beginning of each chapter identifies the icons students will encounter throughout the book. These *chemical icons* identify molecular components of nutrient molecules, making their construction and deconstruction visually and conceptually accessible.

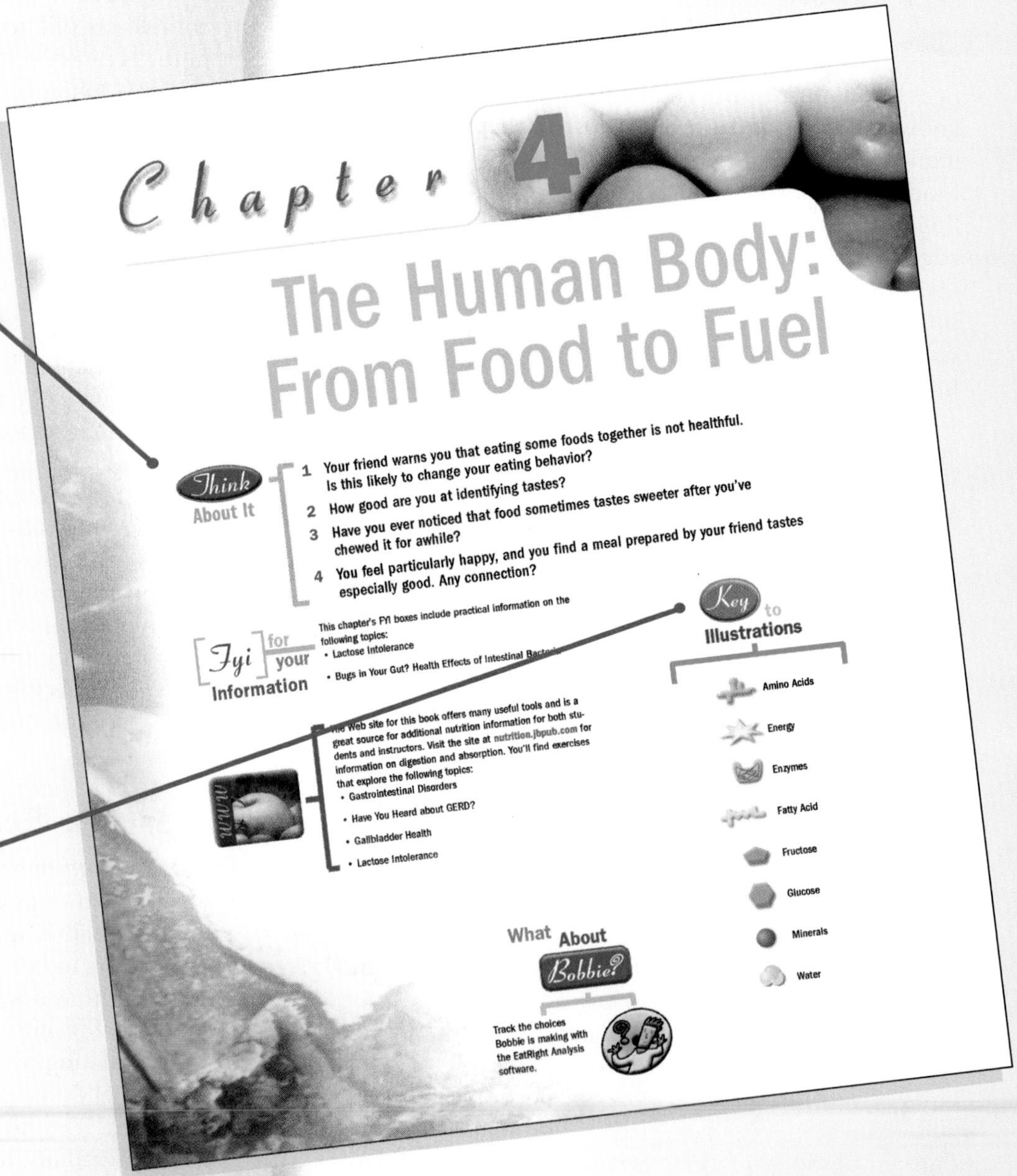

Chapter 4
The Human Body: From Food to Fuel
Think About It
1 Your friend warns you that eating some foods together is not healthful. Is this likely to change your eating behavior?
2 How good are you at identifying tastes?
3 Have you ever noticed that food sometimes tastes sweeter after you've chewed it for awhile?
4 You feel particularly happy, and you find a meal prepared by your friend tastes especially good. Any connection?
Fyi for your Information
This chapter's FYI boxes include practical information on the following topics:
• Lactose Intolerance
• Gastrointestinal Disorders
• Have You Heard about GERD?
• Gallbladder Health
• Lactose Intolerance
Key to Illustrations
Amino Acids
Energy
Enzymes
Fatty Acid
Fructose
Glucose
Minerals
Water
What About Bobbie?
Track the choices Bobbie is making with the EatRight Analysis software.

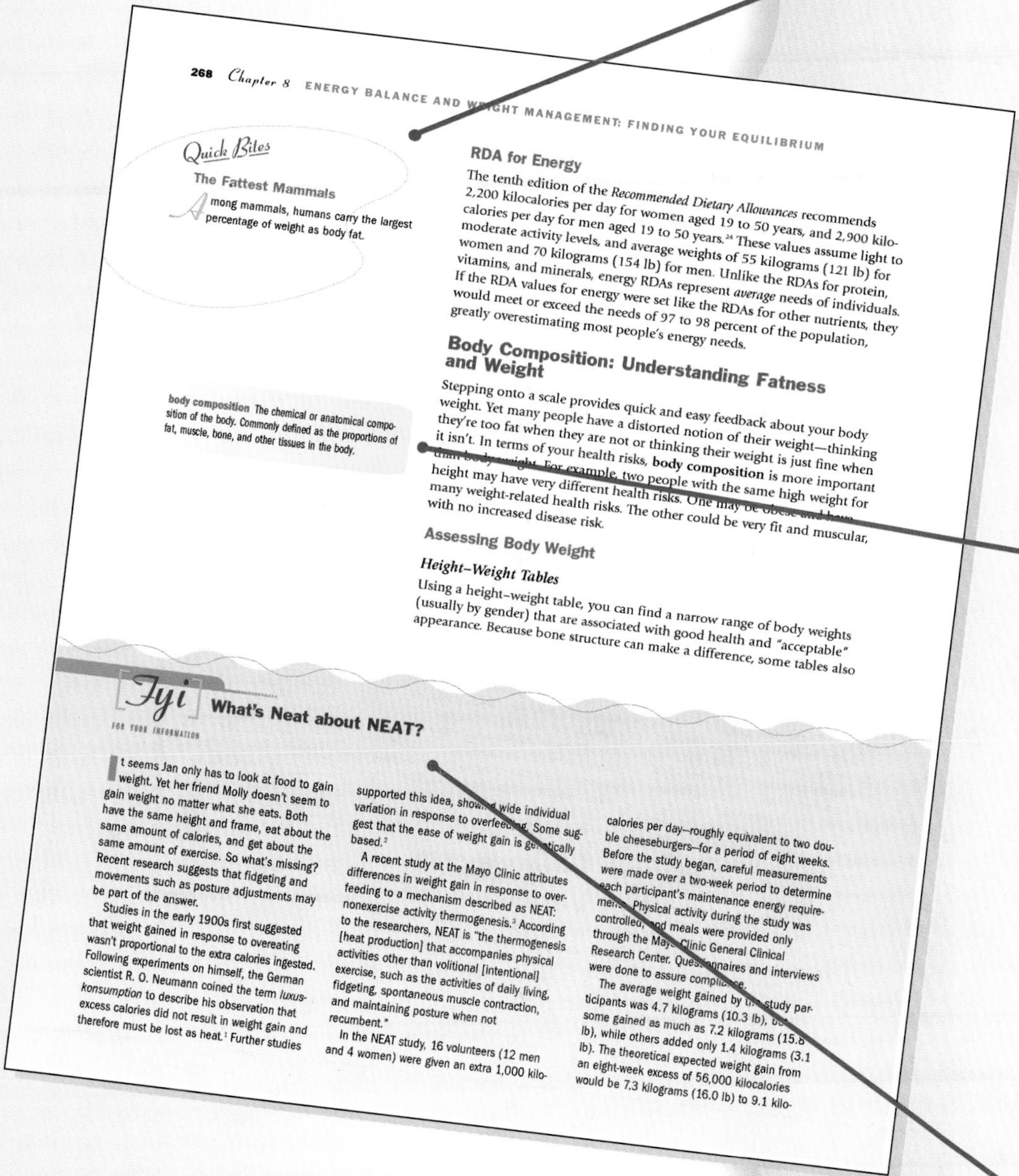

268 *Chapter 8* ENERGY BALANCE AND WEIGHT MANAGEMENT: FINDING YOUR EQUILIBRIUM

Quick Bites

The Fattest Mammals

Among mammals, humans carry the largest percentage of weight as body fat.

RDA for Energy

The tenth edition of the *Recommended Dietary Allowances* recommends 2,200 kilocalories per day for women aged 19 to 50 years, and 2,900 kilocalories per day for men aged 19 to 50 years.[24] These values assume light to moderate activity levels, and average weights of 55 kilograms (121 lb) for women and 70 kilograms (154 lb) for men. Unlike the RDAs for protein, vitamins, and minerals, energy RDAs represent *average* needs of individuals. If the RDA values for energy were set like the RDAs for other nutrients, they would meet or exceed the needs of 97 to 98 percent of the population, greatly overestimating most people's energy needs.

Body Composition: Understanding Fatness and Weight

Stepping onto a scale provides quick and easy feedback about your body weight. Yet many people have a distorted notion of their weight—thinking they're too fat when they are not or thinking their weight is just fine when it isn't. In terms of your health risks, **body composition** is more important than body weight. For example, two people with the same high weight for height may have very different health risks. One may be obese and have many weight-related health risks. The other could be very fit and muscular, with no increased disease risk.

body composition The chemical or anatomical composition of the body. Commonly defined as the proportions of fat, muscle, bone, and other tissues in the body.

Assessing Body Weight

Height–Weight Tables

Using a height–weight table, you can find a narrow range of body weights (usually by gender) that are associated with good health and "acceptable" appearance. Because bone structure can make a difference, some tables also

Fyi FOR YOUR INFORMATION

What's Neat about NEAT?

It seems Jan only has to look at food to gain weight. Yet her friend Molly doesn't seem to gain weight no matter what she eats. Both have the same height and frame, eat about the same amount of calories, and get about the same amount of exercise. So what's missing? Recent research suggests that fidgeting and movements such as posture adjustments may be part of the answer.

Studies in the early 1900s first suggested that weight gained in response to overeating wasn't proportional to the extra calories ingested. Following experiments on himself, the German scientist R. O. Neumann coined the term *luxuskonsumption* to describe his observation that excess calories did not result in weight gain and therefore must be lost as heat.[1] Further studies supported this idea, showing wide individual variation in response to overfeeding. Some suggest that the ease of weight gain is genetically based.[2]

A recent study at the Mayo Clinic attributes differences in weight gain in response to overfeeding to a mechanism described as NEAT: nonexercise activity thermogenesis.[3] According to the researchers, NEAT is "the thermogenesis [heat production] that accompanies physical activities other than volitional [intentional] exercise, such as the activities of daily living, fidgeting, spontaneous muscle contraction, and maintaining posture when not recumbent."

In the NEAT study, 16 volunteers (12 men and 4 women) were given an extra 1,000 kilocalories per day—roughly equivalent to two double cheeseburgers—for a period of eight weeks. Before the study began, careful measurements were made over a two-week period to determine each participant's maintenance energy requirements. Physical activity during the study was controlled, and meals were provided only through the Mayo Clinic General Clinical Research Center. Questionnaires and interviews were done to assure compliance.

The average weight gained by the study participants was 4.7 kilograms (10.3 lb), but some gained as much as 7.2 kilograms (15.8 lb), while others added only 1.4 kilograms (3.1 lb). The theoretical expected weight gain from an eight-week excess of 56,000 kilocalories would be 7.3 kilograms (16.0 lb) to 9.1 kilo-

Quick Bites are sprinkled throughout the book. They offer fun facts about nutrition-related topics such as exotic foods, social customs, origins of phrases, folk remedies, medical history, and so on.

Key terms are in boldface type the first time they are mentioned. Their definitions also appear in the margins near the relevant textual discussion, making it easy for students to review material and terms.

For Your Information offer more in-depth treatment of controversial and timely topics, such as unfounded claims about the effects of sugar, whether athletes need more protein, and megadoses of vitamins.

Key Concepts summarize previous text and highlight important information.

Label to Table helps students apply their new decision-making skills at the supermarket. It walks students through the various types of information that appear on food labels, including government-mandated terminology, misleading advertising phrases, and amounts of ingredients.

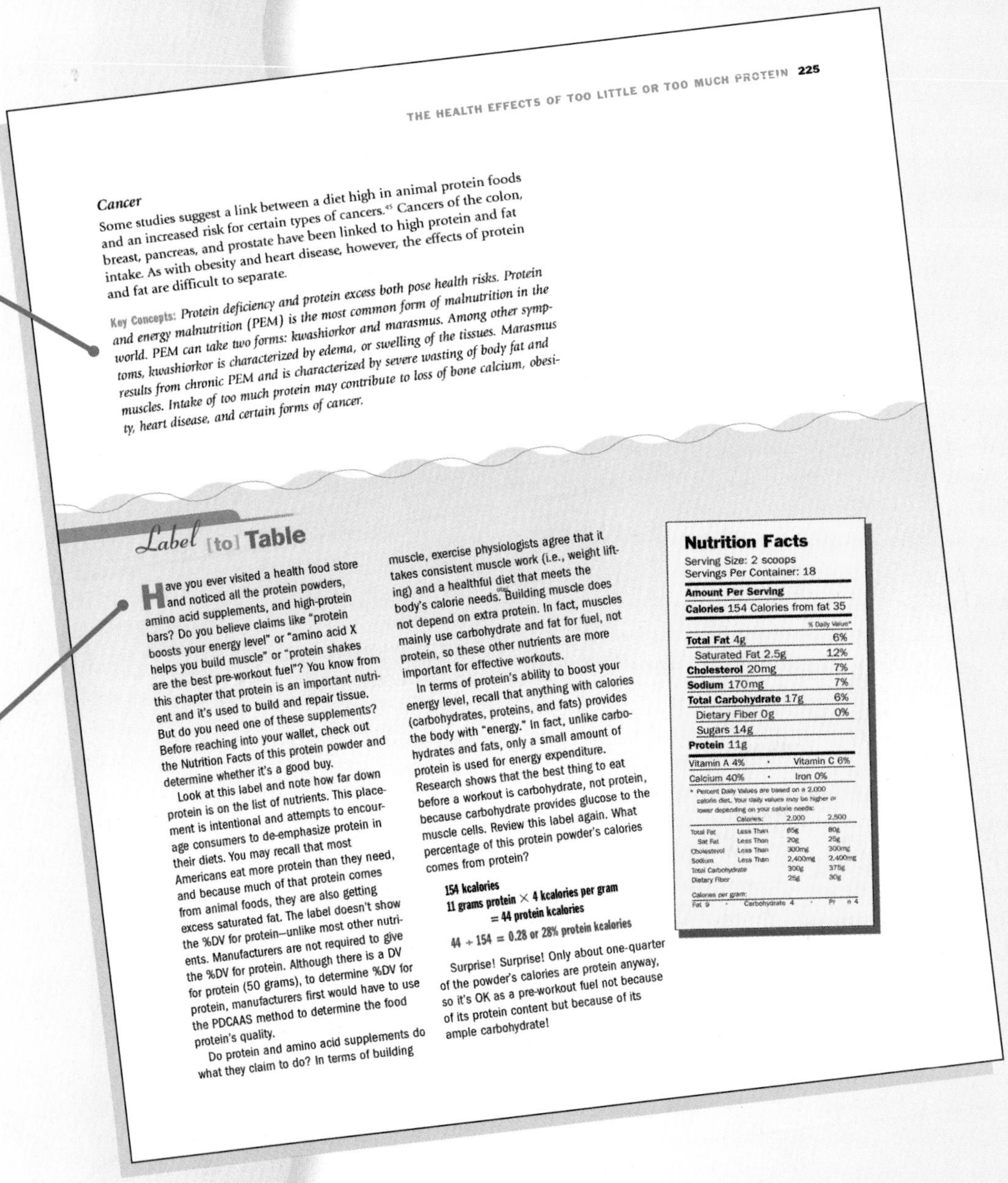

THE HEALTH EFFECTS OF TOO LITTLE OR TOO MUCH PROTEIN 225

Cancer

Some studies suggest a link between a diet high in animal protein foods and an increased risk for certain types of cancers.[45] Cancers of the colon, breast, pancreas, and prostate have been linked to high protein and fat intake. As with obesity and heart disease, however, the effects of protein and fat are difficult to separate.

Key Concepts: *Protein deficiency and protein excess both pose health risks. Protein and energy malnutrition (PEM) is the most common form of malnutrition in the world. PEM can take two forms: kwashiorkor and marasmus. Among other symptoms, kwashiorkor is characterized by edema, or swelling of the tissues. Marasmus results from chronic PEM and is characterized by severe wasting of body fat and muscles. Intake of too much protein may contribute to loss of bone calcium, obesity, heart disease, and certain forms of cancer.*

Label [to] Table

Have you ever visited a health food store and noticed all the protein powders, amino acid supplements, and high-protein bars? Do you believe claims like "protein boosts your energy level" or "amino acid X helps you build muscle" or "protein shakes are the best pre-workout fuel"? You know from this chapter that protein is an important nutrient and it's used to build and repair tissue. But do you need one of these supplements? Before reaching into your wallet, check out the Nutrition Facts of this protein powder and determine whether it's a good buy.

Look at this label and note how far down protein is on the list of nutrients. This placement is intentional and attempts to encourage consumers to de-emphasize protein in their diets. You may recall that most Americans eat more protein than they need, and because much of that protein comes from animal foods, they are also getting excess saturated fat. The label doesn't show the %DV for protein—unlike most other nutrients. Manufacturers are not required to give the %DV for protein. Although there is a DV for protein (50 grams), to determine %DV for protein, manufacturers first would have to use the PDCAAS method to determine the food protein's quality.

Do protein and amino acid supplements do what they claim to do? In terms of building muscle, exercise physiologists agree that it takes consistent muscle work (i.e., weight lifting) and a healthful diet that meets the body's calorie needs. Building muscle does not depend on extra protein. In fact, muscles mainly use carbohydrate and fat for fuel, not protein, so these other nutrients are more important for effective workouts.

In terms of protein's ability to boost your energy level, recall that anything with calories (carbohydrates, proteins, and fats) provides the body with "energy." In fact, unlike carbohydrates and fats, only a small amount of protein is used for energy expenditure. Research shows that the best thing to eat before a workout is carbohydrate, not protein, because carbohydrate provides glucose to the muscle cells. Review this label again. What percentage of this protein powder's calories comes from protein?

154 kcalories
11 grams protein × 4 kcalories per gram = 44 protein kcalories

44 ÷ 154 = 0.28 or 28% protein kcalories

Surprise! Surprise! Only about one-quarter of the powder's calories are protein anyway, so it's OK as a pre-workout fuel not because of its protein content but because of its ample carbohydrate!

Nutrition Facts
Serving Size: 2 scoops
Servings Per Container: 18

Amount Per Serving	
Calories 154 Calories from fat 35	
	% Daily Value*
Total Fat 4g	6%
Saturated Fat 2.5g	12%
Cholesterol 20mg	7%
Sodium 170mg	7%
Total Carbohydrate 17g	6%
Dietary Fiber 0g	0%
Sugars 14g	
Protein 11g	
Vitamin A 4% •	Vitamin C 6%
Calcium 40% •	Iron 0%

* Percent Daily Values are based on a 2,000 calorie diet. Your daily values may be higher or lower depending on your calorie needs:

	Calories:	2,000	2,500
Total Fat	Less Than	65g	80g
Sat Fat	Less Than	20g	25g
Cholesterol	Less Than	300mg	300mg
Sodium	Less Than	2,400mg	2,400mg
Total Carbohydrate		300g	375g
Dietary Fiber		25g	30g

Calories per gram:
Fat 9 • Carbohydrate 4 • Pr n 4

The **Learning Portfolio** at the end of each chapter collects, in one place, all aspects of nutrition information students need to solidify their understanding of the material. The various formats will appeal to students according to their individual learning and studying styles.

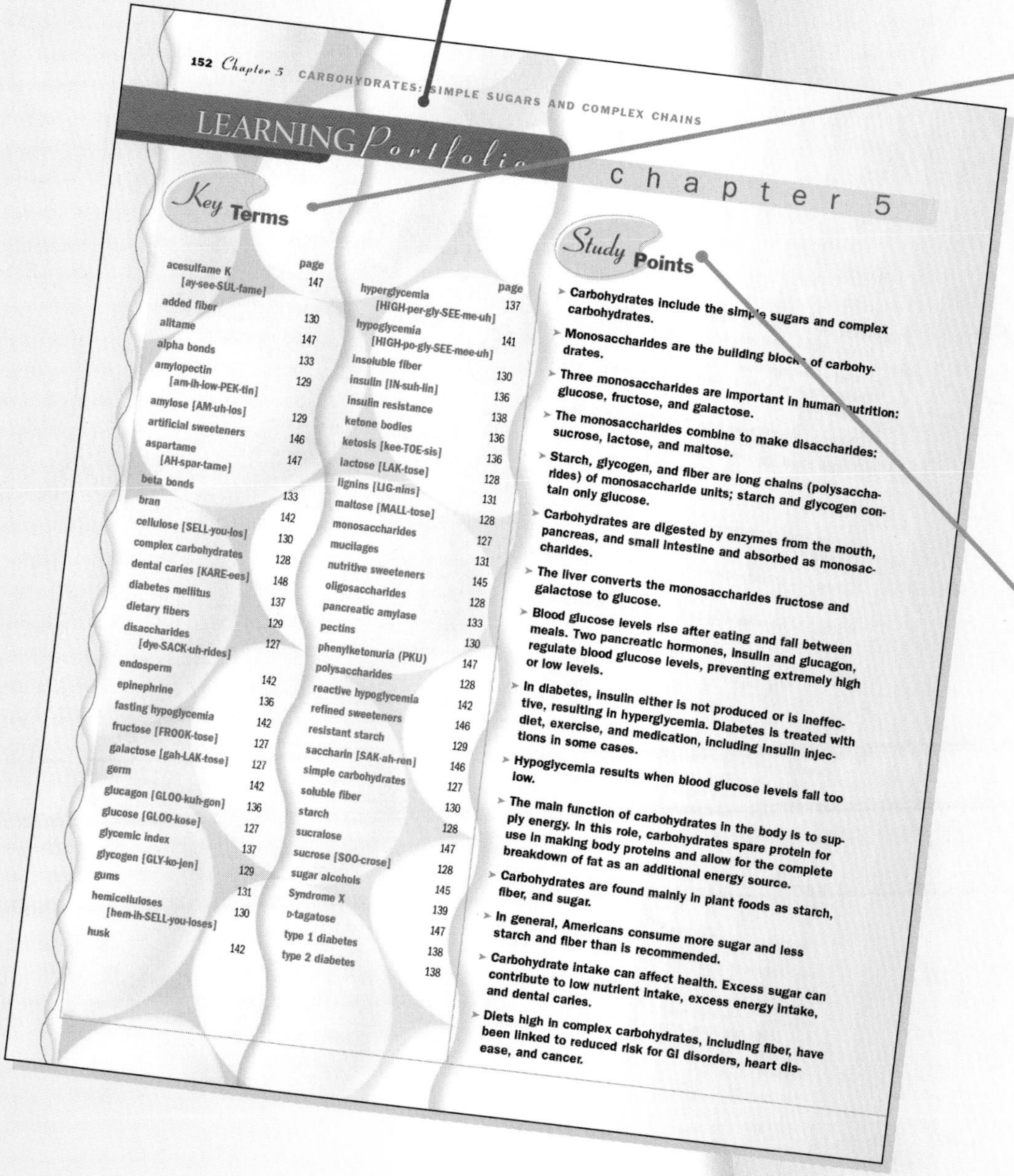
152 Chapter 5 CARBOHYDRATES: SIMPLE SUGARS AND COMPLEX CHAINS

LEARNING Portfolio chapter 5

Key Terms

	page
acesulfame K [ay-see-SUL-fame]	147
added fiber	130
alitame	147
alpha bonds	133
amylopectin [am-ih-low-PEK-tin]	129
amylose [AM-uh-los]	129
artificial sweeteners	146
aspartame [AH-spar-tame]	147
beta bonds	133
bran	142
cellulose [SELL-you-los]	130
complex carbohydrates	128
dental caries [KARE-ees]	148
diabetes mellitus	137
dietary fibers	129
disaccharides [dye-SACK-uh-rides]	127
endosperm	142
epinephrine	136
fasting hypoglycemia	142
fructose [FROOK-tose]	127
galactose [gah-LAK-tose]	127
germ	142
glucagon [GLOO-kuh-gon]	136
glucose [GLOO-kose]	127
glycemic index	137
glycogen [GLY-ko-jen]	129
gums	131
hemicelluloses [hem-ih-SELL-you-loses]	130
husk	142

	page
hyperglycemia [HIGH-per-gly-SEE-me-uh]	137
hypoglycemia [HIGH-po-gly-SEE-mee-uh]	141
insoluble fiber	130
insulin [IN-suh-lin]	136
insulin resistance	138
ketone bodies	136
ketosis [kee-TOE-sis]	136
lactose [LAK-tose]	128
lignins [LIG-nins]	131
maltose [MALL-tose]	128
monosaccharides	127
mucilages	131
nutritive sweeteners	145
oligosaccharides	128
pancreatic amylase	133
pectins	130
phenylketonuria (PKU)	147
polysaccharides	128
reactive hypoglycemia	142
refined sweeteners	146
resistant starch	129
saccharin [SAK-ah-ren]	146
simple carbohydrates	127
soluble fiber	130
starch	128
sucralose	147
sucrose [SOO-crose]	128
sugar alcohols	145
Syndrome X	139
D-tagatose	147
type 1 diabetes	138
type 2 diabetes	138

Study Points

- Carbohydrates include the simple sugars and complex carbohydrates.
- Monosaccharides are the building blocks of carbohydrates.
- Three monosaccharides are important in human nutrition: glucose, fructose, and galactose.
- The monosaccharides combine to make disaccharides: sucrose, lactose, and maltose.
- Starch, glycogen, and fiber are long chains (polysaccharides) of monosaccharide units; starch and glycogen contain only glucose.
- Carbohydrates are digested by enzymes from the mouth, pancreas, and small intestine and absorbed as monosaccharides.
- The liver converts the monosaccharides fructose and galactose to glucose.
- Blood glucose levels rise after eating and fall between meals. Two pancreatic hormones, insulin and glucagon, regulate blood glucose levels, preventing extremely high or low levels.
- In diabetes, insulin either is not produced or is ineffective, resulting in hyperglycemia. Diabetes is treated with diet, exercise, and medication, including insulin injections in some cases.
- Hypoglycemia results when blood glucose levels fall too low.
- The main function of carbohydrates in the body is to supply energy. In this role, carbohydrates spare protein for use in making body proteins and allow for the complete breakdown of fat as an additional energy source.
- Carbohydrates are found mainly in plant foods as starch, fiber, and sugar.
- In general, Americans consume more sugar and less starch and fiber than is recommended.
- Carbohydrate intake can affect health. Excess sugar can contribute to low nutrient intake, excess energy intake, and dental caries.
- Diets high in complex carbohydrates, including fiber, have been linked to reduced risk for GI disorders, heart disease, and cancer.

Key Terms lists all new vocabulary alphabetically with the page number of the first appearance. This arrangement allows students to review any term they do not recall and turn immediately to the definition and discussion of it in the chapter. This approach promotes the acquisition of knowledge, not simply memorization.

Study Points is a bulleted list that summarizes the content of each chapter with a synopsis of each major topic. The points are in the order in which they appear in the chapter, so related concepts flow together.

The **Learning Portfolio** (continued)

Study Questions encourage students to probe deeper into the chapter content, making connections and gaining new insights. Although these questions can be used for pop quizzes, they will also help students to review, especially students who study by writing out material. They can check their work by looking at the Study Question Answers on the *Discovering Nutrition* Web site at **http://nutrition.jbpub.com/discovering.**

What About Bobbie? tracks the eating habits and health-related decisions of a typical college student so that students can apply the material they have learned in the chapter to a typical situation. Following the individual case of Bobbie takes students from the general concepts to the specific application of new information. As a complement to this textual feature, the EatRight Analysis CD allows students to track the various choices Bobbie makes, as well as their own food choices.

Try This! activities are for curious students who like to experiment. These suggestions for hands-on activities encourage students to put theory into practice. It will especially help students whose major learning style is experiential.

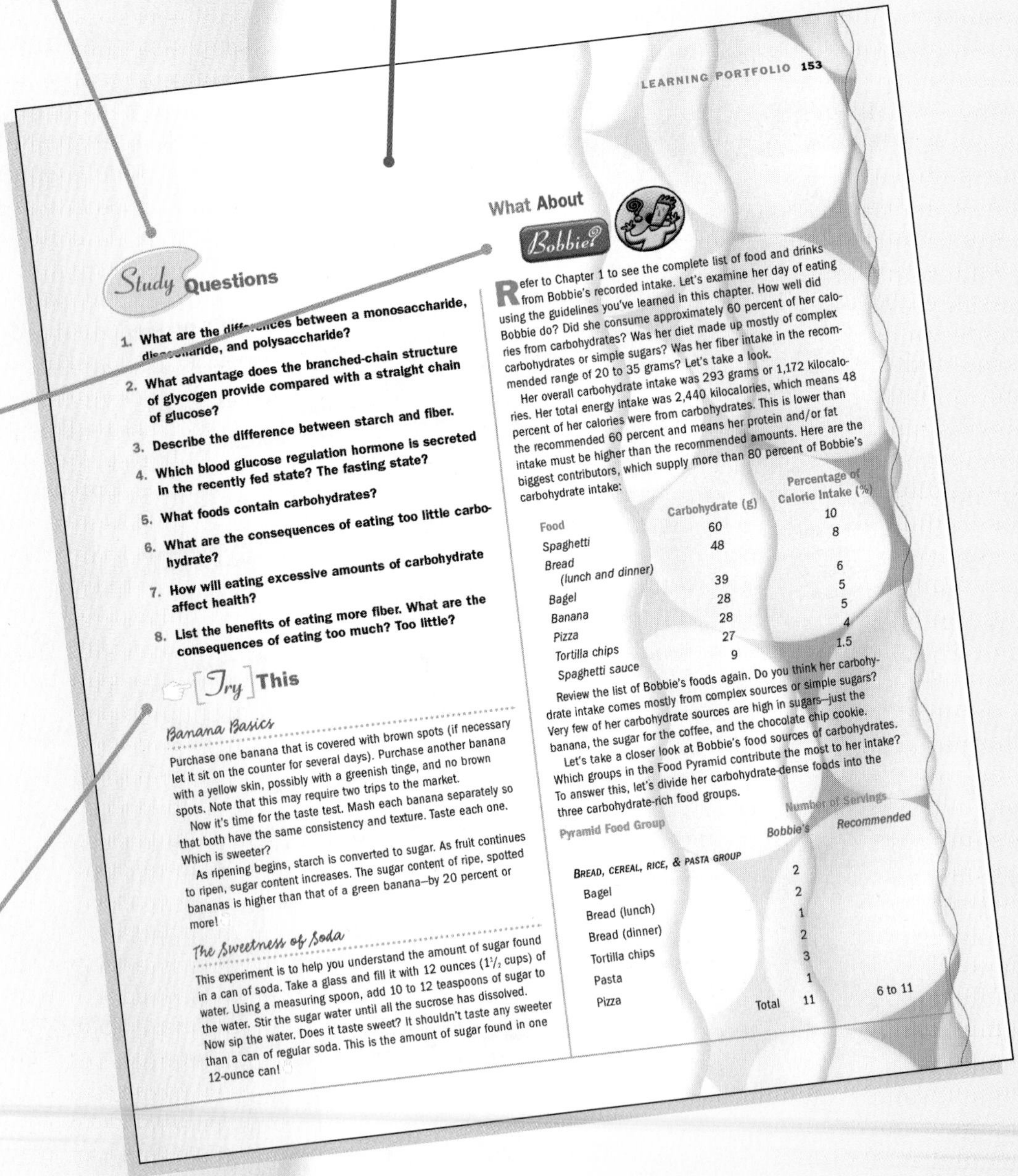

LEARNING PORTFOLIO 153

Study Questions

1. What are the differences between a monosaccharide, disaccharide, and polysaccharide?
2. What advantage does the branched-chain structure of glycogen provide compared with a straight chain of glucose?
3. Describe the difference between starch and fiber.
4. Which blood glucose regulation hormone is secreted in the recently fed state? The fasting state?
5. What foods contain carbohydrates?
6. What are the consequences of eating too little carbohydrate?
7. How will eating excessive amounts of carbohydrate affect health?
8. List the benefits of eating more fiber. What are the consequences of eating too much? Too little?

Try This

Banana Basics

Purchase one banana that is covered with brown spots (if necessary let it sit on the counter for several days). Purchase another banana with a yellow skin, possibly with a greenish tinge, and no brown spots. Note that this may require two trips to the market.

Now it's time for the taste test. Mash each banana separately so that both have the same consistency and texture. Taste each one. Which is sweeter?

As ripening begins, starch is converted to sugar. As fruit continues to ripen, sugar content increases. The sugar content of ripe, spotted bananas is higher than that of a green banana—by 20 percent or more!

The Sweetness of Soda

This experiment is to help you understand the amount of sugar found in a can of soda. Take a glass and fill it with 12 ounces ($1^1/_2$ cups) of water. Using a measuring spoon, add 10 to 12 teaspoons of sugar to the water. Stir the sugar water until all the sucrose has dissolved. Now sip the water. Does it taste sweet? It shouldn't taste any sweeter than a can of regular soda. This is the amount of sugar found in one 12-ounce can!

What About Bobbie?

Refer to Chapter 1 to see the complete list of food and drinks from Bobbie's recorded intake. Let's examine her day of eating using the guidelines you've learned in this chapter. How well did Bobbie do? Did she consume approximately 60 percent of her calories from carbohydrates? Was her diet made up mostly of complex carbohydrates or simple sugars? Was her fiber intake in the recommended range of 20 to 35 grams? Let's take a look.

Her overall carbohydrate intake was 293 grams or 1,172 kilocalories. Her total energy intake was 2,440 kilocalories, which means 48 percent of her calories were from carbohydrates. This is lower than the recommended 60 percent and means her protein and/or fat intake must be higher than the recommended amounts. Here are the biggest contributors, which supply more than 80 percent of Bobbie's carbohydrate intake:

Food	Carbohydrate (g)	Percentage of Calorie Intake (%)
Spaghetti	60	10
Bread (lunch and dinner)	48	8
Bagel	39	6
Banana	28	5
Pizza	28	5
Tortilla chips	27	4
Spaghetti sauce	9	1.5

Review the list of Bobbie's foods again. Do you think her carbohydrate intake comes mostly from complex sources or simple sugars? Very few of her carbohydrate sources are high in sugars—just the banana, the sugar for the coffee, and the chocolate chip cookie.

Let's take a closer look at Bobbie's food sources of carbohydrates. Which groups in the Food Pyramid contribute the most to her intake? To answer this, let's divide her carbohydrate-dense foods into the three carbohydrate-rich food groups.

Pyramid Food Group	Number of Servings: Bobbie's	Recommended
BREAD, CEREAL, RICE, & PASTA GROUP		
Bagel	2	
Bread (lunch)	2	
Bread (dinner)	1	
Tortilla chips	2	
Pasta	3	
Pizza	1	
Total	11	6 to 11

The Integrated Learning and Teaching Package

Integrating the text and ancillaries is crucial to deriving their full benefit. Based on feedback from instructors and students, Jones and Bartlett Publishers offers the following supplements.

Dietary analysis software is an important component of the behavioral change and personal decision-making focus. **EatRight Analysis,** developed by ESHA Research and tailored by the authors, enables students to analyze their diets by calculating their nutrient intake and comparing it to recommended intake levels.

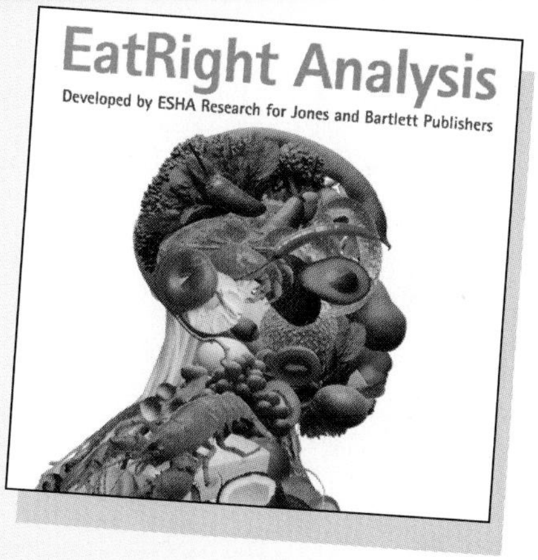

Contact your Nutrition Representative for discount package opportunities.

The **Instructor's ToolKit CD-ROM** is a comprehensive teaching resource available to adopters of the book. It includes:

- PowerPoint Lecture Presentation Slides
- Image Bank: Provides art that can be imported into PowerPoints, tests, or used to create transparencies
- Instructor's Manual: Includes chapter outlines and strategies for teaching difficult concepts
- Computerized TestBank
- Table Bank: Provides tables that can be imported into PowerPoints, tests, or used to create transparencies

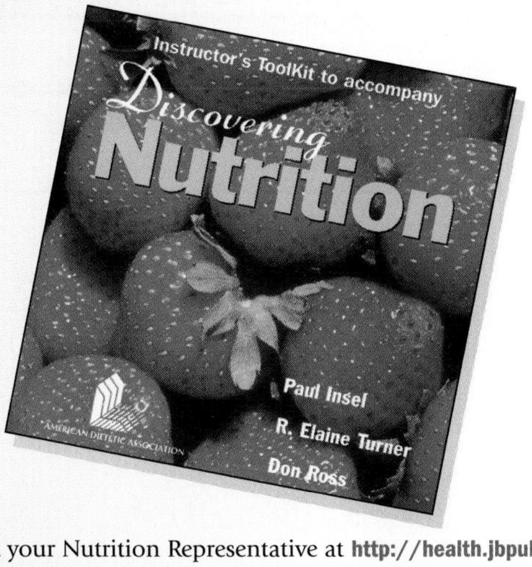

Contact your Nutrition Representative at **http://health.jbpub.com.**

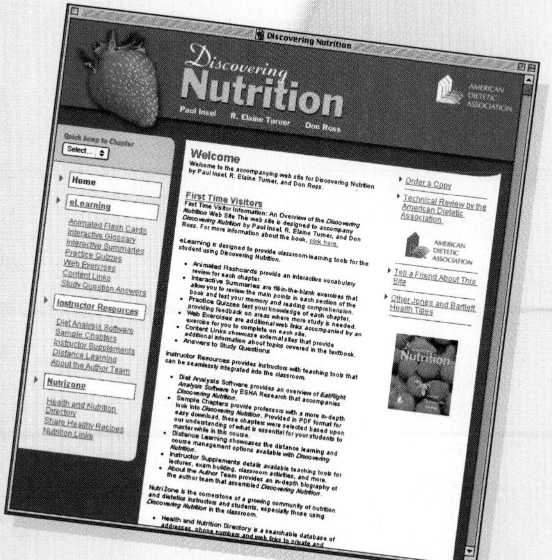

The **Web site** for *Discovering Nutrition*, **http://nutrition.jbpub.com/discovering**, offers students and instructors an unprecedented degree of integration between their text and the online world through many useful study tools, activities, and supplementary health information.

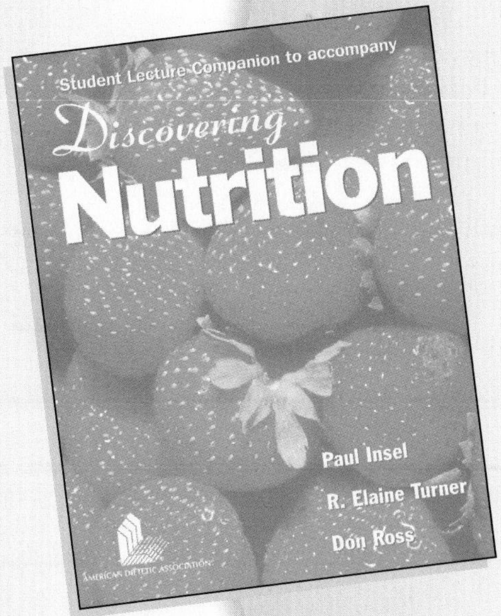

Contact your Nutrition Representative for discount package opportunities.

The **Student Lecture Companion to accompany *Discovering Nutrition*** provides a visual guide that follows *Discovering Nutrition*'s chapter topics and contains a print version of the PowerPoint slides included in the Instructor's ToolKit. Students can concentrate better during lectures and take notes without having to copy down the text from the slides.

Jones and Bartlett Publishers has created a number of customizable, highly interactive teaching and learning Course Cartridges and e-Packs for **Blackboard** and **WebCT** that offer web-based distance learning resources to assist both students and instructors. Instructors can integrate PowerPoint presentations with eLearning interactivities, generate customized exams, and upload additional course materials, while students can receive instant feedback and communicate easily with classmates and instructors.

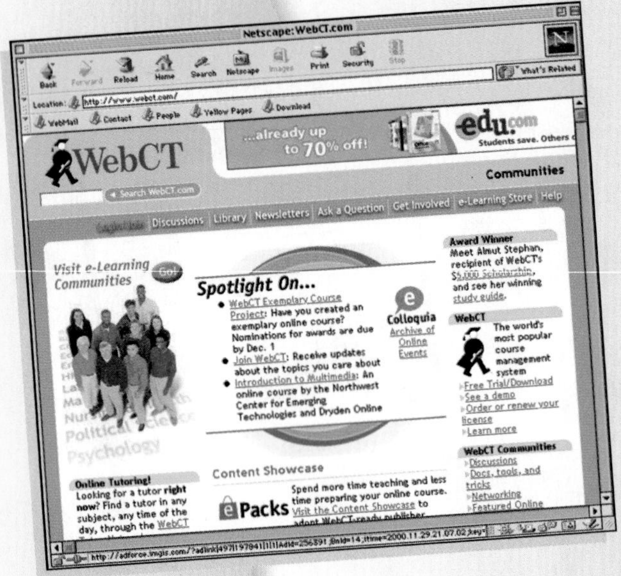

Contact your Nutrition Representative at **http://health.jbpub.com.**

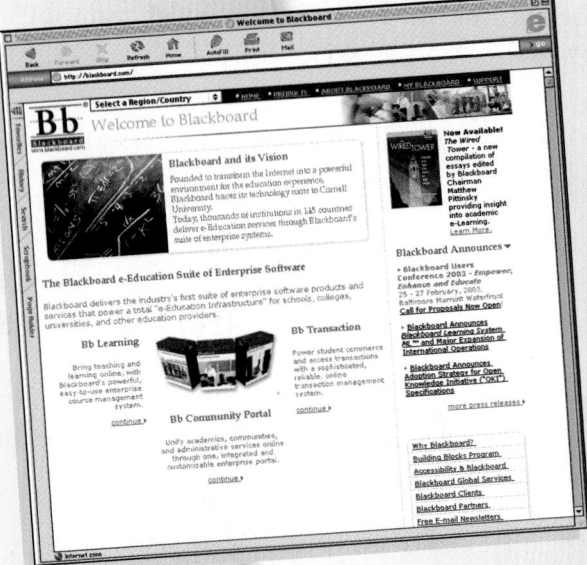

Contact your Nutrition Representative at **http://health.jbpub.com.**

About the Authors

The *Discovering Nutrition* author team represents a culmination of years of teaching and research in psychology and nutrition science. The combined experience of the authors yields a balanced presentation of both the science of nutrition and the components of behavioral change.

Dr. Paul Insel is Clinical Associate Professor of Psychiatry and Behavioral Sciences at Stanford University (Stanford, California). In addition to being the principal investigator on several nutrition projects for the National Institutes of Health (NIH), he is the senior author of the seminal text in health education and has co-authored several best-selling nutrition books.

Dr. R. Elaine Turner is a Registered Dietitian and Associate Professor in the Food Science and Human Nutrition Department at the University of Florida (Gainesville, Florida). Dr. Turner has been teaching courses in introductory and life-cycle nutrition for more than 15 years. Her interests include nutrition labeling and dietary supplement regulations, computer applications in nutrition and education, maternal and infant nutrition, and consumer issues. Dr. Turner was named Undergraduate Teacher of the Year, 2000–2001, for the College of Agricultural and Life Sciences.

Don Ross is director of the California Institute of Human Nutrition (Redwood City, California). For more than 15 years he has created educational materials about health and nutrition for consumers, professionals, and college students. He has special expertise in communicating complicated physiological processes with easily understood graphical presentations. The National Institutes of Health selected his Travels with Cholesterol for distribution to consumers. His multidisciplinary focus brings together the fields of psychology, nutrition, biochemistry, biology, and medicine.

Contributors

The following people contributed to this project:

Janine T. Baer, PhD, RD
University of Dayton
Chapter 11 Sports Nutrition
Chapter 12 Life Cycle: Maternal and Infant Nutrition

Toni Bloom, MS, RD, CDE
Past President of Nutrition Entrepreneurs DPG
Pedagogy

Boyce W. Burge, PhD
Chapter 14 Food Safety and Technology

Eileen G. Ford, MS, RD
Drexel University
Chapter 12 Life Cycle: Maternal and Infant Nutrition

Ellen B. Fung, PhD, RD
University of Pennsylvania
Chapter 10 Water and Minerals

Michael I. Goran, PhD
University of Southern California
Chapter 8 Energy Balance and Weight Management

Nancy J. Gustafson, MS, RD, FADA
Chapter 5 Carbohydrates
Chapter 7 Proteins and Amino Acids

Rita H. Herskovitz, MS
University of Pennsylvania
Chapter 10 Water and Minerals

Nancy I. Kemp, MD
University of California, San Francisco
Chapter 10 Water and Minerals

Sarah Harding Laidlaw, MS, RD, MPA
Chapter 13 Life Cycle: From Childhood through Adulthood

Rick D. Mattes, MPH, PhD, RD
Purdue University
Chapter 1 Food Choices

Maye Musk, MS, RD
Chapter 15 World View of Nutrition

Joyce D. Nash, PhD
Chapter 8 Energy Balance and Weight Management

Rachel Stern, MS, RD, CNS
Chapter 6 Lipids
Spotlight on Alcohol
Chapter 15 World View of Nutrition

Lisa Stollman, MA, RD, CDE, CDN
Chapter 4 The Human Body

Barbara Sutherland, PhD
University of California, Davis
Spotlight on Metabolism

Debra M. Vinci, PhD, RD, CD
Appalachian State University
Chapter 11 Sports Nutrition

Stella L. Volpe, PhD, RD, FACSM
University of Massachusetts
Chapter 8 Energy Balance and Weight Management

Paula Kurtzweil Walter, MS, RD
Federal Trade Commission
Chapter 14 Food Safety and Technology

The authors also would like to acknowledge the valuable contributions from the following people:

Alexandria Miller, PhD, RD/LD
Northeastern State University

Barbara Reynolds, MS, RD
College of the Sequoias

Marcia Nelms PhD, RD
Missouri State University

Pat Brown, MS, RD
Cuesta College

Reviewers

Focus Group

Katie Brown, BS, MS
Central Missouri State University

Christine Goodner, MS, RD
Winthrop University

Nancy Gordon Harris, MS, RD, LDN
East Carolina State University

Mary K. Head, PhD, RD, LD
University of West Virginia

Mary Murimi, PhD
Louisiana Technical University

Barbara A. Stettler, MEd
Bluffton College

Anna Sumabat Turner, MEd
Bob Jones University

Reviewers

Nancy K. Amy, PhD
University of California-Berkeley

Betty B. Alford, PhD, RD, LD
Texas Women's University

Susan I. Barr, PhD, RDN
University of British Columbia

Richard C. Baybutt, PhD
Kansas State University

Beverly A. Benes, PhD, RD
University of Nebraska-Lincoln

Virginia C. Bragg, MS, RD, CD
Utah State University

Melanie Tracy Burns, PhD, RD
Eastern Illinois University

N. Joanne Caid, PhD
College of Agricultural Sciences and Technology

Sai Chidambaram
Canisius College

Holly A. Dieken, PhD, MS, BS, RD
University of Tennessee-Chattanooga

Judy A. Driskell, PhD, RD
University of Nebraska

Liz Emery, MS, RD, CNSD
Drexel University

Christine Goodner, MS, RD
Winthrop University

Margaret Gunther, PhD
Palomar Community College

Shelley R. Hancock, MS, RD, LD
University of Alabama

Nancy Gordon Harris, MS, RD, LDN
East Carolina University

Mary K. Head, PhD, RD, LD
West Virginia University

Deloy G. Hendricks, PhD, CNS
Utah State University

Claire B. Hollenbeck, PhD
San Jose State University

Michael Jenkins
Kent State University

Zaheer Ali Kirmani, PhD, RD, LD
Sam Houston State University

Janet Levins, PhD, RD, LD
Pensacola Junior College

Samantha R. Logan, DrPH, RD
University of Massachusetts

Michael P. Maina, PhD
Valdosta State University

Patricia Z. Marincic, PhD, RD, LD, CLE
College of Saint Benedict/Saint John's University

Melissa J. Martilotta, MS, RD
Pennsylvania State University

Jennifer McLean, MSPH
Corning Community College

Mark S. Meskin, PhD, RD
California State Polytechnic University-Pomona

Stella Miller, BA, MA
Mount San Antonio College

Marilyn Mook, BS, MS
Michigan State University

Mary W. Murimi, PhD
Louisiana Technical University

Katherine O. Musgrave, MS, RD, CAS
University of Maine-Orono

J. Dirk Nelson, PhD
Missouri Southern State College

Nora Norback, MPH, RD, CDE
City College of San Francisco

Anne O'Donnell, MS, MPH, RD
Santa Rosa Junior College

Rebecca S. Pobocik, PhD, RD
Bowling Green State University

Roseanne L. Poole, MS, RD, LD/N
Tallahassee Community College

Amy F. Reeder, MS, RD
University of Utah

Stephen W. Sansone, BS, EdM
Chemekata Community College

Brian Luke Seaward, PhD
University of Colorado-Boulder

Melissa Shock, PhD, RD
University of Central Arkansas

Christine Stapell, MS, RD, LDN
Tallahassee Community College

Bernice Gales Spurlock, PhD
Hinds Community College

Susan T. Saylor, RD, EdD
Shelton State University

Mohammad R. Shayesteh, PhD, RD, LD
Youngstown State University

LuAnn Soliah, PhD, RD
Baylor University

Beth Stewart, PhD, RD
University of Arizona

Karen M. Ulrich, BS
Paul Smith's College of Arts and Sciences

Shahla M. Wunderlich, PhD
Montclair State University

Janelle Walter, PhD
Baylor University

Beverly G. Webber, MS, RD, CD
University of Utah

Erika M. Zablah
Louisiana State University-Baton Rouge

Acknowledgments

We would like to thank all of the instructors and students who were involved in the process of developing the majors edition of *Nutrition,* without whose involvement the creation of *Discovering Nutrition* would not have been possible. We are most grateful to Dr. Nancy Amy (University of California, Berkeley) and Dr. Sally Lederman (Columbia University), whose special nutrition expertise helped us strive for accuracy and precision. Special thanks are also owed to Stan Kubow (McGill University, Montreal, Quebec, Canada), whose extensive knowledge of Canadian nutrition is especially valued by the authors as well as the publisher of this text.

Making this book a reality involved the hard work and dedication of many people whom we would like to take this opportunity to thank. At Jones and Bartlett Publishers, thanks are due to Clayton Jones and Bob Holland for initiating this project; Julie Bolduc for shepherding the manuscript through to completion; and Kris Ellis for giving us help and direction when we needed it and for coordinating the supplemental material that accompanies this book. Thank you to Corinne Hudson, Nathan Schultz, and Ed McKenna for completing the varied tasks a project of this magnitude requires. Thanks are also due to Adam Alboyadjian, Kristin Ohlin, and Kylah McNeill for their efforts to create a Web site that was attractive, accurate, and useful to both students and instructors. At Nesbitt Graphics, thanks are due to Julie DeSilva and Rosemarie Villani for all of their hard work in making the pages come to life.

Finally the authors would also like to thank Michael Maina of Valdosta State University for creating the TestBank and Instructor's Manual; R. Elaine Turner for creating the PowerPoint presentations; and Amy Eades of Eastern Illinois University for sharing and creating the Classroom Activities.

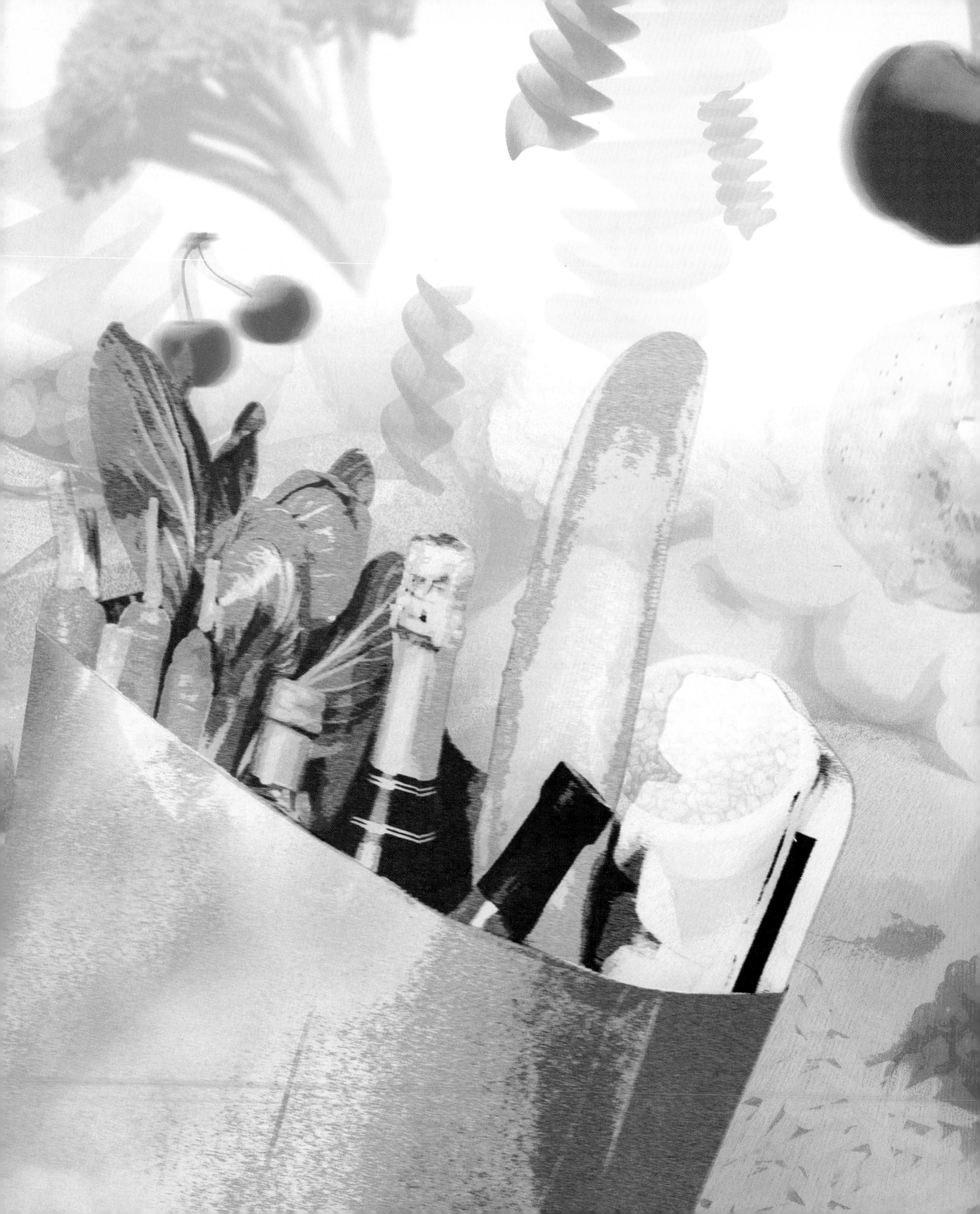

Chapter 1

Food Choices: Nutrients and Nourishment

Think About It

1. How many different foods have you eaten in the last 24 hours? The last week?
2. Do you have a preference for sweets? Chocolate? Ice cream? If so, where do you think it comes from?
3. What do you think is driving the popularity of vitamins and other supplements?
4. Where do you get the majority of your information about nutrition?

Fyi for your Information

This chapter's FYI boxes include practical information on the following topics:

- Do You Speak Metric?
- Evaluating Information on the Internet

WWW

The Web site for this book offers many useful tools and is a great source for additional nutrition information for both students and instructors. For information on nutrients and nourishment, visit the site at **nutrition.jbpub.com/discovering.** You'll find exercises that explore the following topics:

- The French Diet (*bon appetit!*)
- Why Are the Jains Vegetarians?
- Taste and Smell Disorders
- What Do You Eat?
- Ethnic Foods

What About Bobbie?

Track the choices Bobbie is making with the EatRight Analysis software.

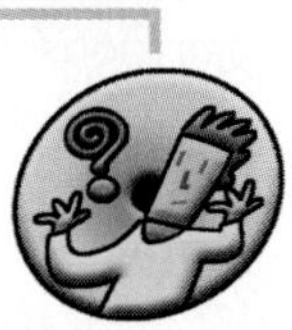

Key to Illustrations

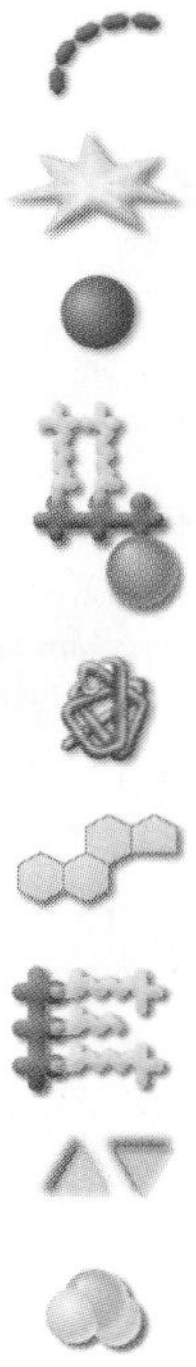

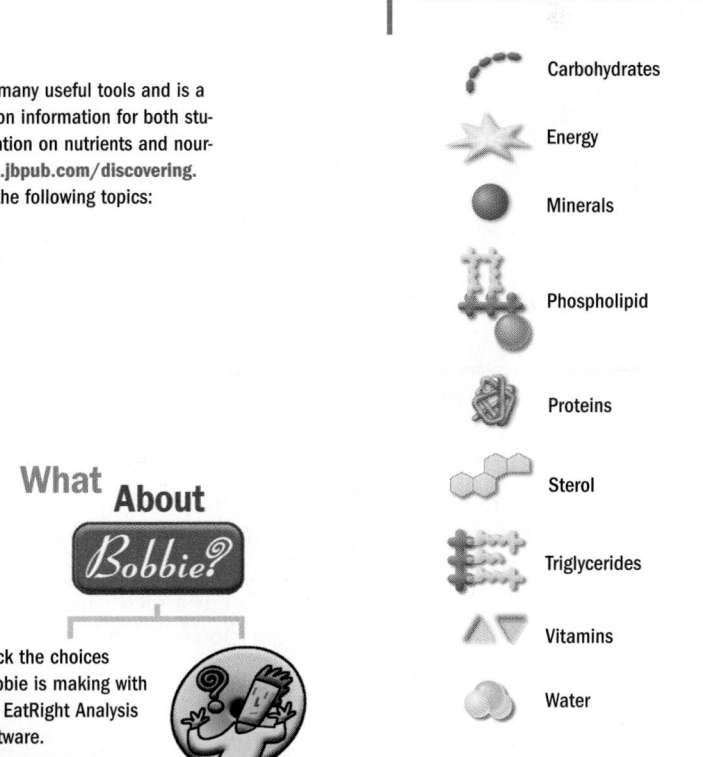

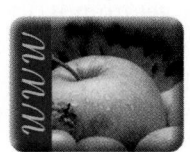

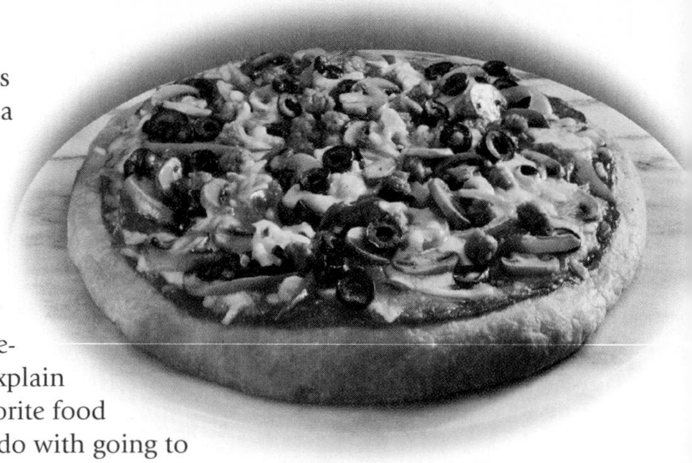

A group of students goes out for pizza every Thursday night. A college freshman greets his new date with a box of chocolates. A 5-year-old imitates her parents after they salt their food. A firefighter who is asked to explain why hot dogs are his favorite food says it has something to do with going to baseball games with his father. A professor recently recruited from a Chinese university feels dissatisfied unless she eats a bowl of rice daily. A parent punishes a misbehaving child by withholding dessert. What do these people have in common? They are all using food for something other than its nutrient value. Can you think of a holiday that is not celebrated with food? For most of us, food is more than a collection of nutrients. Many factors affect what we choose to eat. Many of the foods people choose are nourishing and contribute to good health. The same, of course, may be true of the foods we reject.

nutrition The science of foods and their components (nutrients and other substances) including the relationships to health and disease (actions, interactions, and balances); processes within the body (ingestion, digestion, absorption, transport, functions, and disposal of end products); and the social, economic, cultural, and psychological implications of eating.

neophobia A dislike for anything new or unfamiliar.

The science of **nutrition** helps us improve our food choices by identifying the amounts of nutrients we need, the best food sources of those nutrients, and the other components in foods that may be helpful or harmful. Learning about nutrition will help us make better choices and not only improve our health, but also reduce our risk of disease and increase our longevity. Keep in mind, though, that no matter how much you know about nutrition, you are still likely to choose some foods simply for their taste or just because they make you feel good.

Why Do We Eat the Way We Do?

Do you "eat to live" or "live to eat"? For most of us, the first is certainly true—you must eat to live. But there may be times when our enjoyment of food is more important to us than the nourishment we get from it. Factors such as age, gender, genetic makeup, occupation, lifestyle, family, and cultural background affect our daily food choices. We use food to project a desired image, forge relationships, express friendship, show creativity, and demonstrate our feelings. We cope with anxiety or stress by eating or not eating; we reward ourselves with food for a good grade or a job well done; or, in extreme cases, we punish failures by denying ourselves the benefit and comfort of eating.

Food preferences begin early in life and then change as we interact with parents, friends, and peers. Further experiences with different people, places, and situations often—but not always—cause us to expand or change our preferences. Taste and texture are the two most important things that influence our food choices; next are cost and convenience.[1] What we eat reveals much about who we are.

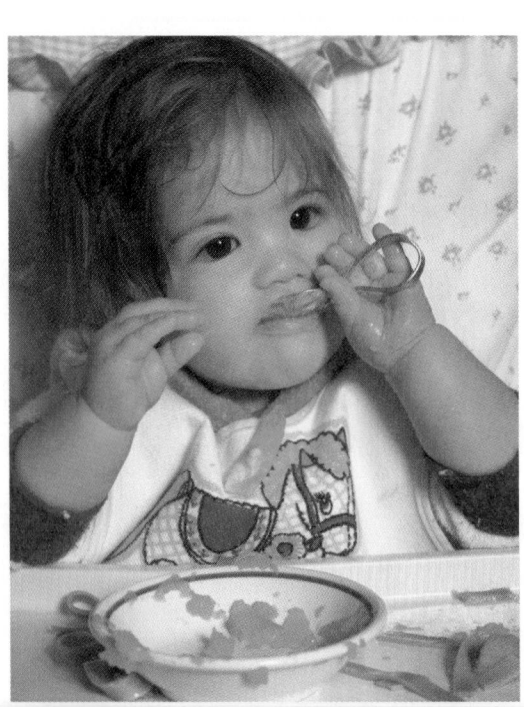

Figure 1.1 **Adventures in eating.** Babies and toddlers are generally willing to try new things.

Age is a factor in food preferences. Young children prefer sweet or familiar foods; babies and toddlers are generally willing to try new things. (See **Figure 1.1**.) Experimental evidence suggests infants exposed to a variety of flavors are even more likely to accept novel foods.[2] Preschoolers typically go through a period of food **neophobia** (a dislike for anything new or unfamiliar); school-age children tend to accept a wider array of foods; and teenagers are strongly influenced by the preferences and habits of their peers. If you track the kinds of foods you have eaten in the past year, you might be surprised to discover how few basic foods are in your diet. By the time we reach adulthood, we have formed a core group of foods we prefer. Of this group, only about 100 basic items account for 75 percent of our food intake.

Think About It 1

Like many aspects of human behavior, food choices are influenced by both inborn (biological) and environmental factors, and it's not always easy to separate them. However, we can look at food preferences in terms of the sensory properties of foods, cognitive factors that influence our choices, and long-term influences like culture. Exploring each of these areas may help you understand why you prefer certain foods. (See **Figure 1.2**.)

flavor The collective experience that describes both taste and smell.

umami [ooh-MA-mee] A Japanese term that describes a delicious meaty or savory sensation. Chemically, this taste detects the presence of glutamate.

Sensory Influences: Taste, Texture, and Smell

In making food choices, we are drawn to what appeals to our senses. People often refer to **flavor** as a collective experience that describes both taste and smell. Texture is also part of the picture.[3] You may prefer foods that have a crisp, chewy, or smooth texture. You may reject foods that feel grainy, slimy, or rubbery. Other sensory characteristics that affect food choice are color, moisture, and temperature.

We are familiar with the classic four tastes—sweet, sour, bitter, and salty—but studies show that there are more. One of these additional taste sensations is **umami**, which is a Japanese term for the taste produced by glutamate.[4] Glutamate is an amino acid (a building block of protein) that is found in monosodium glutamate (MSG). It gives food a distinctive meaty or savory taste (see Chapter 4, "The Human Body," for more information about taste and smell).

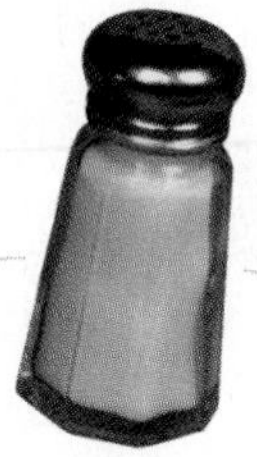

Quick Bites

Sweetness and Salt

Salt can do more than just make your food taste salty. Researchers at the Monell Chemical Senses Center demonstrated that salt also suppresses the bitter flavors in foods. When combined with chocolate, in a chocolate-covered pretzel, for example, salt blocks some of the bitter flavor, making the chocolate taste sweeter. This may explain why people in many cultures salt their fruit.

Cultural
economic
environment
lifestyle
cultural beliefs and traditions
religious beliefs and traditions

Sensory
flavor (taste and smell)
texture
appearance

Cognitive
learned food habits
social factors
emotional needs
nutrition and health beliefs
advertising

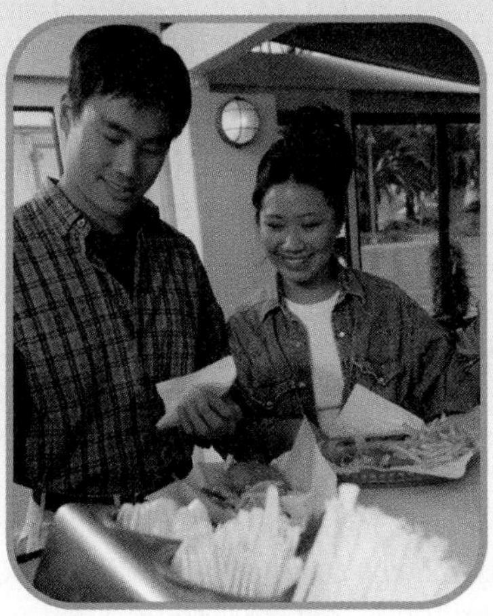

Health Status
physical restrictions due to disease
declining taste sensitivity
age and gender

Genetics
taste sensitivity
preference for sweets
avoidance of bitter
possible "fat tooth"

Figure 1.2 **Factors that affect food choices.** We often select a food to eat automatically, without thought. But in fact, our choices are complex events involving the interactions of a multitude of factors.

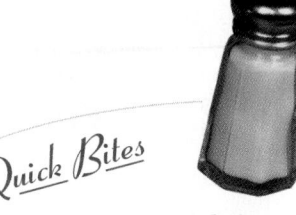

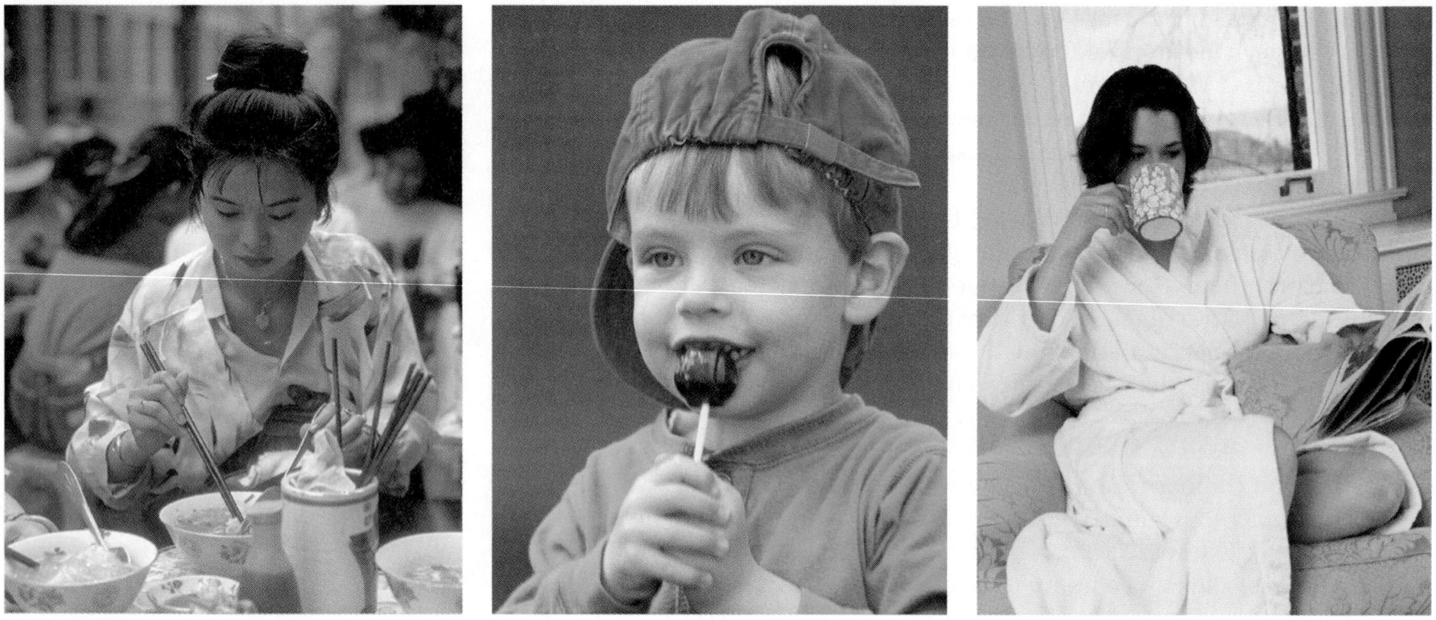

Figure 1.3 **Comfort foods.** Depending on your childhood food experiences, a bowl of traditional soup, a remembered sweet, or a mug of hot chocolate can provide comfort in times of stress.

Cognitive Influences

Along with our experiences, our thoughts and feelings about food influence decisions about what to eat and when. We can call these factors *cognitive* influences because they affect how we think and the decisions we make.

Day-to-Day Influences on Food Choices: Habits

Your eating and cooking habits are likely to reflect what you learned from your parents. We typically learn to eat three meals a day, at about the same times each day. Quite often we eat the same foods, particularly for breakfast (e.g., cereal and milk) and lunch (e.g., sandwiches). This routine makes life convenient, and we don't have to think much about when or what to eat. But we don't have to follow this routine! How would you feel about eating mashed potatoes for breakfast and cereal for dinner? Some people might get a stomachache just thinking about it, while others may enjoy the prospect of doing things differently. Look at your eating habits and see how often you make the same choices every single day.

Comfort/Discomfort Foods

Our desire for particular foods is often based on behavioral motives, even though we are not always aware of them. For some people, food becomes an emotional security blanket. Consuming our favorite foods can make us feel better, relieve stress, and allay anxiety. (See **Figure 1.3**.) Starting with the first days of life, food and affection are intertwined. Infants experience both physical and psychological satisfaction when eating. As we grow older, this experience is continually reinforced. For example, chicken soup and hot tea with honey are favorites when we feel under the weather because Mom and Dad fixed them especially for us. If we were rewarded for good behavior with a particular food (e.g., ice cream, candy, cookies), our positive feelings about that food may persist for a lifetime. And the foods that we associate with positive childhood experiences often continue to generate secure and supportive feelings.

On the other hand, children who have negative associations with certain foods are unlikely to choose those foods as adults. Maybe you avoid a cer-

Quick Bites

What Is an Ice Cream Headache?

After ingesting a cold substance quickly, such as when you take a big bite of ice cream, you may experience what is commonly known as an ice cream headache, or brain freeze. When cold substances touch the back part of the palate, blood vessels, including those that go to the brain, constrict (tighten), resulting in a sharp pain in the mid-frontal part of the brain. About one-third of the population experience this phenomenon.

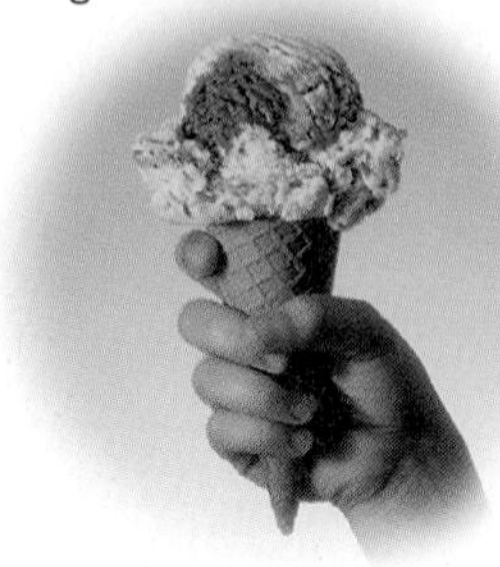

tain food because you know it will make you sick. Chances are that at some point in your childhood, you got sick soon after eating that food, and consequently the two events are linked forever. Repeated power struggles with your parents over a helping of broccoli or zucchini may have turned you away from eating those vegetables. Fortunately, these behaviors can be reversed. Psychologists have shown us that negative associations are easier to extinguish than positive ones. Thus time and the knowledge that vegetables are beneficial may help us overcome negative associations.

Food Cravings

Think About It 2

Chocolates for breakfast? Only if you are one of those people who can't survive more than one waking hour without a chocolate rush. Is the intense desire or craving for a particular food psychological or physiological? It's likely to be both, and these factors may interact to increase the intensity of the desire. Add ice cream to chocolate and you have the top two candidates on the food craver's agenda. The use of chocolate and ice cream as rewards in early childhood often sets the stage for later cravings.

Some people offer a nutritional explanation for food cravings: The body senses a nutrient deficit that triggers the desire for a food rich in that nutrient. Some claim that the practice of eating nonfood items such as dirt, clay, and laundry starch results from nutrient deficits. The craving for and consumption of such substances is called **pica** and is often associated with pregnancy. It has been suggested that iron deficiency drives the pregnant woman's craving so she seeks iron in any form possible, including dirt. Although this is a plausible explanation, current research has not found such a link. Rather, family traditions and cultural acceptance of pica have made it an expected behavior in some groups.[5]

Advertising and Promotion

It may not surprise you that some of the most popular food products are high-fat and high-sugar baked goods and alcoholic beverages. Aggressive and sometimes deceptive advertising programs can influence people to buy foods of poor nutritional quality. On the other hand, we are seeing more innovative and aggressive advertising from the commodity boards that promote milk, meat, cranberries, and other more nutrient-dense products.

Consumers make an estimated 70 percent of their food purchase decisions while shopping rather than before arriving at the market. Accurate nutritional information in the supermarket aisles can improve food choices.[6] Advertising like that in **Figure 1.4**, for example, can be helpful, especially to consumers whose diets require monitoring. In the mid-1980s, Kellogg's launched a print and television ad campaign for All-Bran cereal to suggest that a high-fiber diet would reduce the risk of cancer. Not only did sales of All-Bran increase dramatically in the months that followed, but the sales of all high-fiber cereals increased.[7] When the oat bran craze first hit in the late 1980s, sales of oat bran products by Quaker Oats Company increased 700 percent in one year.

Social Factors

Social factors exert a powerful influence on food choice. By observing their parents, infants and children learn which foods and combinations of foods are appropriate to consume and under what circumstances. Perhaps even

Quick Bites

Dining on Clay

Geophagy, the practice of eating clay, may actually improve nutritional status. When the clay eaten by some West African and black American groups was chemically analyzed, scientists found high levels of calcium, magnesium, potassium, copper, zinc, and iron. Whether our digestive systems can absorb the minerals in the clay remains to be seen, however.

pica The craving for and consumption of nonfood items like dirt, clay, or laundry starch.

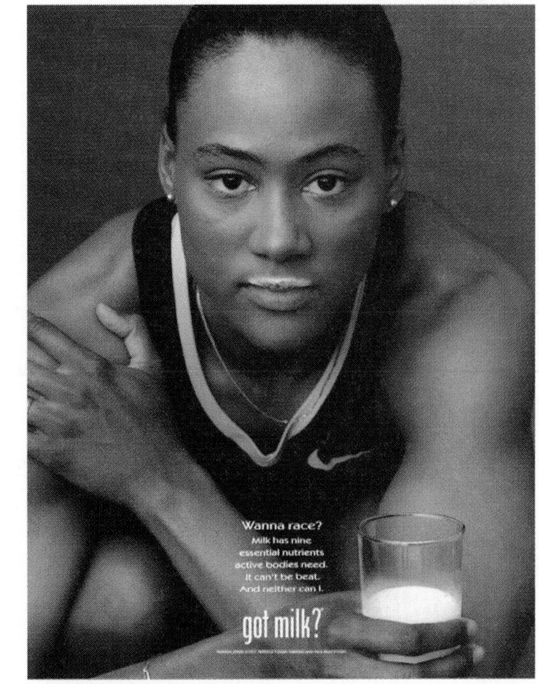

Figure 1.4 **Healthy advertising.** Got milk? is an example of a successful healthy advertising campaign.

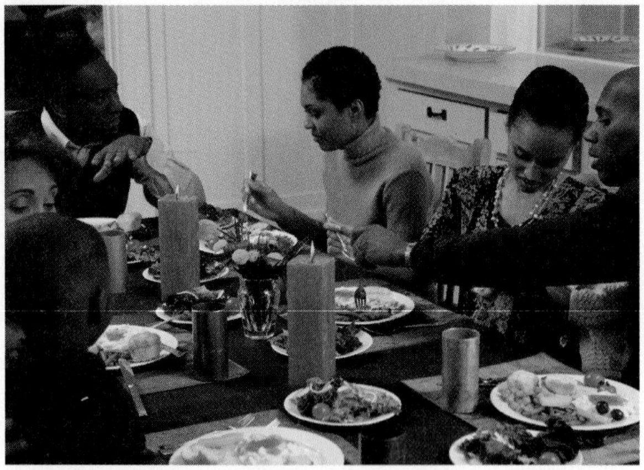

Figure 1.5 **Social facilitation.** Interactions with others can affect your eating behavior.

more influential, though, are the messages gleaned from their peers.[8] Although food neophobia is common among children, it can often be overcome by allowing them to observe another child enjoying a food they have yet to sample. With age and increased social contact, children and teens are likely to adopt more and more of their peers' preferences for foods and for specific preparation and serving methods of those foods: "Mark eats his sandwiches in triangles; that's the way I want mine!"

As **Figure 1.5** illustrates, eating is also a social event that brings together different people for a variety of purposes (e.g., religious or cultural celebrations, business meetings, and family dinners). Thanks to something called **social facilitation**, food intake increases because of the social climate surrounding its consumption.[9] However, social pressures can also restrict our food intake and selection. We might, for example, order nonmeat dishes when dining with a vegetarian.

Social status can also influence food choices. Research in Canada and the United States shows a relationship between nutrient intake and social position. People in lower social positions have diets of inferior quality and are more likely to fall short of recommended nutrient intake standards.[10]

social facilitation Encouragement of the interactions between people.

Nutrition and Health Beliefs

Information about food and nutrition is abundant, as **Figure 1.6** shows. Why do some people ignore health information and indulge themselves with foods that may lead to health problems, while others take the same information and commit themselves to a healthful diet? To examine these questions, we need to consider the health beliefs of consumers, their perceptions of susceptibility to disease, and whether they can take action to prevent or delay its onset.[11] For instance, if people feel vulnerable to disease and believe that dietary change will lead to positive results, they are more likely to heed information about links between dietary choices, dietary fat, and risks for heart disease and cancer. A desire to lose weight can be a powerful force shaping decisions to accept or reject particular foods.[12]

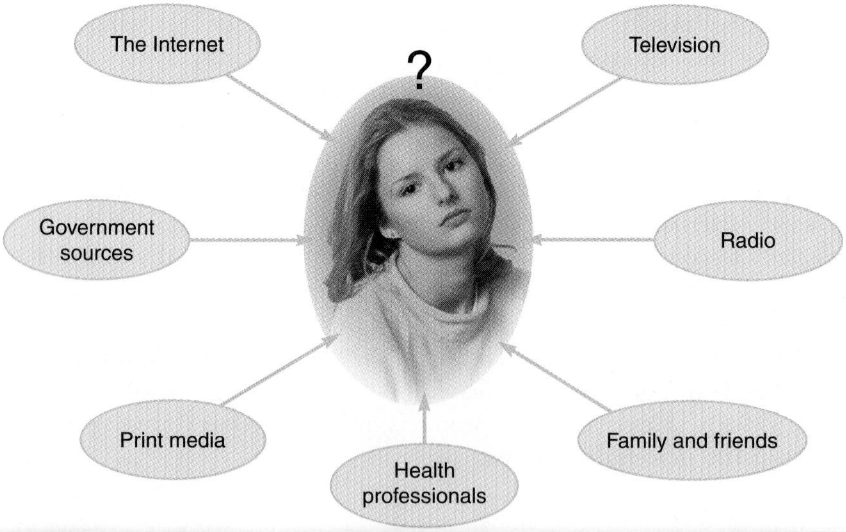

Figure 1.6 **Where do you get your nutrition information?** We are constantly bombarded by food messages. Which sources do you find most influential? Are they also the most reliable?

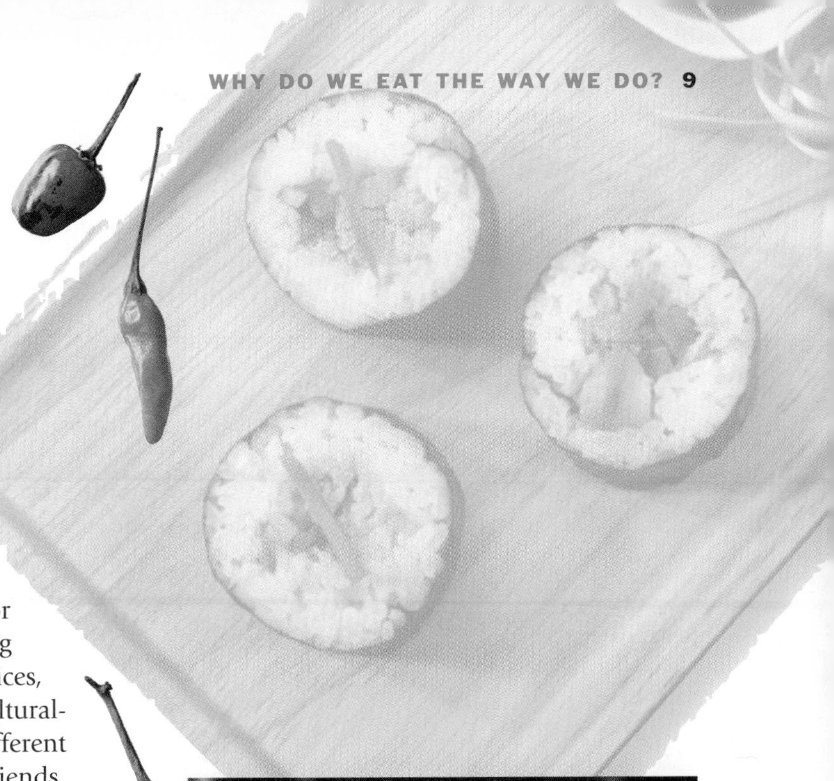

Information about nutrient content on food labels along with health claims that describe links between food components and diseases aid consumers who are trying to make positive choices.

Key Concepts: *Many factors influence our decisions about what to eat and when to eat. The four main factors are taste, texture, cost, and convenience. Habits, experiences, social factors, advertising, and knowledge of relationships between food and health also influence our food decisions.*

Cultural Influences

One of the strongest influences on food preferences is tradition or cultural background. In all societies, no matter how simple or complex, eating is the primary way of initiating and maintaining human relationships. People around us influence our food choices, and we prefer the foods we grew up eating. Sometimes these culturally acquired preferences can seem quite peculiar to those of a different culture. The college student who serves pickled herring to her friends may have learned to enjoy it from her Jewish parents, who introduced it to her as a child in comforting surroundings. Likewise, it is not uncommon for people of Mexican heritage to enjoy eating hot peppers, which were introduced to them early in life in highly gregarious social settings.

To a large extent, culture defines our attitudes. "One man's food is another man's poison." Look at **Figure 1.7**. How does the photo make you feel? Insects, maggots, and entrails are delicacies to some, while just the thought of ingesting them is enough to make others retch. So powerful are cultural forces that if you were permitted only a single question to establish someone's food preferences, a good choice would be "What is your ethnic background?"[13]

Knowledge, beliefs, customs, and habits all are defining elements of human culture.[14] Although genetic characteristics tie people of ethnic groups together, culture is a learned behavior and, consequently, can be modified through education, experience, and social and political trends.[15]

Cultural Beliefs and Traditions

In many cultures, food has symbolic meanings related to family traditions, social status, and even health.[16] Indeed, many folk remedies rely on food. Some of these have gained wide acceptance, such as the use of spices and herbal teas for purposes ranging from allaying anxiety to preventing cancer and heart disease.[17] Traditional medical practices in many cultures follow the belief that nature is composed of two opposing forces (e.g., yin and yang in traditional Chinese medicine). It is typically believed that good health reflects a balance of the two opposing forces. Excesses in either direction cause illness, which then must be treated by giving foods of the opposite force. This idea of balance, accompanied by terms describing illness and foods as either "hot" or "cold," is also found in other Asian cultures, including India and the Philippines, and in Latin American cultures.

Just as cultural distinctions eventually blur when ethnic groups take part in the larger American culture, so do many of the unique expectations about the ability of certain foods to prevent disease, restore health among those with various afflictions, or enhance longevity. These beliefs are still apparent, however, in older, less assimilated groups. Food habits are among the last to change when an immigrant adapts to a new culture.[18]

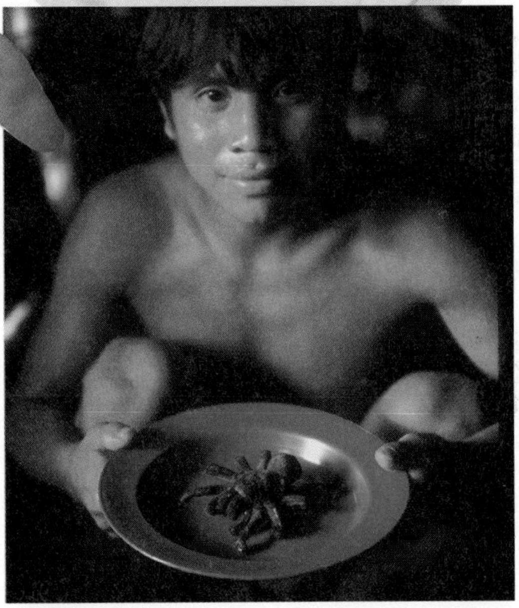

Figure 1.7 **Cultural influences.** What would you do if you were visiting this country? Would you be willing to try this delicacy?

Quick Bites

Nerve Poison for Dinner?

The puffer fish is a delicacy in Japan. Danger is part of its appeal; eating a puffer fish can be life threatening! The puffer fish contains a poison called tetrodotoxin (TTX), which blocks the transmission of nerve signals and can lead to death. Chefs who prepare the puffer fish must have special training and licenses to prepare the fish properly, so diners feel nothing more than a slight numbing feeling.

Religion

Food is an important part of religious rites, symbols, and customs as well as of daily activities that are intended to promote an orderly relationship with supernatural forces. Some religious rules apply to everyday eating, whereas others are concerned with special celebrations.

Christianity, Judaism, Hinduism, Buddhism, and Islam all have distinct dietary laws, but within each religion different interpretations of these laws give rise to variations in dietary practices. For example, Jewish dietary laws specify the foods that are "fit and proper," or *kosher*, to eat. To be kosher, meat must come from clean animals that chew their cud and have cloven hooves. Fish must have fins and scales. Pork, crustaceans and shellfish, and birds of prey are not acceptable. The Orthodox laws of Judaism prohibit eating meat and milk at the same meal or even preparing or serving them with the same dishes and utensils. Islam identifies acceptable foods as *halal* and has rules similar to those of Judaism for slaughtering animals. Islamic faith prohibits the consumption of pork, flesh of clawed animals, alcohol, and other intoxicating drugs. Intoxicating beverages are also prohibited in Buddhism,[19] and the Church of Jesus Christ of Latter Day Saints disapproves of alcoholic and caffeine-containing beverages. Most Hindus are vegetarians and do not eat eggs. The Jain religion (in India) forbids eating meat or animal products (milk, eggs, etc.) and anything grown in darkness (e.g., potatoes or garlic).

Religious rules may also define when and how often we eat. During the holy month of Ramadan, Muslims fast from dawn to sunset. They consume two meals per day, one before the sunrise and one after sunset.[20] Religious laws (e.g., the traditional Catholic practice of substituting fish for meat on Fridays during Lent) also define the types of foods eaten on specific occasions.[21]

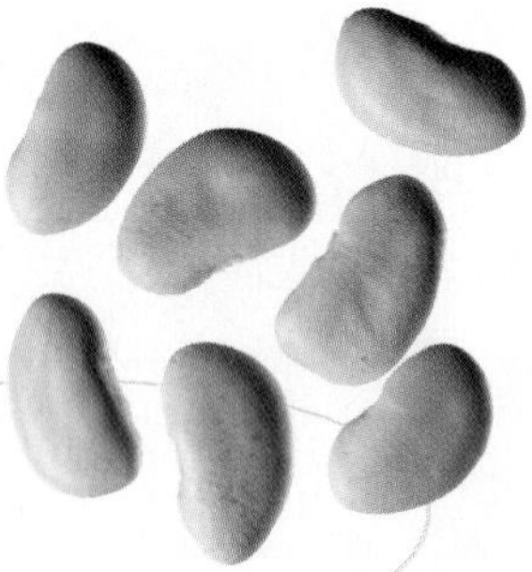

Quick Bites

The Lima Bean

The lima bean has been in cultivation in Peru since 6000 B.C.E. Not so coincidentally, Peru's capital is Lima.

Cultural Cuisine

Diet and culture affect each other. Each contributes to the identity of the other, and both help to define our values, preferences, and practices. As a result, neither is abandoned easily or quickly, even in the face of changing world events. Even so, the question arises: What impact will our increasing mobility have on food choice? Cultural interactions and exposure to various cuisines will undoubtedly increase. Will this ultimately lead to a heightened appreciation and preservation of different culinary practices or the formation of a single new hybrid cuisine?

Key Concepts: *The cultural environments in which people grow up have a major influence on what foods they prefer, what foods they consider edible, and what foods they eat in combination and at what time of day. Many factors work to define a group's culture: economics, geographic location, traditions, and religious beliefs. As people from other cultures immigrate to new lands, they will adopt new behaviors consistent with their new homes. However, food habits are among the last to change.*

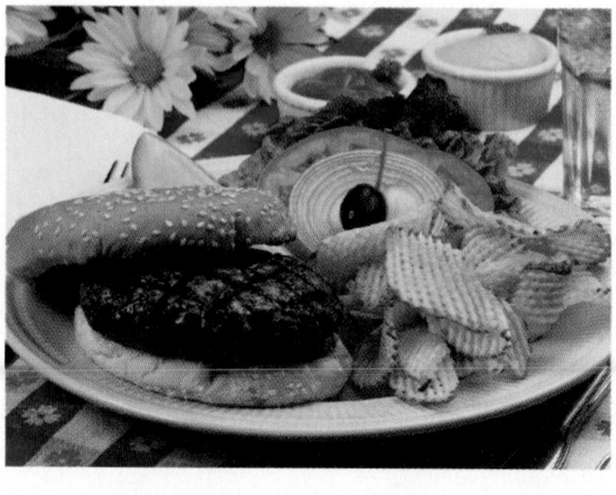

The American Diet

What then is a typical *American diet*? As a country influenced by the practices of both Native Americans and immigrants, there is no easy, single answer to this question. The U.S. diet is as diverse as Americans themselves. Many people around the world imagine that the American diet consists of hamburgers, french fries, and cola drinks! Our fondness for fast food and the marketability of such restaurants overseas make them seem like icons of American culture. And many of the stereotypes are true. The most commonly consumed grain product in the United States is white bread, the favorite meat is beef, and the most frequently eaten vegetable is the potato, usually as french fries. Despite the variety available to us, the American diet is still heavy on meat and potatoes and light on fruits and whole grains. We also are eating more cereals, snack foods, soft drinks, and noncitrus juices than ever before.[22]

So, how healthful is the "American" diet? Although we are bombarded with information about health and nutrition, this doesn't necessarily translate into better food choices. People are not "natural nutritionists"; that is, they don't know instinctively which foods to choose for good health. The majority of the population has never taken a course in nutrition. They probably will never take the time to become well-informed consumers—not just of food, but also of information about food and nutrition.[23] So it is probably not surprising when national surveys indicate that although Americans *know* that nutrition and food choices are important factors in health, few have made the recommended changes (e.g., eating less fat, sugar, and salt and more fruits and vegetables).

You are in a position to gather more information than the average consumer. By taking this course in nutrition, you will be getting the full story: the nutrients we need for good health, the science behind the health messages, and the food choices it will take to implement them. Whether you use this information is up to you, but at least you will be a well-informed consumer!

Key Concepts: *What we think of as "American" cuisine is truly a melting pot of cultural contributions to foods and tastes. Although Americans receive and believe many messages about the role of diet in good health, these beliefs do not always translate into better food choices.*

Quick Bites

America's Favorite Vegetables

When Americans eat vegetables, they are most likely to eat potatoes (especially french fries), tomatoes (usually part of tomato sauce or ketchup), onions, and iceberg lettuce.

Introducing the Nutrients

Although we give food meaning through our culture and experience and make dietary decisions based on many factors, ultimately the reason for eating is to obtain nourishment—nutrition.

Just like your body, food is a mixture of chemicals, some of which are essential for normal body function. These essential chemicals are called **nutrients**. You need nutrients for normal growth and development, for maintaining cells and tissues, for fuel to do physical and metabolic work, and for regulating the hundreds of thousands of body processes that go on inside you every second of every day. Further, food must provide these nutrients; the body either cannot make these **essential nutrients** or cannot make enough of them. There are six classes of nutrients in food: *carbohydrates, lipids* (fats and oils), *proteins, vitamins, minerals,* and *water*. (See **Figure 1.8**.) The minimum diet for human growth, development, and maintenance must supply about 45 essential nutrients.

nutrients Any substances in food that the body can use to obtain energy, synthesize tissues, or regulate functions.

essential nutrients Substances that must be obtained in the diet because the body either cannot make them or cannot make adequate amounts of them.

Definition of Nutrients

In studying nutrition, we focus on the functions of nutrients in the body so that we can see why they are important in the diet. However, to define a nutrient in technical terms, we focus on what happens in its absence. A nutrient is a chemical whose absence from the diet for a long enough time results in a specific change in health; we say that a person has a deficiency

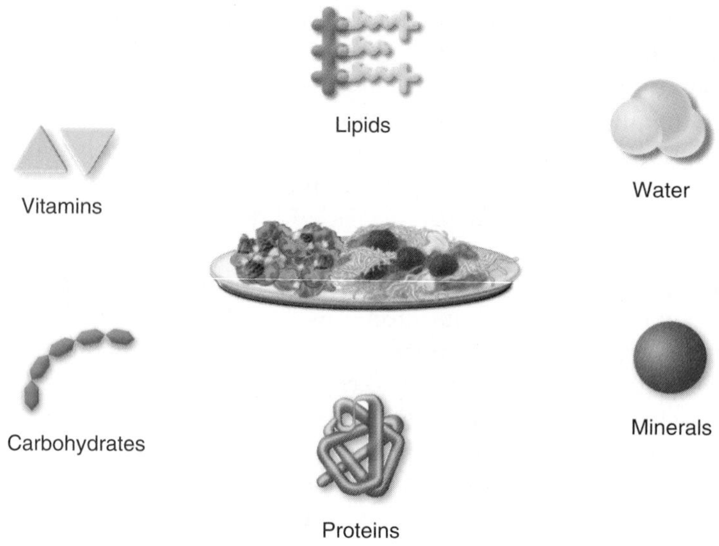

Figure 1.8 **The six classes of nutrients.** Water is our most important nutrient, and we cannot survive long without it. Because our bodies need large quantities of carbohydrate, protein, and fat, they are called macronutrients. Our bodies need comparatively small amounts of vitamins and minerals, so they are called micronutrients.

of that nutrient. A lack of vitamin C, for example, will eventually lead to scurvy. A diet with too little iron will result in iron-deficiency anemia. To complete the definition of a nutrient, it also must be true that putting the essential chemical back in the diet will reverse the change in health, if done before permanent damage occurs. If taken early enough, supplements of vitamin A can reverse the effects of deficiency on the eyes. If not, prolonged vitamin A deficiency can cause permanent blindness.

Nutrients are not the only chemicals in food. Other substances add flavor and color, some contribute to texture, and others, like caffeine, have physiological effects on the body. Some substances in food, like fiber, have important health benefits (as you will discover in Chapter 4, "The Human Body") but do not fit the classical definition of a nutrient. One of the newest areas of research in nutrition is the area of **phytochemicals**. Although these "plant chemicals" are not nutrients, they have important health functions, such as **antioxidant** activity, which may reduce risk for heart disease or cancer.

The six classes of nutrients serve three general functions: They provide fuel or energy, regulate body processes, and contribute to body structures. (See **Figure 1.9**.) While virtually all nutrients can be said to regulate body processes and many contribute to body structures, only the nutrients protein, carbohydrate, and fat are sources of energy. Because the body needs large quantities of carbohydrate, protein, and fat, these are called **macronutrients**; the vitamins and minerals are **micronutrients** because the amounts the body needs are comparatively small.

In addition to their functions, there are several other key differences among the classes of nutrients. First, the chemical composition of nutrients varies widely. One way to divide the nutrient groups is based on whether the compounds contain the element carbon. Substances that contain carbon are **organic** substances; those that do not are **inorganic**. Carbohydrates, lipids, proteins, and vitamins are all organic; minerals and water are not. Structurally, nutrients can be very simple—minerals are single elements (sodium, for example), although we often consume them as larger compounds (sodium chloride, or table salt). Water is also very simple in structure. The organic nutrients have more complex structures—the

phytochemicals Substances in plants that may possess health-protective effects, even though they are not essential for life.

antioxidant A substance that combines with or otherwise neutralizes a free radical, thus preventing oxidative damage to cells and tissues.

macronutrients Nutrients, such as carbohydrate, fat, or protein, that are needed in relatively large amounts in the diet.

micronutrients Nutrients, such as vitamins and minerals, that are needed in relatively small amounts in the diet.

organic [or-GAN-ick] In chemistry, any compound that contains carbon, except carbon oxides (e.g., carbon dioxide) and sulfides and metal carbonates (e.g., potassium carbonate). The term sometimes is used to denote crops that are grown without synthetic fertilizers or chemicals.

inorganic Any substance that does not contain carbon, excepting certain simple carbon compounds such as carbon dioxide and monoxide. Common examples include table salt (sodium chloride) and baking soda (sodium bicarbonate).

carbohydrates, lipids, and proteins we eat are made of smaller building blocks, while the vitamins are elaborately structured compounds.

It is rare for a food to contain just one nutrient. Meat is not just protein any more than bread is solely carbohydrate. Foods contain mixtures of nutrients, although in most cases, protein, fat, or carbohydrate dominates. So while bread is certainly rich in carbohydrates, it also contains some protein, a little fat, and many vitamins and minerals. If it's whole-grain bread you're eating, you also get fiber, not technically a nutrient, but an important compound for good health nonetheless.

Key Concepts: *Nutrients are the essential chemicals in food that the body needs for normal functioning and good health and that must come from the diet because they either cannot be made in the body or cannot be made in sufficient quantities. Six classes of nutrients—carbohydrates, proteins, lipids, vitamins, minerals, and water—can be described by their composition or by their function in the body.*

Carbohydrates

The word **carbohydrate**, or literally "hydrate of carbon," tells you exactly what this nutrient is made of, if you think "water" when you hear the word *hydrate*. Carbohydrates are made of carbon, hydrogen, and oxygen, and are a major

carbohydrate Compounds, including sugars, starches, and dietary fibers, that usually have the general chemical formula $(CH_2O)n$, where *n* represents the number of CH_2O units in the molecule. Carbohydrates are a major source of energy for body functions.

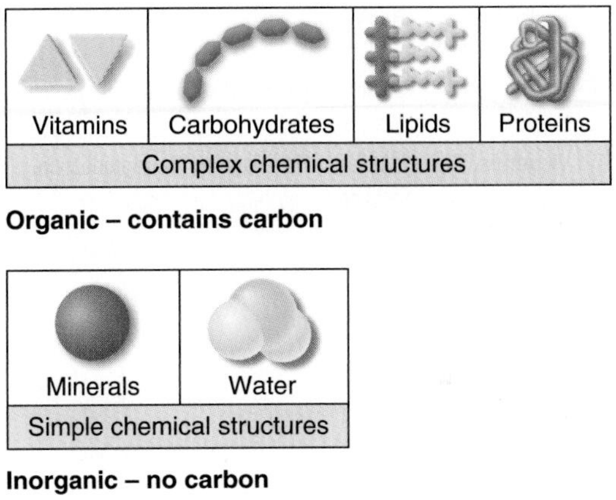

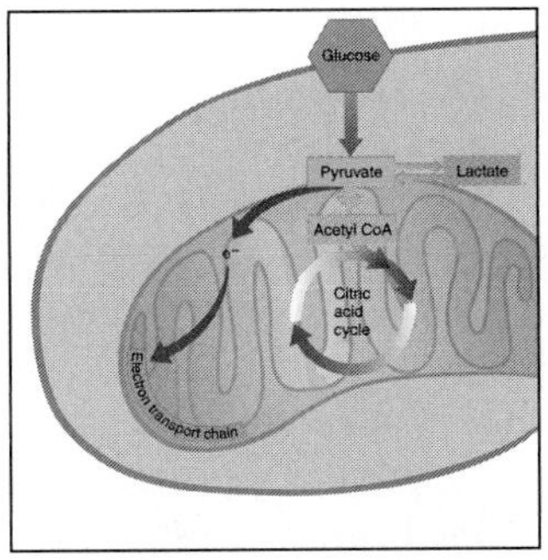

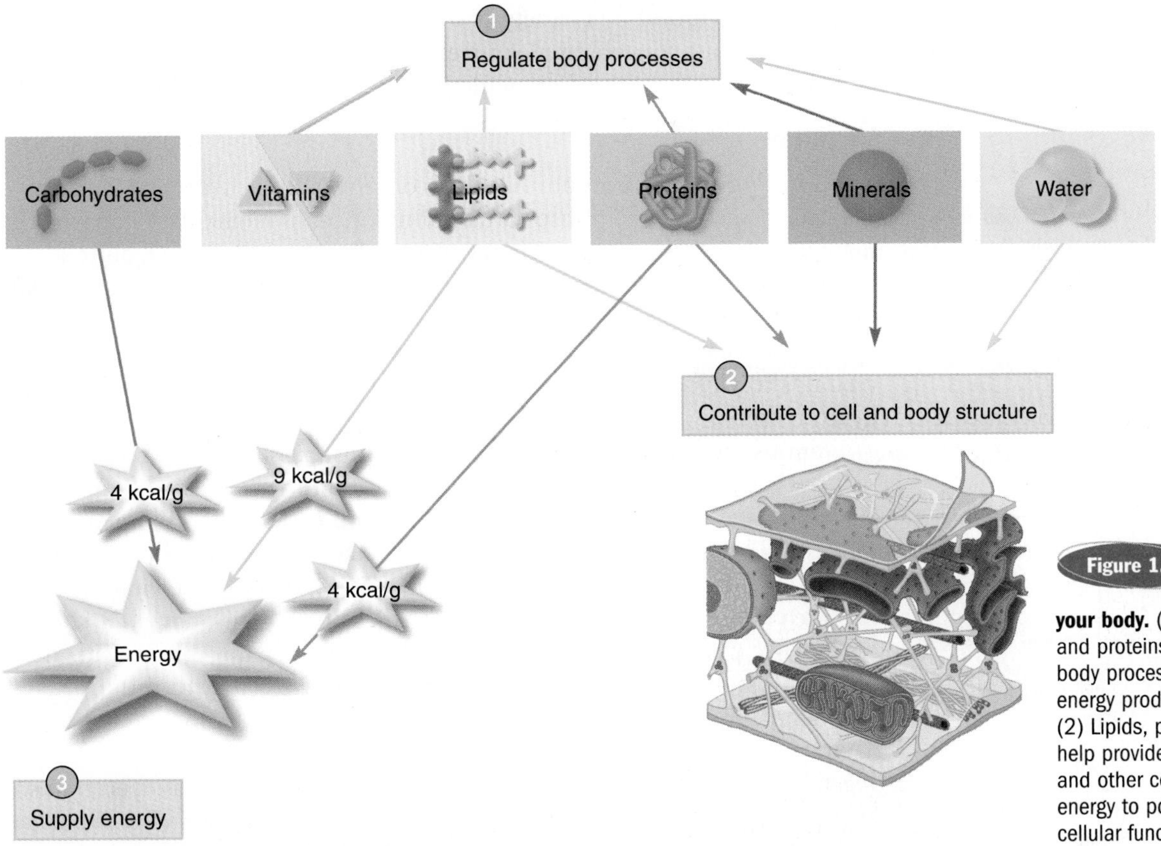

Figure 1.9 **Nutrients have three general functions in your body.** (1) Micronutrients, some lipids and proteins, and water help regulate body processes such as blood pressure, energy production, and temperature. (2) Lipids, proteins, minerals, and water help provide structure to bone, muscle, and other cells. (3) Macronutrients supply energy to power muscle contractions and cellular functions.

circulation Movement of substances through the vessels of the cardiovascular or lymphatic system.

lipids A group of fat-soluble compounds that includes triglycerides, sterols, and phospholipids.

triglycerides Fats composed of three fatty acid chains linked to a glycerol molecule.

hormones Chemical messengers that are secreted into the blood by one tissue and act on cells in another part of the body.

proteins Large, complex compounds consisting of many amino acids connected in varying sequences and forming unique shapes.

amino acids Organic compounds that function as the building blocks of protein.

vitamins Organic compounds necessary for reproduction, growth, and maintenance of the body. Vitamins are required in miniscule amounts.

source of fuel for the body. Dietary carbohydrates are the starches and sugars found in grains, vegetables, legumes (dry beans and peas), and fruits. We also get carbohydrates from dairy products, but practically none from meats. Your body converts most dietary carbohydrates to glucose, a simple sugar compound. It is glucose that we find in **circulation**, providing a source of energy for cells and tissues.[24]

Lipids

The term **lipids** refers to substances we know as fats and oils, but also to fatlike substances in foods, such as cholesterol and phospholipids. Lipids are organic compounds and, like carbohydrates, contain carbon, hydrogen, and oxygen. Fats—or, more correctly, **triglycerides**—are another major fuel source for the body. In addition, triglycerides, cholesterol, and phospholipids have other important functions: providing structure for body cells, carrying the fat-soluble vitamins (A, D, E, and K), and providing the starting material (cholesterol) for making many **hormones**. Dietary sources of lipids include fats and oils we add to foods or cook with, the naturally occurring fats in meats and dairy products, and less obvious plant sources such as coconut, olives, and avocado.

Proteins

Proteins are organic compounds made of smaller building blocks called **amino acids**. Unlike carbohydrates and lipids, amino acids contain nitrogen as well as carbon, hydrogen, and oxygen. Some amino acids also contain the mineral sulfur. The amino acids that we get from dietary protein combine with the amino acids made in the body to make hundreds of different body proteins. Body proteins help build and maintain body structures and regulate body processes. Protein also can be used for energy.

Proteins are found in a variety of foods, but meats and dairy products are among the most concentrated sources. Grains, legumes, and vegetables all contribute protein to the diet, while fruits contribute negligible amounts.[25]

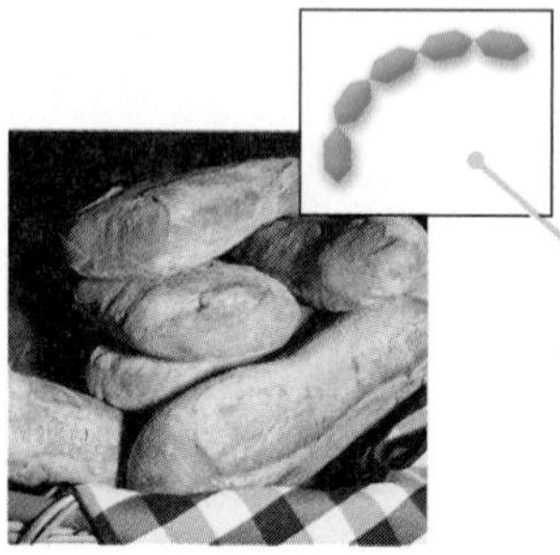

Whenever you see this icon, we'll be talking about **carbohydrates**

Provide:
Energy (4 kcal/g)

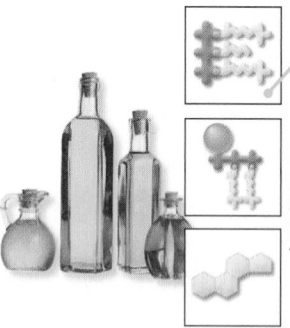

Whenever you see one of these 3 icons, we'll be talking about **lipids**

Provide:
Energy (9 kcal/g)
Structure
Regulation (hormones)
Transport

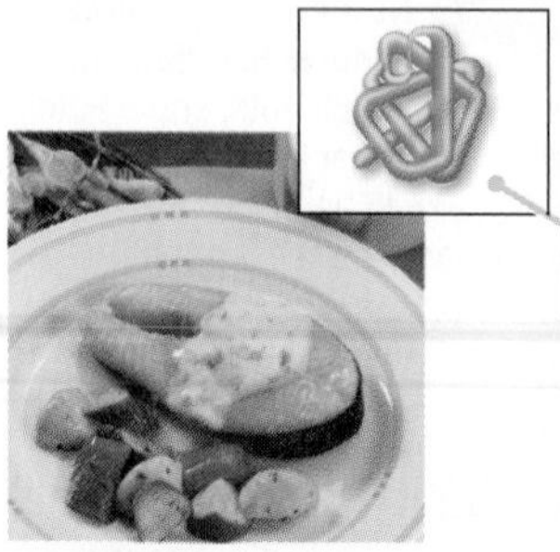

Whenever you see this icon, we'll be talking about **proteins**

Provide:
Energy (4 kcal/g)
Structure
Regulation

Vitamins

Vitamins are organic compounds that contain carbon, hydrogen, and perhaps nitrogen, oxygen, phosphorus, sulfur, or other elements. Vitamins regulate body processes such as energy production, blood clotting, and calcium balance. Vitamins help to keep organs and tissues functioning and healthy. Because vitamins have such diverse functions, a lack of a particular vitamin can have widespread effects. While the body does not break down vitamins to yield energy, vitamins have vital roles in the extraction of energy from carbohydrate, fat, and protein.

Vitamins are usually divided into two groups: fat-soluble and water-soluble. The four fat-soluble vitamins—A, D, E, and K—have very diverse roles. What they have in common is the way they are absorbed and transported in the body and the fact that they are more likely to be stored in larger quantities than the water-soluble vitamins. The water-soluble vitamins include vitamin C and eight B vitamins: thiamin (B_1), riboflavin (B_2), niacin (B_3), pyridoxine (B_6), cobalamin (B_{12}), folate, pantothenic acid, and biotin. Most of the B vitamins are involved in some way with the pathways for energy metabolism.

Vitamins are found in a wide variety of foods, not just fruits and vegetables—although these are important sources—but also meats, grains, legumes, dairy products, and even fats. Choosing a well-balanced diet usually makes vitamin supplements unnecessary. In fact, when taken in large

Think About It 3

doses, vitamin supplements—especially those containing vitamins A, D, B_6, or niacin—can be harmful.

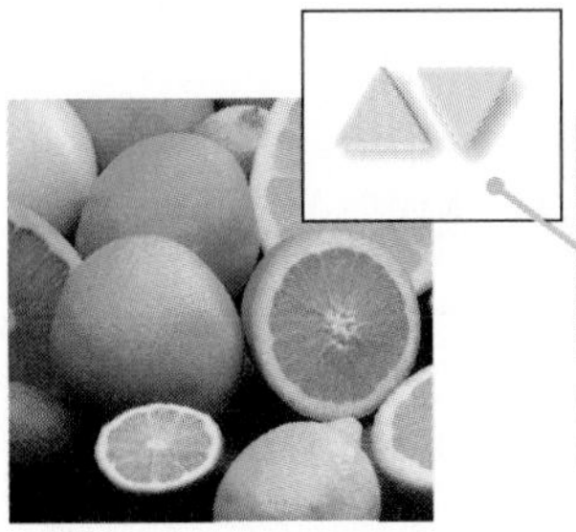

Whenever you see these icons, we'll be talking about **vitamins**

Provide:
Regulation

Minerals

Structurally, **minerals** are simple, inorganic substances. At least 16 minerals are essential to health; among them are sodium, chloride, potassium, calcium, phosphorus, magnesium, and sulfur.[26] Because the body needs these minerals in relatively large quantities compared with other minerals, they are often called **macrominerals**. The body needs the remaining minerals only in very small amounts. These **microminerals**, or **trace minerals**, include iron, zinc, copper, manganese, molybdenum, selenium, iodine, and fluoride. Like vitamins, the functions of minerals are diverse. Minerals can be found in structural roles (e.g., calcium, phosphorus, and fluoride in bones and teeth) as well as regulatory roles (e.g., control of fluid balance and regulation of muscle contraction).

Food sources of minerals are just as diverse. Although we often associate minerals with animal foods such as meats and milk, plant foods are important sources as well. Deficiencies of minerals, except iron and perhaps calcium, are uncommon. A balanced diet provides enough minerals for most people. However, individuals with iron-deficiency anemia may need iron supplements, and others may need calcium supplements if they cannot or will not drink milk or eat dairy products. As is true for vitamins, excessive intake of some minerals as supplements can be toxic.

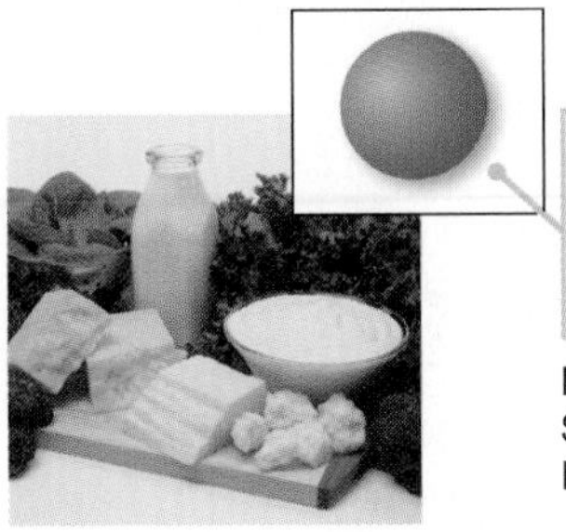

Whenever you see this icon, we'll be talking about **minerals**

Provide:
Structure
Regulation

Water

Next to the mineral elements, water is chemically the simplest nutrient. Water is also the most important nutrient! We can survive far longer without any of the other nutrients in the diet, indeed without food at all, than we can without water. Water has many roles in the body, including temperature control, lubrication of joints, and transportation of nutrients and wastes.

Your body is nearly 60 percent water, so maintaining adequate hydration means regular fluid intake is very important. Water is found not only in beverages, but also in most food products. Fruits and vegetables in particular are high in water content. Through many chemical reactions, the body makes some of its own water, but this is only a fraction of the amount needed for normal function.

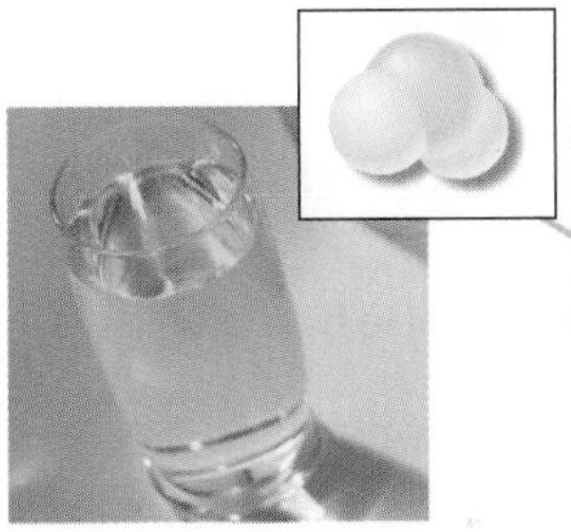

Whenever you see this icon, we'll be talking about **water**

Provides:
Regulation
Structure

Key Concepts: *The body needs larger amounts of carbohydrates, lipids, and proteins (macronutrients) than vitamins and minerals (micronutrients). Carbohydrates, lipids, and proteins provide energy; proteins, lipids, minerals, and water add to body structure; and proteins, vitamins, minerals, and some fatty acids regulate body processes.*

Nutrients and Energy

One of the main reasons we eat food, and the nutrients it contains, is for **energy**. Every cellular reaction, every muscle movement, every nerve impulse requires energy. Three of the nutrient classes—carbohydrates, lipids (triglycerides only), and proteins—are energy sources. When we speak of the energy in foods, we are really talking about the *potential* energy that foods contain. Energy itself is not a food component.

Different scientific disciplines use different measures of energy. In nutrition, we discuss the potential energy in food, or the body's use of energy, in units of heat called **kilocalories** (1,000 calories). One kilocalorie (or kcal)

minerals Inorganic compounds needed for growth and for regulation of body processes.

macrominerals Major minerals required in the diet and present in the body in large amounts compared with trace minerals.

microminerals See *trace minerals.*

trace minerals Trace minerals are present in the body and required in the diet in relatively small amounts compared with major minerals. Also known as microminerals.

energy The capacity to do work. The energy in food is chemical energy, which the body converts to mechanical, electrical, or heat energy.

kilocalories (kcal) [KILL-oh-kal-oh-rees] Units used to measure energy. Food energy is measured in kilocalories (1,000 calories = 1 kilocalorie).

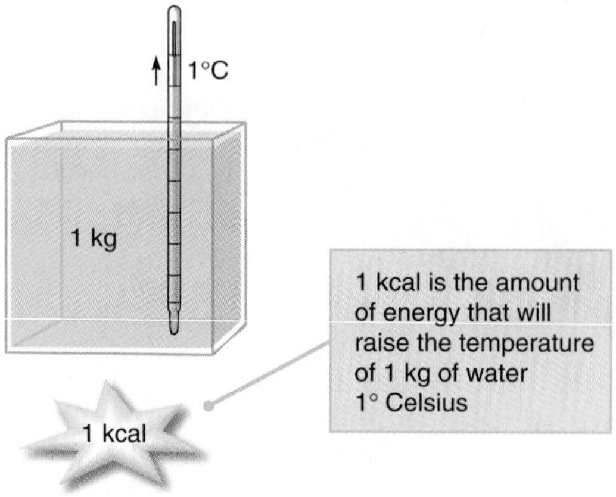

is the amount of energy (heat) it would take to raise the temperature of 1 kilogram (kg) of water by 1 degree Celsius. For now, this may be an abstract concept, but as you learn more about nutrition, you will discover the amount of energy you likely need to fuel your daily activities. And you will also learn about the amounts of potential energy in various foods.

Energy in Foods

Energy is available from foods because foods contain carbohydrate, fat, and protein. These nutrients can be broken down completely (metabolized) to yield energy in a form that cells can use. When completely metabolized in the body, carbohydrate and protein yield 4 kilocalories of energy for every gram (g) consumed; fat yields 9 kilocalories per gram; and alcohol contributes 7 kilocalories per gram. (See **Figure 1.10**.) Therefore, the energy available from a given food or from a total diet is reflected by the amount of each of these substances consumed. Because fat is a concentrated source of energy, adding or removing fat from the diet can have a big effect on available energy.

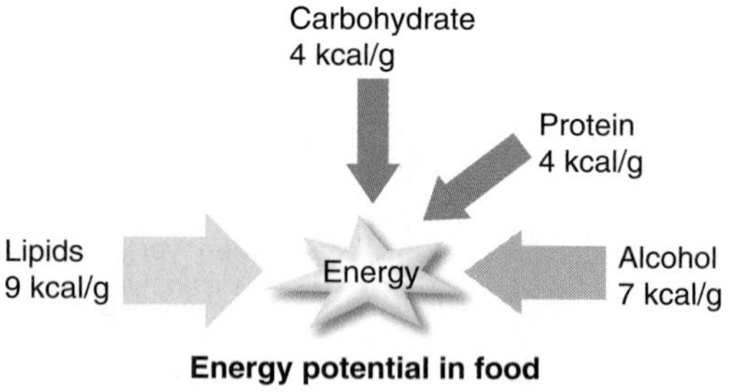

Figure 1.10 **Energy potential in food.** Your body can use carbohydrate, fat, protein, and alcohol as sources of energy.

When Is a Kilocalorie a Calorie?

Many people inappropriately use the terms ***calorie*** and *kilocalorie* interchangeably. To clear up this confusing situation, you should use the term *calorie* as a general term for energy and *kilocalorie* as a specific measurement or unit of that energy. *Calories* is like referring to gas for a car, and *kilocalories* is like referring to gallons of fuel. When in doubt, substitute the word *energy* for calories. The following sentence illustrates the use of *kilocalorie* and *calorie*. Because fat contains 9 *kilocalories* per gram, more than double that of protein or carbohydrate, foods high in fat are rich in *calories* (energy).

You'll find that food labels, diet books, and other sources of nutrition information use the term *calorie*, not *kilocalorie*. Technically, the potential energy in foods is best measured in kilocalories; however, the term *calorie* has become familiar and commonplace.

calorie The general term for energy in food, used synonymously with the term *energy*. Often used instead of *kilocalorie* on food labels, in diet books, and in other sources of nutrition information.

How Can We Calculate the Energy Available from Foods?

To calculate the energy available from food, multiply the number of grams of fat, carbohydrate, and protein by 9, 4, and 4, respectively; then add the results. For example, if we assume that one bagel plus one and a half ounces of cream cheese contains 39 grams of carbohydrate, 10 grams of protein, and 16 grams of fat, we can determine the available energy from each component.

39 g carbohydrate × 4 kcal/g	=	**156 kcal**
10 g protein × 4 kcal/g	=	**40 kcal**
16 g fat × 9 kcal/g	=	**144 kcal**
Total	=	**340 kcal**

To calculate the *percentage* of calories each of these components contributes to the total, divide the individual results by the total, and then multiply by 100. For example, to determine the percentage of calories from fat in this example, divide the 144 fat kilocalories by the total of 340 kilocalories and then multiply by 100 ($144 \div 340 \times 100 = 42\%$).

Be Food Smart: Calculate the Percentages of Calories in Food

Current health recommendations suggest limiting fat intake to about 30 percent of *total* energy intake. This means that during the course of the day, we should strive to eat less than 30 percent of our calories from fat. You can monitor this for yourself in two ways. If you like counting fat grams, you can first determine your suggested maximum fat intake. For example, if you need to eat 2,000 kilocalories each day to maintain your current weight, 30 percent of those calories can come from fat.

$$2{,}000 \text{ kcal} \times 0.30 = 600 \text{ kcal from fat}$$

$$600 \text{ kcal from fat} \div 9 \text{ kcal/g} = 66.7 \text{ g of fat}$$

Therefore, your maximum fat intake should be about 67 grams. You can check food labels to see how many fat grams you typically eat.

Another way to monitor your fat intake is to know the percentage of calories that come from fat in various foods. If the proportion of fat in each food choice throughout the day exceeds 30 percent of calories, then the day's total of fat will be too high as well. Some foods contain virtually no fat calories (e.g., fruits and vegetables), while others are nearly 100 percent fat calories (e.g., margarine, salad dressing). Being aware that a snack like the bagel and cream cheese provides 42 percent of its calories from fat can help you select lower-fat foods at other times of the day.

CALCULATING THE ENERGY AVAILABLE FROM FOODS

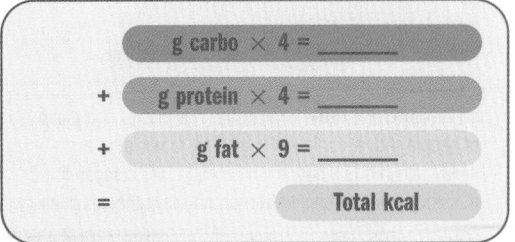

g carbo × 4 = ______
\+ g protein × 4 = ______
\+ g fat × 9 = ______
= Total kcal

Example:

275 g carbohydrate × 4 kcal/g	=	1,100 kcal
75 g protein × 4 kcal/g	=	300 kcal
67 g fat × 9 kcal/g	=	600 kcal (rounded from 603 kcal)
Total	=	2,000 kcal

CALCULATING THE PERCENTAGE OF KILOCALORIES FROM NUTRIENTS

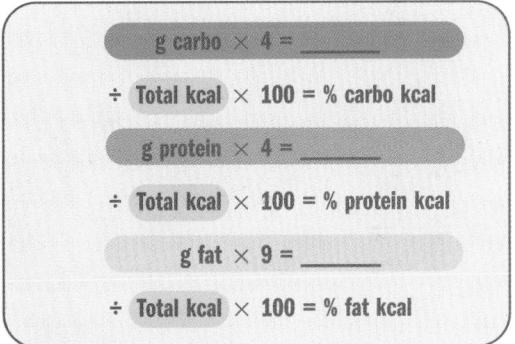

g carbo × 4 = ______
÷ Total kcal × 100 = % carbo kcal
g protein × 4 = ______
÷ Total kcal × 100 = % protein kcal
g fat × 9 = ______
÷ Total kcal × 100 = % fat kcal

Example:

275 g carbohydrate × 4	=	1,100 kcal
1,100 kcal ÷ 2,000 kcal × 100	=	55% carb. kcal
75 g protein × 4	=	300 kcal
300 kcal ÷ 2,000 kcal × 100	=	15% protein kcal
67 g fat × 9	=	600 kcal (rounded from 603 kcal)
600 kcal ÷ 2,000 kcal × 100	=	30% fat kcal

Food Choices Provide Essential Nutrients

The foods we choose do more than provide us with an adequate diet. The balance of energy sources can affect our risk of chronic disease. For example, high-fat diets have been linked to heart disease and cancer. Excess calories contribute to obesity, which also increases disease risk. Other nutrients, such as the minerals sodium, chloride, calcium, and magnesium, affect blood pressure, while lack of the vitamin folate prior to conception and in early pregnancy can cause serious birth defects. Non-nutrient components in the diet (e.g., phytochemicals) may have antioxidant or immune-enhancing properties that also keep us healthy. The choices we make can reduce our disease risk, as well as provide energy and essential nutrients.

Key Concepts: *All cells and tissues need energy to keep the body functioning. Energy in foods and in the body is measured in kilocalories. The carbohydrates, lipids, and proteins in food are potential sources of energy, meaning that the body can extract energy from them. Lipids, specifically the triglycerides in fats, are the most concentrated source of energy, with 9 kilocalories per gram. Carbohydrates and proteins can yield 4 kilocalories per gram, while alcohol can yield 7 kilocalories per gram.*

Applying the Scientific Process to Nutrition

Whether it's identifying essential nutrients, establishing recommended intake levels, or exploring the effects of vitamins on cancer risk, scientific studies are the cornerstone of nutrition. Although we may use creative, artistic talents to choose and serve a pleasing array of foods, the fundamentals of nutrition are developed through the scientific process of observation and inquiry.

The scientific process enables researchers to test the validity of **hypotheses** that arise from observations of natural phenomena. For example, it was common knowledge in the eighteenth century that sailors on long voyages would likely develop scurvy (which we now know results from a deficiency of vitamin C). Scurvy had been recognized since ancient times, and its common symptoms—pinpoint skin hemorrhages, swollen and bleeding gums, joint pain, fatigue and lethargy, and psychological changes such as depression and hysteria—were well known. Native populations discovered

hypotheses Scientists' "educated guesses" to explain phenomena.

epidemiology The science of determining the incidence and distribution of diseases in different populations.

correlations Connections, co-occurring more frequently than can be explained by chance or coincidence, but without a proven cause.

case control study An investigation that uses a group of people with a particular condition, rather than a randomly selected population. These cases are compared with a control group of people who do not have the condition.

experiments Tests to examine the validity of a hypothesis.

plant foods that would cure this illness; among Native Americans these included cranberries in the Northeast and many tree extracts in other parts of the country. From observations such as this come questions that lead to hypotheses, or "educated guesses," about factors that might be responsible for the observed phenomenon. Scientists then test hypotheses using appropriate research designs. Poorly designed research produces useless results or false conclusions.

Epidemiological Studies

An epidemiological study compares disease rates among population groups and attempts to identify related conditions or behaviors such as diet and smoking habits. The observation that scurvy developed during prolonged time at sea is an example of one aspect of **epidemiology**. Another example is the association between dietary intakes of soy and breast cancer rates. While Japanese women have high dietary intakes of soy and low breast cancer rates, American women have comparatively low dietary intakes of soy and high breast cancer rates.

Epidemiological studies provide information about relationships but do not clarify cause and effect. The results of these studies show **correlations**—relationships between two factors. For example, with soy and breast cancer, epidemiological studies show only that populations with higher soy intake (Japanese women) have lower breast cancer rates; they do not establish that soy intake prevents breast cancer. However, epidemiological studies provide clues and insights that lead to animal and human studies that can further clarify diet and disease relationships.

Animal Studies

Animal studies can provide preliminary data that lead to human studies or can be used to study hypotheses that cannot be tested on humans. It was shown in the 1890s that feeding polished (refined) rice to chickens led to a disease similar to beriberi, while a diet of rice with the hull intact did not. It's important to keep in mind that although animal studies give scientists important information that furthers nutrition knowledge, the results of animal studies cannot be transferred directly to humans. Animal studies need to be followed with cell culture studies or human clinical studies to determine specific effects in humans.

Cell Culture Studies

Another way to study nutrition is to isolate specific types of cells and grow them in a laboratory. Scientists can then use these cells to study the effects of nutrients or other components on metabolic processes in the cell. An important area of nutrition research is the effect of specific nutrients and other chemical compounds on gene expression. This area of molecular biology will help us to explain individual differences in chronic disease risk factors and may lead to designing diets based on an individual's genetic profile, rather than on guidelines for the population in general.

Human Studies

The **case control study** and clinical trials are the two primary types of **experiments** used to test hypotheses in humans. Case control studies are small-scale epidemiological studies in which one group of individuals who have a condition (e.g., breast cancer) is compared with a similar group of individuals who do not have the condition. Researchers then identify factors other than the disease in question, such as fruit and vegetable intake, that differ between the two groups. These factors provide researchers with clues about the cause, progression, and prevention of the disease. It is important that the two groups are matched as closely as possible for major characteristics such as age, gender, and race.

Clinical trials are controlled studies where some type of intervention—a nutrient supplement, controlled diet, or exercise program—is used to determine its impact on certain health parameters. These studies include an **experimental group** (the people who are given the intervention) and a **control group** (similar people who are not treated). Scientists measure aspects of health or disease in each group and compare the results.

James Lind's experiments with sailors aboard the *Salisbury* in 1747 are considered to be the first dietary clinical trial. (See **Figure 1.11**.) His observation that oranges and lemons were the only dietary elements that seemed to cure scurvy was an important finding. However, it took more than 40 years before the British Navy began routinely giving all sailors citrus juice or fruit—a practice that led to the nickname "limey" when referring to British sailors. It took nearly 200 years (until the 1930s) for scientists to isolate the compound we call vitamin C and show that it had antiscurvy activity.[27] The chemical name for vitamin C, ascorbic acid, comes from its role as an "antiscorbutic" (antiscurvy) compound.

There are several important elements in a modern clinical trial: random assignment to groups, use of placebos, and the double-blind method. Subjects are assigned randomly—as by the flip of a coin—to the experimental group or the control group. This reduces the risk of introducing bias into either group. People in the experimental group receive the treatment or specific protocol (e.g., consuming a certain nutrient at a specific level). People in the control group do not receive the treatment but usually receive a **placebo**. A placebo is an imitation treatment (such as a sugar pill) that looks the same as the experimental treatment but has no effect. The placebo is also important for reducing bias because subjects do not know if they are receiving the intervention and are less inclined to alter their responses or reported symptoms based on what they think should happen.

When the members of neither the experimental nor the control groups know what treatment they are receiving, we say the subjects are "blinded" to the treatment. If a clinical trial is designed so neither the subjects nor the researchers collecting data are aware of the subjects' group assignments (treatment or placebo), the study is called a **double-blind study**. This reduces the possibility that researchers will see the results they want to see even if these results do not occur. In this case, another member of the research team holds the code for subject assignments and does not participate in the data collection. Double-blind, placebo-controlled clinical trials are considered the "gold standard" of nutrition studies. These studies can show clear cause-and-effect relationships, but often require large numbers of subjects and are expensive and time consuming to conduct.

More on the Placebo Effect

Because the **placebo effect** can exert a powerful influence, research studies must take it into account. For example, when researchers tested the effectiveness of a medication in reducing binge eating among people with bulimia, they used a double-blind study to eliminate the placebo effect.[28] After a baseline number of binge-eating episodes was determined, 22 women with bulimia were given the medication or a placebo. After a

clinical trials Studies that collect large amounts of data to evaluate the effectiveness of a treatment.

experimental group A set of people being studied to evaluate the effect of an event, substance, or technique.

control group A set of people used as a standard of comparison to the experimental group. The people in the control group have characteristics similar to those in the experimental group and are selected at random.

placebo An inactive substance that is outwardly indistinguishable from the active substance whose effects are being studied.

double-blind study A research study set up so that neither the subjects nor the investigators know which study group is receiving the placebo and which is receiving the active substance.

placebo effect A physical or emotional change that is not due to properties of an administered substance. The change reflects participants' expectations.

Key

- Controlled variables
- Experimental variables
- Results
- Conclusions

1. **Observation**
   Sailors on long voyages all became ill with scurvy.
2. **Hypothesis**
   Lack of certain foods causes scurvy.
3. **Experimentation**
   Experiment to test hypothesis.
   Predicts that some dietary element will cure scurvy.

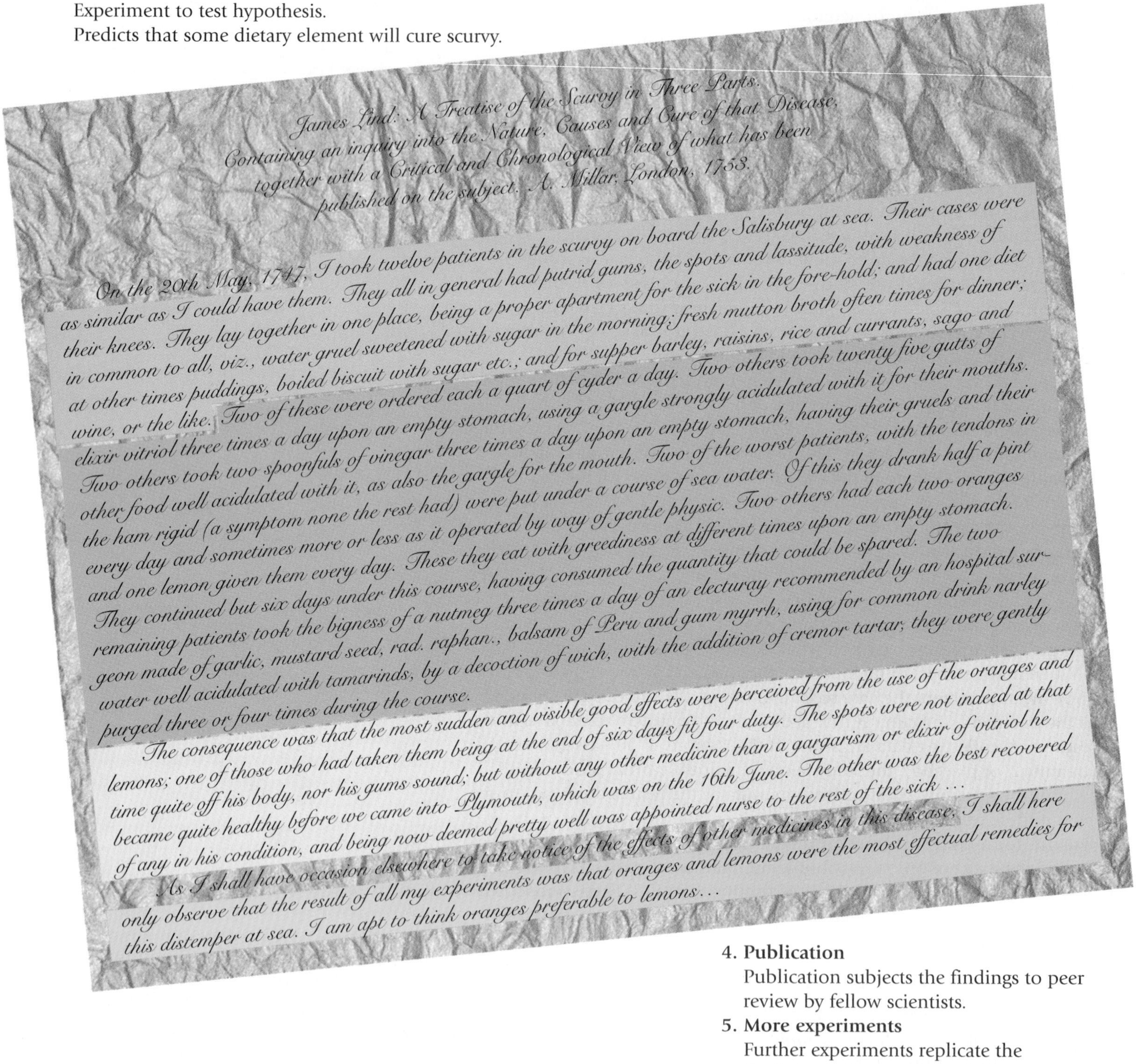

James Lind: A Treatise of the Scurvy in Three Parts.
Containing an inquiry into the Nature, Causes and Cure of that Disease,
together with a Critical and Chronological View of what has been
published on the subject. A. Millar, London, 1753.

On the 20th May, 1747, I took twelve patients in the scurvy on board the Salisbury at sea. Their cases were as similar as I could have them. They all in general had putrid gums, the spots and lassitude, with weakness of their knees. They lay together in one place, being a proper apartment for the sick in the fore-hold; and had one diet in common to all, viz., water gruel sweetened with sugar in the morning; fresh mutton broth often times for dinner; at other times puddings, boiled biscuit with sugar etc.; and for supper barley, raisins, rice and currants, sago and wine, or the like. Two of these were ordered each a quart of cyder a day. Two others took twenty five gutts of elixir vitriol three times a day upon an empty stomach, using a gargle strongly acidulated with it for their mouths. Two others took two spoonfuls of vinegar three times a day upon an empty stomach, having their gruels and their other food well acidulated with it, as also the gargle for the mouth. Two of the worst patients, with the tendons in the ham rigid (a symptom none the rest had) were put under a course of sea water. Of this they drank half a pint every day and sometimes more or less as it operated by way of gentle physic. Two others had each two oranges and one lemon given them every day. These they eat with greediness at different times upon an empty stomach. They continued but six days under this course, having consumed the quantity that could be spared. The two remaining patients took the bigness of a nutmeg three times a day of an electuray recommended by an hospital surgeon made of garlic, mustard seed, rad. raphan., balsam of Peru and gum myrrh, using for common drink narley water well acidulated with tamarinds, by a decoction of wich, with the addition of cremor tartar, they were gently purged three or four times during the course.

The consequence was that the most sudden and visible good effects were perceived from the use of the oranges and lemons; one of those who had taken them being at the end of six days fit four duty. The spots were not indeed at that time quite off his body, nor his gums sound; but without any other medicine than a gargarism or elixir of vitriol he became quite healthy before we came into Plymouth, which was on the 16th June. The other was the best recovered of any in his condition, and being now deemed pretty well was appointed nurse to the rest of the sick …

As I shall have occasion elsewhere to take notice of the effects of other medicines in this disease, I shall here only observe that the result of all my experiments was that oranges and lemons were the most effectual remedies for this distemper at sea. I am apt to think oranges preferable to lemons…

4. **Publication**
   Publication subjects the findings to peer review by fellow scientists.
5. **More experiments**
   Further experiments replicate the findings and extend knowledge.
6. **Theory**
   Scientists consolidate acquired knowledge into a theory that explains the observed phenomenon.

Figure 1.11 **The first clinical trial.** In 1758, physician James Lind reported the careful process of his clinical trial among British sailors afflicted with scurvy.

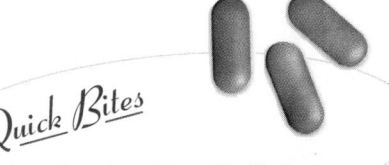

period of time, the number of binge-eating episodes was reassessed. The study found a 78 percent reduction in binge-eating episodes among those taking the medication and a 70 percent reduction in the control group. This showed that the *expectation* that the medication would be effective was nearly as effective as the medication itself. However, a recent review of placebo or no-treatment clinical trials concluded that placebos do not generally have significant effects in studies with objective outcomes, but may have small benefits in studies where the outcome measures were subjective, such as pain intensity.[29] Based on this study, the often-quoted value that one-third of patients show improvement after receiving a placebo is probably an overstatement.

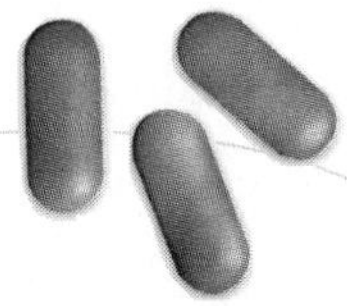

Quick Bites

Swallowing Your Beliefs

Patients' expectations play an important role in their responses to a placebo. In one study, subjects swallowed a pill that contained only a magnet to measure their stomach contractions. Their stomach contractions increased, decreased, or did not change according to what they had been told would happen.

Peer Review of Experimental Results

Once an experiment is complete, scientists publish the results in a scientific journal to communicate new information to other scientists. Generally, before articles are published in scientific journals, other scientists who have expert knowledge of the subject critically review them. **Peer review** ensures that only high-quality research findings are published. Unfortunately, peer-reviewed journals such as the *American Journal of Clinical Nutrition* and the *Journal of the American Dietetic Association* are not the main sources of information presented in the popular media.

peer review An appraisal of research against accepted standards by professionals in the field.

Key Concepts: *The scientific method is used to expand our nutrition knowledge. Hypotheses are formed from observations and are then tested by experiments. Epidemiological studies observe patterns in populations. Animal and cell culture studies can test effects of various treatments. For human studies, placebo-controlled, double-blind clinical trials are the best research tool for determining cause-and-effect relationships.*

From Research Study to Headline

Think About It 4

What about the nutrition and health headlines we see in the newspapers, hear on TV, or read on the Internet daily? Consumers are often confused by what they see as the "wishy-washiness" of scientists—for example, coffee is good, then coffee is bad. Margarine is better than butter…no wait, maybe butter is better after all. These contradictions, despite the confusion they cause, show us that nutrition is truly a science: dynamic, changing, and growing with each new finding.

Each time research findings are summarized and reported, some degree of opinion is introduced into the report. A large-scale clinical trial or a long-term observational report produces mountains of data. Researchers must decide, using their experience and judgment, which data-analysis methods to use and which results to summarize for peer-reviewed publica-

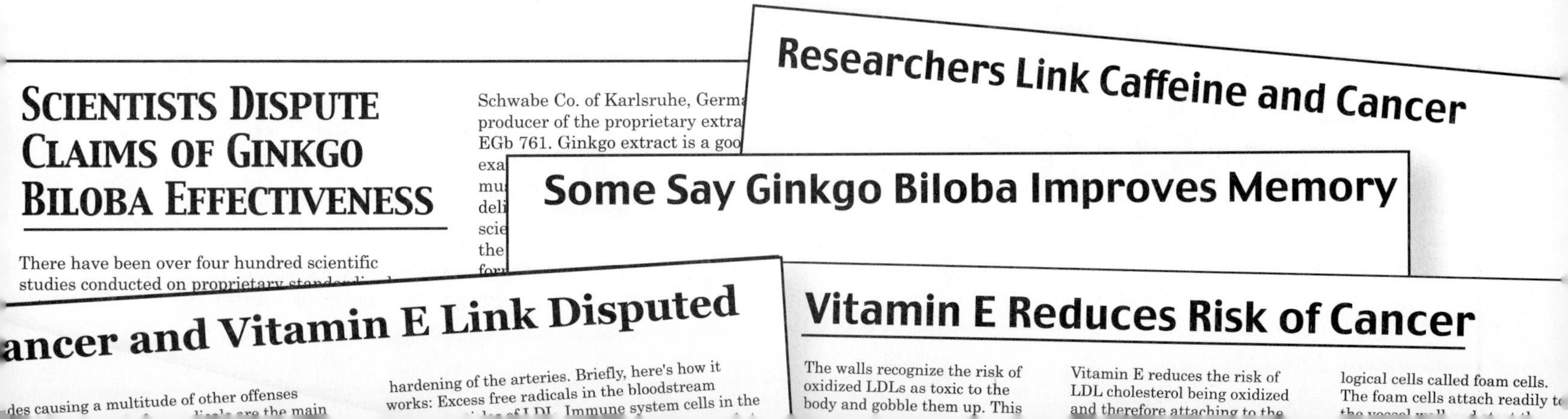

SCIENTISTS DISPUTE CLAIMS OF GINKGO BILOBA EFFECTIVENESS
There have been over four hundred scientific studies conducted on
Schwabe Co. of Karlsruhe, Germ producer of the proprietary extra EGb 761. Ginkgo extract is a goo
Researchers Link Caffeine and Cancer
Some Say Ginkgo Biloba Improves Memory
ancer and Vitamin E Link Disputed
des causing a multitude of other offenses
hardening of the arteries. Briefly, here's how it works: Excess free radicals in the bloodstream
Vitamin E Reduces Risk of Cancer
The walls recognize the risk of oxidized LDLs as toxic to the body and gobble them up. This
Vitamin E reduces the risk of LDL cholesterol being oxidized
logical cells called foam cells. The foam cells attach readily t

tion. The journalist who regularly scans scientific journals for potential headlines decides which studies will get media attention and then summarizes study results in nontechnical terms. A news article becomes a 30-second sound bite that usually is far removed from the original data. In some cases, the study may be distorted, with its results misstated or overstated. (See **Figure 1.12**.)

Sorting Facts and Fallacies in the Media

People tend to believe what they hear repeatedly. Even when it has no basis in fact, a claim can seem credible if heard often enough. For example, do you believe that sugar makes kids hyperactive? There is no *scientific* evidence to support this claim! The public is surrounded by messages from various media: TV, radio, newspapers, magazines, books, and the Internet. Because a larger audience translates into higher ratings or sales and subsequently high advertising rates, the media make money attracting viewers, listeners, and readers. To increase the number of viewers or listeners, media may sensationalize and oversimplify nutrition-related topics. This is particularly true of stories related to obesity, cancer, vitamins and minerals, and food safety. Although news stories may be based on reports in the scientific literature, the media may distort the facts through omission of details.

As you learn about nutrition, you will undoubtedly be more aware not only of your eating and shopping habits but also of nutrition-related information in the media. As you see and hear reports, stop to think carefully about what you are hearing. Headlines and news reports often overstate the findings of a study. You may want to find the scientific article and read it for yourself. At first, reading journal articles will be difficult, but with experience (and growing nutrition knowledge) you will understand more of the information presented. Talk to your instructor for ideas about journal articles that might help you evaluate headlines you are seeing. Two other things to keep in mind: One study does not provide all the answers to our nutrition questions; and if it sounds too good to be true, it probably is!

Your study of nutrition is just beginning. As you learn about the essential nutrients, their functions and food sources, be alert to your food choices and the factors that influence them. When the discussion turns to the role of diet in health, think about your preconceived ideas and evaluate your beliefs in the light of current scientific evidence. Keep an open mind, but also think critically. Most of all, remember that food is more than the nutrients it provides; it is part of the way we enjoy and celebrate life!

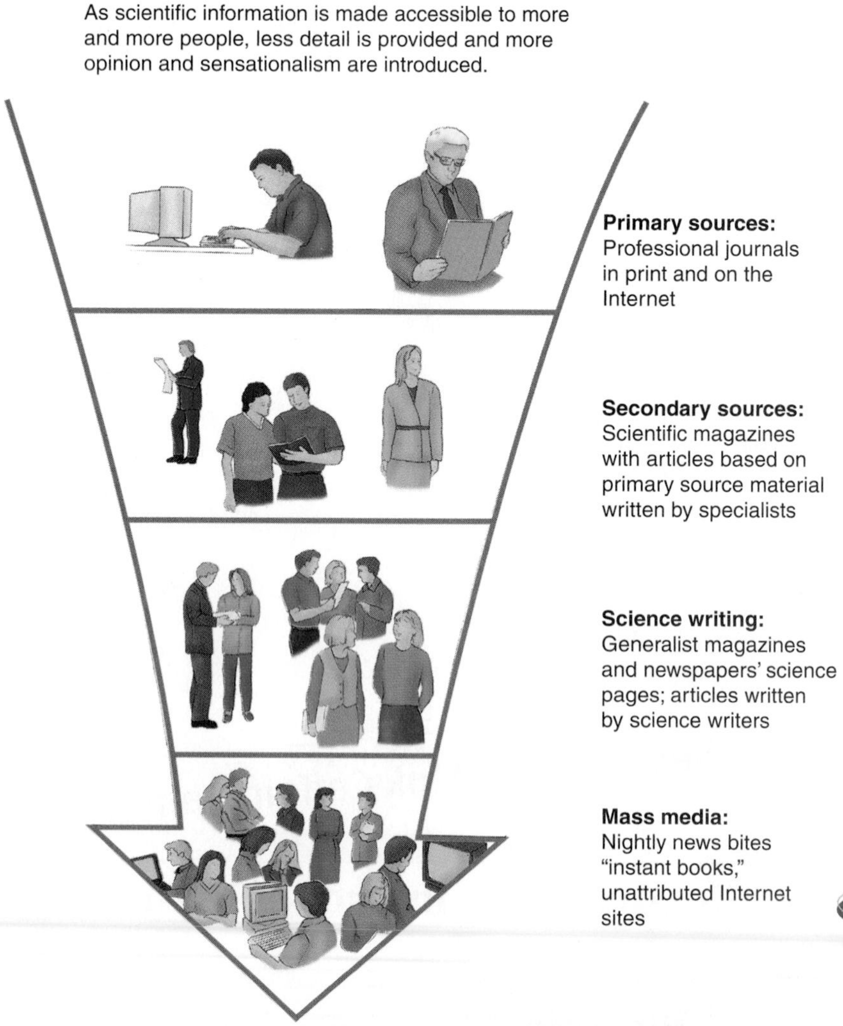
As scientific information is made accessible to more and more people, less detail is provided and more opinion and sensationalism are introduced.
Primary sources: Professional journals in print and on the Internet
Secondary sources: Scientific magazines with articles based on primary source material written by specialists
Science writing: Generalist magazines and newspapers' science pages; articles written by science writers
Mass media: Nightly news bites "instant books," unattributed Internet sites

Figure 1.12 **Sifting facts and fallacies.** From original research to the evening news, each step along the way introduces biases as information is summarized and restated. Whether on television, radio, the Internet, or in print, the best consumer information cites sources for reported facts.

Fyi — FOR YOUR INFORMATION: Do You Speak Metric?

Although the metric system isn't really a language like English or Spanish, in some sense it is the language of science. Nutritionists must be fluent in metrics. Pick up any nutrition journal and you will find units of measurement expressed in terms like kilograms and liters.

The metric system is a decimal-based system of measurement units. Like our monetary system, units are related by factors of 10. There are 10 pennies in a dime, and 10 dimes equal 1 dollar. Calculations involve the simple process of moving the decimal point to the right or to the left.

There are only seven basic units in the metric system. The most common units are the meter (m) to measure length, the kilogram (kg) for mass, the liter (L) for volume, and degree Celsius (°C) for temperature. The metric system avoids the confusing dual use of terms, such as our current use of ounces to measure both weight and volume.

One strategy for learning metric is to find common or familiar associations. For example, when using degrees Celsius you should equate 22 degrees Celsius (22°C) with room temperature, 37 degrees Celsius (37°C) with body temperature, and 0 and 100 degrees Celsius with the freezing and boiling points of water, respectively. A millimeter (1 mm) is about the thickness of a dime, and 2 centimeters (2 cm) is about the diameter of a nickel. Most people already recognize 1-liter and 2-liter soft-drink bottles. When you pick up a 2-pound box of sugar, you are holding a little less than 1 kilogram. A fluid ounce can be tricky because it's a measure of liquid volume, not weight. A 1-liter bottle equals 33.8 fluid ounces.

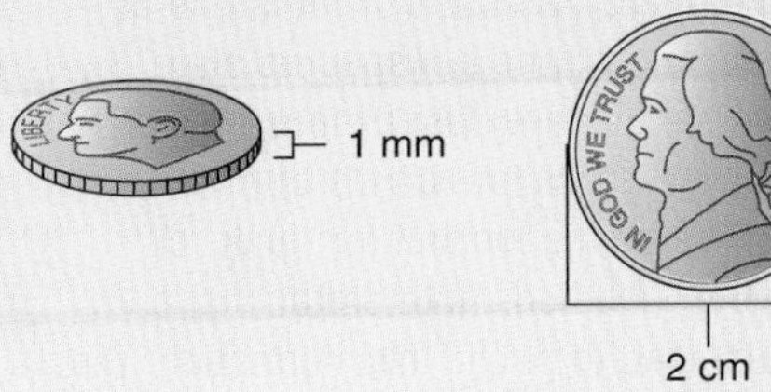

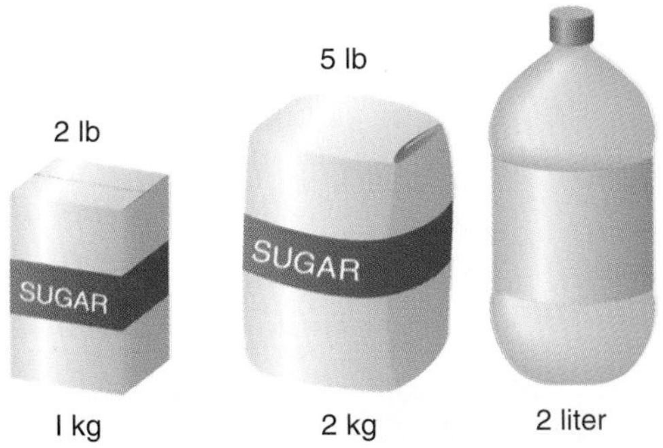

The United States is the only industrialized country in the world not officially using the metric system. Because of its many advantages (e.g., easy conversion between units of the same quantity), the metric system has become the internationally accepted system of measurement.

Many members of the international scientific community use the International System of Units (SI). The SI is the modern metric system and has adopted the joule rather than the calorie to measure food energy. Although we think of the calorie as a measure of energy, it is more accurately a measure of heat. Joules are a measure of work, not heat, and the amount of energy potential in foods is expressed best in kilojoules (kjoules). Each kilocalorie is equivalent to approximately 4.2 (4.184) kilojoules. For example, a 100-kilocalorie glass of juice provides about 420 kilojoules.

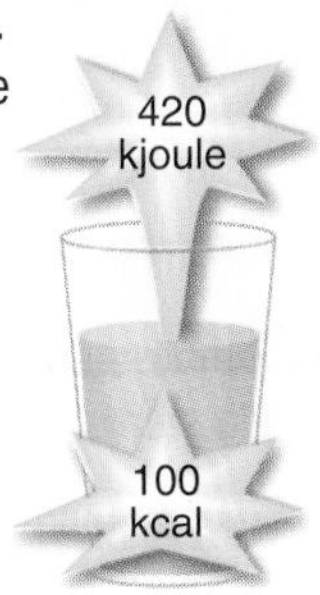

In most cases, familiarity with the following metric units will be sufficient in your study of nutrition.

Measures Commonly Used in Nutrition

	Metric	*English*
Length	1 meter (m)	39.4 inches (in)
	1 centimeter (cm)	0.394 inches (in)
	2.54 centimeters (cm)	1 inch (in)
Weight (mass)	1 kilogram (kg)	2.2 pounds (lb)
	454 grams (g)	1 pound (lb)
	5 grams (g) of salt	about 1 teaspoon (tsp)
Volume	1 liter (L)	1.057 quarts (about 4 cups)
	236 milliliters (mL)	about 1 cup (c)
	15 milliliters (mL)	about 1 tablespoon (tbs)
	5 milliliters (mL)	about 1 teaspoon (tsp)

1 gram = 1,000 milligrams

1 milligram = 1,000 micrograms (μg or mcg)

The Celsius (C) temperature scale should be used instead of the Fahrenheit (F) scale. The following are familiar points:

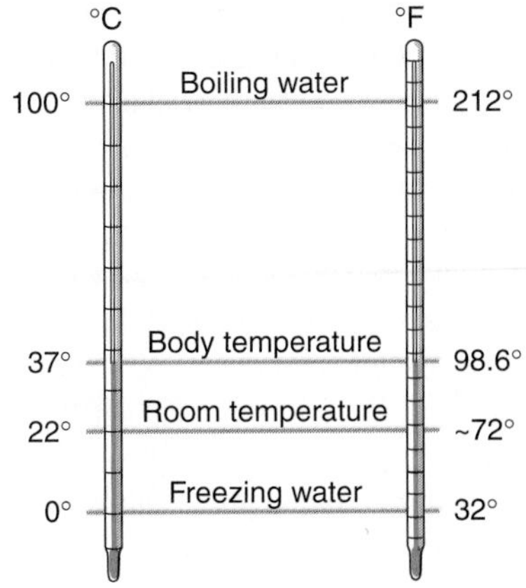

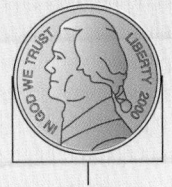

Fyi FOR YOUR INFORMATION

Evaluating Information on the Internet

Surfing the Web has made life easier in many ways. You can buy a car, check stock prices, search out sources for a paper you're writing, chat with like-minded people, and stay up to date on news or sports scores. Hundreds of Web sites are devoted to nutrition and health topics, and you may be asked to visit such sites as part of your course requirements. So, how do you evaluate the quality of information on the Web? Can you trust what you see?

First, it's important to remember that there are no rules for posting on the Internet. Anyone who has the equipment can set up a Web site and post any content he or she likes. Although the Health on the Net Foundation has set up a Code of Conduct for medical and health Web sites, following their eight principles is completely voluntary.[1]

Second, consider the source, if you can tell what it is! Many Web sites do not specify where the content came from, who is responsible for it, or how often it is updated. If the site lists the authors, what are their credentials? Who sponsors the site itself? Educational institutions (.edu), government agencies (.gov), and organizations (.org) generally have more credibility than commercial (.com) sites, where selling rather than educating may be the motive.[2] Identifying the purpose for a site can give you more clues about the validity of its content.

Third, when you see claims for nutrients, dietary supplements, or other products, and results of studies or other information, keep in mind the scientific method and the basics of sound science. Who did the study? What type of study was it? How many subjects? Was it double-blind? Were the results published in a peer-reviewed journal? Think critically about the content, look at other sources, and ask questions of experts before you accept information as truth. What is true of books, magazines, and newspapers also applies to the Internet: Just because it is in print or online doesn't mean it's true.

Finally, be on the lookout for "junk science"—sloppy methods, interpretations, and claims that lead to public misinformation. The Food and Nutrition Science Alliance (FANSA) is a coalition of four professional societies: the American Dietetic Association (ADA), the American Society for Clinical Nutrition (ASCN), the American Society for Nutritional Sciences (ASNS), and the Institute of Food Technologists (IFT). FANSA has developed the "10 Red Flags of Junk Science" to help consumers identify potential misinformation. Use these red flags to evaluate Web sites.

Use the Internet; it's fun and can be educational. Don't forget about the library, though; many scientific journals are not available online. Treat claims as "guilty until proven innocent"—in other words, don't accept what you read at face value until you have evaluated the science behind it. If it sounds too good to be true, it probably is!

The 10 Red Flags of Junk Science

1. Recommendations that promise a quick fix
2. Dire warnings of danger from a single product or regimen
3. Claims that sound too good to be true
4. Simplistic conclusions drawn from a single study
5. Recommendations based on a single study
6. Dramatic statements that are refuted by reputable scientific organizations

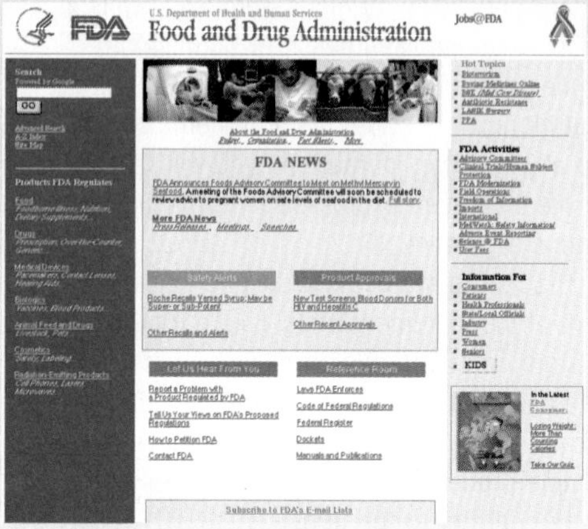

7. Lists of "good" and "bad" foods
8. Recommendations made to help sell a product
9. Recommendations based on studies published without peer review
10. Recommendations from studies that ignore differences among individuals or groups

Source: ADA Serves Up 10 Red Flags to Spot Junk Science. http://www.eatright.org/pr/press021996a.html. Accessed 3/20/02. Reprinted with permission from American Dietetic Association.

Note: *The Journal of the American Dietetic Association* has a list of several reliable Internet resources for dietetics professionals.

[1] http://www.hon.ch/HONcode/Conduct.html. Accessed 3/20/02.

[2] The wheat from the chaff: sorting out nutrition information on the Internet. *J Am Diet Assoc.* 1998;98:1270–1272.

LEARNING Portfolio chapter 1

Key Terms

	page
amino acids	14
antioxidant	12
calorie	16
carbohydrate	13
case control study	18
circulation	14
clinical trials	19
control group	19
correlations	18
double-blind study	19
energy	15
epidemiology	18
essential nutrients	11
experiments	18
experimental group	19
flavor	5
hormones	14
hypotheses	17
inorganic	12
kilocalories (kcal) [KILL-oh-kal-oh-rees]	15
lipids	14
macrominerals	15
macronutrients	12
microminerals	15
micronutrients	12
minerals	15
neophobia	4
nutrients	11
nutrition	4
organic [or-GAN-ick]	12
peer review	21
phytochemicals	12
pica	7
placebo	19
placebo effect	19
proteins	14
social facilitation	8
trace minerals	15
triglycerides	14
umami [ooh-MA-mee]	5
vitamins	14

Study Points

- Most people make food choices for reasons other than nutrient value.
- Taste and texture are the two most important factors that influence food choices.
- In all cultures, eating is the primary way of maintaining social relationships.
- Although Americans know about healthful food choices, their eating habits do not always reflect this knowledge.
- Food is a mixture of chemicals. Essential chemicals in food are called nutrients.
- Carbohydrates, lipids, proteins, vitamins, minerals, and water are the six classes of nutrients found in food.
- Nutrients have three general functions in the body: They serve as energy sources, structural components, and regulators of metabolic processes.
- Vitamins regulate body processes such as energy metabolism, blood clotting, and calcium balance.
- Minerals contribute to body structures and to regulating processes such as fluid balance.
- Water is the most important nutrient in the body. We can survive much longer without the other nutrients than we can without water.
- Energy in foods and the body is measured in kilocalories. Carbohydrates, fats, and proteins are sources of energy.
- Carbohydrate and protein have a potential energy value of 4 kilocalories per gram, and fat provides 9 kilocalories per gram.
- Scientific studies are the cornerstone of nutrition. The scientific method uses observation and inquiry to test hypotheses.
- Double-blind, placebo-controlled clinical trials are considered the "gold standard" of nutrition studies.
- Research designs used to test hypotheses include epidemiological, animal, cell culture, and human studies.
- Information in the public media is not always an accurate or complete representation of the current state of the science on a particular topic.

Study Questions

Answers can be found at nutrition.jbpub.com/discovering.

1. **What are the three main factors that influence our food choices?**
2. **How do our health beliefs affect our food choices?**
3. **List the six classes of nutrients.**
4. **List the 13 vitamins.**
5. **What determines whether a mineral is a macromineral or a micro- (trace) mineral?**
6. **How many kilocalories are in 1 gram of carbohydrate, of protein, and of fat?**
7. **What is an epidemiological study?**
8. **What's the difference between an experimental and control group?**
9. **What's a placebo?**

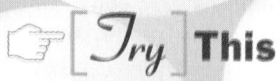

Try This

Try a New Cuisine Challenge

The purpose of this exercise is for you to expand your culinary taste buds and try a new cuisine. Take your local phone book and see how many ethnic restaurants are near campus. Choose a cuisine you are not very familiar with and take some friends along for dinner so you can order and share several dishes. While you're there, don't be afraid to ask questions about the menu, so you can gain a better understanding of the foods, preparation techniques, spices, and even the cultural meaning attached to some of the dishes.

Food Label Puzzle

The purpose of this exercise is to put the individual pieces of the food label together to determine how many kilocalories are in a serving. Take all the foods in your dorm room or apartment that have complete food labels and ask a friend to black out the value for calories on each. Remember that the term *calories* on a food label really is referring to kilocalories. Your job is to determine how many kilocalories are in a serving of each of these foods. You can do this by putting together the individual pieces (carbohydrate, protein, and fat). If you need help, review this chapter and pay close attention to the section on the energy-yielding nutrients. How many kilocalories does each have per gram? You may find that your calculations don't match the numbers on the label. Within labeling guidelines, food manufacturers can round values.

What About Bobbie?

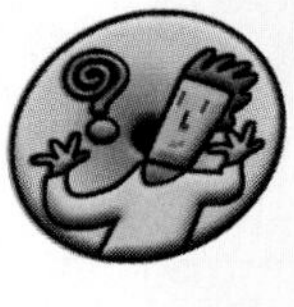

The "What about Bobbie?" feature appears in most chapters. Bobbie is a college student whom you'll follow throughout this text to learn the strengths and weaknesses of her diet. Look for this feature to see how the information you learn in each chapter can be applied to real life.

Bobbie is a 20-year-old college sophomore. She lives in the dorm and has one roommate. She has the standard meal plan with her university, so she eats most of her meals in the cafeteria. Sometimes she'll get a snack from the local coffee shop or a dorm vending machine. Her schedule is fairly typical, with classes spread out in both the morning and afternoon. Occasionally at night, she and her friends will order pizza or go out for ice cream.

Bobbie weighs 155 pounds and is 5 feet, 4 inches tall. She gained 10 pounds her freshman year in college and would like to lose it because she feels that her ideal weight is more like 145 pounds. She exercises infrequently but likes to walk with her friends and take an occasional aerobics class. Here is a typical day of eating for Bobbie:

Sample one-day menu from Bobbie's diet

7:45 A.M.
1 raisin bagel
3 tablespoons light cream cheese
10 fluid ounces regular coffee
2 packets of sugar
2 tablespoons of 2% milk

10:15 A.M.
1 banana

12:15 P.M.
Turkey and cheese sandwich
2 slices sourdough bread
2 ounces sliced turkey lunch meat
2 teaspoons regular mayonnaise
2 teaspoons mustard
2 slices tomato
2 slices dill pickle
shredded lettuce
Salad from cafeteria salad bar
2 cups shredded iceberg lettuce
2 tablespoons each:
shredded carrot
chopped egg
croutons
kidney beans
Italian dressing
12 fluid ounces diet soda
1 small chocolate chip cookie

3:30 P.M.
16 fluid ounces water
1.5 ounces regular tortilla chips
½ cup salsa

6:00 P.M.
Spaghetti with meatballs
1.5 cups pasta
3 ounces ground beef (meatballs)
3 ounces spaghetti sauce with mushrooms
2 tablespoons parmesan cheese
1 piece garlic bread
½ cup green beans
1 teaspoon butter
12 fluid ounces diet soda

10:15 P.M.
1 slice cheese pizza

References

1 Lernmer CM, Mattes R. Cognitive influences on food intake. *Healthline.* June 1999;18:6–7.

2 Gerrish CJ, Mennella JA. Flavor variety enhances food acceptance in formula-fed infants. *Am J Clin Nutr.* 2001;73(6): 1080–1085.

3 Smith DV, Margolskee RF. Making sense of taste. *Scientific American.* 2001;284(3):32–39.

4 Yamaguchi S, Ninomiya K. Umami and food palatability. *J Nutr.* 2000;130:921S–926S.

5 Lacey EP. Broadening the perspective of pica: literature review. *Public Health Reports.* 1990;105(1):29–35.

6 Connell D, Goldberg JP, Folta SC. An intervention to increase fruit and vegetable consumption using audio communications: in-store public service announcements and audiotapes. *J Health Commun.* 2001;6(1):31–43.

7 Levy AS, Stokes RC. Effects of a health promotion advertising campaign on sales of ready-to-eat cereals. *Public Health Reports.* 1987;102(4):398–403.

8 Birch LL. Development of food preferences. *Ann Rev Nutr.* 1999;19:41–62.

9 De Castro JM, Brewer ME. The amount eaten in meals by humans is a power function of the number of people present. *Physiol Behav.* 1991;51:121–125; and Patel KA, Schlundt DG. Impact of moods and social context on eating behavior. *Appetite.* 2001;36(2):111–118.

10 Dubois L, Girard M. Social position and nutrition: a gradient relationship in Canada and the USA. *Eur J Clin Nutr.* 2001; 55(5):366–373.

11 Cockerham WC. *Medical Sociology.* Englewood Cliffs, NJ: Prentice-Hall; 1978.

12 Mooney K, Walbourn L. When college students reject food: not just a matter of taste. *Appetite.* 2001;36(1):41–50.

13 Rozin P. Human food selection: why do we know so little and what can we do about it? *Int J Obes.* 1980;4:333–337.

14 Kittler PG, Sucher KP. *Food and Culture.* 3rd ed. Belmont, CA: Wadsworth; 2001.

15 Fieldhouse P. *Food and Nutrition: Customs and Culture.* UK: Chapman and Hall; 1996.

16 Zeman FJ, Ney DM. Cultural factors in nutrition care. In: Davis KM, ed. *Applications in Medical Nutrition Therapy.* Englewood Cliffs, NJ: Prentice-Hall; 1996:125–138.

17 Sloan AE. America's appetite '96: the top 10 trends to watch and work on. *Food Technology.* 1996;50:55–71.

18 Kittler PG, Sucher KP. Op. cit.

19 Zeman FJ, Ney DM. Op. cit.; Fieldhouse P. Op. cit.; and Kittler PG, Sucher KP. Op. cit.

20 Chiva M. Cultural aspects of meals and meal frequency. *Br J Nutr.* 1997;77(suppl):S21–S28; and Zeman FJ, Ney DM. Op. cit.

21 Fieldhouse P. Op. cit.

22 US Department of Agriculture. Results from the 1994–96 Continuing Survey of Food Intakes by Individuals. http://www.barc.usda.gov/bhnrc/foodsurvey/96result.html. Accessed 3/20/02.

23 Beliefs and attitudes of Americans toward their diet. *Nutrition Insights.* Washington, DC: Center for Nutrition Policy and Promotion, USDA. June 2000;19:1–2.

24 Goran MI. Variation in total energy expenditure in humans. *Obes Res.* 1995;3(suppl 1):59–66.

25 Fuller MF, Garlich PJ. Human amino acid requirements: can the controversy be resolved? *Ann Rev Nutr.* 1994;14:217–241.

26 Food and Nutrition Board. *Recommended Dietary Allowances.* 10th ed. Washington, DC: National Academy Press; 1989.

27 Johnston CS. Vitamin C. In: Bowman BA, Russell RM, eds. *Present Knowledge in Nutrition.* 8th ed. Washington, DC: ILSI Press; 2001.

28 Alger SA, Schwalberg MD, Bigaouette JM, et al. Effect of a tricyclic antidepressant and opiate antagonist on binge-eating behavior in normal weight, bulimic, and obese binge-eating subjects. *Am J Clin Nutr.* 1991;53:865–871.

29 Hrobjartsson A, Gotzsche PC. Is the placebo powerless? An analysis of clinical trials comparing placebo with no treatment. *N Engl J Med.* 2001;344:1594–1602.

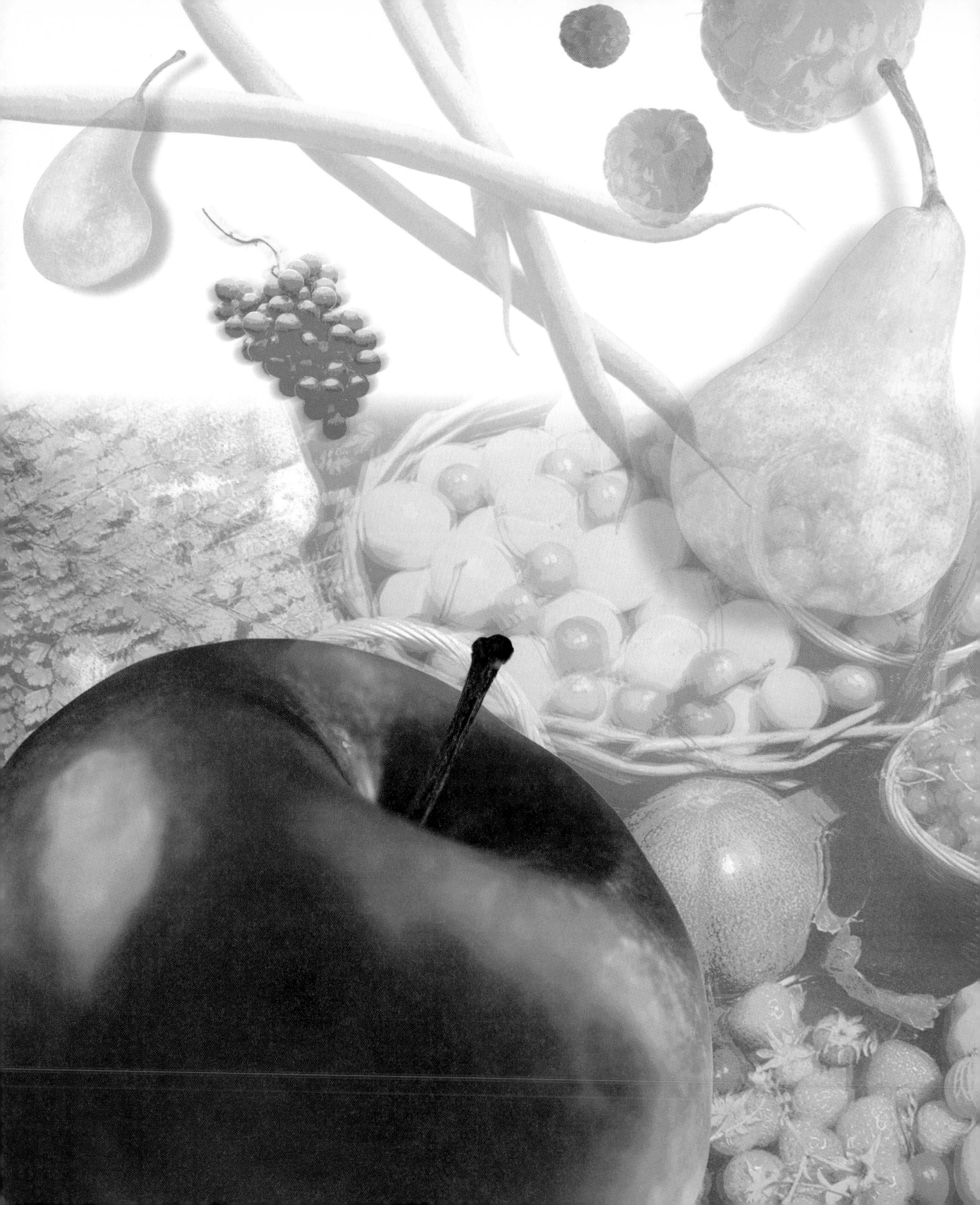

Chapter 2

Nutrition Guidelines: Tools for a Healthful Diet

Think About It

1. Do you and your friends discuss food and diet?
2. Have you ever taken a very large dose of a vitamin or mineral? If so, why? How did you determine whether it was safe?
3. Do you eat the same foods most days, or do you like variety?
4. Which food group in the Food Guide Pyramid makes up the biggest part of your diet?

Fyi for your Information

This chapter's FYI boxes include practical information on the following topics:

- Are All Food Pyramids Created Equal?
- Food Guide Pyramid: Foods, Serving Sizes, and Tips
- Definitions for Nutrient Content Claims on Food Labels

www

The Web site for this book offers many useful tools and is a great source for additional nutrition information for both students and instructors. For information on nutrition guidelines, visit the site at **nutrition.jbpub.com/discovering**. You'll find exercises that explore the following topics:

- Pros and Cons of Food Labeling
- Examining the New DRIs
- The Healthy Eating Index

What About Bobbie?

Track the choices Bobbie is making with the EatRight Analysis software.

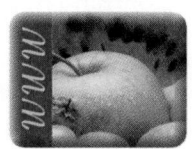

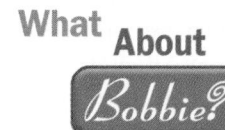

So, you want to be healthier—maybe that's why you are taking this course! If so, you already know that a well-planned diet is one important element of being healthy. Although most of us know that the foods we choose have a major impact on our health, we aren't certain about what choices to make. Choosing the right foods isn't made any easier when we are bombarded by headlines and advertisements: Eat less fat! Get more fiber in your diet! Build strong bones with calcium!

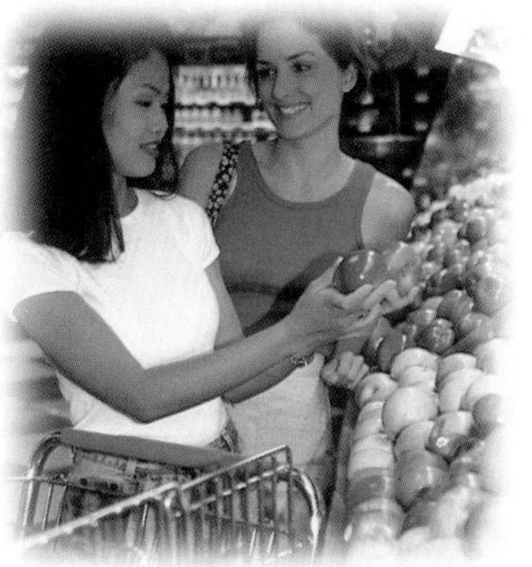

For many Americans, nutrition is simply a lot of hearsay...or maybe the latest slogan coined from last week's news headline. Conversations about nutrition start off with "*They* say you should..." or "Now *they* think that...." Have you ever wondered who "they" are and why "they" are telling you what to eat or what not to eat?

It's no secret that a healthy population is a more productive population, so many of our nutrition guidelines come from the federal government's efforts to improve our overall health. Thus the government is one "they." Many important elements of nutrition policy focus on relieving undernutrition in some population groups. The government requires food manufacturers to add nutrients to certain foods to prevent widespread deficiencies: iodine in salt, vitamin D in milk, and thiamin, riboflavin, niacin, iron, and folic acid in enriched grains. Dietary standards such as the Dietary Reference Intakes make it easier to define adequate diets for large groups of people.

Overnutrition has led to changes in public policy as well. Health researchers have discovered links between diet and high blood pressure, cancer, and heart disease; as a result, nutritionists suggest that we reduce sodium and saturated fat intake. The public's need to know what is in the food supply has led to increased nutrition information on food labels. And public education efforts have resulted in development of teaching tools such as the Food Guide Pyramid.

New information about diet and health will continue to drive public policy. This chapter explores current dietary standards, guidelines, and diet-planning tools. While you're reading, think about your diet and how it measures up to current guidelines and standards.

Quick Bites

Early "Laws of Health"

Galen may be the best-known physician who ever lived. During the second century, Galen expounded his "laws of health"—eat proper foods, drink the right beverages, exercise, breathe fresh air, get enough sleep, have a daily bowel movement, and control your emotions.

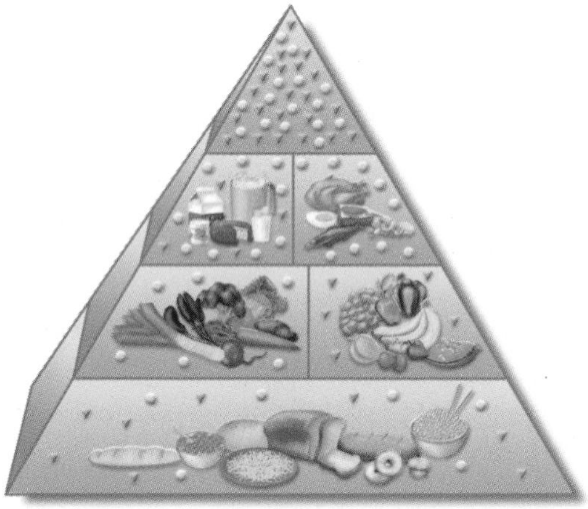

marasmus A type of malnutrition resulting from chronic inadequate consumption of protein and energy that is characterized by wasting of muscle, fat, and other body tissue.

kwashiorkor A type of malnutrition that occurs primarily in young children who have an infectious disease and whose diets supply marginal amounts of energy and very little protein. Common symptoms include poor growth, edema, apathy, weakness, and susceptibility to infections.

undernutrition Poor health resulting from the depletion of nutrients due to inadequate nutrient intake over time. It is now most often associated with poverty, alcoholism, and some types of eating disorders.

overnutrition The long-term consumption of an excess of nutrients. The most common type of overnutrition in the United States is due to the regular consumption of excess calories, fats, saturated fats, and cholesterol.

Linking Nutrients, Foods, and Health

We all know that what we eat affects our health. Nutrition science has made many advances in identifying essential nutrients and the foods in which they are found. Eating foods with all the essential nutrients prevents nutritional deficiencies such as scurvy (vitamin C deficiency) or pellagra (deficiency of the B vitamin niacin). In the United States, few people suffer nutritional deficiencies as a result of dietary inadequacies. More often, Americans suffer from chronic diseases such as heart disease, cancer, hypertension, and diabetes—all linked to overconsumption and lifestyle choices. Think About It 1

The Continuum of Nutritional Status

Your nutritional status can be seen as a point along a continuum, with undernutrition and overnutrition at the extremes. Chronic undernutrition results in the development of nutritional deficiency diseases, as well as conditions of energy and protein malnutrition such as **marasmus** and **kwashiorkor**, and can lead to death. Unlike starvation, **undernutrition** is a condition in which *some* food is being consumed, but the intake is not nutritionally adequate. Although chronic undernutrition and associated deficiency diseases were common in the United States in the 1800s and early 1900s, today they are rare. Undernutrition now is most often associated with extreme poverty, alcoholism, illness, or some eating disorders.

Overnutrition is the chronic consumption of more than is necessary for good health. Specifically, overnutrition is the regular consumption of excess calories, fats, saturated fats, or cholesterol—all of which increase risk for chronic disease. Today, nutrition-related chronic diseases such as coronary heart disease, cancer, stroke, and diabetes are among the 10 leading causes of death in the United States. All of these problems have been linked to dietary excess. (Remember that epidemiological [population] studies can show associations between various factors and diseases, but these correlations do not necessarily indicate cause and effect.)

Between these two extremes lies a region of good health. In 1988, the U.S. Surgeon General wrote, "for the two out of three adult Americans who do not smoke and do not drink excessively, one personal choice seems to influence long-term health prospects more than any other: what we eat."[1] Good food and lifestyle choices, a balanced diet, and regular exercise help to reduce the risk of chronic disease and delay its onset, keeping us in a region of good health for more of our lifetime.

Moderation, Variety, and Balance: Words to the Wise

Living in high-tech America, we expect immediate solutions to long-term problems. It would be nice if we could keep the consequences of overconsumption at bay just by taking a pill, drinking a beverage, or getting a shot. But no magic food, nutrient, or drug exists. Instead, you have to rely on healthful foods, exercise, and lifestyle choices to reduce your risk of chronic disease. Even in the twenty-first century, we will need to follow the same advice we have been hearing for decades—healthful eating requires moderation, variety, and balance.

Moderation

Think About It 2

Not too much or too little of anything—that's what moderation means. Moderation does *not* mean that you have to eliminate high-fat foods from your diet, but rather that you can occasionally include small amounts of them. Moderation also means not taking anything to extremes. You probably know that vitamin E has positive effects, but that doesn't mean that huge doses of this essential nutrient are appropriate for you. It's important to remember that substances that are healthful in small amounts can sometimes be dangerous in large quantities. For example, the body needs zinc for hundreds of chemical reactions, including those that support normal growth, development, and immune function. Too much zinc, however, can cause deficiency of another essential mineral, copper, and can impair immune function.

Food guides convey the message of moderation. Appearing in diverse shapes, international food guides reflect their cultural contexts. Korea, for example, uses the shape of a pagoda. (See **Figure 2.1.**)

Variety

How many *different* foods do you eat on a daily basis? Ten? Fifteen? Would it surprise you that early dietary recommendations in Japan suggested eat-

Quick Bites

How Much Do Doctors and Dentists Know about Nutrition?

Although nutrition is a growing concern for the food industry and the general public, medical and dental schools in the United States seem to be moving in the opposite direction. Currently, only 23 percent of medical and dental schools require that students take a nutrition course. In 1981, 37 percent of these schools required a nutrition course.

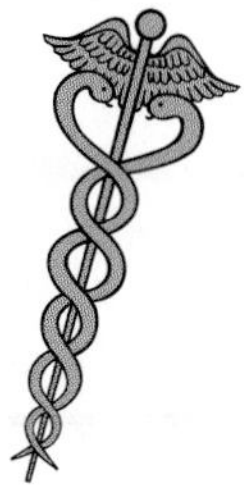

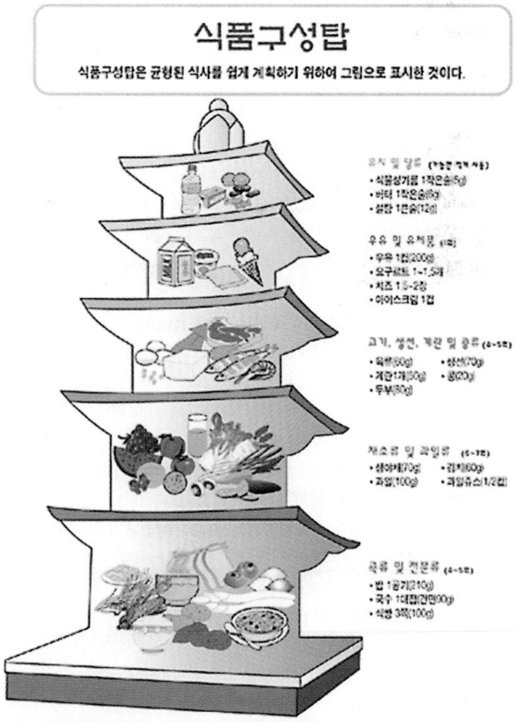

Figure 2.1 **Korean Dietary Guidelines.** Around the world, countries have adopted food guide presentations tailored to their individual cultures as well as physical needs. Both Korea and China use the pagoda shape for their food guides. The United States uses a pyramid and Canada uses a rainbow. Mexico and most European countries use a circular form.
Source: Painter J, Jee-Hyun R, Yeon-Kyung L. Comparison of international food guide pictorial representations. *J Am Diet Assoc.* 2002;102:483–489. ©The American Dietetic Association. Reprinted with permission.

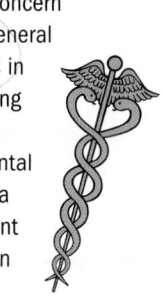

ing 30 different foods each day?[2] Now that's variety! Variety means including lots of different foods in the diet: not just different food groups such as fruits, vegetables, and grains but also different foods from each group. Eating two bananas and three carrots each and every day may give you the minimum number of recommended daily servings for fruits and vegetables, but it doesn't add much variety. Variety is important for a number of reasons. Eating a variety of fruits, for example, will provide a broader mix of vitamins, minerals, and phytochemicals than just including one or two fruits. Choosing a variety of protein sources such as lean meat, fish, and legumes will give a different balance of fats and other nutrients than will always choosing hamburger or steak. Variety can add interest and even mystery to your meals while preventing boredom with your diet. Perhaps most important, variety in your diet helps ensure that you get all the nutrients you need. Studies have shown that people who have varied diets take in more vitamin C and less sodium, sugar, and saturated fat.[3]

Think About It 3

Balance

A healthful diet requires a balance of food groups, energy sources (carbohydrates, protein, and fat), and other nutrients. Your diet is balanced if you choose a variety of foods and eat a moderate amount. Your diet is balanced if the amount of energy (calories) you take in through what you eat equals the amount of energy you expend in daily activities and exercise.

There is no magic diet, food, or supplement. Instead, your overall, long-term food choices can bring you the benefits of a healthful diet. Let's have a look at some general guidance for making those food choices.

Key Concepts: *Food and nutrient intake plays a major role in health and risk of disease. For most Americans, overnutrition is more of a problem than undernutrition. The ideas of moderation, variety, and balance are important concepts in choosing a healthful diet.*

U.S. Department of Agriculture (USDA) The government agency that monitors the production of eggs, poultry, and meat for adherence to standards of quality and wholesomeness. The USDA also provides public nutrition education, performs nutrition research, and administers the WIC program.

U.S. Department of Health and Human Services (DHHS) The principal federal agency responsible for protecting the health of all Americans and providing essential human services. The agency is especially concerned with those Americans who are least able to help themselves.

Dietary Guidelines for Americans The *Dietary Guidelines for Americans* are general goals relating to food intake and diet composition developed by the U.S. Department of Agriculture (USDA) and the Department of Health and Human Services (DHHS). They are intended to reduce the number of Americans who develop chronic diseases such as hypertension, diabetes, cardiovascular disease, obesity, and alcoholism.

Dietary Guidelines

To help citizens improve their food choices and overall health, many countries have developed dietary guidelines—simple, easy to understand statements about food choices. Governments certainly have an interest in keeping their citizens healthier—a healthy population is more productive, and puts less strain on health-care resources. Let's take a look at dietary guidelines for the United States and Canada.

Dietary Guidelines for Americans

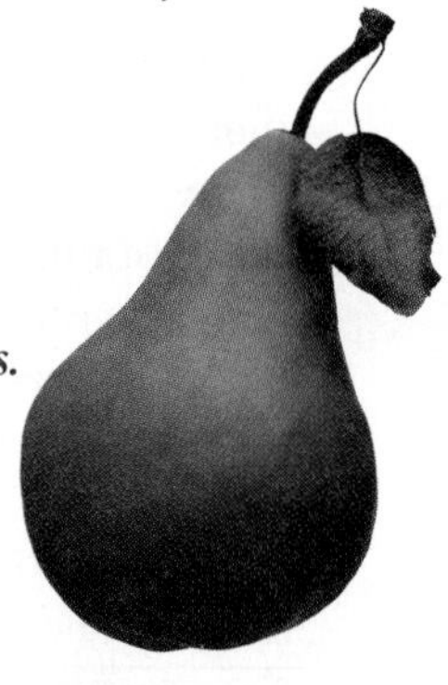

In 1980 the **U.S. Department of Agriculture (USDA)** and **Department of Health and Human Services (DHHS)** jointly released the first edition of the ***Dietary Guidelines for Americans.*** Revised guidelines have been released every five years as scientific information about links between diet and chronic disease is updated. The purpose of the *Dietary Guidelines for Americans* is to provide sound advice for building healthful diets,[4] with special emphasis on dietary factors related to heart disease and cancer, the two leading causes of death in the United States. Released in 2000, the most recent edition of the *Dietary Guidelines for Americans* offers three basic messages to promote food and lifestyle choices that reduce risk for chronic disease: (1) Aim for fitness, (2) Build a healthy base, and (3) Choose sensibly. (See **Figure 2.2**.)

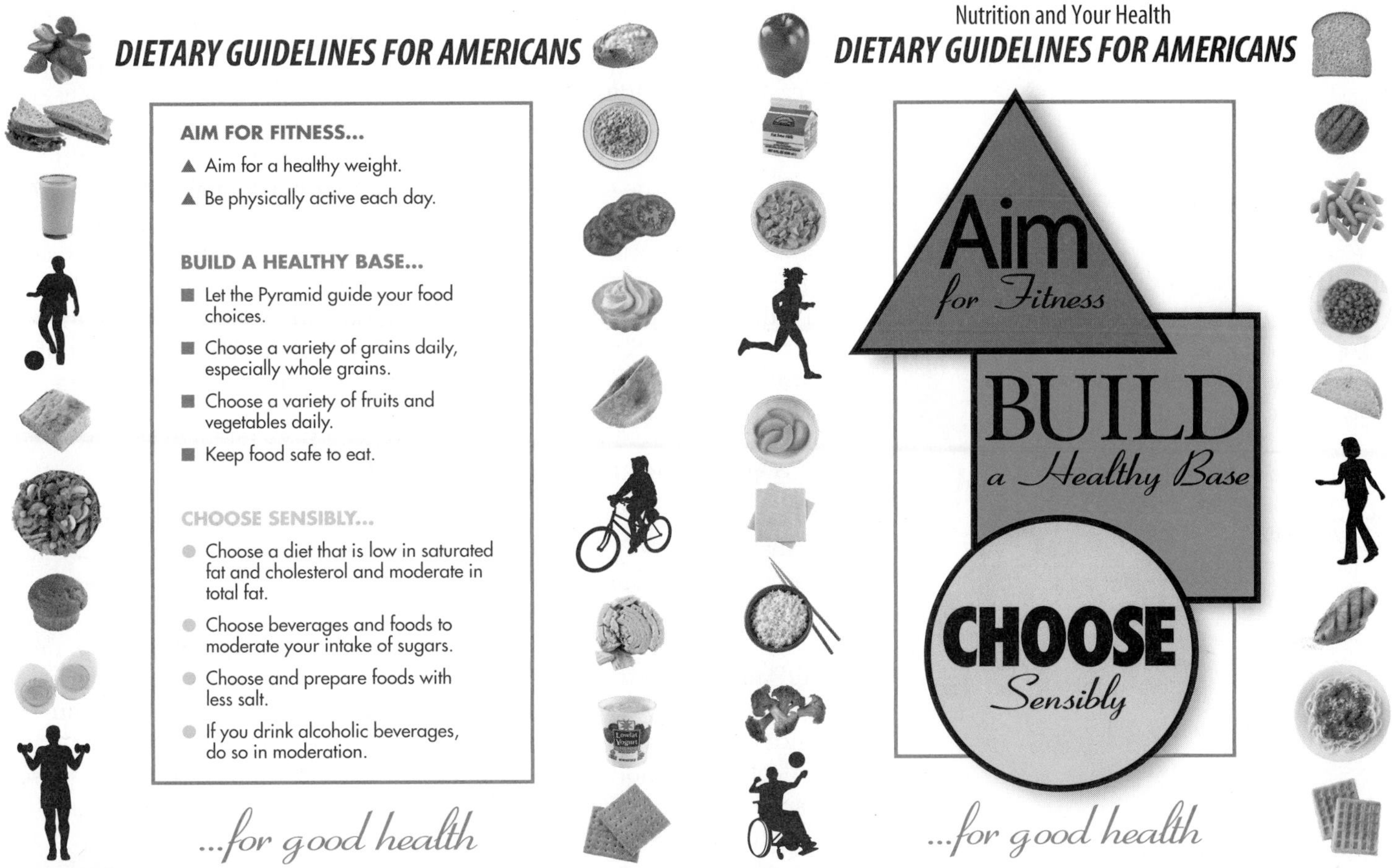
DIETARY GUIDELINES FOR AMERICANS
AIM FOR FITNESS...
▲ Aim for a healthy weight.
▲ Be physically active each day.
BUILD A HEALTHY BASE...
■ Let the Pyramid guide your food choices.
■ Choose a variety of grains daily, especially whole grains.
■ Choose a variety of fruits and vegetables daily.
■ Keep food safe to eat.
CHOOSE SENSIBLY...
● Choose a diet that is low in saturated fat and cholesterol and moderate in total fat.
● Choose beverages and foods to moderate your intake of sugars.
● Choose and prepare foods with less salt.
● If you drink alcoholic beverages, do so in moderation.
...for good health
Nutrition and Your Health
DIETARY GUIDELINES FOR AMERICANS
Aim for Fitness
BUILD a Healthy Base
CHOOSE Sensibly
...for good health

Figure 2.2 ***Dietary Guidelines for Americans.*** Eating is one of life's greatest pleasures. Since there are many foods and many ways to build a healthy diet and lifestyle, there is lots of room for choice. The *Dietary Guidelines for Americans* help you and your family find ways to enjoy food while taking action for good health.
Source: http://www.health.gov/dietaryguidelines/dga2000/10guidelines.pdf. Accessed 3/5/02.

Aim for Fitness

Weight control is important for improving health and reducing chronic disease risk. Obesity has been linked to increased risk of heart disease, many types of cancer, stroke, hypertension, and diabetes. Exercise is an important factor in weight control and overall fitness. The guidelines suggest getting at least 30 minutes of physical activity daily.

Build a Healthy Base

Grains (especially whole grains), fruits, and vegetables should be the foundation of a healthful diet. These foods are rich in carbohydrates, fiber, and many vitamins, minerals, and phytochemicals. Choosing a variety of grains, fruits, and vegetables helps ensure that you get all the nutrients you need. In addition, most plant foods are naturally low in fat and saturated fat. The Food Guide Pyramid (discussed in the next section) promotes a pattern of eating that emphasizes plant foods. Safe handling and preparation of all foods are keys to avoiding foodborne illness. For more information on food safety, see Chapter 14, "Food Safety and Technology."

Quick Bites

How Well Do School Cafeterias Follow Nutrition Guidelines?

Childhood obesity is on the rise, and high-fat school lunches may be part of the problem. Although the USDA mandated in 1995 that schools follow nutrition guidelines and reduce fat and salt in their cafeterias, lunches still average about 40 percent of calories from fat. In addition, according to a 1996 government study, children throw away 42 percent of cooked and 30 percent of raw vegetables. Every year, the government spends $4 billion on school lunches for 26 million children.

Quick Bites

Pass Up the Salt

We require only a few hundred milligrams of sodium each day, but this would be difficult to achieve given our current food supply, and would be unpalatable—so the guideline is to eat less sodium, but not down to the level of actual requirements.

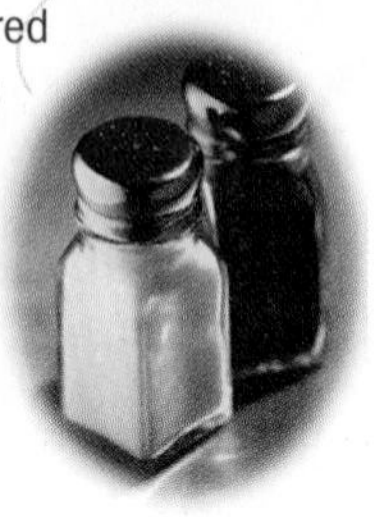

Choose Sensibly

Limiting the amount of fat, sugar, salt, and alcohol in the diet is sensible advice. Reducing saturated fat, cholesterol, and total fat intake can help reduce heart disease and cancer risk. Also, excess fat intake can lead to weight gain and obesity. Sugars and many processed foods that contain added sugar provide energy but have little other nutritional value. Excessive sugar intake accompanied by poor dental hygiene can contribute to tooth decay, and excess calories from sugar may be a factor in obesity. Excess salt (sodium) intake can contribute to high blood pressure in some people. And although studies have shown that a moderate intake of alcohol may have some health benefits, excess alcohol intake contributes to several of the leading causes of death, including accidents, suicide, homicide, and chronic liver disease.

Using the Guidelines in Diet Planning

The *Dietary Guidelines for Americans* are just that: guidelines. They don't identify specific foods to consume or avoid, but instead give advice about the overall composition of the diet. Think about your diet and consider your overall food intake to determine whether it is consistent with the *Dietary Guidelines for Americans*. Choose more fruits, vegetables, and grains to add variety to your diet and also lower your intake of saturated fat, fat, and cholesterol. Eat fewer high-fat toppings and fried foods to help you balance energy intake and expenditure. Use the extra things—sugar, salt, and alcohol—in moderation. Drink water more often than soft drinks; use less salt in your cooking and at the table; and if you choose to drink alcohol at all, use caution.

Sometimes, the lack of specific advice in the *Dietary Guidelines for Americans* causes frustration.[5] Many people like detailed information—how *many* fruits and vegetables? *Which* fat sources to minimize? What does "moderation" really mean? The development of the Food Guide Pyramid as a diet-planning tool has helped resolve many of these questions.

Canada's Guidelines for Healthy Eating

Promoting healthy eating habits among Canadians has been a priority of Health Canada for many years. Health Canada is the federal department responsible for helping the people of Canada maintain and improve their health. In the 1980s, a high priority was given to developing a single set of dietary guidelines that would simplify the *Nutrition Recommendations for Canadians*. (For more on these specific recommendations, see Appendix C.) The result of this effort was *Canada's Guidelines for Healthy Eating*, published in 1991. These five statements are the key messages for healthy Canadians over the age of 2:

- Enjoy a VARIETY of foods.
- Emphasize cereals, breads, other grain products, vegetables, and fruits.
- Choose lower-fat dairy products, leaner meats, and foods prepared with little or no fat.
- Achieve and maintain a healthy body weight by enjoying regular physical activity and healthy eating.
- Limit salt, alcohol, and caffeine.

Dietary guidelines in the United States and Canada address similar issues—less fat; more fruits, vegetables, and grains; less salt; and achieving healthy weights. In addition, both countries have developed graphic depictions of a healthful diet by showing the balance of food groups to be consumed each day. You can read about the U.S Food Guide Pyramid and *Canada's Food Guide* in the next section.

Key Concepts: *Dietary guidelines are a set of statements based on current science that "guide" people toward more healthful choices. Both the United States and Canada have dietary guidelines that embody the basic principles of balance, variety, and moderation.*

Food Groups and Food Guides

For many years, nutritionists and teachers have used **food groups** to illustrate the proper combination of foods in a healthful diet. Even young children can sort food into groups and fill a plate with foods from each group. The foods within each group are similar because of their origins—fruits, for example, all come from the same part of different plants. But from a nutritional perspective, what fruits have in common are the balance of macronutrients and the similarities in micronutrient composition. Even so, the foods in one group may differ significantly in their vitamin and mineral profiles. Some fruits (e.g., citrus, strawberries, and kiwi) are rich in vitamin C, whereas others (e.g., apples and bananas) have very little. Here again, we can see the importance of variety, of not simply including different food groups, but also choosing a variety of foods *within* each group.

food groups Categories of similar foods, such as fruits or vegetables.

Food Guide Pyramid A graphic representation of the number of servings from the five major food groups needed daily to form a healthful diet. A sixth group consists of fats, oils, and sweets—all of which should be consumed sparingly.

A Brief History of Food Group Plans

The USDA published the first guide to using food groups in 1916.[6] Instead of focusing on the problems of fat and sugar intake, this initial guide stressed the importance of consuming enough of these high-energy foods to support daily activity. Because people performed more manual labor in those days, many people were simply not getting enough calories! Canada's Official Food Rules (1942) recommended a weekly serving of liver and regular doses of fish liver oils—good sources of vitamins A and D. More recent food group plans, including the Basic Four that was popular from the 1950s through the 1970s, focus on fruits, vegetables, grains, dairy products, and meats and their substitutes. The Basic Four food plan (dairy, meats, fruits and vegetables, and grains) was usually illustrated as either a circle or a square, with each group having an equal share. The implication was that people should consume equal amounts of food from each group. Nutrition science now tells us that those proportions give us a diet too high in fat and protein for our modern lifestyle—and not high enough in carbohydrates and fiber. Consequently, in the late 1980s and early 1990s, both USDA and Health Canada were working to develop a new graphic image for the food groups.

Components of the Food Guide Pyramid

In 1992 the USDA introduced the **Food Guide Pyramid** (see **Figure 2.3**) to visually represent the variety, moderation, and proportionality needed for a healthful diet.[7] The Pyramid is designed to illustrate the *Dietary Guidelines for Americans* in terms of food groups and recommended numbers of daily servings. The Pyramid shows that the foundation of a healthful diet (the bottom and largest section) is the group made up of bread, cereal, rice, and pasta. Foods in this group are sources of complex carbohydrates and provide important vitamins, minerals, and fiber. Working our way up the

Think About It 4

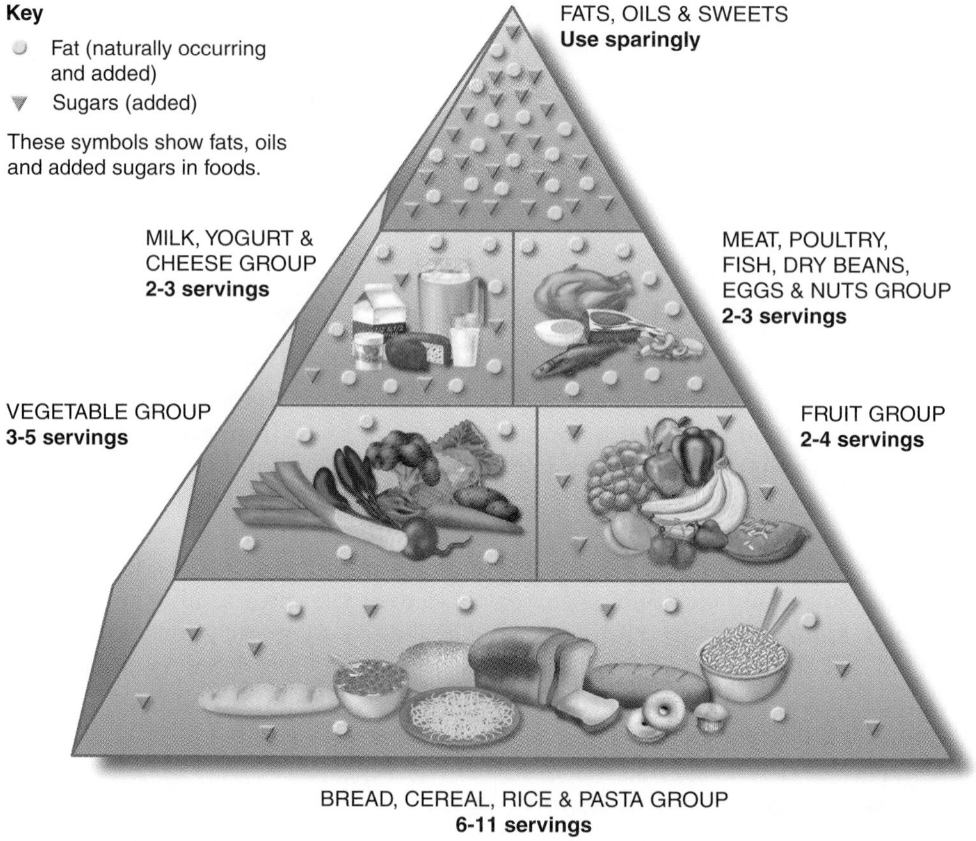

Figure 2.3 **Food Guide Pyramid.** The USDA's Food Guide Pyramid is a research-based guidance system that helps consumers put the *Dietary Guidelines for Americans* into action. The Pyramid shows how many servings to eat from each food group every day. **Source:** U.S. Department of Agriculture. *The Food Guide Pyramid.* Home and Garden Bulletin, No. 252; August 1992, revised October 1996.

Pyramid, we come to the vegetable group and the fruit group. Unlike the Basic Four, the Food Guide Pyramid separates fruits and vegetables because of differences in nutrient composition. Vegetables provide vitamins (such as A, C, and folate), the minerals iron and magnesium, and carbohydrates (including fiber). Fruits are rarely good sources of minerals other than potassium, but many are good sources of vitamins A and C. Taken together, these three groups at the bottom of the Pyramid illustrate that plant foods should make up the bulk of the diet.

Next up are dairy foods, along with meat and meat alternatives (e.g., nuts, eggs, legumes). They are important components of the diet, but we don't need as many servings to obtain the important nutrients from these groups. Dairy products provide protein, vitamins (especially riboflavin and vitamins A and D), and minerals (calcium and phosphorus, in particular). Meats and their substitutes are also good sources of protein, some of the B vitamins, iron, and zinc. The pinnacle of the Pyramid (the smallest section) contains fats and sweets. These are the dietary "extras": oil for cooking, butter or sour cream on potatoes, sugar in tea or coffee, soft drinks, and the like.

The Pyramid's Relationship to the *Dietary Guidelines for Americans*

The Food Guide Pyramid illustrates the *Dietary Guidelines for Americans* in a number of ways. First, the large base of the Pyramid reinforces the advice to choose a variety of grains, vegetables, and fruits each day. Just as the *Guidelines* instruct us to eat less saturated fat, cholesterol, and total fat, the Pyramid shows us that we should eat fewer daily servings of dairy products, meats, and alternatives, and very few added fats. In addition, the ❍ symbols scattered throughout the food groups show where we are likely to encounter fats in foods. You can see that the lower Pyramid groups have less fat, while the top of the Pyramid is more concentrated in fat sources. The ▼ symbol represents added sugars. The highest concentration of sugars is at the top of the Pyramid, in the smallest section, which is in line with the guideline that you should limit your sugar intake.

Canada's Food Guide

Canada's Food Guide (see **Figure 2.4**) is based on the *Guidelines for Healthy Eating* presented earlier, and is intended for people over the age of 4. The "rainbow" side of the *Food Guide* places foods into four groups: Grain Products, Vegetables and Fruit, Milk Products, and Meat and Alternates. It also describes the kinds of foods to choose from each group. For example, under the Vegetables and Fruit group, the *Food Guide* suggests "Choose dark green and orange vegetables and orange fruit more often." Like the U.S. Food Guide Pyramid, *Canada's Food Guide* illustrates that grains, vegetables, and fruits should be the major part of the diet, with milk products and meats in smaller amounts.

The bar side of the *Food Guide* (see Appendix C) shows how many daily servings are recommended from each group and gives examples of serving sizes. For milk products, recommendations are given specific to each age group, and also for pregnant and breastfeeding women. In addition, the *Food Guide* acknowledges that "other foods" in moderation can be incorporated into a healthy diet.

Eating a healthful diet based on the *Food Guide to Healthy Eating* is a cornerstone of *Vitality*, a concept that grew out of Health Canada's strategy to promote healthy weights. The three principles of Vitality—eating well, being active, and feeling good about yourself—aim to enhance people's physical, psychological, and social well-being. (See **Figure 2.5**.) Vitality is

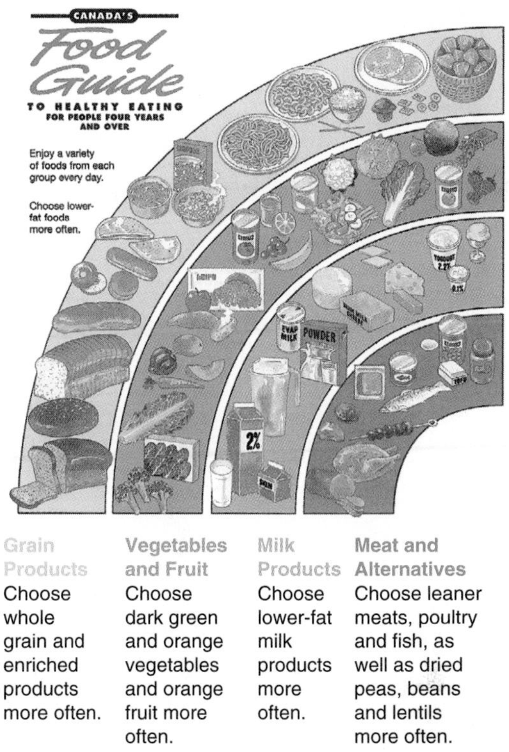
CANADA'S
Food Guide
TO HEALTHY EATING
FOR PEOPLE FOUR YEARS AND OVER
Enjoy a variety of foods from each group every day.
Choose lower-fat foods more often.
Grain Products
Choose whole grain and enriched products more often.
Vegetables and Fruit
Choose dark green and orange vegetables and orange fruit more often.
Milk Products
Choose lower-fat milk products more often.
Meat and Alternatives
Choose leaner meats, poultry and fish, as well as dried peas, beans and lentils more often.

Figure 2.4 ***Canada's Food Guide to Healthy Eating.*** The rainbow portion of *Canada's Food Guide* sorts food into groups from which people can make wise food choices. For the complete guide, see Appendix C.

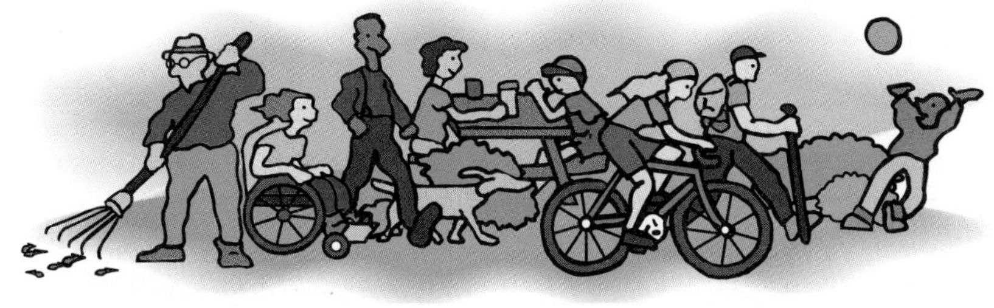

Figure 2.5 **Vitality.** Health Canada promotes the concept of vitality—enjoying eating well, being active, and feeling good about yourself.
Source: http://www.hc-sc.gc.ca/hppb/nutrition/pube/foodguid/eguide8.html. Accessed 3/5/02.

also concerned with creating environments in the community that support healthy choices.

Using the Pyramid or *Food Guide* in Diet Planning

Before you start using the Food Guide Pyramid or *Canada's Food Guide* for diet planning, become familiar with the types of food in each group, the number of recommended servings, and the appropriate serving sizes. The FYI feature "Food Guide Pyramid: Foods, Serving Sizes, and Tips" shows examples of foods and serving sizes for each of the groups. Let's take fruits, for example. According to the Pyramid, our daily diets should include two to four servings of fruits. Suppose you have 6 fluid ounces of orange juice for breakfast and a banana on your cereal. Add an apple for an afternoon snack, and you have already had three servings. Now let's try the grain group. A bowl (approximately 1 cup) of cereal and a slice of toast for

Fyi FOR YOUR INFORMATION

Are All Food Pyramids Created Equal?

Alyson Escobar, M.S., R.D., Center for Nutrition Policy and Promotion

At the moment, several dietary pyramids are competing for the public's attention: the USDA Food Guide Pyramid, the Mediterranean Pyramid, the Asian Pyramid, and the Latin American Pyramid, among others. What do these pyramids, all with seemingly different messages, mean for the American consumer?

The Mediterranean, Asian, and Latin American diet pyramids were produced by Oldways Preservation and Exchange Trust of Cambridge, Massachusetts. Oldways, a nonprofit company, developed these diet pyramids to illustrate traditional food patterns that epidemiological studies have associated with good health.

The USDA Food Guide Pyramid and the Oldways pyramids have much in common. All illustrate eating patterns consistent with current nutritional recommendations, and each can be used to plan diets consisting of different foods. All of these pyramids emphasize eating plenty of grain products, vegetables, and fruits.

Physical activity, moderate consumption of alcoholic beverages, and enjoyment of meals are healthy lifestyle factors suggested by the Oldways pyramids and the *Dietary Guidelines for Americans.*

The USDA's Food Guide Pyramid is based on American eating patterns. Flexibility in food choices is an important objective of the USDA Pyramid. Thus, a person can easily choose to eat "Mediterranean," "Asian," or "Latin American style" within the framework of the USDA Food Guide Pyramid.

In fact, several other pyramids have been developed. The Puerto Rican Pyramid, the Vegetarian Pyramid, and the Soul Food Pyramid all use the USDA Food Guide Pyramid framework but emphasize a different range of foods. These pyramids, used in conjunction with the guidance of the USDA, can help the public choose foods that fit a specific ethnic or cultural diet.

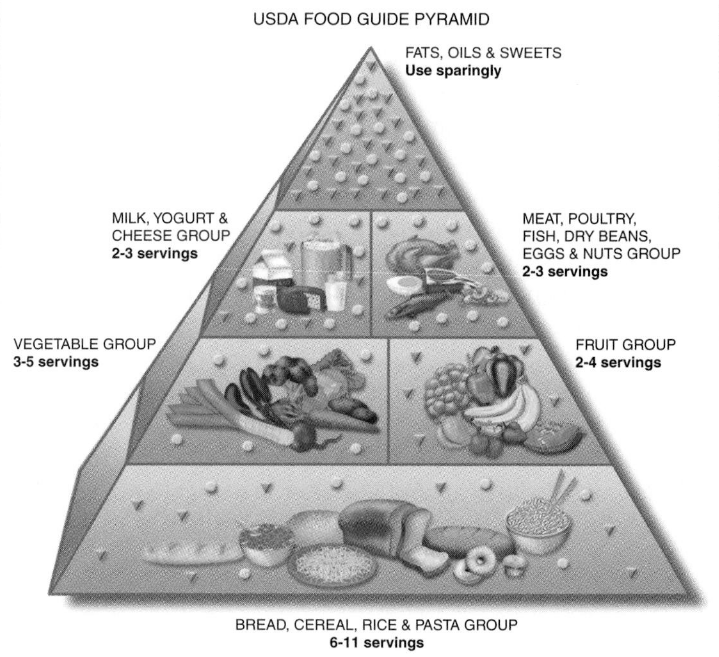

The Oldways pyramids illustrate proportions rather than specific types and amounts of food. They don't recommend serving sizes and numbers of servings of foods. Neither do they specify levels of total fat and saturated fat.

Because they represent cultural eating patterns, the Oldways pyramids include a more limited range of foods than the USDA Food Guide Pyramid. A major difference between the Mediterranean and Asian diet pyramids and the USDA Food Guide Pyramid is their distinction between plant and animal proteins. The Oldways pyramids group plant-based proteins—legumes, soybeans, nuts, and seeds—separately from animal proteins found in meat, poultry, eggs, and dairy products.

Red meat is included only occasionally in both the Mediterranean and Asian pyramids breakfast would be two servings. A sandwich with two slices of bread for lunch adds two more servings. Dinner might include a cup of pasta and two slices of garlic bread. So far, that's eight servings, which is right in the target zone. So, you see, it's not hard to meet the recommendations. **Table 2.1** shows the number of servings appropriate for three calorie-intake levels. This table will give you an idea of how the number of Pyramid servings should vary with different energy needs.

Sometimes it's difficult to figure out how to account for foods that are mixtures of different groups—lasagna, casseroles, or pizza, for example. Try separating such foods into their ingredients (e.g., pizza contains crust, tomato sauce, cheese, and toppings, which might be meats or vegetables) to estimate the number of servings. You should be able to come up with a reasonable approximation. All in all, the Pyramid and *Food Guide* are easy-to-use guidelines that can help you to select a variety of foods.

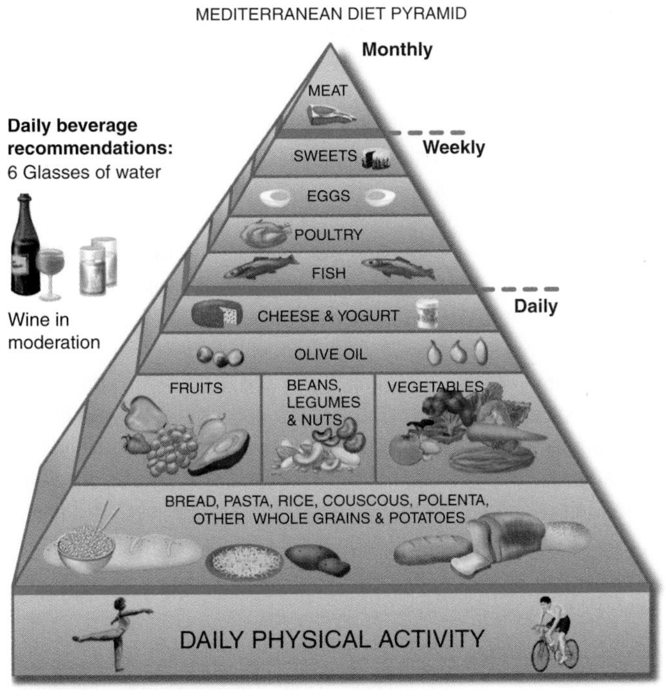

© 2000 Oldways Preservation & Exchange Trust

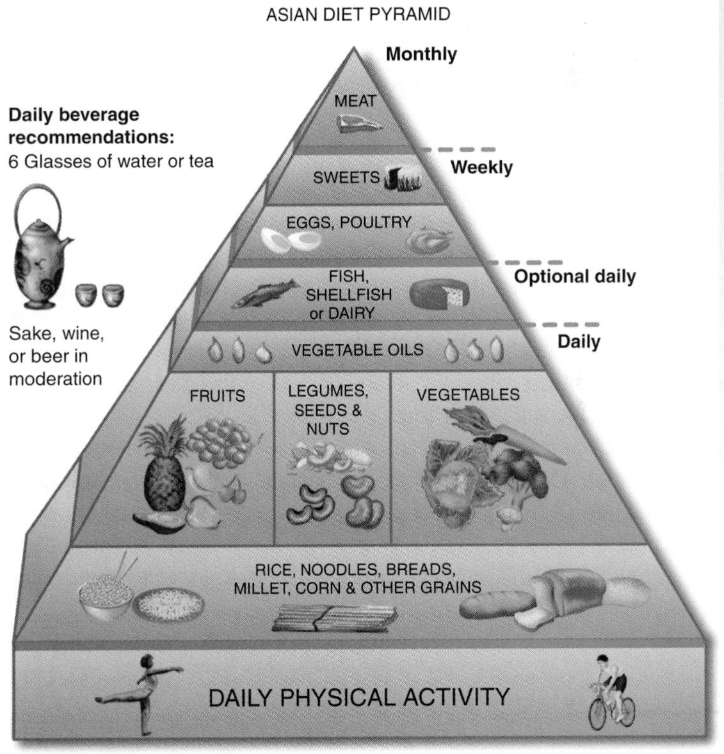

© 2000 Oldways Preservation & Exchange Trust

(a few times a month or less), while poultry and eggs appear slightly more often. The Asian diet pyramid contains limited dairy products, considering them optional and to be eaten in their low-fat forms only. Another important distinction among the pyramids concerns fat. Fat in the Oldways pyramids comes largely from vegetable oils high in monounsaturated fats, such as olive oil in the Mediterranean Pyramid and peanut oil in the Asian Pyramid.

Neither the USDA's Food Guide Pyramid nor the Oldways pyramids can convey all that consumers need to know to make food choices for a healthful diet. The USDA's Food Guide Pyramid is accompanied by additional information, such as the appropriate number of servings from each food group according to an individual's age, gender, and calorie needs.

Source: Adapted from "Are All Food Pyramids Created Equal?" USDA, Nutrition Insights, No. 2; April 1997.

For more information, contact the Center for Nutrition Policy and Promotion, Office of Public Information, at (202) 418-2312, or Oldways Preservation & Exchange Trust, 25 First Street, Cambridge, MA 02141 at (617) 621-3000; fax (617) 621-1230. To receive the handbook *Reaching Consumers with Meaningful Health Messages: A Handbook for Nutrition and Food Communicators,* contact the International Food Information Council, 1100 Connecticut Avenue, NW, Suite 430, Washington, DC 20036.

Fyi — FOR YOUR INFORMATION

Food Guide Pyramid: Foods, Serving Sizes, and Tips

Breads, Cereals, Rice, and Pasta (6–11 servings daily)	Serving Size
Bread	1 slice
English muffin	1/2 muffin
Bagel	1/2 small bagel
Hamburger bun	1/2 bun
Cereal, flake type	1 ounce (approx. 1 cup)
Cereal, granola type	1 ounce (approx. 1/3 cup)
Cereal, cooked	1/2 cup
Rice, cooked	1/2 cup
Noodles, cooked	1/2 cup

Choose grains made with little fat or sugar. Go easy on high-fat and sugary toppings. Choose whole-grain products to increase fiber intake.

Vegetables (3–5 servings daily)	Serving Size
Raw spinach, lettuce, kale, other leafy greens	1 cup
Cooked carrots, green beans, corn, other vegetables	1/2 cup
Baked potato	1 medium
Raw carrots, tomato, cucumber	1/2 cup
French fries	10 pieces

Choose a variety of vegetables to obtain different nutrients. Include dark green leafy vegetables several times each week. Limit fried vegetables and high-fat sauces or toppings to keep fat content low.

Fruit (2–4 servings daily)	Serving Size
Apple, orange, banana	1 medium
Grapes	12
Canned fruit or diced raw fruit	1/2 cup
Fruit juice	3/4 cup
Avocado	1/2 whole

Variety is important here, too. Fresh fruits contain more fiber than canned fruits, fruit sauces, or juice. When choosing a juice, look for "100% juice" on the label.

Milk, Yogurt, and Cheese (2–3 servings daily)	Serving Size
Milk	1 cup
Cottage cheese	2 cups
Yogurt	8 ounces
Natural cheeses (cheddar, Swiss, provolone, etc.)	1 1/2 ounces
Processed cheeses	2 ounces
Ricotta cheese	1/2 cup

For the lowest fat intake, choose skim milk and nonfat yogurt. Look for part-skim or reduced-fat cheeses. Ice cream, ice milk, and frozen yogurt tend to have more fat and sugar and less calcium than other dairy foods.

Meat, Poultry, Fish, Dry Beans, Eggs, and Nuts (2–3 servings daily)	Serving Size
Cooked lean meat, poultry, fish	3 ounces
Cooked ground meat	3 ounces
Bologna or other luncheon meat	2 slices (1 oz)

The following are equivalent to 1 ounce of meat (about ⅓ serving): 1 egg; ½ cup cooked dry beans and peas; 2 tablespoons peanut butter; and ⅓ cup of nuts.

Choose lean meats, skinless poultry, fish, and beans and peas most often. Use lower-fat cooking methods like broiling, grilling, and roasting instead of frying. Egg yolks, liver, and shellfish are higher in cholesterol than other foods in this group. Nuts, seeds, nut butters, and luncheon meats are higher in fat than other choices, so eat them less often.

Fats, Oils, and Sweets	Serving Size
Butter or margarine	Use sparingly
Cooking oil	Use sparingly
Mayonnaise	Use sparingly
Salad dressing (regular)	Use sparingly
Sour cream	Use sparingly
Cream cheese	Use sparingly
Sugar, jam, or jelly	Use sparingly
Honey, syrup	Use sparingly
Soft drink	Use sparingly
Fruit drink	Use sparingly
Chocolate bar	Use sparingly
Sherbet	Use sparingly
Gelatin dessert	Use sparingly

Although fats, oils, and sweets are not a food group, they contribute flavor, texture, and variety to our diet. In a 2,000-kilocalorie diet, no more than 65 grams of fat per day should be eaten on average. For the same 2,000-kilocalorie level, try to keep added sugars to a maximum 10 teaspoons each day.

Source: USDA. *The Food Guide Pyramid.* Home and Garden Bulletin, No. 252; August 1992, revised October 1996.

Table 2.1 **Suggested Numbers of Servings for Three Levels of Energy Intake**

	Energy Intake Level		
Food Group	*Low (about 1,500 kcal)*[a]	*Moderate (about 2,200 kcal)*[b]	*High (about 2,800 kcal)*[c]
		Servings	
Bread/cereals/ rice/pasta	6	9	11
Vegetable	3	4	5
Fruit	2	3	4
Milk/yogurt/cheese	2	2–3	3
Meat/fish/beans/eggs	2	2–3	3
Equivalent amount of meat	(5 ounces)	(6 ounces)	(7 ounces)
Fats/sugars[d]	use sparingly	use sparingly	use sparingly

[a] 1,500 kcal is about right for many sedentary women and some older adults.
[b] 2,200 kcal is about right for most children, teenage girls, active women, and many sedentary men.
[c] 2,800 kcal is about right for teenage boys, many active men, and some very active women.
[d] Although fats and sugars are part of a normal diet, they should be used sparingly, so the Food Guide Pyramid has no recommended number of servings for this group.

Note: Your calorie needs may be higher or lower than those shown. Women need more calories when they are pregnant or breastfeeding.

Source: Adapted from: USDA. *The Food Guide Pyramid.* Home and Garden Bulletin, No. 252; August 1992, revised October 1996.

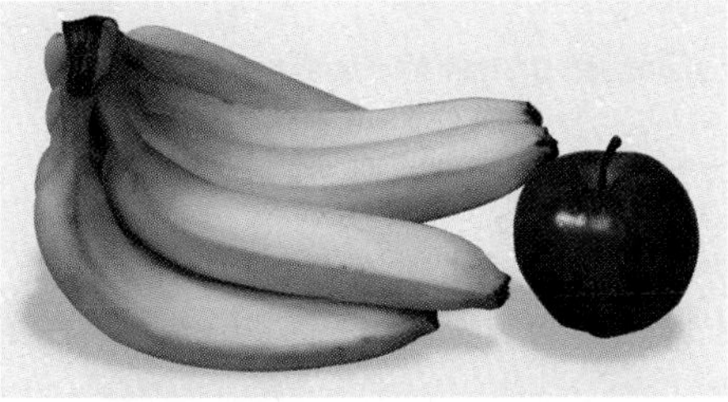

2–4 servings of fruit

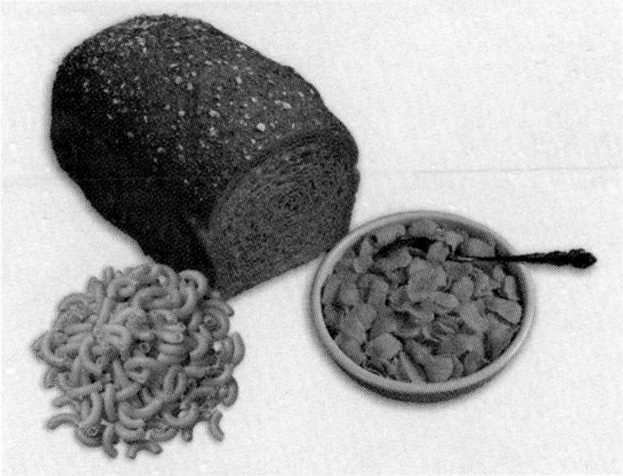

6–11 servings of bread, pasta, rice, and cereal

Key Concepts: *The Food Guide Pyramid is a visual representation of the* Dietary Guidelines for Americans. Canada's Food Guide to Healthy Eating *supports* Canada's Guidelines for Healthy Eating. *These graphic tools show the appropriate balance of food groups in a healthful diet: more grains, vegetables, and fruits and less dairy, meat, and added fats and sugars.*

Exchange Lists

Another tool for diet planning that uses food groups is called the **Exchange Lists for Meal Planning**. Like the Food Guide Pyramid and other food group plans, the Exchange Lists divide foods into groups. Diets can be planned by choosing a certain number of servings, or exchanges, from each group each day. The original purpose of the Exchange Lists was to help people with diabetes plan diets that would provide consistent levels of energy and carbohydrates—both are essential for dietary control of diabetes. For this reason, the foods are organized into groups or lists not only by the type of food (e.g., fruits or vegetables) but also by the amount of macronutrients (carbohydrate, protein, and fat) in each portion. The portions are defined so that each "exchange" has a similar composition. A diet plan would specify the number of exchanges to be consumed from each group

Exchange Lists for Meal Planning Lists of foods that in specified portions provide equivalent amounts of carbohydrate, fat, protein, and energy. Any food in an Exchange List can be substituted for any other without markedly affecting macronutrient intake.

Recommended Dietary Allowances (RDAs) The nutrient intake level that meets the nutrient needs of almost all (97 to 98 percent) individuals in a life-stage and gender group.

Recommended Nutrient Intakes (RNIs) Dietary standards used in Canada.

at each meal, and then the person could pick anything from the lists to fit that plan. For example, 1 fruit exchange is ½ cup of orange juice or 17 small grapes or 1 medium apple or ½ cup of applesauce. All of these exchanges have approximately 60 kilocalories, 15 grams of carbohydrate, 0 grams of protein, and 0 grams of fat. In the Exchange Lists, starchy vegetables such as potatoes, corn, and peas are grouped with breads and cereals instead of with other vegetables because their balance of macronutrients is more like bread or pasta than carrots or tomatoes.

For a complete set of Exchange Lists, see Appendix B.

Key Concepts: *The Exchange Lists are a diet-planning tool that uses the idea of food groups, but defines groups specifically in terms of macronutrient (carbohydrate, fat, and protein) content. Individual diet plans can be developed for people who need to control energy or carbohydrate intake, such as for weight control or management of diabetes mellitus.*

Recommendations for Nutrient Intake: The RDAs and DRIs

So far, the tools we have described (*Dietary Guidelines for Americans,* Canada's *Guidelines for Healthy Eating,* the Food Guide Pyramid, *Canada's Food Guide,* and Exchange Lists) have dealt with whole foods and food groups rather than individual nutrient values; these are what we think about in planning our daily meals and shopping lists. Sometimes, though, we need more specific information about our nutritional needs—a healthful diet is healthful because of the balance of *nutrients* it contains. Before we can choose foods that meet our needs for specific nutrients, we need to know how much of each nutrient we require daily. This is what dietary standards do—they define healthful diets in terms of specific amounts of the nutrients.

Understanding Dietary Standards

Dietary standards are sets of recommended intake values for nutrients. They are a way to tell us how much of each nutrient we should have in our diets. In the United States, we have been using a set of recommended intake values called the **Recommended Dietary Allowances**, or **RDAs**. In Canada, these dietary standards have been called the **Recommended Nutrient Intakes (RNIs)**.

Consider the following scenario. You are running a North Polar research center staffed by 60 people. Because they will not be able to leave the site to get meals, you must provide all of their food. You must keep the group adequately nourished; you certainly don't want anyone to become ill as a result of a nutritional deficiency. How would you (or the nutritionist you hire) start planning? How can you be sure to provide adequate amounts of the essential nutrients? The most important tool would be a set of dietary standards! Essentially the same scenario faces those who plan and provide food for groups of people in more routine circumstances—the military, prisons, and even schools. To assess nutritional adequacy, diet planners can compare the nutrient composition of their food plans to recommended intake values.

A Brief History of Dietary Standards

Health Canada has made recommendations on nutrient requirements since 1938, and the RDAs were first published in 1941. By the 1940s, nutrition scientists had been able to isolate and identify many of the nutrients in food. They were able to measure the amounts of these nutrients in foods and to recommend daily intake levels. The **Food and Nutrition Board** of the National Academy of Sciences assembled a group of nutrition scientists, who reviewed the scientific data to determine appropriate intake levels of the known essential nutrients. These levels then became the first RDA values. Since that time, the Food and Nutrition Board has periodically appointed committees to review the RDAs, and there have been 10 editions of RDAs through 1989. The 1989 RDA values are being replaced by a more comprehensive set of dietary standards called the **Dietary Reference Intakes (DRIs)**. Canadian scientists are participating in the development of the DRI values, and these are replacing the Recommended Nutrient Intakes.

Food and Nutrition Board (FNB) A board within the Institute of Medicine of the National Academy of Sciences. Responsible for assembling the group of nutrition scientists who review available scientific data to determine appropriate intake levels of the known essential nutrients.

Dietary Reference Intakes (DRIs) A framework of dietary standards that includes Estimated Average Requirement (EAR), Recommended Dietary Allowance (RDA), Adequate Intake (AI), and Tolerable Upper Intake Level (UL).

Dietary Reference Intakes

Since the inception of the RDAs and RNIs, we have learned more about the relationships between diet and chronic disease, and nutrient-deficiency diseases have become rare in the United States and Canada. The new DRIs reflect not just dietary adequacy but also optimal nutrition.

Like the RDAs, the DRIs are reference values for nutrient intakes to be used in assessing and planning diets for healthy people. (See **Figure 2.6**.)

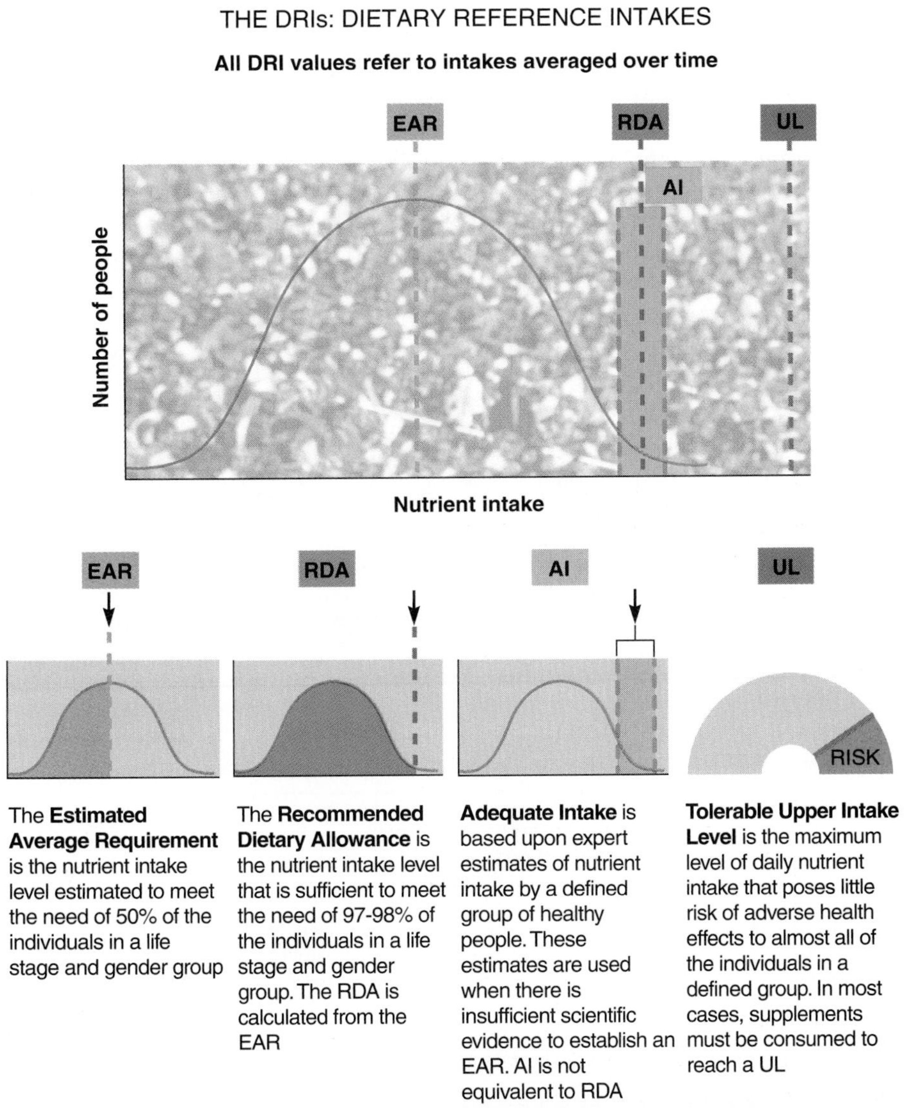
THE DRIs: DIETARY REFERENCE INTAKES
All DRI values refer to intakes averaged over time
EAR
RDA
UL
AI
Number of people
Nutrient intake
EAR
RDA
AI
UL
RISK
The Estimated Average Requirement is the nutrient intake level estimated to meet the need of 50% of the individuals in a life stage and gender group
The Recommended Dietary Allowance is the nutrient intake level that is sufficient to meet the need of 97-98% of the individuals in a life stage and gender group. The RDA is calculated from the EAR
Adequate Intake is based upon expert estimates of nutrient intake by a defined group of healthy people. These estimates are used when there is insufficient scientific evidence to establish an EAR. AI is not equivalent to RDA
Tolerable Upper Intake Level is the maximum level of daily nutrient intake that poses little risk of adverse health effects to almost all of the individuals in a defined group. In most cases, supplements must be consumed to reach a UL

Figure 2.6 **Dietary Reference Intakes.** The Dietary Reference Intakes are a set of dietary standards that include Estimated Average Requirement (EAR), Recommended Dietary Allowance (RDA), Adequate Intake (AI), and Tolerable Upper Intake Level (UL).

requirement The lowest continuing intake level of a nutrient that prevents deficiency in an individual.

Estimated Average Requirement (EAR) The intake value that meets the estimated nutrient needs of 50 percent of individuals in a specific life-stage and gender group.

The Dietary Reference Intakes have four elements: Estimated Average Requirement (EAR), Recommended Dietary Allowance (RDA), Adequate Intake (AI), and Tolerable Upper Intake Level (UL). Underlying each of these values is the definition of a **requirement** as the "lowest continuing intake level of a nutrient that, for a specific indicator of adequacy, will maintain a defined level of nutriture in an individual."[8] In other words, a requirement is the smallest amount of a nutrient you should take in on a regular basis to remain healthy.

Estimated Average Requirement

The **Estimated Average Requirement (EAR)** reflects the amount of a nutrient that would meet the needs of 50 percent of the people in a particular life-stage (age) and gender group. For each nutrient, this requirement is defined using a specific indicator of dietary adequacy. This indicator could be the level of the nutrient or one of its breakdown products in the blood, or the amount of an enzyme associated with that nutrient.[9] The EAR is used to set the RDA, and EAR values can also be used to assess dietary adequacy or plan diets for groups of people.

Recommended Dietary Allowance

The Recommended Dietary Allowance (RDA) is the daily intake level that meets the needs of most people (97 to 98 percent) in a life-stage and gender group. In the DRI values, the RDA is mathematically determined based on the EAR. A nutrient will not have an RDA value if there is not enough scientific data available to set an EAR value.

People can use the RDA value as a target or goal for dietary intake, but comparing your actual intake to the RDA is not very helpful. The RDAs do not define an *individual's* nutrient requirements. Your actual nutrient needs may be much lower than average, and therefore the RDA would be much more than you need. An analysis of your diet might show, for example, that

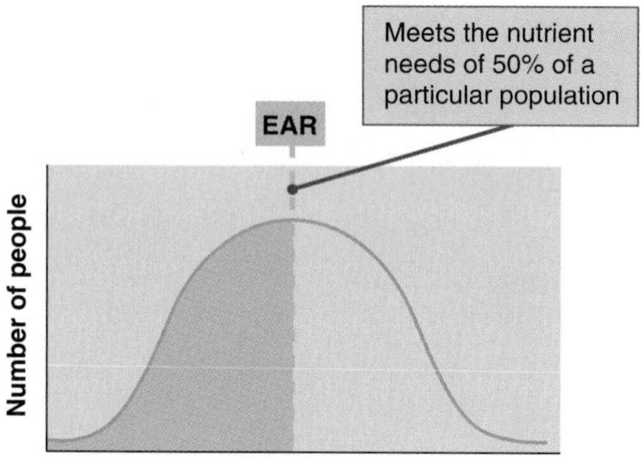

ESTIMATED AVERAGE REQUIREMENT

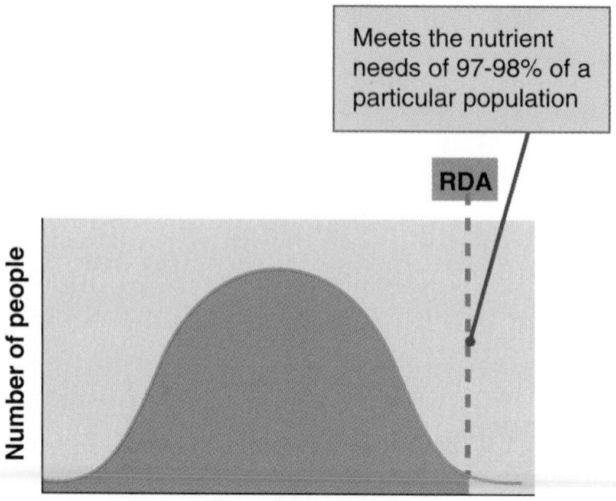

RECOMMENDED DIETARY ALLOWANCE

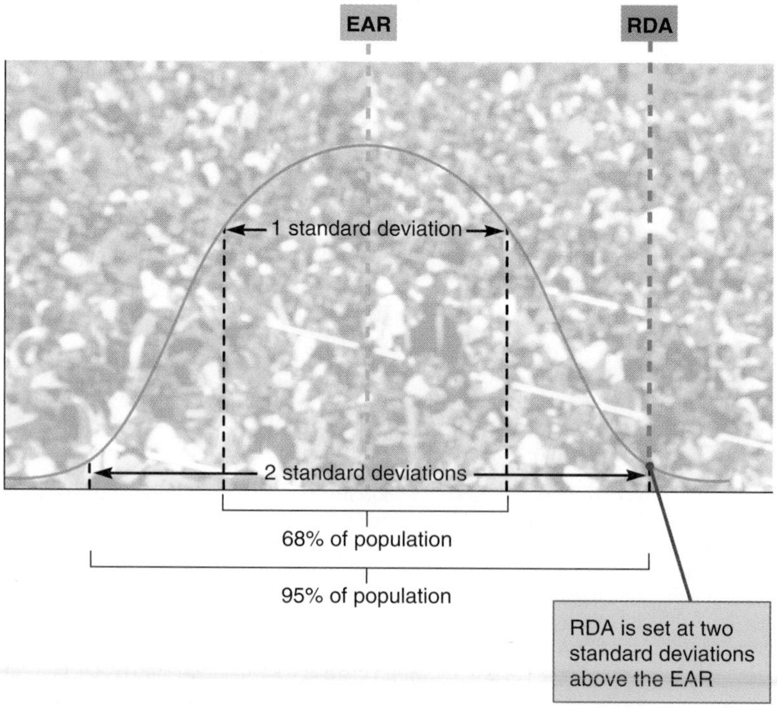

The RDA takes into account about 98% of the population.

you consume 45 percent of the RDA for a certain vitamin, but that might be adequate for your needs. Only specific laboratory or other tests can determine a person's true nutrient requirements and actual nutritional status.

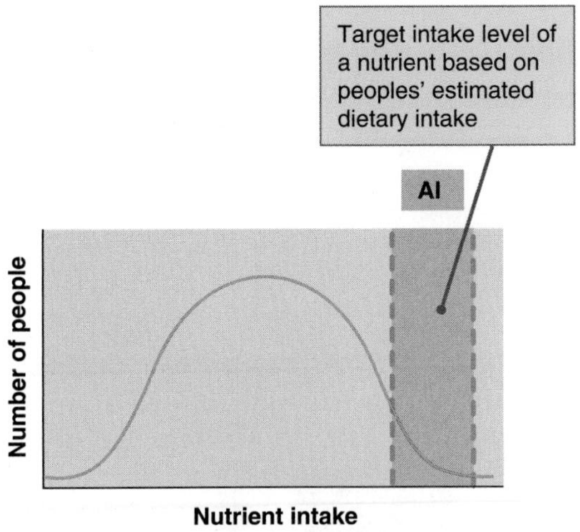

ADEQUATE INTAKE

Adequate Intake

If not enough scientific data are available to set an EAR level, a value called an **Adequate Intake (AI)** is determined instead. AI values are determined in part by observing healthy groups of people and estimating their dietary intake. All the current DRI values for infants are AI levels because there have been too few scientific studies to determine specific requirements in infants. Instead, AI values for infants are usually based on nutrient levels in human breast milk, a complete food for newborns and young infants. Values for older infants and children are extrapolated from human milk and from data on adults. For nutrients with AI instead of RDA values (e.g., calcium, vitamin D), more scientific research is needed to better define nutrient requirements of population groups. AI values can be considered target intake levels for individuals.

Tolerable Upper Intake Level

Finally, **Tolerable Upper Intake Levels (ULs)** have been defined for many nutrients. Consumption of a nutrient in amounts higher than the UL could be harmful. The ULs have been developed partly in response to the growing interest in dietary supplements that contain large amounts of essential nutrients. The UL is not to be used as a target for intake, but rather should be a caution for people who regularly take nutrient supplements.

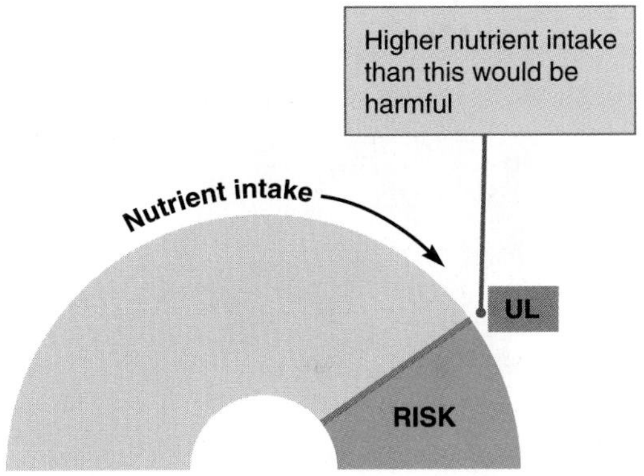

TOLERABLE UPPER INTAKE LEVEL

Use of Dietary Standards

The most appropriate use of DRIs is as tools for planning and evaluating diets for large groups of people. Remember the North Pole scenario at the beginning of this section? If you had planned menus and evaluated the nutrient composition of the foods that would be included and if the nutrient levels of those daily menus averaged or exceeded the RDA/AI levels, you could be confident that your group would be adequately nourished. If you had a very large group—thousands of soldiers, for instance—the EAR would be a more appropriate guide.

Dietary standards are also used to make decisions about nutrition policy. The Special Supplemental Food Program for Women, Infants, and Children (WIC), for example, takes into account the RDAs as it provides food or vouchers for food. The goal of this federally funded supplemental feeding program is to improve the nutrient intake of low-income pregnant and breastfeeding women, their infants, and young children. The guidelines for school lunch and breakfast programs are also based on RDA values.

Often, we use dietary standards as comparison values for individual diets, something you may be doing in class. It can be interesting to see how your daily intake of a nutrient compares to the RDA or AI. However, an intake that is less than the RDA/AI doesn't necessarily mean deficiency; your individual requirement for a nutrient may be less than the RDA/AI value. You can use the RDA/AI values as targets for dietary intake, while avoiding nutrient intake that exceeds the UL.

Adequate Intake (AI) The nutrient intake that appears to sustain a defined nutritional state or some other indicator of health (e.g., growth rate or normal circulating nutrient values) in a specific population or subgroup. AI is used when there is insufficient scientific evidence to establish an EAR.

Tolerable Upper Intake Levels (ULs) The maximum levels of daily nutrient intakes that are unlikely to pose health risks to almost all of the individuals in the group for whom they are designed.

Future of the DRIs

The Food and Nutrition Board continues to develop DRI values in an ongoing review and revision process. As new values become available, nutrition professionals in all settings will be working to adapt existing educational materials, revise nutrient-analysis programs, reevaluate menus and food plans, and change educational strategies. Their first order of business is to understand the science behind the DRIs and the methods used to set each of the values, and then to translate this information into dietary applications.

Key Concepts: *Dietary standards are levels of nutrient intake recommended for healthy people. These standards help the government set nutrition policy and also can be used to guide the planning and evaluation of diets for groups and individuals. Dietary standards for the United States and Canada are being reevaluated and expanded into the Dietary Reference Intakes (DRIs), which focus on optimal health and lowering the risks of chronic disease, rather than simply on dietary adequacy.*

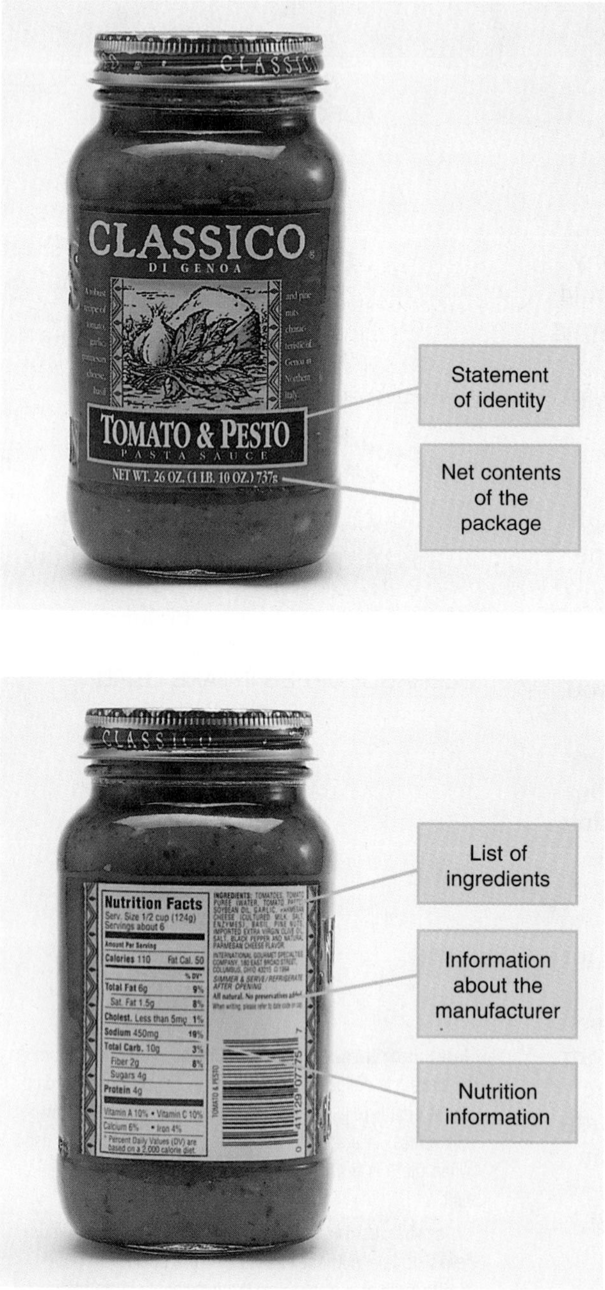

Figure 2.7 **The five mandatory requirements for food labels.** Federal regulations determine what can and cannot appear on food labels.

Food Labels

Now that you understand diet-planning tools and dietary standards, let's focus on your use of these tools—for example, when making decisions at the grocery store. One of the most useful tools in planning a healthful diet is the **food label**.

Specific federal regulations control what can and cannot appear on a food label and what *must* appear on it. The **Food and Drug Administration (FDA)** is responsible for assuring that foods sold in the United States are safe, wholesome, and properly labeled. The Health Products and Food Branch of Health Canada has similar responsibilities. The FDA's jurisdiction does not include meat, meat products, poultry, or poultry products; the USDA regulates these foods.

As information about the role of diet in chronic disease has grown, so has the demand for nutrition labels on all food products. As a result, in 1990 Congress passed the **Nutrition Labeling and Education Act (NLEA)**. Once the necessary regulations had been developed, new "Nutrition Facts" labels began appearing on foods in 1994. As of 1997, 96.5 percent of food products had nutrition labels.[10] Voluntary nutrition labeling was introduced in Canada in 1988, and proposed regulations to make nutrition labeling mandatory were released in 2001. When the proposals are finalized into law in 2002, Canadian nutrition labels will be similar in format to U.S. nutrition labels.

Ingredients and Other Basic Information

The label on a food you buy today has been shaped by many sets of regulations. Nutrition labeling is now required on virtually all packaged foods. As **Figure 2.7** shows, food labels have five mandatory components:

1. a statement of identity
2. the net contents of the package
3. the name and address of the manufacturer, packer, or distributor
4. a list of ingredients
5. nutrition information

The **statement of identity** requirement means that the product must prominently display the common or usual name of the product or identify the food with an "appropriately descriptive term." For example, it would be misleading to label a fruit beverage containing only 10 percent fruit juice as a "juice." The statement of net package contents must accurately reflect the quantity in terms of weight, volume, measure, or numerical count. Information about the manufacturer, packer, or distributor gives consumers a way to contact someone in case they have questions about the product. Ingredients must be listed by common or usual name, in descending order by weight, so the first ingredient listed is the primary ingredient in that food product. Let's compare two cereals:

Cereal A ingredients: Milled corn, sugar, salt, malt flavoring, high-fructose corn syrup

Cereal B ingredients: Sugar, yellow corn flour, rice flour, wheat flour, whole oat flour, partially hydrogenated vegetable oil (contains one or more of the following oils: canola, soybean, cottonseed), salt, cocoa, artificial flavor, corn syrup

In Cereal B, the first ingredient listed is sugar, which means this cereal contains more sugar by weight than any other ingredient. Cereal A's primary ingredient is milled corn. If we were to read the nutrition information, we would find that a 1-cup serving of Cereal A contains 2 grams of sugars, while a similar amount of Cereal B contains 12 grams of sugars. Quite a difference!

As you have probably noticed, when the artificial sweetener aspartame is included in an ingredient list, a warning statement is also included. Also, preservatives that are added to foods must be listed, along with an explanation of their function. Accurate and complete ingredient information is vital for people with food allergies who must avoid certain food components.

food label Labels required by law on virtually all packaged foods with five requirements: (1) a statement of identity; (2) the net contents (by weight, volume, or measure) of the package; (3) the name and address of the manufacturer, packer, or distributor; (4) a list of ingredients; and (5) nutrition information.

Food and Drug Administration (FDA) The federal agency responsible for assuring that foods sold in the United States (except for eggs, poultry, and meat, which are monitored by the USDA) are safe, wholesome, and labeled properly. The FDA sets standards for the composition of some foods, inspects food plants, and monitors imported foods. The FDA is part of the Public Health Service, a component of the Department of Health and Human Services (DHHS).

Nutrition Labeling and Education Act (NLEA) An amendment to the Food, Drug, and Cosmetic Act of 1938. The NLEA made major changes to the content and scope of the nutrition label and to other elements of food labels. Final regulations were published in 1993, and went into effect in 1994.

statement of identity Mandate that commercial food products display prominently the common or usual name of the product or identify the food with an "appropriately descriptive term."

Nutrition Facts A portion of the food label that states the content of selected nutrients in a food in a standard way prescribed by the Food and Drug Administration. By law Nutrition Facts must appear on nearly all processed food products in the United States.

Nutrition Facts Panel

The **Nutrition Facts** panel contains the most important label information for the health-conscious consumer. The Food Marketing Institute's 1997 survey "Shopping for Health" indicated that 54 percent of consumers check the food label before buying a product for the first time. The top three numbers they look for are total fat, calories, and sodium. The Nutrition Facts panel not only is a source of information about the nutritional value of a food product but can also be used to compare similar products.

Let's take a closer look at the elements of the Nutrition Facts panel. It was designed so that the nutrition information would be easy to find on the label. The heading Nutrition Facts stands out clearly. (See **Figure 2.8.**) Just under the heading is information about the serving size and number of servings per container. It is important to note the serving size, because all of the nutrient information that follows is based on that amount of the food, and the listed serving size may be different from what you usually eat. An 8-ounce bag of potato chips may be a "small" snack to a hungry college student, but the manufacturer states the bag really contains eight servings! Serving sizes are standardized according to reference amounts developed by the FDA. Similar products (cereals, for instance) will have similar serving sizes (1 ounce).

The next part of the label shows the calories per serving and the calories that come from fat. This information reveals at a glance whether a food product is high or low in fat. If most of the calories in a product come from

Quick Bites

Truth in Tuna

Due to an old regulation still in the law books, tuna companies can get away with skimping on canned tuna. Legally, a 6-ounce can of solid tuna has to contain only 3.75 ounces of actual tuna. Although the Tuna Foundation has set a voluntary minimum of 4 ounces, not all manufacturers subscribe to the minimum. The FDA is considering making companies use the drained weight on tuna cans, so future labels may be more precise.

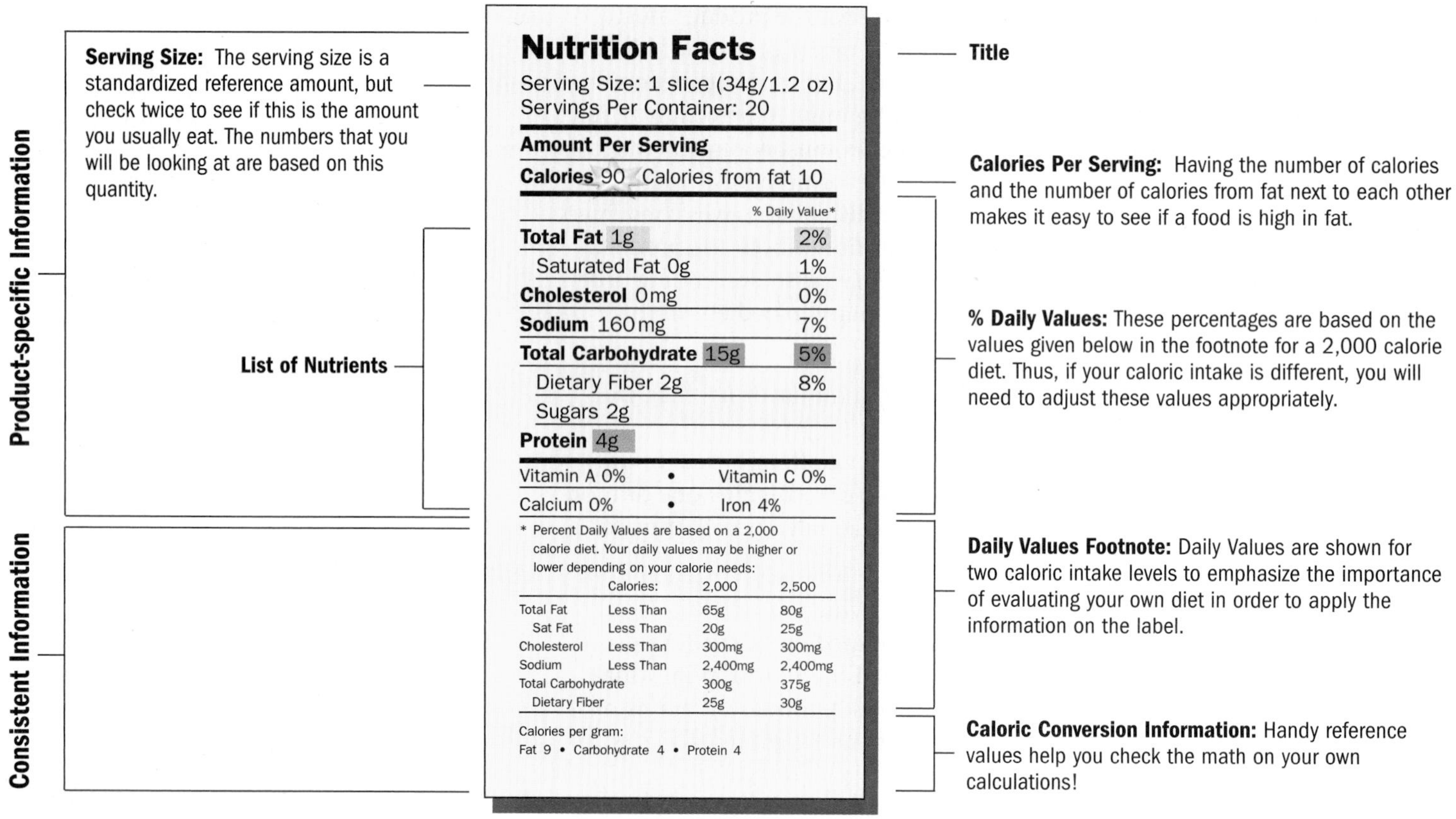
Product-specific Information
Serving Size: The serving size is a standardized reference amount, but check twice to see if this is the amount you usually eat. The numbers that you will be looking at are based on this quantity.
List of Nutrients
Consistent Information
Nutrition Facts
Serving Size: 1 slice (34g/1.2 oz)
Servings Per Container: 20
Amount Per Serving
Calories 90 Calories from fat 10
% Daily Value*
Total Fat 1g 2%
Saturated Fat 0g 1%
Cholesterol 0mg 0%
Sodium 160mg 7%
Total Carbohydrate 15g 5%
Dietary Fiber 2g 8%
Sugars 2g
Protein 4g
Vitamin A 0% • Vitamin C 0%
Calcium 0% • Iron 4%
* Percent Daily Values are based on a 2,000 calorie diet. Your daily values may be higher or lower depending on your calorie needs:
Calories: 2,000 2,500
Total Fat Less Than 65g 80g
Sat Fat Less Than 20g 25g
Cholesterol Less Than 300mg 300mg
Sodium Less Than 2,400mg 2,400mg
Total Carbohydrate 300g 375g
Dietary Fiber 25g 30g
Calories per gram:
Fat 9 • Carbohydrate 4 • Protein 4
Title
Calories Per Serving: Having the number of calories and the number of calories from fat next to each other makes it easy to see if a food is high in fat.
% Daily Values: These percentages are based on the values given below in the footnote for a 2,000 calorie diet. Thus, if your caloric intake is different, you will need to adjust these values appropriately.
Daily Values Footnote: Daily Values are shown for two caloric intake levels to emphasize the importance of evaluating your own diet in order to apply the information on the label.
Caloric Conversion Information: Handy reference values help you check the math on your own calculations!

Figure 2.8 **The Nutrition Facts panel.** Consumers can use the Nutrition Facts panel to compare the nutritional value of different products.

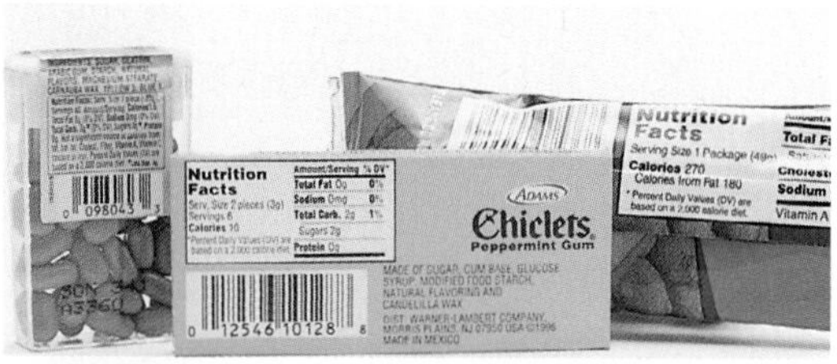

Figure 2.9 **Nutrition Facts on small packages.** When a product package has insufficient space to display a full Nutrition Facts panel, manufacturers may use an abbreviated version.

fat, it is a high-fat food. Following this is a list of the amounts of total fat, saturated fat, cholesterol, sodium, total carbohydrate, dietary fiber, sugars, and protein in one serving. This information is given both in quantity (grams or milligrams per serving) and as a percentage of the Daily Value—a comparison standard specifically for food labels (this standard is described in the next section). Listed next are percentages of Daily Values for vitamins A and C, calcium, and iron, which are the only micronutrients that must appear on all standard labels. Manufacturers may choose to include information about other nutrients, such as potassium, polyunsaturated fat, additional vitamins, or other minerals, in the Nutrition Facts. However, if they make a claim about an optional component (e.g., "good source of vitamin E") or if the food is **enriched** or **fortified**, the manufacturer must include specific nutrition information. This information must be included even when government regulations require enrichment or fortification, such as the fortification of milk with vitamin D to prevent rickets (a bone disease in children that results from vitamin D deficiency) or the fortification of grain products with folic acid to reduce risk of birth defects. Food products that come in small packages (e.g., gum, candy, and tuna) or that have little nutritional value (e.g., diet soft drinks) can have abbreviated versions of the Nutrition Facts on the label, as **Figure 2.9** shows.

Daily Values

Let's come back to the Daily Values part of the label. The **Daily Values (DVs)** are a set of dietary standards used to compare the amount of a nutrient (or other component) in a serving of food to the amount recommended for daily consumption. This information lets consumers see at a glance how a food fits into their diets. Let's say you rely on your breakfast cereal as a major source of dietary fiber intake. Comparing two packages, as in **Figure 2.10**, you find that a serving of corn-flakes cereal has 4 percent of the DV for dietary fiber, but choosing a bran-flakes cereal will give you 20 percent. You don't have to know anything about grams to see which has more! You can find a complete list of Daily Values inside the back cover of this text. Keep in mind that the Daily Values (which were established in 1993) may not exactly match the more recent DRI values, but in most cases, the differences are small.

enriched Refers to grains that have added thiamin, riboflavin, niacin, folic acid, and iron.

fortified Refers to the addition of vitamins or minerals that weren't originally present in a food.

Daily Values (DVs) A single set of nutrient intake standards developed by the Food and Drug Administration to represent the needs of the "typical" consumer, and used as standards for expressing nutrient content on food labels.

nutrient content claims These claims describe the level of a nutrient or dietary substance in the product, using terms such as *good source*, *high*, or *free*.

Nutrient Content Claims

The NLEA and the associated FDA regulations allow food manufacturers to make **nutrient content claims** using a variety of descriptive terms on labels, such as *low fat* and *high fiber*. The FYI feature "Definitions for Nutrient Content Claims on Food Labels" shows a list of terms that may be used. The FDA has made an effort to make the terms meaningful, and the regulations have reduced the number of potentially misleading label statements. Companies can no longer take liberties with label statements, such as printing "cholesterol free" on a can of vegetable shortening—a food that is 100 percent fat and high in saturated fatty acids (a type of fat that raises blood

Nutrition Facts

Serving Size: 1 Cup (28g/1.0 oz.)
Servings Per Container: About 18

Amount Per Serving	Cereal	with ½ cup Skim Milk
Calories	100	140
Fat Calories	0	0
	% Daily Value	
Total Fat 0g	0%	0%
Saturated Fat 0g	0%	0%
Cholesterol 0mg	0%	0%
Sodium 300mg	13%	15%
Potassium 25mg	1%	7%
Total Carbohydrate 24g	8%	10%
Dietary Fiber 1g	4%	4%
Sugars 2g		
Other Carbohydrates 21g		
Protein 2g		
Vitamin A	15%	20%
Vitamin C	25%	25%
Calcium	0%	15%
Iron	45%	45%
Vitamin D	10%	25%
Thiamin	25%	30%
Riboflavin	25%	35%
Niacin	25%	25%
Vitamin B_6	25%	25%
Folate	25%	25%
Vitamin B_{12}	25%	35%

Nutrition Facts

Serving Size: ¾ Cup (30g)
Servings Per Container: About 15

Amount Per Serving	Cereal	with ½ cup Skim Milk
Calories	100	140
Calories from fat	5	5
	% Daily Value	
Total Fat 0.5g	1%	1%
Saturated Fat 0g	0%	0%
Cholesterol 0mg	0%	0%
Sodium 210mg	9%	12%
Potassium 200mg	6%	11%
Total Carbohydrate 24g	8%	10%
Dietary Fiber 5g	20%	20%
Sugars 5g		
Other Carbohydrates 14g		
Protein 3g		
Vitamin A	15%	20%
Vitamin C	0%	2%
Calcium	0%	15%
Iron	45%	45%
Vitamin D	10%	25%
Thiamin	25%	30%
Riboflavin	25%	35%
Niacin	25%	25%
Vitamin B_6	25%	25%
Folate	25%	25%
Vitamin B_{12}	25%	35%

Figure 2.10 **Comparing cereals.** These cereal labels come from different types of breakfast cereal: corn-flakes cereal (left) and bran-flakes cereal (right). What might influence your decision to buy one over the other?

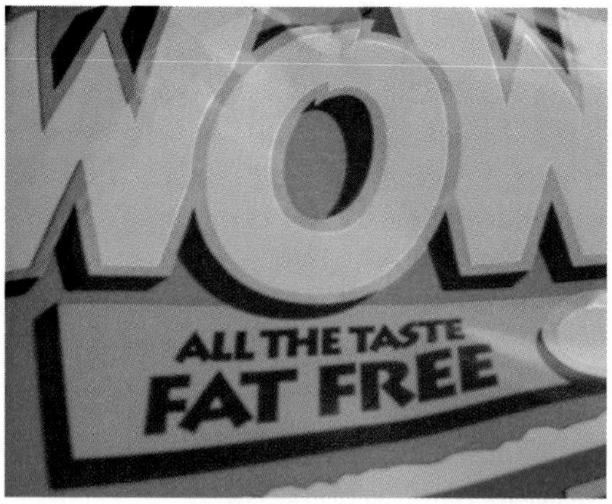

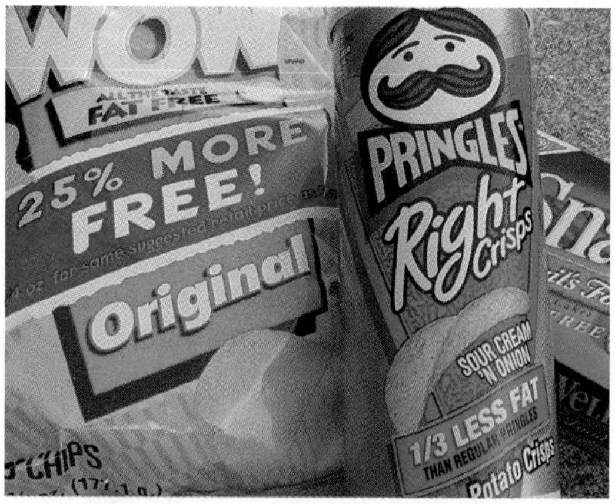

cholesterol levels in the body). This type of statement misleads consumers who associate "cholesterol free" with "heart healthy." Under the NLEA regulations, statements about low cholesterol content can be used only when the product is also low in saturated fat (less than 2 grams per serving).

Health Claims

With the passage of the NLEA, manufacturers also were allowed to add health claims to food labels. Before the NLEA was passed, products making

Fyi FOR YOUR INFORMATION — Definitions for Nutrient Content Claims on Food Labels

Free: Food contains no amount (or trivial or "physiologically inconsequential" amounts). May be used with one or more of the following: fat, saturated fat, cholesterol, sodium, sugar, and calorie. Synonyms include *without, no,* and *zero.*

- ***Fat-free:*** *less than 0.5 g of fat per serving*
- ***Saturated fat free:*** *less than 0.5 g of saturated fat per serving, and no more than 0.5 g of trans fatty acids per serving*
- ***Cholesterol-free:*** *less than 2 mg of cholesterol and 2 g or less of saturated fat per serving*
- ***Sodium-free:*** *less than 5 mg of sodium per serving*
- ***Sugar-free:*** *less than 0.5 g of sugar per serving*
- ***Calorie-free:*** *fewer than 5 calories per serving*

Low: Food can be eaten frequently without exceeding dietary guidelines for one or more of these components: fat, saturated fat, cholesterol, sodium, and calories. Synonyms include *little, few,* and *low source of.*

- ***Low-fat:*** *3 g or less per serving*
- ***Low saturated fat:*** *1 g or less per serving*
- ***Low-cholesterol:*** *20 mg or less and 2 g or less of saturated fat per serving*
- ***Low-sodium:*** *140 mg or less per serving*
- ***Very low sodium:*** *35 mg or less per serving*
- ***Low calorie:*** *40 calories or less per serving*

High: Food contains 20 percent or more of the Daily Value for a particular nutrient in a serving.

Good source: Food contains 10 to 19 percent of the Daily Value for a particular nutrient in one serving.

Lean and extra lean: Describe the fat content of meat, poultry, seafood, and game meat.

- ***Lean:*** *less than 10 g fat, 4.5 g or less saturated fat, and less than 95 mg of cholesterol per serving and per 100 g*
- ***Extra lean:*** *less than 5 g fat, less than 2 g saturated fat, and less than 95 mg of cholesterol per serving and per 100 g*

Reduced: Nutritionally altered product containing at least 25 percent less of a nutrient or of calories than the regular or reference product. (*Note:* A "reduced" claim can't be used if the reference product already meets the requirement for "low.")

Less: Food, whether altered or not, contains 25 percent less of a nutrient or of calories than the reference food. *Fewer* is an acceptable synonym.

such claims were considered drugs, not foods. A **health claim** is a statement that links one or more dietary components to reduced risk of disease—such as a claim that calcium helps reduce the risk of osteoporosis. A health claim must be supported by scientifically valid evidence for it to be approved for use on a food label. In addition, there are specific criteria for the use of claims. For example, a high-fiber food that is also high in fat is not eligible for a health claim. So far, the FDA has approved the following health claims:

health claim Any statement that associates a food or a substance in a food with a disease or health-related condition. The FDA monitors health claims.

- *Calcium and osteoporosis:* Adequate calcium may reduce the risk of osteoporosis.
- *Sodium and hypertension (high blood pressure):* Low-sodium diets may help lower blood pressure.
- *Dietary fat and cancer:* High-fat diets increase risk for some types of cancer.
- *Dietary saturated fat and cholesterol and risk of coronary heart disease (CHD):* Diets high in saturated fat and cholesterol increase risk for heart disease.
- *Fiber-containing grain products, fruits, and vegetables and cancer:* Diets low in fat and rich in high-fiber foods may reduce the risk of certain cancers.

Light: This descriptor can have two meanings:
1. A nutritionally altered product contains one-third fewer calories or half the fat of the reference food. If the reference food derives 50 percent or more of its calories from fat, the reduction must be 50 percent of the fat.
2. The sodium content of a low-calorie, low-fat food has been reduced by 50 percent. Also, *light in sodium* may be used on a food in which the sodium content has been reduced by at least 50 percent.

Note: The term *light* can still be used to describe such properties as texture and color as long as the label clearly explains its meaning (e.g., *light brown sugar* or *light and fluffy*).

More: A serving of food, whether altered or not, contains a nutrient that is at least 10 percent of the Daily Value more than the reference food. This also applies to *fortified, enriched,* and *added* claims, but in those cases, the food must be altered.

Healthy: A *healthy* food must be low in fat and saturated fat and contain limited amounts of cholesterol (less than 60 mg) and sodium (less than 360 mg for individual foods and less than 480 mg for meal-type products). In addition, a single-item food must provide at least 10 percent or more of one of the following: vitamins A or C, iron, calcium, protein, or fiber. A meal-type product, such as a frozen entrée or dinner, must provide 10 percent of two or more of these vitamins or minerals, or protein, or fiber, in addition to meeting the other criteria. Additional regulations allow the term *healthy* to be applied to raw, canned, or frozen fruits and vegetables and enriched grains even if the 10 percent nutrient content rule is not met. However, frozen or canned fruits or vegetables cannot contain ingredients that would change the nutrient profile.

Fresh: Food is raw, has never been frozen or heated, and contains no preservatives. *Fresh frozen, frozen fresh,* and *freshly frozen* can be used for foods that are quickly frozen while still fresh. Blanched foods also can be called fresh.

Percent fat free: Food must be a low-fat or a fat-free product. In addition, the claim must reflect accurately the amount of nonfat ingredients in 100 g of food.

Implied claims: These are prohibited when they wrongfully imply that a food contains or does not contain a meaningful level of a nutrient. For example, a product cannot claim to be made with an ingredient known to be a source of fiber (such as "made with oat bran") unless the product contains enough of that ingredient (e.g., oat bran) to meet the definition for "good source" of fiber. As another example, a claim that a product contains "no tropical oils" is allowed, but only on foods that are "low" in saturated fat, because consumers have come to equate tropical oils with high levels of saturated fat.

Source: Food and Drug Administration, http://www.cfsan.fda.gov/~dms/lab-hlth.html. Accessed 3/20/02.

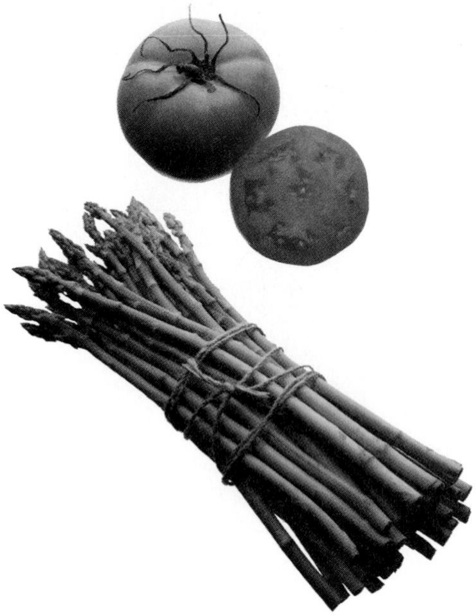

- *Fruits, vegetables, and grain products that contain fiber, particularly pectins, gums, and mucilages, and risk of CHD:* Diets low in fat and rich in these types of fiber may reduce risk of heart disease.
- *Fruits and vegetables and cancer:* Diets low in fat and rich in fruits and vegetables may reduce the risk of certain cancers.
- *Folate and neural tube defects:* Adequate folate intake prior to and early in pregnancy may reduce the risk of neural tube defects (a birth defect).
- *Dietary sugar alcohols and dental caries (cavities):* Foods sweetened with sugar alcohols do not promote tooth decay.
- *Dietary fiber, such as that found in whole oats and psyllium seed husk and CHD:* Diets low in fat and rich in these types of fiber can help reduce the risk of heart disease.
- *Soy protein and CHD:* Foods rich in soy protein as part of a low-fat diet may help reduce the risk of heart disease.
- *Whole-grain foods and CHD or cancer:* Diets high in whole-grain foods and other plant foods and low in total fat, saturated fat, and cholesterol may help reduce the risk of heart disease and certain cancers.
- *Plant sterol/stanol esters and CHD:* Diets low in saturated fat and cholesterol that contain significant amounts of these additives may reduce the risk of heart disease.
- *Potassium and high blood pressure/stroke:* Diets that contain good sources of potassium may reduce the risk of high blood pressure and stroke.

A new health claim may be proposed at any time, so this list will expand.

Structure/Function Claims

Food labels also may contain **structure/function claims** that describe potential effects on body structures or functions, such as bone health, muscle strength, and digestion. As long as the label does not claim to diagnose, cure, mitigate, treat, or prevent a disease, a manufacturer can claim that a product "helps promote immune health" or is an "energizer" if *some* evidence can be provided to support the claim. Currently, structure/function claims on foods must be related to the food's nutritive value. Many scientists are concerned about the lack of a consistent scientific standard for both health claims and structure/function claims. For more on structure/function claims, see Chapter 3, "Complementary Nutrition."

structure/function claims These statements may claim a benefit related to a nutrient-deficiency disease (like *vitamin C prevents scurvy*), or describe the role of a nutrient or dietary ingredient intended to affect a structure or function in humans; for example, *calcium helps build strong bones.*

Using Labels to Make Healthful Food Choices

What's the best way to start using the information on food labels to make food choices? Let's look at a couple of examples. Perhaps one of your goals is to add more iron to your diet. Compare the cereal labels in Figure 2.10. Which cereal contains a higher percentage of the Daily Value for iron? How do they compare in terms of sugar content? What about vitamins and other minerals?

Maybe it's a frozen entrée you're after. Look at the two examples in **Figure 2.11**. Which is the best choice nutritionally? Are you sure? Sometimes the answer is not clear-cut. Product A is higher in sodium, while Product B has more saturated fat. It would be important to know about the rest of your dietary intake before making a decision. Do you already have quite a bit of

Nutrition Facts
Serving Size: 1 Entree (240g)
Servings Per Container: 1

Amount Per Serving	
Calories 400 Calories from fat 150	
	% Daily Value*
Total Fat 16g	25%
Saturated Fat 3.5 g	18%
Cholesterol 10 mg	3%
Sodium 780 mg	33%
Total Carbohydrate 56g	19%
Dietary Fiber 2g	8%
Sugars 2g	
Protein 8g	
Vitamin A 2% •	Vitamin C 4%
Calcium 6% •	Iron 4%

Product A

Nutrition Facts
Serving Size: 1 package (269g)

Amount Per Serving	
Calories 400 Calories from fat 140	
	% Daily Value*
Total Fat 16g	24%
Saturated Fat 8 g	40%
Cholesterol 40 mg	14%
Sodium 690 mg	29%
Total Carbohydrate 48g	16%
Dietary Fiber 2g	9%
Sugars 5g	
Protein 15g	
Vitamin A 10% •	Vitamin C 8%
Calcium 20% •	Iron 15%

Product B

Figure 2.11 **Comparing product labels.** Labels may look similar, but appearances can be deceptive. Compare the amounts of saturated fat and sodium in these two products.

sodium in your diet, or are you likely to add salt at the table? Maybe you never salt your food, so a bit extra in your entrée is OK. If you know that your saturated fat intake is already a bit high, however, Product A might be a better choice. To make the best choice, you should know which substances are most important in terms of your own health risks. The label is there to help you make these types of food decisions.

Key Concepts: *Making food choices at the grocery store is your opportunity to implement the* Dietary Guidelines for Americans *and your Pyramid-planned diet. The Nutrition Facts panel on most packaged foods contains not only the specific amounts of nutrients shown in grams or milligrams, but also comparisons between the amounts of nutrients in a food and the recommended intake values. These comparisons are reported as %DV (Daily Values). The %DV information can be used to compare two products or to see how individual foods contribute to the total diet.*

Label [to] Table Nutrition Labels: Do They Help Us Choose a Healthful Diet?

The Nutrition Labeling and Education Act of 1990 (NLEA) changed food labeling and brought us the Nutrition Facts panel we see on food labels today. One of the NLEA's primary objectives was to help consumers select foods for a healthful diet. Labels were designed to be educational rather than merely informational. Thus, rather than just listing the amounts (e.g., grams and milligrams) for a product's nutrients, Daily Values were developed to make comparisons possible; terms such as *reduced, light, low,* and *free* were defined; and health claims for certain diet–disease relationships were developed. These were dramatic changes from the informational labels of the 1970s and 1980s. But did they work? Does the additional information and the new format encourage more healthful purchases? Policy makers had high hopes for what the changes to nutrition labels would bring. One study predicted four scenarios for behavior change resulting from implementation of the NLEA.[1] Over a period of 20 years, those changes in food choices could lead to a gain of 40,000 to 1.2 million life-years. The potential dollar value of such effects is staggering, ranging from $3 billion to more than $100 billion!

A study of adults found that nutrition labels are useful for people who want to lower the fat content of their diets—an important health goal for most Americans.[2] In this study, adults in Washington state were surveyed by telephone about their use of nutrition labels; their dietary habits as they relate to fat, fruit, and vegetable intake; health behaviors; and demographic characteristics. Women were more likely than men to read nutrition labels and to look at information on serving size, calories, and grams of fat; men were more likely to look at cholesterol information. People under age 35 were more likely to consider serving size, calories from fat, and grams of fat, while those 35 and older read cholesterol information more frequently. Label use was associated with a lower intake of fat, but there was no relation between label use and fruit and vegetable intake. Regular reading of nutrition labels was associated with a reduction in fat intake of at least 5 percent. Although this is lower than the 13 percent figure used by the study that predicted the possible advantages of label use, this level of fat intake reduction would still have significant health benefits for the population as a whole.

In another survey of adults, people who ate diets lower in fat and higher in fruits, vegetables, and fiber were more likely to use labels in deciding what foods to buy. Further, people with high blood cholesterol or hypertension focused their attention on key aspects of the labels—saturated fat and cholesterol or sodium, respectively.[3]

It appears that most label readers still focus on the numbers of grams, calories, or milligrams rather than the %DV. The Washington state study found that while 80 percent of the subjects read nutritional labels, only 39 percent of those label readers used the %DV for fat.[2] It is possible that this information is not well understood by consumers and that the "E" in NLEA (Education) has not been effective or widespread enough to cause consumers to make full use of the information provided. Other surveys indicate that consumers are not clear on the definition of terms such as *low fat* or *cholesterol free.*[4] While these terms are strictly defined in the regulations, the average shopper is not aware of the definitions. Other surveys indicate that interest in labels is waning and that the %DV is not interpreted correctly.[5]

If food labels are going to help the United States realize savings in health-care costs, the average consumer needs to learn more about how to use the valuable information provided on food labels. As the studies have shown, those involved in health education need to focus on educating consumers about food label information. Otherwise, health claims and label statements will just be part of consumers' information overload, rather than a pathway to healthful food choices.

You will find the feature "Label to Table" near the end of most chapters. Use these features to sharpen your critical thinking skills and become an informed consumer who intelligently evaluates nutrition information found on food labels.

1 Zarkin GA, Dean N, Mauskopf JA, Williams R. Potential health benefits of nutrition label changes. *Am J Public Health.* 1993;83:717–724.

2 Neuhouser ML, Kristal AR, Patterson RE. Use of food nutrition labels is associated with lower fat intake. *J Am Diet Assoc.* 1999;99:45–53.

3 Kreuter MW, Brennan LK, Schaff DP, Lukwago SN. Do nutrition label readers eat healthier diets? Behavioral correlates of adults' use of food labels. *Am J Prev Med.* 1997;13:277–283.

4 Resnick ML: *Proceedings of the Human Factors and Ergonomics Society 41st Annual Meeting.* 1997;395–399.

5 Sloan AE. Lessons from labels. *Food Technology.* 1998;52(9):24.

LEARNING *Portfolio* chapter 2

Key Terms

	page
Adequate Intake (AI)	45
Daily Values (DVs)	49
Dietary Guidelines for Americans	32
Dietary Reference Intakes (DRIs)	43
enriched	49
Estimated Average Requirement (EAR)	44
Exchange Lists for Meal Planning	41
Food and Drug Administration (FDA)	47
Food and Nutrition Board (FNB)	43
food groups	35
Food Guide Pyramid	35
food label	47
fortified	49
health claim	51
kwashiorkor	30
marasmus	30
nutrient content claims	49
Nutrition Facts	47
Nutrition Labeling and Education Act (NLEA)	47
overnutrition	30
Recommended Dietary Allowances (RDAs)	42
Recommended Nutrient Intakes (RNIs)	42
requirement	44
statement of identity	47
structure/function claims	52
Tolerable Upper Intake Levels (ULs)	45
undernutrition	30
U.S. Department of Agriculture (USDA)	32
U.S. Department of Health and Human Services (DHHS)	32

Study Points

- Moderation, balance, and variety are general guiding principles for healthful diets.
- The *Dietary Guidelines for Americans* give consumers advice regarding general components of the diet.
- The Food Guide Pyramid is a graphic representation of a food group plan that supports the principles of the *Dietary Guidelines for Americans.*
- Each food group in the Food Guide Pyramid has a recommended number of daily servings. Choose a variety of foods from each group to obtain all the nutrients.
- The Exchange Lists are a diet-planning tool most often used for diabetic or weight-control diets.
- Servings for each food in the Exchange Lists are grouped so that equal amounts of carbohydrate, fat, and protein are provided by each choice.
- Dietary standards are values for individual nutrients that reflect recommended intake levels. These values are used for planning and evaluating diets for groups and individuals.
- The Dietary Reference Intakes are the current dietary standards in the United States. The DRIs consist of four sets of values: EAR, RDA, AI, and UL.
- Nutrition information on food labels can be used to select a more healthful diet.
- Label information not only provides the gram or milligram amounts of the nutrients present, but also gives a percentage of Daily Values so that the consumer can compare the amount in the food and the amount recommended for consumption each day.
- Nutrition information, label statements, and health claims are specifically defined by the regulations that were developed after passage of the Nutrition Labeling and Education Act of 1990.

Study Questions

Answers can be found at nutrition.jbpub.com/discovering.

1. **List the four Dietary Reference Intake categories. How do they differ?**
2. **What is the recommended number of servings for each of the food groups in the Food Guide Pyramid?**
3. **List the ten *Dietary Guidelines for Americans.***
4. **Which food components must be listed on food labels?**
5. **What is the purpose of the "% Daily Value" listed next to most nutrients on a food label?**

[*Try*] This

Are You a Pyramid Pleaser?

Keep a detailed food diary for three days. Make sure to include things you drink, along with the amounts (cups, ounces, tablespoons, etc.) of each food or beverage. Using the serving sizes described in this chapter, determine how many servings from each group of the Food Guide Pyramid you have eaten. Remember that one of your "portions" may equal several "servings" as defined in the Pyramid. Add up the number of servings you ate each day from each Pyramid group and compare the total to the recommended number of servings. How did you do? From which groups did you tend to eat more than is recommended? Were there any groups for which you did not meet the recommendations? Was there a day-to-day variation in the number of servings you ate of each group? Use the results of this activity to plan ways you can improve your diet.

Grocery Store Scavenger Hunt

On your next trip to the grocery store, find a food item that has any number other than a "0" listed for the two vitamins and two minerals required to be listed on the food label %DV. It doesn't matter if you choose a cereal, soup, cracker, or snack item, as long as it has numbers other than "0" for all four items. Once you're home, review the Daily Values (inside the back cover) and calculate the number of milligrams of calcium, iron, and vitamin C found in each serving of your food. Next, take a look at vitamin A: How many International Units (IUs) does each serving of your product have? If you can calculate this, you should have a better understanding of % Daily Values.

What About *Bobbie?*

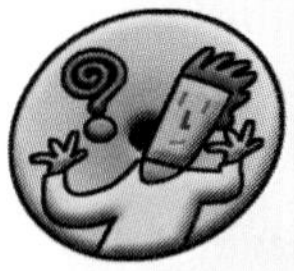

Now that you have learned something about the recommendations for a healthful diet, how do you think Bobbie did? Review her one-day food record in Chapter 1. How closely does Bobbie's intake resemble the Food Guide Pyramid? Do you think she met most of the *Dietary Guidelines?* What about the RDA and AI values? Was her diet balanced enough to meet most of these recommendations?

The following table summarizes the results of a computerized nutrient analysis of Bobbie's diet. You may be completing a similar analysis of your own diet as part of your course requirements. In future chapters, you will explore many of these nutrients further and look at the foods in Bobbie's diet that contributed various nutrients. Keep in mind that this is only a one-day food record and may or may not represent her typical diet.

	Bobbie	RDA/AI	%RDA/AI
Calories	2,440	2,200	111%
Carbohydrates	293 g	—	—
Fiber	24 g	—	—
Fat	99 g	—	—
Cholesterol	263 mg	—	—
Protein	97 g	46 g	211%
Vitamin A	680 mcg	700 mcg	97%
Vitamin D	1 mcg	5 mcg	20%
Vitamin E	9 mg	15 mg	60%
Thiamin	1.8 mg	1.1 mg	164%
Riboflavin	1.9 mg	1.1 mg	173%
Niacin	22 mg	14 mg	157%
Vitamin B_6	1.9 mg	1.3 mg	146%
Folate	471 mcg	400 mcg	118%
Vitamin B_{12}	3.6 mcg	2.4 mcg	150%
Pantothenic acid	3.3 mg	5 mg	67%
Sodium	4,659 mg	—	—
Potassium	2,864 mg	—	—
Calcium	745 mg	1,000 mg	75%
Phosphorus	1,145 mg	700 mg	164%
Magnesium	330 mg	310 mg	106%
Iron	20 mg	18 mg	111%
Zinc	14 mg	8 mg	175%
Copper	1,960 mcg	900 mcg	218%
Manganese	2.8 mg	1.8 mg	156%
Selenium	126 mcg	55 mcg	229%

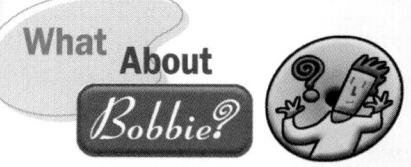

With the Food Guide Pyramid in mind, which food groups are lacking in Bobbie's diet? See if you can classify Bobbie's foods into one of the groups. Some items, like the cheese pizza, have elements of more than one group. Others, like the dill pickle, don't seem to fit anywhere. You may notice that there is only one serving of fruit in her food record—the banana. As for the Milk, Yogurt, and Cheese group, she had 2 tablespoons of milk in her coffee, but no other milk to drink. This milk, combined with the cream cheese, Parmesan cheese, and cheese from one slice of pizza, probably does not meet the minimum suggested servings. Bobbie's diet meets the minimum number of servings from the other food groups. Did she use fats, oils, and sweets sparingly? The servings used were certainly small; future chapters will help you evaluate her fat and sugar intake further.

As for the *Dietary Guidelines for Americans*, since these are recommendations for general patterns of food intake, it would not be fair to evaluate just this single day of eating according to these guidelines. We would need to know much more about Bobbie's usual diet and lifestyle before making this comparison.

References

1 US Department of Health and Human Services. *The Surgeon General's Report on Nutrition and Health.* Washington, DC: US Government Printing Office; 1988.

2 Truswell AS. Dietary goals and guidelines: national and international perspectives. In: Shils ME, Olson JA, Shike M, Ross AC, eds. *Modern Nutrition in Health and Disease.* 9th ed. Baltimore, MD: Williams & Wilkins; 1998.

3 Drewnowski A, Henderson SA, Drisscoll A, Rolls BJ. The Dietary Variety Score: assessing diet quality in healthy young and older adults. *J Am Diet Assoc.* 1997;97:266–271.

4 Keenan DP, Abusabha R. The fifth edition of the *Dietary Guidelines for Americans:* lessons learned along the way. *J Am Diet Assoc.* 2001;101:631–634.

5 Ibid.

6 Davis CA, Britten P, Myers EF. Past, present, and future of the Food Guide Pyramid. *J Am Diet Assoc.* 2001;101:881–885.

7 Dixon LB, Cronin FJ, Krebs-Smith SM. Let the Pyramid guide your food choices: capturing the total diet concept. *J Nutr.* 2001;131(suppl):461S–472S.

8 Institute of Medicine, Food and Nutrition Board. *Dietary Reference Intakes for Calcium, Phosphorus, Magnesium, Vitamin D, and Fluoride.* Washington, DC: National Academy Press; 1997; Institute of Medicine, Food and Nutrition Board. *Dietary Reference Intakes for Thiamin, Riboflavin, Niacin, Vitamin B-6, Folate, Vitamin B-12, Pantothenic Acid, Biotin, and Choline.* Washington, DC: National Academy Press; 1998; Institute of Medicine, Food and Nutrition Board. *Dietary Reference Intakes for Vitamin C, Vitamin E, Selenium, and Carotenoids.* Washington, DC: National Academy Press; 2000; and Institute of Medicine, Food and Nutrition Board. *Dietary Reference Intakes for Vitamin A, Vitamin K, Arsenic, Boron, Chromium, Copper, Iodine, Iron, Molybdenum, Nickel, Silicon, Vanadium, and Zinc.* Washington, DC: National Academy Press; 2001.

9 Yates AA, Schlicker SA, Suitor CW. Dietary Reference Intakes: the new basis for recommendations for calcium and related nutrients, B vitamins and choline. *J Am Diet Assoc.* 1998;98: 699–706.

10 Brecher SJ, Bender MM, Wilkening VL, et al. Status of nutrition labeling, health claims, and nutrient content claims for processed foods: 1997 food label and package survey. *J Am Diet Assoc.* 2000;100:1057–1062.

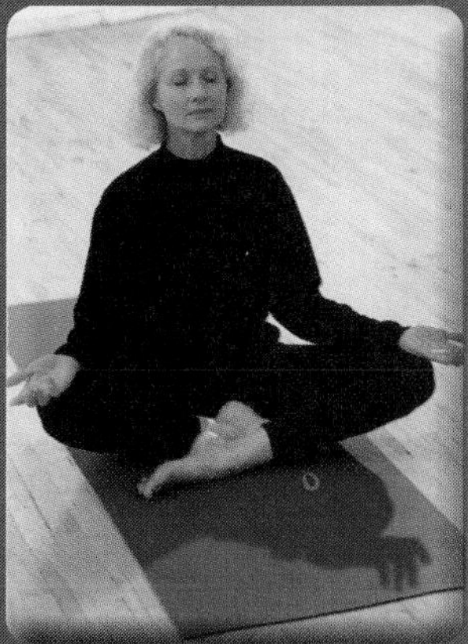
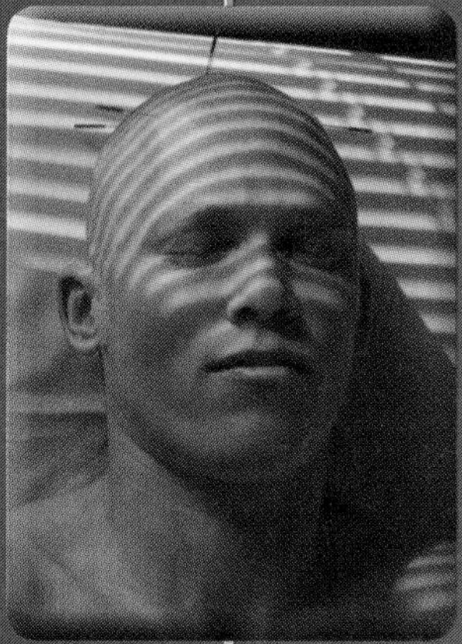
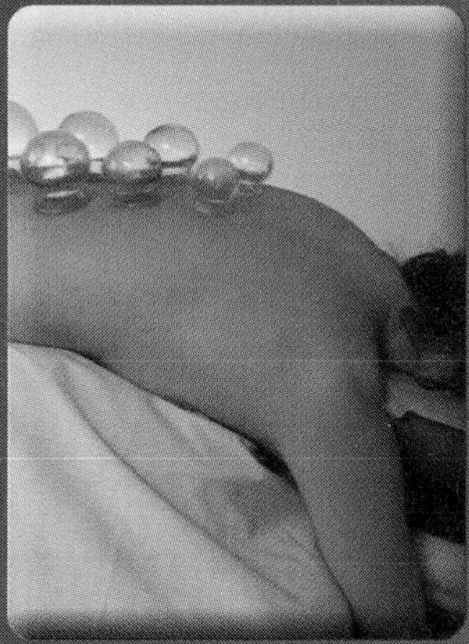
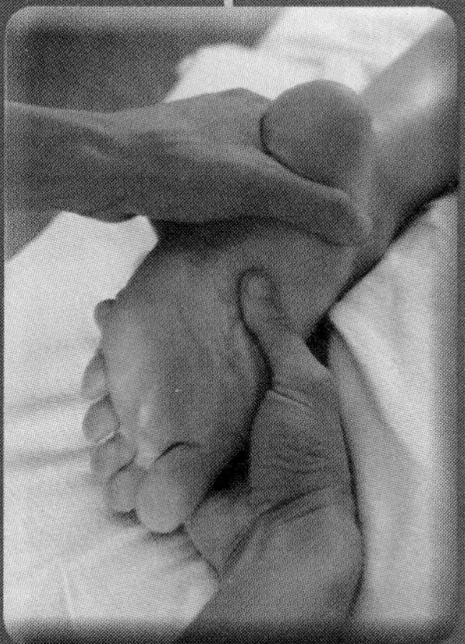
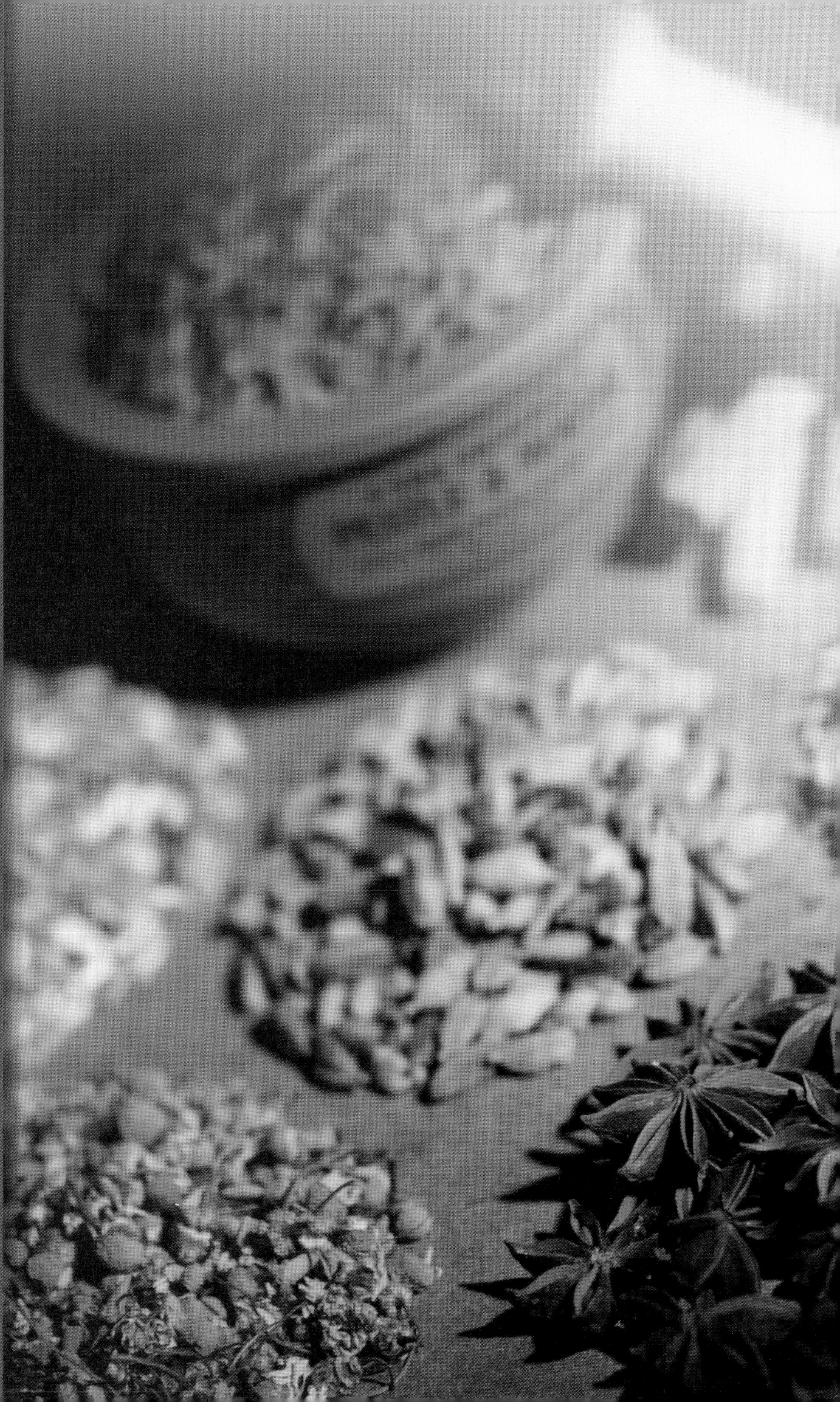

Chapter 3

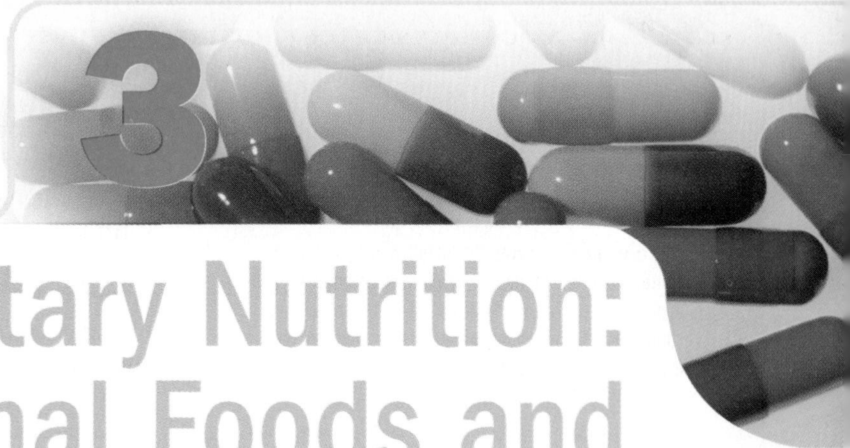

Complementary Nutrition: Functional Foods and Dietary Supplements

Think About It

1. When choosing food, what consideration do you give to health benefits beyond basic nutrition?
2. What are your feelings about the safety of megadose nutrient supplements?
3. Would you ask your physician before taking an herbal supplement?
4. If a friend told you about a new licorice extract that is guaranteed to tone muscles, would you try it?

Fyi for your Information

This chapter's FYI boxes include practical information on the following topics:

- Are Megadoses of Vitamin E Appropriate?
- The Saccharin Story

WWW

The Web site for this book offers many useful tools and is a great source for additional nutrition information for both students and instructors. For information on complementary and alternative nutrition, visit the site at **nutrition.jbpub.com/discovering.** You'll find exercises that explore the following topics:

- The ADA's Dietetics Practice Groups
- The ADA and Diets versus Supplements
- Complementary and Alternative Therapies
- The Office of Dietary Supplements

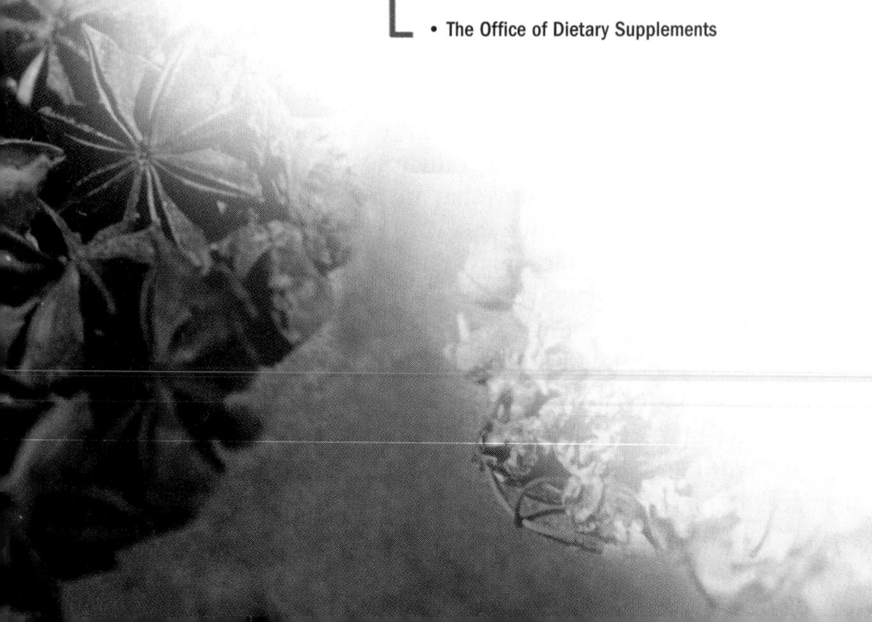

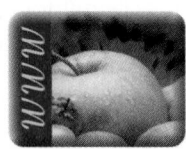

isoflavones Plant chemicals that include genistein and daidzein and may have positive effects against cancer and heart disease. Also called phytoestrogens.

dietary supplements Products taken by mouth and contain dietary ingredients, which may include vitamins, minerals, herbs, or amino acids, as well as other substances such as enzymes, organ tissues, metabolites, extracts, or concentrates.

complementary and alternative medicine (CAM) A broad range of healing philosophies, approaches, and therapies that include treatments and health-care practices not taught widely in medical schools, not generally used in hospitals, and not usually reimbursed by medical insurance companies.

functional food A food that may provide a health benefit beyond basic nutrition.

lycopene One of a family of plant chemicals, the carotenoids. Others in this big family are alpha-carotene and beta-carotene.

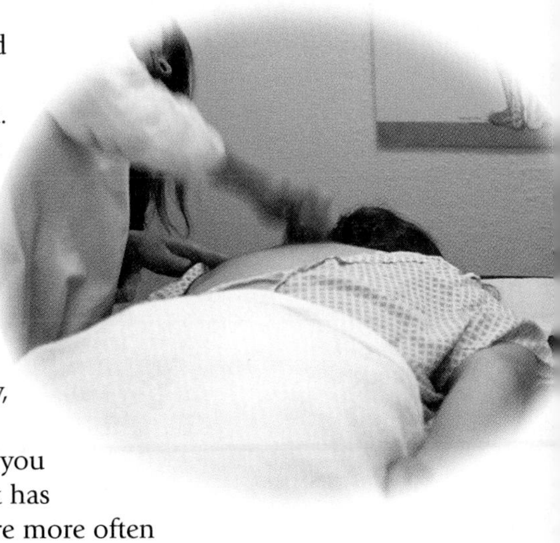

Marcie chooses calcium-fortified foods whenever she has the chance. Seema takes the herb St. John's wort, hoping it will pull her out of the doldrums. Emil swears by the use of creatine in his muscle-building regimen. Jason tries a new energy bar with added ginkgo biloba, hoping it will improve his memory. Others in search of better health turn to massage therapy, magnets, macrobiotic diets, homeopathy, acupuncture, and many other practices.

Any trip to the grocery store will tell you that a new era in product development has begun—one in which food products are more often touted for what they contain (e.g., soy **isoflavones**, vitamins and minerals, herbal ingredients) than for what they lack (e.g., fat, cholesterol). Beverages, energy bars, and teas marketed as foods sit side by side on the shelf with similar products labeled as **dietary supplements**. And the market for dietary supplements—which are much more than the simple vitamins and minerals our parents knew—continues to grow.

This chapter looks at functional foods, dietary supplements, and the role of nutrition in **complementary and alternative medicine (CAM)**. We will look at the claims made for products and therapies in terms of current scientific knowledge; we'll also consider regulatory and safety issues. Making decisions about nutrition and health requires consumers and professionals alike to stay informed and consult reliable sources before trying a new product or embarking on a new health regimen.

Quick Bites

Take out the Bad, Leave in the Good

In Japan, the development of functional foods minimizes undesirable qualities as well as maximizes desirable food factors. This has led to the removal of allergens and the development of hypoallergenic foods.

Functional Foods

What do garlic, tomato sauce, tofu, and oatmeal all have in common? They aren't in the same food group, nor do they have the same nutrient composition. Instead, all of these foods could be considered "functional foods." Although there is not yet a legal definition for the term, a **functional food** is widely considered to be a food that may provide a health benefit beyond basic nutrition.[1] Garlic contains sulfur compounds that may lower low-density lipoprotein (LDL) cholesterol, and tomato sauce is rich in **lycopene**, a compound that may reduce prostate cancer risk. The soy protein in tofu and the fiber in oatmeal can help reduce the risk of heart disease. (See **Figure 3.1**.) Researchers predict a rapidly growing global market for functional foods. Currently, Japan accounts for about half the global sales, but researchers expect the fastest growth in the American market.[2]

Think About It 1

All the functional foods just mentioned get their health-promoting properties from naturally occurring compounds that are not considered nutrients but are called phytochemicals. While the word *phytochemical* itself may sound futuristic, its meaning is simple: "plant chemical." It seems you can't pick up a health magazine these days without seeing an article about phytochemicals. But what do we really mean when we talk about phytochemicals, and why is there so much interest in these compounds?

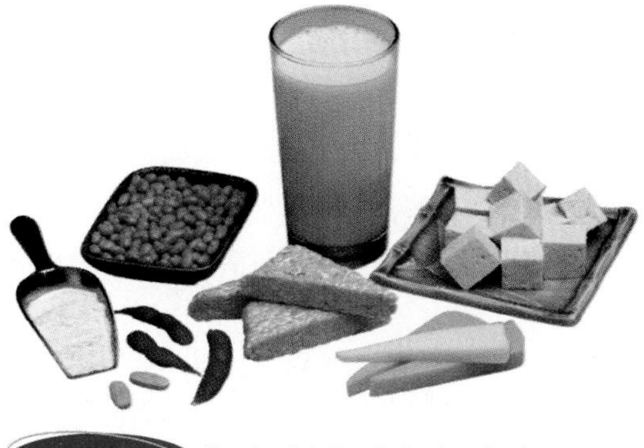

Figure 3.1 **Soy is rich in phytochemicals.** Soybeans contain phytochemicals called isoflavones. High intake of soy products such as tofu is linked to a lower incidence of heart disease and cancer.

Phytochemicals Make Foods Functional

A vitamin is a food substance essential for health. Phytochemicals, in contrast, are substances in plants that may protect our good health, even

though they are not essential for life. Phytochemicals are complex chemicals that vary from plant to plant. They include thousands of compounds, pigments, and natural antioxidants, many of which have been associated with protection from heart disease, hypertension, cancer, and diabetes. **Table 3.1** lists many examples of phytochemicals and their potential benefits.

Plants contain phytochemicals in abundance because these substances are of benefit to the plant itself. For example, an orange has at least 170 distinct phytochemicals. Singly and together, these compounds help plants resist the attacks of bacteria and fungi, the ravages of free radicals, and high levels of ultraviolet light from the sun. When we eat these plants, the phytochemicals end up in our tissues and provide many of the same protections that plants enjoy.

Phytochemicals are part of the reason why the Food Guide Pyramid recommends five servings per day of fruits and vegetables. Of course, fruits and vegetables are also naturally low in fat and calories and tend to be rich in fiber, potassium, and vitamins. In addition, studies show that groups of people who consume more fruits and vegetables tend to have lower rates of common chronic diseases.

Benefits of Phytochemicals

What are some of the benefits of phytochemicals? People who eat tomatoes and processed tomato products take in lycopene, which is associated with a decreased risk of chronic diseases such as cancer and cardiovascular diseases.[3] Scientists believe that the large consumption of soy products in Asian countries contributes to lower rates of cancers of the colon, prostate, uterus, and breast.[4] In fact, a recent study of over 3,000 Chinese women suggests that high soy intake during adolescence may reduce the risk of breast cancer in later life.[5] The foods and herbs with the highest anticancer activity include garlic, soybeans, cabbage, ginger, and licorice, as well as the family of vegetables that includes celery, carrots, and parsley.

How do phytochemicals work to prevent cancer? They neutralize **free radicals** and modify the way hormones affect the body. A number of phytochemicals, including those from soybeans and from the cabbage family, are able to modify estrogen metabolism or block the effect of estrogen on cell growth. Since levels of estrogen and other hormones are in turn closely linked to the development of breast, ovarian, and prostate tumors, it is apparent how phytochemicals might inhibit development of such cancers.

Free radicals (active oxidants) are continually produced in our cells and over time can result in damage to DNA and important cell structures. Eventually, this damage can promote both cancer and cell aging. Many different plant chemicals, such as the pigments in grapes and red wine (see **Figure 3.2**), are able to neutralize or reduce concentrations of free radicals, thus protecting us against the development of both cancer and atherosclerosis.

The phytochemicals in citrus have a number of potential benefits. Pink grapefruit, for instance, contains high levels of beta-carotene and a variety of other carotenoids (plant pigments) with significant antioxidant activity. These compounds are associated with a lower incidence of age-related macular degeneration, the leading cause of blindness in older people. The phytochemicals in whole grains are generally similar to those found in fruits and vegetables and are important in prevention of both cancer and heart disease. One class of grain phytochemicals, the terpenoids, produces a significant reduction in total and LDL cholesterol levels, thus reducing the

Quick Bites

Functional Food Decisions

Are you a health-conscious consumer who seeks out functional foods? According to a 1999 survey, nearly two-thirds of Canadian grocery shoppers reported that their desire to ensure overall good health has replaced balanced nutrition or lowering fat intake as the number one motivating factor to purchase "healthy" foods. In contrast, a 2000 survey found that while over 90 percent of U.S. consumers believe certain foods have health benefits beyond basic nutrition, only one-third add particular foods or ingredients to their diet in an effort to improve or maintain their health.

free radicals Short-lived, highly reactive chemicals often derived from oxygen-containing compounds, which can have detrimental effects on cells, especially DNA and cell membranes.

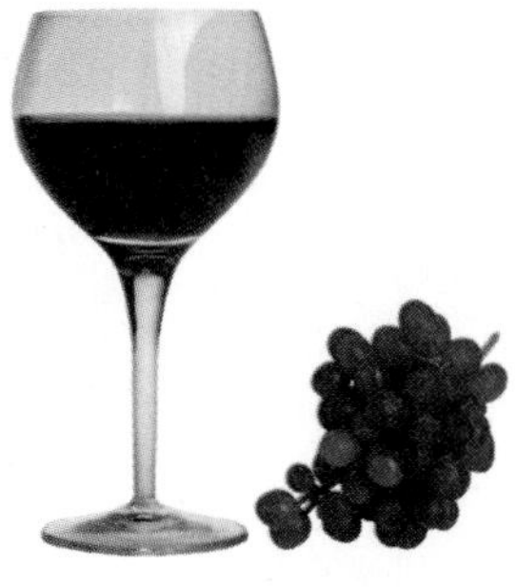

Figure 3.2 Grapes, red wine, and heart disease. Grapes and red wine contain phytochemicals that appear to reduce the risk of heart disease. Studies show that moderate consumption of alcohol independently reduces heart disease risk.

Table 3.1 Phytochemicals and Their Benefits

Foods	Phytochemicals	Possible Benefits
Berries Blueberries, strawberries, raspberries, blackberries, currants, etc.	Anthocyanidins, ellagic acid	Both act as antioxidants, thus as anticancer substances that may help protect cells. Ellagic acid has more than one anticancer activity. Anthocyanidins may also protect against heart disease. Berries are also rich in soluble fiber, which may help reduce cholesterol.
Chili Peppers	Capsaicin, which gives peppers their heat	Little is known about potential health benefits; capsaicin may be an antioxidant or otherwise interfere with cancer development. May help prevent blood clotting. Chili peppers are also rich in vitamin C.
Citrus Fruits Oranges, grapefruit, lemons, limes, etc.	Flavanones such as hesperitin; coumarins; D-limonene (a monoterpene); carotenoids; flavonoids such as tangeretin and nobiletin	D-limonene, in citrus skin, can leach into the juice and may detoxify cancer promoters. Carotenoids may also fight cancer. Flavonoids act as antioxidants and may inhibit blood clotting. These fruits are also rich in vitamin C (a powerful antioxidant), other nutrients, and fiber.
Cruciferous Vegetables Broccoli, broccoli sprouts, Brussels sprouts, kale, cabbage, cauliflower, etc.	Indoles; isothiocyanates such as sulforaphane; carotenoids such as beta-carotene	Long classified as anticancer foods. Sulforaphane may neutralize cancer-causing chemicals that damage cells; also interferes with tumor growth. Broccoli sprouts are particularly rich in the substances that convert into sulforaphane. Indoles act to make estrogen less potent and thus may reduce the risk of breast cancer. These vegetables are also good sources of folate (a B vitamin), vitamin C, fiber, and carotenoids—all cancer fighters.
Flax Seeds, flour	Lignans	Lignans are converted to a form of estrogen in the body and are thought to have some protective effect against cancer. Lignans are not found in flaxseed oil.
Garlic Family Garlic, onions, shallots, leeks, chives, scallions	Allylic sulfides, other sulfur compounds, flavonoids such as quercetin	Add flavor and zest to other good foods. May work against carcinogens and tumors in many ways, lowering risk of colon, stomach, and other cancers. May also benefit the heart. No certainty that cooked onions and garlic work as well as raw. Supplements are unproved and not recommended.
Herbs and Spices Rosemary, sage, thyme, oregano, ginger, cumin, etc.	Carnasol, phenols, curcumin, gingerols, terpenoids, etc.	Major benefit: adding flavor and zest to other good foods. May act as antioxidants and anticancer agents, even in small amounts.
Legumes Lima, kidney, navy, and other beans, lentils, etc.	Isoflavonoids, phytic acid, saponins, phytosterols	Anticancer activity; protection against heart disease. Phytosterols may protect against colon cancer. Beans contain folate (a B vitamin) and other nutrients, as well as soluble fiber, which may reduce blood cholesterol.
Nuts Cashews, almonds, chestnuts, walnuts, etc.	Ellagic acid, saponins	Potential benefits to the heart may come from these chemicals or from the beneficial fats (poly- and monounsaturated) in nuts. High in calories and fat, nuts should be consumed in moderation.

Foods	Phytochemicals	Possible Benefits
Orange and Yellow Fruits and Vegetables; Leafy Greens Apricots, papaya, sweet potatoes, mangoes, carrots, spinach, corn, pumpkin, sweet peppers, etc.	Carotenoids such as beta-carotene, lutein, zeaxanthin	Many anticancer functions; strengthen the immune system; protect the retina from harmful radiation, thus reducing risk of macular degeneration. These fruits and vegetables are also rich in vitamin C, other vitamins, minerals, and fiber.
Red Grapes, Red Wine	Flavonols such as quercetin; resveratrol, anthocyanidins, ellagic acid	Resveratrol may prevent damage to cells and curb tumor growth, reduce risk of skin cancer, and have beneficial effects on blood cholesterol. Quercetin may benefit the heart. Anthocyanidins and ellagic acid are antioxidants. Grapes, grape juice, and wine have different compounds and thus may have different effects.
Soy (Also a Legume) Tofu, soy milk, soybeans, soy protein, etc.	Isoflavonoids such as daidzein and genistein; lignans; saponins; phytosterols	Isoflavonoids and lignans are converted to a kind of estrogen in the body and are thought to have some protective effect against cancer. Saponins and phytosterols also have anti-cancer activity. Different forms of soy have varying amounts of beneficial phytochemicals.
Tea Green, black, oolong, but not herbal tea	Flavonols such as catechins and epigallocatechin gallate (EGCG), plus other flavonoids	Tea, particularly green tea, may reduce the risk of many cancers, according to new research. Flavonols and other flavonoids in tea may combat cancer on several fronts. EGCG is a more powerful antioxidant than vitamin E; both neutralize cell-damaging free radicals. Catechins may protect arteries from plaque buildup. Some evidence suggests that flavonoids in tea may lower blood cholesterol.
Tomatoes	Carotenoids, chiefly lycopene (also found, in much smaller amounts, in red peppers, pink grapefruit, guava, watermelon)	High intake, especially of cooked or processed tomatoes, may reduce risk of prostate and other cancers. Lycopene may fight cancer in several ways, including lowering potency of testosterone. Tomatoes also contain vitamin C and other nutrients.
Whole Grains Whole wheat, oats, barley, rye, brown rice, etc.	Saponins, terpenoids, phytic acid, ellagic acid, phytoestrogens	Saponins may neutralize cancer-causing substances in the intestine. Terpenoids and phytic acid may help reduce heart disease and cancer risk. Also rich in fiber, which helps lower blood cholesterol and may reduce colon cancer risk. Beneficial elements are concentrated in bran and germ; refined grains have little fiber and greatly reduced amounts of beneficial plant chemicals, even when enriched.

Source: *Beyond vitamins: The new nutrition revolution. The wellness guide—a special insert.* UC Berkeley Wellness Letter. *April 1999.*

risk of heart disease. Before you reach for your next slice of bread, it is worth remembering that refined wheat, the source of white flour, has lost more than 99 percent of its phytochemical content, and only four vitamins and one mineral are added back when refined grains are enriched.

Adding Phytochemicals to Your Diet

Since phytochemicals are so beneficial, why can't we just purify the important ones and add them to our diet as supplements, the way we put vitamins back into white flour after processing? The short answer is that we don't know enough about how phytochemicals function.

Many phytochemicals appear to act in concert, both fighting free radicals and blocking the negative effects of hormones. It is not surprising, then, that when a single pure phytochemical, such as beta-carotene, is given as a long-term supplement, only minor benefits are seen. In fact, some studies have shown no health benefits from such purified supplements. Yet there is no doubt that consumption of plant foods containing multiple antioxidants is strongly associated with health benefits. The weight of evidence and experience strongly favors finding a place for a minimum of five servings of fruits and vegetables (see **Figure 3.3**) and an emphasis on whole grains for the six to eleven grain servings recommended each day. Choosing legumes and soy products at least some of the time as alternatives to meat will introduce even more phytochemicals into the diet.

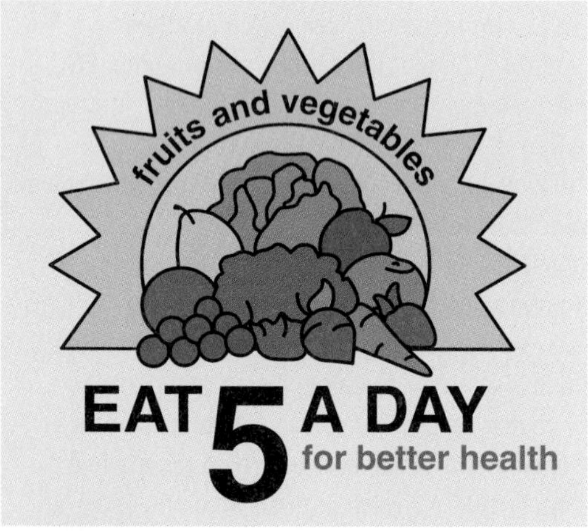

Figure 3.3 **The national 5 a Day for Better Health program.** This program encourages Americans to eat five or more servings of fruits and vegetables every day for better health. It is jointly sponsored by the National Cancer Institute of the U.S. Department of Health and Human Services and the Produce for Better Health Foundation, a nonprofit consumer education foundation representing the fruit and vegetable industry.

Changing your diet to include more functional foods and fewer empty calories needn't be painful if you use your imagination. Sometimes you can have your pizza and eat it too. The next time you indulge, ask for a pizza with minimum cheese and maximum vegetables. The combination of lycopene from tomato sauce, quercetin from onions, glucarates from green peppers, and carotenoids from basil and spinach can turn a potential nutritional train wreck into a phytochemical cornucopia.

Foods Enhanced with Functional Ingredients

Another type of functional food is one that gets its health-promoting properties from what has been added during processing. Calcium-fortified orange juice, breakfast cereals fortified with folic acid, yogurt with live active cultures, and margarines with added plant sterol and plant stanol esters are examples. Health properties come from added nutrients, bacteria, fiber, or other substances. Relatively new on the scene are products that contain herbal compounds, such as those sold in pill form as dietary supplements. The result is a wide variety of products making an often confusing array of label statements and health claims.

Regulatory Issues for Functional Foods

The FDA defines foods as "articles used for food or drink, chewing gum, or articles used for components of any other such article." While this may sound a little confusing, a food is a product that we eat or drink, as well as all the components of that product. This definition distinguishes a food from a drug, which is a substance intended to diagnose, cure, mitigate, treat, or prevent disease. Foods also are distinct from dietary supplements, which are products intended to supplement the diet but which do not represent themselves as a conventional food, meal, or diet. You will learn more about dietary supplements later in this chapter.

Although some manufacturers have tried to market functional products as dietary supplements rather than foods to take advantage of broader enhance your shopping list with nature's functional foods. Second, consider nutrient-fortified products when a particular nutrient is lacking in your diet and you either don't like or can't eat good food sources of that nutrient. For example, if you are allergic to milk and dairy products, consider calcium-fortified orange juice as a nutritious way to get the calcium that you need. Third, *read, read, read* about functional foods, and not just what's on the Internet. Do your homework by looking at scientific articles—your instructor can help you find and interpret studies of functional food components. Finally, be critical of advertising and hype—if it sounds too good to be true, it probably is!

Dietary Supplements: Vitamins and Minerals

Dietary supplements come in various forms—vitamins, minerals, amino acids, herbs, glandular extracts, enzymes, and many others. As a result of recent regulatory changes, the marketplace is seeing an avalanche of new products claiming to do everything from enhancing immune function to improving mood. **Table 3.2** lists many popular supplements, claims, and important cautions. Despite the enticing claims made by many products, vitamins and minerals remain the most popular supplements for Americans.

"Should I take a vitamin (or mineral) supplement?" Apparently many people already have answered that question for themselves: A substantial percentage of Americans regularly take dietary supplements as part of their routine for staying healthy.[10] (See **Figure 3.6**.) We will look at two levels of vitamin and mineral supplementation: (1) moderate doses that are in the range of the Daily Values (DVs) or levels you might eat in a nutrient-rich diet and (2) **megadoses**, or high levels that are typically multiples of the DVs and much greater amounts than diet alone could supply.

megadoses Doses of a nutrient that are 10 or more times the recommended amount.

Moderate Supplementation

Health-care practitioners often recommend moderate nutrient supplementation for people with elevated nutrient needs and people who may not always eat well enough. Some examples include the following:

- *Pregnant and breastfeeding women.* Taking supplemental folic acid prior to and during pregnancy can reduce the incidence of birth defects. During pregnancy, it's hard to meet the increased needs for iron and other nutrients through diet alone. "Morning sickness" makes it even harder. When a woman breastfeeds, some of her nutrient needs are even higher than they were in pregnancy.
- *Women with heavy menstrual bleeding.* Women with high iron losses may need a supplement, but they should not take high doses of iron without a doctor's recommendation. Lab tests can show whether a woman gets enough blood-building nutrients or whether she needs supplements.
- *Children.* A supplement can help balance the diets of picky eaters or children on a food jag (eating only a few specific foods), and it can ease parental worries.
- *Infants.* If their access to sunlight is restricted, infants may need supplemental vitamin D. Doctors also may prescribe fluoride in areas where water is not fluoridated.
- *People with severe food restrictions, either self-imposed or prescribed.* Supplements may help people on a strict weight-loss diet, those

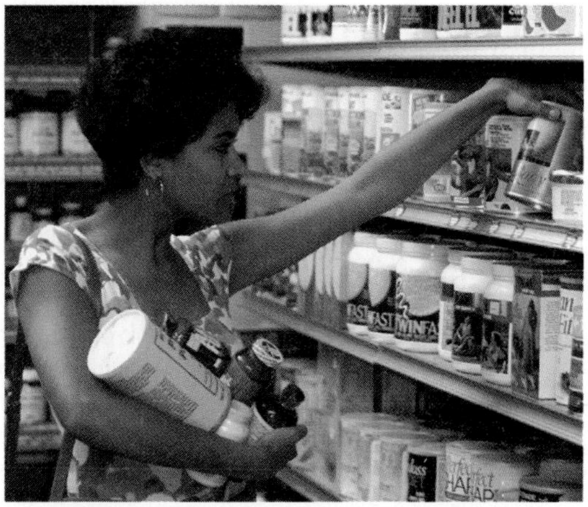

Figure 3.6 **Increasing popularity of dietary supplements.** More than one in four Americans regularly purchase dietary supplements.

Table 3.2 Examples of Dietary Supplements and Their Claims

Supplement	Claimed Benefits	Current Reaserch Caveats
Beta-carotene	Prevents cancer and heart disease and boosts immunity	Diets rich in beta-carotene-containing fruits and vegetables reduce heart disease and cancer risk. Supplements have not been shown to be beneficial. Taking supplements may increase lung cancer risk in smokers.
Chromium picolinate	Builds muscle, prevents and cures diabetes, promotes weight loss	No solid evidence that chromium picolinate supplements perform as claimed or benefit healthy people. Some evidence that they may harm cells.
Coenzyme Q_{10}	Cure-all; prevents heart disease	May have value in pre-existing heart disease, but benefits for healthy people are unproved.
Creatine	Improves athletic performance	May enhance power and strength for some athletes, but is meaningless for casual exercisers and distance athletes.
Echinacea	Cures colds, boosts immunity	Inconsistent evidence of benefit. Products on the market are unstandardized.
Ephedra	Weight control, herbal "high," decongestant	Ephedra raises heart rate and blood pressure and is dangerous for people with diabetes, high blood pressure, heart disease.
Garlic	Lowers blood pressure and blood cholesterol, prevents stomach cancer	Some evidence that garlic reduces cholesterol.
Ginkgo biloba	Improves blood flow and circulatory disorders, and prevents or cures absent-mindedness, memory loss, dementia	Limited benefits for some Alzheimer's patients. No proven benefit for others. Products on the market are unstandardized.
Ginseng	Improves athletic performance, fights fatigue, cures cancer and heart disease	No evidence that ginseng has any beneficial effects. Many products on the market contain no ginseng.
Glucosamine & chondroitin sulfate	Halt, reverse, or cure arthritis	Some evidence of reduced pain, although more studies are needed. Does not reverse arthritis.
Kava	Promotes relaxation and relieves anxiety	May cause liver damage.
Melatonin	Promotes sleep, counters jet lag, improves sex life, etc.	Studies are contradictory relative to sleep/jet lag. No evidence for anti-aging or sex drive claims. No data on long-term safety.
Saw palmetto	May shrink prostate, reduce symptoms of benign prostatic hyperplasia	May improve urinary tract symptoms. No evidence for prevention of prostate cancer. May affect PSA test and diagnosis of prostate cancer.
St. John's wort	Alleviates depression	Studies in Europe suggest efficacy for mild depression. Clinical trial under way in United States. Should not be taken with prescription antidepressants.

Source: Adapted from *The Wellness Guide to Dietary Supplements.* UC Berkeley Wellness Letter; August 1998; and Sarubin A. *The Health Professional's Guide to Popular Dietary Supplements.* Chicago, IL: The American Dietetic Association; 2000.

who have eating disorders, those who have mental illnesses, and those who limit their eating because of social or emotional situations.

- *Strict vegetarians who abstain from animal foods and dairy products.* People who don't eat meat or dairy products may need supplemental vitamin B_{12} and perhaps calcium, zinc, iron, and other minerals.
- *Elders.* Because inadequate stomach acid (which is needed for normal absorption of vitamin B_{12}) is common among older people, elders may need extra vitamin B_{12}. When elders have limited exposure to the sun and their diets lack dairy products, they should take supplements of calcium, vitamin D, and possibly other nutrients to help maintain bone health.

Many people take nutrient supplements to ensure that they meet their nutritional needs. However, taking supplements to "fix" a poor diet is a bad idea. Foods provide not only nutrients but also fiber and other health-promoting phytochemicals. Whenever possible, meet your nutritional needs with food.

Many supplements contain multiple vitamins and minerals. If you are one of those who should take multivitamin/mineral supplements, look for brands that contain at least 20 vitamins and minerals, each no more than 150 percent of its Daily Value. (See **Figure 3.7**.) Some minerals, like calcium, would make a multivitamin/mineral supplement too large to swallow, so people take these supplements separately. Although most products have appropriate nutrient levels, some formulas are irrational and unbalanced, with less than 10 percent of the Daily Value of some nutrients and more than 1,000 percent of others.

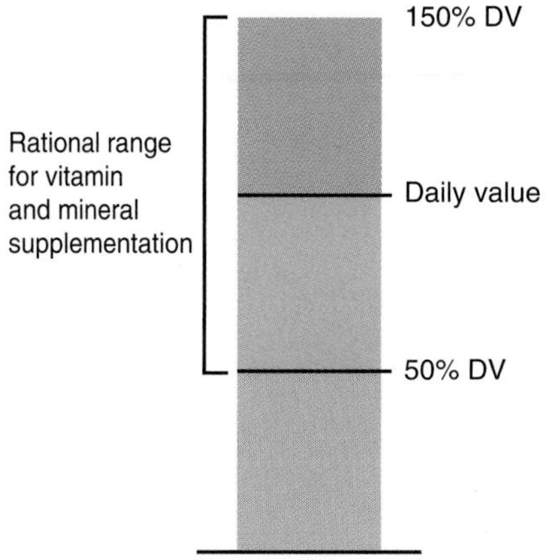

Figure 3.7 **Moderate supplementation.** Health-care practitioners often recommend moderate nutrient supplementation for people with elevated nutrient needs and for people who have consistently poor diets.

Key Concepts: *Vitamin and mineral supplements are popular; however, it is better to obtain nutrients from food. Some conditions and circumstances make it difficult to meet nutritional needs through food alone or to consume enough food to accommodate increases in nutrient needs. Multivitamin/mineral supplements should be well balanced, with doses no greater than about 150% DV of each nutrient.*

Megadoses in Conventional Medical Management

High doses of vitamins and minerals have become so much a part of treating certain illnesses that when physicians prescribe these nutrients, many see themselves as following "standard medical practice" rather than as "practicing nutrition." Here are some situations in which physicians prescribe megadoses.

- When a medication dramatically depletes or destroys the stores or blocks the functions of vitamins or minerals, megadosing can overcome these effects. For example, folic acid and vitamin B_6 are used during long-term treatment with some tuberculosis drugs. B vitamins also may be prescribed along with seizure medications or medicines that block the metabolism of **nucleic acids.**[11]
- People with **malabsorption syndromes** often take large nutrient doses to compensate for nutritive losses and to override intestinal barriers to absorption. Colitis and cystic fibrosis are conditions routinely treated with megadoses.
- Megadoses of vitamin B_{12} can treat pernicious anemia (vitamin B_{12} deficiency), typically caused by malabsorption of B_{12}. Ordinarily,

nucleic acids A family of more than 25,000 molecules found in chromosomes, nucleoli, mitochondria, and cytoplasm of cells.

malabsorption syndromes Conditions that result in imperfect, inadequate, or otherwise disordered gastrointestinal absorption.

an intricate series of steps during digestion prepares B_{12} for normal intestinal absorption; if there is malfunction during any of these steps, the vitamin is lost. Megadoses allow a small amount of the vitamin to diffuse across the intestine, thus overriding the normal mechanism and preventing deficiency.[12]

- A vitamin at megadose levels can have "pharmacological activity"—that is, it acts as a drug. Nicotinic acid (niacin) is the best example. At usual levels (around 10 or 20 milligrams), it functions as a vitamin, but at levels 50 or 100 times higher, it acts as a drug to lower LDL cholesterol and triglycerides. Like any drug, though, it can have serious side effects.[13]

Benefits from high doses of other vitamins are not clear-cut. Researchers have tried prescribing B vitamins, including niacin, for emotional disturbances and mental illnesses; they work well when there's an underlying deficiency, but otherwise results have been mixed and often disappointing. Vitamin E has been tried for some neurological illnesses, to minimize complications of diabetes mellitus, and to reduce the risk of coronary artery disease. Megadoses of vitamin C cannot effectively prevent the common cold or treat cancer, but the vitamin may help prevent other conditions, such as cataracts.[14] Further research into the links between heart disease, homo-

Fyi — FOR YOUR INFORMATION: Are Megadoses of Vitamin E Appropriate?

For decades vitamin E has been touted as a remedy for everything from graying hair to a sluggish libido. While most claims remain unproved, preliminary research shows that large doses bolster immune function as well as help prevent such chronic conditions as heart disease, cancer, and Alzheimer's disease.

Vitamin E ranks as one of the most popular vitamin supplements in the United States, second only to vitamin C.[1] Still, no major health organization has endorsed widespread use of vitamin E supplements because the science on the matter, though encouraging, is still not definitive.

Vitamin E and Heart Disease

Vitamin E may help prevent heart disease, the number one killer of both men and women. Epidemiological studies, animal research, and human clinical trials suggest that the nutrient inhibits oxidation of LDL cholesterol. Cholesterol carried in the blood as part of LDLs (low-density lipoproteins) can be oxidized and contribute to deposits along the artery walls, a condition known as atherosclerosis. For more information about cholesterol, see Chapter 6, "Lipids."

Although the findings are promising, many major health organizations want confirmation by clinical trials before recommending vitamin E supplements. In a recent study of individuals with either cardiovascular disease or diabetes, 400 IU (180 mg) of supplemental vitamin E daily had no apparent effect on cardiovascular events such as heart attack or stroke.[2] Only randomized, placebo-controlled clinical trials can determine whether long-term use of vitamin E—say, over the course of decades—causes side effects that haven't occurred in trials lasting only several years.

Vitamin E and Immunity

Some research suggests that daily doses of vitamin E may help reverse age-related declines in immune function. One study conducted at the Jean Mayer USDA Human Nutrition Research Center on Aging at Tufts University, for example, suggests that vitamin E positively affects the immune system. In the study, people who took 200 milligrams (444 IU) of vitamin E exhibited a substantially better response than people who took either 60 or 800 milligrams (133 or 1,778 IU) of vitamin E. It may be that 200 milligrams was effective because it is just at or below a threshold after which vitamin E confers no benefits to the immune system. This is one of many questions that remain unanswered.[3]

Vitamin E and Alzheimer's Disease

Scientists suspect that vitamin E's antioxidant properties may be useful in treating people with Alzheimer's disease. Research at Columbia University indicates that vitamin E may slow the rate of deterioration in people with moderately severe Alzheimer's disease.[4]

cysteine (an amino acid), and certain B vitamins is needed before specific recommendations for B vitamin supplements can be made.

Megadosing beyond Conventional Medicine: Orthomolecular Nutrition

In 1968 Linus Pauling, the best-known advocate of megadosing, coined the term **orthomolecular medicine**. To him, *orthomolecular* meant achieving the optimal nutrient levels in the body.[15] Few nutritionists argue with the importance of optimum nutrition. In fact, some nutritionists share Pauling's concerns that the typical diet is too refined to provide adequate nutrients and that earlier RDA values may not be high enough to achieve optimal body levels.

orthomolecular medicine The preventive or therapeutic use of high-dose vitamins to treat disease.

Most nutritionists would argue, however, with the high doses Pauling recommended to attain those optimal body levels and with the therapeutic value he and his followers attributed to those doses. Most notably, Pauling's followers continue to recommend vitamin C in levels more than 100 times the Daily Value. (See **Figure 3.8**.) Some advocates of vitamin C recommend even greater doses, relying on intravenous administration to avoid causing diarrhea. Dr. Pauling claimed megadose vitamin C prevented or cured the common cold. Many researchers have attempted to confirm this theory. Although a few found that colds were slightly less severe or less frequent in

These findings prompted the American Psychiatric Association to include the therapeutic use of vitamin E in its 1997 guidelines for the treatment of moderately impaired Alzheimer's patients.[5]

Experts caution, however, that the 2,000-IU (900 mg) dose of vitamin E used in this research should not be taken without a physician's supervision. In addition to the risks of hemorrhagic stroke and decreased ability of blood to clot, vitamin E may also interfere with other medications often administered to people with Alzheimer's disease. The UL for vitamin E is 1,000 milligrams (2,222 IU) of supplemental vitamin E.

Vitamin E and Prostate Cancer

One study has associated vitamin E with a decreased risk of prostate cancer, the most commonly diagnosed cancer in men in the United States.[6] The prostate glands of most older men harbor microscopic areas of cancerous cells that may progress into a cancerous tumor. Because men who took vitamin E experienced a reduction in detectable cancer within two years of taking the supplement, scientists believe that vitamin E may block a prostate's cancerous cells from progressing into malignant masses.

While this study is promising, most experts hesitate to raise hopes until its results are replicated, particularly in groups such as nonsmokers and people of different ethnic backgrounds.

1 Richman A, Witkowski JP. Sixth Annual Dietary Supplement Survey. *Whole Foods.* June 1998:23–28.
2 The Heart Outcomes Prevention Evaluation Study Investigators. Vitamin E supplementation and cardiovascular events in high-risk patients. *N Engl J Med.* 2000;342:154–160.
3 Meydani SN, Meydani M, Blumberg JB, et al. Vitamin E supplementation and in vivo immune response in healthy elderly subjects. *JAMA.* 1997;277:1380–1386; and Chandra RK. Graying of the immune system: can nutrient supplements improve immunity in the elderly? *JAMA.* 1997;277:1398–1399.
4 Sano M, Ernesto C, Thomas RG, et al. A controlled trial of selegiline, alpha-tocopherol, or both as treatment for Alzheimer's disease. *N Engl J Med.* 1997;336:1216–1222.
5 Practice guidelines for the treatment of patients with Alzheimer's disease and other dementias of late life. *Supplement Am J Psychiatry.* 1997;154(suppl 5):1–39.
6 Heinonen OP, Albanes D, Virtamo J, et al. Prostate cancer and supplementation with alpha-tocopherol and beta-carotene: incidence and mortality in a controlled trial. *J Natl Cancer Inst.* 1998;90:440–446.

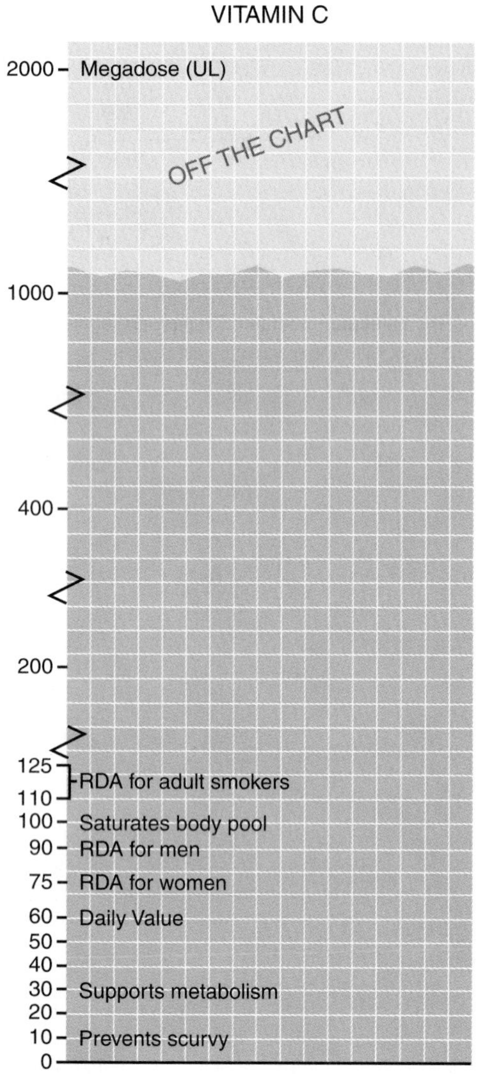

Figure 3.8 Megadoses of vitamin C are much higher intakes than currently recommended.

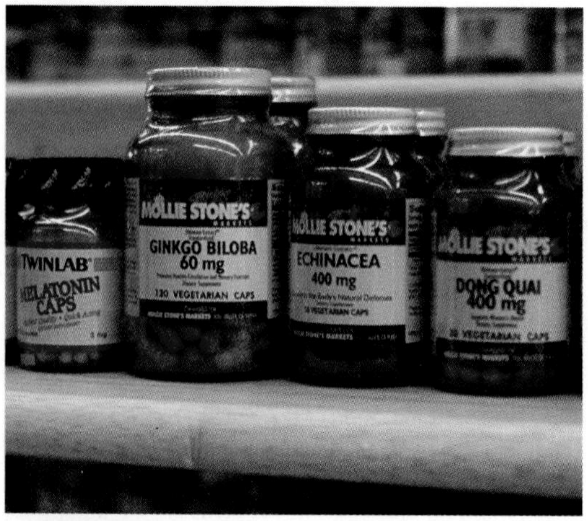

Figure 3.9 **Use of herbal supplements is growing in popularity.** Use of herbal supplements grew more than 16-fold during the last decade.

certain people,[16] most studies found no beneficial effect.[17] The most controversial claim for vitamin C was its purported ability to prevent and treat cancer. Well-controlled studies have now disproved this claim.[18]

Drawbacks of Megadoses

Think About It 2

Megadose vitamins and minerals remain popular. But when taken without recommendation or prescription from a qualified health professional, they can cause problems. Since high doses of a nutrient can act as a drug, with a drug's risk of adverse side effects, people who choose to take megadoses should always check first with their doctors.

Excesses of some nutrients can create deficits of other nutrients. High doses of supplemental minerals, especially calcium, iron, zinc, and copper, can interfere with absorption of the others. In general, it's riskier to megadose with minerals than with vitamins.

It's easy to reach toxic levels if you use high doses of the fat-soluble vitamins A, D, and K. Vitamin E appears relatively safe, even at doses 10 or 20 times the DV, although you should be careful of its tendency to reduce blood clotting. Megadosing with water-soluble vitamin B_6 at 50 to 100 times the DV can cause nerve damage. You may want to review the DRI tables for Tolerable Upper Intake Levels (UL) for vitamins and minerals.

Megadoses often are recommended for sick people, but sick people may be least able to tolerate them. Supplemental iron is very hard on a sensitive digestive system, for example, and high doses of vitamin C can cause diarrhea. Although people who drink a lot of alcohol often are deficient in vitamin A, supplements not much greater than the DV produce undesirable liver changes in alcoholics.[19]

Megadoses can also interfere with medications and treatments. Although some people who take antiseizure medications also may need folic acid supplementation, too much folic acid can allow "breakthrough seizures." Vitamin K interferes with medication to control blood clotting and should be taken only under a doctor's direction. People undergoing surgery should describe their nutritional supplements to their doctor, because high-dose vitamin E, especially if accompanied by blood thinners such as ginkgo biloba, aspirin, or fish oil, can cause bleeding problems in the operating room. Antioxidant nutrients may counteract chemotherapy or radiation aimed at oxidative destruction of cancer cells.

Key Concepts: *High doses (megadoses) of vitamins or minerals turn nutrients into drugs—chemicals with pharmacological activity. While there may be medical reasons for prescribing high-dose supplements, they should be taken under a physician's supervision. Many claims for high-dose supplements, such as claims that vitamin C prevents cancer, are not supported by clinical studies.*

Dietary Supplements: Natural Health Products

Supplementation with herbal and other "natural" products is growing in popularity. (See **Figure 3.9**.) Surveys suggest that the use of herbal products grew from 2.5 percent of adults in 1990 to 12.1 percent in 1997.[20] In the United States, the sale of herbal products skyrocketed from $200 million in 1988 to $5.1 billion in 1997.[21] Health Canada estimates that over 50 percent of Canadians consume natural health products: herbs, vitamins and minerals, and homeopathic products.[22] **Herbal therapy (phytotherapy)** is nothing new, however. Most cultures have long traditions of using plants (and some animal products) to treat illness or sustain health. For centuries there were no other medicines. Even now, most of the world's people depend primarily on herbs for medications; in some remote areas, modern medicines are just not obtainable.

In the Western world, our traditional belief that "natural" is better than "chemical" or "synthetic" has launched the expansion of the herbalism industry.[23] Herbalists reason that natural products are likely to contain a complex of healing ingredients, whereas a purified pharmaceutical product contains only one or two. They believe that when active ingredients are combined with many other plant components, their side effects may be blunted or neutralized. Using herbal medicine sounds simple and easy, but in fact herbalism calls for a great deal of skill. Traditional healers typically serve long apprenticeships and acquire a subjective "feel" for their therapies after much experience. They must learn to judge the safety and potency of individual plants, which vary from season to season, location to location, and with age of the plant and plant part. They must know how to prepare the plant—whether to extract it and with what, or how to make it into a salve or an oral preparation. They must know how to blend it with other herbs and with other therapies. In traditional Chinese medicine, for example, a blend of herbs, sometimes 30 or more, can be used at once; the mixture usually is simmered in water and taken as a tea or "soup." Other herbal traditions use only one or two carefully chosen herbs at a time.

Traditional herbalists know their patients and individualize their herbal remedies accordingly. In the United States that includes knowing results of diagnostic testing; in other cultures it includes recognizing and understanding symptoms. But those who turn to the mass market for herbal supplements rarely receive such attention.

Helpful Herbs, Harmful Herbs

Think About It 3

People who decide to use herbs instead of conventional medicines must choose their practitioners carefully. Herbalists must know their herbs, but they also must know when to tell patients to seek conventional care. People who use both an herbalist and a conventional doctor should tell both practitioners about the other and disclose all treatments.

Until recently, most research on herbs had been published in obscure or foreign-language journals that were hard to locate or read. Traditional herbal medical practices are difficult to study in a controlled manner because they use plants to make teas or soups, a far cry from the purified extracts and herbal blends sold in a supermarket. Nevertheless, for some herbs, researchers have enough data to plan carefully controlled studies. The **National Center for Complementary and Alternative Medicine (NCCAM)** within the National Institutes of Health (NIH) (see **Figure 3.10**) has funded a large study of St. John's wort, based on preliminary evidence that it fights mild depression and sleeplessness.[24] Milk thistle appears helpful for liver disease.[25] Ginkgo biloba appears to help blood circulation, and a preliminary study suggests it may help in treating Alzheimer's disease.[26] Short-term studies indicate that saw palmetto extract improves urinary tract function in men with benign prostate enlargement.[27] Drinking cranberry juice discourages urinary tract infections by inhibiting harmful bacteria from sticking to the urinary tract's lining.[28]

The suggested benefits of other herbs are based not on scientific study but on years of informal observation: Mint helps indigestion; ginger helps nausea and motion sickness; lemon perks appetite; chamomile helps

Quick Bites

Culinary Herbs Are Not Medicinal Herbs—Or Are They?

Herbs used in cooking are called *culinary herbs* to distinguish them from medicinal herbs. But culinary herbs are also rich in phytochemicals. Some examples are beta-carotene in paprika, the antioxidants in rosemary, the mild antibiotic allicin in garlic, and the mild antiviral curcumin in turmeric.

herbal therapy The therapeutic use of herbs and other plants to promote health and treat disease. Also called phytotherapy.

phytotherapy See *herbal therapy.*

National Center for Complementary and Alternative Medicine (NCCAM) An NIH organization established to stimulate, develop, and support objective scientific research on complementary and alternative medicine for the benefit of the public.

NCCAM
National Center for Complementary and Alternative Medicine
National Institutes of Health

Figure 3.10 National Center for Complementary and Alternative Medicine. In 1998, Congress established the NCCAM at the National Institutes of Health (NIH) to stimulate, develop, and support research on CAM for the benefit of the public. The NCCAM is an advocate for quality science, rigorous and relevant research, and open and objective inquiry into which CAM practices work, which do not, and why.

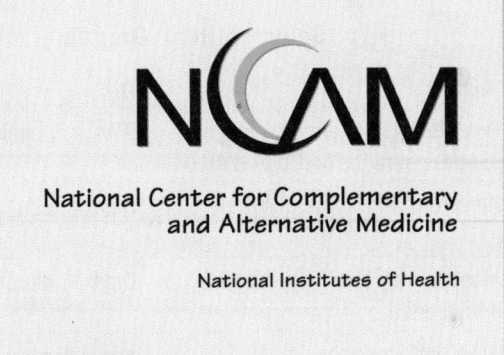

Table 3.3 Popular Herbal Supplements

Ginkgo biloba to combat cerebral vascular insufficiency
Ginseng (Asian) for energy and mood improvement
Garlic to reduce cholesterol and blood pressure; has anticoagulant properties
Echinacea to stimulate the immune system prior to and during the cold and flu season
St. John's wort to treat mild to moderate depression
Saw palmetto to promote prostate health and to treat benign prostatic hyperplasia
Cranberry to treat urinary tract irritations and infections
Valerian as a mild sedative and to treat insomnia
Kava as a tranquilizer and sedative
Milk thistle to detoxify the liver
Feverfew to relieve migraine headaches

insomnia. (See **Table 3.3** for popular supplements and claimed benefits.)

If you're considering using an herb, remember this important rule of thumb: Any herb that is strong enough to help you can be strong enough to hurt you. Like any medicine, herbs can have side effects, and herbs can be contraindicated. For example, the FDA has issued a public health advisory warning of interactions between St. John's wort and some prescription medications, including several used in the treatment of HIV/AIDS.[29] Ginkgo biloba is a blood thinner and has caused harmful bleeding in some people.[30] Just like any other new, unusual substance, herbs can cause sudden allergic reactions.

Herbs can interfere with standard medicines, and they can make people with underlying health problems quite sick. For example, licorice extract—even as a flavoring in chewing tobacco—flushes potassium from the body, raises blood pressure, and can interfere with blood pressure medication.[31] (Most licorice candy is now flavored synthetically; naturally flavored licorice has little effect unless routinely eaten in large amounts.) **Table 3.4** lists some possible interactions of herbs and drugs.

Think About It 4

Some herbs and herbalist treatments are downright dangerous. Some hazardous therapies even use lead or arsenic, known poisons.[32] The herbs yohimbe, ephedra (ma huang), chaparral, and comfrey have been shown to be dangerous.[33] Senna, cascara, and rhubarb are powerful laxatives used in products described as "colon cleansers," "colon purifiers," or even "blood purifiers"; their overuse is as damaging as overuse of conventional laxatives. (See **Table 3.5**.) In June 2001, Health Canada issued an advisory warning consumers not to use products containing ephedra, and in January 2002 issued a voluntary recall of certain products containing ephedra. Also in January 2002, Health Canada advised consumers not to use products containing kava because of European reports of liver toxicity.

Herbal blends marketed for specific conditions, such as "healthy bone formula" or "female blend," do not always make sense in light of current scientific knowledge. For example, pennyroyal and St. John's wort—herbs that should not be used during pregnancy—have shown up in some "prena-

Table 3.4 Selected Herb–Drug Interactions

Herb	Drug	Interaction
Feverfew, garlic, ginger, ginkgo biloba, guarana, and pau d'Arco	Warfarin, aspirin	Increases anticoagulant effect by inhibiting platelet aggregation.
Hawthorn and horse chestnut	Digoxin, diuretics	Affects cardiac function and blood pressure; should not be taken with digoxin and diuretics.
Aloe, senna (laxative), cascara, and licorice	Digoxin, diuretics	Causes electrolyte imbalance; true licorice increases blood pressure. Do not take with diuretics and digoxin.
Kava and valerian	Anxiolytics, narcotics, and alcohol	Increases sedative effects.
St. John's wort	Antidepressants, crixivan (indinavir) and other protease inhibitors, cyclosporine	Should not be taken with prescription antidepressants; risk of hypertensive crisis if taken with antidepressants. St. John's wort makes several prescription medications used in the treatment of AIDS less effective. The herb speeds up activity in a key pathway responsible for breaking down these drugs in the body. When the medications are taken with St. John's wort, blood levels of the drugs decrease because the body breaks them down faster.

Table 3.5 Potential Adverse Effects of Selected Herbs

Herb	Adverse Effects
Chamomile (tea)	Allergic reaction; digestive upset
Chaparral	Liver toxicity
Comfrey	Liver and kidney disease
Echinacea	Allergic reaction; stimulation of immune system: not for use by those with systemic/autoimmune diseases
Ephedra	Insomnia, headaches, nervousness, seizures, increased blood pressure, stroke, death
Ginkgo biloba	Inhibits blood clotting; do not take with aspirin, anticoagulants, vitamin E
Ginseng	Headaches, insomnia, diarrhea, heart palpitations, vaginal bleeding
Kava	Slowed reaction time; scaly dermatitis; liver damage
Licorice	Headaches, fluid retention, increased blood pressure, electrolyte imbalance, heart failure
Pau d'Arco	Severe nausea, vomiting; anemia; bleeding tendencies
Pennyroyal	Liver damage, convulsions, abortions, coma, death; oil is very toxic
St. John's wort	Adverse interactions with antidepressant and HIV/AIDS medications; possible photosensitivity
Senna	Laxative dependency, diarrhea, cramps, electrolyte disturbances
Valerian	Headache, excitability, insomnia

Sources: McGuffin M, Hobbs C, Upton R, Goldberg A. *American Herbal Products Association Botanical Safety Handbook.* Boca Raton, FL: CRC Press; 1997; Sarubin A. *The Health Professional's Guide to Popular Dietary Supplements.* Chicago, IL: American Dietetic Association; 2000; and Foster S, Tyler VE. *Tyler's Honest Herbal: A Sensible Guide to the Use of Herbs and Related Remedies.* Binghamton, NY: Haworth Herbal Press; 1999.

tal formulas." Also, a popular blend used to treat prostate cancer actually had hormonal (estrogenic) activity, which promotes growth of cancer cells.[34]

Quality control is a big issue in herbal medicines. Contaminants have caused acute illness and death.[35] A common problem is poorly standardized strength, or potency. There can be as much as a 17-fold difference in potency of the popular, over-the-counter St. John's wort supplements.[36] One analysis showed that the quantity of active ingredient in ginseng supplements varied from the amount stated on the label by as much as 200-fold.[37]

Manufacturers and practitioners are working with the FDA to establish standards and procedures to ensure potency and to prevent adulteration and contamination. To guarantee quality, each step from field to market must be monitored carefully. However, monitoring the production of herbal supplements poses special challenges. Herbs are grown and harvested in far-flung, sometimes remote areas of the world. Extraction or preparation of the herbs may take place somewhere else. Mixing the herbs and putting them in capsules, tonics, or teas typically takes place in yet another location.

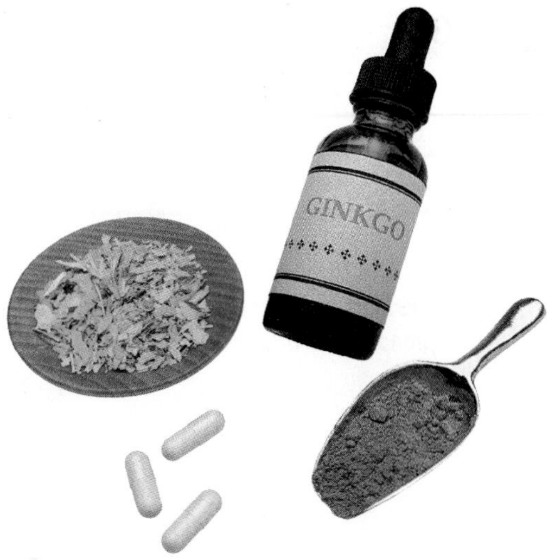

Other Dietary Supplements

The supplement market used to include only vitamins, minerals, and a handful of other products such as brewer's yeast and sea salt. Today there

Quick Bites

Office of Dietary Supplements

The Office of Dietary Supplements (ODS) is a Congressionally mandated office in the National Institutes of Health (NIH). The mission of ODS is to strengthen knowledge and understanding of dietary supplements by evaluating scientific information, stimulating and supporting research, disseminating research results, and educating the public to foster an enhanced quality of life and health for the U.S. population.

are dozens more products, with new ones continuously popping up. Although some are useful, many are of dubious benefit.

Supplement categories now include protein powders, amino acids, carotenoids, **bioflavonoids**, digestive aids, fatty acid formulas and special fats, lecithin and phospholipids, probiotics, products from sharks and other sea animals, algae, human metabolites such as coenzyme Q_{10} and nucleic acids, glandular extracts, garlic products, and fibers such as guar gum. Supplement producers also blend these products with herbs and nutrients, resulting in a countless array of individual and combination supplements sold today. In most cases, labeling and advertising claims go beyond current knowledge about these products.

Key Concepts: *Herbal products are among the many dietary supplements available today. Herbal medicine has a long history in many cultures. Although there is anecdotal support for the use of many herbal products, there is little scientific evidence to back it up. The FDA and manufacturers are working to set standards for production and sale of herbal supplements. It is important to remember that any herb that is strong enough to help you can also be strong enough to hurt you. Before taking any supplements, it's a good idea to consult your health-care practitioner.*

Dietary Supplements in the Marketplace

Although some dietary supplements have druglike actions (e.g., reducing cholesterol levels), government agencies regulate supplements differently from drugs. Manufacturers are allowed to make a wide variety of claims for product effects without having to provide scientific evidence to support those claims. The freedoms of speech and press prevail; in practical terms, almost anything goes. Promotional books, magazine articles, audio- and videotapes, lectures, staged interviews, and messages posted on Internet chat rooms—all are protected by the First Amendment. Their authors have the freedom to inform or to deceive. It's up to the listener or reader to distinguish fact from fiction. (See **Figure 3.11**.)

bioflavonoids Naturally occurring plant chemicals, especially from citrus fruits, that reduce the permeability and fragility of capillaries.

Dietary Supplement Health and Education Act (DSHEA) Legislation that regulates dietary supplements.

The FTC and Supplement Advertising

The Federal Trade Commission (FTC) in the U.S. Department of Commerce is responsible for ensuring that advertisements and commercials are truthful and do not mislead. The agency depends on and encourages self-monitoring by the supplement industry. In pursuing companies that skirt the regulations, the FTC gives priority to cases that seriously put people's health and safety at risk or that affect sick and vulnerable consumers.[38]

The FDA and Supplement Regulation

The Food and Drug Administration has primary responsibility for regulating labeling and content of dietary supplements under the Federal Food, Drug, and Cosmetic Act, as amended by the 1994 **Dietary Supplement Health and Education Act (DSHEA)**.[39] How do you know a product is a "dietary supplement"? Simple. DSHEA defines any product intended to supplement the diet as a dietary supplement and requires that the word *supplement* be clearly stated on the label. Dietary supplements include vitamins, minerals, herbs, and amino acids as well as other substances such as enzymes, organ tissues, metabolites, extracts, or concentrates.

Quick Bites

Pronouncing the Acronym

The Dietary Supplement Health and Education Act of 1994 is better known by its acronym DSHEA, pronounced "da-shay."

Dietary supplements are *not* drugs. A drug is intended to diagnose, cure, mitigate, treat, or prevent disease. Before marketing, drugs must undergo

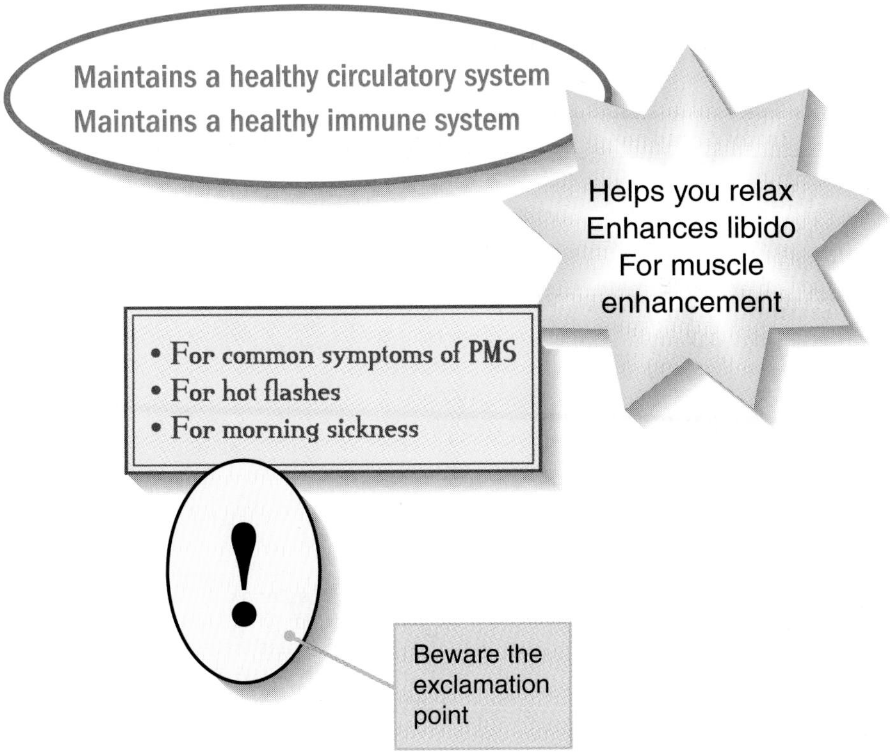
Maintains a healthy circulatory system
Maintains a healthy immune system
Helps you relax
Enhances libido
For muscle enhancement
• For common symptoms of PMS
• For hot flashes
• For morning sickness
!
Beware the exclamation point

Figure 3.11 Dietary supplement label claims. Although claims such as these appear on dietary supplement labels, they do not have to be approved by the FDA. All should be viewed with skepticism.

extensive studies of effectiveness, safety, interactions with other substances, and dosing. The FDA gives formal premarket approval to a drug and monitors its safety after the drug is on the market. None of this is required of dietary supplements. A dietary supplement with a label claiming to cure or treat a specific condition is, in reality, an unauthorized drug.

Dietary supplements are not food additives. For new ingredients in dietary supplements, the manufacturer finds information (usually not scientific proof) to show the supplement is safe if used as directed and submits this information to the FDA 75 days before the supplement is first marketed. However, formal approval by the FDA is not required. New dietary supplements that contain ingredients already in use do not require such advance notification. Unlike pharmaceutical manufacturers, who must prove the safety and efficacy of their products before they sell them, supplement manufacturers can market their products without the FDA's approval. To restrict sale and use of a dietary supplement, the FDA must prove that it isn't safe after it is on the market.

Supplement Labels

Like food labels, supplement labels have mandatory and optional information. Since March 1999 all labels on dietary supplements must include ingredient information and a **Supplement Facts panel**.[40] You'll notice in **Figure 3.12** that the format is similar to the Nutrition Facts on food labels. An important difference is that a Supplement Facts panel includes substances for which no Daily Value has been established. In combination products, the panel separates these substances from established nutrients and displays them at the bottom. Herbal ingredients must list the plant part, such as root or leaf.

Supplement Facts panel Content label that must appear on all dietary supplements.

Serving Size is the manufacturer's suggested serving expressed in the appropriate unit (tablet, capsule, softgel, packet, teaspoonful).

Each Tablet Contains heads the listing of dietary ingredients contained in the supplement.

Each dietary ingredient is followed by the quantity in a serving. For proprietary blends, total weight of the blend is listed, with components listed in descending order by weight.

Dietary ingredients that have no Daily Value are listed below this line.

Botanical supplements must list the part of plant present and its common name (Latin name if common name not listed in *Herbs of Commerce*).

Supplement Facts

Serving Size 1 Tablet

Each Tablet Contains		%DV
Vitamin A	5,000 IU	100%
50% as Beta-Carotene		
Vitamin C	90 mg	150%
Vitamin D	400 IU	100%
Vitamin E	45 IU	150%
Thiamin	1.5 mg	100%
Riboflavin	1.7 mg	100%
Niacin	20 mg	100%
Vitamin B_6	2 mg	100%
Folate	400 mcg	100%
Vitamin B_{12}	6 mcg	100%
Calcium	100 mg	10%
Iron	18 mg	100%
Iodine	150 mcg	100%
Magnesium	100 mg	25%
Zinc	15 mg	100%

Ginseng Root (*Panax ginseng*)	25 mg	*
Ginkgo Biloba Leaf (*Ginkgo biloba*)	25 mg	*
Citrus Bioflavonoids Complex	10 mg	*
Lecithin (*Glycine max*) (bean)	10 mg	*
Nickel	5 mcg	*
Silicon	2 mcg	*
Boron	60 mcg	*

* Daily Value (%DV) not established

%DV indicates the percentage of the Daily Value of each nutrient that a serving provides.

An **asterisk** under %DV indicates that a Daily Value is not established for that ingredient.

List of Ingredients shows the nutrients and other ingredients used to formulate the supplement, in decreasing order by weight.

INGREDIENTS: Dicalcium Phosphate, Magnesium Oxide, Ascorbic Acid, Cellulose, Vitamin A Acetate, Beta-Carotene, Vitamin D, dl-Alpha Tocopherol Acetate, Ginseng Root (*Panax ginseng*), Gelatin, Ginkgo Biloba Leaf (*Ginkgo biloba*), Ferrous Fumarate, Niacinamide, Zinc Oxide, Silicon Dioxide, Lecithin, Citrus Bioflavonoids Complex, Pyridoxine Hydrochloride, Riboflavin, Thiamin Mononitrate, Folic Acid, Potassium Iodine, Boron, Cyanocobalamin, Nickelous Sulfate

Contact Information shows the manufacturer's or distributor's name, address, and zip code.

DISTRIBUTED BY COMPANY NAME
P.O. BOX XXX
CITY, STATE 00000-0000

Figure 3.12 **Supplement Facts panel.** Similar to the Nutrition Facts panel on food labels, the Supplement Facts panel required on dietary supplement labels shows the product composition.

Supplement labels, like food labels, may contain health claims, structure/function claims, and nutrient content claims. However, only a few of the health claims approved for foods are appropriate for dietary supplements. "Adequate calcium may reduce risk of osteoporosis" and "adequate folate intake by women reduces risk of neural tube defects in newborns" are examples of health claims that could appear on supplement labels. The FDA authorizes these claims based on (1) a careful review of the scientific literature (the review is like that done for food labels; see Chapter 2, "Nutrition Guidelines"), (2) an authoritative statement by a scientific body of the U.S. government or the National Academy of Sciences, or (3) a need for qualification to avoid misleading statements. (See **Figure 3.13**.)

"Antioxidants maintain cell integrity," "fiber maintains bowel regularity," and "kava kava promotes relaxation" are examples of structure/function claims that might appear on supplement labels. Structure/function claims also may describe the link between a nutrient and a deficiency disease (like vitamin C and scurvy), as long as the statement also mentions the prevalence of the disease in the United States. Manufacturers can use structure/function claims without FDA authorization and can base their claims on their own review and interpretation of the scientific literature.

Structure/function claims are easy to spot because they are accompanied with the disclaimer "This statement has not been evaluated by the Food and Drug Administration. This product is not intended to diagnose, treat, cure, or prevent any disease." There is often a fine line between structure/function claims and claims that would make the product an unauthorized drug. For example, the claim "promotes urinary tract health" on a bottle of cranberry extract capsules would be allowable, while "prevents urinary tract infections" would not.

Nutrient content claims must be consistent with definitions approved for foods. With few exceptions, nutrient content claims can be made only for a nutrient or dietary substance that has an established Daily Value.

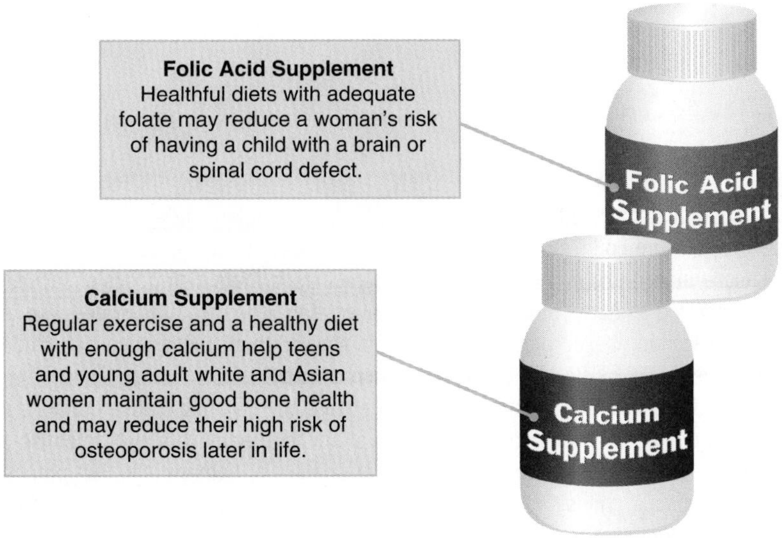
Folic Acid Supplement
Healthful diets with adequate folate may reduce a woman's risk of having a child with a brain or spinal cord defect.
Calcium Supplement
Regular exercise and a healthy diet with enough calcium help teens and young adult white and Asian women maintain good bone health and may reduce their high risk of osteoporosis later in life.
Folic Acid Supplement
Calcium Supplement

Figure 3.13 **Health claims for supplements.** Calcium and folic acid supplements may carry health claims similar to these model statements.
Source: U.S. Food and Drug Administration.

For dietary ingredients without a Daily Value, manufacturers may describe the amount of the ingredient. Examples include simple percentage statements such as "40% *omega*-3 fatty acids, 10 mg per capsule," and comparative percentage claims, such as "twice the *omega*-3 fatty acids per capsule (80 mg) as in 100 mg of menhaden oil (40 mg)."[41]

Canadian Regulations

At present, products considered dietary supplements in the United States are regulated as either foods or drugs under Canada's Food and Drugs Act. However, in December 2001, Health Canada's Natural Health Products Directorate proposed a new category called *natural health products.* Under this proposal, Health Canada would assess each natural health product before authorizing it for sale. The proposal requires manufacturers or distributors of natural health products to supply information about the quantity of medicinal ingredients in the product, the intended use, supporting safety and efficacy data, and evidence of good manufacturing practices. In addition, any adverse reaction must be reported to Health Canada. The Canadian proposals go much farther than DSHEA in terms of assuring safety and efficacy of supplements.

Key Concepts: *Dietary supplements are neither foods nor drugs, and the government regulates their manufacture and sale differently from those of foods, food additives, and drugs. The FTC and FDA monitor advertising and labeling of dietary supplements. A Supplement Facts panel is now required on labels. Canada has proposed regulations for natural health products that will require premarket approval and product licensing.*

Choosing Dietary Supplements

DSHEA has made many improvements, such as the Supplement Facts panel, to help consumers of dietary supplements. By loosening previous

[Fyi] The Saccharin Story

FOR YOUR INFORMATION

The granddaddy of all sugar substitutes is saccharin. Discovered in 1879, it was used during both world wars to sweeten foods, helping to compensate for sugar shortages and rationing. It is 300 times sweeter than sugar.

In 1907 an early attempt to ban saccharin was thwarted when President Theodore Roosevelt proclaimed the top safety official behind the effort to be "an idiot." Safety questions resurfaced in 1911 when a board of federal scientists called the artificial sweetener "an adulterant" that should not be used in foods. This same board later decided to limit saccharin just to products "intended for invalids," a restriction that was lifted after sugar shortages developed during World War I.

In 1958, when Congress passed the Food Additives Amendment to the Food, Drug, and Cosmetic Act, saccharin was one of the ingredients "generally recognized as safe," or GRAS. That same year the saccharin-based product Sweet 'N Low took the public by storm. Food and beverage companies scrambled to offer saccharin-sweetened products, which came to include the diet soda Tab and a plethora of gelatins, candies, and baked goods.

By the early 1970s, studies of rats who had been fed saccharin raised concerns about the sweetener's role in causing bladder cancer, but scientists later suggested that impurities, not saccharin, may have caused the tumors. Then in 1977, a Canadian study looked specifically at the role of saccharin in test animals. Researchers fed rats high doses of saccharin equivalent to 5 percent of their diet. The results again showed that saccharin caused bladder cancer in rats.

Because the Delaney Clause prohibits the use of any food additive shown to cause cancer in animals or humans, the FDA proposed an immediate ban on saccharin. The FDA proposal prompted a public outcry, fueled in part by media reports that the test rats were fed the equivalent of as many as 800 diet sodas a day.[1] Congress responded by passing the Saccharin Study and Labeling Act, which restrictions, DSHEA also has made many more products available to consumers. However, with the resulting array of supplements, it is a challenge for the FDA to effectively monitor claims, quality, and safety. Because manufacturers can market their products without prior approval, you need to be wary. Knowledge of nutrition science is your most valuable tool for evaluating a supplement. Read each label and judge each implied claim in light of what you know. Ask the following questions:

- *Is the quantity enough to have an effect or is it trivial?* Consider amino acids, for example. A product contains 25 milligrams of glycine. How does this compare to the amount of glycine you'd obtain from a diet with 70 grams of protein? Has glycine been added to the product, or is it a component of the gelatin capsule? Is glycine an essential or a nonessential amino acid? What will happen if you take more than you need? Is it a problem if you get less than you need?
- *Is the product new to you?* Learn about it from the many reliable resources listed on the Web site for this book. Evaluate the product in light of scientific research. Has it been studied in humans, rodents, or other animals, or only in cell cultures or *in vitro*? If in humans, was the study controlled to eliminate a placebo effect? For case report studies, could the placebo effect influence the results? Consider also the type of preparation and the route of administration. An injected herbal extract may have a very different effect than the same herb in a pill.
- *Consider the dose used in the study. Is it reasonable and an amount found in over-the-counter products?* For example, serious researchers studied dehydroepiandrosterone (DHEA) and found it may help some immune disorders, but at doses 20 to 50 times greater than the dosage of DHEA sold in healthfood stores.[42] A consumer who chooses to take 20 of these pills daily to match the dosage used in studies

placed a two-year moratorium on any ban of the sweetener while additional safety studies were conducted. Congress has extended the moratorium several times, most recently renewing it until 2002. The law also required that any foods containing saccharin must carry a label that reads "Use of this product may be hazardous to your health. This product contains saccharin, which has been determined to cause cancer in laboratory animals." In 1996 Congress repealed the saccharin notice requirements.

In May 2000, the National Toxicology Program (NTP) removed saccharin from its list of possible human carcinogens. The NTP concluded that the types of tumors caused by saccharin in rats arose from a mechanism that is not relevant to humans. This ruling is in keeping with the opinion of other scientific bodies. The National Cancer Institute (NCI) states in its *Cancer Facts* that "epidemiological studies do not provide clear evidence" of a link between saccharin and human cancer. Regina Ziegler, Ph.D., an NCI epidemiologist, says, "Typical intakes of saccharin at normal levels for adults show no evidence of a public health problem."[2] Other health groups, including the American Medical Association, the American Cancer Society, and the American Dietetic Association, agree that saccharin use is acceptable.

Saccharin remains on the market and continues to have a fairly large appeal as a tabletop sweetener, particularly in restaurants, where it is available in single-serving packets under trade names such as Sweet 'N Low. The familiar warning label on the "pink stuff" may soon be a thing of the past!

1 Henkel J. Sugar substitutes: Americans opt for sweetness and lite. *FDA Consumer,* Nov/Dec 1999.

2 Ibid.

would risk side effects and magnify effects of potential contaminants. Another example is shark cartilage. In the best-controlled study to date of shark cartilage and cancer, the dose was equivalent to about 75 capsules of shark cartilage daily; even at that high dose, patients with advanced cancer were not helped.[43]

- *Can the supplement cross the intestine and travel to its presumed site of action in the body?* The body digests enzyme preparations, for example, along with other proteins. There are little data on the absorption and **bioavailability** of herbal preparations and other types of nonnutrient supplements. Does the product promise too much? A product touted to control hypercholesterolemia, hangnails, psoriasis, and insomnia is unlikely to do much of anything. Neither will a "low-calorie, high-energy" drink. It's possible that the same results can be achieved more cheaply and more enjoyably by eating regular foods. Why take lycopene capsules when you can eat tomatoes, even ketchup? Why take bilberry extract when blueberries (the American equivalent to European bilberries) are delicious and low in calories?
- *Who is selling the product?* Alternative practitioners, dietitians, and even physicians sometimes sell the supplements they recommend[44]—which is a possible conflict of interest that could compromise their objectivity. In **multilevel marketing**, someone at each level in the system takes a commission on the supplements you buy, so expect to pay extra. When you buy a supplement over the phone, by catalogue, or over the Web, you lose the chance to examine it before you buy it.

bioavailability A measure of the extent to which a nutrient becomes available to the body after ingestion and thus is available to the tissues.

multilevel marketing A system of selling in which each salesperson recruits assistants who then recruit others to help them. The person at each level collects a commission on sales made by the later recruits.

U.S. Pharmacopoeia (USP) Established in 1820, the USP is a voluntary, not-for-profit health-care organization that sets quality standards for a range of health-care products.

A good indicator of quality is the **U.S. Pharmacopoeia (USP)** certification mark, which certifies that the product meets the U.S. Pharmacopoeia's standards for quality, strength, purity, packaging, and labeling.[45] In addition, the USP mark certifies that the product contains the dietary supplement ingredient in the designated amount and is manufactured appropriately. Established in 1820, the USP is a voluntary, not-for-profit organization that sets quality standards for a range of health-care products, including prescription and nonprescription medicines, biotechnology drugs, home test kits, medical devices, vitamins and minerals, and dietary supplements. Nationally known food and drug manufacturers have established standards, quality control, and manufacturing practices that they are likely to apply to their dietary supplements as well.

Contact the company with your questions; you'll learn a lot, although maybe not what you expected. The "technical representative" may be unable to give you any more information than a brief readout from a computer database. Some companies respond to queries by sending a long printout of journal citations, most of them inappropriate, without text or even abstracts; many references are in a foreign language. On the other hand, some dietary supplement companies have on-site quality control and on-site nutritionists who are knowledgeable and happy to supply helpful information.

Even the best-intentioned, most carefully considered supplement can prove ineffective or even risky. Take the example of beta-carotene supplements. Even though diets rich in beta-carotene reduce cancer risk, several large well-controlled studies found that beta-carotene supplements had no protective effect. For some groups of people, such as smokers, these supplements actually increased risk.[46] The results disappointed advocates of beta-carotene, but these studies demonstrate the value of carefully controlled studies and the risk of unproved assumptions about dietary supplements.

Fraudulent Products

Some health advocates consider the burgeoning market of dietary supplements an unwelcome return to the "snake oil" era of the late nineteenth and early twentieth centuries, when "magic" potions and cures were sold door to door and at county fairs and markets. Most manufacturers work hard to ensure the quality of their products, yet some supplements on the market are nothing more than a mixture of ineffective ingredients.

In a recent issue of *FDA Consumer*, the agency had this to say about fraudulent products:

> You often can identify fraudulent products by the types of claims made in their labeling, advertising, and promotional literature. Stephen Barrett, M.D., a board member of the National Council Against Health Fraud, points to the following indicators of possible fraud:
>
> - Claims that the product is a secret cure and use of such terms as *breakthrough, magical, miracle cure,* and *new discovery*. "If the product were a cure for a serious disease, it would be widely reported in the media and used by health-care professionals," he says.
> - "Pseudomedical" jargon, such as *detoxify, purify,* and *energize* to describe a product's effects. "These claims are vague and hard to measure," Barrett says. "So, they make it easier for success to be claimed, even though nothing has actually been accomplished," he says.
> - Claims that the product can cure a wide range of unrelated diseases. "No product can do that," he says.
> - Claims that the supplement has only benefits—and no side effects. "A product potent enough to help people will be potent enough to cause side effects," Barrett says.
> - Claims that a product is backed by scientific studies, but with no list of references or references that are inadequate. For instance, if a list of references is provided, the citations cannot be traced, or if they are traceable, the studies are out-of-date, irrelevant, or poorly designed.
> - Accusations that the medical profession, drug companies, and the government are suppressing information about a particular treatment. "It would be illogical," Barrett says, "for large numbers of people to withhold information about potential medical therapies when they or their families and friends might one day benefit from them."[47]

Supplement users who suffer a serious harmful effect or illness that they think is related to supplement use should call a doctor or other health-care provider. Practitioners can report to FDA MedWatch by calling 1-800-FDA-1088 or by going to www.fda.gov/medwatch/report/hcp.htm on the MedWatch Web site. Consumers can call the toll-free MedWatch number or go to www.fda.gov/medwatch/report/consumer/consumer.htm on the MedWatch Web site to report an adverse reaction.

Quick Bites

Jell-O and Your Nails

You may have heard that taking gelatin can make your nails stronger. Not true. Fingernails get their strength from sulfur in amino acids. Gelatin has no sulfur-containing amino acids.

Quick Bites

Mayonnaise Protects against Strokes

Is this claim science or snake oil? Studies show that foods rich in vitamin E help protect against heart disease and stroke. In one study of stroke reduction in postmenopausal women, mayonnaise was the most concentrated food source of vitamin E. But to claim that mayonnaise prevents strokes is unwarranted and overstates the evidence.

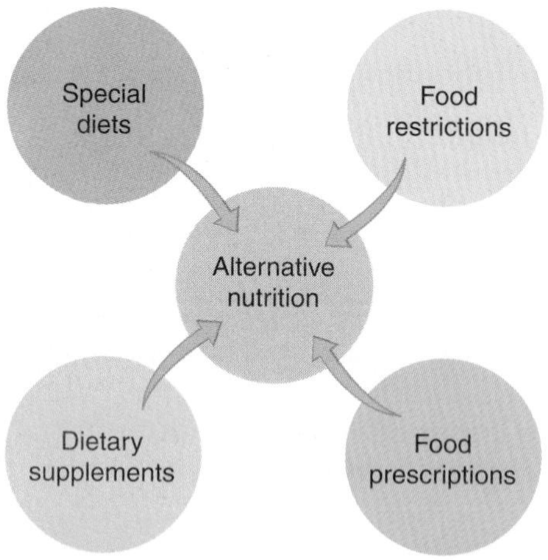

Figure 3.14 **Alternative nutrition practices.** While many mainstream medical practices may involve special dietary regimens, alternative nutrition practices often are overly restrictive, depart from established dietary guidelines, and lack rigorous scientific evidence.

Key Concepts: *When considering a dietary supplement, it is important to consider the product and its claims carefully. Be aware that some products may promise more than they can deliver. A good indicator of quality is the USP notation, but even this does not guarantee that a product will fulfill its claims.*

Complementary and Alternative Medicine

Complementary and alternative medicines (CAM) are therapies and treatments outside the medical mainstream. They tend to be based mainly or solely on observation or anecdotal evidence rather than controlled research. One widely used definition is "treatments or health-care practices neither taught widely in U.S. medical schools nor generally available in U.S. hospitals."[48] This definition, however, may need updating; many medical schools and conventional health-care providers have begun to teach or use these therapies, sometimes with insurance reimbursement.[49]

The term *alternative* suggests practices that replace conventional ones. *Complementary* implies practices that are used *in addition to* conventional ones. For example, using only herbs and megavitamins to treat AIDS would be "alternative," whereas using herbs to combat diarrhea caused by conventional AIDS medications and taking supplements to replace lost vitamins would be "complementary." Many people find the terms *complementary* or *integrative* more acceptable than *alternative,* although all these terms often are used interchangeably. CAM includes a broad range of healing therapies and philosophies. Several among them involve nutrition, including special diet therapies, phytotherapy (herbalism), orthomolecular medicine, and other biologic interventions.

In 1990 about 34 percent of the adult U.S. population used CAM;[50] by 1997 that number had grown to 42 percent.[51] The increases were significant for relaxation techniques, herbal medicine, massage, spiritual healing, megavitamins, self-help groups, folk remedies, energy healing, homeopathy, and acupuncture. The most popular therapies in 1997 were relaxation techniques, herbal medicine, massage, and chiropractic. People seek out CAM for numerous reasons, including fear of aging, personal beliefs, and distrust of institutional medicine.

Where Does Nutrition Fit In?

A number of alternative therapies involve nutrition, and sometimes the line between standard and alternative nutrition is not clear. A variety of health conditions, such as diabetes, gastrointestinal disorders, and kidney disease, require special diets. Alternative nutrition practices include diets to prevent and treat diseases not shown to be diet-related. (See **Figure 3.14**.) What often makes these practices "alternative" is the limited nature of the diet, the lack of rigorous scientific evidence showing effectiveness, and the divergence from established healthy eating patterns such as the Food Guide Pyramid. Other practices outside the nutritional mainstream include reliance on organically grown foods alone and the extensive use of herbal and botanical supplements as well as megadoses of vitamin/mineral supplements that we have already discussed.

Special Diets, Food Restrictions, and Food Prescriptions

Vegetarian Diets

The specifics of vegetarianism are described in Chapter 7, "Proteins and Amino Acids." Most nutritionists consider vegetarianism a routine variation

Quick Bites

The Yin and Yang of Food

The early theory of yin and yang had its genesis during the Yin and Zhou dynasties (1766 B.C.E.–256 B.C.E.). The yin force is passive, downward flowing, and cold. Conversely, the yang force is aggressive, upward rising, and hot. The concept of balance and harmony between these life forces is the basis upon which food and herbs are used as medicine. In traditional Chinese healing methods, disease is viewed as the result of an imbalance of these energies in the body. To balance these energies, according to this view, your diet should balance yin foods and yang foods. Yin (cold) foods include milk, honey, fruit, and vegetables; and yang (hot) foods include beef, poultry, seafood, eggs, and cheese. Foods are also classified as sweet (earth), bitter (fire), sour (wood), pungent (metal), and salty (water). Each class supposedly has specific effects on different parts of the body.

macrobiotic diet A highly restrictive dietary approach applied as a therapy for risk factors or chronic disease in general.

of a normal diet, particularly if the vegetarian's motivation is religious or philosophical, the result of a concern for animals, or an aversion to animal products. When a meat eater goes vegetarian to prevent or cure disease, that's "alternative."

Macrobiotic Diet

Aside from vegetarianism, the **macrobiotic diet** probably is the best-known alternative diet. The original version of this primarily vegetarian diet progressed in 10 increasingly restrictive stages, with the "highest level" consisting of little more than brown rice and water. The diet has since evolved to a simpler one-level regimen based on whole-grain cereals and vegetables, a small amount of fish, no other animal products, and no fruit.[52]

Proponents tout the macrobiotic diet as a cure for a variety of illnesses, most notably cancer. To use it as a cancer treatment, the practitioner individualizes the diet according to Eastern philosophy (yin and yang, whose symbol is shown in **Figure 3.15**) and location of the cancer. Critics say macrobiotic restrictions interfere with legitimate cancer treatment by causing weight loss in people who are already too thin from their illness. The diet is so limited that it just can't meet the increased nutritional needs of the cancer patient. Advocates of macrobiotics, on the other hand, argue that undernutrition may help fight the cancer by starving it.[53] It looks as if neither opinion is correct: Macrobiotic diets appear to have no clear effect, good or bad, on cancer progression or survival.

Compared with the general public, those who follow a macrobiotic diet tend to have healthier blood lipid levels and higher blood levels of phytochemicals, which reflects vegetable intake.[54] However, the diet is low in calcium and vitamin D, which contributes to the risk for osteoporosis. Pediatricians caution against this diet for children.

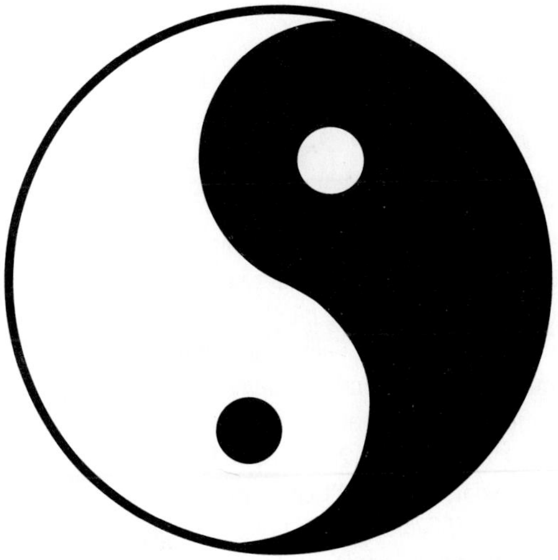

Figure 3.15 **The symbol of yin and yang.** In traditional Chinese medicine, practitioners strive to balance opposing life forces of yin and yang through the use of food and herbs.

Food Restrictions and Food Prescriptions

Societies throughout the world commonly use dietary changes to treat or prevent illness. The specifics vary from place to place, however, which suggests that they are based on cultural factors rather than science.

In recent years we have seen yeast-free diets, dairy-free diets, sugar-free diets, white-flour-free diets, both low-carbohydrate and high-carbohydrate diets, both low-red-meat and high-red-meat diets, caffeine-free diets, salicylate-free diets, and more. We have been advised to load up on molasses, yogurt, honey, vinegar, oysters, mushrooms, and soy nuts. People with subjective symptoms like headaches, fatigue, or back pain have been instructed to avoid irrational lists of "allergenic foods" based on "blood screening." We've also seen illogical instructions on how to combine foods, such as "don't eat applesauce and asparagus at the same meal." For weight loss, we've had grapefruit diets, hard-boiled-egg diets, cottage-cheese diets, water diets, high-fat diets, low-fat diets, and blue-foods-only diets; the list goes on and on.

Such diets come and go. They are not based on science and eventually fall out of style when they don't work. Those few that prove effective and have a scientific basis become integrated into conventional nutrition and diet therapy. (See **Figure 3.16**.)

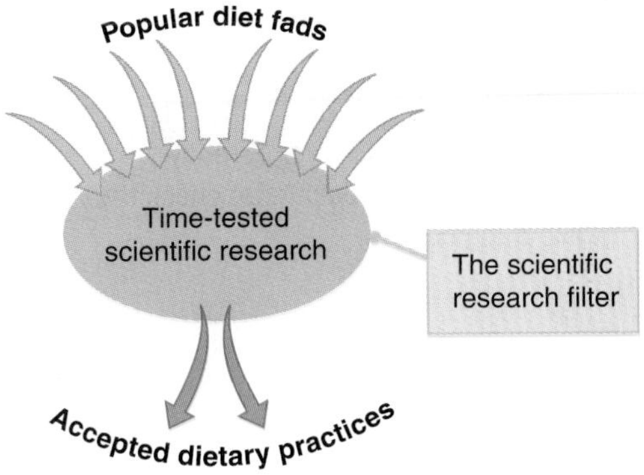

Figure 3.16 **Many apply but few are chosen.** Dietary practices with a scientific basis and proven efficacy are incorporated into conventional nutrition and diet therapy.

Key Concepts: *Many types of diet can be described as alternative. Their origins and claims vary, and their proponents often cannot show that they improve health. Some alternative diets can actually be harmful by restricting foods and thereby lowering the body's intake of necessary nutrients.*

Label [to] Table

If you picked up a multivitamin/mineral container from your drugstore shelf, would you know how to read the label? Look at the following Supplement Facts panel from a basic multivitamin/mineral supplement. Here are some questions that you might have.

1. If you were a 20-year-old woman who knew she wasn't consuming enough calcium, would this supplement allow you to get your recommended intake?
2. If 25 percent of the vitamin A in this supplement comes from beta-carotene, where does the rest come from?
3. What trend do you see in the amounts of B vitamins?
4. What trend do you see in the amounts of bone minerals?
5. What trend do you see in the amounts of antioxidant vitamins?
6. Does the USP statement make this supplement "legitimate"?

Supplement Facts

Daily Multivitamin/Mineral Dietary Supplement

USP Made to U.S. Pharmacopoeia (USP) quality, purity, and potency standards. Laboratory tested to dissolve within 60 minutes.

Serving Size 1 tablet

Each Tablet Contains	% DV	Each Tablet Contains	% DV
Vitamin A 10,000 I.U. 25% as beta-carotene	200%	Iodine 150 mcg	100%
Vitamin C 120 mg	200%	Magnesium 100 mg	25%
Vitamin D 400 IU	100%	Zinc 22.5 mg	150%
Vitamin E 60 IU	200%	Selenium 45 mcg	64%
Vitamin K 25 mcg	31%	Copper 3 mg	150%
Thiamin (vit. B_1) 1.5 mg	100%	Manganese 2.5 mg	125%
Riboflavin (vit. B_2) 1.7 mg	100%	Chromium 100 mcg	83%
Niacin 20 mg	100%	Molybdenum 25 mcg	33%
Vitamin B_6 2 mg	100%	Chloride 36.3 mg	1%
Folate (folic acid) 400 mcg	100%	Sodium less than 5 mg	less than 1%
Vitamin B_{12} 6 mcg	100%	Potassium 40 mg	1%
Biotin 30 mcg	10%	Nickel 5 mcg	*
Pantothenic acid 10 mg	100%	Tin 10 mcg	*
Calcium 162 mg	16%	Silicon 2 mg	*
Iron 9 mg	50%	Vanadium 10 mcg	*
Phosphorus 109 mg	11%	Boron 150 mcg	*

* Daily Value (%DV) not established

Answers to Questions

1. No. This supplement provides only 162 milligrams, and the Adequate Intake (AI) for a 20-year-old woman is 1,000 milligrams. You may need a calcium supplement if you can't eat enough calcium-rich foods.
2. The other 7,500 IU of vitamin A is most likely retinol in the form of retinyl acetate or retinyl palmitate; check the list of ingredients.
3. With the exception of biotin, this supplement provides 100% Daily Value of the B vitamins. And the 30 micrograms of biotin provides 100 percent of the current AI.
4. This supplement contains very low percentages of the Daily Values for calcium, magnesium, and phosphorus (16%, 11%, and 25%, respectively). Adding more of these minerals would make the pill huge and impossible to swallow! A nutritious diet should provide the rest of these minerals.
5. This supplement contains 200 percent of the Daily Value for each of the antioxidant vitamins C and E, and one-fourth (50% DV) of its vitamin A content comes from the antioxidant beta-carotene.
6. By listing the U.S. Pharmacopoeia "stamp of approval," you can be confident that this supplement underwent a test to see how quickly it dissolves. If pills do not dissolve, their contents cannot be absorbed. In this case, the supplement took 60 minutes to dissolve. The USP sets standards for the quality, purity, and potency of supplements.

LEARNING *Portfolio* chapter 3

Key Terms

	page
additives	65
bioavailability	84
bioflavonoids	78
color additive	66
complementary and alternative medicine (CAM)	60
Delaney Clause	67
Dietary Supplement Health and Education Act (DSHEA)	78
dietary supplements	60
direct additives	65
free radicals	61
functional food	60
Generally Recognized as Safe (GRAS)	66
herbal therapy	75
indirect additives	65
isoflavones	60
lycopene	60
macrobiotic diet	86
malabsorption syndromes	71
megadoses	69
multilevel marketing	84
National Center for Complementary and Alternative Medicine (NCCAM)	75
nucleic acids	71
orthomolecular medicine	73
phytotherapy	75
prior-sanctioned substance	67
Supplement Facts panel	79
U.S. Pharmacopoeia (USP)	84

Study Points

- **A functional food is considered to be a food that may provide a health benefit beyond basic nutrition.**
- **Phytochemicals are plant chemicals responsible for the health-promoting properties of functional foods.**
- **Consumption of plant foods containing multiple antioxidants is strongly associated with health benefits. Scientific evidence strongly supports eating five servings of fruits and vegetables daily and emphasizing whole grains.**
- **The federal government reviews the safety of new food additives before they can be used in foods sold on the market.**
- **The Delaney Clause is a controversial food law that prohibits the approval of a food additive if it has been found to cause cancer in humans or laboratory animals, even if massive doses are required to produce the disease.**
- **Dietary supplements encompass vitamins, minerals, herbal products, amino acids, glandular extracts, enzymes, and many other products.**
- **Vitamin and mineral supplements may be warranted in certain circumstances, although the preferred mode of obtaining adequate nutrition is through foods.**
- **Megadose vitamin or mineral therapy has not been proved effective in the treatment of cancer, colds, or heart disease. Moreover, such megadoses act more like drugs than nutrients in the body and should be approached with caution.**
- **Herbal medicine is a traditional form of healing in many cultures. Some herbal medicines have shown enough promise to warrant large-scale clinical studies involving supplements. However, herbal products can have side effects and can interfere with prescription medications.**
- **Dietary supplements are regulated according to the provisions of the Dietary Supplement Health and Education Act of 1994. Unlike drugs and food additives, dietary supplements do not need premarket approval.**
- **Claims for dietary supplements can include health claims, structure/function claims, and nutrient content claims.**
- **Dietary supplements must have a Supplement Facts panel on the label.**
- **Consumers should carefully evaluate claims and evidence for dietary supplements and consult their physician before taking a supplement.**
- **Complementary and alternative medicine (CAM) comprises practices outside the medical mainstream that are becoming increasingly popular. CAM includes a broad range of therapies, many of which include nutrition. People seek them for a variety of reasons, including environmental concerns and a fear of aging.**

Study Questions

Answers can be found at nutrition.jbpub.com/discovering.

1. **What are phytochemicals, and how do they benefit plants and humans?**
2. **Name three chronic diseases that consuming functional foods may help prevent.**
3. **What purpose(s) do food additives serve?**
4. **What is the purpose of the Delaney Clause? What are the complications surrounding this food law?**
5. **What is a macrobiotic diet?**
6. **How do you know a product is a dietary supplement?**
7. **What things should someone do before purchasing supplements?**
8. **If a dietary supplement product label contains the words "High in vitamin E," what type of claim is it making? What other claims can a supplement make?**
9. **What are some of the possible complications involved in using herbal medicines?**

Try This

Finding Functional Beverages

This exercise will familiarize you with the many beverages that contain functional ingredients now available to consumers. Take a trip to your grocery store and spend some time in the beverage aisles. You may want to check out the chilled juice section in addition to the bottled teas and juice beverages. Pick out about 10 different products that have either a nutrient or herbal compound added and try to identify how many have nutrient content claims, health claims, and structure/function claims. Note the prices of these products. How does their nutritional content compare to a 100% fruit juice like orange juice? How does it compare to soda?

Take a Walk on the "Web Side"

This exercise will familiarize you with various Web sites that promote and sell supplements. Log on to the Internet and start doing searches with key words affiliated with supplements. Try *vitamins*, *minerals*, *supplements*, *herbs*, and even some specific terms like *chromium picolinate* and *ginseng*. On the Web sites you visit, how is the nutrition information presented? Do the supplement's benefits sound too good to be true? See if you can spot a fraud. Use the information in the "Fraudulent Products" section of this chapter to identify the accuracy of the product information you find.

References

1 Backgrounder: functional foods. In: *Food Insight Media Guide.* Washington, DC: International Food Information Council Foundation; 1998.

2 Stanton C, Gardiner G, Meehan H, et al. Market potential for probiotics. *Am J Clin Nutr.* 2001;73(suppl 2):476S–483S.

3 Rao AV, Agarwal S. Role of antioxidant lycopene in cancer and heart disease. *J Am Coll Nutr.* 2000;19:563–569.

4 Goldwyn S, Lazinsky A, Wei H. Promotion of health by soy isoflavones: efficacy, benefit and safety concerns. *Drug Metabol Drug Interact.* 2000;17:261–289.

5 Shu XO, Jin F, Dai Q, et al. Soyfood intake during adolescence and subsequent risk of breast cancer among Chinese women. *Cancer Epidemiol Biomarkers Prev.* 2001;10:483–488.

6 Percival SS, Turner RE. Applications of herbs to functional foods. In: Wildman REC, ed. *Handbook of Nutraceuticals and Functional Foods.* Boca Raton, FL: CRC Press; 2001.

7 US Food and Drug Administration. Letter to manufacturers regarding botanicals and other novel ingredients in conventional foods. January 30, 2001. http://www.cfsan.fda.gov/~dms/ds-ltr15.html. Accessed 3/21/02.

8 Food and Drug Administration. Concerns about botanical and other novel ingredients in conventional foods. June 4–5, 2001. http://www.cfsan.fda.gov/~dms/ds-bot5.html. Accessed 3/21/02.

9 Ibid.

10 Blendon RJ, DesRoches CM, Benson JM, et al. Americans' views on the use and regulation of dietary supplements. *Arch Intern Med.* 2001;161(6):805–810.

11 *Physicians' Desk Reference.* 56th ed. Montvale, NJ: Medical Economics Company; 2002.

12 Lederle FA. Oral cyanocobalamin for pernicious anemia: medicine's best kept secret? *JAMA.* 1991;265:94–95.

13 *Physicians' Desk Reference.* 53rd ed. Op. cit.

14 Jacques PF, Taylor A, Hankinson SE, et al. Long-term vitamin C supplement use and prevalence of early age-related lens opacities. *Am J Clin Nutr.* 1997;66:911–916.

15 *Alternative Medicine, Expanding Medical Horizons.* A report to the National Institutes of Health on alternative medical systems and practices in the United States. NIH publication 94-066; December 1994:230–232, 237.

16 Hemila H. Vitamin C intake and susceptibility to the common cold. *Br J Nutr.* 1997;77:59–72.

17 Chalmers TC. Effects of ascorbic acid on the common cold: an evaluation of the evidence. *Am J Med.* 1975;58:532–536.

18 Byers T, Guerrero N. Epidemiologic evidence for vitamin C and vitamin E in cancer prevention. *Am J Clin Nutr.* 1995;62(suppl):1385S–1392S.

19 Leo MA, Lieber CS. Alcohol, vitamin A, and beta-carotene: adverse interactions, including hepatotoxicity and carcinogenicity. *Am J Clin Nutr.* 1999;69:1071–1085.

20 Eisenberg DM, Davis RB, Ettner SL, et al. Trends in alternative medicine use in the United States, 1990–1997: results of a follow-up national survey. *JAMA.* 1998;280:1569–1575.

21 Mahady GB. Global harmonization of herbal health claims. *J Nutr.* 2001;131(suppl 3):1120S–1123S; and Eisenberg DM, Op. cit.

22 Natural Health Products. Health Canada. http://www.hc-sc.gc.ca/english/protection/natural.html. Accessed 2/06/02.

23 Elvin-Lewis M. Should we be concerned about herbal remedies? *J Ethnopharmacol.* 2001;75:141–164.

24 St. John's wort study launched. NIH news release; October 1, 1997.

25 Flora K, Hahn M, Rosen H, Benner K. Milk thistle (*silybum marianum*) for the therapy of liver disease. *Am J Gastroenterol.* 1998;93:139–143.

26 Le Bars PL, Katz MM, Berman N, et al. A placebo-controlled, double-blind, randomized trial of an extract of ginkgo biloba for dementia. North American EGb Study Group. *JAMA.* 1997;278:1327–1332.

27 Wilt TJ, Areef I, Stark G, et al. Saw palmetto extracts for treatment of benign prostatic hyperplasia. *JAMA.*1998;280:1604–1609.

28 Lowe FC, Fagelman E. Cranberry juice and urinary tract infections: what is the evidence? *Urology.* 2001;57:407–413.

29 FDA Public Health Advisory. Risk of drug interactions with St. John's wort, indinavir and other drugs. February 10, 2000. http://www.fda.gov/cder/drug/advisory/stjwort.htm. Accessed 3/21/02.

30 Rosenblatt M, Mindel J. Spontaneous hyphema associated with ingestion of ginkgo biloba extract. *N Engl J Med.* 1997;336:15, 1108.

31 Edwards C. Lessons from licorice. *N Engl J Med.* 1991;325: 1242–1243.

32 Gallagher RE. Arsenic: new life for an old potion. *N Engl J Med.* 1998:339:1389–1390; and Lead poisoning associated with use of traditional ethnic remedies—California, 1991–1992. *MMWR.* 1993;42:521–523.

33 Gordon DW, Rosenthal G, Hart J, et al. Chaparral ingestion: the broadening spectrum of liver injury caused by herbal medications. *JAMA.* 1995;273:489–490.

34 DiPaola RS, Zhang H, Lambert GH, et al. Clinical and biologic activity of an estrogenic herbal combination (PC-SPES) in prostate cancer. *N Engl J Med.* 1998;339:785–791.

35 Anticholinergic poisoning associated with herbal tea—New York City, 1994. *MMWR.*1995;44:193–195; and Plantain adulteration with foxglove. FDA press release; June 12, 1997.

36 Good Housekeeping Consumer Safety Symposium on Dietary Supplements and Herbal Remedies. March 3, 1998; New York, NY.

37 Harkey MR, Henderson GL, Gershwin ME, et al. Variability in commercial ginseng products: an analysis of 25 preparations. *Am J Clin Nutr.* 2001;73(6):1101–1106.

38 Business guide for dietary supplement industry. Washington, DC: Federal Trade Commission press release; November 18, 1998.

39 Dietary Supplement Health and Education Act of 1994. US Food and Drug Administration, Center for Food Safety and Applied Nutrition. December 1, 1995.

40 Kurtzweil P. An FDA guide to dietary supplements. *FDA Consumer.* Sept–Oct 1998, revised January 1999. http://vm.cfsan.fda.gov/~dms/fdsupp.html. Accessed 3/21/02.

41 US Food and Drug Administration. Claims that can be made for conventional foods and dietary supplements. March 20, 2001. http://www.cfsan.fda.gov/~dms/hclaims.html. Accessed 3/21/02.

42 Salvato P, Thompson C, Keister R. Viral load response to augmentation of natural dehydroepiandrosterone (DHEA). Presented at: International Conference on AIDS; July 7–12, 1996; Vancouver, BC, Canada.

43 Miller DR, Anderson GT, Stark JJ, et al. Phase I/II trial of the safety and efficacy of shark cartilage in the treatment of advanced cancers. *J Clin Oncol.* 1998;16:3649–3655.

44 Washburn L. Are doctors' side deals prescription for trouble? *Hackensack (NJ) Sunday Record.* August 22, 1999: A1.

45 USP Dietary Supplementation Verification Program. http://www.usp.org.. Accessed 2/06/02.

46 The Alpha-Tocopherol, Beta-Carotene and Cancer Prevention Study Group. The effect of vitamin E and beta-carotene on the incidence of lung cancer and other cancers in male smokers. *N Engl J Med.* 1994;330:1029–1035.

47 Kurtzweil P. Op. cit.

48 Eisenberg DM, Kessler RC, Foster C, et al. Unconventional medicine in the United States: prevalence, costs, and patterns of use. *N Engl J Med.* 1993;328:246–252.

49 Pelletier KR, Marie A, Krasner M, Haskell WL. Current trends in the integration and reimbursement of complementary and alternative medicine by managed care, insurance carriers, and hospital providers. *Am J Health Promotion.* 1997;12:112–123.

50 Eisenberg DM, Kessler RC, Foster C, et al. Op. cit.

51 Eisenberg DM, Davis RB, Ettner SL, et al. Op. cit.

52 *Alternative Medicine, Expanding Medical Horizons.* Op. cit.

53 Ibid.

54 Ibid.

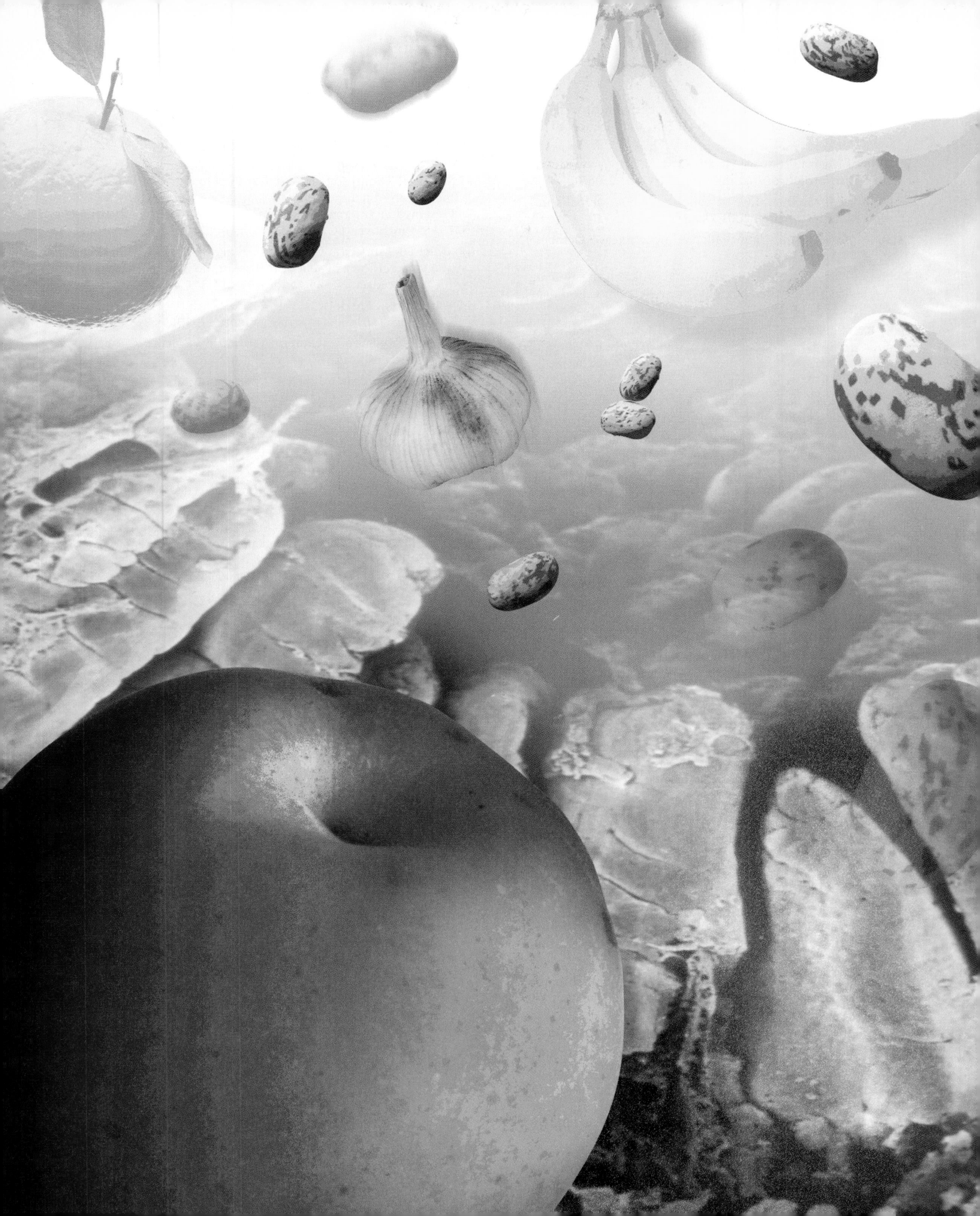

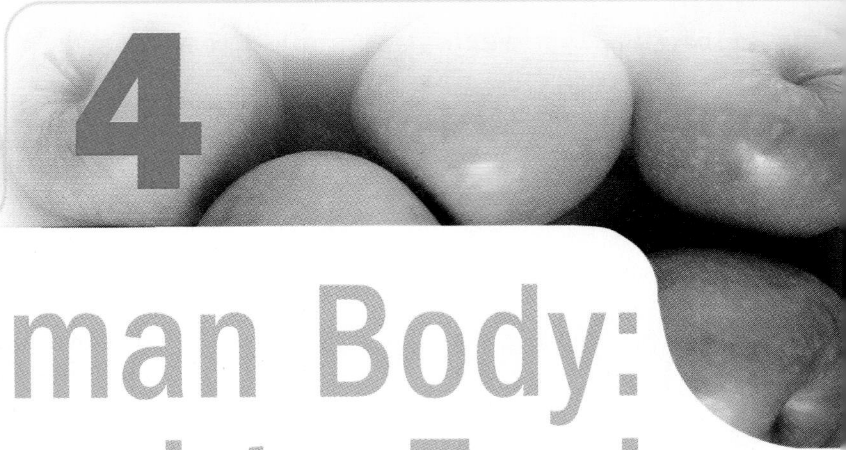

Chapter 4

The Human Body: From Food to Fuel

Think About It

1. Your friend warns you that eating some foods together is not healthful. Is this likely to change your eating behavior?
2. How good are you at identifying tastes?
3. Have you ever noticed that food sometimes tastes sweeter after you've chewed it for awhile?
4. You feel particularly happy, and you find a meal prepared by your friend tastes especially good. Any connection?

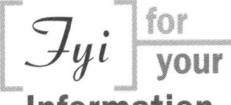

Fyi for your Information

This chapter's FYI boxes include practical information on the following topics:

- Lactose Intolerance
- Bugs in Your Gut? Health Effects of Intestinal Bacteria

www

The Web site for this book offers many useful tools and is a great source for additional nutrition information for both students and instructors. For information on digestion and absorption, visit the site at **nutrition.jbpub.com/discovering**. You'll find exercises that explore the following topics:

- Gastrointestinal Disorders
- Have You Heard about GERD?
- Gallbladder Health
- Lactose Intolerance

What About Bobbie?

Track the choices Bobbie is making with the EatRight Analysis software.

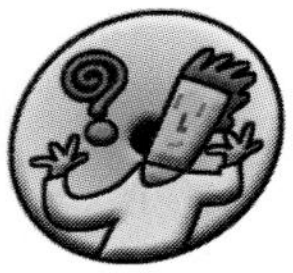

Key to Illustrations

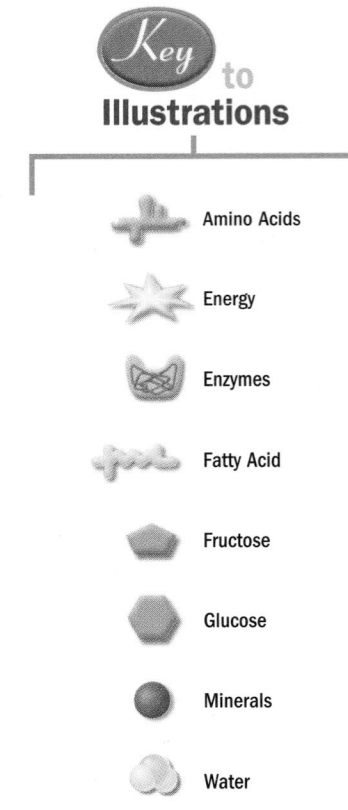

- Amino Acids
- Energy
- Enzymes
- Fatty Acid
- Fructose
- Glucose
- Minerals
- Water

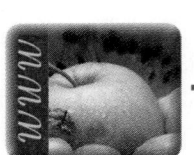

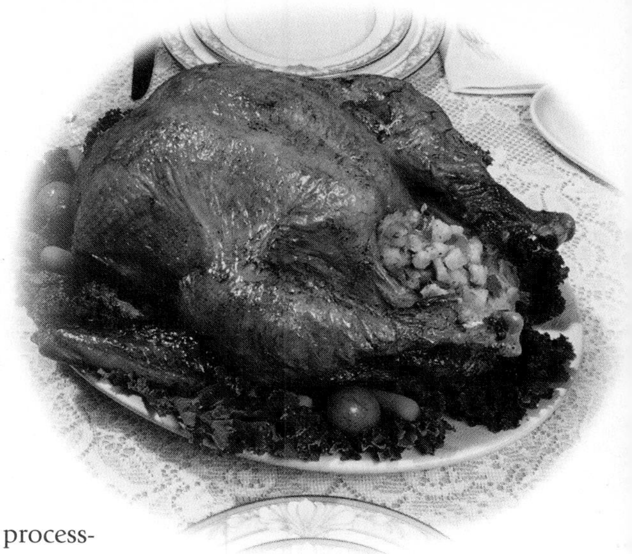

The aroma from a roast turkey floats past your nose. You haven't eaten for six or seven hours. Your mouth waters, anticipating a delicious experience. Your digestive juices are turned on! Is this virtual reality? Not at all! Before you eat a morsel of food, fleeting thoughts from your brain signal your body to prepare for the coming feast.

Your body's mechanisms for processing food and turning it into nutrients are both efficient and elegant. The action unfolds in the digestive tract in two stages: **digestion**—the breaking apart of foods into smaller and smaller units—and **absorption**—the movement of those small units from the gut into the bloodstream or lymphatic system for circulation. Remarkably, your digestive system is designed to digest carbohydrates, proteins, and fats simultaneously, all the while preparing other substances—vitamins, minerals, and cholesterol, for example—for absorption. And the best part is that it doesn't need any help! You may see promotions for enzyme supplements or read diet books that recommend consuming food or nutrient groups separately. There is no scientific basis for most of these claims. Unless you have a specific medical condition, your digestive system is ready, willing, and able to digest and absorb the foods you eat, in whatever combination you eat them. Think About It 1

digestion The process of transforming the foods we eat into units for absorption.

absorption The movement of substances into or across tissues; in particular, the passage of nutrients and other substances into the walls of the gastrointestinal tract and then into the bloodstream.

But go back to the aroma of that roast turkey for a moment. Before digestion and absorption begin, our senses of taste and smell attract us to the foods we are likely to consume.

Taste and Smell: The Beginnings of Our Food Experience

You probably wouldn't eat a food if it didn't appeal in some way to your senses. Odors around us, such as the fragrance of a gardenia or the smell of bread baking, stimulate nerve cells high inside the nose. In the mouth, tastes, as well as texture and temperature, combine with odors to produce a perception of flavor. It is flavor that lets us know whether we are eating a pear or an apple. You recognize flavors mainly through the sense of smell. If you hold your nose while eating chocolate, for example, you will have trouble identifying it—even though you can distinguish the food's sweetness or bitterness. That's because the familiar flavor of chocolate is sensed largely by odor, as is the well-known flavor of coffee. Think About It 2

The sight, smell, thought, taste, and, in some cases, even the sound of food can trigger a set of responses that prepare the digestive tract to receive food.[1] Your mouth begins to water and stomach secretions flow. (See **Figure 4.1**.) If no food is consumed, the response diminishes, but eating prolongs the stimulation of the salivary and gastric cells.

The Gastrointestinal Tract

If, instead of teasing the body with mere sights and smells, we actually sit down to a meal and experience the full flavor and texture of foods, the real

work of the digestive tract begins. In order for the food we eat to nourish our bodies, we need to digest it (break it down into smaller units); absorb it, or move it from the gut into circulation; and finally transport it to the tissues and cells of the body. The digestive process starts in the mouth and continues as food journeys down the gastrointestinal, or GI, tract. At various points along the GI tract, nutrients are absorbed, meaning they move from the GI tract into circulatory systems so they can be transported throughout the body. If there are problems along the way, with either incomplete digestion or inadequate absorption, the cells will not receive the nutrients they need to grow, perform daily activities, fight infection, and maintain health. A closer look at the gastrointestinal tract will help you see just how amazing this organ system is.

gastrointestinal (GI) tract [GAS-troh-in-TES-tin-al] The connected series of organs and structures used for digestion of food and absorption of nutrients; also called the alimentary canal or the digestive tract.

Organization of the GI Tract

The **gastrointestinal (GI) tract**, also known as the alimentary canal, is a long, hollow tube that begins at the mouth and ends at the anus. The specific parts include the mouth, esophagus, stomach, small intestine, large intestine, and rectum. The GI tract works with assisting organs—the salivary glands, liver, gallbladder, and pancreas—to turn food into small molecules that the body can absorb and use. (See **Figure 4.2**.) The GI tract has an amazing variety of functions, including

1. ingestion—the receipt and softening of food
2. transport of ingested food

Figure 4.1 **Are you ready to eat?** In response to the sight and smell of food, as well as other sensory experiences, your body primes its resources to better digest, absorb and use anticipated nutrients.

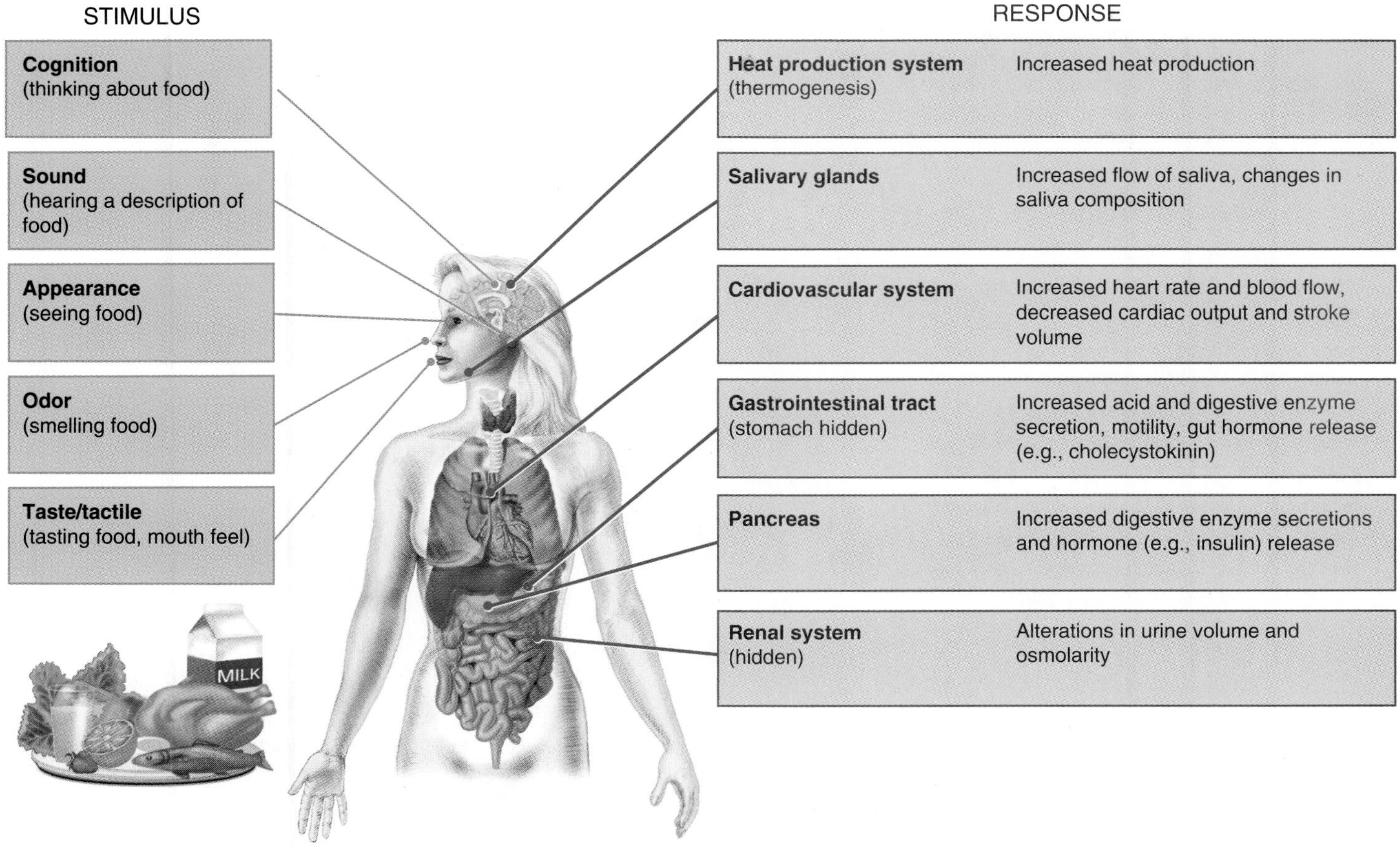

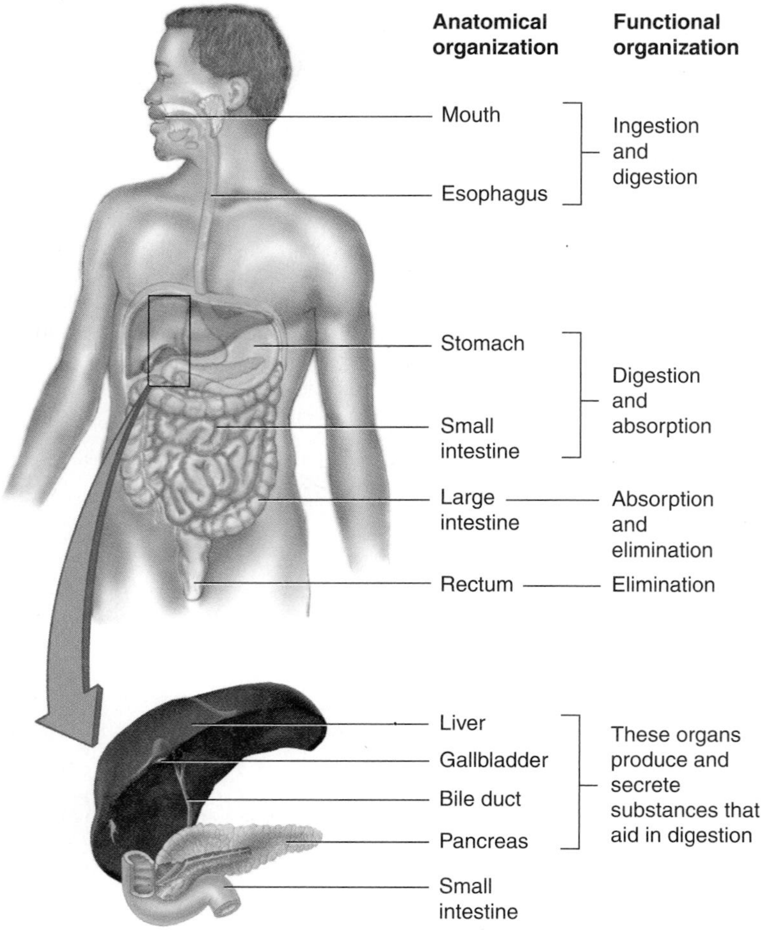

Figure 4.2 **Anatomical and functional organization of the GI tract.** Although digestion begins in the mouth, most digestion occurs in the stomach and small intestine. Absorption takes place primarily in the small and large intestines.

3. secretion of digestive enzymes, acid, mucus, and bile
4. absorption of end products of digestion
5. movement of undigested material
6. **elimination** of digestive waste products

Although it's convenient to describe the GI tract as a hollow tube, its structure is really much more complex. As you can see in **Figure 4.3**, there are several layers to this tube. The innermost layer, called the **mucosa**, is lined with glands and absorptive cells (epithelial cells). Layers of **circular muscle** and **longitudinal muscle** help mix and move food.

At several points along the tract, where one part connects with another (e.g., where the esophagus meets the stomach) the muscles are thicker and form **sphincters**. (See **Figure 4.4**.) By alternately contracting and relaxing, a sphincter acts as a valve and controls the movement of food material so that it goes only in one direction.

Key Concepts: *The gastrointestinal tract consists of the mouth, esophagus, stomach, small intestine, large intestine, and rectum. The function of the GI tract is to ingest, digest, and absorb nutrients, and eliminate waste. The general structure of the GI tract consists of many layers, including the mucosa, the inner lining of glands and absorptive cells. Sphincters are muscular valves along the GI tract that control movement from one part to the next.*

elimination The removal of undigested food from the body.

mucosa [myu-KO-sa] The innermost layer of a cavity. The inner layer of the gastrointestinal tract, also called the intestinal wall. It is composed of epithelial cells and glands.

circular muscle Layers of smooth muscle that surround organs, including the stomach and the small intestine.

longitudinal muscle Muscle fibers aligned lengthwise.

sphincters [SFINGK-ters] Circular bands of muscle fibers that surround the entrance or exit of a hollow body structure (e.g., the stomach) and act as valves to control the flow of material.

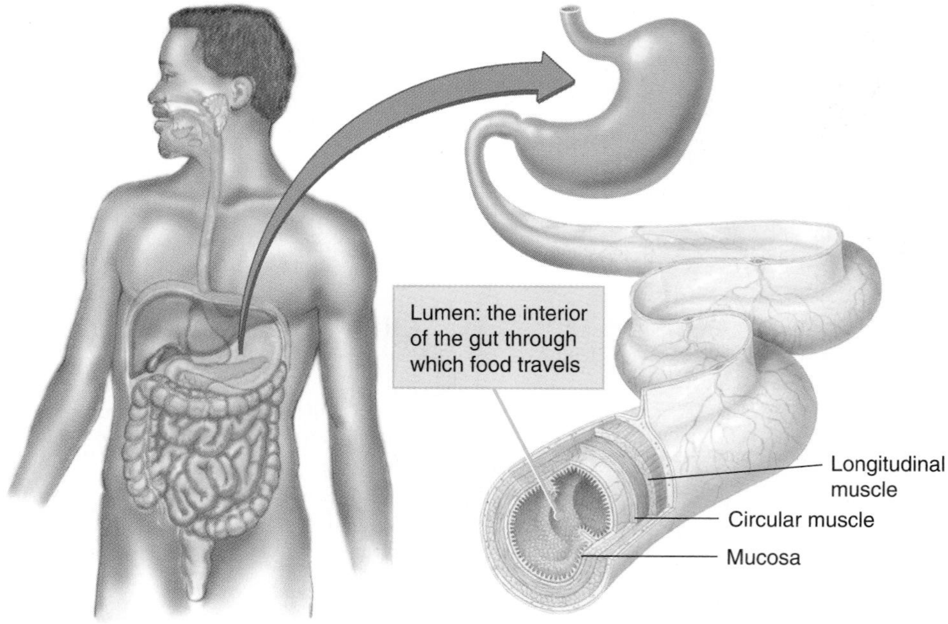

Figure 4.3 **Structural organization of the GI tract wall.** Your intestinal tract is a long hollow tube lined with mucosal cells and surrounded by layers of muscle cells.

Overview of Digestion: Physical and Chemical Processes

The breakdown of food into smaller units and finally into absorbable nutrients involves both chemical and physical processes. The physical process comes first, as food is broken up into smaller pieces. Chewing starts the breakup, and muscular contractions of the GI tract continue it. As the GI tract breaks up food, it mixes the food with various secretions and moves the mixture (called **chyme**) along the tract. Enzymes, along with other chemicals, help complete the breakdown process and promote absorption.

The Physical Movement and Breaking Up of Food

Distinct muscular actions of the GI tract take the food on its long journey. From mouth to anus, waves of muscular contractions, called **peristalsis**, transport food and nutrients along the length of the GI tract. Peristaltic waves from the stomach muscles occur about three times per minute. In the small intestine, circular and longitudinal bands of muscle contract approximately every four to five seconds. Peristaltic contractions of the small intestine often are continuations of contractions that began in the stomach. The large intestine uses slow peristalsis to move the waste products of digestion (feces).

Segmentation, a series of muscular contractions that occur in the small intestine, divides and mixes the chyme. Every few centimeters along the gut wall, alternating constrictions "chop" the contents into smaller portions. Segmentation also increases absorption by bringing chyme into contact with the intestinal wall. **Figure 4.5** shows peristalsis and segmentation.

The Chemical Breakdown of Food

In the chemical process of digestion, enzymes divide nutrients into compounds small enough for absorption.

Enzymes are protein compounds that **catalyze**, or speed up, chemical reactions but are not themselves altered in the process. In digestion, these chemical reactions divide substances into smaller compounds by a process called **hydrolysis** (breaking apart by water), as **Figure 4.6** shows. The function of most digestive enzymes can be identified by their names, which commonly end in *–ase* (amylase, lipase, etc.). For example, the enzyme needed to digest sucr*ose* is sucr*ase*.

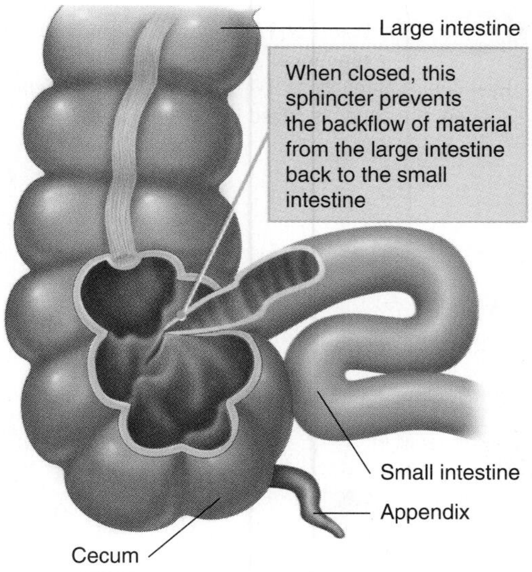
Large intestine
When closed, this sphincter prevents the backflow of material from the large intestine back to the small intestine
Small intestine
Appendix
Cecum

Figure 4.4 **Sphincters in action.** Movement from one section of the GI tract to the next is controlled by muscular valves called sphincters.

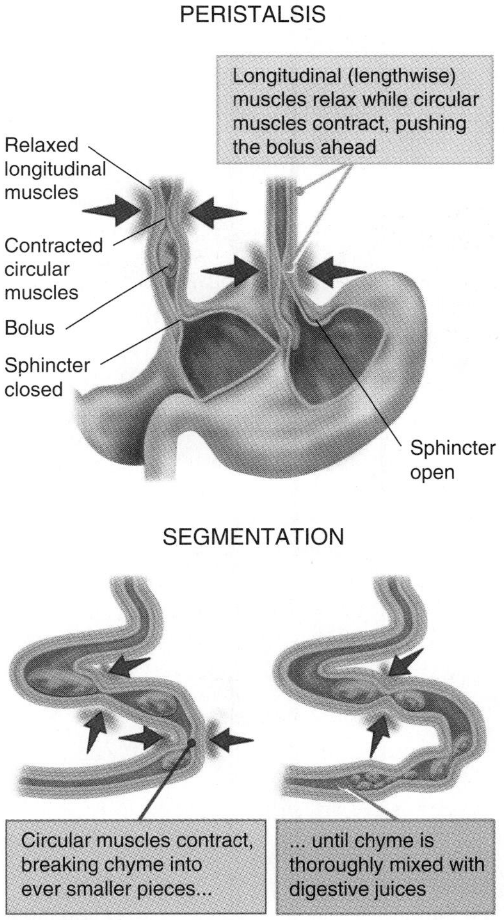
PERISTALSIS
Longitudinal (lengthwise) muscles relax while circular muscles contract, pushing the bolus ahead
Relaxed longitudinal muscles
Contracted circular muscles
Bolus
Sphincter closed
Sphincter open
SEGMENTATION
Circular muscles contract, breaking chyme into ever smaller pieces...
... until chyme is thoroughly mixed with digestive juices

Figure 4.5 **Peristalsis and segmentation.** Peristalsis and segmentation help break up, mix, and move food through the GI tract.

chyme [KIME] A mass of partially digested food and digestive juices moving from the stomach into the small intestine.

peristalsis [per-ih-STAHL-sis] The wavelike, rhythmic muscular contractions of the GI tract that propel its contents down the tract.

segmentation Periodic muscle contractions at intervals along the GI tract that alternate forward and backward movement of the contents, thereby breaking apart chunks of the food mass and mixing in digestive juices.

enzymes [EN-zimes] Proteins in the body that speed up the rate of chemical reactions but are not altered in the process.

catalyze To speed up a chemical reaction.

hydrolysis A reaction that breaks apart a compound through the addition of water.

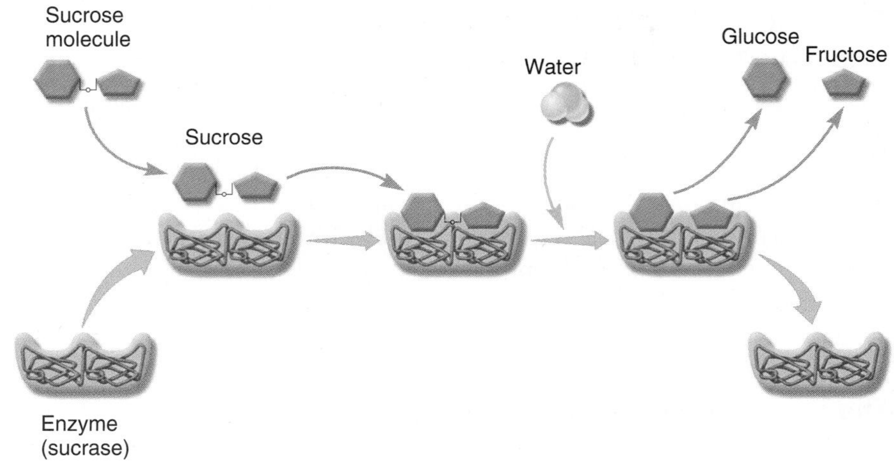

Figure 4.6 **Water and enzymes in chemical reactions.** Enzymes speed up (catalyze) chemical reactions. When water breaks a chemical bond, the action is called hydrolysis.

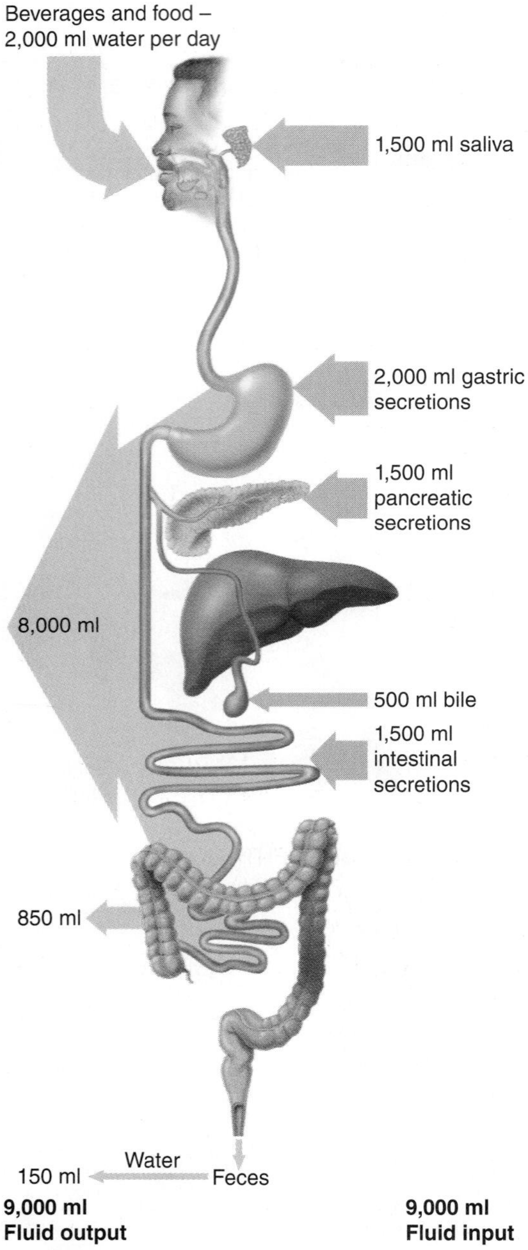

Figure 4.7 **Average daily fluids in the GI tract.** Your GI tract performs a critical balancing act—accepting, secreting, absorbing, and excreting fluids every day.

In addition to enzymes, other chemicals are part of the digestive process. These include acid in the stomach, a neutralizing base in the small intestine, bile that prepares fat for digestion, and **mucus** secreted along the GI tract. This mucus does not break down food but lubricates it and protects the cells that line the GI tract from the strong digestive chemicals. Along the GI tract, fluids containing various enzymes and other substances are added to the consumed food. In fact, the volume of fluid secreted into the GI tract is about 7,000 milliliters (about 6⅔ quarts) per day.[2] **Figure 4.7** shows the average input and output of fluids in the GI tract each day.

Key Concepts: *Digestion involves both physical and chemical activity. Physical activity includes chewing and the movement of muscles along the GI tract that break food into smaller pieces and mix it with digestive secretions. Chemical digestion includes the breaking of bonds in nutrients, such as carbohydrates or proteins, to produce smaller units. Enzymes—proteins that encourage chemical processes—catalyze these reactions.*

Overview of Absorption

Food is broken apart during digestion and moved from the GI tract into circulation and on to the cells. Many of the nutrients—vitamins, minerals and water—do not need to be digested before they are absorbed. But the energy-yielding nutrients—carbohydrate, fat, and protein—are too large to be absorbed intact and must be digested first. At this point, we need to outline how nutrients are moved from the interior, or **lumen**, of the gut through the lining cells (mucosa) and into circulation.

The Roads to Nutrient Absorption

Three main processes allow nutrients to be absorbed from the GI tract into circulation: passive diffusion, facilitated diffusion, and active transport. (See **Figure 4.8**.) Let's take a look at each one in turn.

Passive diffusion is movement of molecules through the cell membrane without the expenditure of energy, by way of special protein channels or intermolecular gaps in the cell membrane. **Concentration gradients** (e.g., a high outside concentration and a low inside concentration of molecules) drive passive diffusion.

Since the cell membrane consists mainly of fat-soluble substances, it welcomes fats and other fat-soluble molecules. Oxygen, nitrogen, carbon diox-

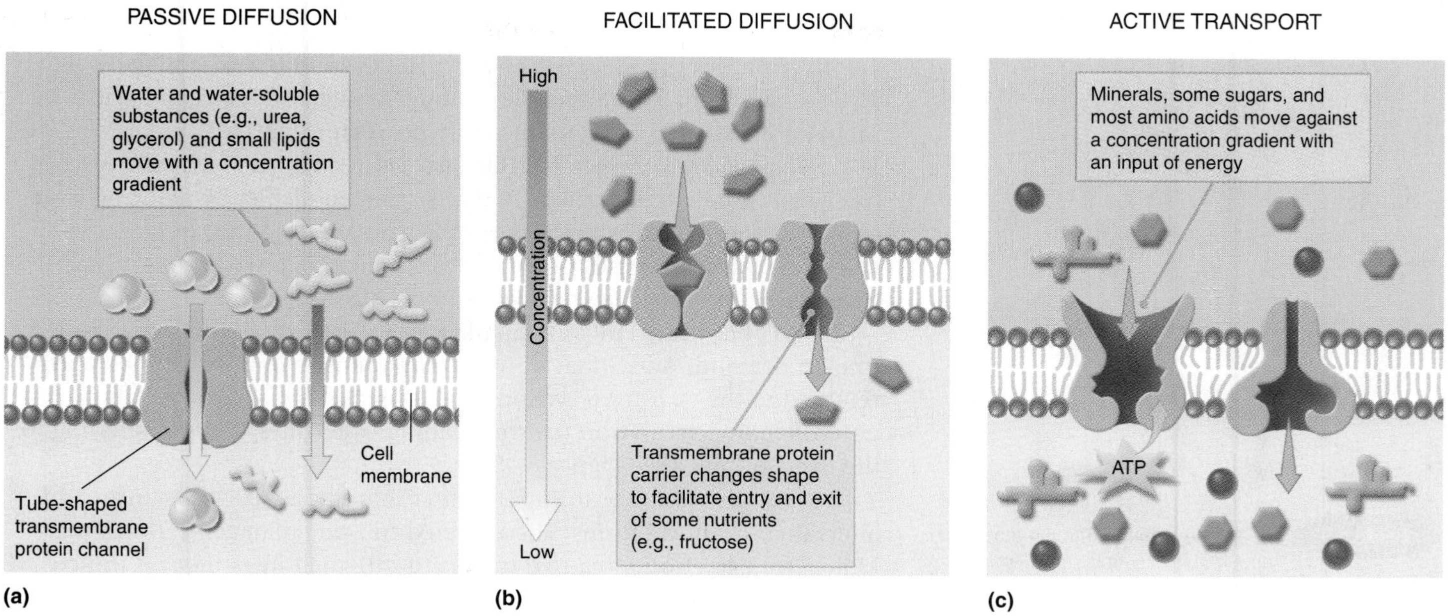

Figure 4.8 **(a) Passive diffusion.** Using passive diffusion, some substances easily move in and out of cells, either through protein channels or directly through the cell membrane.
(b) Facilitated diffusion. Some substances need a little assistance to enter and exit cells. The transmembrane protein helps out by changing shape.
(c) Active transport. Some substances need a lot of assistance to enter cells. Just as in swimming upstream, energy is needed for the substance to get through an unfavorable concentration gradient.

ide, and alcohols are highly soluble in fat and readily dissolve in the cell membrane and diffuse across it. Although water crosses cell membranes easily, most water-soluble nutrients need additional help.

In **facilitated diffusion**, special protein channels help substances cross the cell membrane. The diffusing molecule becomes lightly bound to a protein channel that changes shape to open a pathway for the diffusing molecules to enter or exit the cell.

Some substances need energy to move across a cell membrane, a process called **active transport**. Substances that usually require active transport across some cell membranes include many minerals, several sugars, and most amino acids (simple components of protein).

Key Concepts: *Absorption through the GI cell membranes occurs by one of three basic processes. In passive diffusion, nutrients such as water permeate the intestinal wall without a carrier or energy expenditure. In facilitated diffusion, a protein carrier helps bring substances into the absorptive intestinal cell without expending energy. Active transport requires energy to transport a substance across a cell membrane.*

Assisting Organs

The salivary glands, liver, gallbladder, and pancreas all have critical roles in the digestive process. The GI tract works in concert with these organs, which assist digestion by providing fluid, acid neutralizers, enzymes, and **emulsifiers**.

Salivary Glands

We have three pairs of **salivary glands**, located in or near the mouth, which secrete saliva into the oral cavity. (See **Figure 4.9**.) Saliva moistens food, lubricating it for easy swallowing. Saliva also contains enzymes that begin the process of chemical digestion. We secrete approximately 1,500 milliliters (about 1½ quarts) of saliva each day. The mere sight, smell, or thought of food can start the flow of saliva.

mucus A slippery substance secreted in the GI tract (and other body linings) that protects cells from irritants.

lumen Cavity or hollow channel in any organ or structure of the body.

passive diffusion The movement of substances into or out of cells without the expenditure of energy or the involvement of transport proteins in the cell membrane. Also called simple diffusion.

concentration gradients Differences between the solute concentrations of two solutions.

facilitated diffusion A process by which carrier (transport) proteins in the cell membrane transport substances into or out of cells down a concentration gradient.

active transport The movement of substances into or out of cells against a concentration gradient. Active transport requires energy (ATP) and involves carrier (transport) proteins in the cell membrane.

emulsifiers Agents that blend fatty and watery liquids by promoting the breakup of fat into small particles and stabilizing their suspension in a watery solution.

salivary glands Glands in the mouth that release saliva.

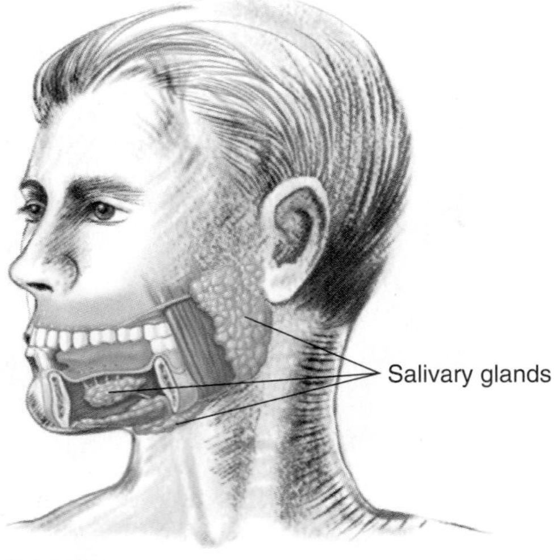
Salivary glands

Figure 4.9 **The salivary glands.** The three pairs of salivary glands supply saliva, which moistens and lubricates food. Saliva also contains salivary enzymes that begin the digestion of starch.

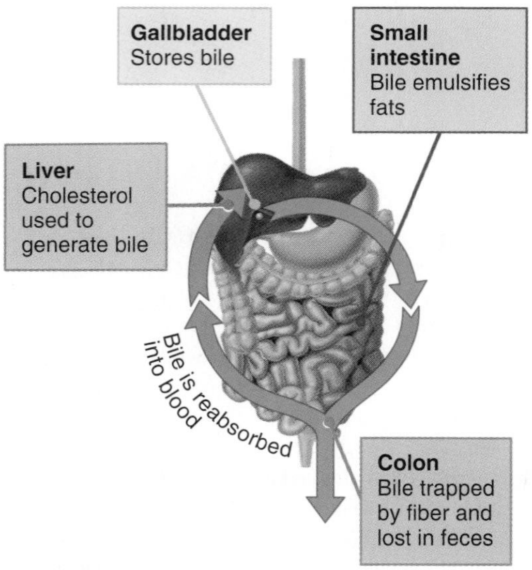
Gallbladder
Stores bile
Small intestine
Bile emulsifies fats
Liver
Cholesterol used to generate bile
Bile is reabsorbed into blood
Colon
Bile trapped by fiber and lost in feces

Figure 4.10 **Enterohepatic circulation.** During this recycling process, bile travels from the liver to the gallbladder and then to the small intestine, where it assists digestion. In the small intestine, most bile is reclaimed and sent back to the liver for reuse.

Liver

The **liver** produces and secretes 600 to 1,000 milliliters of **bile** daily. Bile is a yellow-green, pasty material that contains water, bile salts and acids, pigments, cholesterol, phospholipids (a type of fat molecule), and electrolytes (electrically charged minerals). Bile tastes bitter, which is why the word *bile* has come to denote bitterness. Bile acts as an emulsifier by reducing large globs of fat to smaller globs. This process breaks no bonds in fat molecules, but rather increases the surface area of fat, allowing more contact between fat molecules and enzymes in the small intestine.

Bile is concentrated in your gallbladder and released to the small intestine on demand. After it has done its work, most bile is reabsorbed and returned to the liver for recycling. This recirculation is known as the **enterohepatic circulation** (*entero* meaning "intestines," *hepatic* referring to the liver) of bile. (See **Figure 4.10**.)

The liver also is a detoxification center that filters toxic substances and alters their chemical forms. These altered substances may be sent to the kidney for **excretion** or carried by bile to the small intestine and routed out of the body in feces.

Gallbladder

The primary function of the **gallbladder** is to store and concentrate bile from the liver. A small, muscular, pear-shaped sac nestled in a depression on the right underside of the liver, the gallbladder holds about a quarter of a cup of bile. The gallbladder is a storage stop for bile between the liver and the small intestine. It fills with viscous bile and thickens it, until a hormone released after eating signals the gallbladder to squirt out its colorful contents.

The gallbladder is normally relaxed and full between meals. When dietary fats enter the small intestine, they trigger the contraction of the gallbladder. Like a squeeze bulb, the gallbladder squirts bile through the common bile duct into the upper part of the small intestine. The common bile duct also carries digestive enzymes from the pancreas.

Pancreas

The **pancreas** secretes enzymes that affect the digestion and absorption of nutrients. During the course of a day, the pancreas secretes about 1,500 milliliters of fluid, which contains mostly water, bicarbonate, and digestive enzymes. The pancreas also releases hormones that are involved in other aspects of nutrient use by the body. For example, the pancreatic hormones insulin and glucagon regulate blood glucose levels. The combination of these two functions makes the pancreas one of the most important organs in the digestion and use of food.

Key Concepts: *The salivary glands, liver, gallbladder, and pancreas all make important contributions to the digestive process. The salivary glands release saliva, which contains mucus and enzymes, into the mouth. The liver produces bile, which is stored in the gallbladder and released into the small intestine, where bile helps to prepare fats for digestion. The pancreas secretes liquid containing bicarbonate and several types of enzymes into the small intestine.*

Putting It All Together: Digestion and Absorption

Up to this point, we have focused on structures, mechanisms, and processes to give you a general idea of the workings of the GI tract. Now you're ready for a complete tour, a journey along the GI tract to see what happens and how digestion and absorption are accomplished. Detailed descriptions of specific enzymes and actions on individual nutrients are covered in later chapters.

Mouth

As soon as you put food in your mouth the digestive process begins. As you chew, you break down the food into smaller pieces, increasing the surface area available to enzymes. Saliva contains the enzyme **salivary amylase** (ptyalin), which breaks down starch into small sugar molecules. Food remains in the mouth for just a short time, so only about 5 percent of the starch is completely broken down. The next time you eat a cracker or a piece of bread, chew slowly and notice the change in the way it tastes. It gets sweeter. That's the salivary amylase breaking down the starch into sugar. Salivary amylase continues to work until the strong acid content of the stomach deactivates it. To start the process of fat digestion, the cells at the base of the tongue secrete another enzyme, **lingual lipase**. The overall impact of lingual lipase on fat digestion, though, is small.

Think About It 3

Saliva and other fluids, including mucus, blend with the food to form a **bolus**, a chewed, moistened lump of food that is soft and easy to swallow. When you swallow, the bolus slides past the epiglottis, a valvelike flap of tissue that closes off your air passages so you don't choke. The bolus then moves rapidly through the **esophagus** to the stomach, where it will be digested further. **Figure 4.11** shows the process of swallowing.

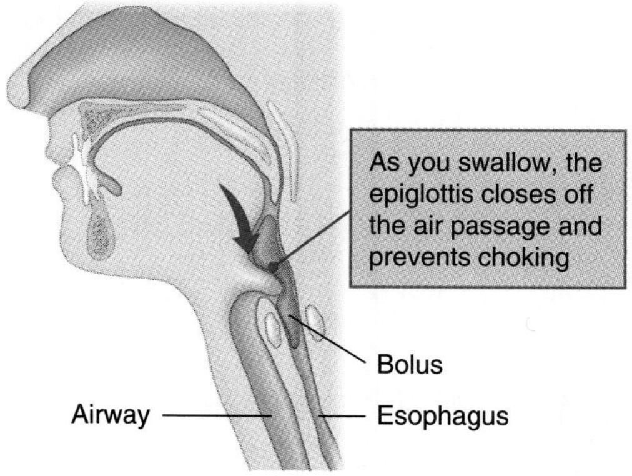
As you swallow, the epiglottis closes off the air passage and prevents choking
Bolus
Airway
Esophagus

Figure 4.11 **Swallowing.** Your epiglottis didn't completely do its job if you have ever choked on a drink that went "down the wrong pipe."

Stomach

The bolus enters the **stomach** through the **esophageal sphincter**, commonly called the cardiac sphincter, which immediately closes to keep the bolus from sliding back into the esophagus. This sphincter needs to close quickly and completely to prevent the acidic stomach contents from backing up into the esophagus, causing pain and tissue damage. **Heartburn** is caused by the movement of acid from the stomach back into the esophagus.

Nutrient Digestion in the Stomach

The stomach cells produce secretions that are collectively called gastric juice. Included in this mixture are water, hydrochloric acid, mucus,

liver The largest glandular organ in the body, it produces and secretes bile, detoxifies harmful substances, and helps metabolize carbohydrates, lipids, proteins, and micronutrients.

bile An alkaline, yellow-green fluid that is produced in the liver and stored in the gallbladder. Bile emulsifies dietary fats, aiding fat digestion and absorption.

enterohepatic circulation [EN-ter-oh-heh-PAT-ik] Recycling of certain compounds between the small intestine and the liver.

excretion The process of separating and removing waste products of metabolism.

gallbladder A pear-shaped sac that stores and concentrates bile from the liver.

pancreas The pancreas secretes enzymes that affect the digestion and absorption of nutrients and releases hormones, such as insulin, which regulate metabolism as well as the way nutrients are used in the body.

salivary amylase [AM-ih-lace] An enzyme that catalyzes the hydrolysis of amylose, a starch. Also called ptyalin.

lingual lipase A fat-splitting enzyme secreted by cells at the base of the tongue.

bolus [BOH-lus] A chewed, moistened lump of food that is ready to be swallowed.

esophagus [ee-SOFF-uh-gus] The food pipe that extends from the pharynx to the stomach.

stomach The enlarged, muscular, saclike portion of the digestive tract between the esophagus and the small intestine, with a capacity of about 1 quart.

esophageal sphincter The opening between the esophagus and the stomach that relaxes and opens to allow the bolus to travel into the stomach, and then closes behind it. Also acts as a barrier to prevent the reflux of gastric contents. Also called the cardiac sphincter.

heartburn Burning pain behind the breastbone area caused by acidic stomach contents backing up into the esophagus.

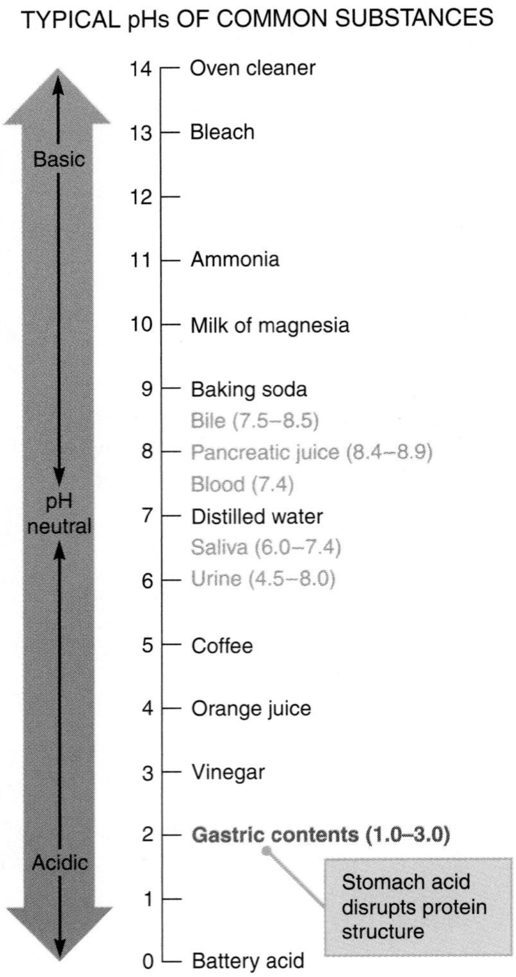

Figure 4.12 **The pH scale.** Because pancreatic juice has a pH around 8, it can neutralize the acidic chyme, which leaves the stomach with a pH around 2.

pepsinogen (the inactive form of the enzyme pepsin), the enzyme gastric lipase, the hormone gastrin, and intrinsic factor.

- **Hydrochloric acid (gastric acid)** makes the stomach contents extremely acidic—a **pH** of 2, compared to a neutral pH of 7. (See the pH scale in **Figure 4.12**.) This acidic environment kills many pathogenic (disease-causing) bacteria that may have been ingested and also aids in the digestion of protein. Mucus secreted by the stomach cells coats the stomach lining, protecting these cells from damage by the strong gastric juice.

  Hydrochloric acid works in protein digestion in two ways. First, it demolishes the functional, three-dimensional shape of proteins, unfolding and breaking them into linear chains; this increases their vulnerability to attacking enzymes. Second, it promotes the breakdown of proteins by converting **pepsinogen**, an enzyme **precursor**, to **pepsin**, its active form.

- Pepsin then begins breaking the links in protein chains, cutting dietary proteins into smaller and smaller pieces.

- Stomach cells also produce an enzyme called **gastric lipase**. It has a minor role in the digestion of lipids, specifically butterfat.

- **Gastrin**, another component of gastric juice, is a hormone that stimulates gastric secretion and movement.

- **Intrinsic factor** is a substance necessary for the absorption of vitamin B_{12} that occurs further down the GI tract, near the end of the small intestine. In the absence of intrinsic factor, only about $\frac{1}{50}$ of ingested vitamin B_{12} is absorbed.

After you swallow, salivary amylase continues to digest carbohydrates. About an hour later, acidic stomach secretions become well mixed with the food. This increases the acidity of the food and effectively blocks further salivary amylase activity.

Do you sometimes feel your stomach churning? The stomach works to continue mixing food with GI secretions and produce the semiliquid chyme. To accomplish this, the stomach has an extra layer of muscles. These diagonal muscles, along with the circular and longitudinal muscles, contract and relax to mix food completely. When the chyme is ready to leave the stomach, about 30 to 40 percent of carbohydrate, 10 to 20 percent of protein, and less than 10 percent of fat have been digested.[3] The stomach slowly releases the chyme through the **pyloric sphincter** and into the small intestine. When closed, the pyloric sphincter prevents the chyme from returning to the stomach. (See **Figure 4.13**.)

The stomach normally empties in one to four hours, depending on the types and amounts of food eaten. Carbohydrates speed through the stomach in the shortest time, followed by protein and fat. Thus, the higher the fat content of a meal, the longer it will take to leave the stomach.

Nutrient Absorption in the Stomach

Although much digestion has been accomplished by the time chyme leaves the stomach, very little absorption has occurred. The stomach absorbs weak acids, such as alcohol and aspirin, and only a few fat-soluble compounds. Chyme moves on to the small intestine, the digestive and absorptive workhorse of the gut.

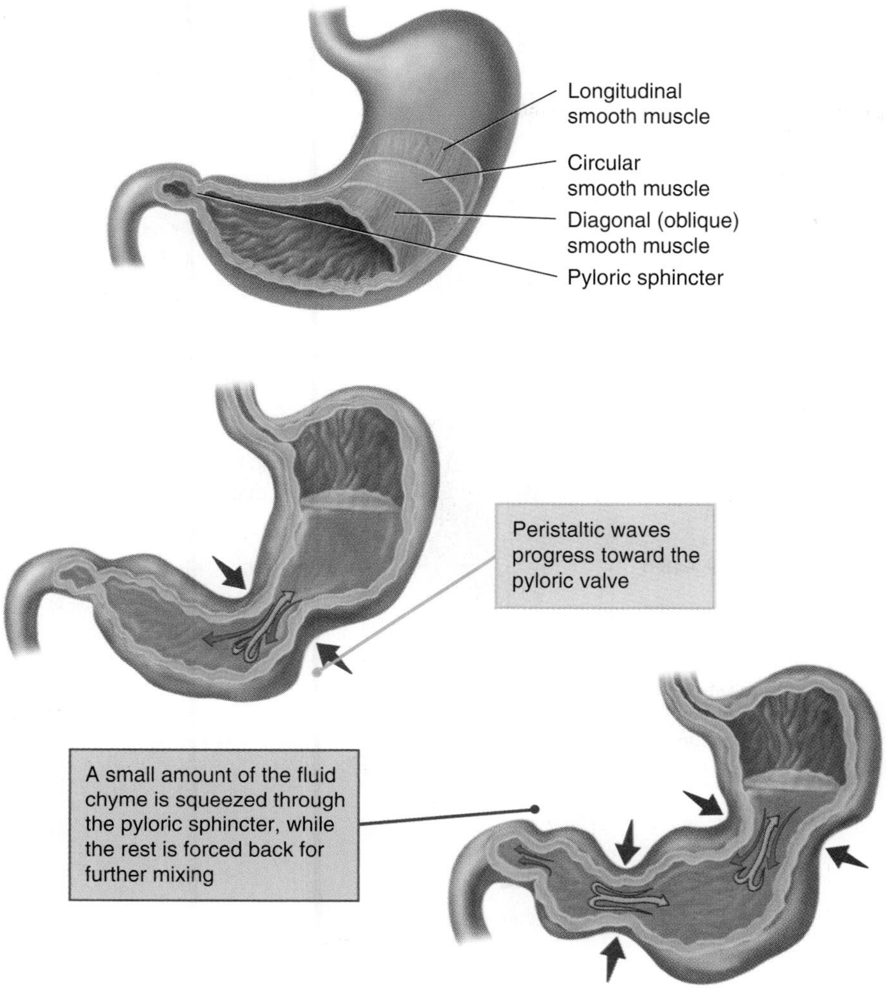
Longitudinal smooth muscle
Circular smooth muscle
Diagonal (oblique) smooth muscle
Pyloric sphincter
Peristaltic waves progress toward the pyloric valve
A small amount of the fluid chyme is squeezed through the pyloric sphincter, while the rest is forced back for further mixing

Figure 4.13 **The stomach.** The stomach churns and mixes food with gastric secretions.

Small Intestine

The **small intestine** completes the digestion of protein, fat, and nearly all carbohydrate, and absorbs most nutrients. As you can see in **Figure 4.14**, the small intestine is a tube approximately 10 to 12 feet (about 3 meters) long, divided into three parts:

- **duodenum** (the first 10 to 12 inches, or 25 to 30 centimeters)
- **jejunum** (about 4 feet, or about 120 centimeters)
- **ileum** (about 5 feet, or about 150 centimeters)

Most digestion occurs in the duodenum, where the small intestine receives **digestive secretions** from the pancreas, gallbladder, and its own glands. The remainder of the small intestine primarily absorbs previously digested nutrients.

Nutrient Digestion in the Small Intestine

In the duodenum, bicarbonate from the pancreas neutralizes the acidic chyme from the stomach. This is important because the enzymes of the small intestine need a more neutral environment to work effectively. Pancreatic juice contains a variety of digestive enzymes that help to digest fats, carbohydrates, and proteins. Secretions from the intestinal wall cells add enzymes to complete carbohydrate digestion.

hydrochloric acid A very strong acid of chloride and hydrogen atoms made by stomach glands and secreted into the stomach. Also called gastric acid.

gastric acid See *hydrochloric acid.*

pH A measurement of the hydrogen ion concentration, or acidity, of a solution.

pepsinogen The inactive form of the enzyme pepsin.

precursor A substance that is converted into another active substance. Enzyme precursors also are called proenzymes.

pepsin A protein-digesting enzyme produced by the stomach.

gastric lipase An enzyme in the stomach that primarily breaks down butterfat.

gastrin [GAS-trin] A hormone released from the walls of the stomach and duodenum that stimulates gastric secretions and motility.

intrinsic factor A protein released from cells in the stomach wall that binds to and aids in absorption of vitamin B_{12}.

pyloric sphincter [pie-LORE-ic] A circular muscle that forms the opening between the duodenum and the stomach. It regulates the passage of food into the small intestine.

small intestine The tube (approximately 3 meters [10 ft] long) where the digestion of protein, fat, and carbohydrate is completed and where the majority of nutrients are absorbed. The small intestine is divided into three parts: the duodenum, the jejunum, and the ileum.

duodenum [doo-oh-DEE-num, or doo-AH-den-um] The portion of the small intestine closest to the stomach. The duodenum is 25 to 30 cm (10 to 12 in.) long and wider than the remainder of the small intestine.

jejunum [je-JOON-um] The middle section of the small intestine (about 120 cm [4 ft] long), lying between the duodenum and ileum.

ileum [ILL-ee-um] The terminal segment of the small intestine (about 150 cm [5 ft] long), which opens into the large intestine.

digestive secretions Substances released at different places in the GI tract to speed the breakdown of ingested carbohydrates, fats, and proteins.

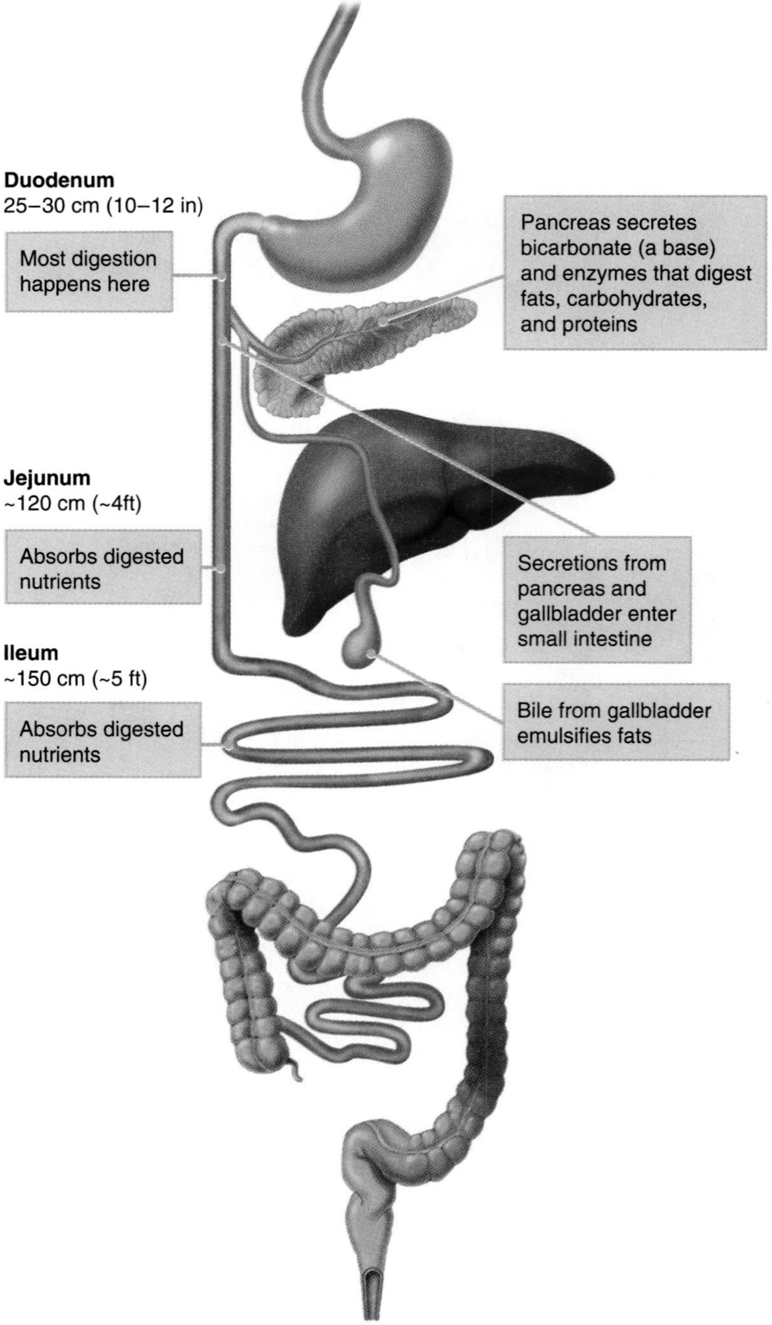
Duodenum
25–30 cm (10–12 in)
Most digestion happens here
Pancreas secretes bicarbonate (a base) and enzymes that digest fats, carbohydrates, and proteins
Jejunum
~120 cm (~4ft)
Absorbs digested nutrients
Secretions from pancreas and gallbladder enter small intestine
Ileum
~150 cm (~5 ft)
Absorbs digested nutrients
Bile from gallbladder emulsifies fats

Figure 4.14 **The small intestine.** The duodenum is mainly responsible for digesting food; the jejunum and ileum primarily deal with the absorption of nutrients. In addition to receiving the digestive juices from assisting organs, the duodenum secretes mucus, enzymes, and hormones to aid digestion. All along the intestinal walls, nutrients are absorbed into blood and lymph. Undigested materials are passed on to the large intestine.

villi Small fingerlike projections that blanket the folds in the lining of the small intestine. Singular is *villus*.

microvilli Minute, hairlike projections that extend from the surface of absorptive cells facing the intestinal lumen.

The presence of fat in the duodenum stimulates the release of stored bile by the gallbladder. Lipids ordinarily do not mix with water, but bile acts as an emulsifier, keeping lipid molecules mixed with the watery chyme and digestive secretions. Without the action of bile, lipids might not come into contact with pancreatic lipase, and digestion would be incomplete.

With the pancreatic and intestinal enzymes working together, digestion progresses nicely, leaving smaller protein, carbohydrate, and lipid compounds ready for absorption. Other nutrients, such as vitamins, minerals, and cholesterol, are not digested and generally are absorbed unchanged.

Just as the small intestine accomplishes much of the nutrient digestion, it is also responsible for most nutrient absorption. Its structure makes the process of absorption efficient and complete. In most cases, more than 90 percent of ingested carbohydrate, fat, and protein is absorbed. To see how this is possible, we need to examine the structure of the small intestine.

Absorptive Structures of the Small Intestine

The small intestine packs a gigantic surface area into a small space. As you can see in **Figure 4.15**, the interior surface of the small intestine is wrinkled into folds, tripling the absorptive surface area. These folds are carpeted with fingerlike projections called **villi** that expand the absorptive area another 10-fold. Each cell lining the surface of each villus is covered with a "brush border" containing as many as 1,000 hairlike projections called **microvilli**. The microvilli increase the surface area another 20 times. Taken together, the folds plus the villi and microvilli yield a 600-fold increase in surface area. In fact, your 10-foot- (3-meter-) long intestine has an absorptive surface area of more than 300 square yards (250 or more square meters)—equivalent to the surface of a tennis court!

Nutrient Absorption in the Small Intestine

As nutrients journey through the small intestine, they are trapped in the folds and projections of the intestinal wall and absorbed through the microvilli into the lining cells. Depending on your diet, each day your small intestine absorbs several hundred grams of carbohydrate, 60 or more grams of fat, 50 to 100 grams of amino acids, and 7 to 8 liters of water. But the total absorptive capacity of the healthy small intestine is far greater. It actually has the capacity to absorb as much as several kilograms of carbohydrate, 500 grams of fat, 500 to 700 grams of amino acids, and 20 or

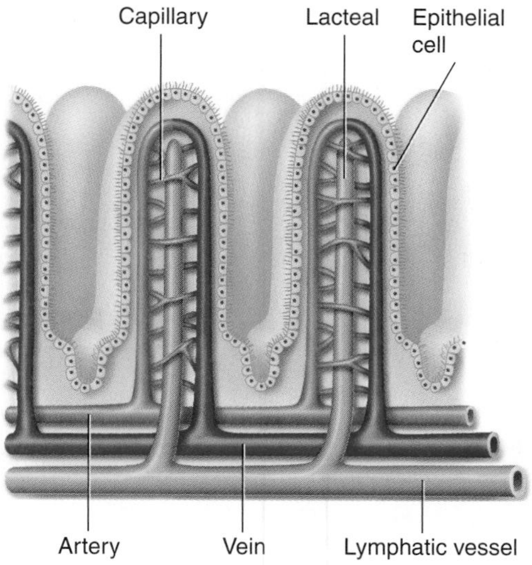
Capillary
Lacteal
Epithelial cell
Artery
Vein
Lymphatic vessel

Anatomy of the villi.

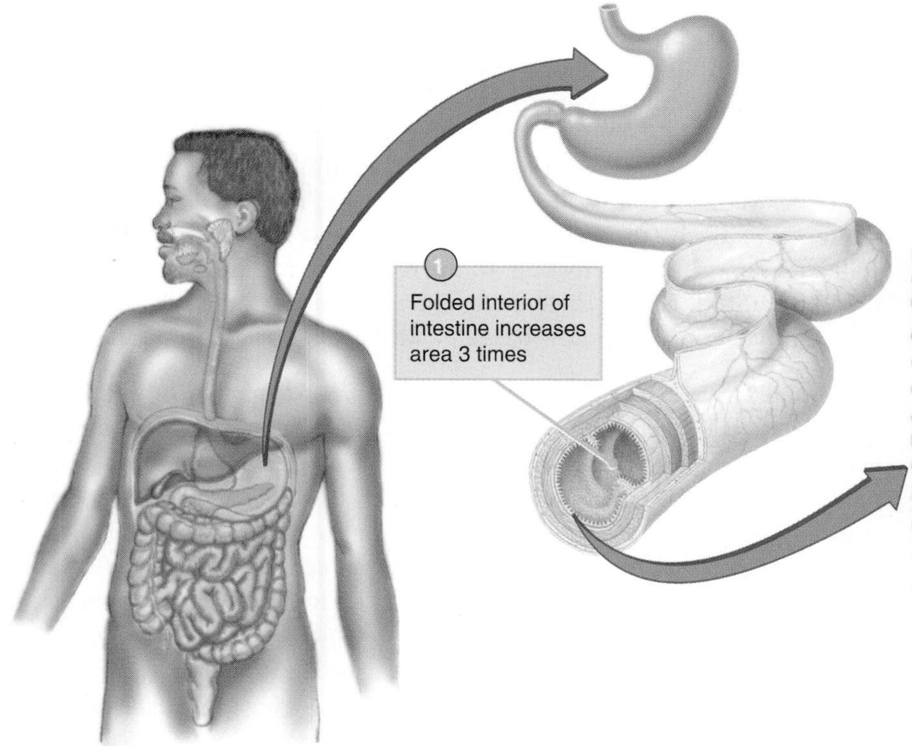
1
Folded interior of intestine increases area 3 times

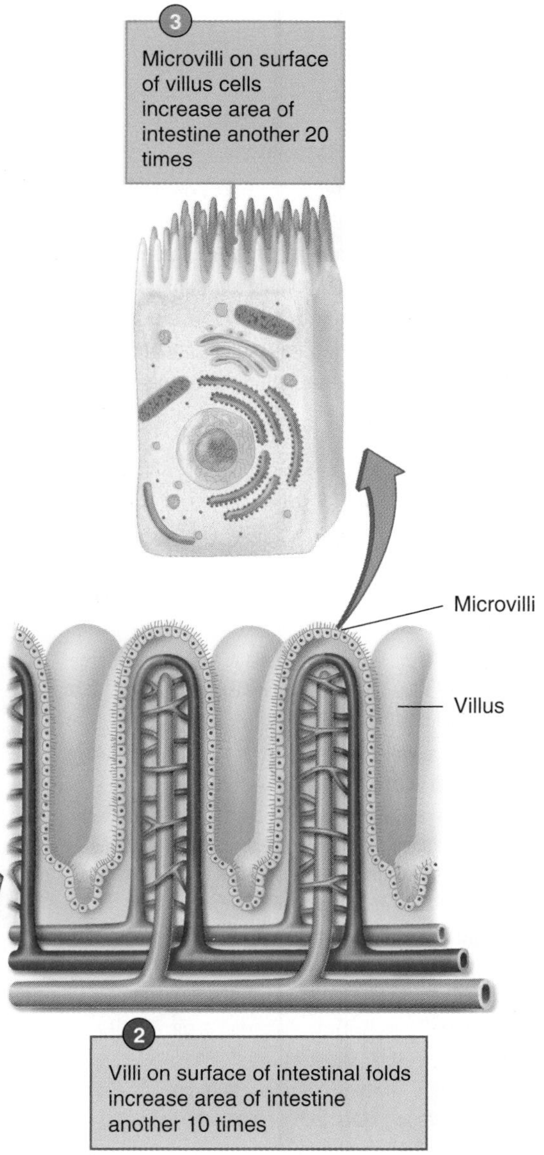
3
Microvilli on surface of villus cells increase area of intestine another 20 times
Microvilli
Villus
2
Villi on surface of intestinal folds increase area of intestine another 10 times

Figure 4.15 **The absorptive surface of the small intestine.** To maximize the absorptive surface area, the small intestine is folded and lined with villi. You have a surface area the size of a tennis court packed into your gut.

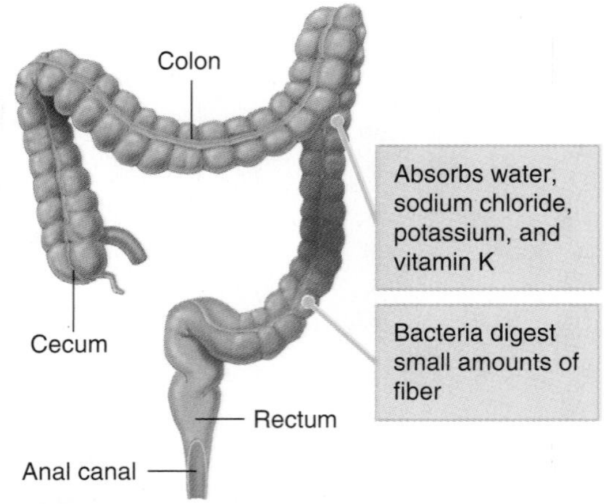

Figure 4.16 **The large intestine.** As the large intestine absorbs water, it forms undigested materials into feces for elimination.

more liters of water per day.[4] Approximately 85 percent of the water absorption by the gut occurs in the jejunum.[5]

Nutrients absorbed through the intestinal lining pass into the interior of the villi. Each villus contains blood vessels (veins, arteries, and capillaries) and a **lymph** vessel (known as a **lacteal**) that transport nutrients to other parts of your body. Water-soluble nutrients are absorbed directly into the bloodstream. Fat-soluble lipid compounds are absorbed into the lymph rather than directly into the blood.

The small intestine suffers constant wear and tear as it propels and digests the chyme. The intestinal lining is renewed continually as the mucosal cells are replaced every two to five days. When the chyme completes its 3- to 10-hour journey through the small intestine, it passes through the **ileocecal valve**, the connection to the large intestine.

Large Intestine

The chyme's next stop is the **large intestine**. As **Figure 4.16** shows, this 5-foot-long tube includes the cecum, **colon**, **rectum**, and anal canal. As chyme fills the cecum, a local reflex signals the ileocecal valve to close, preventing material from reentering the ileum of the small intestine.

Digestion in the Large Intestine

The peristaltic movements of the large intestine are sluggish compared with those of the small intestine. Normally 18 to 24 hours are required for material to travel its length. During that time, the colon's large population of bacteria digests small amounts of fiber,[6] providing a negligible number of calories daily. Of more significance are the other substances formed by this bacterial activity, including several vitamins, short-chain fatty acids, and various gases that contribute to **flatulence**.[7] Other than bacterial action, no further digestion occurs in the large intestine.

Nutrient Absorption in the Large Intestine

Nutrient absorption in the large intestine is minimal, limited to water, sodium, chloride, potassium, and some of the vitamin K produced by bacteria. Although the colon's bacteria also produce vitamin B_{12}, it is not absorbed. The colon dehydrates the watery chyme, removing and absorbing most of the fluid. Of the approximately 1,000 milliliters of material that enters the large intestine, only about 150 milliliters remain for elimination as feces. The semisolid feces, consisting of roughly 60 percent solid matter (e.g., dietary fiber, bacteria, and digestive secretions) and 40 percent water, then pass into the rectum. In the rectum, strong muscles hold back the waste until it is time to defecate. The rectal muscles then relax, and the anal sphincter opens to allow passage of the stool out the anal canal.[8]

Key Concepts: *Digestion begins in the mouth with the action of salivary amylase. Food material next moves down the esophagus to the stomach, where it mixes with gastric secretions. Protein digestion begins with the action of pepsin, while salivary amylase action ceases due to the low pH level of the stomach. The liquid material (chyme) next moves to the small intestine. Here, secretions from the gallbladder, pancreas, and intestinal lining cells complete the digestion of carbohydrates, proteins, and fats. The end products of digestion, along with vitamins, minerals, water, and other compounds, are absorbed through the intestinal wall and into circulation. Undigested material and some liquid move on to the large intestine, where water and electrolytes are absorbed, leaving waste material to be excreted as feces.*

Quick Bites

Short Bowel Syndrome

Patients who suffer from short bowel syndrome commonly have difficulty absorbing fat-soluble vitamins. To enhance absorption, treatment includes taking a fat-soluble vitamin supplement that easily mingles with water. These patients may also need to take intramuscular shots of B_{12} because they are unable to absorb this water-soluble vitamin.

lymph Fluid that travels through the lymphatic system, made up of large fat particles and fluid drained from the areas between cells.

lacteal A small lymphatic vessel in the interior of each intestinal villus that picks up fat-soluble compounds from intestinal cells.

ileocecal valve The sphincter at the junction of the small and large intestines.

large intestine The tube (about 150 cm [5 ft] long) extending from the ileum of the small intestine to the anus. The large intestine includes the appendix, cecum, colon, rectum, and anal canal.

colon The portion of the large intestine extending from the cecum to the rectum. It is made up of four parts—the ascending, transverse, descending, and sigmoid colons.

rectum The muscular final segment of the intestine, extending from the sigmoid colon to the anus.

flatulence The presence of excessive amounts of air or other gases in the stomach or intestines.

Circulation of Nutrients

After foods are digested and nutrients are absorbed, they are transported via the vascular and lymphatic systems to specific destinations throughout the body. Let's take a closer look at how each of these circulatory systems delivers nutrients to the places they are needed.

Vascular System

The **vascular system**, or blood circulatory system, is a network of veins and arteries through which the blood carries nutrients. (See **Figure 4.17**.) The heart is the pump that keeps the blood circulating through the body. Water-soluble nutrients are absorbed directly from intestinal cells into tiny capillary tributaries of the bloodstream, which carries them to the liver before they are dispersed throughout the body. Blood carries oxygen from the lungs and nutrients from the GI system to all body tissues. Once the destination cells have used the oxygen and nutrients, carbon dioxide and

vascular system A network of veins and arteries through which the blood carries nutrients. Also called the blood circulatory system.

Quick Bites

The Clever Colon

Though it has been presumed that the colon has no digestive function, recent research shows that the human colon can be an important digestive site in patients who are missing significant sections of their intestines. These patients can actually absorb energy from starch and nonstarch polysaccharides in the colon.

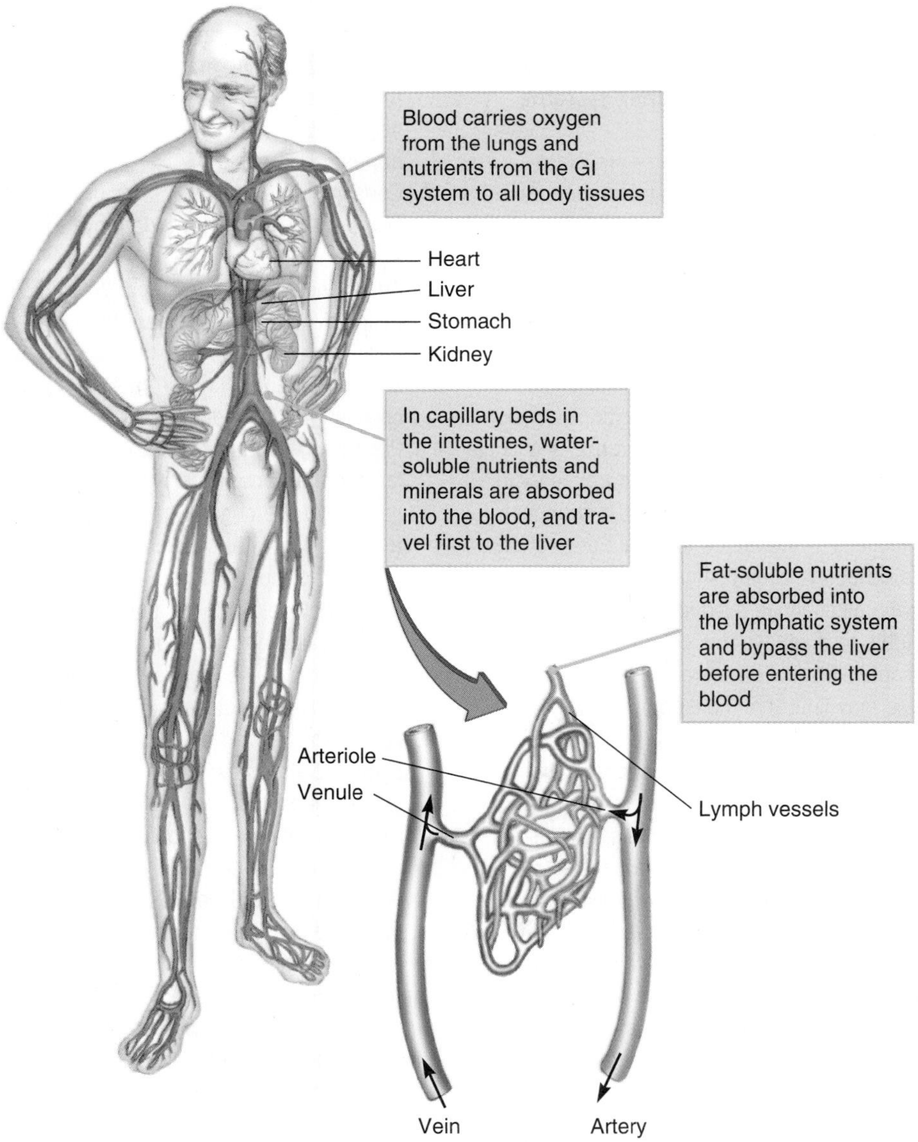
Blood carries oxygen from the lungs and nutrients from the GI system to all body tissues
Heart
Liver
Stomach
Kidney
In capillary beds in the intestines, water-soluble nutrients and minerals are absorbed into the blood, and travel first to the liver
Fat-soluble nutrients are absorbed into the lymphatic system and bypass the liver before entering the blood
Arteriole
Venule
Lymph vessels
Vein
Artery

Figure 4.17 **Circulation.** The vascular system disperses oxygen and nutrients throughout the body. The lymphatic system carries fat-soluble nutrients from the GI tract to the vascular system. Nutrients carried by the lymphatic system bypass the liver before entering the bloodstream.

lymphatic system A system of small vessels, ducts, valves, and organized tissue (e.g., lymph nodes) through which lymph moves from its origin in the tissues toward the heart.

waste products are picked up by the blood and transported to the lungs and kidneys, respectively, for excretion.

Lymphatic System

Most fat-soluble nutrients are absorbed into the **lymphatic system**, which plays an important role in nutrition. Its vessels pick up and transport most end products of fat digestion. After a fatty meal, lymph can become as

Fyi Lactose Intolerance

FOR YOUR INFORMATION

If you drink a milkshake and soon afterward experience bloating, gas, abdominal pain, and diarrhea, the problem could be lactose intolerance—the incomplete digestion of the lactose in milk due to low levels of the intestinal enzyme lactase. Lactose is the primary carbohydrate in milk and other dairy foods. Nondairy foods—such as instant breakfast mixes, cake mixes, mayonnaise, luncheon meats, medications, and vitamin supplements—also may contain small amounts of lactose. Lactase enzyme is necessary to digest lactose in the small intestine. If lactase is deficient, undigested lactose enters the large intestine, where it is broken down by colonic bacteria, producing short-chain organic acids and gases (hydrogen, methane, carbon dioxide).

With the exception of a rare congenital disorder in which infants are born without lactase, infants have sufficiently high levels of lactase. However, lactase activity declines with weaning in many racial/ethnic groups. This normal, genetically controlled decrease in lactase activity, called lactose maldigestion, is prevalent among Asians, Native Americans, and African Americans. However, among U.S. Caucasians and people from northern and central Europe, lactose maldigestion is far less common because lactase activity tends to persist into adulthood. Lactose maldigestion occurs in about 25 percent of the U.S. population and in 75 percent of the worldwide population.

In addition to primary lactose intolerance, lactose intolerance can be secondary to diseases or conditions (e.g., inflammatory bowel disease such as Crohn's disease or celiac disease, gastrointestinal surgery, and certain medications) that injure the intestinal mucosa where lactase is secreted. Secondary lactose maldigestion is temporary, and lactose digestion improves once the underlying causative factor is corrected.

Lactose intolerance is far less prevalent than commonly believed. Many factors unrelated to lactose, including strong beliefs, can contribute to this condition. Studies have demonstrated that among self-described lactose-intolerant individuals, one-third to one-half develop few or no gastrointestinal symptoms following intake of lactose under well-controlled, double-blind conditions.

Self-diagnosis of lactose intolerance is a bad idea because it could lead to unnecessary dietary restrictions, expense, nutritional shortcomings, and failure to detect or treat a more serious gastrointestinal disorder. If lactose maldigestion is suspected, tests are available to diagnose this condition.

People with real or perceived lactose intolerance may limit their consumption of dairy foods unnecessarily and jeopardize their intake of calcium and other essential nutrients. A low intake of calcium is associated with increased risk of osteoporosis (porous bones), hypertension, and colon cancer.

With the exception of the few individuals who are sensitive to very small amounts of lactose, avoiding all lactose is neither necessary nor recommended because some lactase is still being produced. Lactose maldigesters need to determine the amount of lactose they can comfortably consume at any one time.

Here are some strategies for including milk and other dairy foods in your diet without developing symptoms:

1. Initially, consume small servings of lactose-containing foods such as milk (e.g., ½ cup). Gradually increase the serving size until symptoms begin to appear, then back off.
2. Consume lactose with a meal or foods (e.g., milk with cereal) to improve tolerance.
3. Adjust the type of dairy food. Whole milk may be tolerated better than low-fat milk, and chocolate milk may be tolerated better than unflavored milk. Many cheeses (e.g., cheddar, Swiss, Parmesan) contain considerably less lactose than does milk. Aged cheeses generally have negligible amounts of lactose. Yogurts with live, active cultures are another option; these bacteria will digest lactose. Sweet acidophilus milk, yogurt milk, and other nonfermented dairy foods may be tolerated better than regular milk by lactose maldigesters.
4. Lactose-hydrolyzed dairy foods and/or commercial enzyme preparations (e.g., lactase capsules, chewable tablets, solutions) are another option. Lactose-reduced (70 percent less lactose) and lactose-free (99.9 percent less lactose) milks are available, although at a higher cost than regular milk.

Lactose maldigestion need not be an impediment to including milk and other dairy foods in the diet to help meet the needs for calcium and other essential nutrients.

much as 1 to 2 percent fat. We'll discuss the specific process for absorption of lipids into the lymphatic system in Chapter 6, "Lipids."

The lymphatic system is a network of vessels that drain lymph, the clear fluid formed in the spaces between cells. Lymph moves through its system, eventually to empty into the bloodstream near the neck. Unlike nutrients absorbed directly into the vascular system, nutrients absorbed into the lymphatic system bypass the liver before entering the bloodstream.

Distribution of lactose intolerance worldwide.

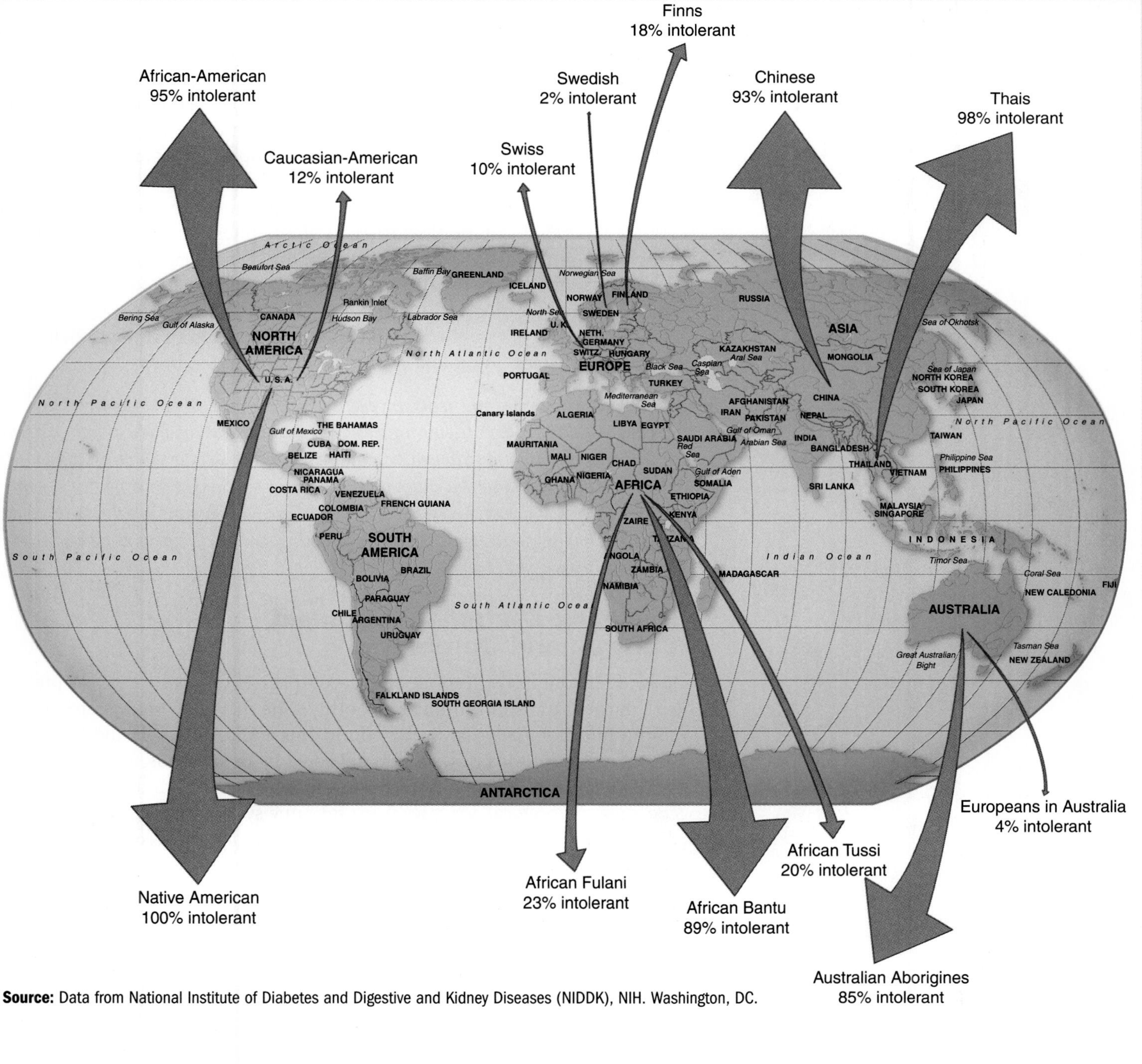

Source: Data from National Institute of Diabetes and Digestive and Kidney Diseases (NIDDK), NIH. Washington, DC.

Unlike the vascular system, the lymphatic system has no pumping organ. The major lymph vessels contain one-way valves; and when vessels are filled with lymph, smooth muscles in the vessel walls contract and pump the lymph forward. The succession of valves allows each segment of the vessel to act as an independent pump. Lymph also is moved along by skeletal muscle contractions that squeeze the vessels.

The lymphatic system also performs an important cleanup function. Proteins and large particulate matter in tissue spaces cannot be absorbed directly into the blood capillaries, but they easily enter the lymphatic system, which carries them away for removal. This removal process is essential—without it a person would die within 24 hours from buildup of fluid and materials around the cells.[9]

Excretion and Elimination

Excretion regulates the concentrations of minerals and other substances in the body and removes the waste products of metabolism. Do not confuse the metabolic waste removed by excretion with digestive waste removed by elimination. Metabolic waste arises from all the chemical reactions that take place in cells throughout the body. Digestive waste never passes into cells—it is the unabsorbed "leftovers" that pass along and out of the GI tract.

The primary organs of excretion are the lungs and kidneys. The lungs excrete water and carbon dioxide. The kidneys filter the blood and excrete substances to remove waste and maintain the body's water and ion balance. The kidneys excrete salts; nitrogen-containing wastes such as urea; small amounts of other substances; and water. This watery mix is called urine. The kidneys vary the amount and concentration of urine to help maintain constant physiological conditions within the body.

Key Concepts: *Absorbed nutrients are carried by either the vascular or lymphatic system. Water-soluble nutrients are absorbed directly into the bloodstream, carried to the liver, and then distributed around the body. Fat-soluble vitamins and large lipid molecules are absorbed into the lymphatic vessels and carried by this system before entering the vascular system. The main excretory organs are the lungs and kidneys. The lungs excrete carbon dioxide and water. The kidneys excrete salts, metabolic wastes, and water.*

Signaling Systems: Command, Control, and Defense

How does your body keep the complex processes of digestion, absorption, and nutrient transport running smoothly? The nervous system, your body's communication network, carries commands and feedback to and from tissues throughout the body. Signals delivered by the nervous system can trigger the release of hormones—chemical messengers that control and coordinate biological activities. Your immune system also involves a coordinated interplay of signals. It feeds back and coordinates complex communication signals as part of the defense against invading microorganisms.

Nervous System

Nerves carry information back and forth between tissues and the brain. Chemicals called neurotransmitters send signals to either excite or suppress nerves, thereby stimulating or inhibiting activity in various parts of the body.

The **central nervous system (CNS)** regulates GI activity in two ways. The **enteric nervous system** is a local system of nerves in the gut wall that is stimulated both by the chemical composition of chyme and by the stretching of the GI lumen that results from food in the GI tract. This stimulation leads to nerve impulses that enhance secretions and muscle movement along the tract. The enteric nervous system plays an essential role in controlling movement, blood flow, water and electrolyte transport, and acid secretion in the GI tract. A branch of the **autonomic nervous system** (the portion of the CNS that controls organ function) responds to the sight, smell, and thought of food. Via the vagus nerve, this branch of the CNS carries signals to and from the GI tract and also enhances GI movement and secretion. In the past, treatments for some ulcers and other GI ailments included severing the vagus nerve, a measure that brought temporary, but not long-term, relief from pain.

Hormonal System

Hormones also are involved in GI regulation. Hormones are chemical messengers that generally are produced at one location and travel in the bloodstream to affect another location in the body.

Gastrointestinal hormonal signals increase or decrease GI motility and secretions and influence your appetite by sending signals to the central nervous system. Some GI hormones function as growth factors for the gastrointestinal mucosa and pancreas.

Taken together, nerve cells and hormones coordinate the movement and secretions of the GI tract so that enzymes are released when and where they are needed. Chyme moves at a rate that will make digestion and absorption most efficient.

Immune System

To identify and attack foreign invaders, your body has a finely tuned, elaborate defense system, the immune system. When a food causes an allergic response, you see the results of the immune system in action. Allergic responses may be mild (e.g., a rash) or life threatening (e.g., breathing difficulties). Usually when particular foods "disagree" with us, the response is due to a lack of digestive enzymes or spoiled food, not an allergy.

Different types of white blood cells carry out the immune response. Some travel the bloodstream to areas of invasion, attacking and ingesting pathogens. **Natural killer cells** attack virus-infected cells and cells that have turned cancerous. **Macrophages**, or "big eaters," take up stations in tissues and act as scavengers, devouring pathogens and worn-out cells. At various places in the lymphatic system there are lymph nodes where macrophages congregate and filter bacteria and other substances from lymph.

There are many different types of **lymphocytes**, which travel in both the bloodstream and lymphatic system. Some produce antibodies. Others remember a prior invader, enabling the body to mount a rapid response should the same invader appear again. Upon recognizing an invasion, helper cells trigger the mass production of killer cells. Killer cells destroy infected body cells, and other lymphocytes mark viruses for destruction by macrophages. When the danger is over, suppressor cells halt the immune response.

All cells in the body have markers on their surfaces that identify them as "self" to the defenders. Invading microorganisms also display surface mark-

central nervous system (CNS) Comprising the brain and the spinal cord, the central nervous system transmits signals that control muscular actions and glandular secretions along the entire GI tract.

enteric nervous system A network of nerves located in the gastrointestinal wall.

autonomic nervous system The part of the central nervous system that regulates the automatic responses of the body; comprises the sympathetic and parasympathetic systems.

natural killer cells Nonspecific lymphocytes that spontaneously attack and kill cancer cells and cells infected by microorganisms. They are "natural" killers because they do not need to recognize a specific antigen in order to attack and kill.

macrophages Large immune system cells that function as patrol cells and engulf and kill foreign invaders.

lymphocytes White blood cells that are primarily responsible for immune responses. Present in the blood and lymph.

antigens Substances that stimulate the immune system to produce antibodies. Antigens often are foreign substances such as invading bacteria or viruses.

antibodies Infection-fighting protein molecules in blood or secretory fluids that tag, neutralize, and help destroy pathogenic microorganisms (e.g., bacteria, viruses) or toxins.

acrolein A pungent decomposition product of fats, generated from dehydrating the glycerol component of fats; responsible for the coughing attacks caused by the fumes released by burning fat. This toxic water-soluble liquid vaporizes easily and is highly flammable.

ers, which the defenders identify as foreign or "nonself." Nonself markers that trigger the immune response are known as **antigens**.

Antibodies have complementary surface markers that work with antigens like a lock and key. The antibody locks onto the antigen, triggering the series of events designed to destroy the invading pathogen.

Key Concepts: *Both hormonal and nervous system signals regulate gastrointestinal activity. Nerve cells in both the enteric and autonomic nervous systems control muscle movement and secretions. Key hormones coordinate GI movement and secretion for optimal digestion and absorption of nutrients. During an immune response, the immune system mobilizes several types of white blood cells. Antigens mark invaders for destruction by antibodies.*

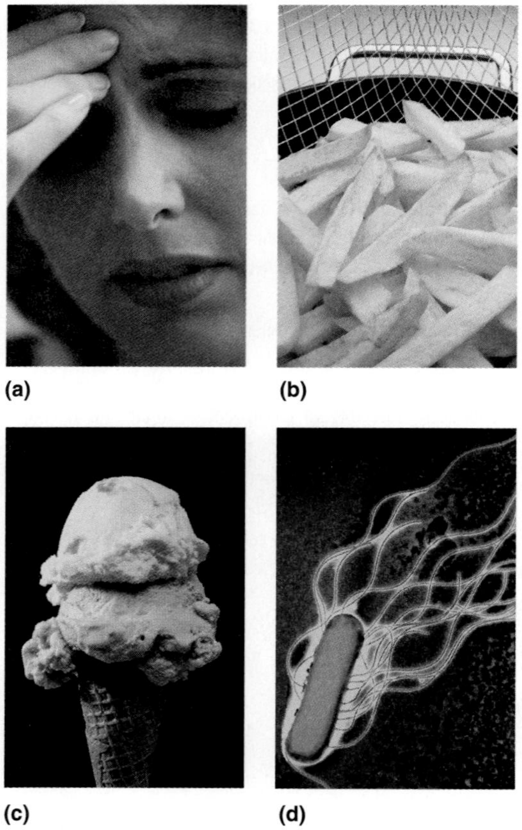

Figure 4.18 **Negative factors for digestion.** Several factors can reduce digestive secretions that interfere with digestion and absorption. Such factors include (a) stress, (b) high-temperature fat frying, (c) cold foods, and (d) bacteria.

Influences on Digestion and Absorption

Psychological Influences

The taste, smell, and presentation of foods can have a positive effect on digestion. Just the thought of food can trigger saliva production and peristalsis. Stressful emotions such as depression and fear can have the reverse effect (see **Figure 4.18**); they stimulate the brain to activate the autonomic nervous system. This results in decreased gastric acid secretion, reduced blood flow to the stomach, inhibition of peristalsis, and reduced propulsion of food.[10] The next time you sit down to a holiday meal, notice how you feel at the sight of your family's traditional foods as well as smells from your childhood. Happiness and positive memories add to the enjoyment of food, whereas unhappiness can bring on a poor appetite or stomach upset.

Think About It 4

Chemical Influences

The type of protein you eat and the way it is prepared affect digestion. Plant proteins tend to be less digestible than animal proteins. Cooking food usually denatures protein (uncoils its three-dimensional structure), which increases digestibility. Cooking meat softens its connective tissue, making chewing easier and increasing the ability of digestive enzymes to break the meat down into absorbable nutrients. Food processing produces chemicals that may influence digestive secretions. For example, whereas meat extracts may stimulate digestion, frying foods in fat at very high temperatures produces small amounts of **acrolein**,[11] a chemical that decreases the flow of digestive secretions. The physical condition of a food sometimes causes problems with digestion. Cold foods may cause intestinal spasms in people who suffer from irritable bowel syndrome or Crohn's disease. Stomach contents can affect absorption. When food is consumed on an empty stomach, it has more contact with gastric secretions and will be absorbed faster than if it were consumed on a full stomach.

Bacterial Influences

In the healthy stomach, hydrochloric acid kills most bacteria. In conditions where there is a lower concentration of hydrochloric acid, more bacteria can survive and multiply. Harmful bacteria can cause gastritis, an inflammation of the stomach lining, and peptic ulcer—a wound in the mucous membranes lining the stomach or duodenum. Bacteria that cause foodborne illness can resist the germicidal effects of hydrochloric acid, so they survive to wreak havoc on the digestive process.

Quick Bites

Gastrointestinal Flora Abound

Your entire body has about 100 trillion cells, but this is only one-tenth the number of protective microorganisms normally living in your body. More than 500 bacterial species live in your GI tract.

The large intestine has the largest population of helpful bacteria. Bacterial activity can form several vitamins and digest small amounts of cellulose, producing a small amount of energy. These bacteria also synthesize gases, such as hydrogen, ammonia, and methane, as well as acids and various substances that contribute to the odor of feces. If the digestion and absorption of food in the small intestine are incomplete, the debris enters the large intestine, where bacterial action produces excessive gas and possibly bloating and pain.

Key Concepts: *Psychological, chemical, and bacterial factors can influence the processes of digestion and absorption. Emotions can influence GI motility and secretion. The temperature and form of food can also affect digestive secretions. Although stomach acid kills many types of bacteria, some are resistant to acid and cause foodborne illness. Helpful bacteria in the large intestine can cause bloating and gas if they receive and begin to digest food components that are normally digested in the small intestine.*

Quick Bites

Halt! Who Goes There?

Be they friend or foe, antibiotics kill microorganisms in your GI tract, frequently causing diarrhea. About half of pharmaceutical drugs have gastrointestinal side effects.

constipation Infrequent and difficult bowel movements, followed by a sensation of incomplete evacuation.

Nutrition and GI Disorders

"I have butterflies in my stomach." "It was a gut-wrenching experience." Our language contains many references to the connection between emotional distress and the GI tract. Most of us have experienced intestinal cramping right before a big date or job interview or a queasy stomach in response to something very disgusting. Through its many neurochemical connections with the gut, the brain exerts a profound influence on GI function. Nearly all GI disorders are influenced to some degree by emotional state. On the other hand, a number of illnesses that were once attributed largely to emotional stress, such as peptic ulcer disease, have been shown to be caused primarily by infection and other physical causes. **Figure 4.19** shows some common ailments that affect the GI tract.

Although stress management might help and medical intervention might be required, we can prevent and manage most GI disorders with diet. For instance, adding fiber-rich foods (see **Table 4.1**) and water to the diet reduces intestinal pressure, decreases the time food byproducts remain in the colon, and promotes bowel regularity. You can avoid most problems and keep your GI tract operating at peak efficiency if you regularly eat a healthful diet, exercise, and maintain a healthy weight.

Constipation

When the colon's muscle contractions are slow or sluggish, the stool moves too slowly. This delay causes the colon to absorb too much water and produces the hard and dry stools of **constipation**.

A diet low in fiber and water and high in fats is the most common cause of constipation. Soluble fiber dissolves easily in water and takes on a soft, gel-like texture in the intestines. Insoluble fiber passes almost

Figure 4.19 **Common GI ailments.** Beans are familiar culprits in what is perhaps the most common GI ailment–gas. Rice is the only starch that does not cause gas.

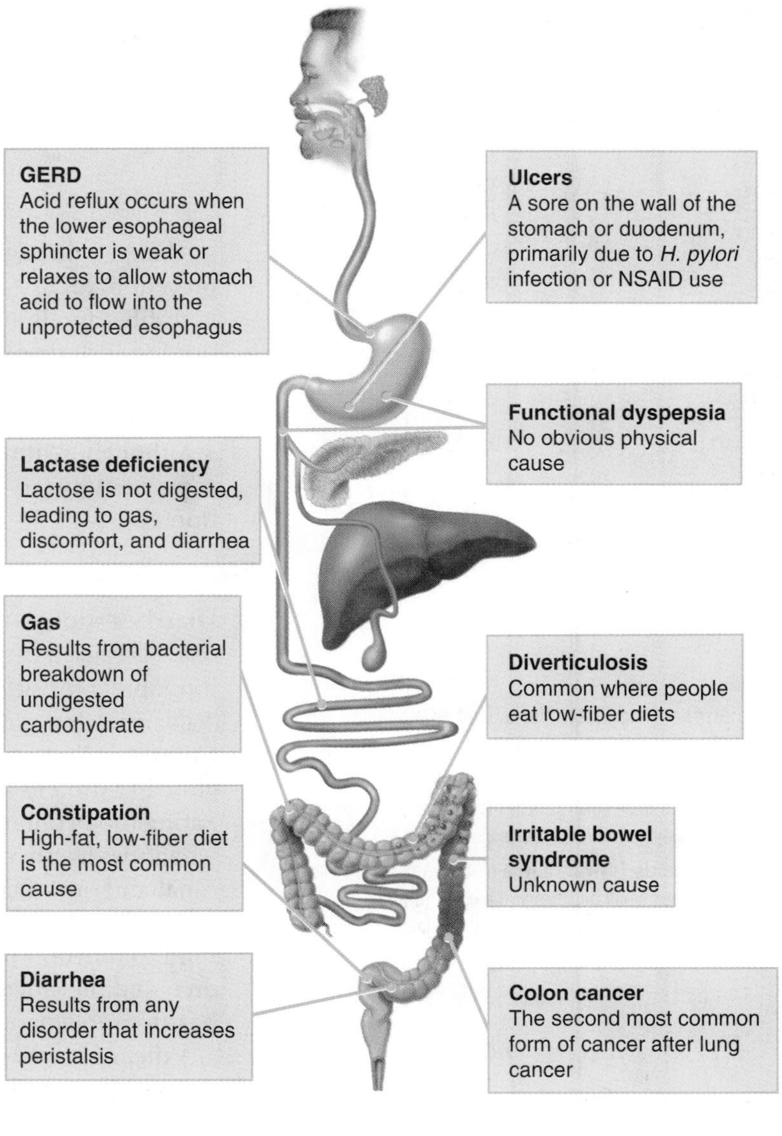

GERD
Acid reflux occurs when the lower esophageal sphincter is weak or relaxes to allow stomach acid to flow into the unprotected esophagus
Ulcers
A sore on the wall of the stomach or duodenum, primarily due to *H. pylori* infection or NSAID use
Functional dyspepsia
No obvious physical cause
Lactase deficiency
Lactose is not digested, leading to gas, discomfort, and diarrhea
Gas
Results from bacterial breakdown of undigested carbohydrate
Diverticulosis
Common where people eat low-fiber diets
Constipation
High-fat, low-fiber diet is the most common cause
Irritable bowel syndrome
Unknown cause
Diarrhea
Results from any disorder that increases peristalsis
Colon cancer
The second most common form of cancer after lung cancer

Table 4.1 Dietary Fiber in Foods

Food Group	Serving Size	Fiber (g)
Legumes		
Kidney beans	1/2 cup	8
Lentils	1/2 cup	5
Split peas	1/2 cup	4.4
Fruit		
Dried plums	1/2 cup	6.0
Apple with skin	1 medium	3.1
Peach with skin	1 medium	2.3
Vegetables		
Broccoli	1 cup	4.6
Carrot, raw	1 medium	2.3
Tomato	1 medium	2.3
Grains		
Wheat-bran cereal	1 ounce	8
Bulgur wheat	1/2 cup, cooked	5.3
Whole-wheat bread	1 slice	2–3
Brown rice	1/2 cup, cooked	1.7
Spaghetti, enriched white	1/2 cup, cooked	1.1
White bread	1 slice	0.5
White rice	1/2 cup, cooked	0

unchanged through the intestines. The bulk and soft texture of fiber help prevent hard, dry stools that are difficult to pass. People who eat plenty of high-fiber foods are not likely to become constipated. High-fiber diets also need to include plenty of liquids to prevent dehydration. Also, regular exercise helps keep all the body's muscles healthy, including the GI tract muscles, and will help promote regularity.

Although treatment depends on the cause, severity, and duration, in most cases dietary changes help relieve symptoms and prevent constipation.

Diarrhea

Diarrhea—loose, watery stools that occur more than three times in one day—is caused by digestion products moving through the large intestine too rapidly for sufficient water to be reabsorbed.

Diarrhea is a symptom of many disorders that cause increased peristalsis. Culprits include stress, intestinal irritation or damage, and intolerance to gluten (a protein in wheat), fat, or lactose (the natural sugar in milk). Eating food contaminated with bacteria or viruses often causes diarrhea when the digestive tract speeds the offending food along the alimentary canal and out of the body.

Diarrhea can cause dehydration, which means the body lacks enough fluid to function properly. Dehydration is particularly dangerous in children and the elderly, and it must be treated promptly to avoid serious health problems.

A diet of broth, tea, and toast and avoidance of lactose, caffeine, and sorbitol (a carbohydrate found in fruits and also used as a sweetener in

diarrhea Watery stools due to reduced absorption of water.

diverticulosis [dy-vur-tik-yoo-LOH-sis] A condition that occurs when small pouches (diverticula) push outward through weak spots in the colon.

diverticulitis [dy-vur-tik-yoo-LY-tis] A condition that occurs when small pouches in the colon (diverticula) become infected or irritated. Also called left-sided appendicitis.

some sugar-free products) can reduce diarrhea until it subsides. As stools form, you can gradually introduce more foods. Pectin, a form of dietary fiber, may be helpful, along with foods high in potassium—if they are tolerated—to replace lost electrolytes. Fluid replacement is also important to avoid dehydration.

Diverticulosis

Like an inner tube that pokes through weak places in a tire, the colon develops small pouches that bulge outward through weak spots as people age. (See **Figure 4.20**.) Known as **diverticulosis**, this condition afflicts about half of all Americans aged 60 to 80 and almost everyone over age 80. Although it usually causes few problems, in 10 to 25 percent of these people, the pouches become infected or inflamed—a condition called **diverticulitis**.

Diverticulosis and diverticulitis are common in developed or industrialized countries—particularly the United States, England, and Australia—where low-fiber diets are common. Diverticular disease is rare in countries of Asia and Africa, where people eat high-fiber, vegetable-based diets.

A low-fiber diet can make stools hard and difficult to pass. If the stool is too hard, muscles must strain to move it. This is the main cause of increased pressure in the colon, which causes weak spots to bulge outward.

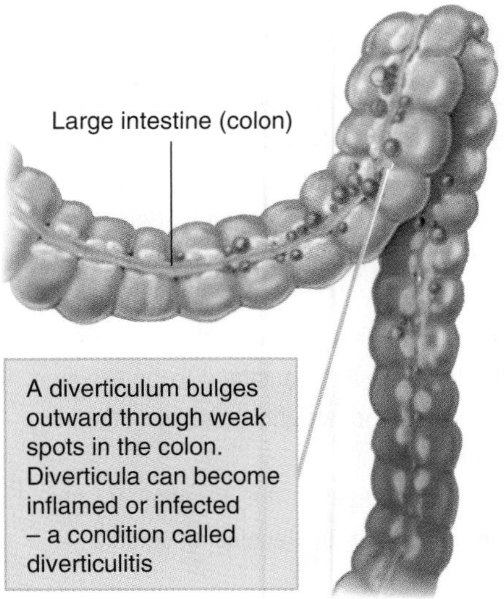
Large intestine (colon)
A diverticulum bulges outward through weak spots in the colon. Diverticula can become inflamed or infected – a condition called diverticulitis

Figure 4.20 **Diverticulosis.** In industrialized nations, diverticulosis is common in older people. It is unusual in developing countries where people eat high-fiber diets.

Fyi — FOR YOUR INFORMATION: Bugs in Your Gut? Health Effects of Intestinal Bacteria

Unseen and unnoticed, millions and millions of bacteria call your GI tract home. Although we often associate bacteria with illness, the right kinds of bacteria in the gut actually protect us from disease. The normal bacterial population of the gut, specifically strains of lactobacilli and bifidobacteria, have been linked to improved digestion, enhanced GI immune function, improved lactose tolerance, and even reduced risk of colon cancer. So how can we be good hosts to our intestinal guests, keeping them well fed and happy? The answer may be in food products and dietary supplements known as probiotics and prebiotics.

Probiotics are foods (or supplements) that contain live microorganisms such as *Lactobacillus acidophilus*. Such lactic-acid-producing bacteria have been used for centuries to break milk down into yogurt, cheeses, and other products. The bacteria convert lactose into lactic acid, which causes the milk to gel and imparts a tart flavor to the product. The resulting product has a much longer shelf life than fresh milk and is associated with good health and longevity in many societies.

The term *prebiotic* describes an indigestible food product that stimulates the growth and/or activity of "good" gut bacteria. For example, it is thought that the composition of breast milk strongly favors the growth of lactobacilli and bifidobacteria in the newborn gut. Some scientists have found bifidobacteria to be the dominant species in breast-fed infants, while the bacterial population of bottle-fed infants is more diverse. The reduced incidence of GI infections in breast-fed infants has been attributed to the dominance of bifidobacteria. Substances that may be effective prebiotics include fructooligosaccharides, galactooligosaccharides, and inulin.

So how does feeding your gut improve your health? Intestinal bacteria metabolize both indigestible and incompletely digested food material. Some types of bacteria produce compounds that may reduce risk of colon cancer. For example, acids produced by colon bacteria change the pH of the colon, and this may interfere with carcinogenesis. "Good" bacteria can digest the lactose that enters the colon of a person with lactose intolerance, reducing symptoms and discomfort. Successful colonization of helpful bacteria allows them to outnumber (and out-eat) disease-causing bacteria, thus reducing the likelihood of foodborne illness.

Fermented milk products such as yogurt or kefir are one way to keep your gut happy. Look for a seal recently adopted by the National Yogurt Association to identify products that contain a minimum of 100 million live lactic acid bacteria per gram of yogurt. Not all brands of yogurt contain live, active cultures. Probiotics in supplement form must have sufficient numbers of live bacteria to be useful; currently, identification and standardization procedures are lacking. Prebiotics such as fructooligosaccharides are the subject of intense and promising research. Although results are preliminary, food and supplement sources of prebiotics may be another useful way to improve gut microflora and overall health.

Table 4.2 Benefits of Dietary Fiber

1. It has a positive impact on weight control because it delays gastric emptying and enhances a feeling of fullness.
2. It improves glucose tolerance by delaying the movement of carbohydrates into the small intestine.
3. It removes cholesterol by binding with bile in the intestine and causing it to be excreted.
4. It increases stool weight, thus promoting regularity.
5. It may protect against the development of colorectal cancer by decreasing colonic transit time.
6. It decreases pressure within the colon.

Increasing the amount of fiber in the diet may reduce symptoms of diverticulosis and prevent complications such as diverticulitis. Fiber keeps stools soft and lowers pressure inside the colon so bowel contents can move through easily (**Table 4.2**).

Until recently, many doctors suggested avoiding foods with small seeds, such as tomatoes or strawberries, because they believed that particles could lodge in the pouches and cause inflammation. However, this is now a controversial point, and no evidence supports this recommendation.

If cramps, bloating, and constipation are problems, the doctor may prescribe a short course of pain medication. However, many medications cause either diarrhea or constipation, undesirable side effects for people with diverticulosis.

Gastroesophageal Reflux

Gastroesophageal reflux disease (GERD) occurs when the sphincter between the esophagus and stomach is weak or relaxes inappropriately, allowing the stomach's contents to flow back into the esophagus. Unlike the stomach, the esophagus has no protective mucous lining, so acid can quickly damage it, causing pain. GERD has a variety of causes, and many treatment strategies involve lifestyle and nutrition.

gastroesophageal reflux disease (GERD) Tissue damage to the esophagus due to the reflux of gastric contents.

irritable bowel syndrome (IBS) A disruptive state of intestinal motility with no known cause.

Doctors recommend avoiding foods and beverages that can weaken the esophageal sphincter, including chocolate, peppermint, fatty foods, coffee, and alcoholic beverages. Foods and beverages that can irritate a damaged esophageal lining, such as citrus fruits and juices, tomato products, and pepper, also should be avoided.

Decreasing both the portion size and the fat content of meals may help. High-fat meals remain in the stomach longer than low-fat meals. This creates back pressure on the esophageal sphincter. Eating meals at least two to three hours before bedtime may reduce reflux problems by allowing partial emptying and a decrease in stomach acidity. Elevating the head of the bed on 6-inch blocks or sleeping on a specially designed wedge reduces heartburn by allowing gravity to minimize reflux of stomach contents into the esophagus.

In addition, cigarette smoking weakens the esophageal sphincter, and being overweight often worsens symptoms. Smokers have various reasons to stop, including GERD, and many overweight people find relief when they lose weight.

Irritable Bowel Syndrome

About 20 percent of people in Western countries suffer from **irritable bowel syndrome (IBS)**,[12] a poorly understood condition that causes abdominal pain, altered bowel habits (such as diarrhea or constipation), and cramps. Often IBS is just a mild annoyance, but for some people it can be disabling.

The cause of IBS remains a mystery, but emotional stress and specific foods clearly aggravate the symptoms in most sufferers.[13] Beans, chocolate, milk products, and large amounts of alcohol are frequent offenders. Fat in any form (animal or vegetable) is a strong stimulus of colonic contractions after a meal. Caffeine causes loose stools in many people, but it is more likely to affect those with IBS. Women with IBS may have more symptoms during their menstrual periods, suggesting that reproductive hormones can increase IBS symptoms.

The good news about IBS is that although its symptoms can be uncomfortable, it does not shorten life span or progress to more serious illness. IBS can usually be controlled with diet and lifestyle modifications, as well as judicious use of medication if needed. Psychiatric treatment, biofeedback, and Transcendental Meditation (a deep relaxation technique) have all been reported to alleviate symptoms in some patients.[14]

Colon Cancer

After lung cancer, colon cancer is the second most common form of cancer in the United States.[15] A diet high in animal fat and low in dietary fiber, which is the typical American diet today, has been linked to colon cancer.[16] A review of the relationships between diet, exercise, and colon cancer suggests that diets high in vegetables and regular physical activity are the most significant factors in reducing risk. Strong evidence shows that physical activity can reduce the risk of colon cancer by up to 50 percent.[17] Some scientists hypothesize that fiber (from vegetables) might bind to potential carcinogens and cause them to be excreted before they can cause harm; others suggest that, in enhancing the movement of materials through the GI tract, exercise or a high-fiber diet reduces the time that carcinogens have to come in contact with colon cells. Other scientists suggest that high levels of antioxidants present in foods such as fruits, grains, and vegetables may help protect the GI tract and delay the development of stomach, colon, and rectal cancer.[18] Alternatively, the breakdown products of fiber produced by colonic bacteria, including acids that lower colon pH, might make carcinogens inactive.

Although these logical reasons point to a beneficial effect of fiber, a major study of women fails to support the protective effect of dietary fiber against colorectal cancer.[19] However, a recent study of 400,000 men and women across nine European countries shows as much as a 40 percent reduction in risk.[20]

flatus Lower intestinal gas that is expelled through the rectum.

Gas

Everyone has gas and eliminates it by burping or passing it through the rectum. Gas is made primarily of odorless vapors. Flatulence has an unpleasant odor because bacteria in the large intestine release small amounts of gases that contain sulfur. Although having gas is common, it can be uncomfortable and embarrassing.

Gas in the stomach is commonly caused by swallowing air. We all swallow small amounts of air when we eat and drink. However, eating or drinking rapidly, chewing gum, smoking, or wearing loose dentures can cause us to take in more air. Burping, or belching, is the way most swallowed air leaves the stomach. The remaining gas moves into the small intestine, where it is partially absorbed. A small amount travels into the large intestine for release through the rectum. (The stomach also releases carbon dioxide when stomach acid and bicarbonate mix, but most of this gas is absorbed into the bloodstream and does not enter the large intestine.)

Frequent passage of rectal gas may be annoying, but it's seldom a symptom of serious disease. **Flatus** (lower intestinal gas) composition depends to a great extent on your carbohydrate intake and the activity of the colon's bacterial population.

Most foods that contain carbohydrates can cause gas. By contrast, fats and proteins cause little gas. In the large intestine, bacteria partially break down undigested carbohydrate, producing hydrogen, carbon dioxide, and,

Quick Bites

Flatulence Facts

Researchers studying pilots and astronauts during the 1960s made some interesting discoveries. The average person inadvertently swallows air with food and drink, and subsequently expels approximately one pint of gas per day, composed of 50 percent nitrogen. Another 40 percent is composed of carbon dioxide and the products of aerobic bacteria in the intestine.

ulcer A craterlike lesion that occurs in the lining of the stomach or duodenum; also called a peptic ulcer to distinguish it from a skin ulcer.

functional dyspepsia Chronic pain in the upper abdomen not due to any obvious physical cause.

in about one-third of people, methane. Eventually these gases exit through the rectum.

Foods that produce gas in one person may not cause gas in another. Some common bacteria in the large intestine can destroy the hydrogen that other bacteria produce. The balance of the two types of bacteria may explain why some people have more gas than others.

Sugars that commonly cause gas are (1) raffinose and stachyose, found in large quantities in beans, (2) fructose, a common sweetener in soft drinks and fruit drinks, (3) lactose, and (4) sorbitol.

Most starches, including potatoes, corn, noodles, and wheat, produce gas as they are broken down in the large intestine. Rice is the only starch that does not cause gas.

Soluble fiber, found in oat bran, beans, peas, and most fruits, is broken down in the large intestine, where digestion causes gas. On the other hand, insoluble fiber, found in wheat bran and some vegetables, passes essentially unchanged through the intestines and produces little gas.

Ulcers

A gnawing, burning pain in the upper abdomen is the classic sign of a peptic **ulcer**, which also can cause nausea, vomiting, loss of appetite, and weight loss. A peptic ulcer is a sore that forms in the duodenum (the beginning of the small intestine) or the lining of the stomach.

Ulcers used to be blamed on stress, particularly in people with "intense" personalities. Diet was also thought to be important, with spicy foods often cast as a major villain. But much to the amazement of most of the medical community, research over the last 10 years has confirmed that infection with the bacterium *Helicobacter pylori* actually causes most ulcers. Use of nonsteroidal anti-inflammatory drugs (NSAIDs), such as aspirin, ibuprofen, and naproxen sodium, is also a common cause of ulcers.

H. pylori causes 80 percent of stomach ulcers and more than 90 percent of duodenal ulcers. These bacteria weaken the protective mucous coating, allowing acid to penetrate to the sensitive lining beneath. Both the acid

Label [to] Table

As you've learned in this chapter, fiber is one of the few things you do not digest fully. Instead, fiber moves through the GI tract, and most of it leaves the body in feces. If it's not digested, then why all the fuss about eating more fiber? You'll learn in Chapter 5, "Carbohydrates," that a healthy intake of fiber may lower your risk of cancer and heart disease and help with bowel regularity. So how do you know which foods have fiber? You have to check out the food label!

This Nutrition Facts panel is from the label on a loaf of whole-wheat bread. The highlighted sections show you that every slice of bread contains 3 grams of fiber. The 12% listed to the right of that refers to the Daily Values below. Look at the Daily Values at the bottom of the label, and note that there are two numbers listed for fiber. One (25 g) is for a person who consumes about 2,000 kilocalories per day, and the other (30 g) is for a 2,500-kilocalorie level. It should be no surprise that if you are consuming more calories, you should also be consuming more fiber. The 12% Daily Value is calculated using the 2,000-kilocalorie fiber guideline as follows:

$$\frac{\text{3 grams fiber per slice}}{\text{25 grams Daily Value}} = .12\text{, or }12\%$$

This means if you make a sandwich with two slices of whole-wheat bread, you're getting 6 grams of fiber and almost one-fourth (24% Daily Value) of your fiber needs per day. Not bad! Be careful, though—many people inadvertently buy wheat bread thinking that it's as high in fiber as whole-wheat bread, but it's not. Whole-wheat bread contains the whole (complete) grain, but wheat bread is usually made of refined wheat flour that has been stripped of its fiber. Check the label before you buy your next loaf of bread!

and the bacteria irritate the lining and cause a sore, or ulcer. *H. pylori* is able to survive in stomach acid because it secretes enzymes that neutralize the acid. This mechanism allows *H. pylori* to make its way to the "safe" area—the protective mucous lining. Once there, the bacterium's spiral shape helps it burrow through the mucous lining.[21]

NSAIDs cause ulcers by interfering with the GI tract's ability to protect itself from acidic stomach juices. Normally the stomach and duodenum employ three defenses against digestive juices: mucus that coats the lining and shields it from stomach acid, the chemical bicarbonate that neutralizes acid, and blood circulation that aids in cell renewal and repair. NSAIDs hinder all these protective mechanisms; with the defenses down, digestive juices can cause ulcers by damaging the sensitive lining of the stomach and duodenum. Fortunately, NSAID-induced ulcers usually heal once the person stops taking the medication.

If you had ulcers in the 1950s, you probably were told to quit your high-stress job and switch to a bland diet. Today, ulcer sufferers usually are treated with a program of antibiotics that can eradicate most cases of *H. pylori*.[22] Although personality and life stress are no longer considered significant factors in the development of most ulcers, relapse after treatment is more common in people who are emotionally stressed or suffering from depression.

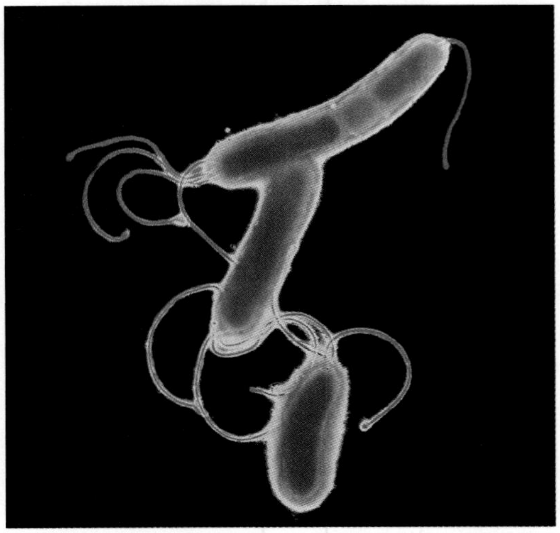

Helicobacter pylori.

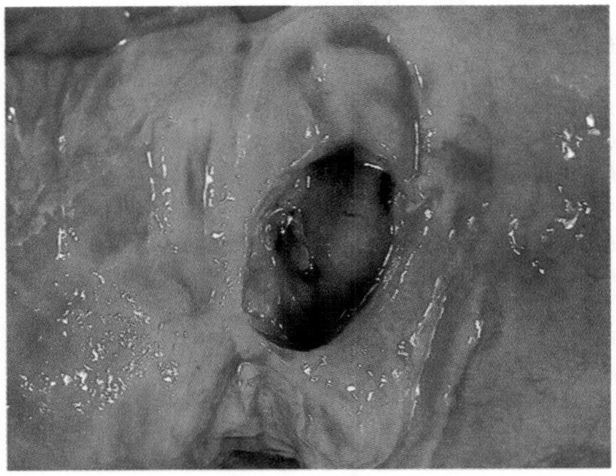

Stomach ulcer.

Functional Dyspepsia

Chronic pain in the upper abdomen that has no obvious physical cause (such as inflammation of the esophagus, peptic ulcer, or gallstones) is referred to as **functional dyspepsia**. As with IBS, the cause of functional dyspepsia is unknown. Hypersensitivity to GI stimuli, abnormal GI motility, and psychosocial problems have all been suggested as causes of dyspepsia.[23] *H. pylori* may also be a factor in some cases of functional dyspepsia.

The treatment of functional dyspepsia includes drugs that speed up the movement of food through the upper part of the intestinal tract, products that decrease stomach acid production, and antibiotics. Just as with IBS,

Nutrition Facts

Serving Size: 1 slice (43g)
Servings Per Container: 16

Calories 100
Calories from Fat 15

Amount Per Serving	% Daily Value*	Amount Per Serving	% Daily Value*
Total Fat 2g	**3%**	**Sodium** 230 mg	**9%**
Saturated Fat 0g	**0%**	**Total Carbohydrate** 18g	**6%**
Polyunsaturated Fat 0g		Dietary Fibers 3g	**12%**
Monounsaturated Fat 0g		Sugars 2g	
Cholesterol 0mg	**0%**	**Protein** 5g	

Vitamin A 0% • Vitamin C 0% • Calcium 6% • Iron 6%
Thiamin 10% • Riboflavin 4% • Niacin 10% • Folate 10%

* Percent Daily Values are based on a 2,000 calorie diet. Your daily values may be higher or lower depending on your calorie needs:

		2,000	2,500
	Calories:	2,000	2,500
Total Fat	Less Than	65g	80g
Sat Fat	Less Than	20g	25g
Cholesterol	Less Than	300mg	300mg
Sodium	Less Than	2,400mg	2,400mg
Total Carbohydrate		300g	375g
Dietary Fiber		25g	30g

INGREDIENTS: STONE GROUND WHOLE WHEAT FLOUR, WATER, HIGH FRUCTOSE CORN SYRUP, WHEAT GLUTEN, WHEAT BRAN. CONTAINS 2% OR LESS OF EACH OF THE FOLLOWING: YEAST, SALT, PARTIALLY HYDROGENATED SOYBEAN OIL, HONEY, MOLASSES, RAISIN JUICE CONCENTRATE, DOUGH CONDITIONERS (MAY CONTAIN ONE OR MORE OF EACH OF THE FOLLOWING: MONO- AND DIGLYCERIDES, CALCIUM AND SODIUM STEAROYL LACTYLATES, CALCIUM PEROXIDE), WHEAT GERM, WHEY, CORNSTARCH, YEAST NUTRIENTS (MONOCALCIUM PHOSPHATE, CALCIUM SULFATE, AMMONIUM SULFATE).

stress-reduction techniques such as meditation and biofeedback can often improve the symptoms of functional dyspepsia.

Key Concepts: *GI disorders generally produce uncomfortable symptoms such as abdominal pain, gas, bloating, and change in elimination patterns. Some GI disorders, such as diarrhea, are generally symptoms of some other illness. Although medications are useful in reducing symptoms, many GI disorders are treatable with changes in diet, especially the addition of adequate fiber and fluids.*

As you have seen, the gastrointestinal tract is the key to turning food and its nutrients into nourishment for our bodies. (See **Figure 4.21**.) A healthy GI tract is an important factor in our overall health and well-being.

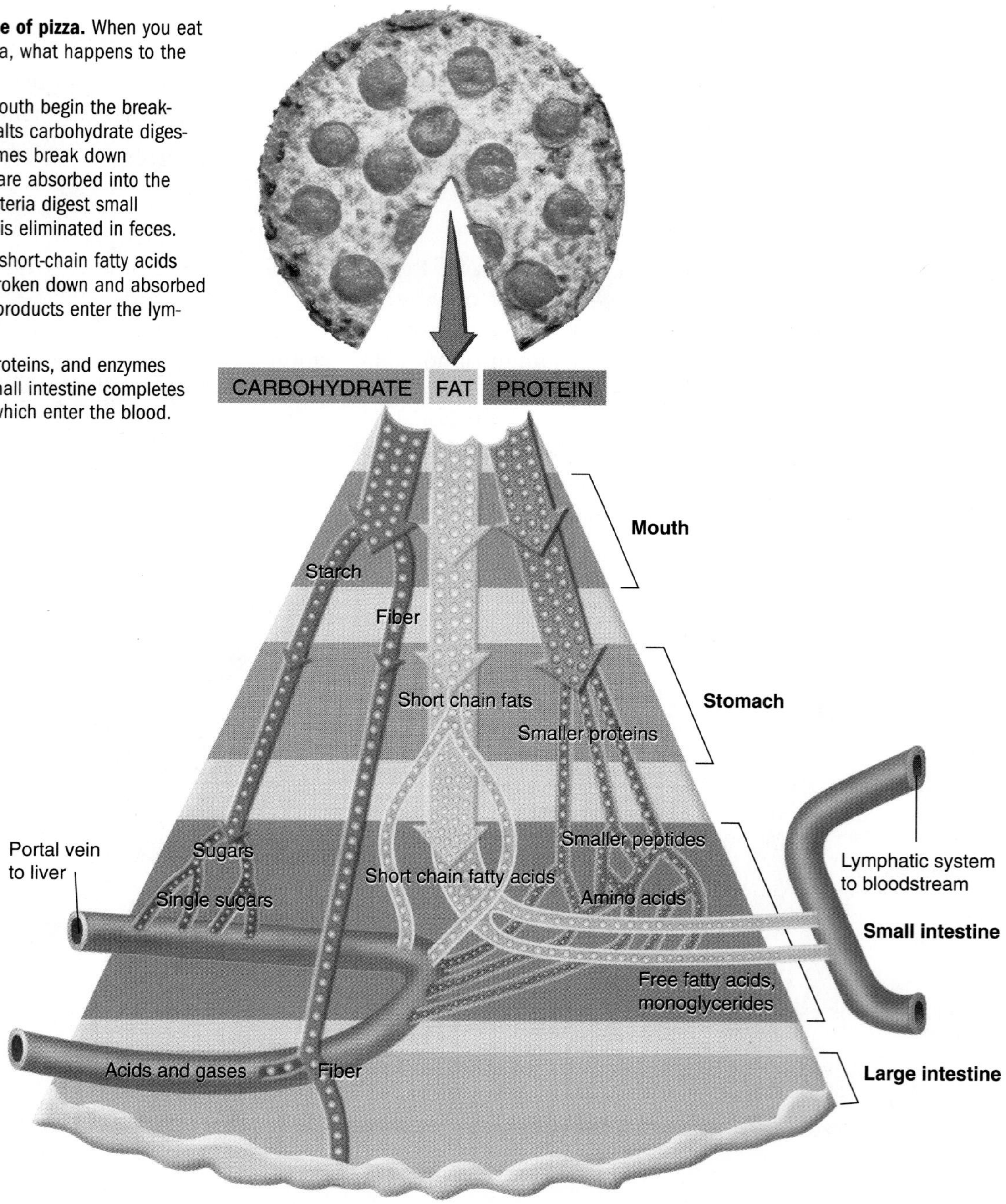

Figure 4.21 **Fate of a piece of pizza.** When you eat a piece of pizza, what happens to the carbohydrate, fat, and protein?

Carbohydrate. Enzymes in the mouth begin the breakdown of starch. Stomach acid halts carbohydrate digestion. In the small intestine, enzymes break down carbohydrate, and the products are absorbed into the blood. In the large intestine, bacteria digest small amounts of fiber. The remainder is eliminated in feces.

Fat. The stomach absorbs a few short-chain fatty acids into the blood. But most fat is broken down and absorbed in the small intestine, where its products enter the lymphatic system.

Protein. Stomach acid unfolds proteins, and enzymes begin protein breakdown. The small intestine completes the breakdown to amino acids, which enter the blood.

LEARNING Portfolio chapter 4

Key Terms

	page
absorption	94
acrolein	112
active transport	99
antibodies	112
antigens	112
autonomic nervous system	111
bile	101
bolus [BOH-lus]	101
catalyze	97
central nervous system (CNS)	111
chyme [KIME]	97
circular muscle	96
colon	106
concentration gradients	99
constipation	113
diarrhea	114
digestion	94
digestive secretions	103
diverticulitis [dy-vur-tik-yoo-LY-tis]	114
diverticulosis [dy-vur-tik-yoo-LOH-sis]	114
duodenum [doo-oh-DEE-num, or doo-ODD-num]	103
elimination	96
emulsifiers	99
enteric nervous system	111
enterohepatic circulation [EN-ter-oh-heh-PAT-ik]	101
enzymes [EN-zimes]	97
esophageal sphincter	101
esophagus [ee-SOFF-uh-gus]	101
excretion	101
facilitated diffusion	99
flatulence	106
flatus	117
functional dyspepsia	119
gallbladder	101
gastric acid	103
gastric lipase	103
gastrin [GAS-trin]	103
gastroesophageal reflux disease (GERD)	116
gastrointestinal (GI) tract [GAS-troh-in-TES-tin-al]	95
heartburn	101
hydrochloric acid	103
hydrolysis	97
ileocecal valve	106
ileum [ILL-ee-um]	103
intrinsic factor	103
irritable bowel syndrome (IBS)	116
jejunum [je-JOON-um]	103
lacteal	106
large intestine	106
lingual lipase	101
liver	101
longitudinal muscle	96
lumen	99
lymph	106
lymphatic system	108
lymphocytes	111
macrophages	111
microvilli	105
mucosa [mu-KO-sa]	96
mucus	99
natural killer cells	111
pancreas	101
passive diffusion	99
pepsin	103
pepsinogen	102
peristalsis [per-ih-STAHL-sis]	97
pH	103
precursor	103
pyloric sphincter [pie-LORE-ic]	103
rectum	106
salivary amylase [AM-ih-lace]	101
salivary glands	99
segmentation	97
small intestine	103
sphincters [SFINGK-ters]	96
stomach	101
ulcer	118
vascular system	107
villi	104

Study Points

- **The GI tract is a tube that can be divided into regions: the mouth, esophagus, stomach, small intestine, large intestine, and rectum.**
- **Digestion and absorption of the nutrients in foods occur at various sites along the GI tract.**
- **Digestion involves both physical processes (e.g., chewing, peristalsis, and segmentation) and chemical processes (e.g., the hydrolytic action of enzymes).**
- **Absorption is the movement of molecules across the lining of the GI tract and into circulation.**
- **The major mechanisms involved in nutrient absorption are passive diffusion, facilitated diffusion, and active transport.**
- **In the mouth, food is mixed with saliva for lubrication. Salivary amylase begins the digestion of starch.**
- **Acid and enzyme secretions from the stomach lower the pH of stomach contents and begin the digestion of proteins.**
- **The pancreas and gallbladder secrete material into the small intestine to help with digestion.**
- **Most chemical digestion and nutrient absorption occur in the small intestine.**
- **Electrolytes and water are absorbed from the large intestine. Remaining material, waste, is excreted as feces.**
- **Both the nervous system and hormonal system regulate GI tract processes.**
- **Numerous factors affect GI tract functioning, including psychological, chemical, and bacterial factors.**
- **Problems that occur along the GI tract can affect digestion and absorption of nutrients. Dietary changes are important in the treatment of GI disorders.**

Study Questions

Answers can be found at nutrition.jbpub.com/discovering.

1. **The contents of which organ have the lowest pH? What organ produces an alkaline or basic solution to buffer this low pH?**
2. **What is the purpose of mucus in the GI tract? What would happen if it didn't line the stomach?**
3. **Where in the GI tract does the majority of nutrient digestion and absorption take place?**
4. **List the organs (in order) that make up the GI tract.**
5. **Name three "assisting" organs that are not part of the GI tract but are needed for proper digestion. What are their roles in digestion?**
6. **What is gastroesophageal reflux?**

Try This

The Saltine Cracker Experiment

This experiment will help you understand the effect of salivary amylase. Remember, salivary amylase is the starch-digesting enzyme produced by the salivary glands. Chew two saltine crackers until a watery texture forms in your mouth. You have to fight the urge to swallow so you can pay attention to the taste of the crackers. Do you notice a change in the taste?

The crackers first taste salty and "starchy," but as amylase is secreted it begins to break the chains of starch into sugar. As it does this, the saltines begin to taste sweet like animal crackers!

What About Bobbie?

Because both fluid and fiber are important for a healthy gastrointestinal tract, let's check out Bobbie's intake of these. Refresh yourself with her day of eating (see Chapter 1). How do you think Bobbie did in terms of fiber? She did pretty well! At 24 grams of fiber, she's just right in the recommended range of 20 to 35 grams per day. Here are her best fiber sources:

Food	Fiber Grams
Spaghetti (pasta)	*3.5*
Tortilla chips	*3*
Banana	*3*
Salsa	*2*
Green beans	*2*

Are you surprised by the tortilla chips and the amount of fiber they add? Don't misinterpret this to mean that tortilla chips are a great source of fiber. There are two reasons why the chips rank so high. First, the other grain choices were not whole wheat and therefore didn't contribute a lot of fiber. Second, her afternoon snack consisted of over 200 kilocalories of tortilla chips.

What could Bobbie have done differently if she wanted to reach the high end of the recommended range? Here are a few small changes that would add more fiber.

- By choosing a whole-wheat bagel, she'd add 4 grams of fiber.
- By having her sandwich on whole-wheat bread, she'd add at least 3 grams of fiber.
- By substituting the 2 tablespoons of croutons with 2 more tablespoons of kidney beans, she'd add 1.5 grams of fiber.
- If she ate another piece of fruit as a snack sometime during the day, it would add 1 to 3 grams of fiber.

Now let's look at Bobbie's fluid intake. Remember, when you increase your fiber intake, you need to increase your fluid intake so you don't become constipated. Here's a list of Bobbie's drinks:

Breakfast—10 ounces coffee

Snack—none

Lunch—12 ounces diet soda

Snack—16 ounces water

Dinner—12 ounces diet soda

Snack—none

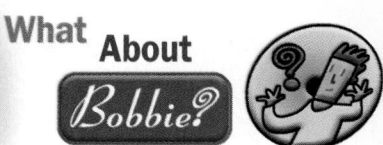

How do you think she did? Her total fluid intake is 50 ounces (about 1,500 mL), which, along with the fluids found in her foods, may be enough to meet her recommended fluid intake. (See Chapter 10, "Water and Minerals.") However, three of her four beverages contain caffeine—a diuretic that causes water loss. So her overall intake of fluids may not be enough to handle her fiber intake and keep her GI contents moving smoothly.

What suggestions do you have that will increase Bobbie's fluid intake? Any of the following would work:

- Carry a water bottle to sip throughout the day.
- Wash down the morning banana snack with a cup or two of water.
- Consider decaffeinated coffee or decaffeinated soda.
- Drink more water with the tortilla chips in the afternoon.
- Add another beverage at dinner.
- Drink water with the piece of pizza at night.

References

1 Mattes RD. Physiologic responses to sensory stimulation by food: nutritional implications. *J Am Diet Assoc.* 1997;97:406–410.

2 Klein S, Cohn SM, Alpers DH. The alimentary tract in nutrition. In: Shils ME, Olson JA, Shike M, Ross AC, eds. *Modern Nutrition in Health and Disease.* 9th ed. Baltimore: Williams & Wilkins; 1998:605–629.

3 Guyton AC, Hall JE. *Textbook of Medical Physiology.* 10th ed. Philadelphia: W.B. Saunders; 2000.

4 Yamada T, Alper DH. *Textbook of Gastroenterology.* New York: JB Lippincott; 1995.

5 Klein S, Cohn SM, Alpers DH. The alimentary tract in nutrition. Op. cit.

6 Scheppach W, Luehrs H, Menzel T. Beneficial health effects of low-digestible carbohydrate consumption. *Br J Nutr.* 2001;85 (suppl 1):S23–S30.

7 Guyton AC, Hall JE. Op. cit.

8 Yamada T, Alper DH. Op. cit.

9 Guyton AC, Hall JE. Op. cit.

10 Mahan LK, Escott-Stump S. *Krause's Food Nutrition and Diet Therapy.* 10th ed. Philadelphia: W.B. Saunders; 2000.

11 *Toxicological Profile for Acrolein.* Atlanta, GA: US Public Health Service, US Department of Health and Human Services, Agency for Toxic Substances and Disease Registry (ATSDR); 1989.

12 Ringel Y, Sperber AD, Drossman DA. Irritable bowel syndrome. *Annu Rev Med.* 2001;52:319–338.

13 Clouse RE. Anxiety and gastrointestinal illness. *Psychiatr Clin North Am.* 1988;11:399–417; Dancey CP, Taghavi M, Fox RJ. The relationship between daily stress and symptoms of irritable bowel: a time-series approach. *J Psychosom Res.* 1998;44:537–45; and Jarrett M, Heitkemper M, Cain KC, et al. The relationship between psychological distress and gastrointestinal symptoms in women with irritable bowel syndrome. *Nurs Res.* 1998;47:154–161.

14 Mine K, Kanazawa F, Hosoi M, et al. Treating nonulcer dyspepsia considering both functional disorders of the digestive system and psychiatric conditions. *Dig Dis Sci.* 1998;43: 1241–1247; and Lembo T, Munakata J, Merz H, et al. Evidence for the hypersensitivity of lumbar splanchnic afferents in irritable bowel syndrome. *Gastroenterology.* 1994;107:1686–1696.

15 *Prevention of Colon Cancer.* American Cancer Society; 1998.

16 Slattery ML, Boucher KM, Caan BJ, et al. Eating patterns and risk of colon cancer. *Am J Epidemiol.* 1998;148:4–16.

17 Peters HP, De Vries WR, Vanberg-Henegouwen GP, Akkermans LM. Potential benefits and hazards of physical activity and exercise on the gastrointestinal tract. *Gut.* 2001;48:435–439.

18 Halliwell B, Zhao K, Whiteman M. The gastrointestinal tract: a major site of antioxidant action? *Free Radic Res.* 2001;33: 819–830.

19 Fuchs CS, Giovannucci EL, Coldiz GA, et al. Dietary fiber and the risk of colorectal cancer and adenoma in women. *N Engl J Med.* 1999;340:169–176.

20 Bingham S, Day N. European prospective investigation of cancer and nutrition (EPIC). Presented at the European Conference on Nutrition and Care; June 21–24, 2001; Lyon, France.

21 *Helicobacter pylori* in peptic ulcer disease. NIH Consensus Statement. 1994;12:1–23.

22 Williamson JS. *Helicobacter pylori:* current chemotherapy and new targets for drug design. *Curr Pharm Des.* 2001;7:355–392.

23 Wiklund J, Butler-Wheelhouse P. Psychosocial factors and their role in symptomatic gastroesophageal reflux disease and functional dyspepsia. *Scand J Gastroenterol.* 1996;220(suppl): 94–100.

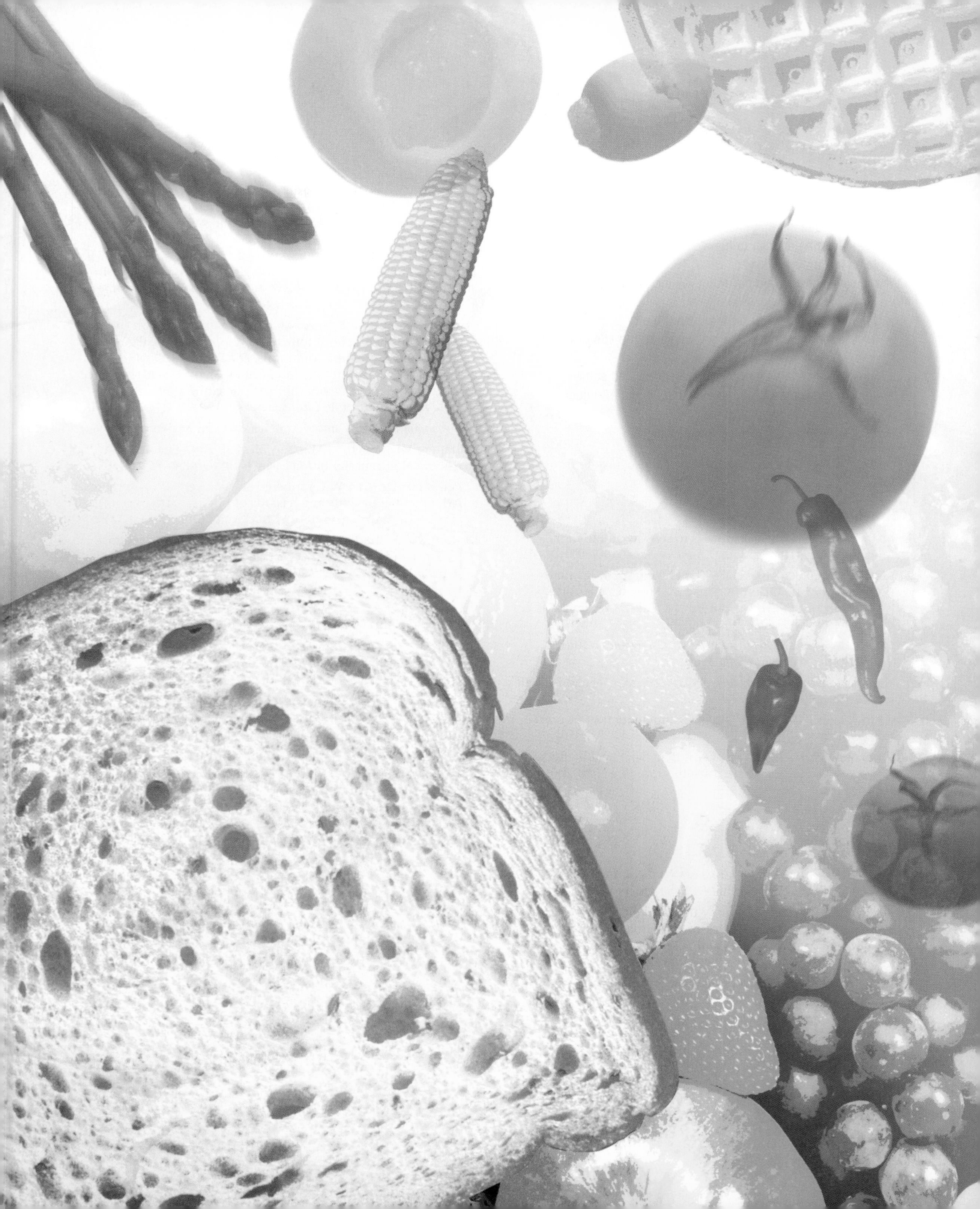

Chapter 5

Carbohydrates: Simple Sugars and Complex Chains

Think About It

1. When you think of the word *carbohydrate,* what foods come to mind?
2. How satisfied are you with your fiber intake?
3. Many people choose honey instead of white sugar because they think it's more "natural" and therefore more nutritious. What do you think?
4. Do you prefer artificial sweeteners to sugar? Explain your preference.

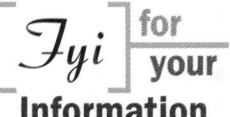

Fyi for your Information

This chapter's FYI boxes include practical information on the following topics:

- The Glycemic Index of Foods: Useful or Useless?
- Unfounded Claims against Sugars

www

The Web site for this book offers many useful tools and is a great source for additional nutrition information for both students and instructors. For information on carbohydrates, visit the site at **nutrition.jbpub.com/discovering.** You'll find exercises that explore the following topics:

- Aspartame: Your Friend or Foe?
- Are You in the Carbohydrate Zone?
- Constant Craving?

Key to Illustrations

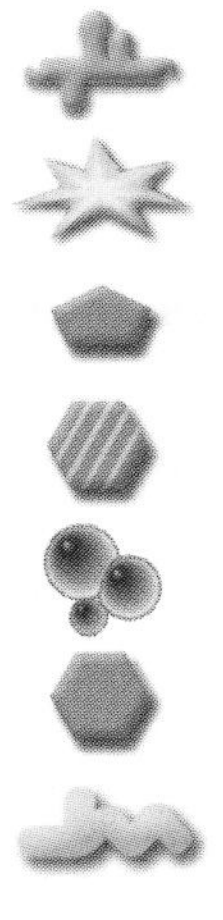

- Amino Acids
- Energy
- Fructose
- Galactose
- Gas
- Glucose
- Short-Chain Fatty Acids

What About Bobbie?

Track the choices Bobbie is making with the EatRight Analysis software.

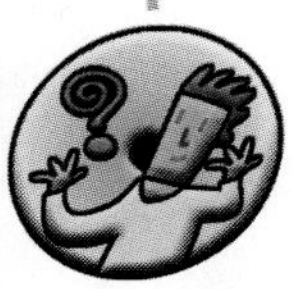

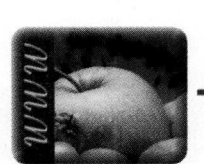

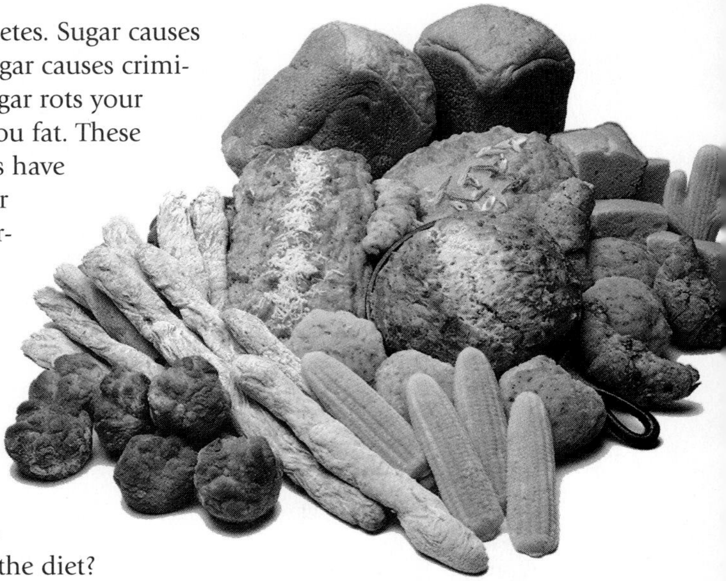

Sugar causes diabetes. Sugar causes hyperactivity. Sugar causes criminal behavior. Sugar rots your teeth. Starches make you fat. These and many other claims have been made about sugar and starch—dietary carbohydrates—over the years. But where do these claims come from? What is myth and what is fact? What links, if any, are there between carbohydrates in your diet and health? Are carbohydrates important in the diet?

Most of the world's people depend on carbohydrate-rich plant foods for daily sustenance. Carbohydrates contain 4 kilocalories per gram, and in some countries they supply 80 percent or more of daily calorie intake. Rice provides the bulk of the diet in Southeast Asia, as does corn in South America, cassava in certain parts of Africa, and wheat in Europe and North America. (See **Figure 5.1**.) Besides providing energy, foods rich in carbohydrates, such as whole grains, legumes, fruits, and vegetables, are also good sources of vitamins, minerals, dietary fiber, and phytochemicals that can help lower the risk of chronic diseases.

Think About It 1

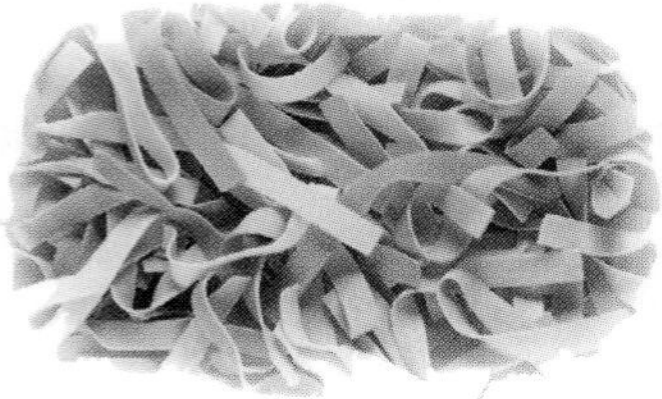

Quick Bites

Is Pasta a Chinese Food?

Noodles were used in China as early as the first century; Marco Polo did not bring them to Italy until the 1300s.

Carbohydrates Capture Energy from the Sun

Plants produce carbohydrates (and oxygen) through photosynthesis—using carbon dioxide from the air, water from the soil, and energy from the sun.[1] The two main types of carbohydrates in food are simple carbohydrates (sugars) and complex carbohydrates (starches and dietary fiber).

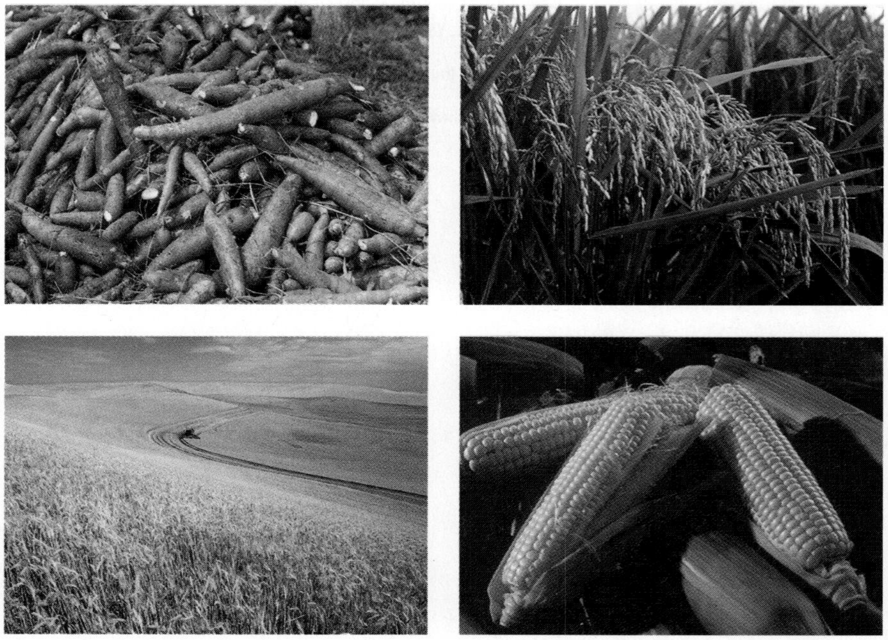

Figure 5.1 **Cassava, rice, wheat, and corn.** These carbohydrate-rich foods are dietary staples in many parts of the world.

Simple Sugars: Monosaccharides and Disaccharides

Simple carbohydrates are naturally present as simple sugars in fruits, milk, and other foods. Plant carbohydrates also can be refined to produce sugar products such as table sugar or corn syrup. The two main types of sugars are monosaccharides and disaccharides. **Monosaccharides** consist of a single sugar molecule (*mono* meaning "one" and *saccharide* meaning "sugar"). **Disaccharides** consist of two sugar molecules chemically joined together (*di* meaning "two"). Monosaccharides and disaccharides give various degrees of sweetness to foods.

simple carbohydrates Sugars composed of a single sugar molecule (a monosaccharide) or two joined sugar molecules (a disaccharide).

monosaccharides Single sugar units. The common monosaccharides are glucose, fructose, and galactose.

disaccharides [dye-SACK-uh-rides] Carbohydrates composed of two monosaccharide units chemically linked. They include sucrose (common table sugar), lactose (milk sugar), and maltose.

glucose [GLOO-kose] A common monosaccharide that is a component of disaccharides (sucrose, lactose, and maltose) and various complex carbohydrates; present in the blood and also known as dextrose.

fructose [FROOK-tose] A common monosaccharide naturally present in honey and many fruits. Also called levulose or fruit sugar.

galactose [gah-LAK-tose] A monosaccharide that has a structure similar to glucose; usually joined with other monosaccharides.

Monosaccharides: The Single Sugars

The most common monosaccharides in the human diet are

- glucose
- fructose
- galactose

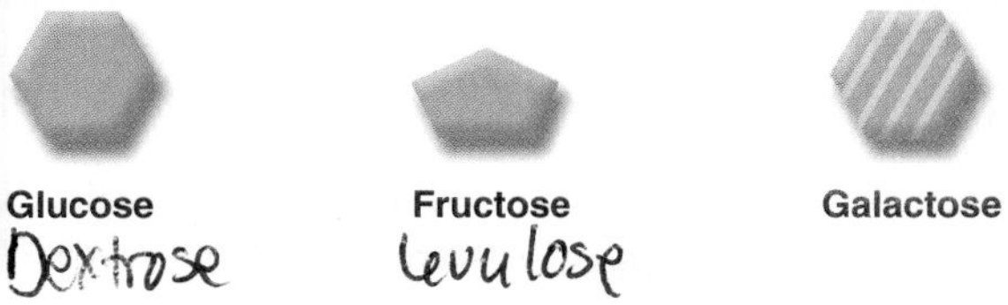

Glucose

The monosaccharide glucose is the most abundant simple carbohydrate unit in nature. Also referred to as dextrose, **glucose** plays a key role in both foods and the body. Glucose gives food a mildly sweet flavor. It doesn't usually exist as a monosaccharide in food but is instead joined to other sugars to form disaccharides, starch, or dietary fiber. Glucose makes up at least one of the two sugar molecules in every disaccharide.

In the body, glucose supplies energy to cells. The body closely regulates blood glucose (blood sugar) levels to assure a constant fuel source for vital body functions. Glucose is virtually the only fuel used by the brain, except during prolonged starvation when the glucose supply is low.

Fructose

Also called levulose or fruit sugar, **fructose** tastes the sweetest of all the sugars—it is what commonly sweetens colas and other soft drinks. It occurs naturally in fruits and vegetables. Although the sugar in honey is about half fructose and half glucose, fructose is the primary source of the sweet taste. Food manufacturers use high-fructose corn syrup as an additive to sweeten many foods, including soft drinks, desserts, candies, jellies, and jams. Fructose currently provides about 5 percent of people's energy intake in the United States.[2]

Galactose

Galactose rarely occurs as a monosaccharide in food. It usually is chemically bonded to glucose to form lactose, the primary sugar in milk.

Disaccharides: The Double Sugars

Disaccharides consist of two monosaccharides linked together. The following disaccharides (see **Figure 5.2**) are important in human nutrition:

- sucrose (common table sugar)
- lactose (major sugar in milk)
- maltose (product of starch digestion)

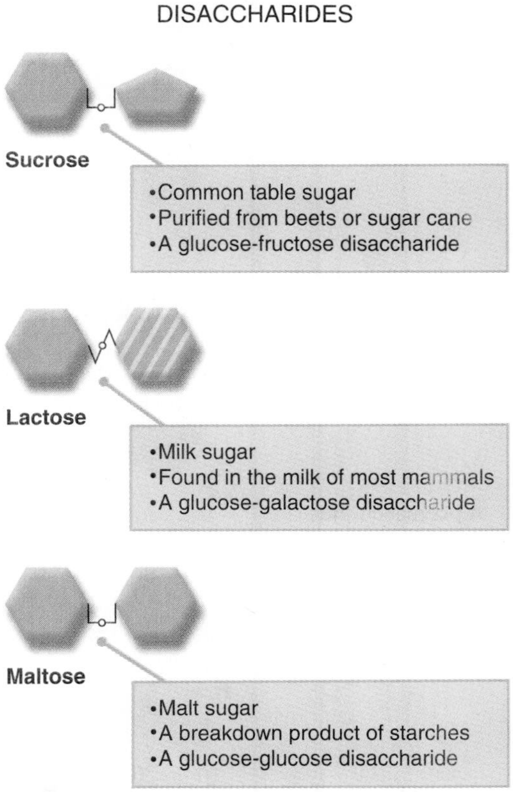

Figure 5.2 **The disaccharides: sucrose, lactose, and maltose.** The three monosaccharides pair up in different combinations to form the three disaccharides.

sucrose [SOO-crose] A disaccharide composed of glucose and fructose; also known as table sugar.

lactose [LAK-tose] A disaccharide composed of glucose and galactose; also called milk sugar.

maltose [MALL-tose] A disaccharide composed of two glucose molecules; sometimes called malt sugar. Maltose seldom occurs naturally in foods but is formed whenever long molecules of starch break down.

complex carbohydrates Chains of more than two monosaccharides. May be oligosaccharides or polysaccharides.

oligosaccharides Short carbohydrate chains composed of 3 to 10 sugar molecules.

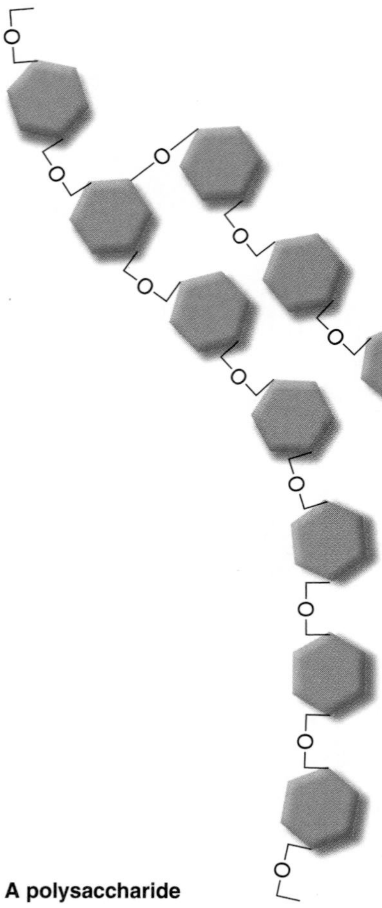

A polysaccharide

Sucrose

Sucrose, most familiar to us as table sugar, is made up of one molecule of glucose and one molecule of fructose. Sucrose provides some of the natural sweetness of honey, maple syrup, fruits, and vegetables. Manufacturers use a refining process to extract sucrose from the juices of sugar cane or sugar beets. Full refining removes impurities; white sugar and powdered sugar are so highly refined they are virtually 100 percent sucrose. When a food label lists sugar as an ingredient, the term refers to sucrose.

Lactose

Lactose, or milk sugar, is composed of one molecule of glucose and one molecule of galactose. Lactose gives milk and other dairy products a slightly sweet taste. Human milk has a higher concentration of lactose than cow's milk, so human milk tastes sweeter than cow's milk.

Maltose

Maltose is composed of two glucose molecules. Maltose seldom occurs naturally in foods, but forms whenever long molecules of starch break down. Human digestive enzymes in the mouth and small intestine break starch down into maltose. When you chew a slice of fresh bread, you may detect a slightly sweet taste as starch breaks down into maltose. Starch also breaks down into maltose in germinating seeds. Maltose is fermented in the production of beer.

Key Concepts: *Carbohydrates can be categorized as simple or complex. Simple carbohydrates include monosaccharides and disaccharides. The monosaccharides glucose, fructose, and galactose are single sugar molecules. The disaccharides sucrose, lactose, and maltose are double sugar molecules.*

Complex Carbohydrates

Complex carbohydrates are chains of more than two sugar molecules. Short carbohydrate chains are called **oligosaccharides** (*oligo* meaning "scant") and contain 3 to 10 sugar molecules. Long carbohydrate chains, known as **polysaccharides** (*poly* meaning "many"), can contain hundreds or even thousands of monosaccharide units. Some polysaccharides form straight chains, while others branch off in all directions. These structural differences affect how the polysaccharide behaves in water and with heating. The way the monosaccharides are linked to form the polysaccharides makes them digestible (e.g., starch) or indigestible (e.g., dietary fiber).

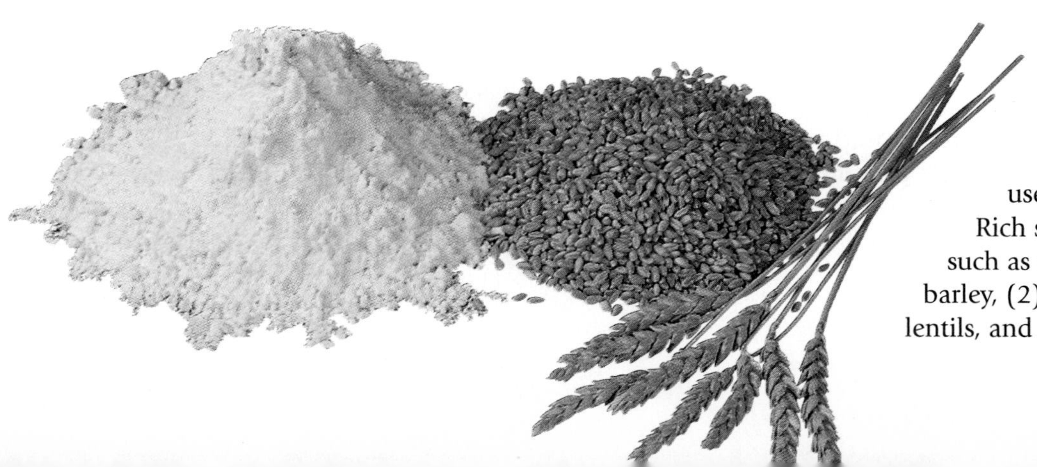

Starch

Plants store energy as **starch** for use during growth and reproduction. Rich sources of starch include (1) grains such as wheat, rice, corn, oats, millet, and barley, (2) legumes such as peas, beans, and lentils, and (3) tubers such as potatoes, yams, and cassava. Starch gives food a moist, gelatinous texture. For example, it makes the inside of a baked potato moist, thick, and almost sticky. The starch in flour absorbs moisture and thickens gravy.

Starch takes two main forms in plants: amylose and amylopectin. **Amylose** is made up of long, unbranched chains of glucose molecules, while **amylopectin** is made up of branched chains of glucose molecules. (See **Figure 5.3**.) There is usually three to four times as much amylopectin in plants as amylose, although this proportion can vary.[3]

Although the body easily digests most starches, a small portion of the starch in plants may remain enclosed in cell structures and escape digestion in the small intestine. Starch that is not digested is called **resistant starch**.[4] Some legumes, such as white beans, contain large amounts of resistant starch.[5]

Glycogen

Living animals, including humans, store carbohydrate in the form of **glycogen**, also called animal starch. When we slaughter animals for meat, their tissue enzymes break down most glycogen within 24 hours. While some organ meats, such as kidney, heart, and liver, contain small amounts of carbohydrate, meat from muscle contains none.[6] Since plant foods also contain no glycogen, it is a negligible carbohydrate source in our diets. Glycogen does, however, play an important role in our bodies, providing glucose when blood glucose levels get low.

Glycogen is composed of long, highly branched chains of glucose molecules. Its structure is similar to that of the plant starch amylopectin, but glycogen is much more highly branched. (See **Figure 5.3**.) When we need extra glucose, glycogen is broken down rapidly into single glucose molecules. But, since enzymes can only attack the ends of glycogen chains, the highly branched structure of glycogen offers an increased number of sites for enzyme activity.

Most glycogen is stored in skeletal muscle and the liver. In muscle cells, glycogen provides a supply of glucose for strenuous muscular activity. Liver cells use glycogen to regulate blood glucose levels. Normally, the body can store only about 200 to 500 grams of glycogen at a time.[7] Some athletes "load" carbohydrates by gradually tapering off rigorous training and emphasizing high-carbohydrate meals for a few days to one week before they compete. This can increase the amount of stored glycogen by about 50 percent, providing a competitive edge for marathon running and other endurance events.[8] (See Chapter 11, "Sports Nutrition.")

Dietary Fibers

Dietary fibers give plant cell walls their structure and also are found inside plant cells. All types of plant foods—including fruits, vegetables, legumes, and whole grains—contain fiber. Dietary fibers often resemble starches, but human digestive enzymes cannot break down fiber.[9] Dietary fibers include oligosaccharides and the nonstarch polysaccharides cellulose, hemicellulose, pectins, gums, and mucilages. Other types of dietary fiber, such as lignins, cutins, and waxes, are not polysaccharides. Food manufacturers add certain fibers to food products to thicken and stabilize them.

In the past, dietary fibers have been classified based on results of different methods to analyze fibers or by certain physical properties. The terms

polysaccharides Long carbohydrate chains composed of more than 10 sugar molecules. Polysaccharides can be straight or branched.

starch The major storage form of carbohydrate in plants; starch is composed of long chains of glucose molecules in a straight (amylose) or branching (amylopectin) arrangement.

amylose [AM-uh-los] A straight-chain polysaccharide composed of glucose units.

amylopectin [am-ih-low-PEK-tin] A branched-chain polysaccharide composed of glucose units.

resistant starch Starch that is not digested.

glycogen [GLY-ko-jen] A very large, highly branched polysaccharide composed of multiple glucose units. Sometimes called animal starch, glycogen is the primary storage form of glucose in animals.

dietary fibers The nondigestible carbohydrates and lignin found intact in plants.

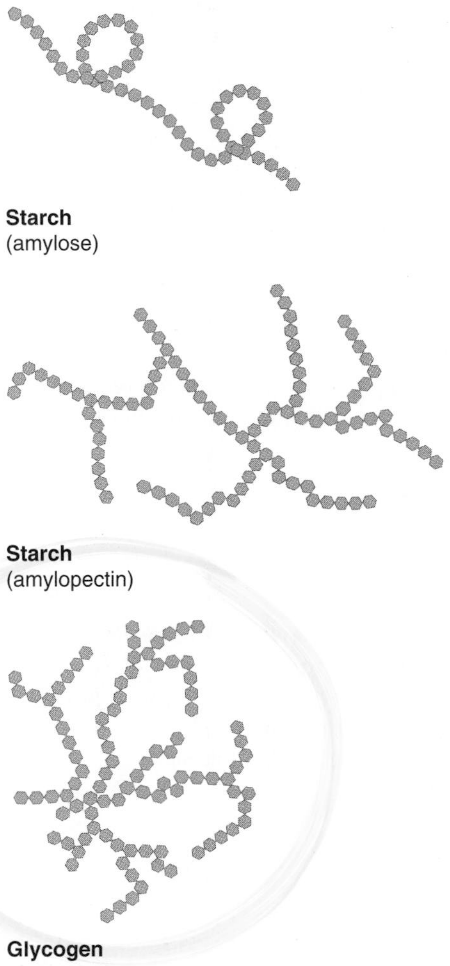

Figure 5.3 **Starch and glycogen.** Plants have two main types of starch—amylose, which has long unbranched chains of glucose, and amylopectin, which has branched chains. Animals store glucose in highly branched chains called glycogen.

soluble fiber Dietary fiber components that dissolve in water, including pectins, gums, mucilages, and some hemicelluloses.

insoluble fiber Dietary fiber components that do not dissolve in water, including cellulose, lignin, and some hemicelluloses.

added fiber The isolated nondigestible carbohydrates added to foods, which have beneficial physiological effects in humans.

soluble fiber and **insoluble fiber** reflect the ability of different fibers to dissolve in water.[10] As part of its review of fiber for the development of recommended intake levels, the Food and Nutrition Board has developed new definitions for dietary fiber and **added fiber**.[11] While dietary fiber is present naturally in plants, added fiber refers to isolated nondigestible carbohydrates added to foods. Both types have beneficial physiological effects that include laxation (fecal bulking and softening; increased frequency; and/or regularity) and positive adjustments of blood cholesterol or blood glucose levels.

Only plant foods contain dietary fiber. Foods rich in dietary fiber include whole-grain foods such as brown rice, rolled oats, and whole-wheat breads and cereals; legumes such as kidney beans, garbanzo beans (chickpeas), peas, and lentils; fruits; and vegetables. (See **Table 5.1**.) Cereal grains, such as wheat bran, promote normal bowel function and regularity. Psyllium, derived from the husk of blonde psyllium seed, is a fiber used in the laxative Metamucil. The fiber from psyllium and oats has been shown to help lower blood cholesterol levels[12] and is being added to some breakfast cereals for this purpose. (For more on this, see the later section on "Carbohydrates and Health.")

Table 5.1 Foods Rich in Dietary Fiber

Fruits	
Apples	Grapefruit
Bananas	Mango
Berries	Oranges
Cherries	Pears
Cranberries	
Vegetables	
Asparagus	Green peppers
Broccoli	Red cabbage
Brussels sprouts	Spinach
Carrots	Sprouts
Nuts and Seeds	
Almonds	Sesame seeds
Peanuts	Sunflower seeds
Pecans	Walnuts
Legumes	
Most legumes	
Grains	
Brown rice	Wheat-bran cereals
Oat bran	Whole-wheat breads
Oatmeal	

Source: Adapted from Shils ME, Olson JA, Shike M, Ross AC, eds. *Modern Nutrition in Health and Disease.* 9th ed. Philadelphia: Lippincott Williams & Wilkins; 1999.

Oligosaccharides

Dried beans, peas, and lentils contain the two most common oligosaccharides—raffinose and stachyose.[13] Raffinose is formed from three monosaccharide molecules—one galactose, one glucose, and one fructose. Stachyose is formed from four monosaccharide molecules—three galactose and one fructose. The body cannot break down raffinose or stachyose, but they are readily metabolized by intestinal bacteria and are responsible for the familiar gaseous effects of foods such as beans.

Human milk contains more than one hundred different oligosaccharides, which vary according to how long a woman has been pregnant, how long she has been nursing, and her genetic makeup.[14] For breast-fed infants, oligosaccharides work as dietary fiber does in adults—making stools easier to pass. Some of these oligosaccharides also protect infants from disease-causing agents by binding to them in the intestine. Oligosaccharides in human milk may also provide sialic acid, which is essential for normal brain development.[15]

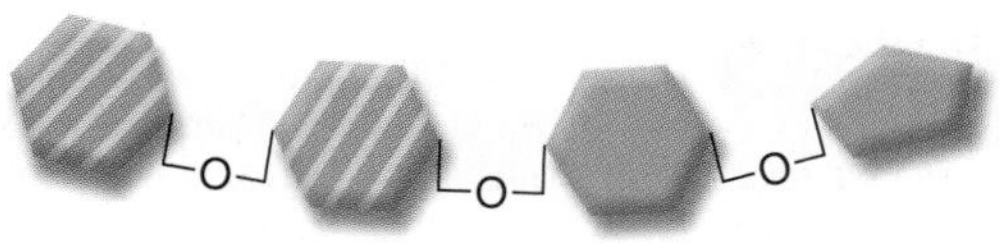

Stachyose

Cellulose

In plants, **cellulose** makes the walls of cells strong and rigid. It forms the woody fibers that support tall trees. It also forms the brittle shafts of hay and straw and the stringy threads in celery. Cellulose is made up of long, straight chains of glucose molecules. (See **Figure 5.4**.)

Hemicelluloses

The **hemicelluloses** are a diverse group of polysaccharides that vary from plant to plant. They are mixed with cellulose in plant cell walls.[16] Hemicelluloses are composed of a variety of monosaccharides with many branching side chains. The outer bran layer on many cereal grains is rich in hemicelluloses, as are whole-grain cereals and food products.

Pectins

Found in all plants, but especially in fruits, **pectins** are gel-forming polysaccharides. In fruits, pectin acts like a cement that gives the fruit body and

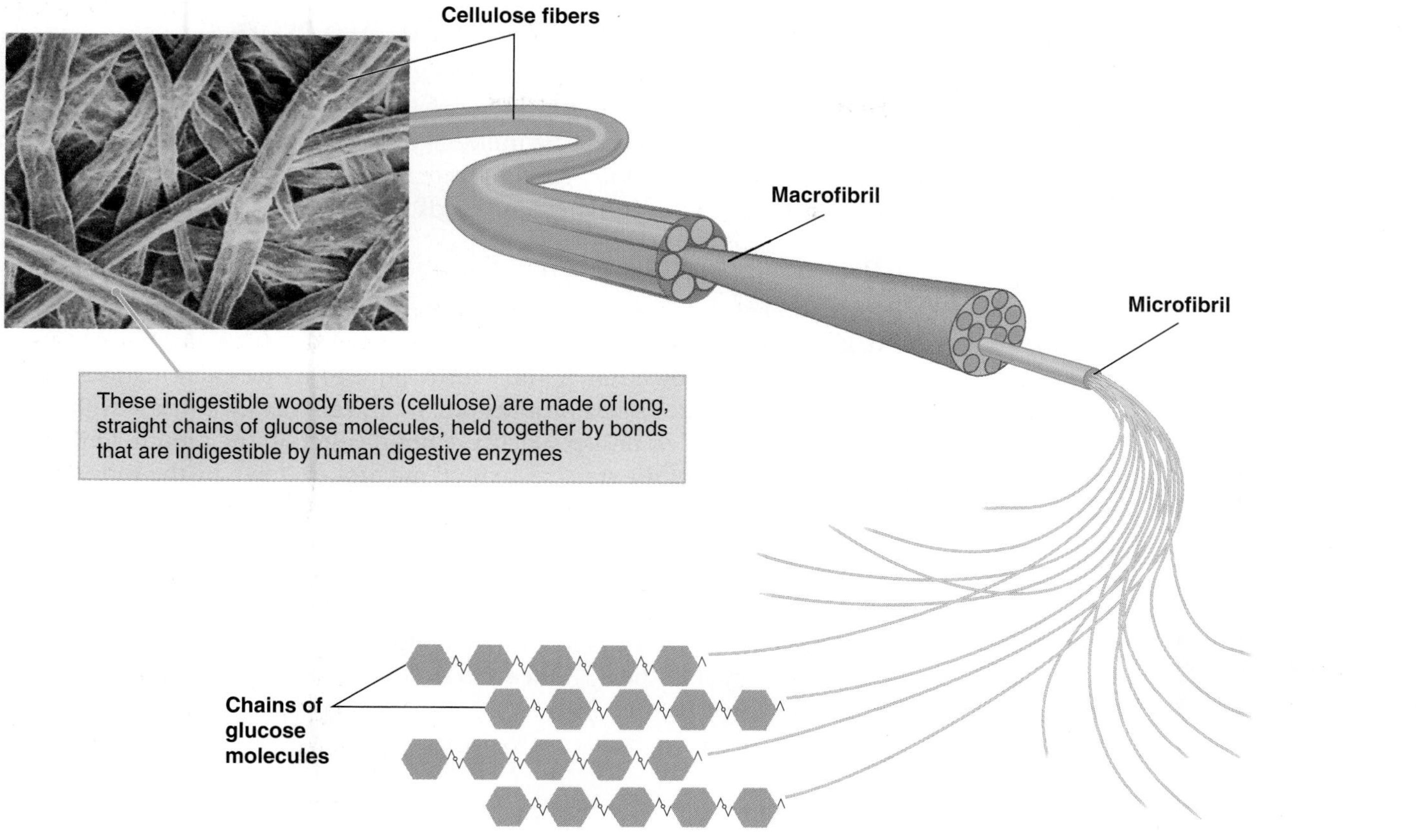
Cellulose fibers
Macrofibril
Microfibril
These indigestible woody fibers (cellulose) are made of long, straight chains of glucose molecules, held together by bonds that are indigestible by human digestive enzymes
Chains of glucose molecules

Figure 5.4 **The structure of cellulose.** Cellulose forms the indigestible, fibrous component of plants and is part of grasses, trees, fruits, and vegetables.

helps keep its shape. When fruit becomes overripe, pectin breaks down into monosaccharides, and the fruit becomes mushy. Mixed with sugar and acid, pectin forms a gel that the food industry uses to add firmness to jellies, jams, sauces, and salad dressings.

Gums and Mucilages

Like pectin, **gums** and **mucilages** are thick, gel-forming fibers that help hold plant cells together. The food industry uses plant gums (gum arabic, guar gum, locust bean gum, and xanthan gum, for example) and mucilages (such as carrageenan) to thicken, stabilize, or add texture to foods such as salad dressings, puddings, pie fillings, candies, sauces, and even drinks.

Lignins

Not actually carbohydrates, **lignins** are indigestible substances that make up the woody parts of vegetables such as carrots and broccoli and the seeds of fruits such as strawberries.

Key Concepts: *Complex carbohydrates include starch, glycogen, and dietary fiber. Starch is composed of straight or branched chains of glucose molecules and is the storage form of energy in plants. Glycogen is composed of highly branched chains of glucose molecules and is the storage form of energy in animals. Dietary fibers include many different substances that cannot be digested by enzymes in the human intestinal tract and are found in plant foods such as whole grains, legumes, vegetables, and fruits.*

cellulose [SELL-you-los] A straight-chain polysaccharide composed of hundreds of glucose units linked by beta bonds. It is indigestible by humans and is a component of dietary fiber.

hemicelluloses [hem-ih-SELL-you-loses] A group of large polysaccharides in dietary fiber that are fermented more easily than cellulose.

pectins Dietary fibers that are found in fruits.

gums Dietary fibers that contain galactose and other monosaccharides; found between plant cell walls.

mucilages Gel-forming dietary fibers containing galactose, mannose, and other monosaccharides; found in seaweed.

lignins [LIG-nins] Dietary fibers that are not a carbohydrate.

Carbohydrate Digestion and Absorption

Although glucose is a key building block of carbohydrates, you can't exactly find it on the menu at your favorite restaurant or campus hangout. You must first drink that chocolate milkshake or eat the hamburger bun so your body can convert the food carbohydrate into glucose in the body. So let's see what happens to carbohydrate foods you eat!

Digestion: Breaking Down Carbohydrates to Single Sugars

Refer to **Figure 5.5** for an overview of the digestive process. Carbohydrate digestion begins in the mouth, where the starch-digesting enzyme salivary amylase breaks down starch into shorter polysaccharides and maltose. Chewing stimulates saliva production and mixes salivary amylase with food. Disaccharides, unlike starch, are not digested in the mouth. Only about 5 percent of the starches in food are broken down by the time the food is swallowed.

When carbohydrate enters the stomach, the acidity of stomach juices eventually halts the action of salivary amylase by causing the enzyme (a protein) to lose its shape and function. This stops carbohydrate digestion, which will restart in the small intestine. Certain fibers, such as pectin, provide a feeling of fullness and tend to delay digestive activity by slowing stomach emptying.

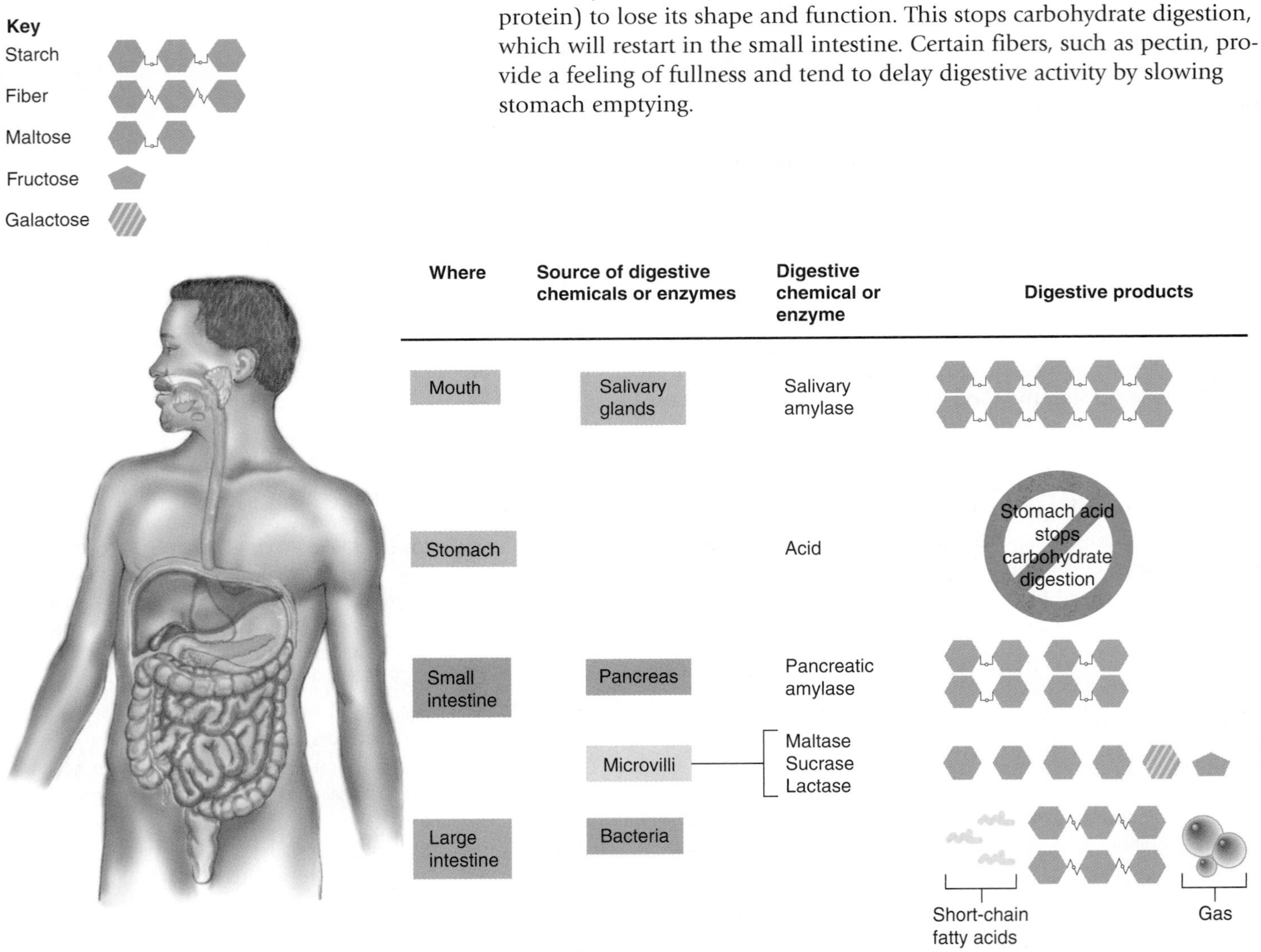

Figure 5.5 **Carbohydrate digestion.** Most carbohydrate digestion takes place in the small intestine.

Most carbohydrate digestion takes place in the small intestine. As stomach contents enter the small intestine, the pancreas secretes pancreatic amylase through the pancreatic duct and into the small intestine. **Pancreatic amylase** continues the digestion of starch, breaking it into the disaccharide maltose.

Meanwhile, enzymes attached to the brush border (microvilli) of the mucosal cells lining the intestinal tract go to work. (See Chapter 4, "The Human Body," for a detailed explanation of the complex structure of the small intestine.) These digestive enzymes break disaccharides into monosaccharides for absorption. The enzyme maltase splits maltose into two glucose molecules. The enzyme sucrase splits sucrose into glucose and fructose. The enzyme lactase splits lactose into glucose and galactose.

The bonds that link glucose molecules in complex carbohydrates are called glycosidic bonds. The two forms of these bonds, **alpha bonds** and **beta bonds**, have important differences. (See **Figure 5.6**.) Human enzymes easily break alpha bonds, making glucose available from the polysaccharides starch and glycogen. Cellulose, which is an indigestible polysaccharide found in dietary fiber, contains long chains of glucose molecules linked by beta bonds, which the body's enzymes cannot break. Beta bonds also link the galactose and glucose molecules in the disaccharide lactose, but the enzyme lactase is specifically tailored to attack this small molecule. People with a sufficient supply of the enzyme lactase can break these bonds. But when lactase is lacking, the beta bonds remain unbroken and lactose remains undigested until bacteria in the colon can attack it. (See Chapter 4, "The Human Body," for more on lactose maldigestion.)

Enzymes are highly specific; they speed up only specific reactions and work only on certain molecules. Humans lack the digestive enzymes to break down the oligosaccharides raffinose and stachyose. The commercial product Beano is an enzyme preparation. When taken right before eating beans or other gas-forming vegetables, Beano helps break oligosaccharides into monosaccharides so the body can absorb them.

Indigestible carbohydrate remains intact as it enters the large intestine. This carbohydrate may be dietary fiber or resistant starch, or the small intestine may have lacked the necessary enzymes to break it down. In the large intestine, bacteria partially ferment (break down) these undigested carbohydrates, producing gas and a few short-chain fatty acids.[17] These fatty acids are absorbed into the colon and are used for energy by the colon cells. In addition, these fatty acids may have other health effects, such as reducing blood cholesterol levels[18] and helping to protect against colon cancer.[19]

Not all fiber is fermented in the large intestine. Some fibers soften the stool and make it easier to pass, while other fibers add bulk to stools. These unfermented fibers pass essentially unchanged through the intestines and produce little gas.

Absorption: The Small Intestine Swings into Action

Monosaccharides are absorbed into the mucosal cells lining the small intestine. Glucose, galactose, and fructose molecules travel to the liver through the portal vein, where galactose and fructose are converted to glucose. The liver stores and releases glucose as needed to maintain constant

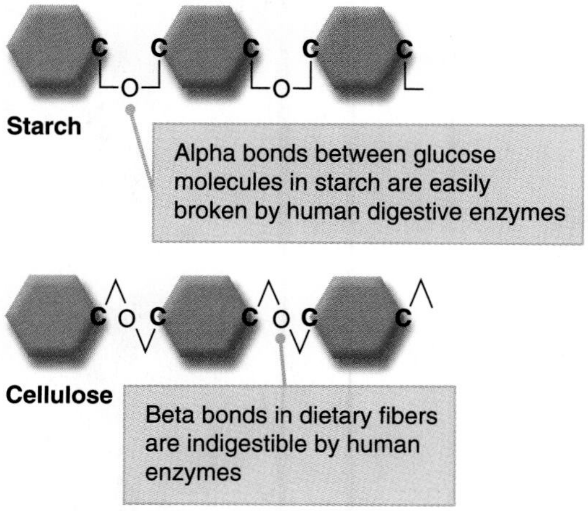
Starch
Alpha bonds between glucose molecules in starch are easily broken by human digestive enzymes
Cellulose
Beta bonds in dietary fibers are indigestible by human enzymes

Figure 5.6 **Alpha bonds and beta bonds.** Human digestive enzymes easily can break the alpha bonds in starch, but they cannot break the beta bonds in cellulose.

pancreatic amylase Starch-digesting enzyme secreted by the pancreas.

alpha bonds Chemical bonds linking monosaccharides, which can be broken by human intestinal enzymes, releasing the individual monosaccharides. Starch, maltose, and sucrose contain alpha bonds.

beta bonds Chemical bonds linking monosaccharides, which sometimes cannot be broken by human intestinal enzymes. Lactose contains digestible beta bonds, and cellulose contains nondigestible beta bonds.

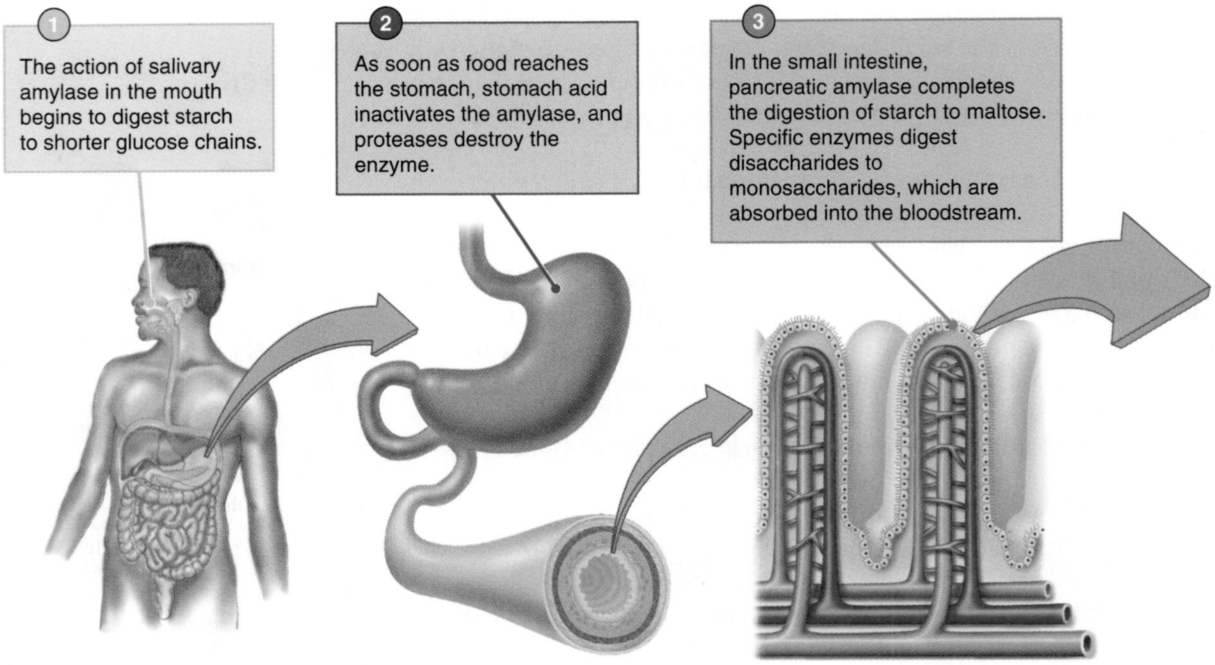
1
The action of salivary amylase in the mouth begins to digest starch to shorter glucose chains.
2
As soon as food reaches the stomach, stomach acid inactivates the amylase, and proteases destroy the enzyme.
3
In the small intestine, pancreatic amylase completes the digestion of starch to maltose. Specific enzymes digest disaccharides to monosaccharides, which are absorbed into the bloodstream.

Figure 5.7 **Travels with carbohydrate.** (1) Carbohydrate digestion begins in the mouth. (2) Stomach acid halts carbohydrate digestion. (3) Carbohydrate digestion resumes in the small intestine, where monosaccharides are absorbed. (4) The liver converts fructose and galactose to glucose, which it can assemble into chains of glycogen, release to the blood, or use for energy.

blood glucose levels. **Figure 5.7** illustrates digestion and absorption of carbohydrates.

Key Concepts: *Carbohydrate digestion takes place primarily in the small intestine, where digestible carbohydrates are broken down and absorbed as monosaccharides. Bacteria in the large intestine partially ferment indigestible carbohydrates such as resistant starch and certain types of fiber, producing gas and a few short-chain fatty acids that can be absorbed by the large intestine and used for energy. The liver converts absorbed monosaccharides into glucose.*

Carbohydrates in Action

Through the processes of digestion and absorption, our varied diet of carbohydrates from vegetables, fruits, grains, and milk becomes glucose. Glucose has one major role—to supply energy for the body.

Glucose Is Your Primary Fuel

Cells throughout the body depend on glucose for energy to drive chemical processes. Although most, but not all, cells can also burn fat for energy, the body needs some glucose to burn fat efficiently.

When we eat food, our bodies immediately use some glucose to maintain normal blood glucose levels. We store excess glucose as glycogen in liver and muscle tissue.

Using Glucose for Energy

Glucose is the primary fuel for most cells in the body and the preferred fuel for the brain, red blood cells, and nervous system, as well as for the fetus

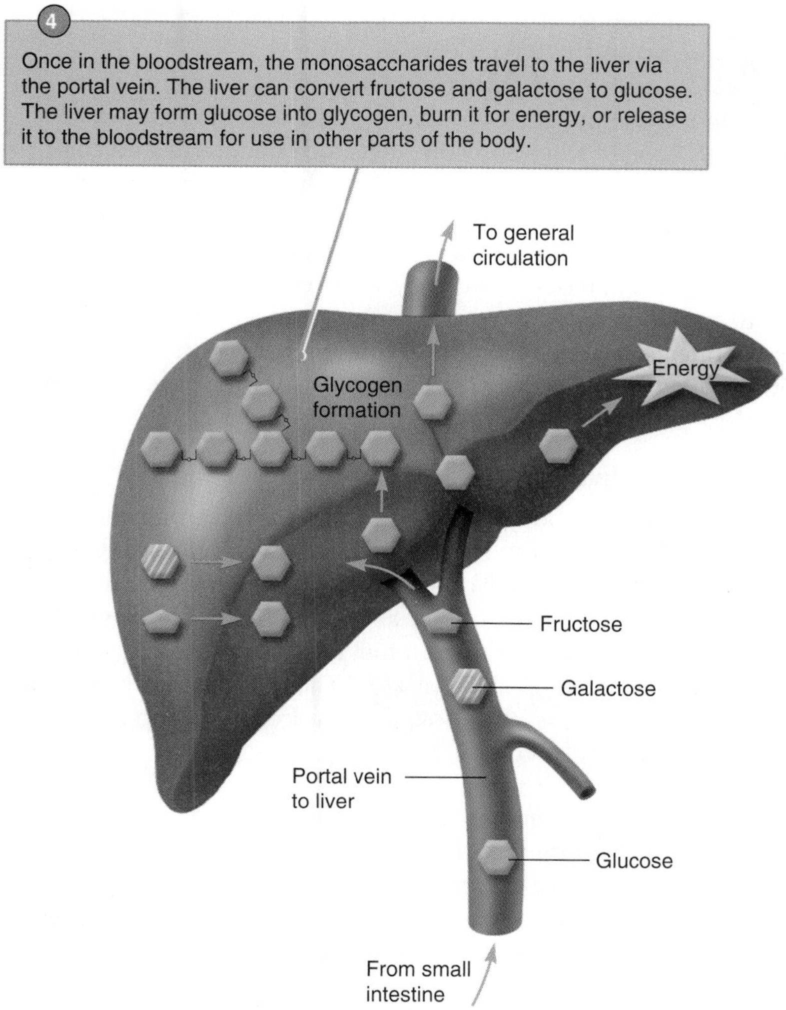
4
Once in the bloodstream, the monosaccharides travel to the liver via the portal vein. The liver can convert fructose and galactose to glucose. The liver may form glucose into glycogen, burn it for energy, or release it to the bloodstream for use in other parts of the body.
To general circulation
Energy
Glycogen formation
Fructose
Galactose
Portal vein to liver
Glucose
From small intestine

and placenta in a pregnant woman. Even when fat is burned for energy, a small amount of glucose is needed to metabolize fat completely. To obtain energy from glucose, glucose from the blood must be taken up by cells. Once glucose enters cells, a series of metabolic reactions breaks it down into carbon dioxide and water, releasing energy in a form the cells can use.[20]

Sparing Body Protein

If carbohydrate is not available, both proteins and fats can be used for energy. Although most cells can break down fat for energy, brain cells and developing red blood cells require a constant supply of glucose.[21] (After an extended period of starvation, the brain adapts and is able to use some byproducts of fat breakdown for part of its energy needs.) What happens if glucose stores (glycogen in liver and muscles) are depleted and the diet supplies no carbohydrate? To maintain blood glucose levels and supply glucose to the brain, the body can make glucose from body proteins. Dietary carbohydrate spares body proteins from being broken down and used to make glucose.

Preventing Ketosis

Even when fat provides fuel for the body, cells require a small amount of carbohydrate to completely break down fat to release energy. When no carbohydrate is available, the liver cannot break down fat completely for energy and instead produces small compounds called **ketone bodies**.[22] Most cells can use ketone bodies for energy.

When cells produce ketone bodies faster than the body can use them, these compounds build up in the blood, causing a condition known as **ketosis**. This can happen when someone diets too strenuously and consumes only small amounts of carbohydrates or when someone cannot metabolize blood glucose normally. Starvation, diabetes mellitus, and chronic alcoholism are the most common causes. Ketosis interferes with the balance of acids and bases in the body, causing the blood to become too acidic. Because the body loses water excreting excess ketones in the urine, ketosis often causes dehydration. To prevent ketosis, the body needs at least 50 to 100 grams of carbohydrate per day.[23] (See the "Spotlight on Metabolism" for more details on ketosis.)

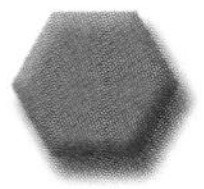

Glucose

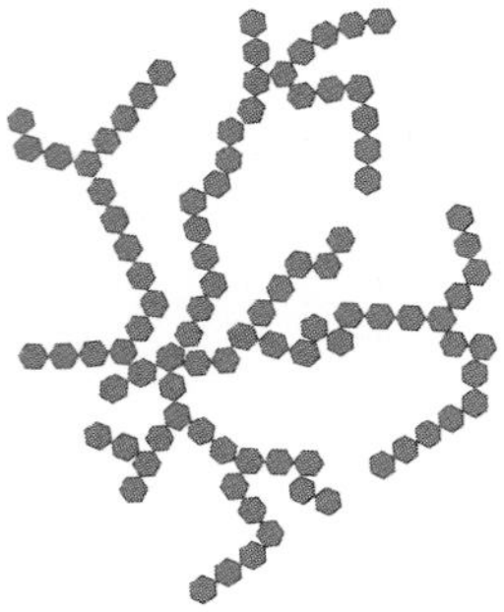

Glycogen

Storing Glucose as Glycogen

To store excess glucose, the body assembles it into the long, branched chains of glycogen. Glycogen can be broken down quickly, releasing glucose for energy as needed. Liver glycogen stores are used to maintain normal blood glucose levels and account for about one-third of body glycogen stores. Muscle glycogen stores are used to fuel muscle activity and account for about two-thirds of body glycogen stores.[24] The body can store only limited amounts of glycogen—usually enough to last from a few hours to one day, depending on activity level.[25]

Key Concepts: *Glucose circulates in the blood to provide immediate energy to cells. The body needs adequate carbohydrate intake so that body proteins are not broken down to fulfill energy needs. The body requires some carbohydrate to completely break down fat and prevent the buildup of ketone bodies in the blood. The body stores excess glucose in the liver and muscle as glycogen.*

ketone bodies Molecules formed from fat when cells do not have enough available carbohydrate to break down fat completely. Sometimes improperly called ketones.

ketosis [kee-TOE-sis] Abnormally high concentration of ketone bodies in body tissues and fluids.

insulin [IN-suh-lin] Produced by the pancreas, this hormone stimulates the uptake of blood glucose into cells, the formation of glycogen in the liver, and various other processes.

glucagon [GLOO-kuh-gon] Produced by the pancreas, this hormone promotes the breakdown of liver glycogen to glucose, and so increases blood glucose levels.

epinephrine A hormone released in response to stress or sudden danger, epinephrine raises blood glucose levels to ready the body for "fight or flight." Also called adrenaline.

Regulating Blood Glucose Levels

The body closely regulates blood glucose (also known as blood sugar) to maintain an adequate supply of glucose for cells. If blood glucose levels drop too low, a person becomes shaky and weak. If blood glucose levels rise too high, a person becomes sluggish and confused and may have difficulty breathing.

Two hormones produced by the pancreas tightly control blood glucose levels.[26] When blood glucose levels rise after a meal, the pancreas releases the hormone insulin into the blood. **Insulin** acts like a key, "unlocking" the cells of the body and allowing glucose to enter and fuel them. Insulin works on receptors on the surface of cells, increasing their attraction for glucose and increasing glucose uptake by cells. Insulin also stimulates liver and muscle cells to store glucose as glycogen. As glucose enters cells to deliver energy or be stored as glycogen, blood glucose levels return to normal. (See **Figure 5.8**.)

When an individual has not eaten in a while and blood glucose levels begin to fall, the pancreas releases another hormone called **glucagon**. Glucagon stimulates the body to break down stored glycogen, releasing glucose into the bloodstream. Glucagon also stimulates the synthesis of glucose from protein. Another hormone, **epinephrine** (also called adrenaline), exerts effects similar to glucagon to ensure that all body cells have adequate energy for emergencies. Released by the adrenal glands in response to sudden stress or danger, epinephrine is called the "fight-or-flight" hormone.

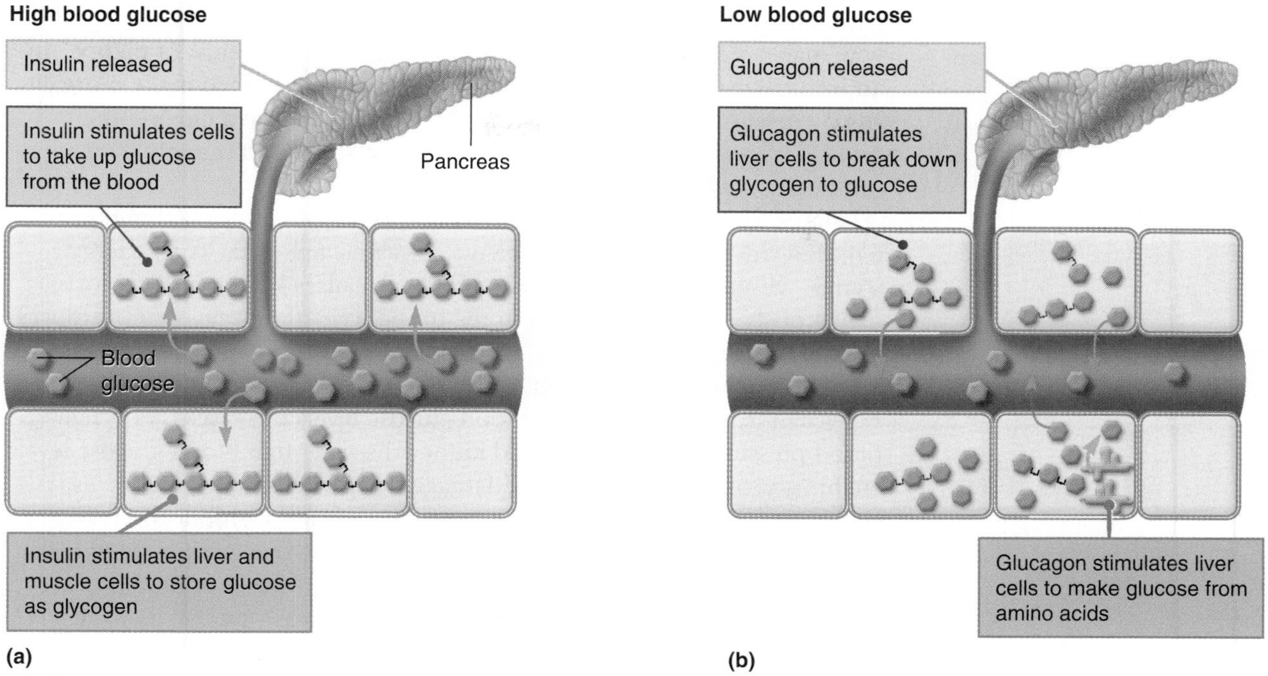

Figure 5.8 **Regulating blood glucose levels.** Insulin and glucagon have opposing actions. (a) Insulin acts to lower blood glucose levels, and (b) glucagon acts to raise them.

Different foods vary in their effect on blood glucose regulation. Foods rich in simple carbohydrates or starch but low in fat or fiber tend to be digested and absorbed rapidly. This rapid absorption causes a corresponding large and rapid rise in blood glucose levels.[27] The body reacts to this rise by pumping out extra insulin, which rapidly lowers blood glucose levels. Other foods, especially foods rich in dietary fiber, resistant starch, or fat, cause a lesser blood glucose response with smaller swings in blood glucose levels.

The **glycemic index** measures the effect of a food on blood glucose levels. Foods with a high glycemic index cause a faster and higher rise in blood glucose than foods with a low glycemic index. Although some experts disagree on the usefulness of the glycemic index for humans, diets that emphasize foods with a low glycemic index may offer important health benefits.[28] For more about this debate, see the FYI feature "The Glycemic Index of Foods: Useful or Useless?"

glycemic index A measure of the effect of food on blood glucose levels.

diabetes mellitus A chronic disease in which uptake of blood glucose by body cells is impaired, resulting in high glucose levels in the blood and urine.

hyperglycemia [HIGH-per-gly-SEE-me-uh] Abnormally high concentration of glucose in the blood.

High Blood Glucose: Diabetes Mellitus

When people have **diabetes mellitus**, their bodies either do not produce enough insulin or do not use insulin properly. If diabetes mellitus is not treated and controlled, it causes elevated blood glucose levels. Among Americans, diabetes mellitus is the seventh leading cause of death. While 22 million Americans have diabetes, only 14 million are aware they have it. About 1 in 20 people will develop diabetes sometime during their life.[29] Although scientists don't completely understand the causes of diabetes, both genetics and environmental factors (obesity and lack of exercise, for example) appear to be involved.

Consequences of Diabetes

Hyperglycemia, or an abnormally high blood glucose level, is the hallmark of diabetes mellitus. (See **Figure 5.9**.) Even though blood glucose is overly

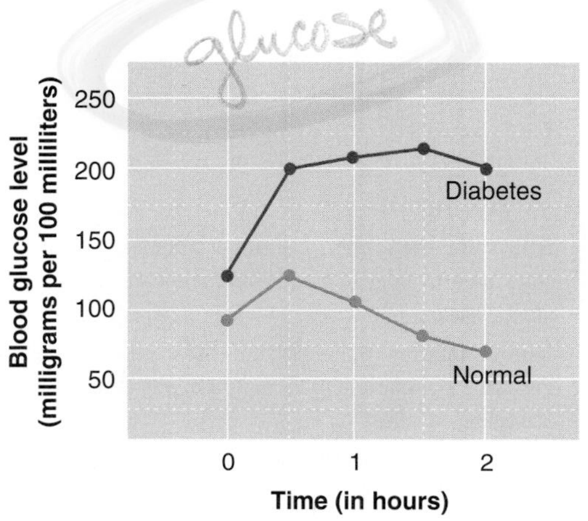

Figure 5.9 **Glucose tolerance test.** A glucose tolerance test measures the level of glucose in the blood following consumption of a standard dose of glucose. Glucose tolerance tests are used to diagnose diabetes.

abundant, it is unable to enter starving cells and fuel their needs. This is why diabetes is called the disease of "starvation in the midst of plenty." In an ironic twist of fate, these starving cells signal the liver to make more glucose, worsening the hyperglycemia. The kidneys are taxed beyond their capacities to reabsorb glucose, and the excess spills into the urine, where it can be detected by urine glucose tests.

Unable to use glucose, cells turn to other energy sources—fat and protein. But this leads to other problems. Excessive use of fat as an energy source, without available glucose in the cell, causes ketosis and acidosis, dangerously high acidity levels in the blood. Use of muscle proteins causes muscle wasting and weakness. Abnormalities in fat and protein metabolism often accompany hyperglycemia.[30]

Over time, abnormally high blood glucose levels increase risk of high blood pressure, heart disease, and kidney disease. High blood glucose levels enable glucose to react with and damage body proteins and tissues, especially in the eyes, kidneys, nerves, and blood vessels. Complications of diabetes can contribute to degenerative conditions such as peripheral vascular disease (disease of blood vessels outside the heart), deterioration of the eye and eventual blindness, kidney disease, and progressive nerve damage. Diabetes is responsible for 50 percent of all amputations of the lower extremities and 25 percent of all kidney failure in adults.[31] Diabetes is also the leading cause of blindness in adults.[32] People with diabetes are two to four times more likely to develop heart disease than people without diabetes.

Forms of Diabetes

There are two main forms of diabetes:

- Type 1, previously known as insulin-dependent diabetes mellitus (IDDM) or juvenile-onset diabetes; in type 1 diabetes, the pancreas is unable to produce insulin.
- Type 2, previously known as non-insulin-dependent diabetes mellitus (NIDDM) or adult-onset diabetes; in type 2 diabetes, cells become resistant to insulin.

Type 2 diabetes is far more common, accounting for 90 to 95 percent of diabetes cases. Another type of diabetes, gestational diabetes, occurs during pregnancy. (See Chapter 12, "Life Cycle: Maternal and Infant Nutrition," for more information on gestational diabetes.)

Type 1 diabetes usually occurs in people under the age of 30 and often develops suddenly. Symptoms include excessive thirst, frequent urination, nausea, and rapid weight loss.[33] When blood glucose levels rise, glucose spills into the urine, taking water with it and causing frequent urination and increased thirst. Although blood glucose levels are high, insulin is lacking and so glucose cannot get into cells to be burned for energy, causing weight loss and feelings of hunger.

People with type 1 diabetes require lifelong, daily insulin injections balanced with a healthful diet and regular exercise to maintain blood glucose levels in the normal range. Since exercise lowers blood glucose levels, individuals must consider the timing of exercise in addition to food intake and insulin injections to avoid lowering blood glucose levels too far.

In **type 2 diabetes**, glucose has trouble entering body cells because either the pancreas cannot produce enough insulin or cells in the body become resistant to the action of insulin. Although obesity is the cause of **insulin resistance** in most people with type 2 diabetes, genetic factors may play a

type 1 diabetes Type 1 diabetes occurs when the pancreas loses its ability to make insulin; also called juvenile-onset diabetes.

type 2 diabetes Type 2 diabetes occurs when cells lose the ability to respond normally to insulin; also called adult-onset diabetes.

insulin resistance Reduction in the ability of cells to respond to the action of insulin and take up glucose.

role for some lean individuals with this type of diabetes. Type 2 diabetes usually develops in overweight individuals aged 45 and older.

Diet and exercise are the primary management tools for type 2 diabetes, and weight loss often restores normal glucose metabolism.[34] Exercise increases the sensitivity of body cells to insulin, so the body needs less insulin to let glucose into cells. If diet and exercise fail to maintain blood glucose levels in the normal range, people with type 2 diabetes sometimes need medications to either increase insulin production or improve glucose uptake by cells. In some cases, insulin is needed to normalize blood glucose levels. (See **Figure 5.10**.)

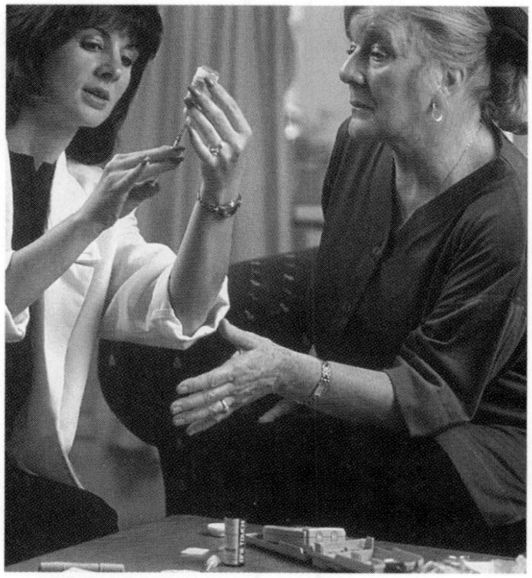

Figure 5.10 **Insulin injections.** In type 1 diabetes and some cases of type 2 diabetes, people need daily insulin injections to normalize blood glucose levels.

Risk Factors for Diabetes

Some people are at higher risk than others of developing diabetes. **Table 5.2** lists the risk factors for type 1 and type 2 diabetes. Any person with a family history of diabetes has an increased risk. Diabetes also occurs more frequently in Native Americans, Hispanic Americans, and African Americans.

Because it tends to run in families, the major risk factor for type 1 diabetes appears to be genetics. The risk of developing type 2 diabetes increases progressively as body fat increases, especially around the midsection. Compared to a normal-weight person, an obese person can have 40 times the risk of type 2 diabetes.[35] Most, but not all, people diagnosed with type 2 diabetes are obese when the diagnosis is made.

In recent years, scientists have recognized a cluster of risk factors dubbed **Syndrome X**. Like diabetes, Syndrome X involves impaired uptake of glucose by cells, but it also includes high blood pressure and high blood levels of insulin, fat, and cholesterol. Combined, these factors increase the risk of type 2 diabetes and heart disease by several fold. As many as 30 percent of adult males and 15 percent of postmenopausal women have Syndrome X.[36]

Syndrome X A cluster of risk factors for heart disease associated with insulin resistance. These risk factors include high blood pressure and high blood levels of insulin, fat, and cholesterol.

Contrary to popular thought, high sugar or high carbohydrate intake does not by itself cause diabetes. In fact, current dietary recommendations for individuals with diabetes emphasize diets rich in complex carbohydrates (including fiber) and low in fat.[37] Although in the past, dietary

Table 5.2 Risk Factors for Type 1 and Type 2 Diabetes Mellitus

Who is at greater risk for type 1 diabetes?
- Siblings of people with type 1 diabetes
- Children of parents with type 1 diabetes

Who is at greater risk for type 2 diabetes?
- People with high blood pressure
- People with a family history of diabetes
- People who are overweight
- People who do not exercise regularly
- People with low HDL or high triglyceride levels in the blood
- Certain racial and ethnic groups (e.g., African Americans, Hispanic Americans, Asian and Pacific Islanders, and Native Americans)
- Women who have had gestational diabetes, a form of diabetes that occurs in about 4 percent of pregnancies, or who have had a baby who weighed 9 pounds or more at birth

Source: American Diabetes Association. Position statement: screening for diabetes. *Diabetes Care.* 2002;25(suppl 1): S21–S24. Reprinted by permission.

treatment of diabetes eliminated simple sugars from the diet, current recommendations allow individuals with diabetes to include moderate amounts of simple sugars in their diet as long as sugar intake does not contribute to excess energy intake and obesity.[38]

The best prevention for both type 2 diabetes due to obesity and Syndrome X is a healthful diet and regular exercise. Reducing excess body fat will improve glucose tolerance and reduce related risk factors for heart disease. Regular exercise will improve carbohydrate and lipid metabolism and

Fyi — FOR YOUR INFORMATION

The Glycemic Index of Foods: Useful or Useless?

The glycemic index classifies foods based on their potential to raise blood glucose levels. Foods with a high glycemic index cause a faster and higher rise in blood glucose than a similar amount of carbohydrate from a low-glycemic-index food. Although simple in concept, the glycemic index has been the subject of heated debate among scientists. Some claim it is a valuable and easy-to-use concept that can help in the treatment of diabetes and can reduce risk for several chronic diseases. Others contend that it has no clinical benefit, and is impractical to use.

What Factors Affect the Glycemic Index of a Food?

The glycemic index of a food is not always easy to predict. You probably would expect a high-sugar food like ice cream to have a high glycemic index. But ice cream actually has a low index, since the fat in it slows sugar absorption. On the other hand, you might expect complex carbohydrate foods like bread or potatoes to have a low index. In fact, the starch in white bread and cooked potatoes is readily digested and absorbed, so each has a high value. The type of carbohydrate, the cooking process, and the presence of fat and dietary fiber all affect a food's glycemic index.[1] Table A lists several high-glycemic-index foods along with lower-glycemic-index alternatives.

Why Do Some Researchers Believe the Glycemic Index Is Useful?

People whose diets are rich in carbohydrates with low glycemic indexes may realize significant health benefits. A diet that emphasizes low-glycemic-index foods decreases the risk of developing type 2 diabetes[2] and, in people with diabetes, improves blood glucose control.[3] Such diets also may reduce the risk of colon cancer[4] and heart disease.[5]

Why Do Some Researchers Believe the Glycemic Index Is Useless?

Some researchers believe the glycemic index is not useful and question the quality of the research that shows benefits.[6] They point out that other dietary and behavioral changes, such as weight reduction, yield much stronger benefits. Also, since we eat meals of mixed foods rather than one food at a time, knowing the glycemic index of individual foods is not helpful. Determining the glycemic index of the infinite combinations of food that people eat would be impossible, not to mention impractical! In fact, we don't even know the glycemic index of most foods, and have no reliable way to predict it based on a food's sugar, starch, or fiber content.

Many scientists believe these unknowns make the glycemic index too difficult and complex for most people to use effectively.

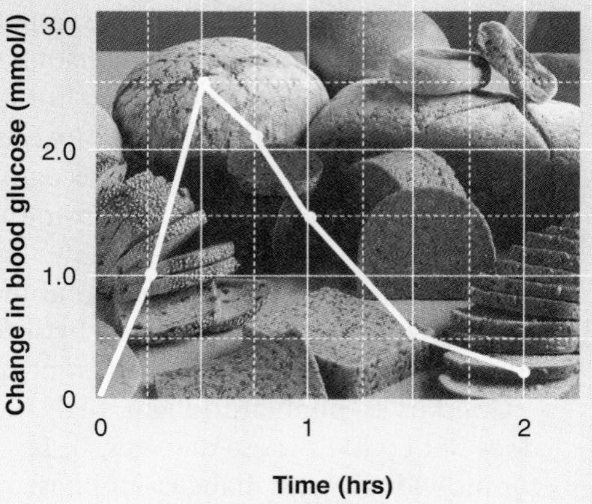

HIGH GLYCEMIC INDEX

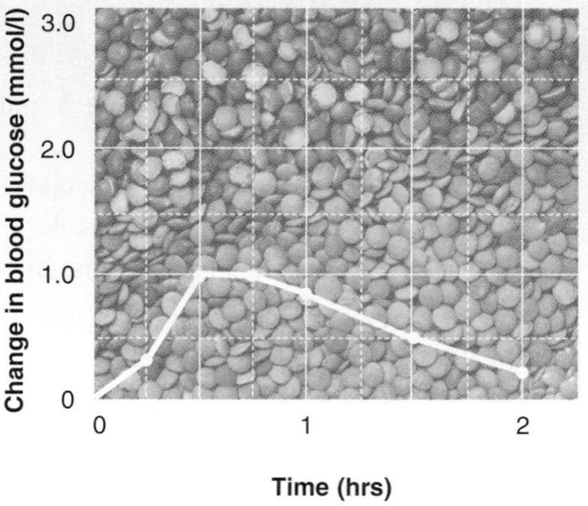

LOW GLYCEMIC INDEX

increase insulin sensitivity. (See **Figure 5.11**.) In addition, exercise improves blood flow to the extremities, bringing blood pressure down to normal levels and reducing risk of heart disease.

hypoglycemia [HIGH-po-gly-SEE-mee-uh] Abnormally low concentration of glucose in the blood.

Low Blood Glucose: Hypoglycemia

Excess insulin results in low blood glucose, or **hypoglycemia**. Too much glucose enters cells, lowering blood glucose levels too far. When blood glucose levels drop too low, nervousness, irritability, hunger, headache,

The American Diabetes Association seems to concur. For people with diabetes, it states that "from a clinical perspective first priority should be given to the total amount of carbohydrate consumed rather than the source of carbohydrate."[7]

So, What's the Bottom Line?

Studies of the benefits of a diet rich in low-glycemic-index carbohydrates are promising. But before this concept can be widely applied, there is more work to be done. Until that day comes, we should rely on the advice of the *Dietary Guidelines for Americans:* choose a variety of grains, fruits, and vegetables, with an emphasis on whole grains and other high-fiber foods.

1 World Health Organization. *Carbohydrates in Human Nutrition: Report of a Joint FAO/WHO Expert Consultation, Rome, 1997.* FAO Food and Nutrition Paper 66; 1997.

2 Salmeron J, Manson JE, Stampfer MJ, et al. Dietary fiber, glycemic load, and risk of non-insulin-dependent diabetes mellitus in women. *JAMA.* 1997; 277:472–477; and Salmeron J, Ascherio A, Rimm EB, et al. Dietary fiber, glycemic load, and risk of NIDDM in men. *Diabetes Care.* 1997;20:545–550.

3 Miller JB. Importance of glycemic index in diabetes. *Am J Clin Nutr.* 1994;59(suppl):747S–752S.

4 Slattery ML, Benson J, Berry TD, et al. Dietary sugar and colon cancer. *Cancer Epidemiol Biomarkers Prev.* 1997;6:677–685.

5 Frost G, Leeds A, Trew G, et al. Insulin sensitivity in women at risk of coronary heart disease and the effect of a low glycemic diet. *Metabolism.* 1998;47:1245–1251.

6 Coulston AM, Reaven GM. Much ado about (almost) nothing. *Diabetes Care.* 1997;20:241–243.

7 Franz MJ, Horton ES, Bantle JP, et al. Nutrition principles for the management of diabetes and related complications [technical review]. *Diabetes Care.* 1994;17:490–518.

Table A **Sample Substitutions for High-Glycemic-Index Foods**

High-Glycemic-Index Food	*Low-Glycemic-Index Alternative*	*High-Glycemic-Index Food*	*Low-Glycemic-Index Alternative*
Bread, wheat	Oat bran, rye, or pumpernickel bread	Plain cookies and crackers	Cookies made with dried fruits and whole grains such as oats
Processed breakfast cereal	Unrefined cereal such as oats (either muesli or oatmeal)	Cakes and muffins	Cakes and muffins made with fruit, oats, or whole grains
		Bananas	Apples
		Potatoes	Pasta or legumes

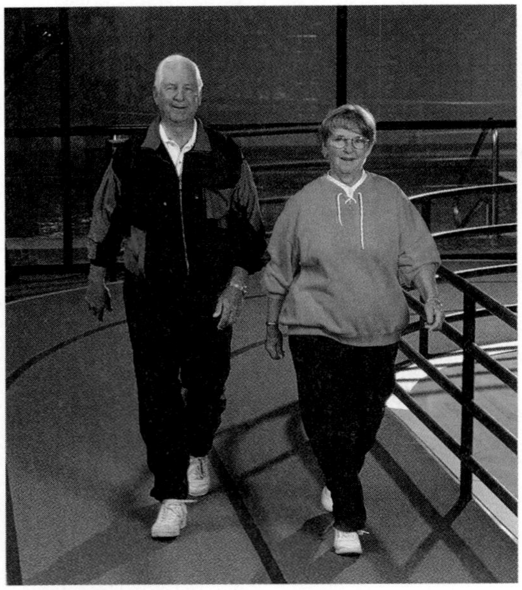

Figure 5.11 **Diabetes management.** Exercise, diet, and weight loss can have a significant impact on blood glucose levels for people with type 2 diabetes.

Quick Bites

Carbohydrate Companions

The word *companion* comes from the Latin word *companio*, meaning "one who shares bread."

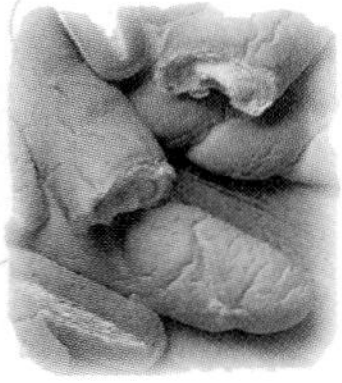

reactive hypoglycemia A type of hypoglycemia that occurs about one hour after eating carbohydrate-rich food. The body overreacts and produces too much insulin in response to food, rapidly decreasing blood glucose levels.

fasting hypoglycemia A type of hypoglycemia that occurs because the body produces too much insulin even when no food is eaten.

germ The innermost part of a grain that can grow into a new plant. The germ is rich in protein, oils, vitamins, and minerals.

endosperm The middle portion of a grain kernel; high in starch to provide food for the growing plant embryo.

bran The layers of protective coating around the grain kernel that are rich in dietary fiber and nutrients.

husk The inedible covering of grain; also known as the chaff.

shakiness, rapid heartbeat, and weakness can develop. A further drop in blood glucose levels can cause coma and death.

A person with diabetes can develop hypoglycemia in response to an overdose of insulin or vigorous exercise. In nondiabetic individuals, two types of hypoglycemia occur. **Reactive hypoglycemia** occurs about one hour after eating carbohydrate-rich food. The body overreacts and produces too much insulin in response to food. Individuals can prevent reactive hypoglycemia by eating frequent, smaller meals to smooth out blood glucose responses to food. **Fasting hypoglycemia** occurs because the body produces too much insulin even when no food is eaten. Pancreatic tumors can cause fasting hypoglycemia.

Key Concepts: *In healthy individuals, two hormones produced by the pancreas closely regulate blood glucose levels. Insulin allows glucose to enter cells and stimulates storage of glucose as glycogen, lowering blood glucose levels. Glucagon stimulates the release of glucose from glycogen and the formation of glucose from protein. Some individuals lack the ability to regulate blood glucose levels properly, resulting in diabetes (characterized by hyperglycemia, high blood glucose) or hypoglycemia (low blood glucose). Individuals with type 1 diabetes cannot make insulin; individuals with type 2 diabetes are resistant to the action of insulin or make inadequate amounts.*

Carbohydrates in Your Diet

What foods supply our dietary carbohydrates? **Figure 5.12** shows many foods rich in carbohydrates. The food groups in the lower part of the Food Guide Pyramid are our main dietary sources of carbohydrates: Grains and vegetables provide starches and fibers; fruits provide sugars and fibers. Additional sugar (mainly lactose) is found in dairy foods, while complex carbohydrates are also found in the legumes included in the meat and meat alternatives group. Sugars of all types are found at the tip of the Pyramid as sweeteners, beverages, jams, jellies, candy, and so forth.

Recommendations for Carbohydrate Intake

The *Surgeon General's Report on Nutrition and Health* recommends that carbohydrate contribute about 55 to 60 percent of daily calories for individuals older than 2 years.[39] For the average American who eats about 2,000 kilocalories daily, a daily carbohydrate intake of 275 to 300 grams meets this recommendation. The Daily Value for carbohydrates is 300 grams, representing 60 percent of the calories in a 2,000-kilocalorie diet. The number of servings of food groups recommended for adults by the Food Guide Pyramid—6 to 11 servings of breads, cereals, rice, and pasta; 2 to 4 servings of fruits; 3 to 5 servings of vegetables; and 2 to 3 servings of milk—would provide this amount of carbohydrate.

The *Dietary Guidelines for Americans* offer general goals for intake of sugars and complex carbohydrates.[40] One goal states "choose beverages and foods to moderate your sugar intake." Other goals include "choose a variety of grains daily, especially whole grains" and "choose a variety of fruits and vegetables daily." These goals are reflected in the Food Guide Pyramid.

Other recommendations suggest that added sugars (excluding natural sugars in foods like fruits and milk) should provide no more than 10 percent of daily energy intake. For an adult consuming about 2,000 kilocalories daily, this amounts to about 50 grams or less of added sugar daily.

Considering that a *single* can of soft drink contains 35 to 40 grams of sugar, it's not surprising that Americans generally consume more added sugar than recommended. Health experts also suggest we get about 10 to 13 grams of dietary fiber per 1,000 kilocalories, or about 20 to 35 grams of fiber daily for adults.[41] The Daily Value for fiber is 25 grams.

How Much Carbohydrate Do You Eat?

Think About It 2

Adult Americans currently consume about 50 percent of their energy intake as carbohydrate.[42] Dietary fiber intake averages about 15 grams daily,[43] about half the recommended amount. Thus, Americans are not eating enough total carbohydrate or dietary fiber. Carbohydrate intake also tends to reflect the quality of a person's diet. A recent study shows that people with high intakes of carbohydrate have better diets than people with low carbohydrate intakes.[44]

Natural sugars in milk, fruits, and grains make up about half of our sugar intake; refined sugars added to foods make up the other half. Consumption of sugars in the United States rose 15 percent between 1971 and 1991 and currently averages a little over 100 grams of sugar per person per day—equivalent to about ½ cup of sugar daily.[45] This value may be a little misleading, because it is based on food disappearance data (sugar that disappears from the food supply rather than sugar actually consumed) and includes sugar lost in processing or wasted, such as sugar poured out when the juice is drained from canned fruit. Actual sugar intake is lower and may be closer to the recommended maximum 10 percent of energy intake from added sugars.[46] However, the rapid increase in popularity of soft drinks and the addition of sugar in low-fat and fat-free foods probably mean that our sugar intake remains higher than what nutritionists recommend.

Increasing Your Complex Carbohydrate Intake

The Food Guide Pyramid emphasizes grains, vegetables, and fruits as the foundation of a healthful diet.[47] While naturally low in fat, these foods are rich in complex carbohydrates, both starches and fibers. Legumes are rich in both protein and complex carbohydrates.

Whole kernels of grains consist of four parts: germ, endosperm, bran, and husk. (See **Figure 5.13**.) The **germ**, the innermost part at the base of the kernel, is the part that grows into a new plant. It is rich in protein, oils, vitamins, and minerals. The **endosperm** is the middle portion (and largest part) of the grain kernel. It is high in starch to provide food for the growing plant embryo. The **bran** is composed of layers of protective coating around the grain kernel and is rich in dietary fiber. The **husk** is an inedible covering.

When grains are refined, making white flour from wheat, for example, or making white rice from brown rice, the process removes the outer husk and bran layers and sometimes the inner germ of the grain kernel. Since the bran and germ portions of the grain contain much of the dietary fiber, vitamins, and minerals, the nutrient content of whole grains is far superior to that of refined grains. Although food manufacturers enrich white flour to replace lost iron, thiamin, riboflavin, and niacin, they usually do not add back lost dietary fiber and nutrients such as vitamin B_6, calcium, phosphorus, potassium, magnesium, and zinc. Read labels carefully to choose foods that contain whole grains. Terms like *whole wheat, whole grain, rolled oats,* and *brown rice* indicate that the entire grain kernel is included in the food.

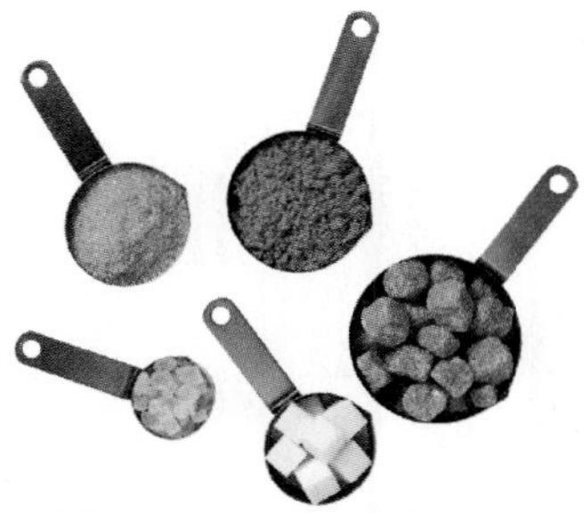

Table sugar, corn syrup, and brown sugar are rich in sucrose, a simple carbohydrate.

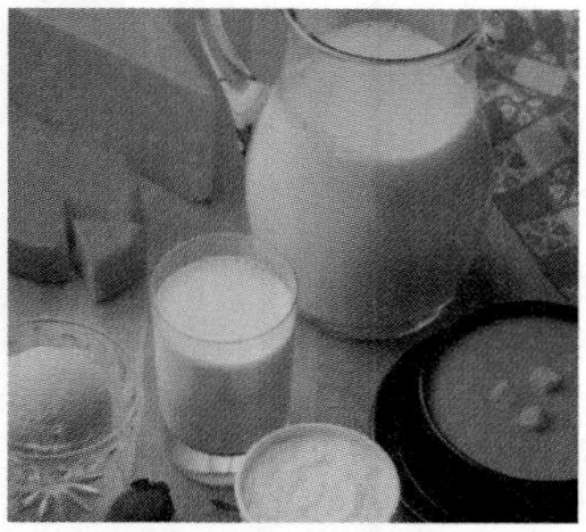

Milk and milk products are rich in lactose, a simple carbohydrate.

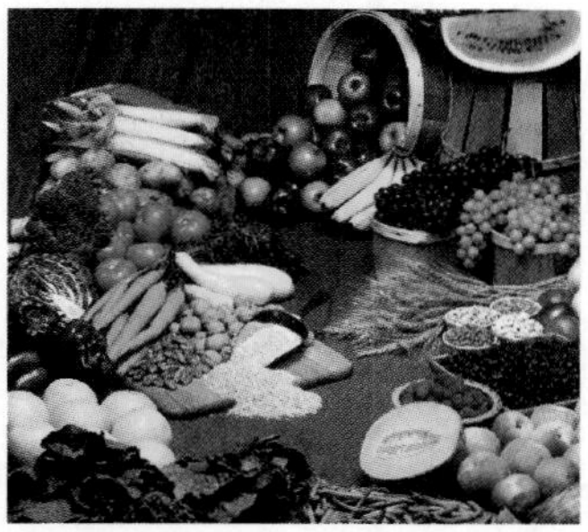

Fruits and vegetables provide simple sugars, starch, and fiber.

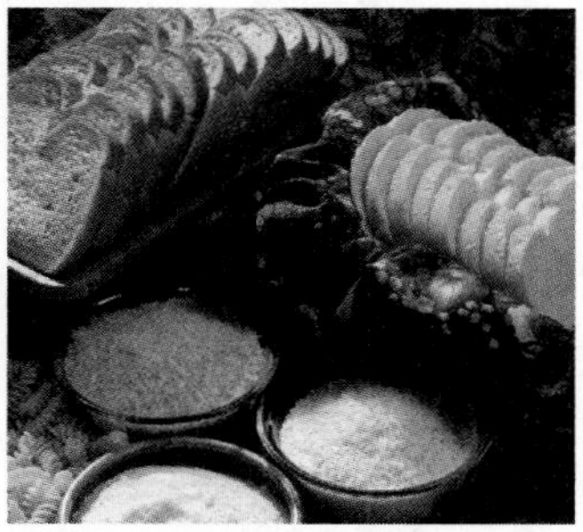

Bread, flour, cornmeal, rice, and pasta are rich in starch and, sometimes, dietary fiber.

Figure 5.12 **Carbohydrate sources from the Food Guide Pyramid.** Foods lower on the Food Guide Pyramid generally have a higher carbohydrate density. The sugars, sweets, and soft drinks in the top of the Pyramid should be consumed sparingly.

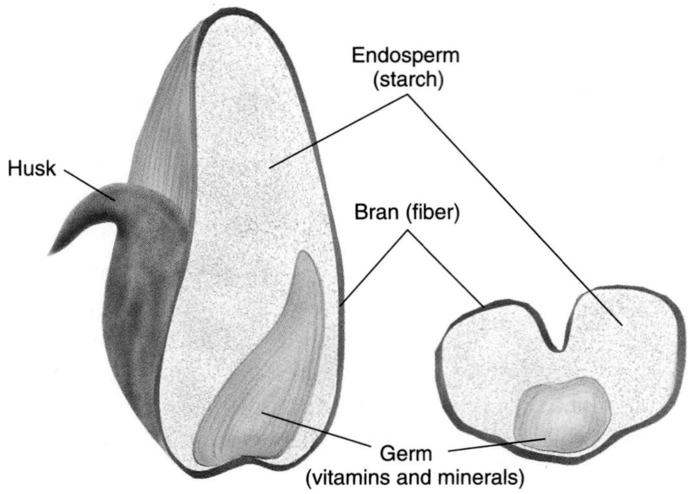

Figure 5.13 **Anatomy of a kernel of grain.** Whole kernels of grains consist of four parts: germ, endosperm, bran, and husk.

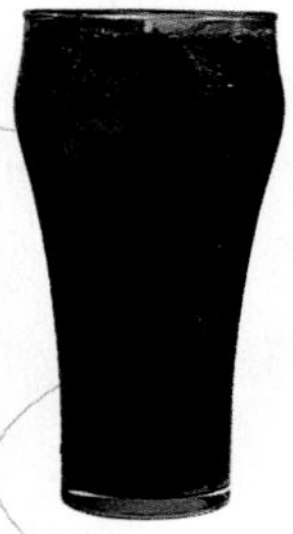

Quick Bites

Liquid Candy

Soft drinks are the biggest source of refined sugars for Americans. Soft drinks provide 44 percent of the 34 teaspoons of sugar that 12- to 19-year-old boys consume every day. Girls of this age group average about 24 teaspoons of sugar each day, 40 percent from soft drinks.

To emphasize complex carbohydrates (including fiber) in your diet:

- Eat more breads, cereals, pasta, rice, fruits, vegetables, and legumes.
- Eat fruits and vegetables with the peel, if possible. The peel is high in fiber.
- Add fruits to muffins and pancakes.
- Add legumes like pinto, navy, kidney, and black beans and lentils to casseroles and mixed dishes as a meat substitute.
- Substitute whole-grain flour for all-purpose flour in recipes whenever possible.
- Use brown rice instead of white rice.
- Substitute oats for flour in crumb toppings.
- Choose high-fiber cereals.
- Choose whole fruits rather than fruit juices.

When increasing your fiber intake, do so gradually and drink plenty of fluids to allow your body to adjust. Add just a few grams a day; otherwise, abdominal cramps, gas, bloating, and diarrhea or constipation may result. Parents and caregivers should also emphasize foods rich in complex carbohydrate and dietary fiber for children older than 2 years, but must take care that these foods do not fill a child up before energy and nutrient needs are met. **Table 5.3** lists various foods that are high in simple and complex carbohydrates.

Although health food stores, pharmacies, and even grocery stores sell many types of fiber supplements, most experts agree that you should get fiber from food rather than from a supplement. Foods rich in dietary fiber contain a variety of fibers as well as vitamins, minerals, and other phytochemicals that offer important health effects themselves.

Table 5.3 **High-Carbohydrate Foods**

High in Complex Carbohydrates	High in Simple Carbohydrates
Bagels	**Naturally Present**
Tortillas	Fruits
Cereals	Fruit juices
Crackers	Skim milk
Rice cakes	Plain nonfat yogurt
Legumes	
Corn	**Added**
Potatoes	Angel food cake
Peas	Soft drinks
Squash	Sherbet
Popcorn	Syrups
	Sweetened nonfat yogurt
	Candy
	Jellies
	Jams
	Gelatin
	High-sugar breakfast cereals
	Cookies
	Frosting

Moderating Your Sugar Intake

Most of us enjoy the taste of sweet foods, and there's no reason why we should not. But for some individuals, habitually high sugar intake crowds out foods that are higher in complex carbohydrates, vitamins, and minerals.

To moderate sugars in your diet:

- Use less of all added sugars, including white sugar, brown sugar, honey, and syrups.
- Limit use of soft drinks, high-sugar breakfast cereals, candy, ice cream, and sweet desserts.
- Use fresh or frozen fruits and fruits canned in natural juices or light syrup for dessert and to sweeten waffles, pancakes, muffins, and breads.

Read ingredient lists carefully. Food labels list the total grams of sugar in a food, which includes sugars naturally present in foods and sugars added to foods. Many terms for added sweeteners appear on food labels. Foods likely to be high in sugar list some form of sweetener as the first, second, or third ingredient on labels. **Table 5.4** lists various forms of sugar used in foods.

Sugar substitutes such as artificial sweeteners can help you lower sugar intake, but foods with artificial sweeteners may not provide less energy than similar products containing nutritive sweeteners. Rather than sugar, other energy-yielding nutrients, such as fat, are the primary source of the calories in these foods. Also, as artificial sweetener use in the United States has increased, so has sugar consumption—an interesting paradox!

Table 5.4 Forms of Sugar Used in Foods

Brown rice syrup	Invert sugar
Brown sugar	Lactose
Concentrated fruit juice sweetener	Levulose
Confectioners' sugar	Maltose
Corn syrup	Mannitol
Dextrose	Maple sugar
Fructose	Molasses
Galactose	Natural sweeteners
Glucose	Raw sugar
Granulated sugar	Sorbitol
High-fructose corn syrup	Turbinado sugar
	White sugar
	Xylitol

Key Concepts: *Dietary guidelines recommend that you get 55 to 60 percent of your calorie intake every day from carbohydrates, with less than 10 percent of calories coming from added sugars. You also should aim for a fiber intake of 20 to 35 grams per day. If you are like most Americans, you need to increase intake of complex carbohydrates and decrease intake of sugars to meet these recommendations. To increase complex carbohydrates (starches and fibers) in the diet, emphasize whole grains, legumes, fruits, and vegetables. To moderate sugar consumption, limit use of high-sugar foods such as high-sugar breakfast cereals, soft drinks, candies, jellies, jams, and some desserts.*

nutritive sweeteners Substances that make foods sweet and can be absorbed and yield energy in the body.

sugar alcohols Compounds formed from monosaccharides; commonly used as nutritive sweeteners.

Nutritive Sweeteners

Because **nutritive sweeteners** are digestible carbohydrates, they provide energy. Nutritive sweeteners include monosaccharides, disaccharides, and **sugar alcohols** from either natural or refined sources. White sugar, brown sugar, honey, maple syrup, glucose, fructose, xylitol, sorbitol, and mannitol are just some of the many nutritive sweeteners used in foods. One slice of angel food cake, for example, contains about 5 teaspoons of sugar. Fruit-flavored yogurt contains about 7 teaspoons of sugar. Even two sticks of chewing gum contain about 1 teaspoon of sugar. Whether sweeteners are added to foods or present naturally, all are broken down in the small intestine and absorbed as monosaccharides. Since all the absorbed monosaccharides end up as glucose, the body cannot tell whether these monosaccharides came from honey or table sugar. **Figure 5.14** compares the sweetness of sweeteners.

Think About It 3

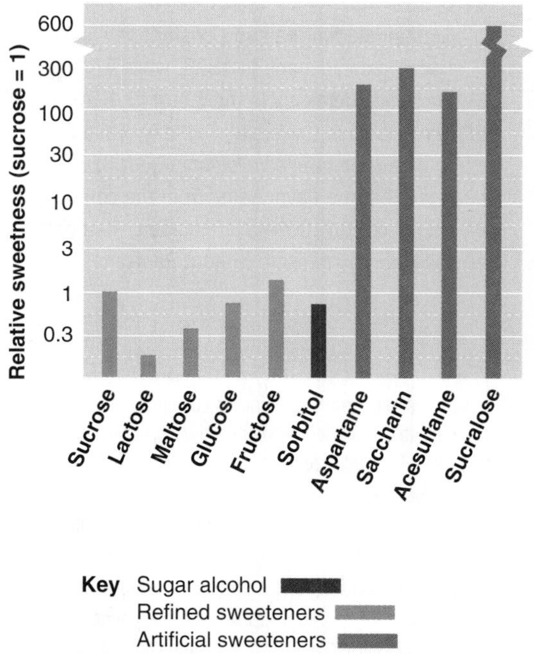

Figure 5.14 Comparing the sweetness of sweeteners. Artificial sweeteners are much sweeter than table sugar.

Natural sweeteners Natural sweeteners such as honey and maple syrup contain monosaccharides and disaccharides that make them taste sweet. Honey contains a mix of fructose and glucose—the same two monosaccharides that make up sucrose. Bees make honey from the sucrose-containing nectar of flowering plants. Real maple syrup contains primarily sucrose and

Quick Bites

Why Is Honey Dangerous for Babies?

Honey should never be fed to infants younger than 1 year of age because it can contain spores of the bacterium *Clostridium botulinum.* Infants do not produce as much stomach acid as older children and adults, so these spores can germinate in an infant's GI tract and cause botulism, a deadly foodborne illness.

is made by boiling and concentrating the sap from sugar maple trees. Most maple-flavored syrups sold in grocery stores, however, are made from corn syrup with maple flavoring added.

Many fruits also contain sugars that impart a sweet taste. Usually the riper the fruit, the higher its sugar content—a ripe pear tastes sweeter than an unripe one.

Refined sweeteners **Refined sweeteners** are monosaccharides and disaccharides that have been extracted from plant foods. White table sugar is sucrose extracted from either sugar beets or sugar cane. Molasses is a byproduct of the sugar-refining process. Most brown sugar is really white table sugar with molasses added for coloring and flavor.

Manufacturers make high-fructose corn syrup by treating cornstarch with acid and enzymes to break the starch into glucose. Then different enzymes convert much of the glucose to fructose. High-fructose corn syrup tastes 1.5 times sweeter than table sugar and costs less to produce. An increase in high-fructose corn syrup in soft drinks and other processed foods accounts for much of the increased use of sweeteners in the United States since the 1970s.[48]

Sugar Alcohols The sugar alcohols sorbitol, xylitol, and mannitol occur naturally in foods and are additives in sugar-free products like gum and mints. Although these sweeteners are not as sweet as sucrose, they do have the advantage of being less likely to cause tooth decay. The body does not digest and absorb sugar alcohols fully, so they provide only 2 kilocalories per gram compared with the 4 kilocalories per gram that other sugars provide. When sugar alcohols are used as the sweetener, the product may be free of sugar (sucrose), but it is not free of calories. Check the label to be sure.

Artificial Sweeteners

Gram for gram, most **artificial sweeteners** are many times sweeter than nutritive sweeteners. Thus, food manufacturers can use much less artificial sweetener to sweeten foods. Although some artificial sweeteners do provide energy, the amounts used are so small that their energy contribution is minimal. Think About It 4

The most common artificial sweeteners in the United States are saccharin, aspartame, acesulfame K, and sucralose. Cyclamates, banned in the United States in 1969 because of cancer concerns, are still used in Canada and many other countries. For people who want to decrease their intake of sugar and energy while still enjoying sweet foods, artificial sweeteners offer an alternative. Also, artificial sweeteners do not contribute to tooth decay.

Saccharin Discovered in 1879 and used in foods ever since then, **saccharin** tastes about 300 times sweeter than sucrose. In the 1970s research indicated that very large doses of saccharin were associated with bladder cancer in laboratory animals. As a result, in 1977 the Food and Drug Administration (FDA) proposed banning saccharin from use in food. Widespread protests by consumer and industry groups, however, led Congress to impose a moratorium on the saccharin ban. Every few years, the moratorium was extended, and products containing saccharin had to display a warning label about saccharin and cancer risk in animals. In 2000, convincing evidence of safety led to saccharin's removal from the National Toxicology Program's list of potential cancer-causing agents, and the U.S. Congress repealed the warning

Quick Bites

The Discovery of Saccharin

A German student named Constantine Fahlberg discovered saccharin in 1879, while working with organic chemicals in the lab of Ira Remsen at Johns Hopkins University. One day, while eating some bread, he noticed a strong sweet flavor. He deduced that the flavor came from the compound on his hands, $C_6H_4CONHSO_2$. Fahlberg then patented saccharin by himself, without Remsen.

refined sweeteners Substances composed of monosaccharides and disaccharides that have been extracted and processed from other foods.

artificial sweeteners Substances that impart sweetness to foods but supply little or no energy to the body; also called non-nutritive or alternative sweeteners.

saccharin [SAK-ah-ren] An artificial sweetener that tastes about 300 to 700 times sweeter than sucrose. Neither digested nor absorbed, saccharin contributes no calories to the diet.

label requirement.[49] In Canada, although saccharin is banned from food products, it can be purchased in pharmacies and carries a warning label.

Aspartame The artificial sweetener **aspartame** is a combination of the two amino acids phenylalanine and aspartic acid. When digested and absorbed, it provides 4 kilocalories per gram. However, aspartame is so many times sweeter than sucrose that the amount used to sweeten foods contributes virtually zero calories to the diet, and it does not promote tooth decay. The FDA approved aspartame for use in some foods in 1981 and for use in soft drinks in 1983. More than 90 countries allow aspartame in products such as beverages, gelatin desserts, gums, and fruit spreads. Because heating destroys the sweetening power of aspartame, aspartame cannot be used in products that require cooking.

Some groups believe aspartame could cause high blood levels of the amino acid phenylalanine. However, high-protein foods such as meats contain much more phenylalanine than foods sweetened with aspartame. The amounts of phenylalanine in aspartame-sweetened foods are not high enough to cause concern for most people. However, people with a genetic disease called **phenylketonuria (PKU)** cannot properly metabolize the amino acid phenylalanine, so they must carefully monitor their phenylalanine intake from all sources, including aspartame.

Although some people report headaches, dizziness, seizures, nausea, or allergic reactions with aspartame use, scientific studies have failed to confirm these effects, and most experts believe aspartame is safe for healthy people.[50] The FDA sets a maximum allowable daily intake of aspartame of 50 milligrams per kilogram of body weight. This amount of aspartame equals the amount in sixteen 12-ounce diet soft drinks for adults and eight diet soft drinks for children.

Acesulfame K Marketed under the brand name Sunette, **acesulfame K** is about 200 times sweeter than table sugar. The FDA approved its use in the United States in 1988. Acesulfame K provides no energy because the body cannot digest it. Food manufacturers use acesulfame K in chewing gum, powdered beverage mixes, nondairy creamers, gelatins, and puddings. Heat does not affect acesulfame K, so it can be used in cooking.

Sucralose Known under the trade name Splenda, **sucralose** was approved for use in the United States in 1998 and has been used in Canada since 1992. Sucralose is made from sucrose, but the resulting compound is nonnutritive and about 600 times sweeter than sugar. Sucralose has been approved for use in a wide variety of products, including baked goods, beverages, gelatin desserts, frozen dairy desserts, and many others. It also can be used as a "table-top sweetener" and added directly to food by consumers.

Other Artificial Sweeteners Other artificial sweeteners such as alitame and D-tagatose are awaiting approval by the FDA for use in the United States.[51] **Alitame** is composed of two amino acids plus another nitrogen-containing compound and tastes 2,000 times sweeter than sucrose. **D-tagatose** is derived from lactose and has the same sweetness of sucrose with only one-half the energy.

Key Concepts: *Sweeteners add flavor to foods. Nutritive sweeteners provide energy, whereas artificial sweeteners provide little or no energy. The body cannot tell the difference between sugars derived from natural and refined sources.*

aspartame [AH-spar-tame] An artificial sweetener composed of two amino acids. It is 200 times sweeter than sucrose and sold by the trade name NutraSweet.

phenylketonuria (PKU) An inherited disorder that causes a lack of the enzyme that metabolizes phenylalanine.

acesulfame K [ay-see-SUL-fame] An artificial sweetener that is 200 times sweeter than common table sugar (sucrose). Because it is not digested and absorbed by the body, acesulfame contributes no calories to the diet and yields no energy when consumed.

sucralose An artificial sweetener made from sucrose. Sucralose is non-nutritive and about 600 times sweeter than sugar.

alitame An artificial sweetener composed of two amino acids and a nitrogen compound. Alitame tastes 2,000 times sweeter than sucrose. The compound is awaiting FDA approval.

D-tagatose An artificial sweetener derived from lactose that has the same sweetness as sucrose with only half the calories. The compound is awaiting FDA approval.

Quick Bites

Sugar Overload

In many affluent countries, sugar consumption is nearly 100 pounds per capita per year. The United States averages 80 pounds of sugar per person per year. Americans consume an average of 40 gallons of soft drinks per person per year.

dental caries [KARE-ees] Destruction of the enamel surface of teeth caused by acids that are created when bacteria break down sugars in the mouth.

Carbohydrates and Health

Carbohydrates contribute both positively and negatively to health. Fiber helps to keep the gastrointestinal tract healthy and, along with other complex carbohydrates, may reduce the risk of heart disease and cancer. Excess sugar can contribute to poor nutrient intake and tooth decay.

Sugar and Nutrient Intake

Foods high in sugar are popular in American diets. These empty-calorie foods (e.g., candy, soft drinks, sweetened gelatin, and some desserts) provide energy but contain little or no dietary fiber, vitamins, or minerals. Studies link the rising prevalence of obesity in children to consumption of sugar-sweetened drinks.[52] On average, Americans drink 53 gallons of soda per year—40 percent more than two decades ago.[53] Consider that one 12-ounce soft drink contains 10 to 12 teaspoons of sugar. Would you add that much sugar to a glass of iced tea?

People with high energy needs, such as active teenagers and young adults, can afford to get a bit more of their calories from high-sugar foods. People with low energy needs, such as some elderly or sedentary people or people trying to lose weight, cannot afford as many calories from high-sugar foods. Most people can include moderate amounts of sugar in their diet and still meet other nutrient needs.

Sugar and Dental Caries

High sugar intake contributes to **dental caries**, or cavities. (See **Figure 5.15**.) When bacteria in your mouth feed on sugars, they produce acids that eat away tooth enamel and dental structure, causing dental caries. Although these bacteria quickly metabolize sugars, they feed on any carbohydrate, including starch.

The longer a carbohydrate remains in the mouth, the more likely it is to promote dental caries. Foods that stick to your teeth, such as caramel, licorice, crackers, sugary cereals, and cookies, are more likely to cause dental caries than foods that are quickly washed out of your mouth. If you sip high-sugar beverages such as soft drinks over an extended period of time, you will be more likely to have problems with dental caries. A baby should never be put to bed with a bottle, because the warm milk or juice may remain in the mouth all night, providing a ready source of carbohydrate for bacteria to break down.

Snacking on high-sugar foods throughout the day provides continuous carbohydrates that nourish the bacteria in your mouth, promoting the formation of dental caries. Good dental hygiene, adequate fluoride, and a well-balanced diet for strong tooth formation can help prevent dental caries.[54]

Complex Carbohydrates and Obesity

A diet rich in complex carbohydrates promotes a healthy body weight and lowers the risk of obesity. Foods rich in complex carbohydrates usually are low in fat and energy. They offer a greater volume of food for fewer calories, take longer to eat, and are filling. Once eaten, foods high in dietary fiber take longer to leave the stomach and they attract water, adding to the feeling of fullness. Consider, for example, three apple products with the same energy but different complex carbohydrate content: a large apple (5 grams fiber), 1/2 cup applesauce (2 grams fiber), and 3/4 cup of apple juice (0.2 grams fiber). Most of us would find the whole apple more filling and satisfying than the applesauce or apple juice.

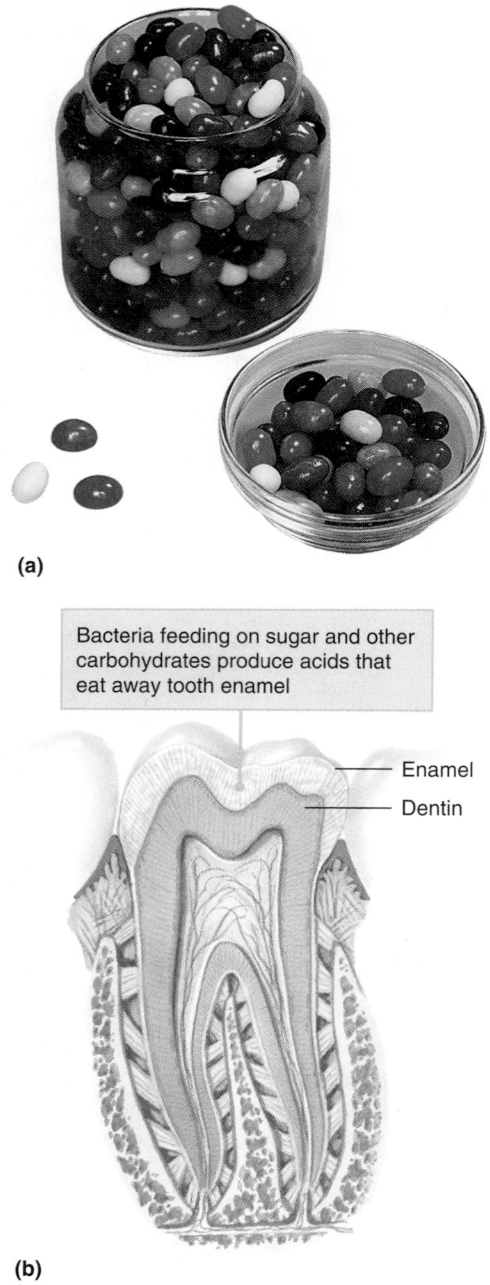
(a)
Bacteria feeding on sugar and other carbohydrates produce acids that eat away tooth enamel
Enamel
Dentin
(b)

Figure 5.15 **Dental health.** (a) To help prevent dental caries, avoid continuous snacking on high-sugar foods, especially those that stick to the teeth. (b) Good dental hygiene, adequate fluoride, and proper nutrition help maintain healthy teeth. A well-balanced diet contains vitamins and minerals crucial for healthy bones and teeth.

Complex Carbohydrates and Type 2 Diabetes

People who consume plenty of complex carbohydrates have a low incidence of type 2 diabetes.[55] A high intake of complex carbohydrates decreases the risk of becoming obese, and obesity greatly increases the risk for developing type 2 diabetes. High intake of certain types of fiber also delays stomach emptying and keeps blood glucose levels stable—effects that are helpful for healthy people as well as for people with type 2 diabetes. Current dietary recommendations for people with type 2 diabetes advise a high intake of complex carbohydrates and dietary fiber.[56]

Complex Carbohydrates and Cancer

A diet rich in complex carbohydrates lowers risk of certain kinds of cancer.[57] These benefits may be attributed to components other than just fiber. Foods rich in complex carbohydrates usually contain hundreds of phytochemicals, which together with vitamins and minerals such as vitamin E and selenium may play important roles in cancer prevention. For more on dietary fiber and cancer, see Chapter 4, "The Human Body."

[Fyi] Unfounded Claims against Sugars

FOR YOUR INFORMATION

Sugar has become the vehicle used by some diet zealots to create a new soapbox. Cut sugar to trim fat! Bust sugar! Break the sugar habit! These battle cries falsely demonize sugar as a dietary villain. But what are the facts?

Sugar and Obesity

Many people believe that sugar is fattening and causes obesity. Sugar is a carbohydrate, and carbohydrates provide 4 kilocalories per gram. High fat—not sugar—intakes are associated with a greater risk of obesity.[1] Fat is a more concentrated source of energy and provides 9 kilocalories per gram. However, many foods high in sugar, such as doughnuts and cookies, are also high in fat. Excess energy intake from any source will cause obesity, but sugar by itself is no more likely to cause obesity than starch or protein. The increased availability of low-fat and fat-free foods has not reduced obesity rates in the United States; in fact, incidence of obesity is still climbing. Some speculate that consumers equate fat-free with calorie-free and eat more of these foods, not realizing that fat-free foods often have a higher sugar content, which makes any calorie savings negligible.

Sugar and Heart Disease

Risk factors for heart disease include a genetic predisposition, smoking, high blood pressure, high blood cholesterol levels, diabetes, and obesity. Sugar by itself does not cause heart disease.[2] However, if intake of high-sugar foods contributes to obesity, then risk for heart disease increases. In addition, excessive intake of refined sugar can alter blood lipids in carbohydrate-sensitive people, increasing their risk for heart disease. However, a high fat intake is more likely to promote obesity than a high sugar intake. Thus, total fats, saturated fat, cholesterol, and obesity have a significantly more important relationship to heart disease than sugar.

Sugar and Behavior

Parents continue to talk about kids "bouncing off the walls" at birthday parties because of "all that sugar." So, what's going on? Most likely, the event (a party, trick-or-treating for Halloween, a carnival) is enhancing kids' normal levels of excitement and enthusiasm. From a brain chemistry perspective, carbohydrates actually have a calming effect by increasing production of the sleep-inducing chemical serotonin! Well-controlled research studies have found no link between sugar and hyperactivity, so blame the excitement of the party, but not the sugar, for kids' "wild" behavior.[3]

In 1978 Dan White gunned down the mayor of San Francisco and blamed the act on his emotional state—created, he said, by eating too many Hostess Twinkies. This legal strategy became known as the Twinkie defense. Claims that sugar causes criminal behavior in adults are unfounded. Studies show no association between high sugar intake and aggressive behavior.[4]

1 Lichtenstein AH, Kennedy E, Barrier P, et al. Dietary fat consumption and health. *Nutr Rev.* 1998;56:S3–S19.

2 World Health Organization (WHO). *Carbohydrates in Human Nutrition: Report of a Joint FAO/WHO Expert Consultation, Rome, 1997.* FAO Food and Nutrition Paper 66; 1997.

3 White JW, Wolraich M. Effect of sugar on behavior and mental performance. *Am J Clin Nutr.* 1995;62:S242–S249; and Wolraich ML, Lindgren SD, Stumbo PJ, et al. Effects of diets high in sucrose or aspartame on the behavior and cognitive performance of children. *N Engl J Med.* 1994;330:301–307.

4 White JW, Wolraich M. Op. cit.

Complex Carbohydrates and Cardiovascular Disease

High blood cholesterol levels increase risk for heart disease. Diets rich in fiber can lower blood cholesterol levels by 20 percent or more.[58] If you reduce your blood cholesterol level 1 percent, you can decrease your risk of heart disease by 2 percent, so high fiber intake can decrease risk of heart disease by 40 percent or more.

Fibers from certain sources, such as oat bran, legumes, and psyllium, can lower blood cholesterol levels. Your body uses cholesterol to make bile, which is secreted into the intestinal tract to aid fat digestion. Most bile is reabsorbed and recycled. In the gastrointestinal tract, fiber can bind bile and reduce the amount available for reabsorption. With less reabsorbed bile, the body makes up the difference by removing cholesterol from the blood and making more bile. The short-chain fatty acids produced from bacterial breakdown of fiber in the large intestine also may prevent cholesterol formation.[59]

Studies also show a relationship between high intake of whole grains and low risk of heart disease.[60] Whole grains contain not only fiber but also antioxidants and other compounds that may protect against cellular damage that promotes heart disease. It is likely that the combination of compounds found in grains, rather than any one component, explains the protective effects against heart disease.[61]

Label [to] Table

This label highlights all of the carbohydrate-related information you can find on a food label. Look at the center of the Nutrition Facts label and you'll see the Total Carbohydrates along with two of the carbohydrate "subgroups"—Dietary Fiber and Sugars. Recall that carbohydrates are classified into simple carbohydrates and the two complex carbohydrates starch and fiber.

Using this food label, you can determine all three of these components. There are 19 total grams of carbohydrate, with 14 grams coming from sugars and 0 grams from fiber. This means the remaining 5 grams must be from starch, which is not required to be listed separately on the label. Without even knowing what food this label represents, you can decipher that it contains a high proportion of sugar (14 of the 19 grams) and is probably sweet. If this is a fruit juice, that level of sugar would be expected; but if this is cereal, you'd be getting a lot more sugar than complex carbohydrates and probably wouldn't be making the best choice!

Do you see the 6% listed to the right of "Total Carbohydrate"? This doesn't mean that the food item contains 6% of its calories from carbohydrate. Instead, it refers to the Daily Value for carbohydrates listed at the bottom of the label. You can see there that a person consuming 2,000 kilocalories per day should consume 300 grams of carbohydrates each day. This product contributes 19 grams per serving, which is just 6% of the recommended 300 grams per day. Note that the % Daily Value for fiber is 0% because this food item lacks fiber.

The last highlighted section on this label, at the bottom of some Nutrition Facts labels, is the number of calories in a gram of carbohydrate. Recall that carbohydrates contain 4 kilocalories per gram. Armed with this information and the product's calorie information, can you calculate the percentage of calories that come from carbohydrate?

Here's how:

19 g carbohydrate × 4 kcal per g = 76 carbohydrate kcal

76 carbohydrate kcal ÷ 154 total kcal = 0.49 or 49% carbohydrate kcal

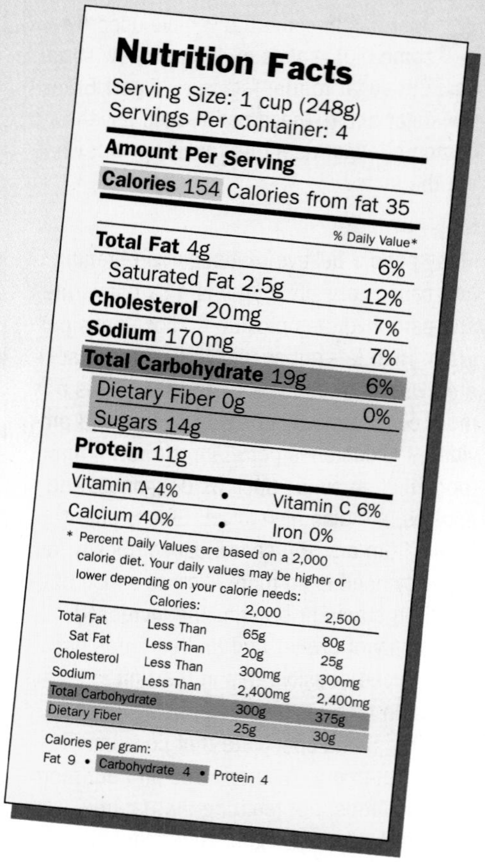

Nutrition Facts
Serving Size: 1 cup (248g)
Servings Per Container: 4
Amount Per Serving
Calories 154 Calories from fat 35
% Daily Value*
Total Fat 4g 6%
Saturated Fat 2.5g 12%
Cholesterol 20mg 7%
Sodium 170mg 7%
Total Carbohydrate 19g 6%
Dietary Fiber 0g 0%
Sugars 14g
Protein 11g
Vitamin A 4% • Vitamin C 6%
Calcium 40% • Iron 0%
* Percent Daily Values are based on a 2,000 calorie diet. Your daily values may be higher or lower depending on your calorie needs:
Calories: 2,000 2,500
Total Fat Less Than 65g 80g
Sat Fat Less Than 20g 25g
Cholesterol Less Than 300mg 300mg
Sodium Less Than 2,400mg 2,400mg
Total Carbohydrate 300g 375g
Dietary Fiber 25g 30g
Calories per gram:
Fat 9 • Carbohydrate 4 • Protein 4

Dietary Fiber and Gastrointestinal Disorders

Eating plenty of dietary fiber, especially the types found in cereal grains, helps promote healthy gastrointestinal functioning. Diets rich in fiber add bulk and increase water in the stool, softening the stool and making it easier to pass. Fiber also speeds passage of food through the intestinal tract, promoting regularity. If fluid intake is also ample, high fiber intake helps prevent and treat constipation, hemorrhoids (swelling of rectal veins), and diverticular disease (development of pouches on the intestinal wall). For more about fiber and GI disorders, see Chapter 4, "The Human Body."

Negative Health Effects of Excess Dietary Fiber

Despite its health advantages, high fiber intake can cause problems, especially for people who drastically increase their fiber intake in a short period of time. If you increase your fiber intake, you also need to increase your water intake to prevent the stool from becoming hard and impacted. A sudden increase in fiber intake also can cause increased intestinal gas and bloating. You can prevent these problems both by increasing fiber intake gradually over several weeks and by drinking plenty of fluids.

Just as fiber binds cholesterol, it can also bind small amounts of minerals in the GI tract and prevent them from being absorbed. Fiber binds the minerals zinc, calcium, magnesium, and iron. For people who get enough of these minerals, however, the recommended amounts of dietary fiber do not affect mineral status significantly.[62]

Some people, such as young children and the elderly who eat high-fiber diets, may feel full before meeting energy and nutrient needs. Because of a limited stomach capacity, they must be careful that fiber intake does not interfere with their ability to consume adequate energy and nutrients.

Key Concepts: *High sugar intake leads to dental caries and can contribute to nutrient deficiencies by replacing other more nutritious foods in the diet. High intake of complex carbohydrates offers many health benefits. Diets high in starch and dietary fiber decrease risk of obesity, type 2 diabetes, cancer, cardiovascular disease, and gastrointestinal disorders. Increase fiber intake gradually while drinking plenty of fluids; children and the elderly with small appetites should take care that energy needs are still met.*

Quick Bites

Fierce Fiber and Flatulence

The Jerusalem artichoke surpasses even dry beans in its capacity for facilitating flatulence. This artichoke contains large amounts of indigestible carbohydrate. After passing through the small intestine undigested, the fiber is attacked by gas-generating bacteria in the colon.

LEARNING Portfolio chapter 5

Key Terms

	page
acesulfame K [ay-see-SUL-fame]	147
added fiber	130
alitame	147
alpha bonds	133
amylopectin [am-ih-low-PEK-tin]	129
amylose [AM-uh-los]	129
artificial sweeteners	146
aspartame [AH-spar-tame]	147
beta bonds	133
bran	142
cellulose [SELL-you-los]	131
complex carbohydrates	128
dental caries [KARE-ees]	148
diabetes mellitus	137
dietary fibers	129
disaccharides [dye-SACK-uh-rides]	127
endosperm	142
epinephrine	136
fasting hypoglycemia	142
fructose [FROOK-tose]	127
galactose [gah-LAK-tose]	127
germ	142
glucagon [GLOO-kuh-gon]	136
glucose [GLOO-kose]	127
glycemic index	137
glycogen [GLY-ko-jen]	129
gums	131
hemicelluloses [hem-ih-SELL-you-loses]	131
husk	142
hyperglycemia [HIGH-per-gly-SEE-me-uh]	137
hypoglycemia [HIGH-po-gly-SEE-mee-uh]	141
insoluble fiber	130
insulin [IN-suh-lin]	136
insulin resistance	138
ketone bodies	136
ketosis [kee-TOE-sis]	136
lactose [LAK-tose]	128
lignins [LIG-nins]	131
maltose [MALL-tose]	128
monosaccharides	127
mucilages	131
nutritive sweeteners	145
oligosaccharides	128
pancreatic amylase	133
pectins	131
phenylketonuria (PKU)	147
polysaccharides	129
reactive hypoglycemia	142
refined sweeteners	146
resistant starch	129
saccharin [SAK-ah-ren]	146
simple carbohydrates	127
soluble fiber	130
starch	129
sucralose	147
sucrose [SOO-crose]	128
sugar alcohols	145
Syndrome X	139
D-tagatose	147
type 1 diabetes	138
type 2 diabetes	138

Study Points

- Carbohydrates include the simple sugars and complex carbohydrates.
- Monosaccharides are the building blocks of carbohydrates.
- Three monosaccharides are important in human nutrition: glucose, fructose, and galactose.
- The monosaccharides combine to make disaccharides: sucrose, lactose, and maltose.
- Starch, glycogen, and fiber are long chains (polysaccharides) of monosaccharide units; starch and glycogen contain only glucose.
- Carbohydrates are digested by enzymes from the mouth, pancreas, and small intestine and absorbed as monosaccharides.
- The liver converts the monosaccharides fructose and galactose to glucose.
- Blood glucose levels rise after eating and fall between meals. Two pancreatic hormones, insulin and glucagon, regulate blood glucose levels, preventing extremely high or low levels.
- In diabetes, insulin either is not produced or is ineffective, resulting in hyperglycemia. Diabetes is treated with diet, exercise, and medication, including insulin injections in some cases.
- Hypoglycemia results when blood glucose levels fall too low.
- The main function of carbohydrates in the body is to supply energy. In this role, carbohydrates spare protein for use in making body proteins and allow for the complete breakdown of fat as an additional energy source.
- Carbohydrates are found mainly in plant foods as starch, fiber, and sugar.
- In general, Americans consume more sugar and less starch and fiber than is recommended.
- Carbohydrate intake can affect health. Excess sugar can contribute to low nutrient intake, excess energy intake, and dental caries.
- Diets high in complex carbohydrates, including fiber, have been linked to reduced risk for GI disorders, heart disease, and cancer.

Chapter 6

Lipids: Not Just Fat

Think About It

1. How important is fat to the foods you find tasty?
2. What's your view about the value of body fat?
3. What's your take on the differences between fat and cholesterol?
4. What's your understanding of "good" versus "bad" cholesterol?

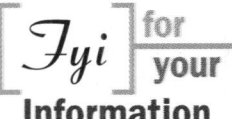

Fyi for your Information

This chapter's FYI boxes include practical information on the following topics:

- Fats on the Health Food Store Shelf
- Which Spread for Your Bread?
- Does "Reduced Fat" Reduce Calories? It Depends on the Food

www

The Web site for this book offers many useful tools and is a great source for additional nutrition information for both students and instructors. For information on lipids, visit the site at **nutrition.jbpub.com/discovering.** You'll find exercises that explore the following topics:

- Olestra: Snack without the Guilt?
- Fat, Low-Fat, No Fat?
- Fat Intake and Cancer
- Around the World with Lipids

What About Bobbie?

Track the choices Bobbie is making with the EatRight Analysis software.

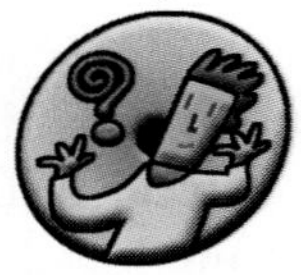

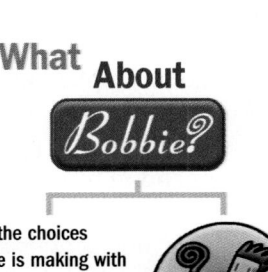

Key to Illustrations

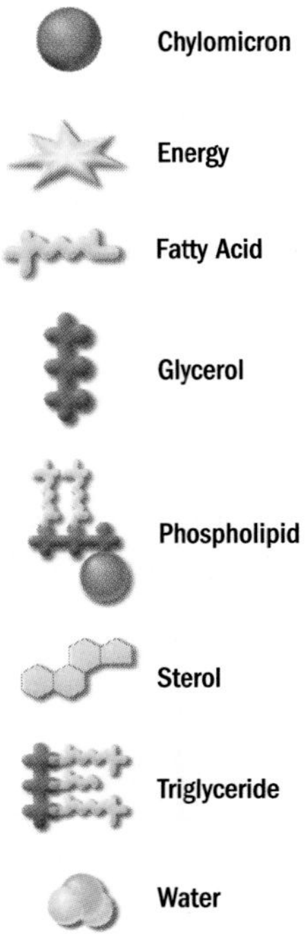

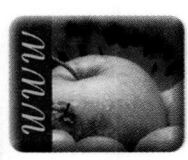

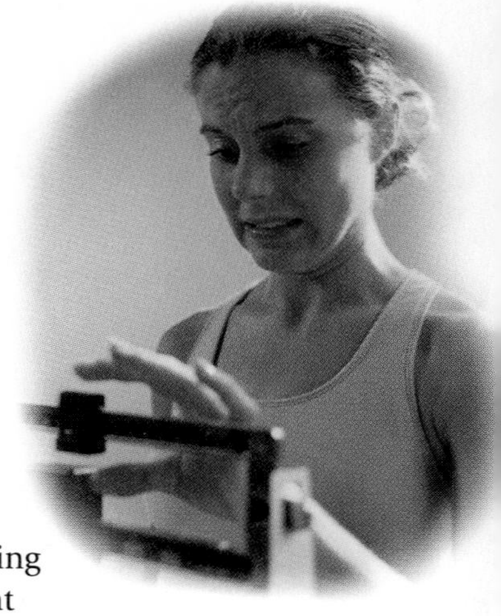

Consider two friends, Maria and Rachel, both on weight-loss diets. Maria swears by a new diet program that allows you to eat all the fat you want, but no high-carbohydrate "starchy" foods, and it's working—she's already lost 10 pounds! Then there's Rachel, whose goal in life is an intake of zero grams of fat. She's fat-obsessed—always buying "fat-free" this or that, and driving her friends nuts with information about the number of fat grams in everything they eat. As you listen to the two of them compare dieting stories, you start to wonder which one has the right approach to fat consumption or even if there is a right approach. On the one hand, it seems that as each day goes by, you hear more and more about Americans' high-fat diets and high rates of obesity and heart disease. On the other hand, is a "no-fat" diet healthy? Are all the low-fat and no-fat products really better choices nutritionally?

Fat is an essential nutrient that provides energy and helps transport fat-soluble nutrients to destinations throughout the body. Triglycerides, the fats we associate with fried foods, cream cheese, vegetable oil, or salad dressing, are one type of a larger group of compounds called lipids. Cholesterol, another lipid, is familiar to most Americans, but you may not realize that your body makes cholesterol and that dietary cholesterol makes only a small contribution to the total amount in your body. All lipids have important roles, but at the same time, too much triglyceride or too much cholesterol can lead to heart and circulatory problems.

Fats contribute greatly to the flavor and texture of foods. When food manufacturers remove fat to produce a low-fat product, they often have to boost the flavor with sugar, sodium, or other additives to create a tasty product. This means that fat-free foods sometimes aren't any lower in calories than regular food—so Rachel can't eat the whole box of fat-free cookies and still expect to lose weight! Think About It 1

phospholipids Compounds that consist of a glycerol molecule bonded to two fatty acid molecules and a phosphate group with a nitrogen-containing component. Phospholipids have both water-soluble and fat-soluble regions, which makes them good emulsifiers.

sterols A category of lipids that includes cholesterol. Sterols are hydrocarbons with several rings in their structures.

fatty acids Compounds containing a long hydrocarbon chain with a carboxyl group (—COOH) at one end and a methyl group ($-CH_3$) at the other end.

chain length The number of carbons that a fatty acid contains. Foods contain fatty acids with chain lengths of 4 to 24 carbons, and most have an even number of carbons.

What Are Lipids?

The term *lipids* applies to a variety of substances, including triglycerides, **phospholipids,** and **sterols**. Triglycerides are the most abundant lipid. In the body, fat cells store triglycerides in adipose tissue. In foods, we call triglycerides "fats and oils," with fats usually being solid and oils being liquid at room temperature. Overall, however, the choice of terms—*fat, triglyceride, oil*—is somewhat arbitrary, and these words often are used interchangeably. In this chapter, when we use the word *fat,* we are referring to *triglycerides*.

About 2 percent of dietary lipids are phospholipids. They are found in foods of both plant and animal origin, and the body can make them. Unlike other lipids, phospholipids are soluble in both fat and water. These versatile molecules play crucial roles as major components of cell membranes and in blood and body fluids, where they help keep fats suspended.

Only a small percentage of our dietary lipids are sterols, yet one infamous member, cholesterol, causes much public concern. The body makes cholesterol, which is an important component of cell membranes and a precursor of sex hormones, adrenal hormones (e.g., cortisol), vitamin D, and bile acids.

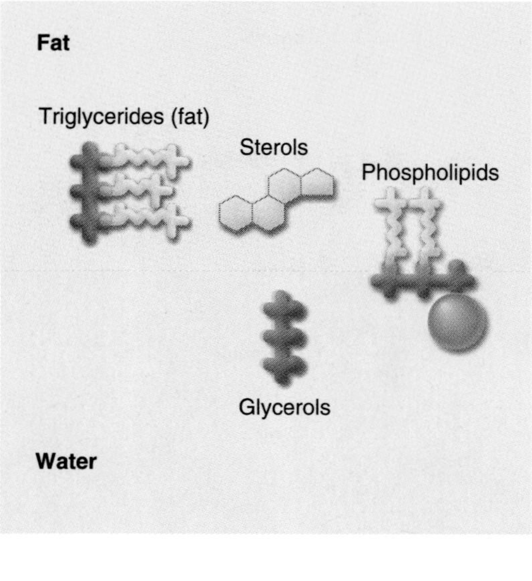

Fatty Acids Are Key Building Blocks

Fatty acids determine the characteristics of a fat, such as whether it is solid or liquid at room temperature. The basic structure of a fatty acid is a chain of carbon atoms with a carboxyl (acid) group (–COOH) at one end and a methyl group (–CH_3) at the other end. (See **Figure 6.1**.) Fatty acids that are not attached to other compounds are sometimes called "free" fatty acids. Some free fatty acids have their own distinct flavor. Butyric acid gives butter its flavor. Caproic, caprylic, and capric acids, all named after the Greek word for *goat*, have the undesirable "goaty" flavors and odors their names suggest. These "goaty" fatty acids contribute to the strong unpleasant odor of spoiled foods.

Chain Length

Fatty acids differ in **chain length** (the number of carbons in the chain). Foods contain fatty acids with chain lengths of 4 to 24 carbons, and most have an even number of carbons. Fatty acids are grouped as short-chain (less than 6 carbons), medium-chain (6 to 10 carbons), and long-chain (12 or more carbons). (See **Figure 6.2**.) The shorter the carbon chain, the more liquid the fatty acid becomes (the lower its melting point).

Figure 6.1 **Butyric acid.** Butyric acid is a fatty acid found in butter fat. Like all fatty acids, it has a methyl end (–CH_3) and an acid (carboxyl) end (–COOH).

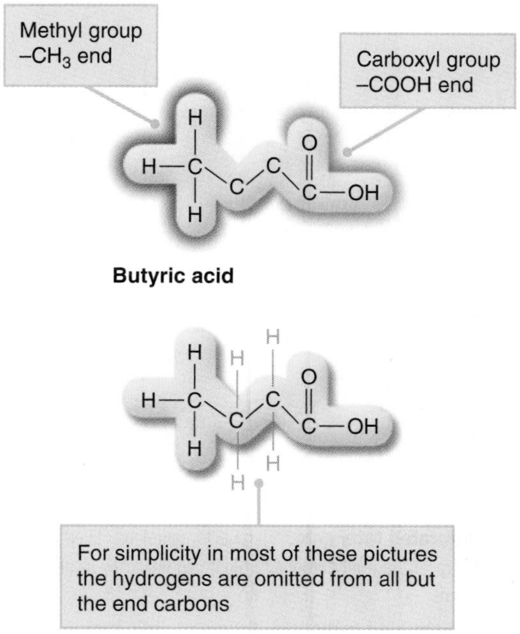

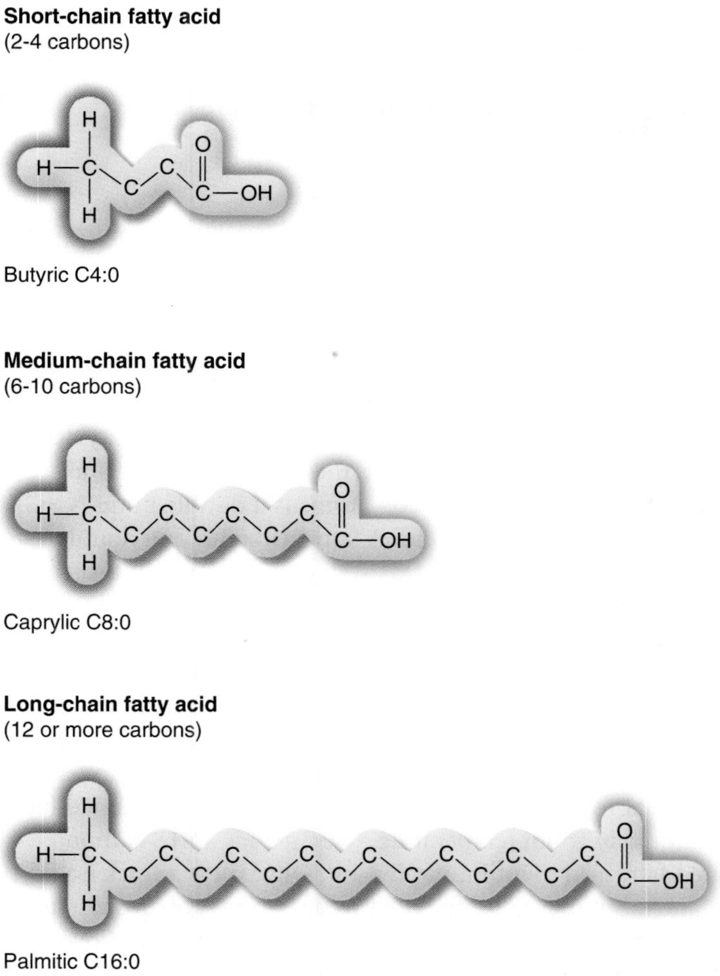

Figure 6.2 **Fatty acid chain lengths.** Fatty acids can be classified by their chain length as short-, medium-, and long-chain fatty acids.

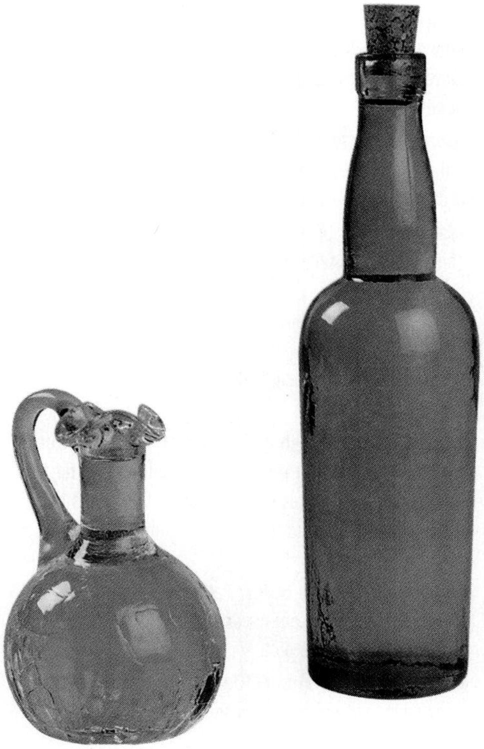

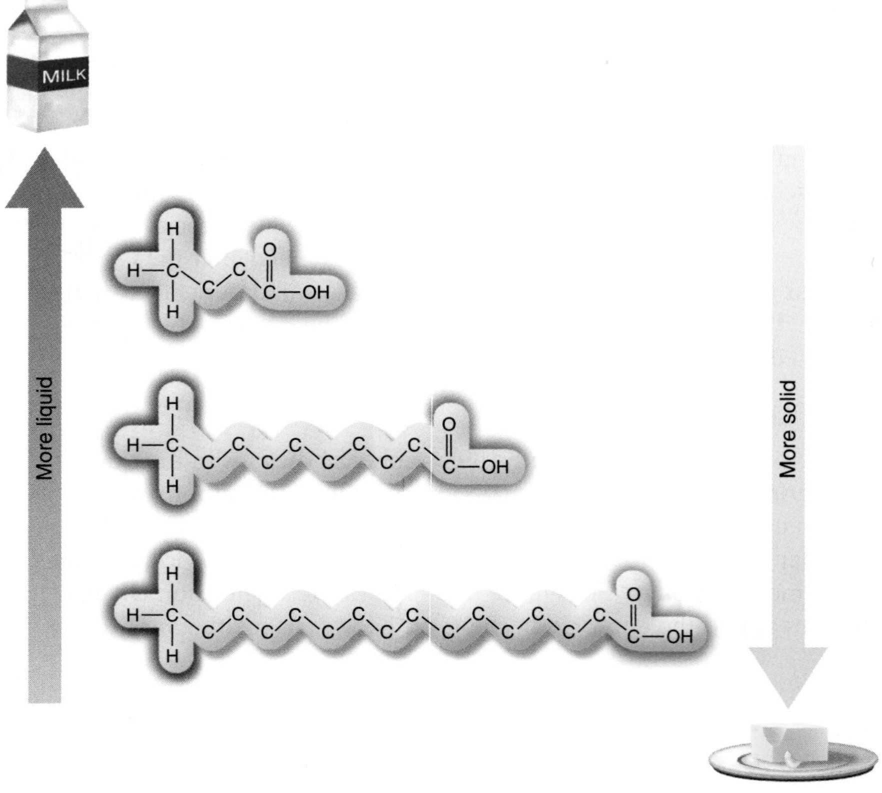

Figure 6.3 **Fatty acid chain lengths and liquidity.** As chain lengths of saturated fatty acids increase, fats tend to become more solid at room temperature.

saturated fatty acid A fatty acid completely filled by hydrogen, with all carbons in the chain linked by single bonds.

unsaturated fatty acid The carbon chain contains one or more double bonds.

monounsaturated fatty acid The carbon chain contains one double bond.

polyunsaturated fatty acid The carbon chain contains two or more double bonds.

linoleic acid [lin-oh-LAY-ik] An essential *omega*-6 fatty acid that contains 18 carbon atoms and 2 carbon–carbon double bonds (18:2); a thin liquid at room temperature.

conjugated linoleic acid (CLA) A polyunsaturated fatty acid in which the position of the double bonds has moved, so that a single bond alternates with two double bonds.

***alpha*-linolenic acid [Al-fah-lin-oh-LEN-ik]** An essential *omega*-3 fatty acid that contains 18 carbon atoms and 3 carbon–carbon double bonds (18:3).

***cis* fatty acid** Unsaturated fatty acid with a bent carbon chain. Most naturally occurring unsaturated fatty acids are *cis* fatty acids.

***trans* fatty acid** Unsaturated fatty acid with a straighter chain than a *cis* fatty acid, usually as a result of hydrogenation; *trans* fatty acids are more solid than *cis* fatty acids.

hydrogenation [high-dro-jen-AY-shun] A chemical reaction in which hydrogen atoms are added to a fat; hydrogenation produces more saturated fatty acids and converts some unsaturated fatty acids from a *cis* form to a *trans* form.

nonessential fatty acids Fatty acids that your body can make when they are needed. It is not necessary to consume them in the diet.

essential fatty acids (EFAs) Fatty acids that the body needs but cannot synthesize and must obtain from the diet.

(See **Figure 6.3**.) Shorter fatty acids also are more water-soluble, a property that affects their absorption in the digestive tract.

Saturation

The carbons in a fatty acid chain are attached to each other and to hydrogen atoms. If all the bonds between the carbon atoms in a fatty acid chain are single bonds (C–C), then the fatty acid is called a **saturated fatty acid**. Hydrogen atoms completely fill (saturate) all the other available bonding sites. If one or more bonds between carbon atoms is a double bond (C=C), the fatty acid is an **unsaturated fatty acid**. A fatty acid with one double bond is a **monounsaturated fatty acid (MUFA)**; one with two or more double bonds is a **polyunsaturated fatty acid (PUFA)**. **Figure 6.4** illustrates the three types of fatty acids.

Even though we refer to olive oil, for example, as a monounsaturated fat, food fats are a mixture of fatty acid types. Foods rich in saturated fatty acids tend to be solid at room temperature. (See **Figure 6.5**.) For example, stearic acid is an 18-carbon saturated fatty acid abundant in chocolate and meat fats, which are solid at room temperature. Food fats rich in unsaturated fatty acids tend to be liquid at room temperature. Oleic acid is an 18-carbon monounsaturated fatty acid plentiful in olive oil. Olive oil is a thick liquid at room temperature, but may solidify under refrigeration. Polyunsaturated **linoleic acid** is the major fatty acid of soybean oil, which is a thin liquid at room temperature. One form of linoleic acid, **conjugated linoleic acid (CLA)**, is under study for potential anticancer benefits.[1] Another polyunsaturated fatty acid, ***alpha*-linolenic acid** (don't confuse linolenic with linoleic), is abundant in flaxseed oil, a very thin liquid at room temperature.

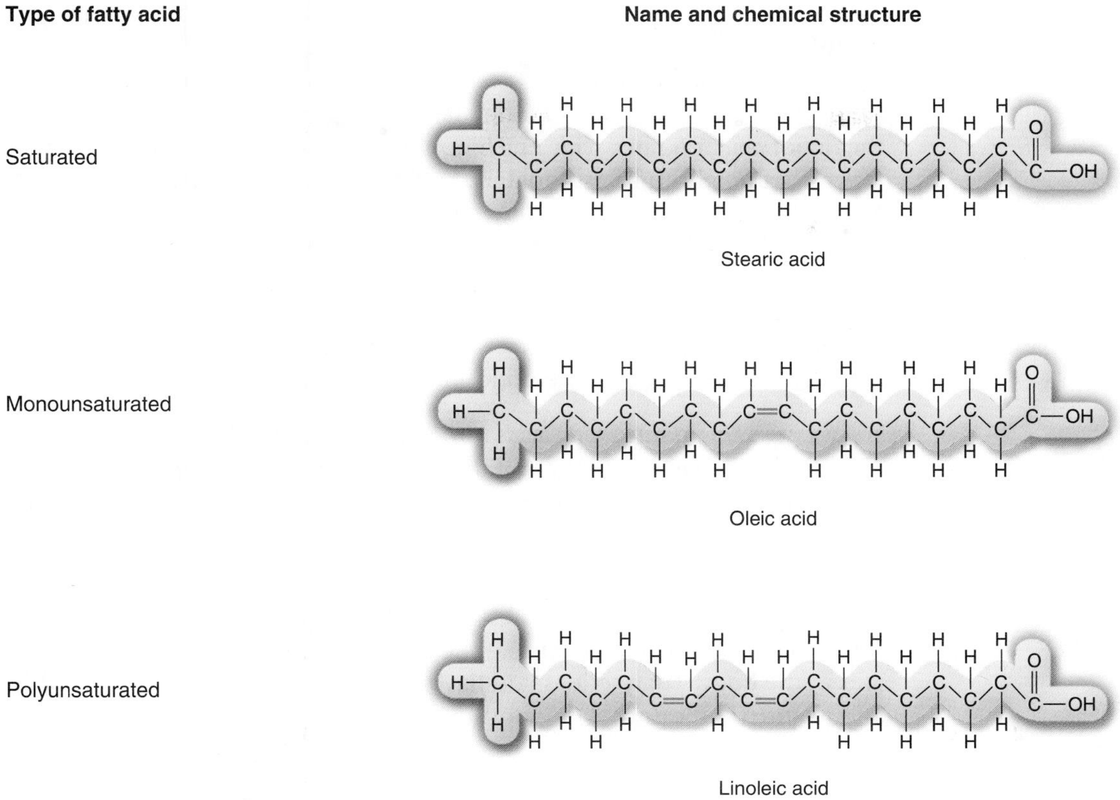
Type of fatty acid
Name and chemical structure
Saturated
Stearic acid
Monounsaturated
Oleic acid
Polyunsaturated
Linoleic acid

Figure 6.4 **Saturated, monounsaturated, and polyunsaturated fatty acids.** Hydrogens saturate the carbon chain of a saturated fatty acid. Unsaturated fatty acids have fewer hydrogens and have one (mono) or more (poly) carbon–carbon double bonds.

Key Concepts: *The term* lipids *refers to a group of substances that includes triglycerides, phospholipids, and sterols. Fatty acids are key building blocks of both triglycerides and phospholipids. Fatty acids are carbon chains of varying lengths. Fatty acids filled with hydrogen are called saturated, while those with missing hydrogen are unsaturated fatty acids.*

Cis versus *Trans*

Otherwise identical unsaturated fatty acids can have different shapes. The carbon chain of a ***cis* fatty acid** is bent, and the chain of a ***trans* fatty acid** is straighter. (See **Figure 6.6**.) Most naturally occurring unsaturated fatty acids are *cis* fatty acids. While cow's milk contains small amounts of *trans* fatty acids, a commercial process called **hydrogenation** creates most *trans* fatty acids in our diets. Hydrogenation adds hydrogen to an unsaturated fatty acid, making it more saturated. This process also straightens the fatty acid to a *trans* configuration. Because *trans* fatty acids have been implicated in raising blood cholesterol levels, they have become a health concern.

Nonessential and Essential Fatty Acids

The body is a good chemist, synthesizing many fatty acids as needed. Because it is not essential to have these fatty acids in your diet, they are called **nonessential fatty acids**. Don't confuse "nonessential" with "unimportant"—you must have an adequate supply of nonessential fatty acids, either by making or eating them.

Because the body cannot make all types of fatty acids it needs, some must come from food. These fatty acids are called **essential fatty acids (EFAs)**.

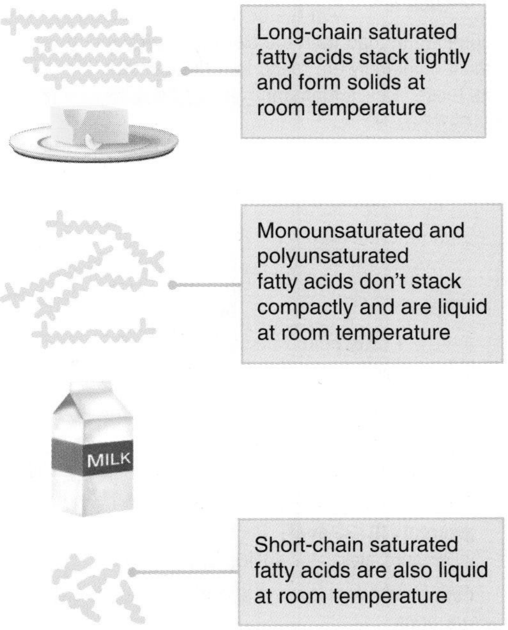
Long-chain saturated fatty acids stack tightly and form solids at room temperature
Monounsaturated and polyunsaturated fatty acids don't stack compactly and are liquid at room temperature
MILK
Short-chain saturated fatty acids are also liquid at room temperature

Figure 6.5 **Liquid or solid at room temperature?** Short-chain and unsaturated fatty acids cannot pack tightly together and tend to be more liquid than long-chain saturated fatty acids.

(See **Figure 6.7**.) There are two families of essential fatty acids—***omega*-3** and ***omega*-6**. These numbers refer to the location of the first double bond in these unsaturated fatty acids, counting from the carbon in the methyl (*omega*) end. *Alpha*-linolenic is the major *omega*-3 fatty acid, and linoleic is the major *omega*-6 fatty acid. Arachidonic acid, a longer *omega*-6 fatty acid, was once thought to be essential, but our bodies can make it from linoleic acid.

Essential fatty acids are precursors to hormonelike compounds called **eicosanoids**. Eicosanoids formed from the *omega*-6 fatty acid arachidonic acid can increase blood pressure, heart rate, blood clotting, immune response, and inflammation. Eicosanoids formed from the *omega*-3 fatty acid *alpha*-linolenic acid have opposing "heart healthy" effects.

Key Concepts: *Unsaturated fatty acids can have* cis *or* trans *double bonds. The body can make many, but not all, types of the fatty acids it needs. A fatty acid the body can make is a nonessential fatty acid, and one that must come from the diet is an essential fatty acid.*

Triglycerides

Triglycerides are the major lipid in the diet and in the body. Triglycerides add flavor and texture (and calories!) to foods and are an important source of energy.

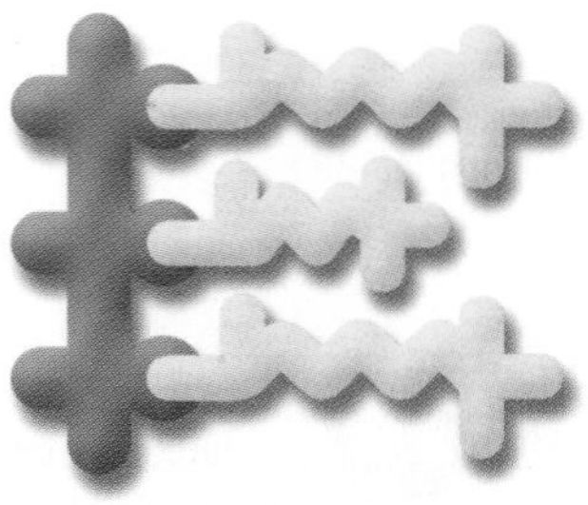

A generic triglyceride

Triglyceride Structure

Most fatty acids in food and in the body exist as part of a triglyceride molecule.

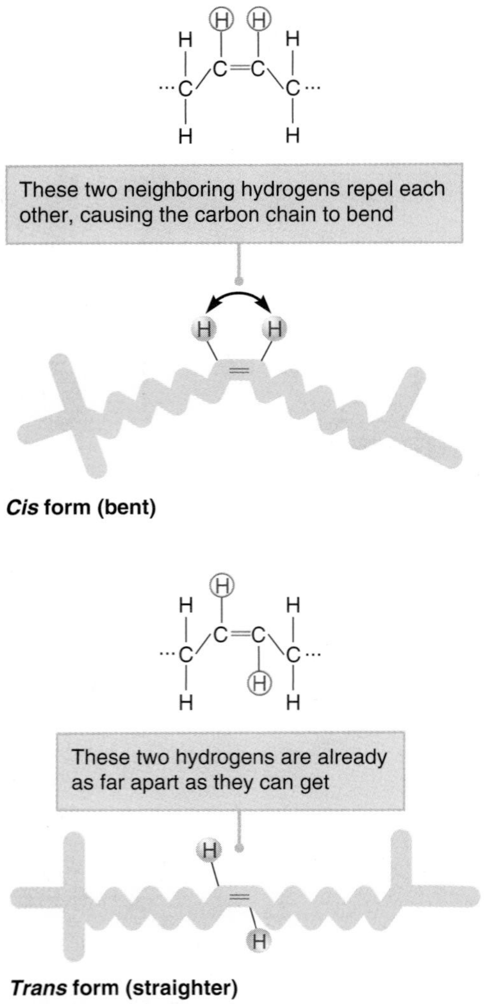

Figure 6.6 ***Cis* and *trans* fatty acids.** Fatty acids with the bent *cis* form are more common in food than the *trans* form. *Trans* fatty acids most commonly are found in hydrogenated fats, such as those in stick margarine, shortening, and deep-fat-fried foods.

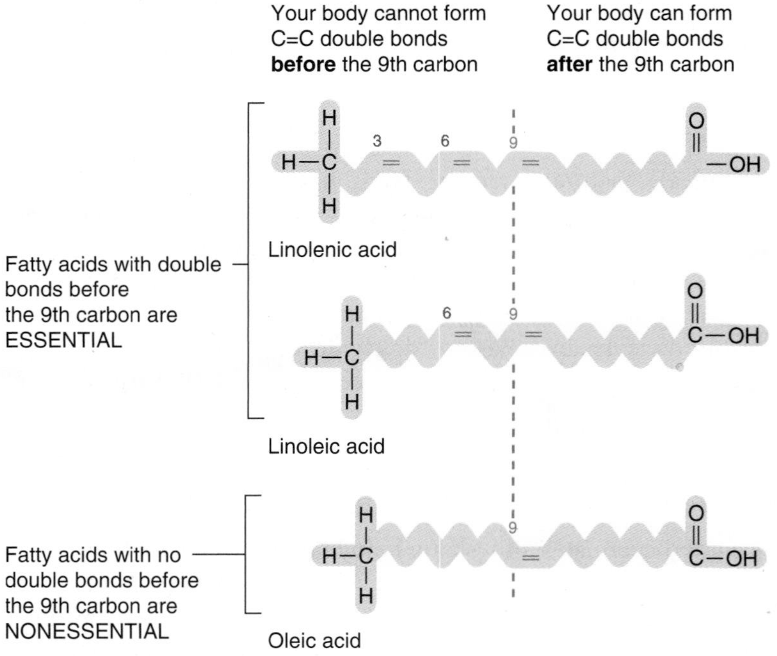

Figure 6.7 **Essential and nonessential fatty acids.** Your body makes some types of fatty acids, but others are essential in your diet.

***omega*-3 fatty acid** An essential fatty acid; *alpha*-linolenic acid is the major type.

***omega*-6 fatty acid** An essential fatty acid; linoleic acid is the primary type.

eicosanoids A class of hormonelike substances formed in the body from long-chain essential fatty acids.

glycerol [GLISS-er-ol] The backbone of mono-, di-, and triglycerides; alone, it is a thick, smooth liquid.

diglyceride A molecule of glycerol combined with two fatty acids.

monoglyceride A molecule of glycerol combined with one fatty acid.

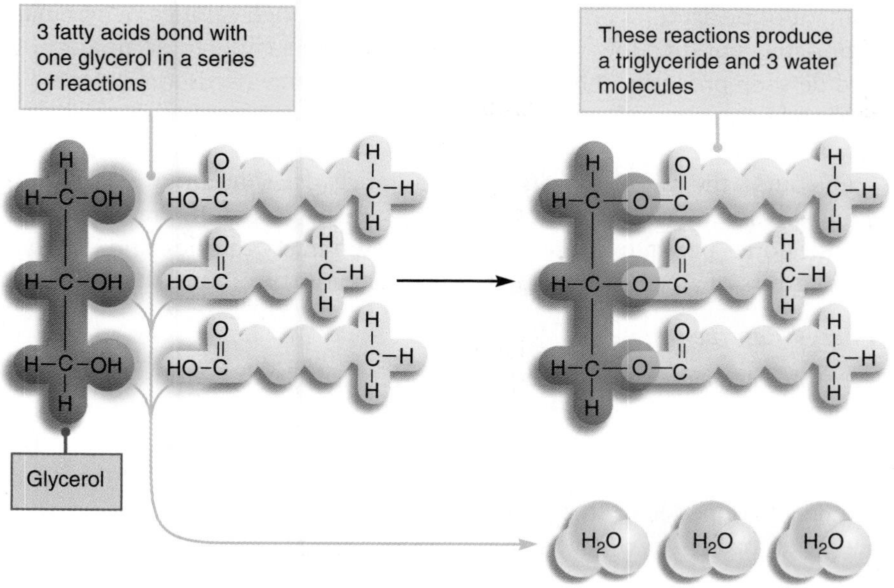

Figure 6.8 **Forming a triglyceride.** Reactions attach three fatty acids to a glycerol backbone to form a triglyceride. These reactions release water.

A triglyceride consists of three fatty acids attached to a glycerol backbone. Alone, **glycerol** is a thick, smooth liquid often used by the food industry. **Figure 6.8** illustrates the formation of a triglyceride.

Two fatty acids attached to a glycerol form a **diglyceride**. A **monoglyceride** has one fatty acid attached to glycerol. Our foods contain relatively small amounts of mono- and diglycerides, mostly as food additives used for their emulsifying or blending qualities.

Triglyceride Functions

Although some of us, like Rachel at the beginning of this chapter, think of fat as something to avoid, fat is a key nutrient with important body functions. **Figure 6.9** shows the functions of triglycerides.

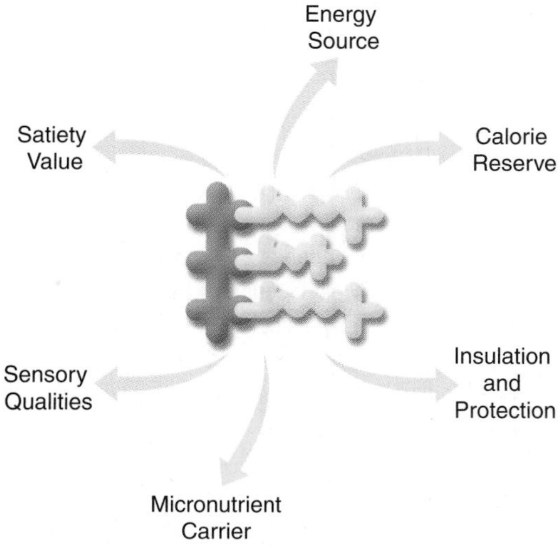

Figure 6.9 **Functions of triglycerides.** Fat performs a number of essential functions in the body.

Energy Source

Fat is a rich and efficient source of calories. Under normal circumstances, dietary and stored fats supply about 60 percent of the body's resting energy needs. Like carbohydrate, fat is *protein-sparing*; that is, fat is burned for energy, saving valuable proteins for their important roles as muscle tissue, enzymes, antibodies, and the like. Different body tissues prefer different sources of calories. While muscle tissue at rest prefers to burn fat (see **Figure 6.10**), brain cells rely almost exclusively on glucose except during prolonged starvation. During physical activity, glucose and glycogen join fat in supplying energy to muscles.

High-fat foods are higher in calories than high-protein or high-carbohydrate foods. One gram of fat contains 9 kilocalories, compared with only 4 kilocalories in a gram of carbohydrate or protein, or 7 kilocalories per gram of alcohol. For example, a tablespoon of corn oil (pure fat) has 120 kilocalories, whereas a tablespoon of sugar (pure carbohydrate) has only 50 kilocalories.

We welcome the high caloric density of fat when our energy needs are high. An infant, for example, who needs ample energy for fast growth but whose stomach can hold only a limited amount of food, needs the high-fat

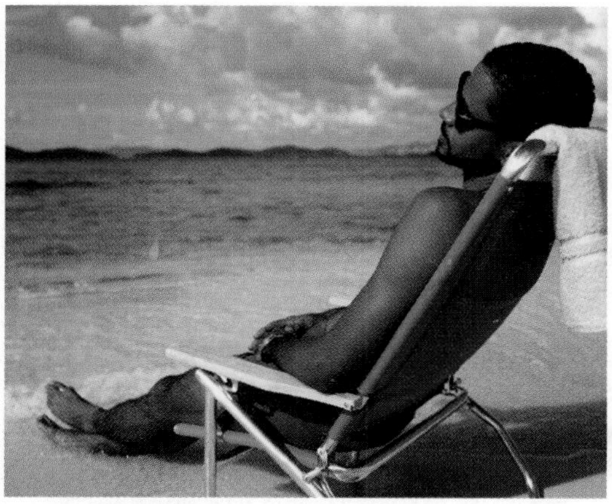

Figure 6.10 **Fat is an important energy source.** When at rest, muscles prefer to use fat for fuel.

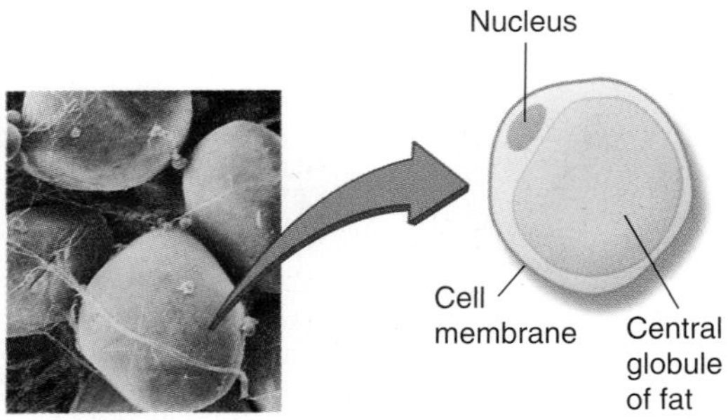

Figure 6.11 **Adipose cells store fat.** Adipocytes (fat cells) in adipose (fat) tissue store fat as an energy reserve. These are simple cells with just a nucleus, cell membrane, and fat droplet.

Quick Bites

The Marvelous Storage Efficiency of Fat

Why do you think we don't store all our extra energy as readily available glycogen? It would take more than 6 pounds of glycogen to store the same energy as 1 pound of fat. Just imagine how much bulkier we would be! How cumbersome it would be to move about! That's why only a very small portion of the body's energy reserve is glycogen.

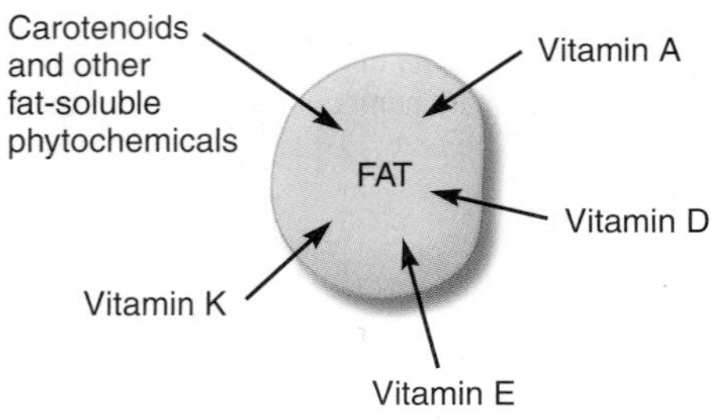

Figure 6.12 **Fat is a micronutrient carrier.** Fat holds more than just energy. It also carries important nutrients, such as fat-soluble vitamins and carotenoids.

adipocytes Fat cells.

adipose tissue Body fat tissue.

visceral fat Fat stores that cushion body organs.

subcutaneous fat Fat stores under the skin.

lanugo [lah-NEW-go] Soft, downy hair that covers a normal fetus from the fifth month but is shed almost entirely by the time of birth. It also appears on semi-starved individuals who have lost much of their body fat, serving as insulation normally provided by body fat.

content of breast milk or infant formula to get enough calories. When inappropriately put on a low-fat diet, infants and young children do not grow and develop properly. Other people with high-energy needs are athletes, those who are physically active in their jobs, or people regaining weight lost due to illness.

Of course, the caloric density of fat has a negative side, and we don't welcome it when we are trying to maintain a healthy weight. In practical terms, 9 kilocalories per gram makes it easy to eat too many calories, and dietary fat in excess of a person's energy needs is a major contributor to obesity.

Energy Reserve

We store excess dietary fat as body fat to get us through periods of calorie deficit. Because fat is calorie-dense, it can store a lot of energy in a small space. The fat is stored inside fat cells called **adipocytes**, which form body fat tissue, technically called **adipose tissue**. (See **Figure 6.11**.) Hibernating animals have perfected this process; the fat stores they build in autumn can see them through a winter's fast.

Insulation and Protection

Fat tissue usually accounts for about 15 to 30 percent of body weight. Part of this is **visceral fat**, adipose tissue around organs. Visceral fat cushions and shields delicate organs, especially the kidneys. Women have extra fat, most noticeably in the breasts and hips, to help shield reproductive organs and to guarantee adequate calories during pregnancy. Other fat tissue is **subcutaneous**, lying under the skin, where it protects and insulates the body. Perhaps nowhere is fat's structural role more dramatic than in the brain, which is 60 percent fat.[2]

Can one have too little body fat? Just ask someone whose body fat has been depleted by illness. It hurts to sit and it hurts to lie down. For people without enough body fat, cool temperatures are intolerable and even room temperature may be uncomfortably cool. Women stop menstruating and become infertile. Children stop growing. Skin deteriorates from pressure sores or from fatty acid deficiency and may become covered with fine hair called **lanugo**. Illness, involuntary starvation, and famine can deplete fat to this extent, as can excessive dieting and exercise. *Think* About It 2

Carrier of Fat-Soluble Compounds

Dietary fats dissolve and transport micronutrients such as fat-soluble vitamins (A, D, E, and K) and fat-soluble phytochemicals (carotenoids, for example). (See **Figure 6.12**.) Dietary fats carry fat-soluble substances through the digestive process, improving intestinal absorption, or bioavailability.[3] For example, the body absorbs more lycopene, the healthful red-colored phytochemical in tomatoes, if the tomatoes are served with oil or salad dressing.

Removing a food's lipid portion—for example, removing butterfat from milk—also removes fat-soluble vitamins. In most dairy products, manufacturers replace vitamin A. Refining wheat grain to white flour extends shelf life but removes the lipid-rich germ portion. Vitamin E is lost with the germ and is not replaced. Processing fats may destroy fat-soluble vitamins; for example, some vitamin E is lost in processing vegetable oils.

Sensory Qualities

Fat contributes greatly to the flavor, odor, and texture of food. Simply put, it makes food taste good. (See **Figure 6.13**.) Flavorful chemicals dissolve in the fat of a food; heat sends them into the air, producing mouth-watering odors that perk up appetites. Fats have a rich, satisfying feeling in the mouth. In liquid form, they're uniquely efficient at stimulating taste buds.[4] Fats make baked goods tender and moist. And fats can be heated to high temperatures for frying, which seals in flavors and cooks food quickly. These are all good qualities, but too good for many people who find high-fat foods irresistible and eat too much of them. Alas, fat's most appealing attributes are also serious drawbacks to maintaining a healthful diet.

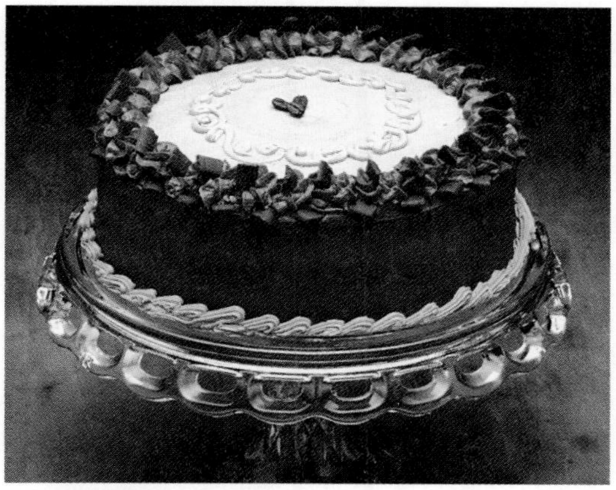

Figure 6.13 Fat imparts a rich texture and smooth mouth feel to food.

Triglycerides in Food

Dietary triglycerides are found in a variety of fats and oils as well as in foods that contain them, such as salad dressing or baked goods. Some food fats are obvious, such as butter, margarine, cooking oil, and the fat along a cut of meat or under the skin of chicken. Less noticeable food fats are found in baked goods, snack foods, nuts, and seeds.

Fats and oils are complex mixtures, but we often classify them simplistically by their saturation—saturated, monounsaturated, or polyunsaturated—depending on their overall fatty acid content. (See **Figure 6.14**.) Canola oil, for example, often is classified as a monounsaturated fat. Most fatty acids in canola oil are monounsaturated oleic acid, although about 10 percent is polyunsaturated *alpha*-linolenic acid.

oxidation Oxygen attaches to the double bonds of unsaturated fatty acids. Oxidation causes fats to become rancid.

Sources of Omega-3 Fatty Acids

Generally, polyunsaturated fatty acids are found in plant foods. Soybean oil, canola oil, and walnuts contain *alpha*-linolenic acid, an essential *omega*-3 fatty acid. However, the most generous source is flaxseed (or linseed) oil, which is over 50 percent *alpha*-linolenic. Longer-chain *omega*-3s, EPA and DHA, are found in fatty fish (e.g., salmon, tuna, or mackerel) and in fish oil supplements. These supplements should not be taken without medical supervision because of their potent effects.[5] See the FYI feature "Fats on the Health Food Store Shelf."

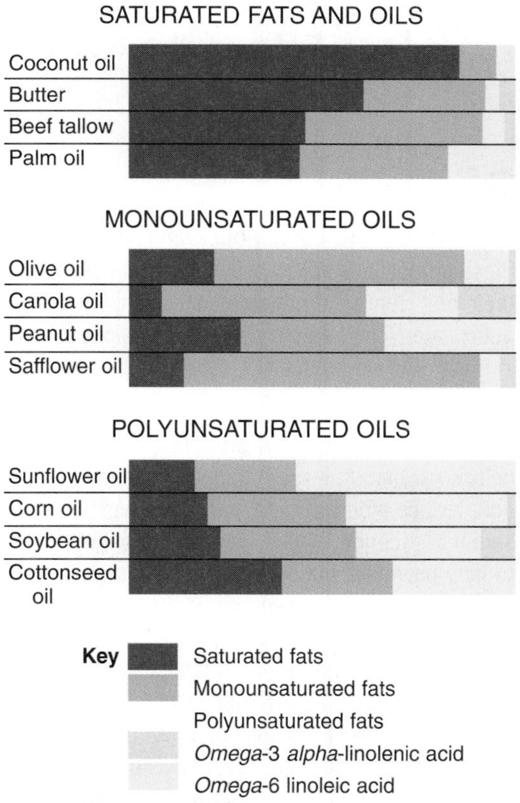

Figure 6.14 **The diversity of fats.** Fats contain a mix of saturated and unsaturated fatty acids. Depending on which type of fatty acid is most prevalent, the fat is classified as saturated, monounsaturated, or polyunsaturated.
Source: Adapted from *Nutrition Today*, May/June 1996;31(3).

Sources of Omega-6 Fatty Acids

Good sources of the *omega*-6 fatty acid linoleic acid include seeds, nuts, and the richest source, common vegetable oils. Arachidonic acid, a longer *omega*-6 fatty acid found in some meats, is less common.

Commercial Processing of Fats

In earlier times, people could obtain concentrated fats and oils only through simple processing: rendering fats from meats and poultry, skimming or churning the butterfat from milk, skimming the oil from ground nuts, or pressing a few oil-rich plant parts such as coconuts or olives.

In the 1920s new technology began producing pure vegetable oils.[6] Processing vegetable oils reduces waste, prevents spoilage during normal use, and increases the worldwide availability of calorie-rich oils. Processing removes damaging free fatty acids and certain destructive enzymes. Processing also adds antioxidants such as vitamin E to delay rancidity and extend shelf life. Without protection, unsaturated fats exposed to air undergo **oxidation** and rapidly turn rancid. People fortunately avoid bad-tasting rancid fats. Oxidized fats damage body tissues, particularly blood vessels.[7] Exposure to light increases the rate of oxidation and shortens shelf life.

Unfortunately, processing also has a negative side. To achieve stability and uniform taste, processing removes potentially healthful phospholipids, plant sterols, and other phytochemicals; and a significant portion of the natural vitamin E is lost. Oils have become so familiar that we often forget they are highly processed, highly refined foods. Further processing of oils into solid fats such as margarine or shortening also produces some undesirable changes, such as increasing the proportion of *trans* fatty acids.

To get a liquid vegetable oil to act like a solid fat, hydrogenation adds hydrogen to unsaturated fatty acids. This process produces a harder, more saturated fat that is more effective for making baked goods and snack foods and one that spreads like butter. (Most of us recoil at the thought of putting pure corn oil on toast!) While hydrogenation protects the fat from oxidation and rancidity, it also straightens the fatty acids to become *trans* fatty acids. This, combined with the increase in saturated fatty acids, might lead you to wonder if margarine is indeed a better alternative to butter. (See the FYI feature "Which Spread for Your Bread?")

Key Concepts: *Triglycerides are formed when a glycerol molecule combines with three fatty acids. Dietary triglycerides add texture and flavor to food and are a concentrated source of calories. The body stores excess calories as adipose tissue. While storing energy, adipose tissue also insulates the body and cushions its organs. The fats in food carry valuable fat-soluble nutrients into the body and help with their absorption.*

[Fyi] Fats on the Health Food Store Shelf

FOR YOUR INFORMATION

Many claims made for lipid products sold as supplements may not hold up under scientific scrutiny. You may not even recognize these products as lipids, especially because their long, complicated names are often abbreviated. The amount of lipid and calories in most of these products is quite small.

EPA and DHA in Fish Oil Capsules

These *omega*-3 fatty acids are thought to help lower blood pressure, reduce inflammation, reduce blood clotting, and lower high serum triglyceride levels.[1] They were thought to help psoriasis, but studies proved disappointing.[2] EPA (eicosapentaenoic acid) and DHA (docosahexaenoic acid) usually make up only about one-third of the fatty acids in fish oil capsules, and research studies often use multiple doses. These should not be taken without close medical supervision, because their blood-thinning properties can cause bleeding. Because fish oil is highly unsaturated, antioxidant vitamins are included to prevent oxidation. Another problem, though not health related, is that fish oil capsules often leave a fishy aftertaste.

Flaxseed Oil Capsules

Flaxseed oil, or linseed oil, is an unusually good source of *omega*-3 *alpha*-linolenic acid, which accounts for about 55 percent of its fatty acids. Like fish oil, flaxseed oil is highly unsaturated and thus very susceptible to rancidity. Capsules protect the oil from oxygen, but limit the dose. A half-tablespoon of canola oil has about as much *omega*-3 as a capsule of flaxseed oil, but adds more calories. DHA and EPA are considered more potent *omega*-3 fatty acids than *alpha*-linolenic.

GLA in Borage, Evening Primrose, or Black Currant Seed Oil Capsules

These oils contain 9 to 24 percent GLA (*gamma*-linolenic acid), an *omega*-6 derivative of linoleic acid. Studies of GLA's effects on skin diseases, heart conditions, and other disorders have been disappointing.[3]

Medium-Chain Triglycerides Oil

Medium-chain triglycerides (MCT) can be purchased as such or found as ingredients in "sports" drinks and foods. They are marketed to athletes as a noncarbohydrate source of quick, concentrated energy; however, although readily absorbed, they have no specific performance benefits. A tablespoon of MCT contains about 100 kilocalories.

Lecithin Oil or Granules

Lecithin supplements are a mixture of phospholipids derived from soybeans. They often are

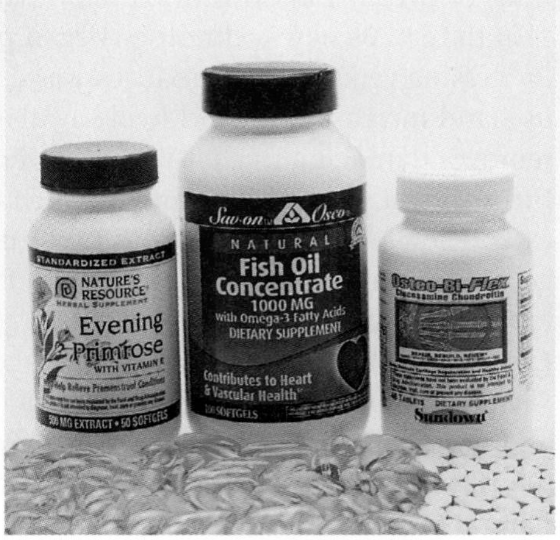

Phospholipids

Like triglycerides, phospholipids contain glycerol and fatty acids. However, phospholipids also contain other substances that give them entirely different properties and functions. Our bodies can make phospholipids, so we do not need them in our diets.

Phospholipid Structure

A phospholipid looks like a triglyceride, except that one fatty acid is replaced by another compound. Phospholipids are diglycerides—two fatty acids attached to a glycerol backbone. A **phosphate group** with a nitrogen-containing component occupies the third attachment site.

The phosphate–nitrogen component of phospholipids is soluble in water, so a phospholipid is compatible with both fat and water: The fatty acids in its diglyceride area attract fats, and the phosphate–nitrogen component attracts water-soluble substances. **Figure 6.15** shows the structure of a phospholipid.

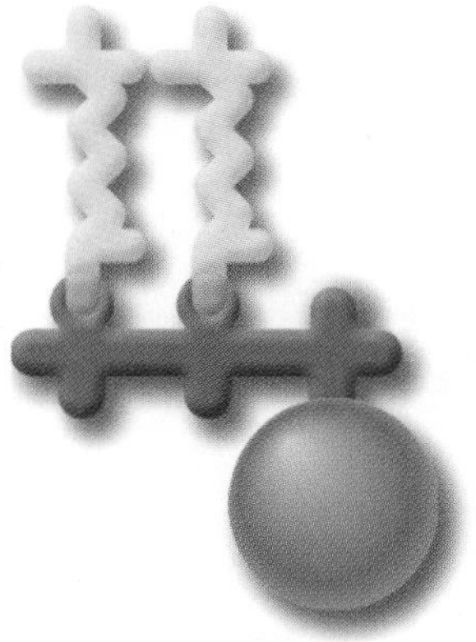

A generic phospholipid

phosphate group A chemical group that contains phosphate ($-PO_4$) attached to a larger molecule. Attaching a phosphate group, along with two fatty acids, to a glycerol backbone forms a phospholipid.

promoted as emulsifiers that lower cholesterol, but since dietary phospholipids are broken down by the enzyme lecithinase in the intestine, they cannot have this effect. They may be useful as a source of choline. Since choline is the precursor of acetylcholine (a neurotransmitter), lecithin is promoted for treating Parkinson's and Alzheimer's diseases, which are associated with low levels of acetylcholine in the brain. Unfortunately, these efforts have met with little success.[4]

Monolaurin Capsules

Monolaurin is a type of lauric acid, a 12-carbon fatty acid found in coconut oil. Lauric acid is said to protect against infection, but the amount in these capsules is probably too small to be significant.

CLA

Conjugated linoleic acid (CLA) is linoleic acid with a different pattern of chemical bonds. It is promoted as an aid for reducing body fat, among other claims, but the effects of supplementation are largely unstudied.

DHEA

Dehydroepiandrosterone (DHEA) is a testosterone precursor formed from cholesterol. It is present in the body in large quantities during adolescence, peaks in the 20s, and gradually declines with age. Many elderly people have low levels, and levels also dip during serious illnesses. With only a few exceptions, attempts to use DHEA for illnesses or to slow aging have been disappointing. Researchers generally use doses many times greater than those in over-the-counter supplements, levels that may cause hairiness in women and, more seriously, a risk of liver problems.[5]

Squalene Capsules and Shark Liver Oil

Squalene, an intermediary compound in the synthesis of cholesterol in the body, and shark liver oil, which contains squalene, are said to help liver, skin, and immune function. The basis for these claims is unclear.

1 Connor SL, Connor WE. Are fish oils beneficial in disease prevention and treatment? *Am J Clin Nutr.* 1997;66:S1020-S1031.

2 Soyland E, et al. Effect of dietary supplementation with very-long-chain n-3 fatty acids in patients with psoriasis. *N Engl J Med.* 1993;328:1812–1816.

3 Berth-Jones J, Graham-Brown RAC. Placebo-controlled trial of essential fatty acid supplementation in atopic dermatitis. *Lancet.* 1993;341:1557–1560.

4 Mauron J, Leathwood P. Dietary phosphatidylcholine as a precursor of brain acetylcholine. In: Horisberger H, Bracco U, eds. *Lipids in Modern Nutrition.* New York: Raven Press; 1987:133–145.

5 Khaw KT. Dehydroepiandrosterone, dehydroepiandrosterone sulphate and cardiovascular disease. *J Endocrinol.* 1996;150:S149–S153.

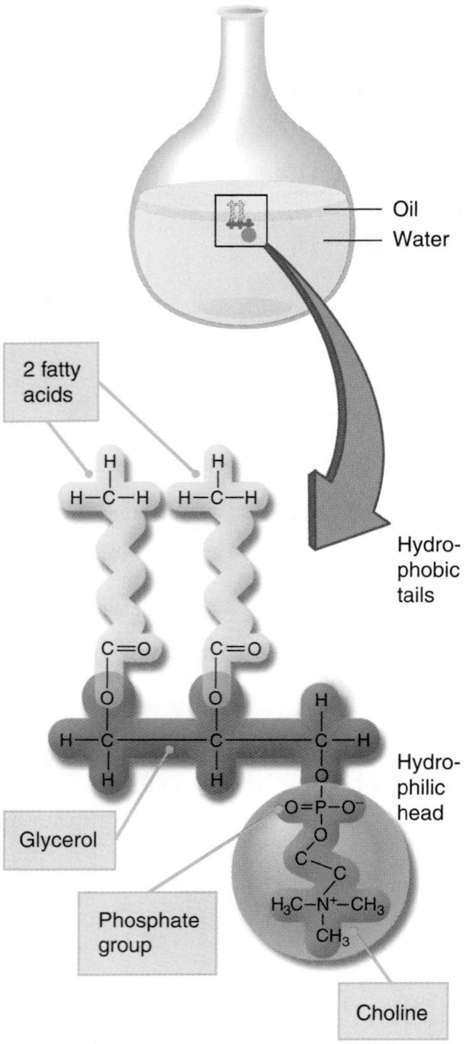

Figure 6.15 **Phospholipid.** A phospholipid is compatible with both oil and water. This is a useful property for transporting fatty substances in the body's watery fluids.

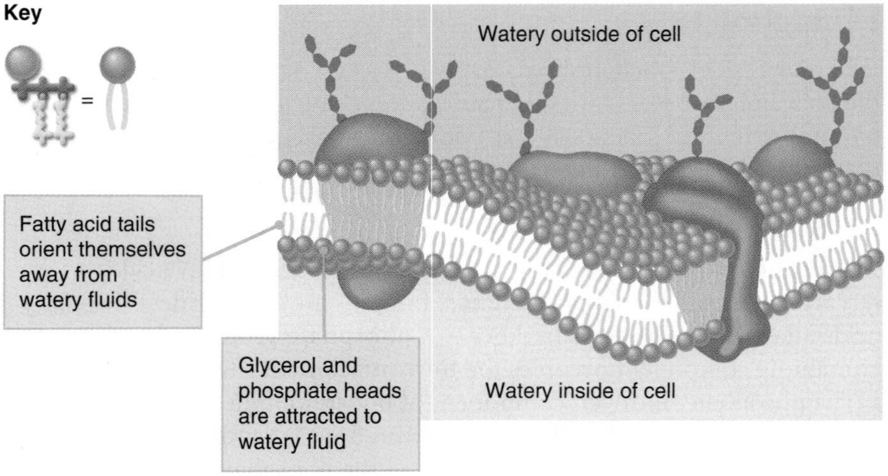

Figure 6.16 **Cell membranes are phospholipid bilayers.** Although proteins and other substances are embedded in cell membranes, these membranes primarily consist of phospholipids.

Phospholipid Functions

Because phospholipids have both water-soluble and fat-soluble parts, they are ideal emulsifiers (compounds that help keep fats suspended in a watery environment). In foods, phospholipids can keep oil and water mixed. This same property makes phospholipids a perfect structural element for cell membranes—able to communicate with the watery environments of blood and cell fluids, yet with a lipid portion that allows other lipids to enter and exit cells.

Cell Membranes

Phospholipids are major components of cell membranes. Cell membranes are a double layer of phospholipids that selectively allow both fatty and water-soluble substances into the cell. (See **Figure 6.16**.) They also store fatty acids temporarily, donating them when the body has short-term energy needs or must make regulatory chemicals (e.g., eicosanoids). One phospholipid, phosphatidylcholine, whose **choline** component eventually becomes part of the major neurotransmitter acetylcholine, plays an especially important role in nerve cells. By keeping fatty acids, choline, and other biologically active substances bound in phospholipids and freeing them only as needed, the body can regulate them closely.

Lipid Transport

The ability of phospholipids to combine both fatty and watery substances comes in handy throughout the body. In the stomach, dietary phospholipids help break fats into tiny particles for easier digestion. In the intestine, phospholipids from bile continue emulsifying. And in the watery environment of blood, phospholipids coat the surface of the lipoproteins that carry lipid particles to their destinations in the body.

Emulsifiers (Lecithin)

In the body and in foods of animal origin, phosphatidylcholine is also called **lecithin**. However, for food additives or supplements, the term *lecithin* is used for a mix of phospholipids derived from plants (usually soybeans). Understandably, this inconsistent terminology has caused confusion.

Quick Bites

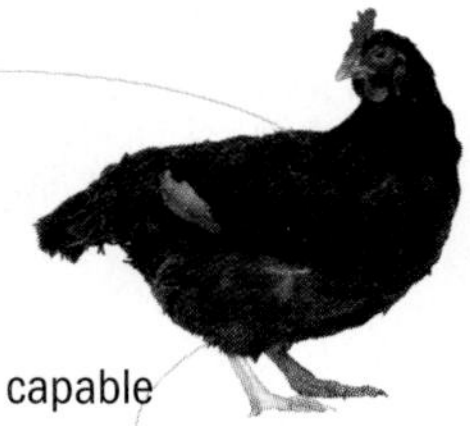

The Power of Yolk

A single raw egg yolk is capable of emulsifying many cups of oil. Cooks take advantage of the natural emulsifying ability of egg yolk phospholipids to emulsify and stabilize preparations such as mayonnaise (oil and vinegar emulsion) or hollandaise sauce (butter and lemon juice emulsion). Food producers use phospholipid emulsifiers in processed foods, which today provide much of our intake.

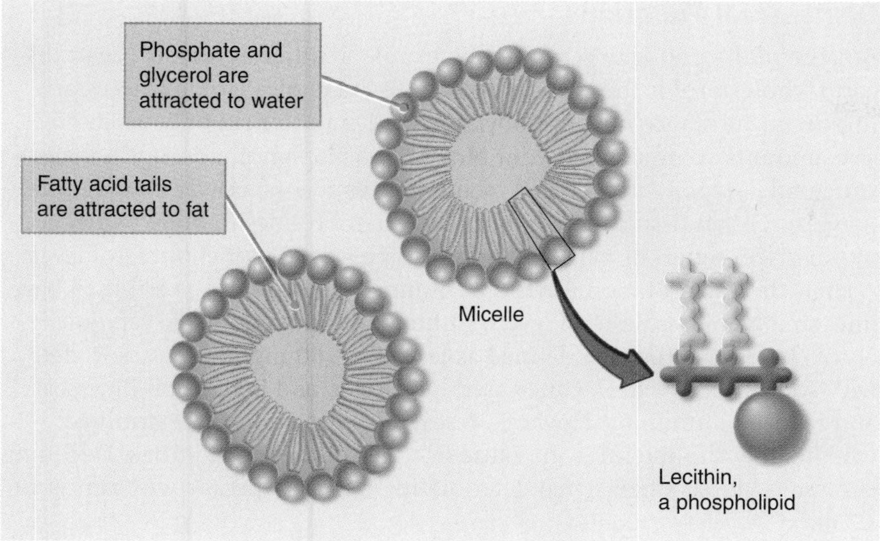

Figure 6.17 **Lecithin and emulsification.** Lecithin, a phospholipid, forms water-soluble packages called *micelles* that suspend fat-soluble compounds in watery mediums. In a micelle, the lecithin molecules form into a water-soluble ball with a fatty core. The water-soluble head of each lecithin molecule points outward in contact with the watery medium, while the fat-soluble tails point inward in contact with the fatty core.

The food industry uses lecithin as an emulsifier to combine two ingredients that don't ordinarily mix, such as oil and water. (See **Figure 6.17**.) In high-fat powdered products (e.g., dry milk, milk replacers, and coffee creamers), lecithin helps mix fatty compounds with water. Lecithin in salad dressing, chili, and sloppy-joe mixes allows the ingredients to mix well and remain mixed, avoiding separation. Lecithin is even added to chewing gum to increase shelf life, prolong flavor release, and prevent the gum from sticking to teeth and dental work.

choline A nitrogen-containing compound that is part of the phospholipid lecithin. Choline also is part of the neurotransmitter acetylcholine. The body can synthesize choline from the amino acid methionine.

lecithin In the body, a phospholipid with the nitrogen-containing component choline. In foods, lecithin is a blend of phospholipids with different nitrogen-containing components.

Phospholipids in Food

Phospholipids occur naturally throughout the plant and animal world, although in much smaller amounts than triglycerides. They are most abundant in egg yolks, liver, soybeans, and peanuts. While food processing often removes some phospholipids, other phospholipids are common food additives. Overall, a typical diet contains only about 2 grams per day. Because your body can make phospholipids, they are not a dietary essential.

Key Concepts: *Phospholipids are diglycerides (glycerol plus two fatty acids) with a phosphate–nitrogen compound attached at the third attachment point of glycerol. This structure makes phospholipids compatible with both fat and water. Phospholipids are major components of cell membranes and act as emulsifiers. Phospholipids also store fatty acids for release into the cell, and they are a source of choline. Because the body can make phospholipids, they are not needed in the diet.*

Sterols

Think About It 3

Although sterols are lipids, they are quite different from triglycerides and phospholipids. While triglycerides and phospholipids have a glycerol backbone and fingerlike fatty acid structures, sterols have a multiple-ring structure. (See **Figure 6.18**.) Unlike triglycerides and phospholipids, most sterols contain no fatty acids.

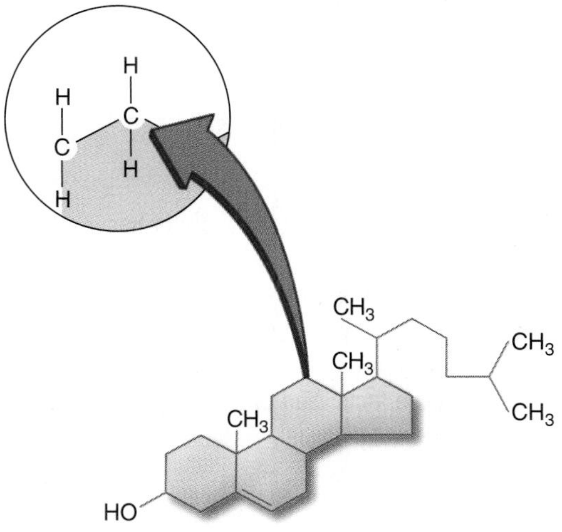

Cholesterol

Figure 6.18 **Sterols.** Sterols are multi-ring structures. Because of cholesterol's role in heart disease, it has become the best-known sterol.

Cholesterol Functions

Because of the publicity generated by its role in **atherosclerosis** (heart disease), **cholesterol** is the best-known sterol. But cholesterol is a necessary, important substance in your body; it becomes a problem only when excessive amounts accumulate in your blood. Like phospholipids, it is a major structural component of all cell membranes and is especially abundant in nerve and brain tissue. In fact, most cholesterol resides in body tissue, not in the blood serum or plasma that is routinely tested for cholesterol levels.

High cholesterol blood levels are common, but it is also possible to have undesirably low cholesterol levels. Although it's not common, very low levels of cholesterol (usually defined as less than 160 mg/dL) are associated with some kinds of stroke; increased lung, liver, and behavioral illnesses; and reduced immunity.[8] However, researchers have not yet determined whether low cholesterol is the cause or result of these conditions. Declining cholesterol levels often signal deteriorating health in people with cancer or AIDS.[9]

atherosclerosis [ath-e-roh-scle-ROH-sis] The accumulation of fatty plaques inside artery walls. These plaques cause vessel walls to become thick and hardened.

cholesterol [ko-LES-te-rol] A waxy lipid (sterol) whose chemical structure contains multiple hydrocarbon rings.

[Fyi] FOR YOUR INFORMATION

Which Spread for Your Bread?

Okay, it's time to see if you can put some of your new knowledge about lipids to work. You're standing in front of the dairy case ready to pick out the best spread. But, wow! So many choices. Of course, there's butter, the traditional spread—wholesome, natural, and creamy; sometimes there's just no substitute for the real thing. Margarine is the choice of many and has come to be more familiar than butter to some consumers. Then what's this "vegetable oil spread"? Here's one that says it "helps promote healthy cholesterol levels."

Butter

When it comes to heart health, butter has some serious disadvantages: (1) Butter is high in cholesterol-raising saturated fat, (2) it contains cholesterol, and (3) like other fats, it's high in calories.

Here are the facts: one tablespoon of butter provides the following:

- 100 kcals
- 11 g fat
- 8 g saturated fat
- 30 mg cholesterol
- 85 mg sodium
- 8% Daily Value for vitamin A

The ingredients are simple: "cream, salt, annatto (added seasonally)." Annatto is a natural coloring (a carotenoid) that is used to keep the color of butter consistent, despite what dairy cows might have been grazing on.

If you like the taste of butter, but want a bit less saturated fat and cholesterol, you can buy "whipped butter." The ingredients are the same, with the exception of incorporated air, and the reduction in calories, fat, saturated fat, cholesterol, and sodium is 30 to 40 percent.

Margarine

Margarine was developed to be a substitute for butter. Made from vegetable oils, it appears to be more healthful; as a plant-derived food, it's certainly cholesterol-free, and vegetable oils contain more unsaturated fatty acids than butter. Inconveniently, though, unsaturated oils are liquid, and without extra processing, margarine would run right off any slice of bread. Hydrogenated oils are needed to produce a spreadable consistency. But, as you know, hydrogenation increases the number of saturated and *trans* fatty acids in a fat, and both of these are associated with higher blood cholesterol levels.

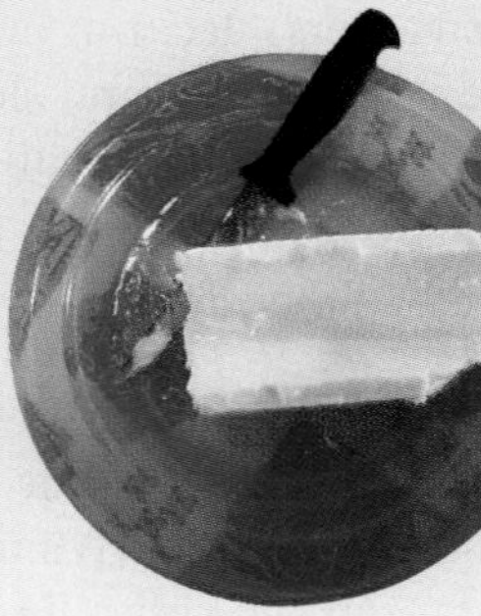

Looking at the label of a standard stick margarine, you'll find the following per tablespoon:

- 100 kcals
- 11 g fat
- 2 g saturated fat
- 3.5 g polyunsaturated fat
- 3.5 g monounsaturated fat
- 0 mg cholesterol
- 115 mg sodium
- 10% Daily Value for vitamin A

So compared with butter, margarine has the same amount of calories and fat (a fact unknown to many consumers!), less saturated fat and cholesterol, and a bit more sodium and vitamin A. The PUFA and MUFA content of butter is not listed, because these are not required elements of the Nutrition Facts label.

Turning to the list of ingredients, we find "liquid soybean oil, partially hydrogenated soybean oil, water, whey, salt, soy lecithin, and vegetable mono- and diglycerides (emulsifiers), sodium benzoate (a preservative),

Cholesterol also is a precursor of important substances. For example, your body can use cholesterol to make vitamin D. Cholesterol also is the precursor of five major classes of sterol hormones: progesterone, glucocorticoids, mineralocorticoids, androgens, and estrogens. (See **Figure 6.19**.) When making testosterone (an androgen) from cholesterol, our bodies form an intermediate compound called DHEA (dehydroepiandrosterone). DHEA has become a popular nutritional supplement, marketed with the largely unfulfilled promise that it will boost potency and restore youth.

The liver uses cholesterol to manufacture bile acids, which are secreted in bile. The gallbladder stores and concentrates the bile. On demand, the gallbladder releases the bile into the small intestine, where bile acids emulsify dietary fats.

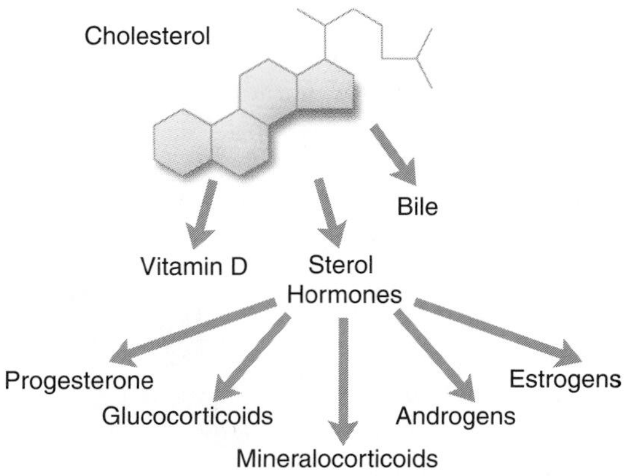

Figure 6.19 **Cholesterol has important roles.** Cholesterol is a precursor of vitamin D and sterol hormones. The liver uses cholesterol to make bile.

Cholesterol Synthesis

Because your body can make cholesterol, you do not need cholesterol in your diet. While researchers believe all cells synthesize some cholesterol,

vitamin A palmitate, beta carotene (color)." Nothing terribly unusual, especially now that you know what lecithin and mono- and diglycerides are.

Spreads and Other Butter Imitators

Beyond the traditional stick margarine, there are a growing number of "light," "soft," "whipped," "squeeze," "spray," and "spread" products. These items do not fit the legal definition of "margarine," and so the term *vegetable oil spread* is generally used. In terms of ingredients, these products have more liquid oil and water, and less partially hydrogenated oil. More emulsifiers may be needed, along with flavors (including salt) and colors. The result typically is fewer calories, less saturated fat, and still no cholesterol.

Some products tout the inclusion of canola or olive oil for more healthful MUFA. Others indicate "no *trans* fatty acids" and have no hydrogenated oils on the list. Two new spreads, and at least one in development, contain plant sterols that reduce intestinal absorption of cholesterol.[1] More expensive than most spreads, these products have been treading a thin regulatory line between food regulations and dietary supplement regulations. A third product, still under development, will contain the soluble fiber psyllium, also meant to lower cholesterol absorption.[2]

Cholesterol-Lowering Margarines

Stanols are plant sterols similar in structure to cholesterol. Ingested plant sterols compete with and inhibit cholesterol absorption. Studies show that consumption of stanols reduces total blood cholesterol levels and LDL cholesterol levels,[3] while HDL cholesterol levels increased or remained unchanged.[4] The new "cholesterol-lowering" margarines, Benecol and Take Control, contain plant sterols. Consumption of 3 grams of stanol per day, which is equivalent to three pats, can effectively improve lipid profiles and may reduce cardiovascular risk.[5]

Making Choices

The spread you choose may depend on your purpose. There are times, and foods, where nothing but real butter will do. If you've ever tried baking cookies with a soft, reduced-fat spread, you know the outcome . . . and probably will use butter, margarine, or vegetable shortening next time.

Remember, your goal is to limit total fats as well as saturated and *trans* fatty acids. Using less butter or margarine overall will do that. Choosing a margarine or spread with liquid vegetable oil as the first ingredient (meaning that the amount of hydrogenated oil is less) will reduce not only saturated fat, but *trans* fatty acids as well. Moderation is the key—making choices that consider your whole diet will help you stay in line with heart-healthy recommendations.

1 Haumann BF. Widening array of spreads awaits shoppers. *Inform.* Jan 1998;6–13.

2 Ibrahim Y. Rocky path to market for edible foe of cholesterol. *New York Times.* January 31, 1999;D4 (col. 1).

3 Jones PJ, Ntanios FY, Raeini Sarjaz M, Vanstone CA. Cholesterol-lowering efficacy of a sitostanol-containing phytosterol mixture with a prudent diet in hyperlipidemic men. *Am J Clin Nutr.* 1999;69: 1144–1150; Gylling H, Miettinen TA. Cholesterol reduction by different plant stanol mixtures and with variable fat intake. *Metabolism.* 1999;48:575–580; and Avery JK. Making the most of cholesterol-lowering margarines. *Cleve Clin J Med.* 2001;68:194–196.

4 Gylling H, Miettinen TA. Op. cit.

5 Jones PJ, MacDougall DE, Ntanios F, Vanstone CA. Dietary phytosterols as cholesterol-lowering agents in humans. *Can J Physiol Pharmacol.* 1997;75: 217–227.

Quick Bites

Would you pay more for cholesterol-free mushrooms?

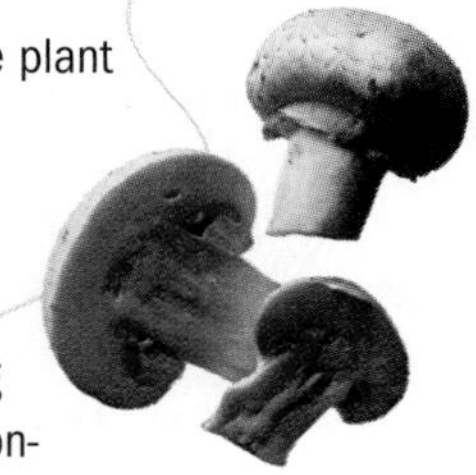

Several years ago, some plant foods were promoted with labels claiming they were "cholesterol free." As you might expect, the FDA found this misleading since plant foods never contain cholesterol unless an animal product like butter or egg has been added. Regulations no longer allow the implication that cholesterol has been removed from a naturally cholesterol-free food. Rather than saying "cholesterol-free mushrooms," labels must now say "mushrooms, a cholesterol-free food."

the liver is the primary cholesterol-manufacturing site, and the intestines contribute appreciable amounts. In fact, your body produces at least 1,000 milligrams of cholesterol per day, far more than is found in the average diet. This attests to cholesterol's biological importance. In the lens of the eye, which has a high concentration of cholesterol, on-site cholesterol synthesis may be essential for preventing cataracts.[10] Animal studies suggest that the brain makes almost all the cholesterol incorporated into it during development.[11] Increasing dietary cholesterol reduces synthesis somewhat, but not by an equivalent amount.[12] When we eat frequent small meals our bodies produce less cholesterol than when we eat a few large meals. Fasting markedly reduces cholesterol production.[13]

Sterols in Food

Only foods of animal origin contain cholesterol. The brain has the highest cholesterol content, liver and other organ meats are high, and muscle tissue contains moderate amounts. Egg yolks are high in cholesterol, with about 218 milligrams per large egg (the egg white contains no cholesterol), and

Table 6.1 Cholesterol in Selected Foods (in milligrams)

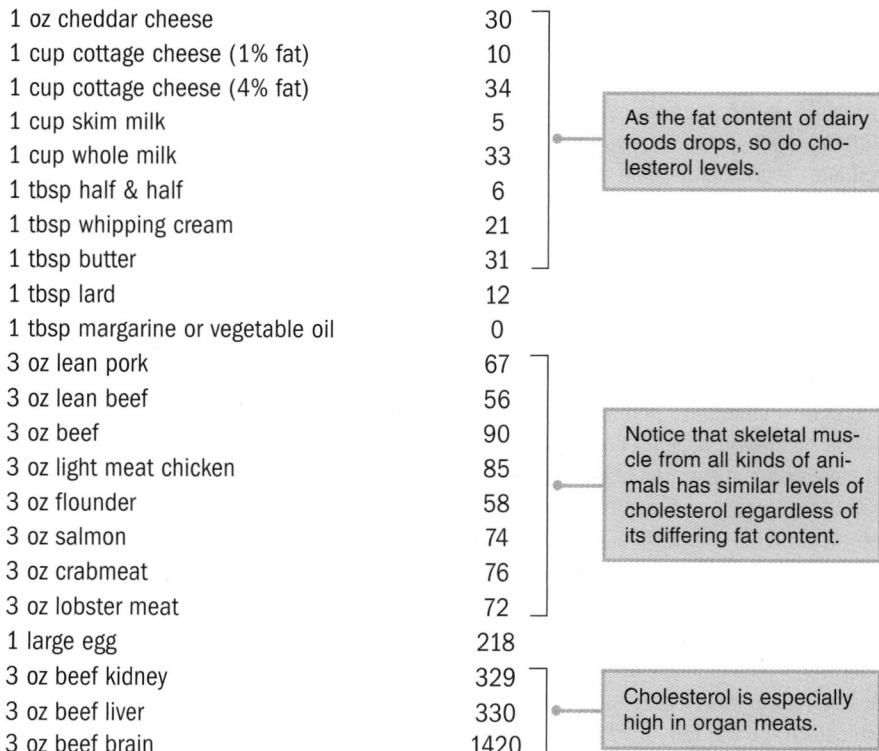

	Approximate Cholesterol	
1 oz cheddar cheese	30	
1 cup cottage cheese (1% fat)	10	
1 cup cottage cheese (4% fat)	34	
1 cup skim milk	5	As the fat content of dairy foods drops, so do cholesterol levels.
1 cup whole milk	33	
1 tbsp half & half	6	
1 tbsp whipping cream	21	
1 tbsp butter	31	
1 tbsp lard	12	
1 tbsp margarine or vegetable oil	0	
3 oz lean pork	67	
3 oz lean beef	56	
3 oz beef	90	
3 oz light meat chicken	85	Notice that skeletal muscle from all kinds of animals has similar levels of cholesterol regardless of its differing fat content.
3 oz flounder	58	
3 oz salmon	74	
3 oz crabmeat	76	
3 oz lobster meat	72	
1 large egg	218	
3 oz beef kidney	329	
3 oz beef liver	330	Cholesterol is especially high in organ meats.
3 oz beef brain	1420	

The values here give only a general idea of amounts in foods. Cholesterol values are quite variable, differing by times of the year, the animal's origin, species, or breed, processing, and more. One thing is always true, though: Cholesterol is never found in plant foods.

Source: Based on figures from US Department of Agriculture, Agricultural Research Service. *USDA Nutrient Database for Standard Reference*, Release 13; 1999.

breast milk is moderately high, suggesting the importance of cholesterol during early growth and development.[14] Dairy products also contain cholesterol, which is found in the butterfat portion. **Table 6.1** lists the amounts of cholesterol in some common foods.

Aside from cholesterol and vitamin D, there are few dietary sterols of nutritional significance. Whale liver and plants contain the cholesterol precursor **squalene**. Although whale liver is not a common item in grocery stores, squalene capsules are sold as dietary supplements with the unproved claim that squalene speeds healing. Plants contain a number of other sterols (**phytosterols**) that are poorly absorbed. Because phytosterols reduce intestinal absorption of cholesterol, they have attracted much interest and recently have been introduced as a cholesterol-lowering food ingredient.

squalene A cholesterol precursor found in whale liver and plants.

phytosterols Sterols found in plants. Phytosterols are poorly absorbed by humans and reduce intestinal absorption of cholesterol. They recently have been introduced as a cholesterol-lowering food ingredient.

Key Concepts: *Sterols have ring structures and contain no fatty acids. Cholesterol is the best-known sterol, and other sterols are hormones or hormone precursors. Cholesterol is an important precursor compound and is a key component of cell membranes. High levels of blood cholesterol are a heart disease risk. Cholesterol is found only in foods of animal origin; because the body can make all it needs, cholesterol is not a dietary essential.*

Digestion and Absorption

Like the other macronutrients (carbohydrates and proteins), most lipids are broken into smaller compounds for absorption. (See **Figure 6.20**.) However, because lipids generally are not water-soluble and digestive secretions are all water-based, the body has to treat lipids a bit differently.

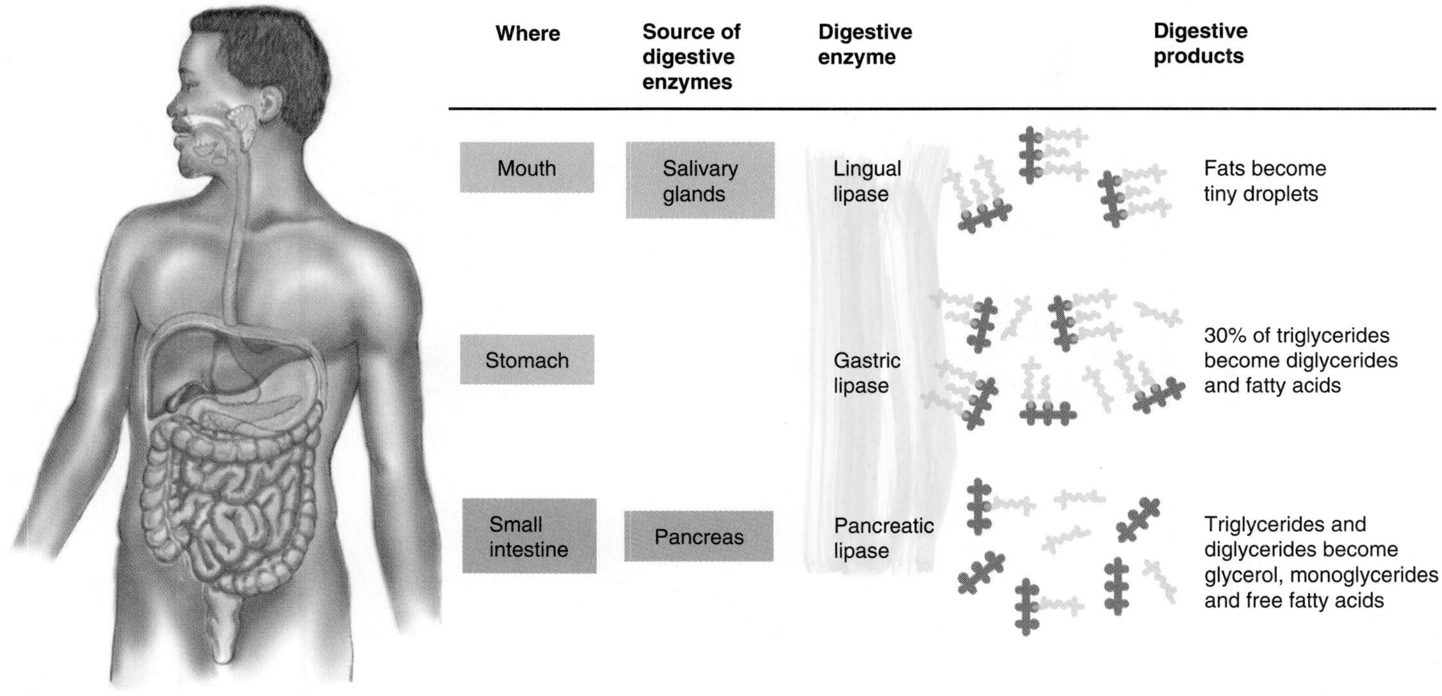
Where
Source of digestive enzymes
Digestive enzyme
Digestive products
Mouth
Salivary glands
Lingual lipase
Fats become tiny droplets
Stomach
Gastric lipase
30% of triglycerides become diglycerides and fatty acids
Small intestine
Pancreas
Pancreatic lipase
Triglycerides and diglycerides become glycerol, monoglycerides and free fatty acids

Figure 6.20 **Triglyceride digestion.** Most triglyceride digestion takes place in the small intestine.

Digestion of Triglycerides and Phospholipids

Triglycerides are not soluble in water, but the enzymes that digest them are found only in a watery environment. Don't worry! Your digestive system is equal to the task. Physical actions (chewing, peristalsis, and segmentation), combined with various emulsifiers, allow digestive enzymes to do their work. The digestion of triglycerides and phospholipids is similar and breaks these molecules down to their component parts—fatty acids, glycerol, and, in the case of phospholipids, a component containing phosphate and

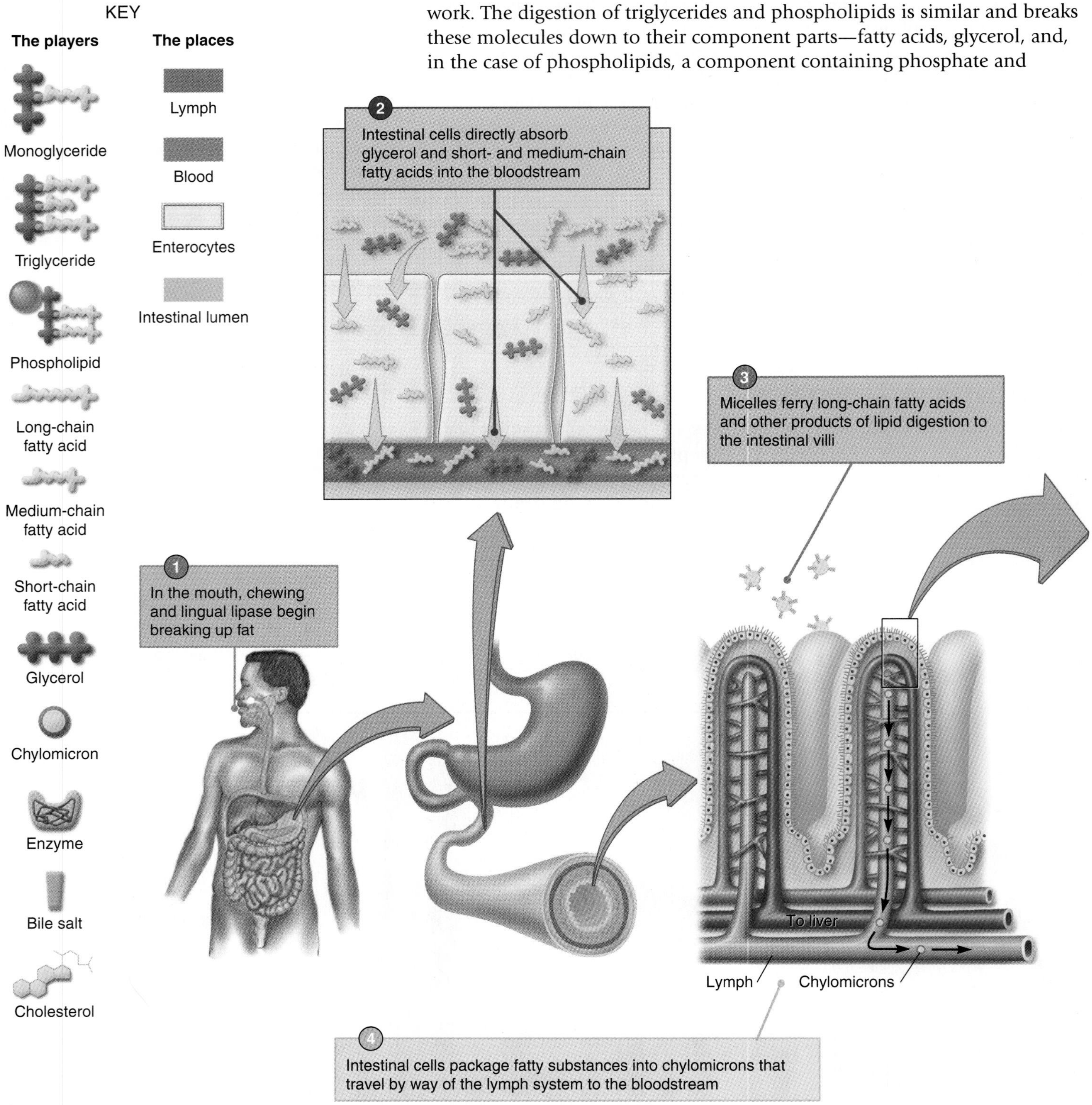
KEY
The players
Monoglyceride
Triglyceride
Phospholipid
Long-chain fatty acid
Medium-chain fatty acid
Short-chain fatty acid
Glycerol
Chylomicron
Enzyme
Bile salt
Cholesterol
The places
Lymph
Blood
Enterocytes
Intestinal lumen
1 In the mouth, chewing and lingual lipase begin breaking up fat
2 Intestinal cells directly absorb glycerol and short- and medium-chain fatty acids into the bloodstream
3 Micelles ferry long-chain fatty acids and other products of lipid digestion to the intestinal villi
To liver
Lymph
Chylomicrons
4 Intestinal cells package fatty substances into chylomicrons that travel by way of the lymph system to the bloodstream

Figure 6.21 **Digestion and absorption of lipids.** Minimal fat digestion takes place in the mouth and stomach. In the small intestine, bile salts and lecithin break up and disperse fatty lipids in tiny globules. Enzymes attack these globules, breaking down triglycerides and phospholipids to fatty acids and other component parts. Bile salts surround these products of fat digestion, forming water-soluble micelles that carry fat to intestinal cells.

nitrogen.

In the mouth, a combination of chewing and the work of lingual lipase starts the digestive process rolling, with the small amount of dietary phospholipid providing emulsification. In the stomach, gastric lipase joins in, and the stomach's churning and contractions keep the fat dispersed. Diglycerides that form in the breakdown process become emulsifiers, too. After two to four hours in the stomach, digestion has broken down about 30 percent of dietary triglycerides to diglycerides and free fatty acids.[15]

Fat in the small intestine stimulates the gallbladder to contract, sending bile down the bile duct. The pancreas releases pancreatic juice rich in pancreatic lipase, which joins bile just before they enter the small intestine and mix with the watery chyme.

Bile contains a large quantity of bile salts and the phospholipid lecithin. These key elements emulsify fat, breaking globules into smaller pieces so water-soluble pancreatic lipase can attack the surface. Emulsification increases the total surface area of fats by as much as 1,000-fold.[16] (Many common household detergents use emulsification to remove grease from dishes or clothing.) Pancreatic juice contains enormous amounts of pancreatic lipase. Within minutes, it breaks down nearly all accessible triglycerides to monoglycerides and free fatty acids. (See **Figure 6.21**.)

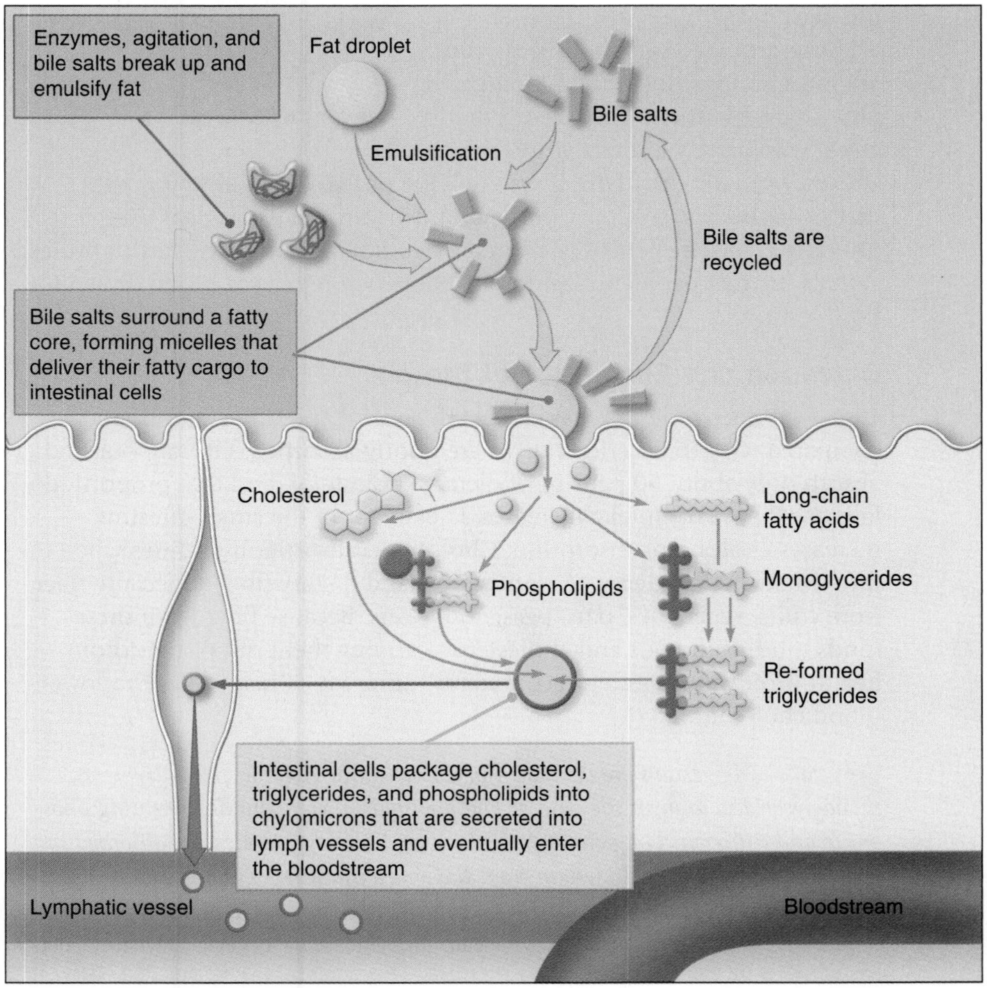

Lipid Absorption

In the small intestine, bile salts surround monoglycerides and free fatty acids, forming **micelles**—water-soluble globules with a fatty core. Micelles carry monoglycerides and long-chain fatty acids through the watery intestinal environment to the surfaces of the microvilli, even penetrating the recesses between individual microvilli. Here, the monoglycerides and long-chain fatty acids immediately diffuse into the intestinal cells, and the bile salts return to the interior of the small intestine to form another micelle. The last section of the small intestine absorbs bile salts for recycling. The bile salts return via the portal vein to the liver, where they are once again secreted into the bile. This bile recycling pathway—the liver to the intestine and the intestine to the liver—is called enterohepatic circulation. Figure 4.10 in Chapter 4, "The Human Body," illustrates enterohepatic circulation.

micelles Tiny emulsified fat packets. They are composed of emulsifier molecules (phospholipids) oriented with their fat-soluble part facing inward and their water-soluble part facing outward toward the surrounding aqueous environment.

lipoprotein A complex that transports lipids in the lymph and blood. Lipoproteins consist of a central core of triglycerides and cholesterol surrounded by a shell composed of proteins, cholesterol, and phospholipids. The various types of lipoproteins differ in size, composition, and density.

chylomicron [kye-lo-MY-kron] A large lipoprotein formed in intestinal cells following the absorption of dietary fats. A chylomicron has a central core of triglycerides and cholesterol surrounded by phospholipids and proteins.

Inside intestinal cells, monoglycerides and fatty acids re-form triglycerides. These triglycerides, as well as cholesterol and phospholipids, join protein carriers to form a **lipoprotein**. When this assemblage leaves the intestinal cell, it is called a **chylomicron**. Chylomicrons make their way to the interior of the villi, where they enter the lymph system, which eventually empties into veins in the neck.

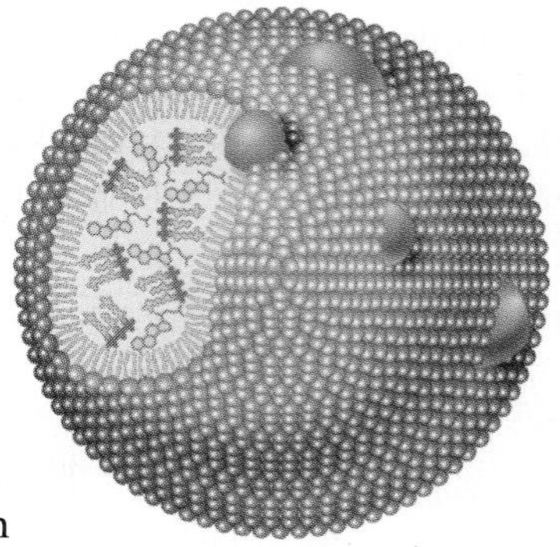

Chylomicron

Short- and medium-chain fatty acids are more water-soluble than long-chain fatty acids. Intestinal cells absorb them, along with glycerol, directly into the bloodstream, bypassing the lymph system. One or two hours after you eat, dietary fat begins to appear in the bloodstream. Fat levels peak after 3 to 5 hours, and fats are generally cleared by 10 hours. That's why health professionals instruct people to fast for 12 hours before having blood drawn for lipid testing.

Digestion and Absorption of Sterols

Digestion does little to break down cholesterol and other sterols, and, compared with triglycerides, these are poorly absorbed. Overall, our bodies absorb only about 50 percent of dietary cholesterol, and that proportion falls as cholesterol intake increases. Dietary fat in the small intestine increases cholesterol absorption. Cholesterol absorption declines when the intestine contains plenty of plant sterols and dietary fiber, especially fiber from fruits, vegetables, oats, peas, and beans. Because fiber from these foods binds bile acids and cholesterol, carrying them out of the colon, health professionals often recommend eating foods rich in fiber to lower blood cholesterol.

Quick Bites

How do cholesterol-lowering medications work?

One class of cholesterol-lowering medications, the "bile-acid sequestrants," works by combining bile acid and cholesterol in the intestine to form compounds that the body cannot absorb. Since this cholesterol is then lost in the feces, cholesterol must be taken from the blood to make more bile, thus lowering the blood cholesterol level.

Key Concepts: *Digestion breaks most lipids down into glycerol, free fatty acids, monoglycerides, and, in the case of phospholipids, a compound containing phosphate and nitrogen. Long-chain fatty acids and monoglycerides are absorbed primarily into the lymphatic system from the small intestine, while glycerol, short-chain, and medium-chain fatty acids are absorbed directly into the blood. Sterols are mostly unchanged by digestion and their absorption is relatively poor.*

Lipids in the Body

The digestive tract is not the only place where lipids need special handling to move in a water-based environment. To travel in the bloodstream, lipids must be specially packaged into lipoprotein carriers.

Lipoproteins have a lipid core of triglycerides and cholesterol esters (cholesterol linked to fatty acids) surrounded by a shell of phospholipids with embedded proteins and cholesterol. They can carry water-insoluble lipids through the watery environment of the bloodstream. There are several main classes of lipoproteins and many subclasses. These differ mainly by size, density, and the composition of their lipid cores. In general, as the percentage of triglyceride drops, the density increases. A lipoprotein with a small core that contains little triglyceride is much more dense than a lipoprotein with a large core composed mostly of triglycerides. To get a feel for relative sizes, you can think of the different lipoproteins as a huge beach ball, softball, baseball, golf ball, and ¾-inch steel ball bearing. (See **Figure 6.22**.)

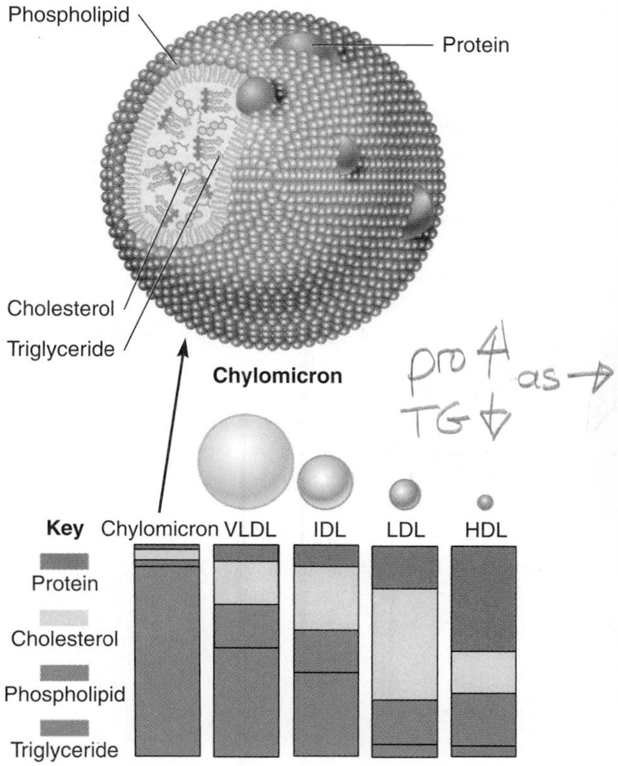

Figure 6.22 Lipoprotein sizes and composition. Lipoproteins become less dense as they increase in size. LDL is about double the size of HDL. VLDL is about 60 times larger than HDL. Chylomicrons range from 500 to 1000 times larger than HDL.

Chylomicrons

Chylomicrons formed in the intestinal tract enter the lymphatic system, which empties into the bloodstream at the jugular veins of the neck. When chylomicrons enter the bloodstream, they are large, fatty lipoproteins—think of a beach ball 3 to 6 feet in diameter. Chylomicrons are about 90 percent fat, but as they circulate through the capillaries, they gradually give up their triglycerides. An enzyme located on the capillary walls, called **lipoprotein lipase**, attacks the chylomicrons and removes triglyceride, breaking it into free fatty acids and glycerol. These components enter adipose cells as needed, where they are reassembled into triglycerides. Alternatively, they may remain in circulation, with the free fatty acids bound to albumin, a water-soluble protein. After about 10 hours, little is left of a circulating chylomicron but cholesterol-rich remnants. It's as if the air was let out of our beach ball, shrinking it to about the size of a softball 4½ inches in diameter. The liver picks up these chylomicron remnants and uses them as raw material to build very-low-density lipoproteins.

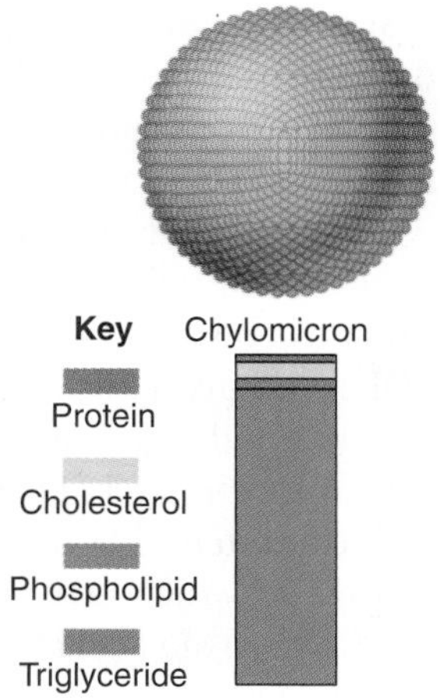

lipoprotein lipase The major enzyme responsible for the breakdown of lipoproteins and triglycerides in the blood.

very-low-density lipoproteins (VLDL) The triglyceride-rich lipoproteins formed in the liver. VLDL enters the bloodstream and is gradually acted upon by lipoprotein lipase, releasing triglyceride to body cells.

Very-Low-Density Lipoprotein

The liver and intestines assemble **very-low-density lipoproteins (VLDL)** with a triglyceride-rich core—for relative size, think of a softball. VLDL has a very low density because it is nearly two-thirds fat. As with chylomicrons, lipoprotein lipase splits off and breaks down triglycerides as VLDL circulates through the capillaries. As VLDL loses triglycerides, it becomes denser, gradually becoming an IDL, or intermediate-density lipoprotein. Our softball has shrunk to about the size of a baseball, 2¾ inches in diameter.

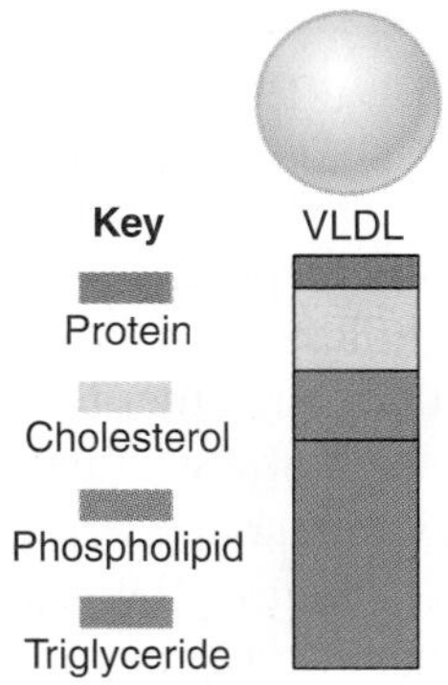

intermediate-density lipoproteins (IDL) The lipoproteins formed when lipoprotein lipase strips some of the triglycerides from VLDL.

low-density lipoproteins (LDL) The cholesterol-rich lipoproteins that result from the breakdown and removal of triglycerides from intermediate-density lipoprotein. LDL cholesterol sometimes is called "bad cholesterol."

high-density lipoproteins (HDL) The blood lipoproteins that contain high levels of protein and low levels of triglycerides. Synthesized primarily in the liver and small intestine, HDL picks up cholesterol released from dying cells and other sources and transfers it to other lipoproteins. HDL cholesterol sometimes is called "good cholesterol."

Intermediate-Density Lipoprotein

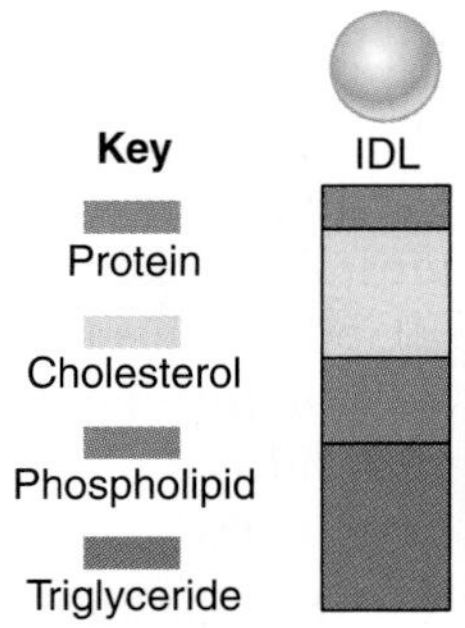

Intermediate-density lipoproteins (IDL) are about 40 percent fat. As IDL travels through the bloodstream, it acquires cholesterol from another lipoprotein (HDL, see below), and circulating enzymes remove some phospholipids. IDL returns to the liver, where liver cells convert it to low-density lipoproteins.

Low-Density Lipoprotein

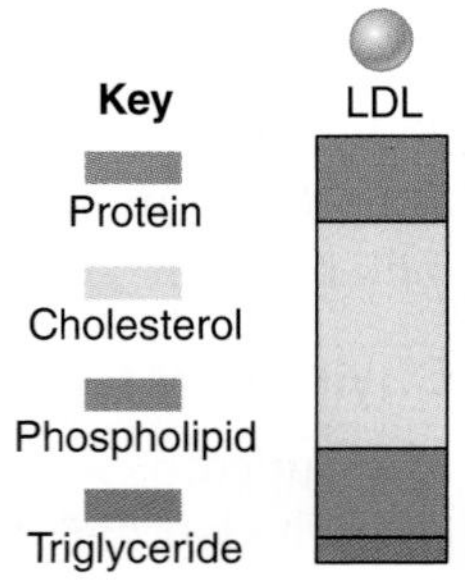

Low-density lipoproteins (LDL) deliver cholesterol to body cells, which use it to synthesize membranes, hormones, and other vital compounds. LDL is more than half cholesterol and cholesterol esters; triglycerides make up only 6 percent. For a relative size, think of a golf ball about $1\frac{5}{8}$ inches in diameter.

Special receptors on the cell walls bind low-density lipoproteins, which the cell engulfs and ingests. Once inside, the cell breaks down LDL, releasing LDL's load of cholesterol.

When the LDL receptors on liver cells bind LDL, they help control blood cholesterol levels.[17] Saturated fats appear to block these receptors, which explains why saturated fats tend to raise blood cholesterol levels.[18] A lack of LDL receptors reduces the uptake of cholesterol, forcing it to remain in circulation at dangerously high levels.

Because elevated LDL levels are associated with artery and heart disease, LDL cholesterol has acquired the nickname of "bad cholesterol." The process by which LDL affects the blood vessels takes place over a number of years. When smoking, diabetes, high blood pressure, or infections injure blood vessel walls, the body's emergency repair team swings into action. It mobilizes white blood cells, which travel to the site of the injury, where they bury themselves in the blood vessel wall. Certain white blood cells bind and ingest LDL, especially altered (oxidized) LDL, which degrades and releases cholesterol. Over several decades, cholesterol accumulates as plaque thickens and narrows the artery, a condition known as atherosclerosis. The antioxidant vitamin E and several carotenoids reduce the oxidation of LDL and may interfere with cholesterol accumulation and plaque buildup.

Think About It 4

High-Density Lipoprotein

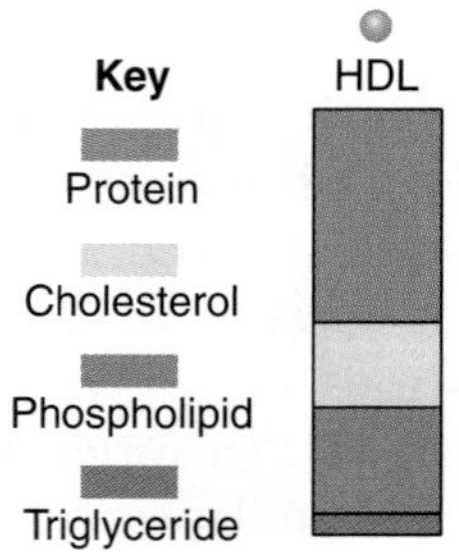

The liver and intestines make **high-density lipoproteins (HDL)**. HDL is about 5 percent triglyceride, similar to LDL. On the other hand, HDL is only about 20 percent cholesterol, much less than LDL, which is more than 50 percent cholesterol. HDL has a higher protein content than any other lipoprotein. For a relative size, think of a steel ball bearing about $\frac{3}{4}$ inches in diameter.

Because HDL appears to protect against atherosclerosis, HDL cholesterol has earned the nickname "good cholesterol." In the bloodstream, HDL picks up cholesterol from arterial plaques, reducing their accumulation. HDL also picks up cholesterol released by dying cells and from cell membranes as they are renewed. HDL hands off cholesterol to other lipoproteins, especially IDL, which return cholesterol to the liver for recycling. Low HDL levels increase risk for atherosclerotic heart disease, while high HDL levels have a protective effect. Some people (only about 1 percent of the population) have extremely high HDL levels and so have extremely low rates of heart disease and stroke.[19]

Key Concepts: *Lipoprotein carriers transport lipids in the blood. Chylomicrons, formed in the intestinal mucosal cells, transport lipids from the digestive tract into circulation. VLDL carries lipids from the liver to the other body tissues, delivering triglycerides and gradually becoming IDL. The liver takes up IDL and assembles LDL, the main carrier of cholesterol. High blood levels of LDL, the "bad cholesterol," have been shown to be a risk factor for heart disease. Circulating HDL picks up cholesterol and sends it back to the liver for recycling or excretion. A relatively high level of HDL, the "good cholesterol," reduces risk for heart disease.*

Lipids in the Diet

Now that you know something about lipids and their importance in the body, you can see that Rachel's no-fat approach to life has serious flaws. However, too much dietary fat can contribute unwanted calories, and high intake of fat has been linked to heart disease. Read on for a discussion of the recommended amounts and balance of lipids in a healthful diet.

Recommended Intakes

Most health policy agencies recommend reducing intake of total fat, saturated fat, and cholesterol. As interest in the relationship between fat intake and health grew in the 1970s and 1980s, the American Heart Association (AHA), the National Cholesterol Education Program (NCEP) of the National Institutes of Health, and the *Dietary Guidelines for Americans* set intake guidelines for lipids.

The Daily Values on food labels reflect these older recommendations. Based on a 2,000-kilocalorie diet, the Daily Value is 65 grams (29 percent of calories) for fat, 20 grams (9 percent of calories) for saturated fat, and 300 milligrams for cholesterol. While some suggest that all healthy Americans 2 years of age and older follow these recommendations, others suggest phasing in the reduction in fat intake up to the age of 5 years.[20]

For people with elevated blood cholesterol levels, the NCEP's Therapeutic Lifestyle Changes recommend daily intakes of less than 7 percent of calories from saturated fat and less than 200 milligrams of dietary cholesterol. It also allows up to 35 percent of daily calories from total fat, provided most is from unsaturated fat, which doesn't raise cholesterol levels. To boost the LDL-lowering power of the diet, the NCEP also encourages consumption of foods that contain plant stanols and sterols or are rich in dietary fiber. In addition, the NCEP stresses weight control and physical activity, both of which improve various heart disease risk factors. Weight control, for example, enhances LDL lowering and raises HDL, while physical activity improves HDL and, for some, LDL. **Figure 6.23** shows the NCEP dietary recommendations.

Are we meeting fat intake goals? Dietary surveys, including the large National Health and Nutrition Examination Survey of 1988–1994 (NHANES III), report that average fat intake is 34 percent of calories, down from 36 percent 10 years earlier and down markedly from 45 percent in 1965. See "What About Bobbie?" at the end of the chapter to see how to calculate the percentage of calorie intake from fat.

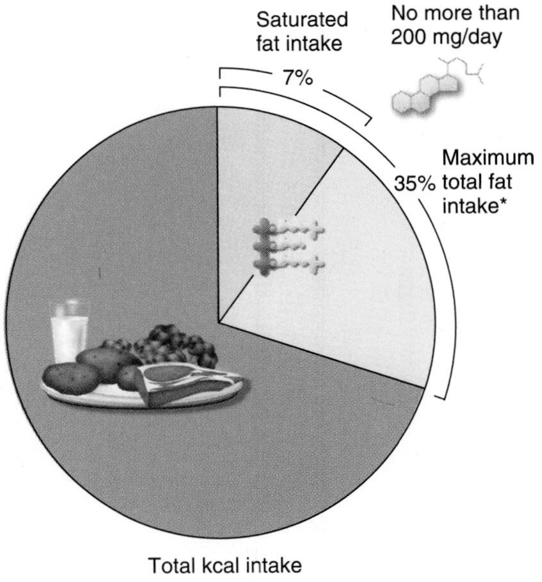

Figure 6.23 NCEP intake recommendations. The NCEP dietary recommendations are part of the Therapeutic Lifestyle Changes for the treatment of elevated blood cholesterol level. These changes also include weight management and increased physical activity.

fat consumption has ↓'d but not incidence of ♡ dse

Table 6.2 AHA Dietary Guidelines

The American Heart Association Dietary Guidelines are designed to assist individuals in achieving and maintaining:

A Healthy Eating Pattern Including Foods from All Major Food Groups

- Consume a variety of fruits and vegetables and grain products, including whole grains.
- Include fat-free and low-fat dairy products, fish, legumes, poultry, and lean meats.

A Healthy Body Weight

- Match intake of energy to overall energy needs; limit consumption of foods with a high caloric density and/or low nutritional quality.
- Maintain a level of physical activity that achieves fitness and balances energy expenditure with energy intake; for weight reduction, expenditure should exceed intake.

A Desirable Blood Cholesterol and Lipoprotein Profile

- Limit the intake of foods with a high content of saturated fatty acids and cholesterol.
- Substitute grains and unsaturated fatty acids from vegetables, fish, legumes, and nuts.

A Desirable Blood Pressure

- Limit the intake of salt to less than 6 grams per day.
- Limit alcohol consumption.
- Maintain a healthy body weight and a dietary pattern that emphasizes vegetables, fruits, and low-fat or fat-free dairy products.

Source: *Circulation.* 2000;102:2296–2311.

Although the percentage of calories from fat dropped, average calorie intake increased, which means Americans actually are consuming more total grams of fat. Desserts, hamburgers, and french-fried potatoes are the largest contributors to fat intake, according to the NCEP.[21] While fat intake from meats has fallen significantly since 1970, fat from salad and cooking oils and shortenings has risen dramatically.[22] In addition, the percentage of fat from fast foods and ethnic foods has increased more than 10-fold.[23]

Released in 2000, new AHA guidelines (see **Table 6.2**) focus on overall eating patterns rather than specific percentages of dietary fat—an approach similar to the 2000 *Dietary Guidelines for Americans*. The four main goals of the new guidelines are to help Americans (1) achieve an overall healthy eating pattern, (2) achieve and maintain an appropriate body weight, (3) achieve and maintain a desirable blood cholesterol profile, and (4) achieve and maintain a desirable blood pressure. One of the most significant changes in the new guidelines is a recommendation to consume two weekly servings of fatty fish, such as tuna or salmon.

Essential Fatty Acid Requirements

Although too much fat in the diet is not healthful, we still need to get enough fat to meet our need for essential fatty acids. To fulfill our need for *omega*-6 fatty acids, linoleic acid should provide about 2 percent of our calories. Average U.S. consumption is much more than that. Two teaspoons of corn oil, which is a little over half linoleic acid, would supply more than 2 percent of the calories in a 2,000-kilocalorie diet.

Because science has only recently recognized the importance of *omega*-3 fatty acids, we know less about our requirements. Researchers suggest that we eat a minimum of 3 grams of *omega*-3 fatty acids each day (about 1.3 percent of calories for a 2,000-kilocalorie diet).[24] The recommended ratio of *omega*-3 fatty acids to *omega*-6 fatty acids in the diet is 1 to 2.3.[25] To meet these recommendations for *omega*-3 fatty acids, we would need about 2 tablespoons of vegetable oil per day along with four meals containing fatty fish each week—a threefold increase in current U.S. fish consumption!

Omega-6 and *Omega*-3 Imbalance

Before commercial processing, large quantities of vegetable oils were unavailable, so the *omega*-6 linoleic acid was hard to come by. There is a small amount in whole grains and smaller amounts in fruits and vegetables that also contain very small amounts of *omega*-3s. Today, linoleic acid is widely available. In contrast, availability of *omega*-3s in the food supply is relatively unchanged. As a result, the ratio of *omega*-3 to *omega*-6 in the American diet has fallen. The low intake of *omega*-3 fatty acids in relation to the high intake of *omega*-6 fatty acids has caused concerns about an unhealthy imbalance in the eicosanoids these fatty acids produce.

Role of Fat Substitutes

In response to the public health challenge to provide lower-fat foods, the food industry pursued low-fat, low-calorie goodies that still taste good. There are now many types of **fat substitutes**, and more than 15,000 fat-reduced foods have made it to the marketplace.[26]

fat substitutes Compounds that imitate the functional and sensory properties of fats, but contain less available energy than fats.

olestra A fat substitute made from a sucrose backbone with six to eight fatty acids attached. The fatty acid arrangement prevents breakdown by the digestive enzyme lipase, so the fatty acids are not absorbed. Olestra can withstand heat and is stable at frying temperatures. Trade name is Olean.

Fat Substitutes: What Are They Made Of?

Some fat substitutes are carbohydrates: generally starches and fibers like vegetable gums, cellulose, maltodextrins, and Oatrim. Some are more digestible than others, but all provide far fewer than the 9 kilocalories per gram of fat. They also bind water and incorporate it into foods, further diluting calories. With their moist, thick textures, they mimic fat's richness and smooth "mouth feel."

Proteins are the raw ingredients of other fat substitutes. Food manufacturers modify egg whites and whey from milk so they become thick and smooth and hold water. Because this protein and water combination has fewer calories per gram than fat, it cuts calories. However, high heat changes protein structures, thus changing the properties of these substitutes and limiting their usefulness. Manufacturers used the protein-based product Simplesse in frozen desserts, but it was not well accepted by consumers.

The most high-tech fat replacers—and the most controversial—are the lipids (or "fat-based" substitutes, as the industry calls them). This group includes Olean, Caprenin, and Salatrim (or Benefat). Caprenin is a blend of medium-chain fatty acids and a 22-carbon fatty acid. Salatrim is primarily a blend of 18-carbon stearic acid and short-chain fatty acids. For both Caprenin and Salatrim, the fatty acids are arranged on glycerol in a way that inhibits digestion. They provide about half the calories of fat, though this is only an estimate because people differ in their ability to digest them. Manufacturers use them in reduced-fat candies and baked goods.

One advantage of lipid-based fat substitutes is their ability to withstand heat. That's fortunate for **olestra** (Olean), because few food ingredients have had to take as much heat from consumer advocacy groups. Olestra has a sucrose (instead of glycerol) backbone, with six to eight fatty acids attached (instead of triglyceride's three). (See **Figure 6.24**.) Manufacturers can alter the characteristics of the fatty acids—their number, length, arrangement, and saturation, for example—to vary properties such as melting point and consistency. Digestive enzymes do not recognize the fatty acid arrangement, so olestra is not broken down and absorbed. This makes olestra calorie-free, even though its fatty acids give it the flavor and cooking performance of fat. It is stable even at frying temperatures.

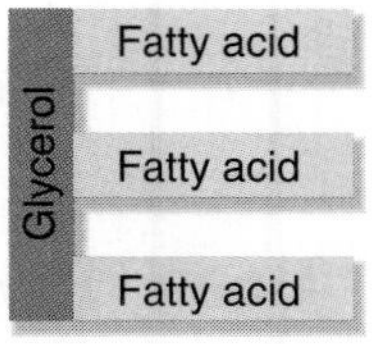

A triglyceride has three fatty acids attached to a glycerol backbone

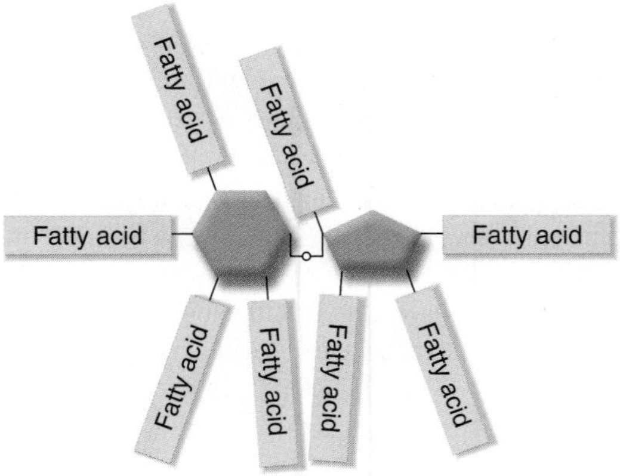

Olestra has six to eight fatty acids attached to a sucrose backbone

Figure 6.24 **The structure of olestra is unlike the structure of a triglyceride.** Olestra adds the savory qualities of fat, but your digestive enzymes cannot break it down.

The Olestra Controversy: Are Fat Substitutes Safe?

Consumers have expressed few safety concerns about carbohydrate- and protein-based fat substitutes. Most concerns center on olestra, which aroused controversy long before it received FDA approval as a food additive in January 1996. The approval process itself was lengthy and controversial,[27] and olestra continues to evoke strong, conflicting opinions.[28]

Unfortunately, olestra is a solvent for fat-soluble nutrients. While in the GI tract, olestra absorbs fat-soluble nutrients and carries them out of the body. The manufacturer replaces fat-soluble vitamins, but critics counter that healthful phytochemicals like the carotenoids are lost and not replaced.

Since the GI tract does not absorb olestra, some people suffer fat malabsorption symptoms—diarrhea, gas, and cramps. The FDA requires a label warning: "This Product Contains Olestra. Olestra may cause abdominal cramping, and loose stools. Olestra inhibits the absorption of some vitamins and other nutrients. Vitamins A, D, E, and K have been added." Olestra critics want this label displayed more prominently and want the warning to be more explicit about nutrient loss; olestra proponents disagree.

The FDA, concerned about malabsorption and nutrient loss, limits olestra's use to a few snack foods. Critics would like to see olestra eliminated, while the industry wants to expand usage. Among people who eat snacks containing olestra, researchers expect an average intake of about 10 grams daily, the amount in a 1-ounce serving of snack chips. These snackers would save about 80 kilocalories daily. Heavy snackers who eat olestra

Fyi Does "Reduced Fat" Reduce Calories? It Depends on the Food

FOR YOUR INFORMATION

Experts often tell us to reduce fat in our diets to help reduce risk for heart disease, cancer, and obesity. Given that fat is our most concentrated source of calories, we would expect a reduced-fat or low-fat food to have fewer calories than its unmodified counterpart. But is this always true?

Sometimes low-fat and fat-free foods make a big difference in calories.[1]

Food	Kcalories
1 oz American cheese	105
1 oz reduced-fat cheese product	75
2 oz bologna	180
2 oz fat-free bologna	40
1 tbsp mayonnaise	100
1 tbsp low-fat mayonnaise/dressing	25

But sometimes they make almost no difference at all.[2]

Food	Kcalories
½ cup canned vegetable soup	80
½ cup fat-free vegetable soup	90
2 chocolate cookies (30 g)	140
2 reduced-fat chocolate cookies (30 g)	120
2 tbsp peanut butter	190
2 tbsp reduced-fat peanut butter	190
3 oz country-style steak-fried potatoes	110
3 oz low-fat steak-fried potatoes	110
2 tbsp butterscotch caramel topping	130
2 tbsp fat-free caramel topping	130

Many fat-reduced products contain added sugar. Although sugar has fewer calories per gram than fat, the amount added may negate any difference in calories. If fat is your concern, low-fat or fat-free products make sense. But if you're trying to reduce fat *and* calories, modified products may not be a big help. So, be a smart shopper—check the label before you check out with a cartload of fat-free foods.

Sources

[1]Adapted from *Food Insight*, Sep/Oct 1997;2–3. Published by the International Food Information Council, Washington, D.C.

[2]Adapted from *Tufts University Health & Nutrition Letter*, March 1998;4–5. Published by Tufts University, Medford, Mass.

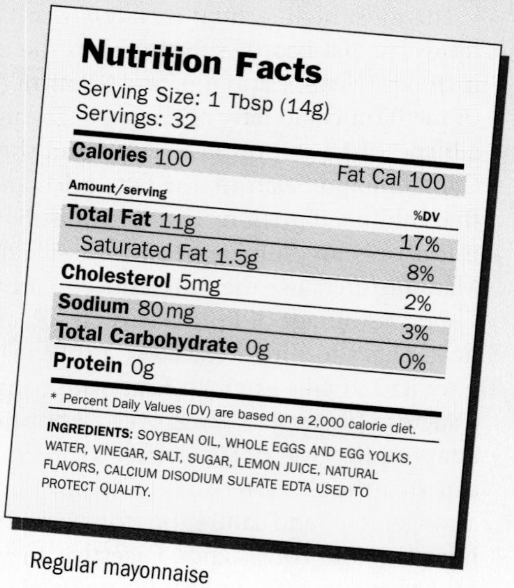
Nutrition Facts
Serving Size: 1 Tbsp (14g)
Servings: 32
Calories 100
Fat Cal 100
Amount/serving
%DV
Total Fat 11g
17%
Saturated Fat 1.5g
8%
Cholesterol 5mg
2%
Sodium 80mg
3%
Total Carbohydrate 0g
0%
Protein 0g
* Percent Daily Values (DV) are based on a 2,000 calorie diet.
INGREDIENTS: SOYBEAN OIL, WHOLE EGGS AND EGG YOLKS, WATER, VINEGAR, SALT, SUGAR, LEMON JUICE, NATURAL FLAVORS, CALCIUM DISODIUM SULFATE EDTA USED TO PROTECT QUALITY.

Regular mayonnaise

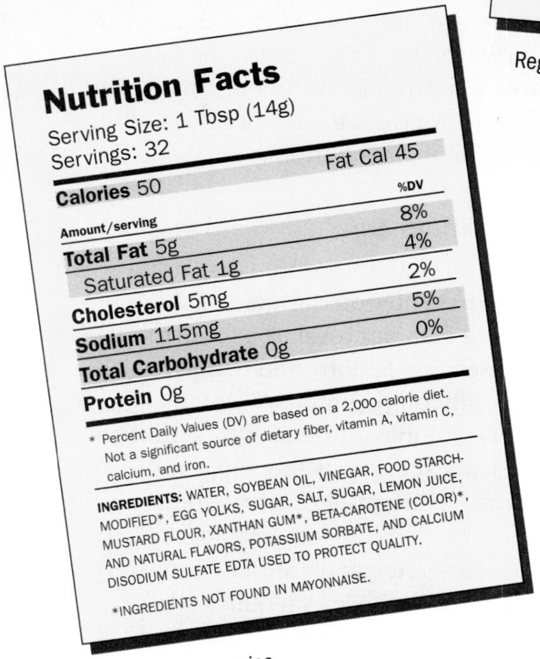
Nutrition Facts
Serving Size: 1 Tbsp (14g)
Servings: 32
Fat Cal 45
Calories 50
%DV
Amount/serving
8%
Total Fat 5g
4%
Saturated Fat 1g
2%
Cholesterol 5mg
5%
Sodium 115mg
0%
Total Carbohydrate 0g
Protein 0g
* Percent Daily Values (DV) are based on a 2,000 calorie diet. Not a significant source of dietary fiber, vitamin A, vitamin C, calcium, and iron.
INGREDIENTS: WATER, SOYBEAN OIL, VINEGAR, FOOD STARCH-MODIFIED*, EGG YOLKS, SUGAR, SALT, SUGAR, LEMON JUICE, MUSTARD FLOUR, XANTHAN GUM*, BETA-CAROTENE (COLOR)*, AND NATURAL FLAVORS, POTASSIUM SORBATE, AND CALCIUM DISODIUM SULFATE EDTA USED TO PROTECT QUALITY.
*INGREDIENTS NOT FOUND IN MAYONNAISE.

Light mayonnaise

products are expected to get about 20 grams. Market surveillance (as mandated by the FDA) evaluates customer experience and safety of olestra in the marketplace. Analysis of the data found no ill health effects beyond what would be expected in the general population.[29]

The power of suggestion, brought on by adverse publicity and the label warning, may be responsible for some consumers' digestive discomfort after eating olestra-containing chips. In fact, in a large double-blind study of volunteers eating olestra-containing chips or regular chips, more people had indigestion after eating the regular chips. Will using olestra subtly encourage people to eat more? In another study, when subjects ate unlabeled olestra-containing potato chips, they ate fewer total calories and less fat than when they ate unlabeled regular potato chips. But when they knew the chips they were eating were fat-free, the subjects ate more.[30] If consumers overeat olestra-containing snacks, they may be more likely to suffer side effects.

Do Fat Substitutes Save Calories? Do They Reduce Total Fat Intake?

Considering the American population as a whole, the answer to these questions seems to be no. American fat and calorie intakes have not gone down over the past few years, a time when the fat-substitute market has been growing rapidly. It is clear that fat substitutes won't help if people treat them simply as an excuse to eat more. Nor should "low-fat foods" be confused with "low-calorie foods"; the calories saved by eating low-fat foods are often negligible.[31]

Key Concepts: *Americans are making progress toward lowering their intake of fat, saturated fat, and cholesterol. It appears, though, that progress has slowed over the past few years, with more people eating more fat and calories, despite the increased availability of a wide variety of fat substitutes and lower-fat foods.*

Lipids and Health

Moderation and balance are the keys to a healthful diet. **Figure 6.25** lists sources of fatty acids. If your diet is consistently high in fat, you may have several problems. High-fat diets are typically high in calories and contribute to weight gain and obesity. High intakes of fat and saturated fat increase risk for heart disease, and high-fat diets have been inconsistently linked to several types of cancer.[32] If you follow the dietary recommendations discussed previously in this chapter, you should reduce your risk for these conditions.

Obesity

Obesity is defined as the excessive accumulation of body fat leading to a body weight in relation to height that is substantially greater than some accepted standard. The National Institutes of Health estimates that 55 percent of American adults are overweight or obese, and the rates are climbing, especially among children and teens.

Eating large amounts of dietary fat contributes to this obesity epidemic. Fat is a dense source of calories (see **Table 6.3**), it makes food taste good, and it's often unnoticed or "hidden" in restaurant and convenience foods. Standard advice to Americans trying to maintain or attain normal weight usually includes cutting back on fats and fatty foods, along with increasing physical activity and eating fewer calories. For more on obesity and weight management, see Chapter 8, "Energy Balance and Weight Management."

BASIC FATTY ACIDS

Saturated
Animal products (including dairy products), palm and coconut oils, and cocoa butter.

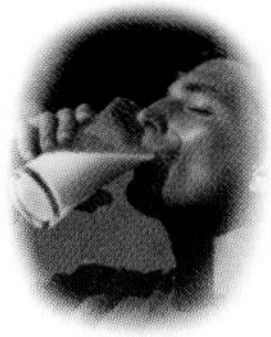

Polyunsaturated
Sunflower, corn, soybean, and cottonseed oils.

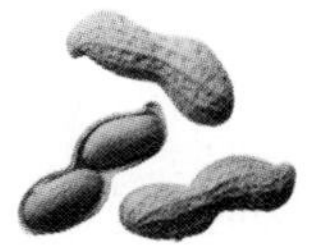

Monounsaturated
Most nuts and olive, canola, peanut, and safflower oils.

TRANS FATTY ACIDS

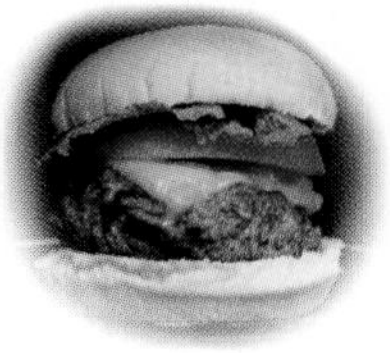

Stick margarine (not soft or liquid margarine) and many fast foods and baked goods.

ESSENTIAL FATTY ACIDS

***Omega*-3 fatty acids**

Alpha-linolenic acid
Canola oil, soybeans, olive oil, many nuts (e.g., walnuts, peanuts, filberts, pistachios, pecans, almonds), seeds, and purslane (a green, leafy vegetable).

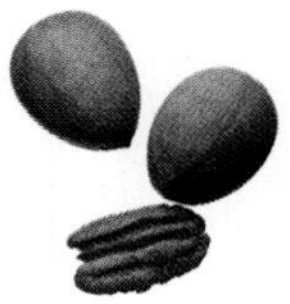

DHA and EPA
Fish such as mackerel, tuna, salmon, herring, trout, and cod liver oil. The fish with the lowest amount of total fat include Atlantic cod, haddock, and pink salmon. Other fish high in omega-3 but also high in total fat are sardines and bluefish. Human milk.

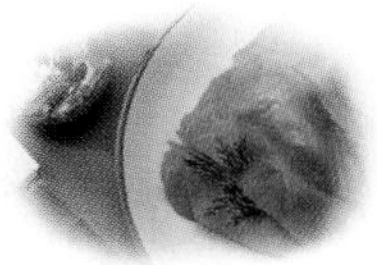

***Omega*-6 fatty acids**

Linoleic acid
Plants (flax) and some vegetable oils (soybean and canola oil).

Figure 6.25 **Overview of dietary sources of fatty acids.**
Source: *Cancer Smart.* Scientific American. July, 1998;4(3):9.

obesity Excessive accumulation of body fat leading to a body weight in relation to height that is substantially greater than some accepted standard.

Table 6.3 **Fat Can Markedly Increase Calories in Food**

	Approximate Kcalories	Approximate Fat (g)
4 oz fried potatoes	209	9.4
4 oz boiled potatoes	98	0.1
$^{1}/_{2}$ c creamed cottage cheese	108	4.7
$^{1}/_{2}$ c 1% low-fat cottage cheese	82	1.2
$^{1}/_{2}$ c green beans + 1 tsp butter	69	5.9
$^{1}/_{2}$ c green beans without butter	18	0.1
3 oz T-bone steak, untrimmed	253	18.0
3 oz T-bone steak, trimmed	182	8.8
$^{1}/_{2}$ c vanilla ice cream	150	8.0
$^{1}/_{2}$ c low-fat vanilla ice cream	100	2.0

Source: Based on data from U.S. Department of Agriculture, Agricultural Research Service. *USDA Nutrient Database for Standard Reference*, Release 13; 1999.

hypercholesterolemia High blood cholesterol (total cholesterol).

cardiovascular disease General term for all disorders affecting the heart and blood vessels.

Heart Disease

In the early 1960s researchers identified high blood cholesterol, or **hypercholesterolemia**, along with smoking and high blood pressure, as principal risk factors for **cardiovascular disease**. They understood that a high-fat, high-cholesterol diet tends to raise blood cholesterol, and that high blood cholesterol levels promote atherosclerosis. Atherosclerosis leads to artery disease and often causes heart attacks.

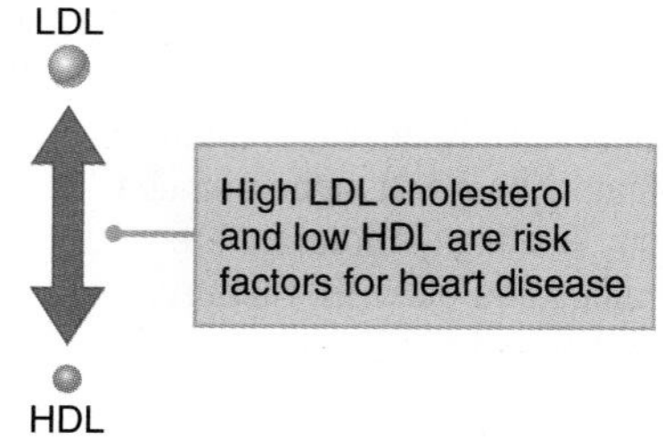
LDL
High LDL cholesterol and low HDL are risk factors for heart disease
HDL

Recently, the cholesterol–heart disease picture has become more complicated. Total cholesterol levels do not tell the entire story. The levels of LDL and HDL cholesterol predict health risks more accurately than total cholesterol levels do. High LDL cholesterol levels are a greater risk than high total cholesterol, with some kinds of LDL being more dangerous than others. Low HDL cholesterol levels increase the risk of heart disease, as do high levels of triglycerides and other newly discovered blood lipids.[33] For example, high levels of lipoprotein a [Lp(a)], a low-density lipoprotein, seem especially harmful. High levels of Lp(a) prevent the normal breakup of blood clots that cause heart attack or stroke. Lp(a) is associated with heart attack, but it's still unclear if and how it is influenced by diet.[34] Some viral and bacterial infections also may damage blood vessels, thus initiating atherosclerosis.[35]

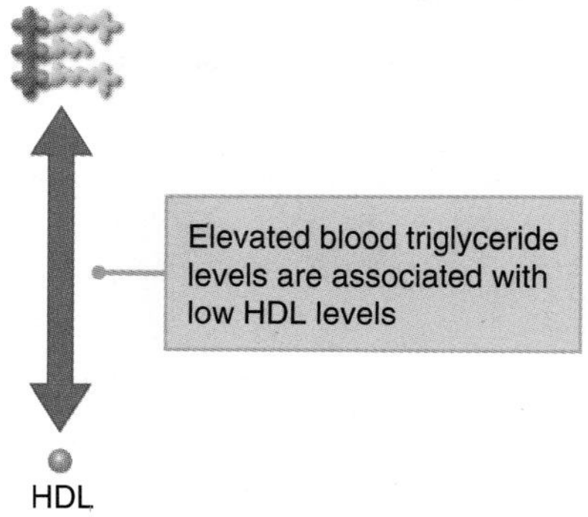
Elevated blood triglyceride levels are associated with low HDL levels
HDL

In May 2001, the NCEP released new guidelines for reducing heart disease risk. Changes from earlier guidelines include (1) treating high cholesterol more aggressively in people with diabetes, (2) testing all adults over age 20 for cholesterol levels every five years, (3) defining low HDL as being less than 40 mg/dL, rather than the earlier value of 35 mg/dL, (4) intensifying the use of nutrition, physical activity, and weight control in the treatment of elevated blood cholesterol levels, (5) identifying a "metabolic syndrome" of risk factors (Syndrome X, see Chapter 5, "Carbohydrates") linked to insulin resistance that often occur together and dramatically increase risk of heart attack, and (6) treating people with elevated triglycerides more aggressively.[36] **Table 6.4** shows triglyceride levels and levels of total and LDL cholesterol considered desirable, borderline high, and high according to the new NCEP guidelines.

Table 6.4 Adult Blood Cholesterol and Triglyceride Levels

Total Cholesterol	
Desirable	< 200
Borderline high	200–239
High	≥ 240

LDL Cholesterol	
Optimal	< 100
Near optimal/above optimal	100–129
Borderline high	130–159
High	160–189
Very high	≥ 190

Triglyceride	
Normal	< 150
Borderline high	150–199
High	200–499
Very high	≥ 500

HDL Cholesterol
Low < 40
High ≥ 60

Note: All units are mg/dL.

Sources: National Cholesterol Education Program. *Third Report of the Expert Panel on Detection, Evaluation, and Treatment of High Blood Cholesterol in Adults (Adult Treatment Panel III).* Washington, DC: US Department of Health and Human Services; 2001. NIH publication 01-3305.

Reducing Risk of Heart Disease: Lifestyle Factors

Some risks for developing atherosclerosis are beyond our control—like being male or getting older. But there are many risk factors we can control. What steps can you take? Avoid or quit smoking. Manage weight and control blood pressure. Make physical activity part of your daily life to help keep weight normal and promote overall heart health. After age 20, have your total, LDL, and HDL cholesterol levels measured every five years.

Reducing Risk of Heart Disease: Dietary Factors

Some years ago, many health experts advised people to emphasize polyunsaturated oils in their diets. You seldom will hear this advice today. Replacing saturated fat with *omega*-6-rich polyunsaturated oils like corn oil may decrease total cholesterol and LDL cholesterol, but it also lowers healthful HDL cholesterol. Polyunsaturated fatty acids in vegetable oils also oxidize easily and provide too much *omega*-6 fatty acid in relation to *omega*-3. Newer research shows that monounsaturated fats like olive oil lower total and LDL cholesterol without lowering HDL.[37]

Earlier diet advice also emphasized minimizing dietary cholesterol—few egg yolks, no liver or organ meats, and no seafood (the amount of cholesterol in seafood was later found to have been overestimated). Lowering cholesterol intake does help some people, but for most, lower blood levels aren't guaranteed, and lowering saturated fat intake is more effective.

Today, nutritionists recommend lowering total fat intake, lowering saturated fat, and keeping body weight normal. Within total fat limits, monounsaturated oils should be the fat source of choice. For people who respond to a reduced-cholesterol diet, lowering dietary cholesterol is a good idea. Eating fruits, vegetables, legumes, and grains that contain fiber helps lower cholesterol levels, too. These foods also have antioxidant nutrients and B vitamins such as folic acid that may also reduce the risk of heart disease.

Quick Bites

NCEP Tips for Healthful Eating Out

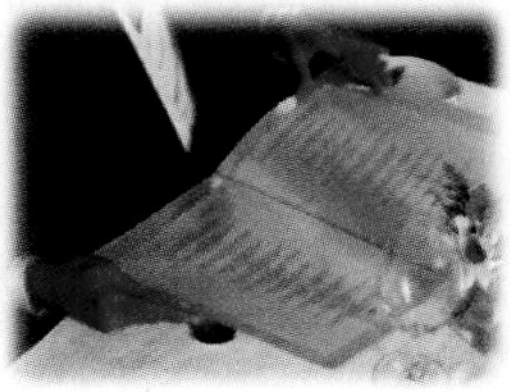

- Choose restaurants that have low-fat, low-cholesterol menu items.
- Don't be afraid to ask for foods that follow your eating pattern.
- Select poultry, fish, or meat that is broiled, grilled, baked, steamed, or poached rather than fried.
- Choose lean deli meats like fresh turkey or lean roast beef instead of higher-fat cuts like salami or bologna.
- Look for vegetables seasoned with herbs or spices rather than butter, sour cream, or cheese. Ask for sauces on the side.
- Order a low-fat dessert like sherbet, fruit ice, sorbet, or low-fat frozen yogurt.
- Control serving sizes by asking for a small serving, sharing a dish, or taking some home.
- At fast-food restaurants, go for grilled chicken and lean roast beef sandwiches or lean plain hamburgers (but remember to hold the fatty sauces), salads with low-fat salad dressing, low-fat milk, and low-fat frozen yogurt. Pizza topped with vegetables and minimum cheese is another good choice.

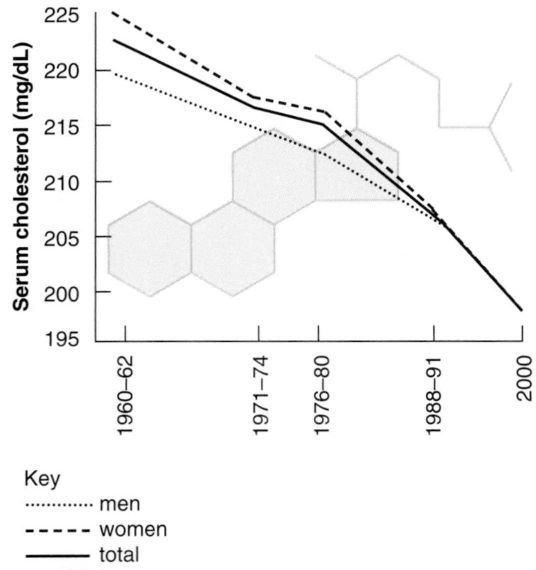

Figure 6.26 **Trends in age-adjusted (mean) serum cholesterol.** Although mean cholesterol levels of adults have fallen significantly, cardiovascular disease remains the leading cause of death in the United States and Canada.
Source: CDC, NCHS, NHESI, NHANES I, NHANES II, NHANES III (Phase 1, 1988–91).

Since its inception in 1985, the National Cholesterol Education Program has made population-wide dietary recommendations. Here are the latest recommendations:

- Choose foods low in saturated fat.
- Choose foods low in total fat.
- Choose foods high in starch and fiber.
- Choose foods low in cholesterol.
- Be more physically active.
- Maintain a healthy weight, and lose weight if you are overweight.

Beyond Cholesterol

Death from coronary heart disease has fallen dramatically, by more than 50 percent over the past 30 years. That drop seems related to a 28 percent drop in average cholesterol levels from 1976 to 1994 (see **Figure 6.26**), which in turn parallels a reduced consumption of cholesterol and a lower percentage of calories from fat.[38]

But have less fat and cholesterol made us more heart healthy? Or do falling death rates reflect better treatment of heart attacks and existing heart disease? Although preventive efforts, such as diet, are important, several studies suggest that treatment has been the more important factor in reducing deaths from heart disease.[39]

Since most heart attacks occur in people with average to moderately high blood cholesterol levels, researchers are exploring other factors that may produce these heart attacks.[40] They also are exploring why many people with high blood cholesterol levels don't develop heart disease. Looking beyond fat and cholesterol, these researchers have found that other important dietary factors are involved.

Antioxidants In the blood, oxygen can damage low-density lipoproteins. Once oxidized, they are deposited in the inner layer of the blood vessels, and the process of building up plaque begins.[41] A diet high in vitamin E and other antioxidants appears to inhibit oxidation and subsequent atherosclerosis.[42]

Homocysteine High levels of the amino acid homocysteine may contribute to heart disease by promoting atherosclerosis, excessive blood clotting, or blood vessel rigidity. Folic acid and vitamins B_6 and B_{12} can help reduce destructive levels of homocysteine. Scientists believe that a diet rich in these vitamins helps prevent blood vessel damage from homocysteine.[43]

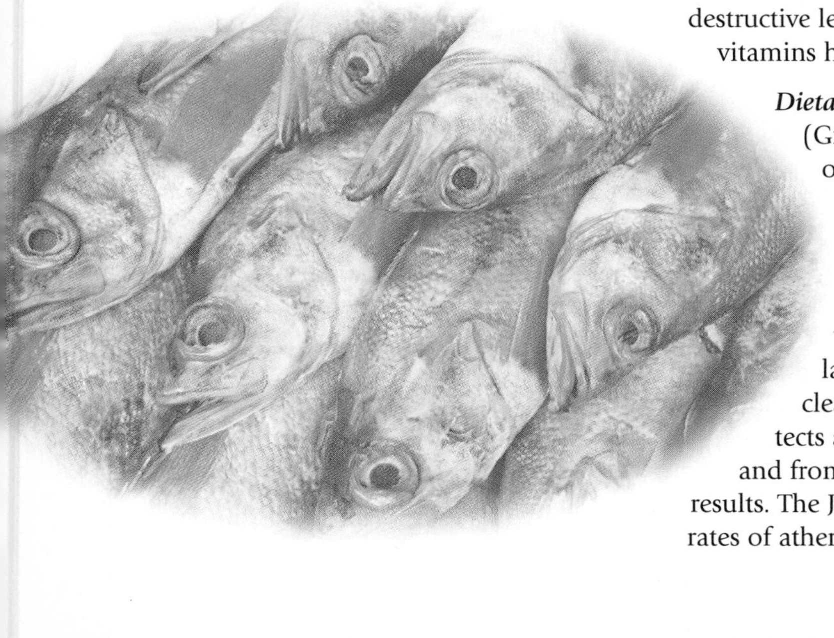

Dietary Omega-3 *Fatty Acids* In the 1970s a study of the Inuits (Greenland Eskimos) focused attention on the beneficial effects of EPA and DHA, the *omega*-3 fatty acids in fish fats.[44] Researchers were puzzled: Here was a group of people with a high intake of fat, saturated fat, and cholesterol from marine mammals and fish. Yet, they had little evidence of atherosclerosis. The Inuits were compared with the Danes, among whom atherosclerosis was common and whose diet was similarly high in fat, but from meats and dairy products. It became clear the high EPA and DHA content of fish in the Inuit diet protects against heart disease, discouraging blood cells from clotting and from sticking to artery walls. Studies of other groups show similar results. The Japanese, for example, with their generous fish intake, have low rates of atherosclerosis. Many other studies point in the same direction;

some show that as few as two or three servings of fish weekly can be protective.

Interest in *omega*-3 fatty acids has expanded recently. Increasing evidence suggests that consuming *omega*-3s from fish and fish oils protects against heart disease and its many complications.[45] The Nurses' Health Study also shows that higher consumption of fish or *omega*-3 fatty acids reduces the risk of stroke caused by blood clots.[46] Scientists are investigating whether *omega*-3s may help some chronic inflammatory conditions such as rheumatoid arthritis,[47] asthma,[48] or psoriasis, but research in these areas has had some disappointing results.[49] All in all, however, there are enough positive results to encourage further study and recommend regular consumption of fish for EPA and DHA, as well as plant foods with *omega*-3 *alpha*-linolenic acid.[50]

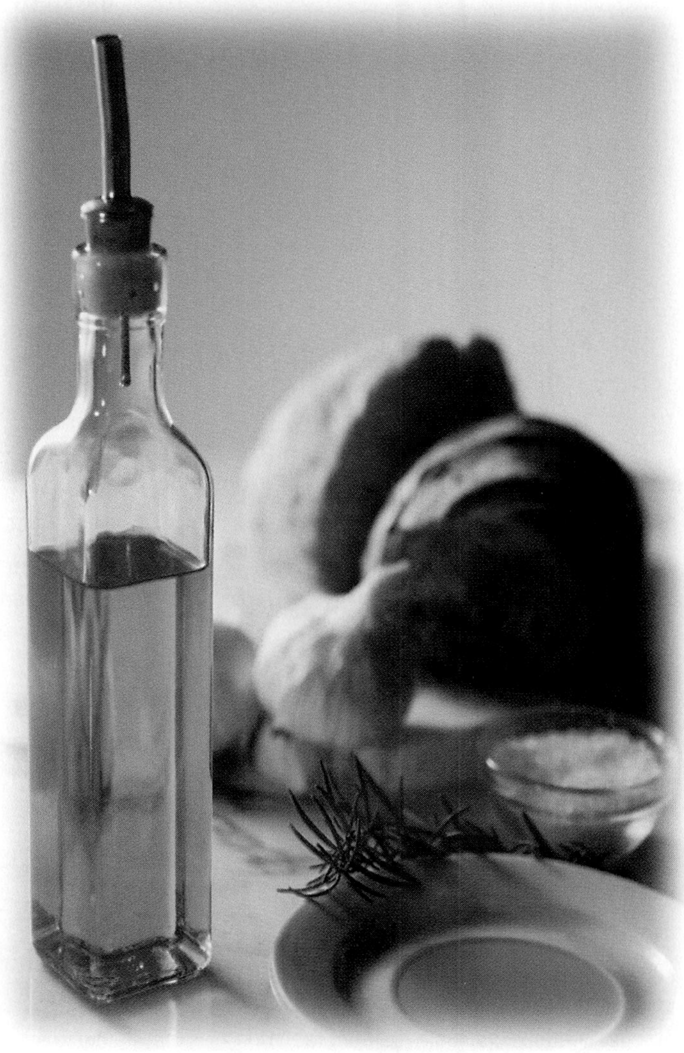

Dietary Fiber As described in Chapter 5, "Carbohydrates," fiber can bind to bile acids in the gastrointestinal tract, so these bile acids are excreted in the feces rather than recycled and reused. Additional bile acids then must be made from cholesterol, lowering the total amount in the body. Intestinal bacteria can partially digest dietary fibers, and the resulting short-chain fatty acids are linked to reduced cholesterol synthesis.[51]

The French Paradox How can the French eat rich cheeses and fatty meats but still have low rates of heart disease? They also have relatively high intakes of red wine and grapes, both rich in antioxidant phytochemicals.[52] Antioxidants and moderate alcohol consumption may offset some of the adverse effects of poor food choices and help protect against heart disease. Recent studies associate moderate alcohol consumption with a substantial decrease in heart disease risk.[53]

The Mediterranean Diet How can Greeks, Turks, and others around the Mediterranean eat a diet high in fat but still have low rates of heart disease? The focus here is on the source of the fat—olive oil, which is rich in monounsaturated fatty acids. Their diet pattern—ample fresh fruits, vegetables, pasta, and grains, small amounts of meat and poultry, and generous use of olive oil—has gained support among many nutritionists.[54]

Other Phytochemicals Along with antioxidants, other plant chemicals affect heart disease risk. Two widely studied phytochemical groups are isoflavones in soybeans and lignins in flaxseed, whole grains, and some fruits. These are also referred to as phytoestrogens—plant compounds with hormonelike effects. In November 1999, the FDA approved a health claim for food labels about the role of soy protein in reducing the risk of cardiovascular disease. The proposal was based on studies showing that eating 25 grams of soy protein per day has a cholesterol-lowering effect.[55]

Cancer

The evidence linking dietary fat to cancer is inconclusive. The case looks strong when we compare cancer rates between countries: Overall cancer rates generally are higher in countries with high fat intake and lower in countries where people eat less fat. But in population studies within those countries, the evidence linking fat to cancer is weaker. The Nurses' Health Study followed over 121,000 women for 14 years and found no evidence that higher total fat intake was associated with an increased risk of breast cancer.[56] These results call into question theories that link dietary fat with other cancers. Red meat intake, but not total fat, may be related to colon cancer, and high consumption of red meat and dairy products may be related to prostate cancer. Calorie intake may be a more important factor than fat intake.[57]

Development of Cancer

Cancer develops in a multistage process that occurs over many years. There are typically three phases of development:

1. *initiation,* when something alters a cell's genetic structure and prepares it to act abnormally during later stages
2. *promotion,* a reversible stage when a chemical or other factor encourages initiated cells to become active
3. *progression,* when promoted cells multiply and may invade surrounding healthy tissue

Evidence suggests that between 30 and 40 percent of cancers are due to poor food choices and physical inactivity, although the role of nutrition and diet in cancer development is complex. Some dietary factors may act as

Label [to] Table

The Nutrition Facts panel shown here highlights all of the lipid-related information you can find on a food label. Look at the top of the label, where it states that this product contains 35 "Calories from fat." Do you know how you can estimate this number from another part of the label? Recall that each gram of fat contains 9 kilocalories (or look at the bottom of the label). If this food item has 4 grams of fat, then it should make sense that there are approximately 36 kilocalories provided by fat. In this case, because the manufacturer listed only 35 you can assume that the 4 grams of fat on the label is rounded up from the actual total fat content of 3.9 grams (3.9 grams of fat × 9 kilocalories per gram = 35 kilocalories of fat).

"Total Fat" is the second thing you'll see, along with saturated fat. Recall that fats are classified into three types: saturated, monounsaturated, and polyunsaturated. Manufacturers are required to list only saturated fat on the label, but they can voluntarily list the others. Using this food label, you can estimate the amount of unsaturated fat by simply looking at the highlighted sections. There are 4 total grams of fat, and 2.5 of them are saturated. That means the remaining 1.5 grams are either polyunsaturated or monounsaturated. Without even knowing what food item this label represents, you can see that it contains more saturated fat than unsaturated fat (2.5 grams vs. 1.5 grams). This is typical of a food that contains fat from an animal source or tropical oil.

Do you see the 6% to the right of "Total Fat"? This does not mean that the food item contains 6% of its calories from fat. In fact, this food item contains 23% of its calories from fat (35 fat kilocalories ÷ 154 total kilocalories = 0.23, or 23% fat). The 6% refers to the Daily Values found below. You can see that a person who consumes 2,000 kilocalories per day could consume up to 65 grams of fat per day. This product contributes just 4 grams per serving, which is 6% of that amount (4 ÷ 65 = 0.06, or 6%). Note that the % Daily Value for saturated fat is 12%, so just a few servings of this food can contribute quite a bit of saturated fat to your diet. Cholesterol is also highlighted on this label (20 mg), along with its Daily Value contribution (7%).

Nutrition Facts

Serving Size: 1 cup (248g)
Servings Per Container: 4

Amount Per Serving	
Calories 154 Calories from fat 35	
% Daily Value •	
Total Fat 4g	6%
Saturated Fat 2.5g	12%
Cholesterol 20mg	7%
Sodium 170mg	7%
Total Carbohydrate 19g	6%
Dietary Fiber 0g	0%
Sugars 14g	
Protein 11g	

Vitamin A 4% • Vitamin C 6%
Calcium 40% • Iron 0%

• Percent Daily Values are based on a 2,000 calorie diet. Your daily values may be higher or lower depending on your calorie needs:

	Calories:	2000	2,500
Total Fat	Less Than	65g	80g
Sat Fat	Less Than	20g	25g
Cholesterol	Less Than	300mg	300mg
Sodium	Less Than	2,400mg	2,400mg
Total Carbohydrate		300g	375g
Dietary Fiber		25g	30g

Calories per gram:
Fat 9 • Carbohydrate 4 • Protein 4

promoters; many others may have protective roles, blocking the cellular changes in one of the developmental stages.

When scientists induce cancer in laboratory rodents, high intakes of fat, calories, and *omega*-6 fatty acids all appear to promote tumor growth.[58] Just how relevant these studies are to humans is unclear, and any conclusions about the relationship between dietary fats and cancer remain controversial.

Diet and Cancer Risk Reduction

To reduce your cancer risk, eat a moderately low-fat diet and increase your consumption of fruits, vegetables, and whole grains. Sounds familiar, right? The same antioxidant properties that may reduce atherosclerosis can also affect cancer development. In addition to having antioxidant effects, nutrients and other phytochemicals may inhibit multiplication of cancer cells, alter enzymes, inhibit the conversion of chemicals into toxins, and alter hormone metabolism.

In 2002, the American Cancer Society released new Nutrition and Physical Activity Guidelines for Cancer Prevention.[59] The new guidelines put more emphasis on physical activity and weight control, and also make suggestions for how communities can provide opportunities for Americans to be physically active. There are four major recommendations for individual choices. Notice how similar these guidelines are to those for reducing the risk of heart disease.

1. Eat a variety of healthful foods, with an emphasis on plant sources.
   - Eat five or more servings of a variety of vegetables and fruits each day.
   - Choose whole grains in preference to processed (refined) grains and sugars.
   - Limit consumption of red meats, especially those high in fat and processed.
   - Choose foods that help you to maintain a healthful weight.
2. Adopt a physically active lifestyle.
   - For adults: at least 30 minutes of moderate activity per day for five or more days of the week.
   - For children and adolescents: at least 60 minutes per day of moderate to vigorous activity at least five days of the week.
3. Maintain a healthful weight throughout life.
   - Balance caloric intake with physical activity.
   - Lose weight if currently overweight or obese.
4. If you drink alcoholic beverages, limit consumption.
   - Limit intake to no more than two drinks per day for men and one drink per day for women. Regular consumption of even a few drinks per week has been associated with an increased risk of breast cancer in women.

Key Concepts: *Excessive fat intake has been linked to obesity, heart disease, and cancer. There is a major public heath effort to reduce intake of fat, saturated fat, and cholesterol. Cholesterol-lowering diets have changed over the years, with somewhat less emphasis on reducing dietary cholesterol and more on reducing fats and saturated fats and increasing fruits, vegetables, and whole grains. The evidence linking dietary fats with cancer is less clear, but many other dietary factors are important in reducing risk.*

Quick Bites

What Does the Color of Beef Fat Reveal?

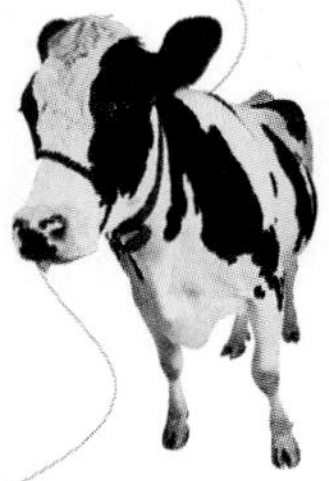

Yellow-tinged fat indicates that a steer was grass fed. White fat suggests that the animal was fed corn or cereal grain, at least during its final months. Thus, steak surrounded by pearly white fat should be more tender and, consequently, more expensive.

LEARNING Portfolio chapter 6

Key Terms

	page
adipocytes	164
adipose tissue	164
alpha-linolenic acid [Al-fah-lin-oh-LEN-ik]	160
atherosclerosis [ath-e-roh-scle-ROH-sis]	170
cardiovascular disease	184
chain length	158
cholesterol [ko-LES-te-rol]	170
choline	169
chylomicron [kye-lo-MY-kron]	176
cis fatty acid	160
conjugated linoleic acid (CLA)	160
diglyceride	162
eicosanoids	162
essential fatty acids (EFAs)	160
fat substitutes	180
fatty acids	158
glycerol [GLISS-er-ol]	162
high-density lipoproteins (HDL)	178
hydrogenation [high-dro-jen-AY-shun]	160
hypercholesterolemia	184
intermediate-density lipoproteins (IDL)	178
lanugo [lah-NEW-go]	164
lecithin	169
linoleic acid [lin-oh-LAY-ik]	160
lipoprotein	176
lipoprotein lipase	177
low-density lipoproteins (LDL)	178
micelles	176
monoglyceride	162
monounsaturated fatty acid	160
nonessential fatty acids	160
obesity	183
olestra	180
omega-3 fatty acid	162
omega-6 fatty acid	162
oxidation	165
phosphate group	167
phospholipids	158
phytosterols	173
polyunsaturated fatty acid	160
saturated fatty acid	160
squalene	173
sterols	158
subcutaneous fat	164
trans fatty acid	160
unsaturated fatty acid	160
very-low-density lipoproteins (VLDL)	177
visceral fat	164

Study Points

- **There are three main classes of lipids: triglycerides, phospholipids, and sterols.**
- **Fatty acids are components of both triglycerides and phospholipids.**
- **Saturated fatty acids have no double bonds between carbon atoms in their carbon chains; monounsaturated fatty acids have one double bond; and polyunsaturated fatty acids have more than one double bond in their carbon chains.**
- **Two polyunsaturated fatty acids, linoleic acid and *alpha*-linolenic acid, are essential and must be supplied in the diet. Phospholipids and sterols are made in the body and do not have to be supplied in the diet.**
- **Essential fatty acids are precursors of hormonelike compounds called eicosanoids. These compounds regulate many body functions, including blood pressure, heart rate, inflammation, and immune response.**
- **Triglycerides are food fats and storage fats. They are composed of glycerol and three fatty acids.**
- **In the body, triglycerides are an important source of energy. Stored fat provides an energy reserve.**
- **Phospholipids are made of glycerol, two fatty acids, and a compound containing phosphate and nitrogen.**
- **Phospholipids are components of cell membranes and lipoproteins. Having both fat- and water-soluble components allows them to be effective emulsifiers in foods and in the body.**
- **Cholesterol is found in cell membranes and is used to synthesize vitamin D, bile acids, and steroid hormones. High levels of blood cholesterol are associated with increased heart disease risk.**
- **For people with elevated blood cholesterol levels, the NCEP recommends daily intakes of (1) no more than 35 percent of calories as fat, provided most is unsaturated fat, (2) no more than 7 percent of calories as saturated fat, and (3) no more than 200 milligrams of cholesterol.**
- **Diets high in fat and saturated fat tend to increase blood levels of LDL cholesterol and increase risk for heart disease.**
- **Excess fat in the diet is linked to obesity, heart disease, and some types of cancer.**

Study Questions

Answers can be found at nutrition.jbpub.com/discovering.

1. **How is it that different oils can contain a mixture of polyunsaturated, monounsaturated, and saturated fats?**
2. **What does the hardness or softness of a fat typically signify?**
3. **What is the most common form of lipid found in food?**
4. **What are the positive and negative consequences of hydrogenating a fat?**
5. **List the many functions of triglycerides.**
6. **Describe the difference between LDL and HDL in terms of cholesterol and protein composition.**
7. **List the recommendations for intake of fat, saturated fat, polyunsaturated fat, monounsaturated fat, and cholesterol.**
8. **What foods contain cholesterol?**
9. **Name the two essential fatty acids.**

[Try] This

The Fat = Fullness Challenge

The goal of this experiment is to see whether fat affects your desire to eat between meals. Do this experiment for two consecutive breakfasts. Each meal is to include only the foods listed below. Try to eat normally for the other meals of the day and eat around the same time of day. Each of these breakfasts has approximately the same calories, but one has a high percentage of them from fat, the other from carbohydrate. After each breakfast, take note of how many hours pass before you feel hungry again.

Day 1 (~455 kcal)	Day 2 (~460 kcal)
One 3-oz bagel with 3 tbsp of jelly	*2 eggs fried with a minimal ($< \frac{1}{2}$ tbsp) amount of butter/margarine*
	2 pieces of whole wheat bread with 1 tbsp of butter/margarine or $\frac{2}{3}$ tbsp of peanut butter

The Salad Dressing Experiment

You can learn a lot from oil-and-vinegar dressing! The purpose of this experiment is twofold. First, you will understand better what it means to say that lipids are insoluble (or not water-soluble). Second, you will be able to experience how fat acts based on its density. Go to your local grocery store and purchase a seasoning packet for Italian (oil and vinegar) dressing. Make sure you also purchase the amount of oil (any type is fine) and vinegar (any type is fine) you need based on the directions. Once home, prepare the dressing. Shake the dressing as if you were to pour it on a salad and then let it stand. What happens to the dressing? What explains this action? Once the dressing settles, which ingredient is found on top—the oil or the vinegar? What property of fat explains this?

What About Bobbie?

Let's take a look at Bobbie's fat intake. Review her day of eating (Chapter 1) and pay special attention to the foods you know contain fat. Do you think she ate above or below 30 percent of total calories from fat? Did she eat more saturated or unsaturated fat? How about her cholesterol intake? Do you think she came in below the guideline?

Bobbie's total fat intake was 98 grams. Here are the foods that contributed the most fat:

Food	Fat (g)
Meatballs	*17*
Salad dressing	*14*
Tortilla chips	*11*
Pizza	*11*
Garlic bread	*10*
Cream cheese	*8*
Mayonnaise	*7*

Bobbie's diet has 36 percent of its calories from fat, which is higher than recommended.

$$98 \text{ g fat} \times 9 \text{ kcal/g} = 882 \text{ kcal fat}$$

$$882 \text{ kcal fat} \div 2{,}440 \text{ total kcal} = 0.36, \text{ or } 36\% \text{ kcal from fat}$$

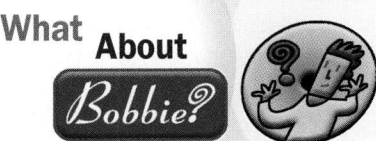

Are you surprised her fat intake is so high? Her intake doesn't look too unusual, but you can see how the "extras" along the way add up. Look at the list of fat-containing foods again. Do you think her diet is higher in saturated or unsaturated fat? Well, three of the foods listed are animal products (meatballs, pizza, and cream cheese), so you know they contribute to the amount of saturated fat. Both the tortilla chips and garlic bread contain a mixture of saturated and unsaturated fats, and the Italian dressing contains mostly unsaturated fat. Her overall saturated fat intake is 32 grams. That's about 12 percent of her caloric intake, which is more than the Daily Value (9 percent).

If Bobbie wanted to lower her saturated fat and total fat intake, what changes could she make? Here are some suggestions.

Bobbie can lower her saturated fat intake by:

- topping her bagel with peanut butter instead of cream cheese
- decreasing the number of meatballs on her pasta
- snacking on pizza less often

Bobbie can lower her overall fat intake by:

- using cream cheese on only half her bagel and using jelly on the other half
- using only mustard on her sandwich, not mustard and mayonnaise
- reducing the amount of tortilla chips she eats by half and having a piece of fruit in their place
- reducing the amount of Italian dressing she puts on her salad (2 tbsp contain 14 grams of fat and almost 140 kilocalories!)
- having a plain piece of bread with dinner, not the garlic bread made with butter or margarine

In terms of cholesterol, how do you think Bobbie did? She consumed 263 milligrams in this day. If she follows the above tips to lower her saturated fat intake, she'll find her overall cholesterol intake will be cut in half!

References

1 Devery R, Miller A, Stanton C. Conjugated linoleic acid and oxidative behavior in cancer cells. *Biochem Soc Trans.* 2001;29:341–344.

2 Crawford MA. The role of essential fatty acids in neural development: implications for perinatal nutrition. *Am J Clin Nutr.* 1993;57:S703–S710.

3 Erdman JW, Bierer TL, Gugger ET. Absorption and transport of carotenoids. *Ann NY Acad Sci.* 1993;691:76–85.

4 Bilger B. The flavor of fat. *The Sciences.* Nov/Dec 1997;10.

5 National Cholesterol Education Program (NCEP). *Detection, Evaluation, and Treatment of High Blood Cholesterol in Adults.* Washington, DC: National Institutes of Health; 1993.

6 Wan PJ, Hron RJ. Extraction solvents for oilseeds. *Inform.* 1998;9(7):707–709.

7 Seidner DL. Clinical uses for omega-3 polyunsaturated fatty acids and structured triglycerides. *Support Line.* 1994;16(3):7–11.

8 Neaton JD, Blackburn H, Jacobs D, et al. Serum cholesterol level and mortality findings for men screened in the Multiple Risk Factor Intervention Trial. Multiple Risk Factor Intervention Trial Research Group. *Arch Intern Med.* 1992;152:1490–1500.

9 Cheblowski RT, Grosvenor M, Lillington L. Dietary intake and counseling, weight management, and the course of HIV infection. *J Am Diet Assoc.* 1995;95:428–432.

10 Cendella RJ. Cholesterol and cataracts. *Surv Ophthalmol.* 1996;40:320–337.

11 Morell P, Jurevics H. Origin of cholesterol in myelin. *Neurochem Res.* 1996;21:463–470.

12 Jones PJH. Regulation of cholesterol biosynthesis by diet in humans. *Am J Clin Nutr.* 1997;66:438–446.

13 Ibid.

14 Strauss E. One-eyed animals implicate cholesterol in development. *Science.* 1998;280:1528–1529.

15 Jones PJH, Kubow S. Lipids, sterols and their metabolites. In: Shills ME, Olson JA, Shike M, Ross CA, eds. *Modern Nutrition in Health and Disease.* 9th ed. Philadelphia: Lippincott Williams & Wilkins; 1999:67–94.

16 Guyton AC, Hall JE. *Textbook of Medical Physiology.* 10th ed. Philadelphia: W.B. Saunders; 2000.

17 Brown MS, Goldstein JL. A receptor-mediated pathway for cholesterol homeostasis. *Science.* 1986;232:34–47.

18 Dietschy JM, Turley SD, Spady DK. Role of liver in the maintenance of cholesterol and low density lipoprotein homeostasis in different animal species, including humans. *J Lipid Res.* 1993;34:1637–1659.

19 National Cholesterol Education Program. Op. cit.

20 Williams CL, Bollella M, Boccia L, et al. Dietary fat and children's health. *Nutrition Today.* 1998;33(4):144–155.

21 High blood cholesterol: what's known, what's new, what's ahead. *Heart Memo.* Summer 1998;5–17.

22 US Department of Agriculture, Economic Research Service. *Food Review.* Sept/Dec 1997.

23 Popkin BM, Siega-Riz AM, Haines PS, Janhs L. Where's the fat? Trends in U.S. diets 1965–1996. *Prev Med.* 2001;32:245–254.

24 Kris-Etherton PM, Taylor DS, Yu-Poth S, et al. Polyunsaturated fatty acids in the food chain in the United States. *Am J Clin Nutr.* 2000;71(suppl):179S–188S.

25 Ibid.

26 Calorie Control Council. Consumer demand for less fat remains strong. *Calorie Control Commentary.* Fall 1996;3; and Taubes T. The soft science of dietary fat. *Science.* 2001;291: 2536–2545.

27 Blackburn H. Olestra and the FDA. *N Engl J Med.* 1996;334.

28 Jacobsen M, Corcoran L. Olestra. *Nutrition Action Healthletter.* March 1998;9–11; and Callaway CW. Role of fat-modified foods in the American diet. *Nutrition Today.* 1998;33(4):156–163.

29 Allgood GS, Kuter DJ, Roll KT, et al. Postmarketing surveillance of new food ingredients: results from the program with the fat replacer olestra. *Regul Toxicol Pharmacol.* 2001;33: 224–233.

30 Miller DL, Casteollanos VH, Shide DJ, et al. Effect of fat-free potato chips with and without nutrition labels on fat and energy intakes. *Am J Clin Nutr.* 1998;68:282–290.

31 Are reduced-fat foods keeping Americans healthier? *Tufts University Health & Nutrition Letter.* 1998;16(1):4–5.

32 Zock PL. Dietary fats and cancer. *Curr Opin Lipidol.* 2001;12:5–10; and Smith-Warner SA, Spiegelman D, Adami HO, et al. Types of dietary fat and breast cancer: a pooled analysis of cohort studies. *Int J Cancer.* 2001;92:767–774.

33 Hoeg JM. Evaluating coronary heart disease risk. *JAMA.* 1997;277:1387–1390.

34 Bostrom AG, Cupples A, Jenner JL. Elevated plasma lipoprotein(a) and coronary heart disease in men aged 55 years and younger: a prospective study. *JAMA.* 1996;276:544–548.

35 Mlot C. Chlamydia linked to atherosclerosis. *Science.* 1996;272:1422; and Zhou YF, Leon MB, Waclawiw MA, et al. Association between prior cytomegalovirus infection and the risk of restonsis after coronary atherectomy. *N Engl J Med.* 1996;335:624–630.

36 National Cholesterol Education Program. *Third Report of the Expert Panel on Detection, Evaluation, and Treatment of High Blood Cholesterol in Adults (Adult Treatment Panel III).* Washington, DC: US Department of Health and Human Services; 2001. NIH publication 01-3305.

37 Kris-Etherton PM, Pearson TA, Wan Y, et al. High-monounsaturated fatty acid diets lower both plasma cholesterol and triacylglycerol concentrations. *Am J Clin Nutr.* 1999;70:1009–1015.

38 National Cholesterol Education Program (NCEP). Op. cit.

39 Rosamond WD, Chambless LE, Folsom AR, et al. Trends in the incidence of myocardial infarction and in mortality due to coronary heart disease, 1987 to 1994. *N Engl J Med.* 1998;339:861–867.

40 National Heart, Lung, and Blood Institute. Emerging risk factors—science's agenda for the next century. *Heart Memo.* Summer 1998;15.

41 Witzum JL. The oxidation hypothesis of atherosclerosis. *Lancet.* 1994;344:793–795.

42 Hodis HN, Mack WJ, LaBree L, et al. Serial coronary angiographic evidence that antioxidant vitamin intake reduces progression of coronary artery atherosclerosis. *JAMA.* 1995;273: 1849–1854.

43 Epstein FH. Homocysteine and atherothrombosis. *N Engl J Med.* 1998;338:1042–1060.

44 Bang HO, Dyerberg J. The composition of food consumed by Greenlandic Eskimos. *Acta Med Scand.* 1973;200:69–73.

45 Mori TA, Beilin LJ. Long-chain omega-3 fatty acids, blood lipids, and cardiovascular risk reduction. *Curr Opin Lipidol.* 2001;12:11–17; and Harris WS, Isley WL. Clinical trial evidence for the cardioprotective effects of omega-3 fatty acids. *Curr Atheroscler Rep.* 2001;3:174–179.

46 Iso H, Rexrode KM, Stampfer MJ, et al. Intake of fish and omega-3 fatty acids and risk of stroke in women. *JAMA.* 2001;285:304–312.

47 Adam O. Anti-inflammatory diet in rheumatic diseases. *Eur J Clin Nutr.* 1995;49:703–717.

48 Lewis RA, Austen K, Soberman RJ. Leukotrienes and other products of the 5-lipoxygenase pathway. *N Engl J Med.* 1990;323;645–655.

49 Soyland E, Funk J, Rajka G, et al. Effect of dietary supplementation with very-long-chain n-3 fatty acids in patients with psoriasis. *N Engl J Med.* 1993;328:1812–1816.

50 Neaton JD, Blackburn H, Jacobs D, et al. Op. cit. and Rosenberg IH. Fish—food to calm the heart. *N Engl J Med.* 2002;346:1102–1103.

51 Anderson JW. Short-chain fatty acids and lipid metabolism. In: Cummings JH, Rombeau JL, Sakata T, eds. *Physiological and Clinical Aspects of Short Chain Fatty Acids.* New York: Cambridge University Press; 1995:509–523.

52 Drewnowski A, Henderson SA, Shore AB. Diet quality and dietary diversity in France: implications for the French paradox. *J Am Diet Assoc.* 1996;96:663–669.

53 Klatsky AL. Should patients with heart disease drink red wine? *JAMA.* 2001;285:2004–2006.

54 Katan MB, Grundy SM, Willett WC. Beyond low fat diets. *N Engl J Med.* 1997;337:563–566.

55 US Department of Health and Human Services, Food and Drug Administration. *New Health Claim Proposed for Relationship of Soy Protein and Coronary Heart Disease.* Rockville, MD: National Press Office; 1998. FDA Talk Paper.

56 Holmes MD, Hunter DJ, Colditz GA, et al. Association of dietary intake of fat and fatty acids with risk of breast cancer. *JAMA.* 1999;281:914–920.

57 Byers T, Nestle M, McTiernan A, Doyle C, Currie-Williams A, Gansler T, Thun M; and the American Cancer Society 2001 Nutrition and Physical Activity Guidelines Advisory Committee. American Cancer Society Guidelines on Nutrition and Physical Activity for Cancer Prevention (2002): Reducing risk of cancer with healthy food choices and physical activity. *CA Cancer J Clin.* 2002;52:92–119.

58 Jonnalagadda SS, Mustad VA, Shaomei Y, et al. Effects of individual fatty acids on chronic diseases. *Nutrition Today.* 1996;31:90–107.

59 Byers T, Nestle M, McTiernan A, et al. Op. cit.

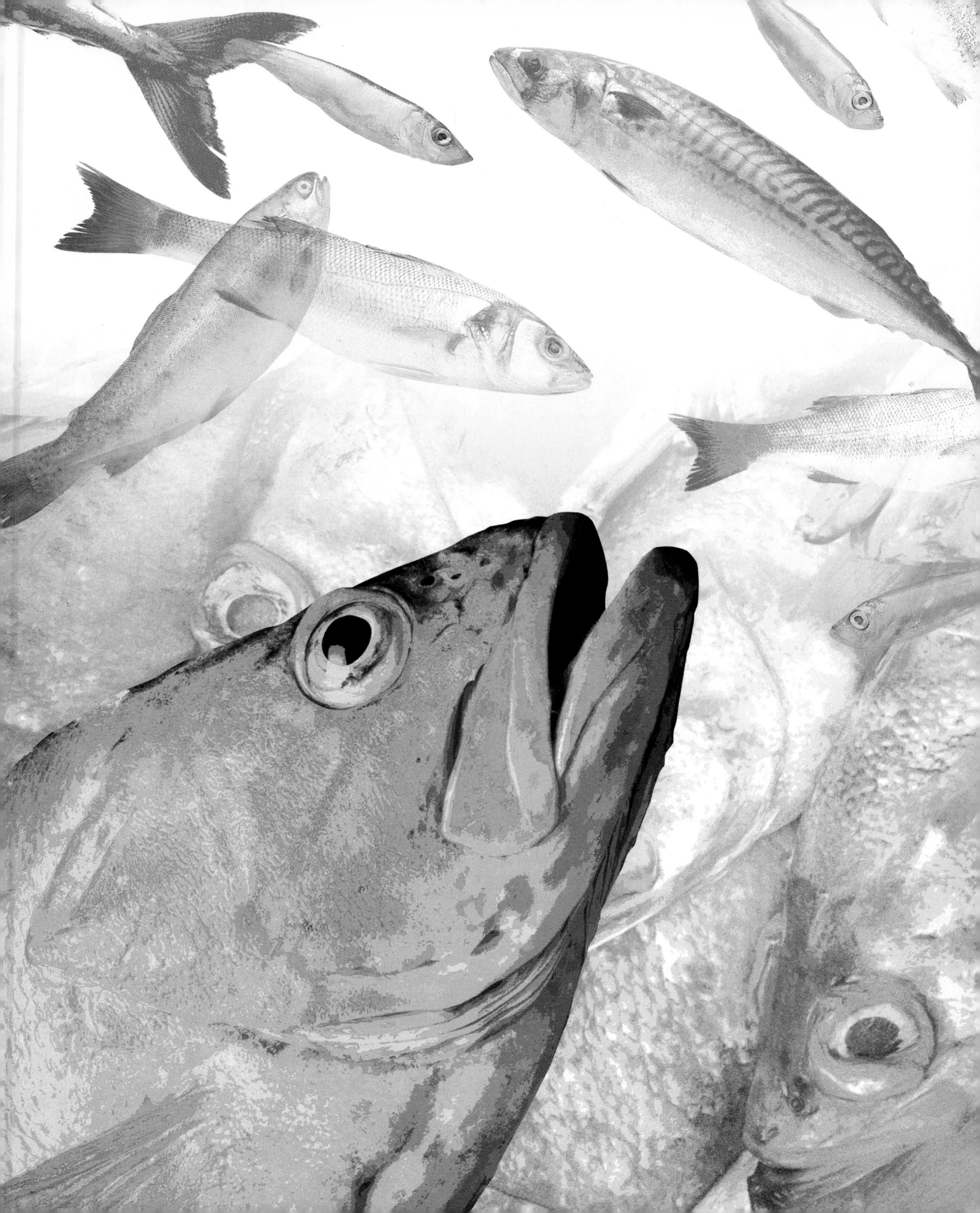

Chapter 7

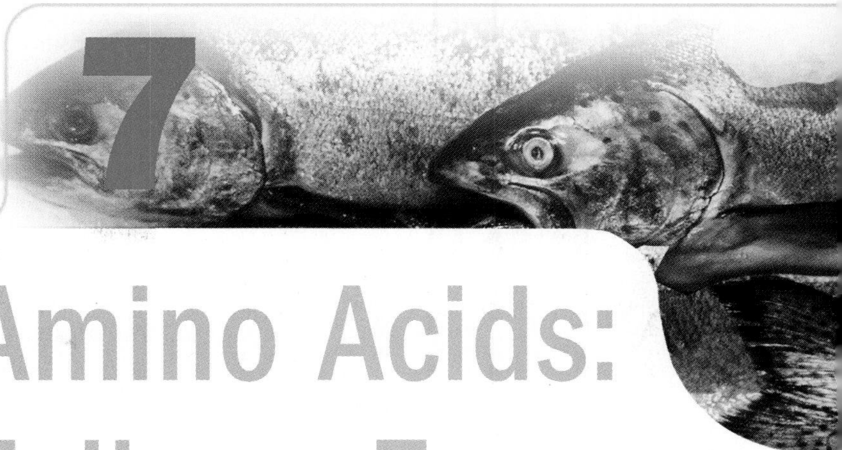

Proteins and Amino Acids: Function Follows Form

Think About It

1. What's your understanding of the term *protein-sparing*?
2. What percentage of your energy intake do you think comes from protein?
3. What's your view of amino acid supplements? What do you see as benefits and risks?
4. Have you ever considered a vegetarian diet?

Fyi for your Information

This chapter's FYI boxes include practical information on the following topics:

- Scrabble Anyone?
- Do Athletes Need More Protein?
- High-Protein Plant Foods

WWW

The Web site for this book offers many useful tools and is a great source for additional nutrition information for both students and instructors. For information on proteins and amino acids, visit the site at **nutrition.jbpub.com/discovering**. You'll find exercises that explore the following topics:

- Protein Supplements
- Different Proteins, Different Benefits
- Around the World with Proteins
- Insulin in 3-D

Key to Illustrations

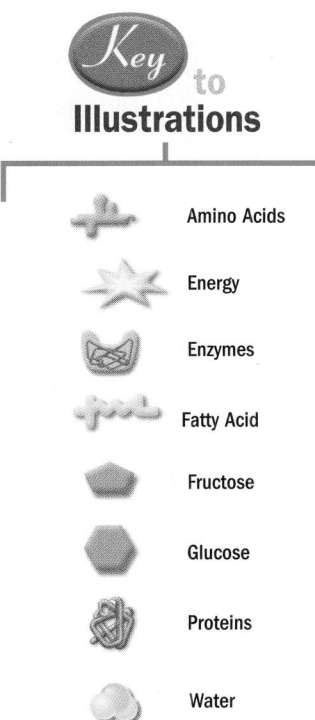

- Amino Acids
- Energy
- Enzymes
- Fatty Acid
- Fructose
- Glucose
- Proteins
- Water

What About Bobbie?

Track the choices Bobbie is making with the EatRight Analysis software.

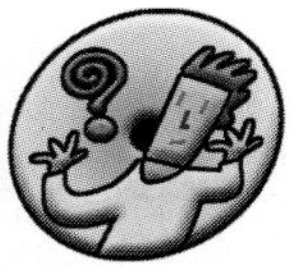

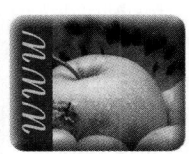

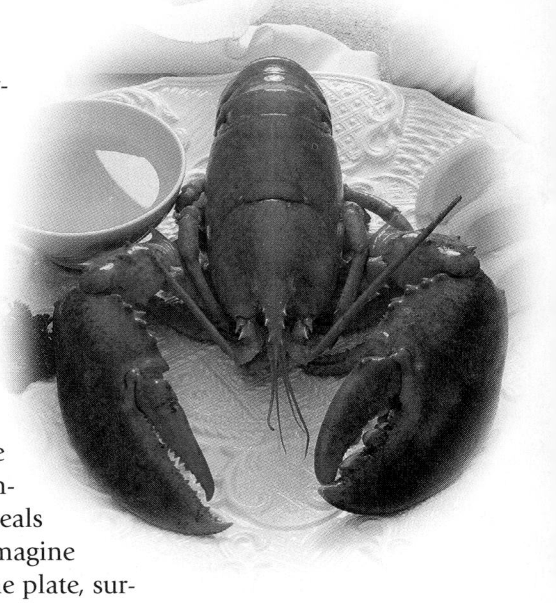

Think of your favorite meal—perhaps a holiday feast, the foods you always ask for on your birthday, or something from a special restaurant. What are you imagining? If you're like most Americans, you've probably conjured up something along the lines of steak and baked potato; lobster with corn on the cob; turkey with dressing, mashed potatoes, and all the trimmings; or maybe something more simple—a juicy hamburger and fries. What do all these meals have in common? In each case you imagine a meat or fish item at the center of the plate, surrounded by various grain or vegetable accompaniments.

From a young age, we're told that meat is an important source of protein and that protein helps us grow big and strong. Many traditional diets emphasize meat as the most important part of the meal and protein as the most important nutrient. But do such meals meet your body's needs? Would a different style of eating be more healthful? For example, what about adding a small amount of meat to a stir-fry of vegetables over rice? Or what about eliminating meat entirely from the diet? What makes the most sense nutritionally?

From the body's perspective, protein is certainly extremely important. Protein is part of every cell, is needed in thousands of chemical reactions, and keeps us "together" structurally. But, as you are about to learn, the human body is so good at using the protein we feed it that our actual needs for dietary protein are relatively small—meat doesn't need to be at the center of the plate to keep you healthy!

Quick Bites

A Bugburger Anyone?

Did you know that bugs provide 10 percent of the protein consumed worldwide? What creepy crawler would you choose for your dinner plate? A grasshopper is 15 to 60 percent protein. Pound for pound, spiders have more protein than any other bug.

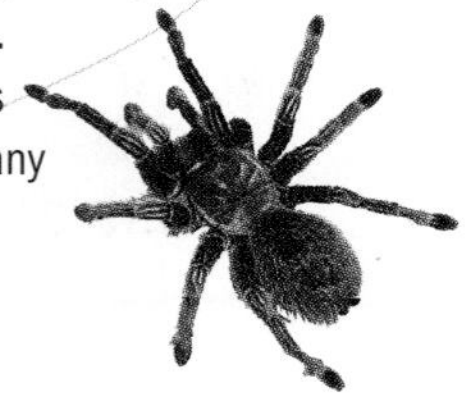

Why Is Protein Important?

The word *protein* was coined by the Dutch chemist Gerardus Mulder in 1838 and comes from the Greek word *protos*, meaning "of prime importance." Mulder discovered that proteins are a major component of all plant and animal tissues, second only to water. Today we know these intricately constructed molecules are vital to many aspects of health and play an essential role in every living cell. Our bodies constantly assemble, break down, and use proteins, so we count on our diet to provide enough protein each day to replace what is being used. When we eat more protein than we need, the excess is either used to make energy or stored as fat.

Most people associate protein with animal foods like beef, chicken, fish, or milk. However, plant foods such as dried beans and peas, grains, nuts, seeds, and vegetables also provide protein. Many protein-rich plant foods are also rich in vitamins and minerals. These plant foods usually are low in fat and calories.

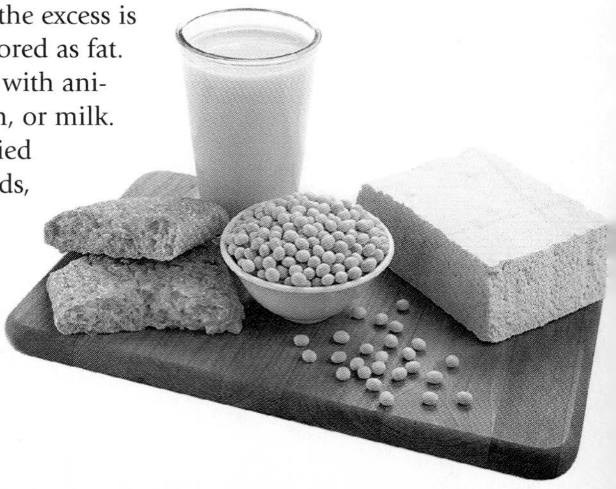

People living in poverty may suffer from a shortage of both protein and energy in the diet. When the diet lacks protein, the body breaks down body tissue such as muscle and uses it as a protein source. This causes loss, or **wasting**, of muscle, organs, and other tissues. Protein deficiency also affects the immune system, making people more vulnerable to infection, and impairs digestion and absorption of nutrients. In the United States and other industrialized countries, most people are able to get more than enough protein to meet the body's needs. In fact, a more common problem in these areas is excess intake of protein.

Amino Acids Are the Building Blocks of Protein

Just as glucose is the basic building block of carbohydrates, amino acids are the basic building blocks of protein. Proteins are sequences of amino acids. Your body has 20 different amino acids to choose from when building these sequences. Nine of these amino acids are called **essential amino acids** because your body cannot make them and must get them in the diet. Your body can manufacture the remaining 11, called **nonessential amino acids**, when enough nitrogen, carbon, hydrogen, and oxygen are available. Nonessential amino acids do not need to be supplied in your diet.

Sometimes, certain nonessential amino acids become essential. Tyrosine and cysteine are both considered **conditionally essential amino acids**. Under normal circumstances, your body makes tyrosine from the essential amino acid phenylalanine, and cysteine from the essential amino acid methionine. When your intake of phenylalanine and methionine is low, however, your body needs tyrosine and cysteine from your diet to free phenylalanine and methionine for protein formation. **Table 7.1** lists the essential, nonessential, and conditionally essential amino acids.

Tyrosine becomes an essential amino acid for individuals with the rare genetic disorder phenylketonuria (PKU). A person with PKU lacks an enzyme needed to convert phenylalanine to tyrosine, so tyrosine must be supplied in the diet. Phenylalanine intake must be carefully controlled because excess phenylalanine can build up and contribute to irreversible brain damage.[1] When babies with PKU receive treatment starting at birth,

wasting The breakdown of body tissue such as muscle and organ for use as a protein source when the diet lacks protein.

essential amino acids Amino acids the body cannot make at all or cannot make in sufficient quantities to meet the body's needs. Essential amino acids must be supplied in the diet.

nonessential amino acids Amino acids the body can make if supplied with adequate nitrogen. Nonessential amino acids do not need to be supplied in the diet.

conditionally essential amino acids Amino acids that are normally made in the body (nonessential) but become essential under certain circumstances, such as during critical illness.

Table 7.1 Essential, Nonessential, and Conditionally Essential Amino Acids

Essential	Nonessential	Conditionally Essential
Histidine	Alanine	
Isoleucine	Arginine	Arginine
Leucine	Asparagine	
Lysine	Aspartic acid	
Methionine	Cysteine	Cysteine
Phenylalanine	Glutamic acid	
Threonine	Glutamine	Glutamine
Tryptophan	Glycine	
Valine	Proline	
	Serine	
	Tyrosine	Tyrosine

their IQ development is unaffected. Without treatment, they suffer severe mental retardation.

Other amino acids also can become essential under certain circumstances. The amino acid glutamine is the main fuel for rapidly dividing cells and plays a key role in transporting nitrogen between organs.[2] Although normally considered nonessential, glutamine can become essential if the body's need increases substantially, such as when a person suffers trauma or becomes critically ill.[3] The amino acid arginine also can become essential when people are ill or experiencing severe physiological stress.[4]

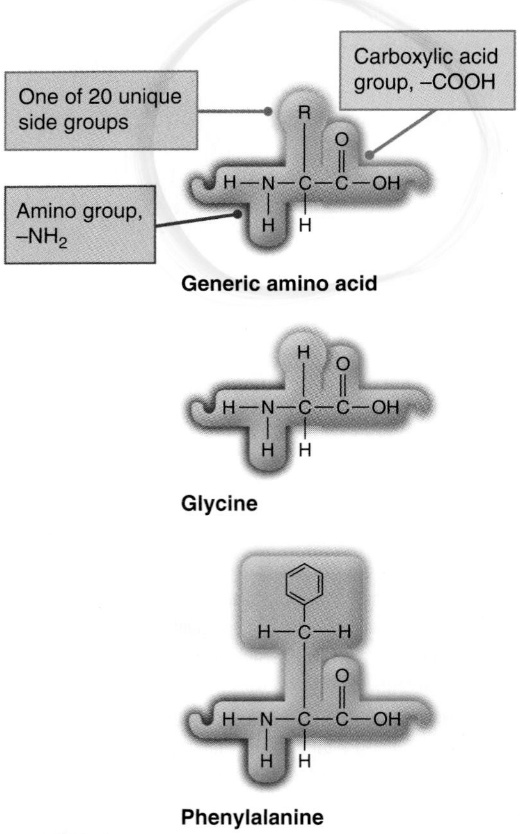

Figure 7.1 **Structure of an amino acid.** All amino acids have a similar structure. Attached to a carbon atom is a hydrogen (H), an amino group ($-NH_2$), an acid group (–COOH), and a side group (R). The side group gives each amino acid its unique identity.

Amino Acids Are Identified by Their Side Groups

Amino acids (with the exception of proline) have a central carbon atom with one hydrogen atom (H), one carboxylic acid group (–COOH), one amino (nitrogen-containing) group ($-NH_2$), and one side group unique to each amino acid (R). The side group gives each amino acid its identity. It can vary from a simple hydrogen atom, as in glycine, to a complex ring of carbon and hydrogen atoms, as in phenylalanine. The variations in side groups mean that individual amino acids differ in shape, size, composition, electrical charge, and pH. When amino acids link together to form a protein, these characteristics work together to determine that protein's specific function. **Figure 7.1** shows the structure of an amino acid.

Key Concepts: *Amino acids, which consist of a central carbon atom bonded to a hydrogen, a carboxyl group, an amino group, and a side group, are the building blocks of protein. Essential amino acids cannot be made by the body and must be supplied in the diet. Nonessential amino acids can be made in the body, given an adequate supply of nitrogen, carbon, hydrogen, and oxygen.*

Protein Structure: Unique Three-Dimensional Shapes and Functions

Proteins are very large molecules. Just as we combine letters of the alphabet in different sequences to form an infinite variety of words, the body combines amino acids in different sequences to form a nearly infinite variety of proteins. For this reason, protein molecules are more varied than those of either carbohydrates or lipids.

Amino Acid Sequence

Amino acids link in specific sequences to form strands of protein (often called peptides) up to hundreds of amino acids long. Each amino acid is joined to the next by a **peptide bond**. (See **Figure 7.2**.) A **dipeptide** is two amino acids joined by a peptide bond, while a **tripeptide** is three amino acids joined by peptide bonds. The term **oligopeptide** refers to a chain of 4 to 10 amino acids, while a **polypeptide** contains more than 10 amino acids.[5] Proteins in the body and in the diet are long polypeptides, most with hundreds of linked amino acids.

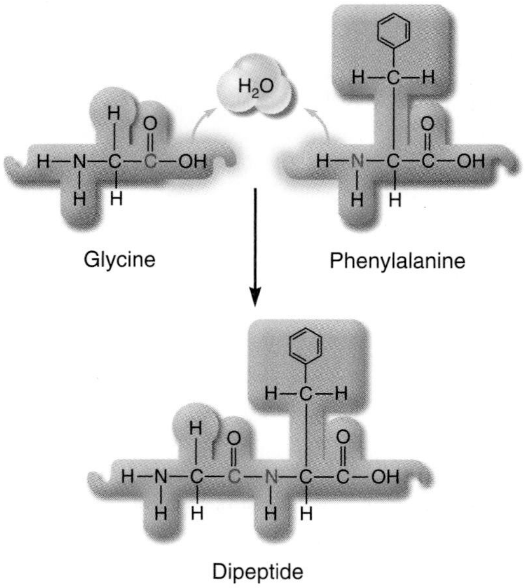

Figure 7.2 **Forming a peptide bond.** When two amino acids join together, the acid group of one amino acid is matched with the carboxyl group of another. When amino acids are joined, the reaction forms a peptide bond and releases water.

Protein Shape

As a cell assembles amino acids into a protein, the protein assumes a unique three-dimensional shape that stems from the sequence and properties of its amino acids. This three-dimensional shape determines the protein's function and the way it interacts with other molecules. For example, **Figure 7.3** illustrates the unique folded and twisted shape of **hemoglobin**, the iron-carrying protein in red blood cells. In the lungs, hemoglobin binds oxygen and releases carbon dioxide. Hemoglobin then delivers oxygen to other tissues and picks up carbon dioxide for the return trip to the lungs.

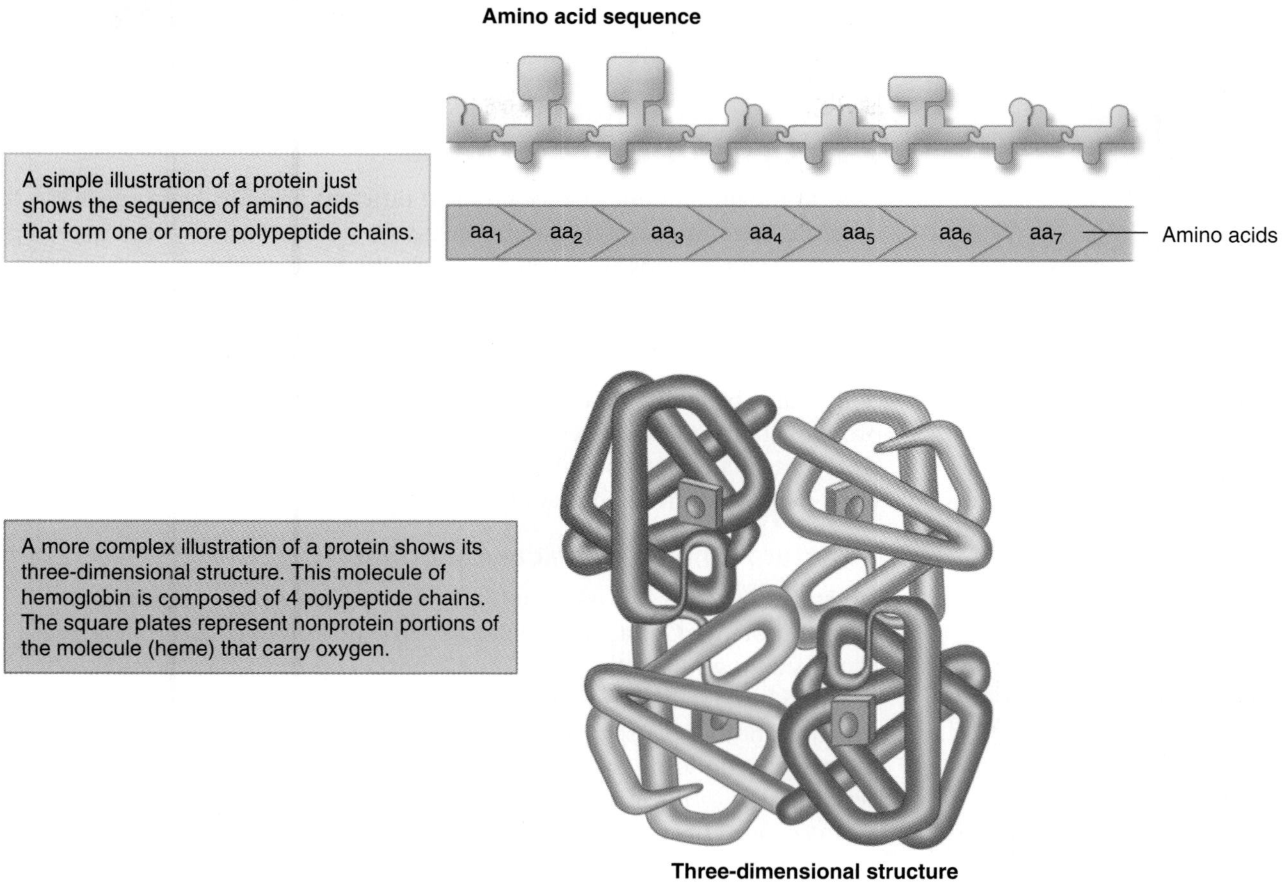
Amino acid sequence
A simple illustration of a protein just shows the sequence of amino acids that form one or more polypeptide chains.
aa1 aa2 aa3 aa4 aa5 aa6 aa7
Amino acids
A more complex illustration of a protein shows its three-dimensional structure. This molecule of hemoglobin is composed of 4 polypeptide chains. The square plates represent nonprotein portions of the molecule (heme) that carry oxygen.
Three-dimensional structure

Figure 7.3 **Protein structure.** The simplest depiction of a protein reveals its unique sequence of amino acids. Each protein becomes folded, twisted, and coiled into a shape all its own. This shape defines how a protein functions in your body.

Protein Denaturation: Destabilizing a Protein's Shape

The chemical links that hold a protein's three-dimensional shape can be disrupted. Changes in the acidity or alkalinity of the protein's environment, high temperatures, alcohol, oxidation, and agitation can all cause a protein to unfold and lose its shape (denature), as shown in **Figure 7.4**. Since a protein's shape determines its function, denatured proteins lose their ability to function properly.

If you've ever cooked an egg, you've witnessed protein **denaturation**. As the egg cooks, some of its protein bonds break. As these proteins unfold, they bump into and bind to each other. Eventually, as these interconnections increase, the liquid egg coagulates to form a solid. Egg white proteins denature and stiffen as they are whipped, and milk proteins denature and curdle when acid is added.

If an egg is eaten raw, its avidin protein can bind to the B vitamin biotin in the digestive tract, making the vitamin unavailable for absorption. Cooking the egg denatures the avidin and destroys its affinity for biotin. Denaturation is the first step in breaking down protein for digestion. Stomach acids denature protein, uncoiling the structure into a simple amino acid chain that digestive enzymes can start breaking apart.

Key Concepts: *Proteins are large molecules made up of amino acids joined in various sequences. Amino acids are joined by peptide bonds. Each protein assumes a unique three-dimensional shape depending on the sequence of its amino acids and*

peptide bond The bond between two amino acids formed when a carboxyl (–COOH) group of one amino acid joins an amino ($–NH_2$) group of another amino acid, releasing water in the process.

dipeptide Two amino acids joined by a peptide bond.

tripeptide Three amino acids joined by peptide bonds.

oligopeptide Four to 10 amino acids joined by peptide bonds.

polypeptide More than 10 amino acids joined by peptide bonds.

hemoglobin [HEEM-oh-glow-bin] The oxygen-carrying protein in red blood cells that consists of four heme groups and four globin polypeptide chains. The presence of hemoglobin gives blood its red color.

denaturation A change in the three-dimensional structure of a protein resulting in an unfolded polypeptide chain that cannot fulfill the protein's function. Treatment with heat, acid, alkali, or extreme agitation can denature most proteins.

properties of their side groups. Acid, alkali, heat, alcohol, and agitation can disrupt chemical forces that stabilize proteins, causing the proteins to denature, or lose their shape.

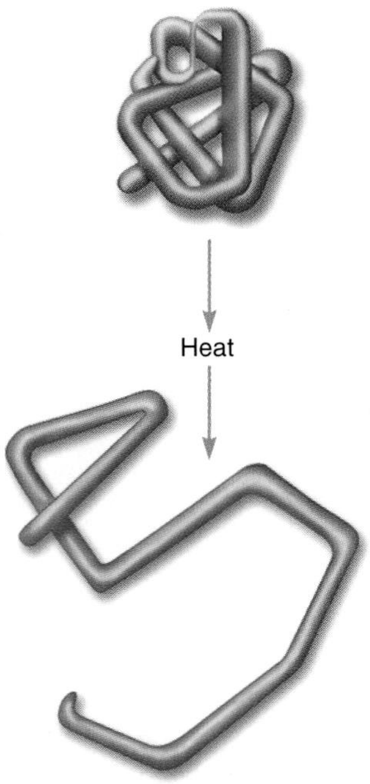

Figure 7.4 **Denaturation.** Heat, pH, oxidation, and mechanical agitation are some of the forces that can destabilize a protein, causing it to unfold and lose its functional shape.

Functions of Body Proteins

Each of the human body's thousands of different proteins has a specific function determined by its unique shape. Proteins act as enzymes, speeding up chemical reactions, and as hormones, which are a kind of chemical messenger. Antibodies made of protein protect us from foreign substances. Proteins maintain fluid balance by pumping molecules across cell membranes and attracting water. They maintain the acid and base balance of body fluids by taking up or giving off hydrogen ions as needed. Finally, proteins transport many key substances, such as oxygen, vitamins, and minerals, to target cells throughout the body. **Figure 7.5** illustrates the functions of proteins in the human body.

Structural and Mechanical Functions

Structures such as bone, skin, and hair owe their physical properties to unique proteins. **Collagen**, which under the microscope looks like a densely packed long rod, is the most abundant protein in mammals and gives skin and bone their elastic strength. Hair and nails are made of **keratin**, which is another dense protein made of coiled shapes. Because protein is essential for building these structures, protein deficiencies during a child's development can be disastrous.

Motor proteins turn energy into mechanical work. In fact, these proteins are the final step in converting our food into physical work. When you bike down a road or up a mountain, you are using your stored food energy to power your muscles. Acting like tiny "motors," protein filaments slide past each other as they shorten (contract) your muscle. As you pump the pedals,

Fyi — Scrabble Anyone?

FOR YOUR INFORMATION

Key

Amino Acid		Scrabble Tile
Glutamic acid	Glu	E
Isoleucine	Ile	I
Asparagine	Asn	N
Serine	Ser	S
Threonine	Thr	T
Lysine	Lys	K
Arginine	Arg	R

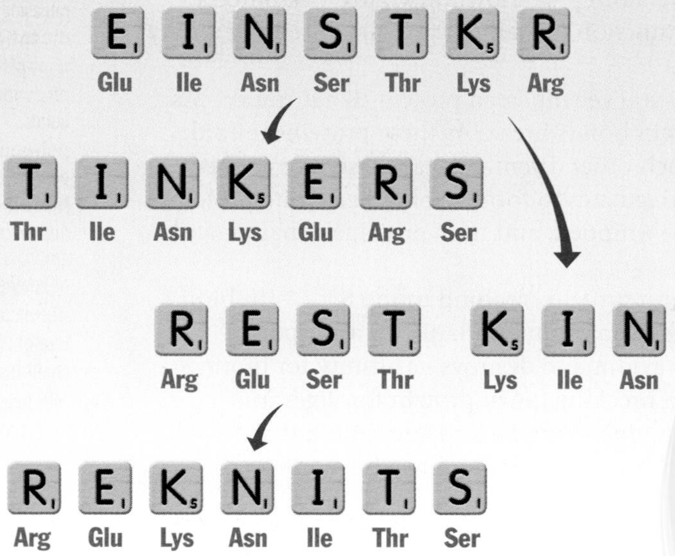

Scrabble Tile = Amino Acid
Word = Protein Chain

Making a meaningful word from available Scrabble tiles is a good analogy for the making of a functional protein chain from available amino acids. Just as we can make many different words from the same tiles, cells can make many different proteins from the same amino acids.

If your cells have all 20 amino acids at their disposal, these can be arranged in a bewildering number of combinations to create tens of thousands of different protein chains, just as all the letters of the alphabet can be used to make an almost unlimited number of words.

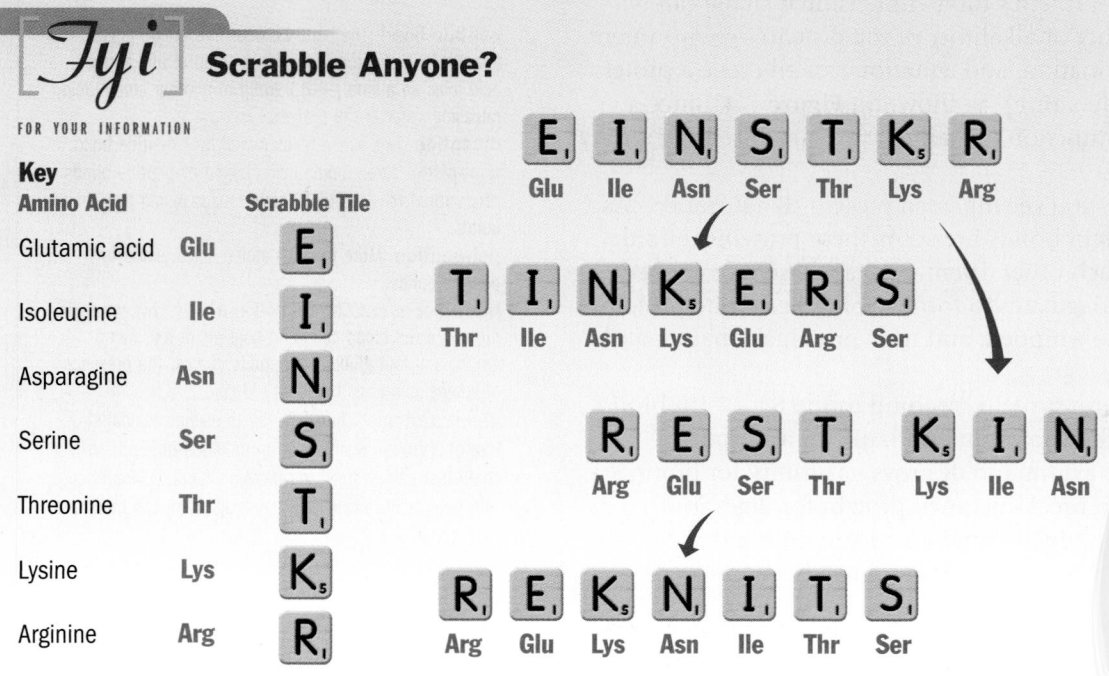

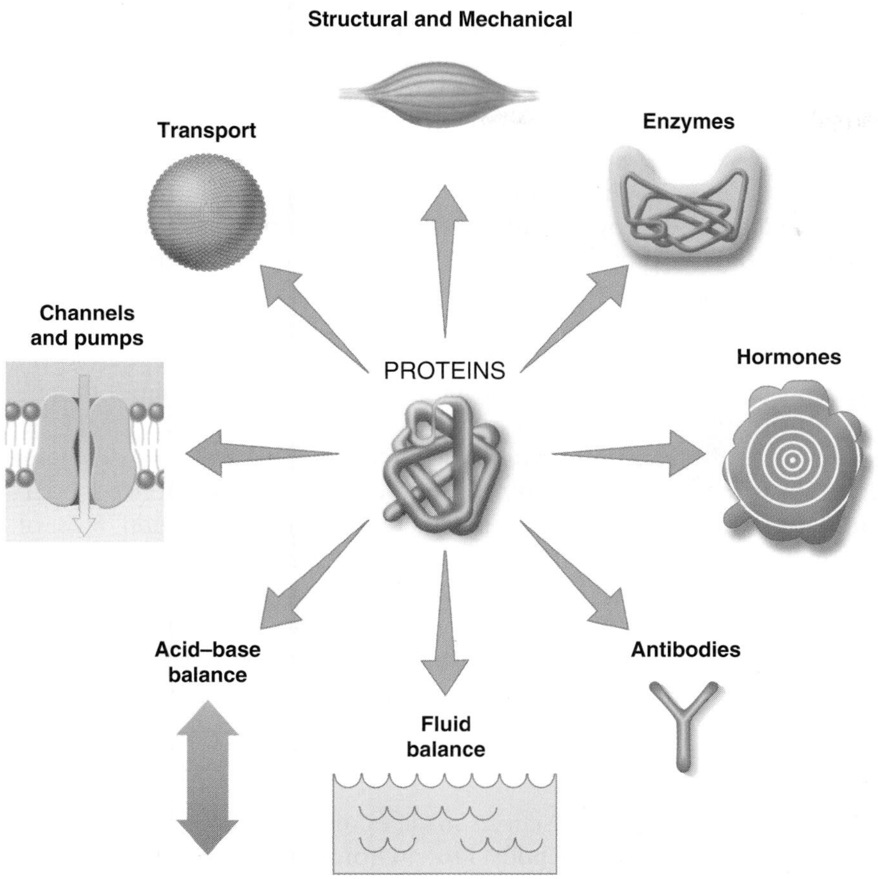

Figure 7.5 **Functions of proteins.** There are many different types of proteins, each with its particular role in the body.

collagen The most abundant fibrous protein in the body, it is the major constituent of connective tissue, forms the foundation for bones and teeth, and helps maintain the structure of blood vessels and other tissues.

keratin A water-insoluble fibrous protein that is the primary constituent of hair, nails, and the outer layer of the skin.

motor proteins Proteins that use energy and convert it into some form of mechanical work. Motor proteins are active in processes such as cell division, muscle contraction, and sperm movement.

antibodies [AN-tih-bod-eez] Large blood proteins produced by white blood cells after exposure to a particular antigen (e.g., a protein on the surface of a virus or bacterium). Each type of antibody specifically binds to and helps eliminate its matching antigen from the body. Once formed, antibodies circulate in the blood and help protect the body against subsequent infection.

immune response A coordinated set of steps, including production of antibodies, that the immune system takes in response to an antigen.

proteins turn that energy bar you ate into work! Similarly, specialized motor proteins also are involved in cell division, sperm movement, and other processes.

Immune Function

Proteins play an important role in the immune system, which is responsible for fighting infection and invasion by foreign substances. **Antibodies** are blood proteins that attack and inactivate bacteria and viruses that cause infection. When your diet does not contain enough protein, your body cannot make as many protein antibodies as it needs. Your immune response is weakened, and your risk of infection and illness increases. Each protein antibody has a specific shape that allows it to attack and destroy a specific foreign invader. Once your immune system learns how to make a certain kind of antibody, your body can protect itself by quickly making that antibody the next time the same germ invades.

Viruses, like those that cause the common cold, take over cells in order to replicate. In a series of steps known as the **immune response**, your body mobilizes its defenses. As part of the defense strategy, you produce protein antibodies that bind to the virus, marking it for destruction. Even when the virus is gone, special cells retain a memory of this virus so that a faster immune response can be mounted against future invasions. When people are immunized for a disease such as measles or mumps, they are actually

Quick Bites

How to Beat the Stiffest Egg Whites

Whenever you want the greatest possible lightness or fluffiness, beat egg whites alone. A single drop of yolk or fat may reduce the foam's maximum volume by as much as two-thirds. Also avoid plastic bowls because plastics tend to retain fatty material on their surfaces.

getting a small amount of dead or inactivated virus in the injection. The dead virus cannot cause infection, but it does allow the body to make antibodies to the disease.

Enzymes

Enzymes are proteins that catalyze, or speed up, chemical reactions without being used up or destroyed in the process. (See **Figures 7.6a** and **7.6b**.) Every cell contains thousands of types of enzymes, each with its own purpose. During digestion, for example, enzymes help break down carbohydrates, proteins, and fats into monosaccharides, amino acids, and fatty acids so the body can absorb them. Enzymes release energy from these nutrients to fuel thousands of body processes. Enzymes also trigger the reactions that build muscle and tissue.

Our foods also contain enzymes, which cooking inactivates, or denatures. Stomach acid denatures the enzymes in raw foods. You may notice special purified enzymes being sold as supplements to enhance digestion. Most of the time, stomach acid denatures these enzymes, so they are unable to function in the intestinal tract. However, some enzyme supplements are coated with a special substance to protect them from stomach acid. For example, a specially coated tablet form of the enzyme lactase can help people with lactose intolerance. Such coated enzymes temporarily help break down foods in the small intestine but eventually are digested themselves.

Hormones

Hormones are chemical messengers made in one part of the body but act on cells in other parts of the body. Protein hormones perform many important regulatory functions. Insulin, for example, is a protein hormone that plays a key role in regulating the amount of glucose in the blood. It is released from the pancreas in response to a rise in blood glucose levels and works to lower those levels. (See Chapter 5, "Carbohydrates.")

Figure 7.6a Enzymes catalyze (speed up) reactions that make or change substances (reactants).

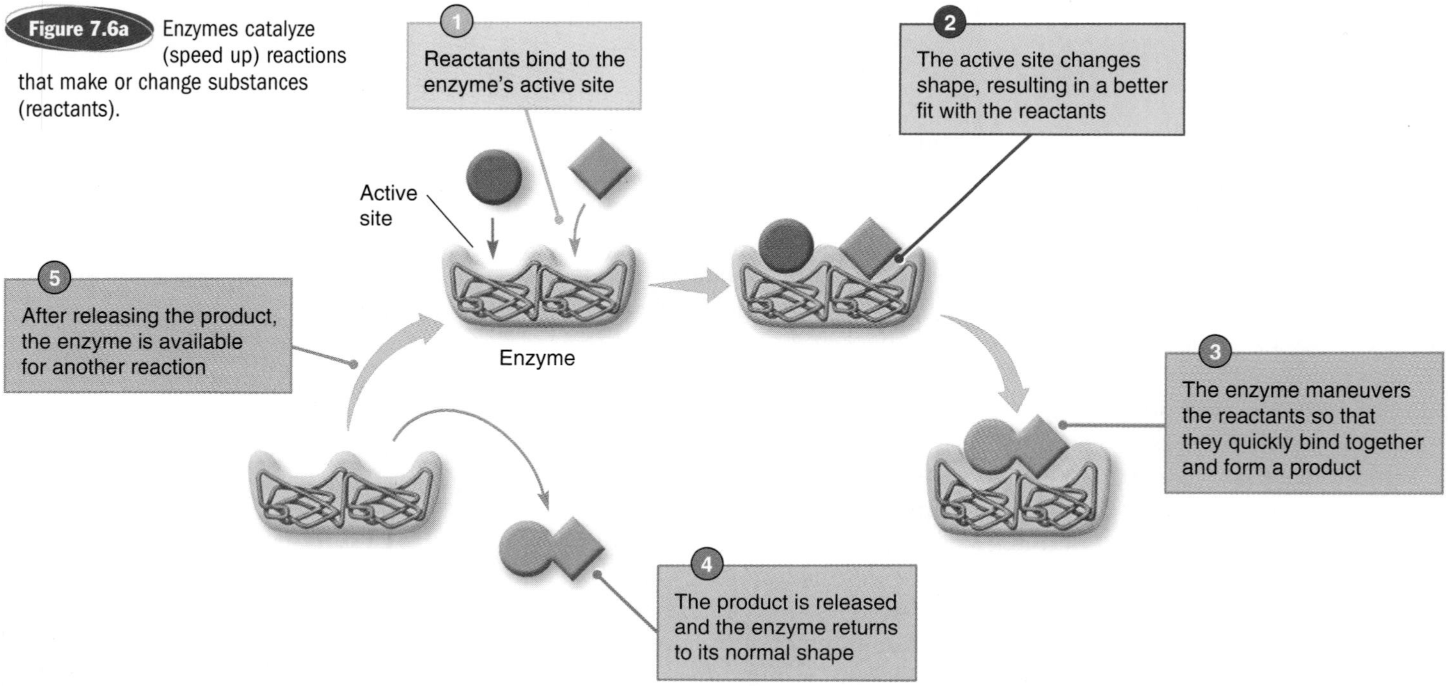
1
Reactants bind to the enzyme's active site
2
The active site changes shape, resulting in a better fit with the reactants
3
The enzyme maneuvers the reactants so that they quickly bind together and form a product
4
The product is released and the enzyme returns to its normal shape
5
After releasing the product, the enzyme is available for another reaction
Active site
Enzyme

People with type 1 diabetes must take insulin injections to control blood glucose levels. If people with diabetes tried to take insulin as a pill, it would be denatured and digested just like any other protein.

Acid–Base Balance

Measured on a scale of 0 to 14, pH indicates the concentration of hydrogen ions in a substance. The higher the concentration of hydrogen ions, the lower the pH. Acids, with a high concentration of hydrogen ions, have a pH lower than 7; bases, with a low concentration of hydrogen ions, have a pH higher than 7. The lower the pH, the stronger the acid. The higher the pH, the stronger the base. The body works hard to keep the pH of the blood near 7.4, or nearly neutral. We can tolerate only small blood pH fluctuations without disastrous consequences. Only a few hours with a blood pH above 8.0 or below 6.8 will cause death.

Proteins help maintain stable pH levels in body fluids by serving as **buffers**; they pick up extra hydrogen ions when conditions are acidic, and they donate hydrogen ions when conditions are alkaline. If proteins are not available to buffer acidic or alkaline substances, the blood can become too acidic or too alkaline, resulting in either **acidosis** or **alkalosis**.

buffers Compounds that can take up and release hydrogen ions to keep the pH of a solution constant. The buffering action of proteins and bicarbonate in the bloodstream plays a major role in maintaining the blood pH at 7.35 to 7.45.

acidosis An abnormally low blood pH (below about 7.35) due to increased acidity.

alkalosis An abnormally high blood pH (above about 7.45) due to increased alkalinity.

Transport Functions

Many substances pass in and out of cells through proteins that cross cell membranes and act as channels and pumps. Some protein channels allow substances to flow rapidly through the membranes without an input of energy. Other channels are protein pumps that use energy to drive substances across membranes.

Proteins also act as carriers, transporting many important substances in the bloodstream for delivery throughout the body. Lipoproteins, for example, package proteins with lipids so that lipid particles can be carried in the blood. Other proteins carry fat-soluble vitamins and certain other vitamins and miner-

Figure 7.6b Enzymes catalyze reactions that break down molecules.

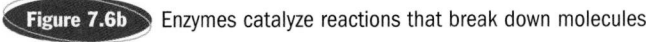

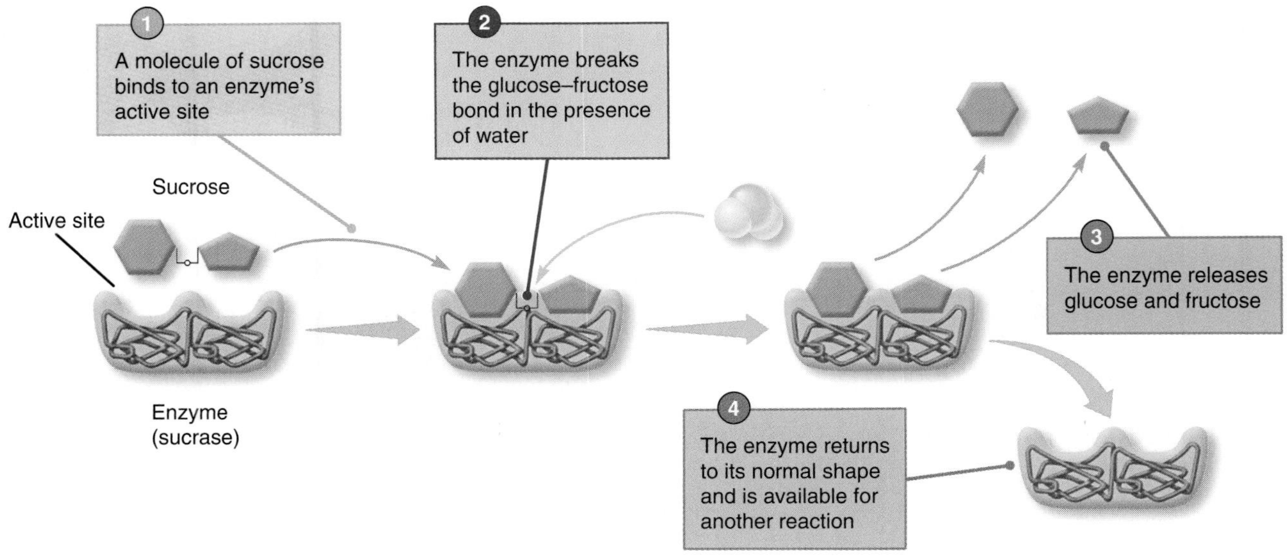
1
A molecule of sucrose binds to an enzyme's active site
2
The enzyme breaks the glucose–fructose bond in the presence of water
Sucrose
Active site
3
The enzyme releases glucose and fructose
Enzyme (sucrase)
4
The enzyme returns to its normal shape and is available for another reaction

als. Since protein carries vitamin A in the blood, protein deficiency contributes to vitamin A deficiency. The protein transferrin carries iron in the blood.

Fluid Balance

Fluids in the body are found inside cells (**intracellular fluid**) or outside cells (**extracellular fluid**). There are two types of extracellular fluid—fluid between cells (intercellular fluid, or **interstitial fluid**) and fluid in the blood (**intravascular fluid**). These interior and exterior fluid levels must stay in balance for body processes to work properly.

Proteins in the blood help to maintain appropriate fluid levels in the vascular system. (See **Figure 7.7**.) When your heart beats, the force pushes fluid and nutrients from the capillaries out into the fluid surrounding the cells. But blood proteins like albumin and globulin are too large to leave the capillary beds. These proteins remain in the capillaries, where they attract fluid to replace what has been pushed out. This system maintains a balance of fluids in the vascular system.

If the diet lacks enough protein to maintain normal levels of blood proteins, fluid will leak into the surrounding tissue and cause swelling, also called **edema**. Children with protein malnutrition often suffer from severe edema. Reestablishing a diet adequate in protein and energy will allow the edema to subside.

intracellular fluid The fluid in the body's cells, usually high in potassium and phosphate and low in sodium and chloride. It constitutes about two-thirds of total body water.

extracellular fluid The fluid located outside of cells. It is composed largely of the liquid portion (plasma) of the blood and the fluid between cells in tissues (interstitial fluid), with fluid in the GI tract, eyes, joints, and spinal cord contributing a small amount. It constitutes about one-third of body water.

interstitial fluid [in-ter-STISH-ul] The fluid between cells in tissues. Also called intercellular fluid.

intravascular fluid The fluid portion (plasma) of the blood contained in arteries, veins, and capillaries. It accounts for about 15 percent of the extracellular fluid.

edema Swelling caused by the buildup of fluid between cells.

Source of Energy and Glucose

Although your body prefers to burn carbohydrate and fat for energy, if necessary it can use protein for energy or to make glucose. Thus, carbohydrate and fat are protein-sparing: They spare amino acids from being burned for energy and allow them to be used for protein synthesis. Think About It 1

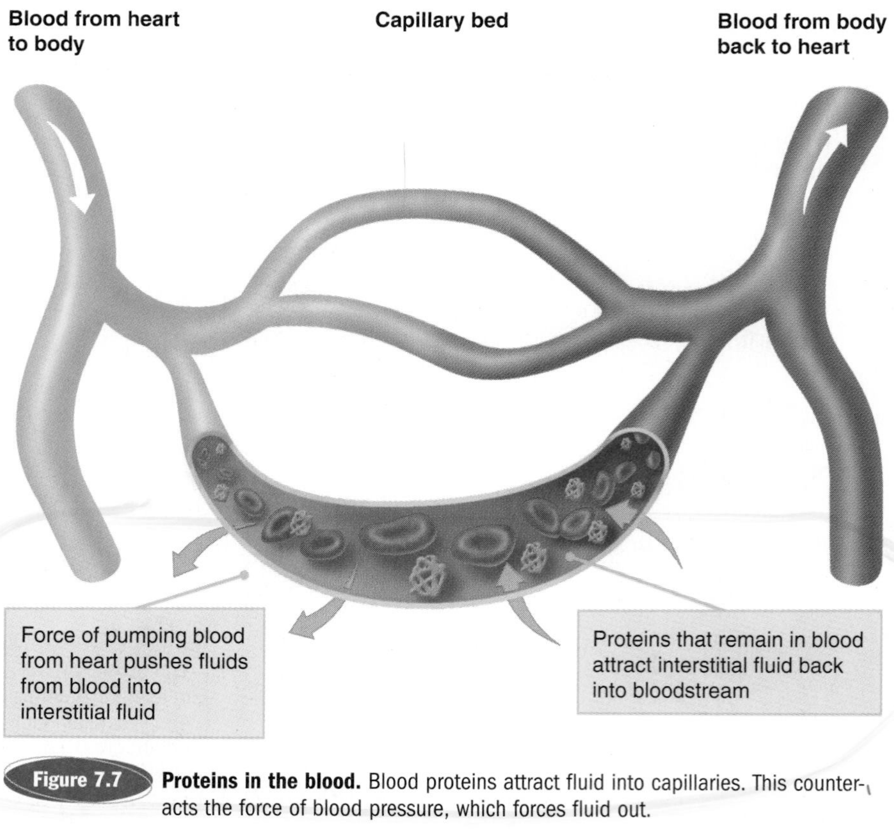

Blood from heart to body
Capillary bed
Blood from body back to heart
Force of pumping blood from heart pushes fluids from blood into interstitial fluid
Proteins that remain in blood attract interstitial fluid back into bloodstream

Figure 7.7 **Proteins in the blood.** Blood proteins attract fluid into capillaries. This counteracts the force of blood pressure, which forces fluid out.

If the diet does not provide enough energy for vital functions, the body will sacrifice its own protein from enzymes, muscle, and other tissues to make energy and glucose for use by the brain, lungs, and heart. This is what happens in cases of starvation. (See the "Spotlight on Metabolism.")

When the body uses its own protein for energy, it first breaks the protein into individual amino acids. To then release energy from an amino acid, the body first removes the nitrogen group—a process called **deamination**. It can use the remaining carbon skeleton for energy or to make glucose.

If your diet contains more protein than you need for protein synthesis, your body converts most of the excess to glucose or stores it as fat. So taking protein supplements or eating high-protein diets as a means of increasing muscle mass may instead add to body fat.

deamination The removal of the amino group ($-NH_2$) from an amino acid.

proteases Enzymes that break down protein into peptides and amino acids.

proenzymes Inactive precursors of enzymes.

Key Concepts: *In the body, proteins perform numerous vital functions that are determined by each protein's shape. Protein antibodies protect the body from infection and illness. As enzymes, proteins speed up chemical reactions; as hormones, they are chemical messengers. Proteins also maintain fluid balance and acid–base balance and transport substances throughout the body. If needed, protein can also be used as a source of energy or glucose.*

Protein Digestion and Absorption

Before your body can make a body protein from food protein, it must digest and absorb the protein you eat. **Figure 7.8** shows the process of protein digestion and absorption.

Protein Digestion

The first step in using dietary protein is breaking down its long polypeptide chains into amino acids. As with the other energy-yielding nutrients, digestion of protein requires enzymes from a number of sources. Cells produce and secrete most **proteases** (protein-digesting enzymes) as **proenzymes**, inactive forms of the enzymes, for later activation in the intestine. If a cell produced active forms of a protease, it could digest itself and break down its own cellular protein. Delaying the activation of proteases protects the integrity of cells.

Quick Bites

Softening Tough Meat

Cooking tough meat in liquid for hours helps dissolve the source of its toughness, fibrous protein called connective tissue.

In the Stomach

Digestion of protein begins in the stomach. Here, hydrochloric acid (HCl) denatures a protein, unfolding it and making the amino acid chain more accessible to the action of enzymes. Glands in the stomach lining produce the proenzyme pepsinogen, the inactive precursor of the enzyme pepsin. When pepsinogen comes in contact with hydrochloric acid, it is converted to the active enzyme pepsin. Gastric juices must be acidic for this enzyme to be active. By the time dietary protein leaves the stomach, pepsin has broken it down into individual amino acids and peptides of various lengths. Pepsin is responsible for about 10 to 20 percent of protein digestion.[6]

In the Small Intestine

From the stomach, amino acids and polypeptides pass into the small intestine, where most protein digestion takes place. In the small intestine, activated proteases from the pancreas and intestinal lining cells break down large peptides into smaller peptides. Pancreatic enzymes completely digest only a small percentage of proteins into individual amino acids; enzymes on the surface of the small intestine split the remaining larger polypeptides into tripeptides and dipeptides, and some are even split all the way into amino acids. The intestinal cells absorb these smaller units and break down virtually all the remaining dipeptides and tripeptides into individual amino acids for absorption into the bloodstream.

Amino Acid and Peptide Absorption

More than 99 percent of protein enters the bloodstream as individual amino acids. Peptides are rarely absorbed, and whole proteins that escape digestion hardly ever are. The absorption of only a few molecules of whole

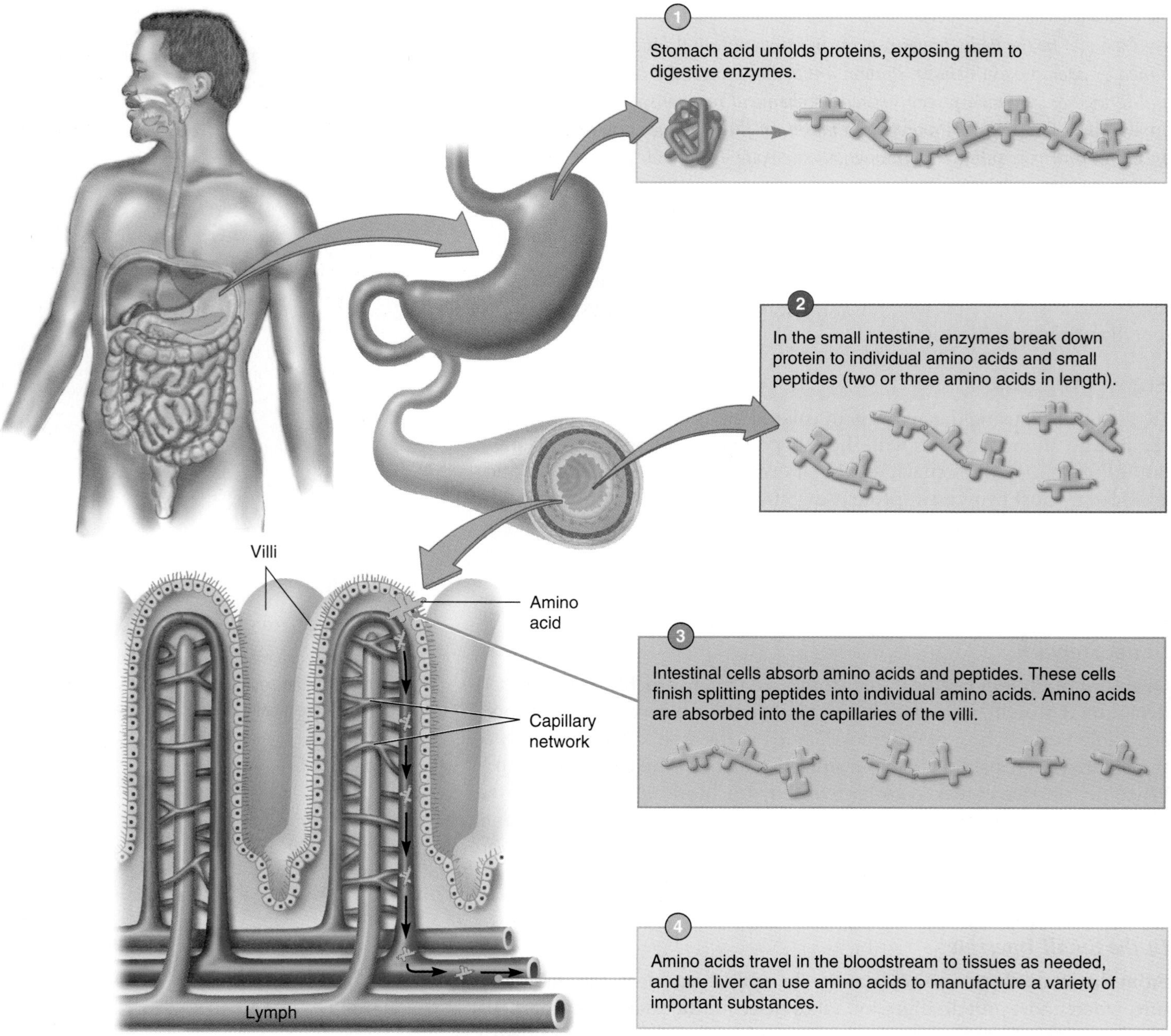
1
Stomach acid unfolds proteins, exposing them to digestive enzymes.
2
In the small intestine, enzymes break down protein to individual amino acids and small peptides (two or three amino acids in length).
Villi
Amino acid
3
Intestinal cells absorb amino acids and peptides. These cells finish splitting peptides into individual amino acids. Amino acids are absorbed into the capillaries of the villi.
Capillary network
4
Amino acids travel in the bloodstream to tissues as needed, and the liver can use amino acids to manufacture a variety of important substances.
Lymph

Figure 7.8 **Digestion and absorption of protein.** Digestion breaks down protein to amino acids and small peptides for absorption.

protein can cause a severe allergic reaction or immune dysfunction.[7] Once absorbed, most amino acids and the few absorbed peptides travel via the portal vein to the liver, which releases them into general circulation. Intestinal cells retain some amino acids to synthesize enzymes and make new cells.

Undigested Protein

Any parts of proteins not digested and absorbed in the small intestine continue through the large intestine and pass out of the body in the feces. Normally, the body efficiently digests and absorbs protein. Diseases of the intestinal tract, however, decrease the efficiency of absorption and increase protein losses in the feces.[8] People with **celiac disease**, for example, cannot properly digest gluten—a protein found in wheat, rye, and oats. Unless treated with a gluten-free diet, people with celiac disease show poor growth, weight loss, and other symptoms resulting from poor absorption of protein and other nutrients. People who suffer from **cystic fibrosis** have fewer protein-digesting enzymes than normal in the small intestine, resulting in poor digestion and absorption of protein and other nutrients.[9]

celiac disease [SEA-lee-ak] A disease that involves an inability to digest gluten, a protein found in wheat, rye, oats, and barley. If untreated, it causes flattening of the villi in the intestine, leading to severe malabsorption of nutrients. Symptoms include diarrhea, fatty stools, swollen belly, and extreme fatigue.

cystic fibrosis An inherited disorder that causes widespread dysfunction of the exocrine glands, resulting in chronic lung disease, abnormally high levels of electrolytes (e.g., sodium, potassium, chloride) in sweat, and deficiency of pancreatic enzymes needed for digestion.

Key Concepts: *Protein digestion begins in the stomach, where the enzyme pepsin breaks proteins into smaller peptides. Digestion continues in the small intestine, where proteases break polypeptides into smaller peptide units, which are then absorbed into cells where additional enzymes complete digestion to amino acids. So that cells do not digest themselves, proteases (protein-digesting enzymes) are synthesized and secreted as inactive proenzymes.*

Proteins in the Body

Once in the bloodstream, amino acids are transported throughout the body and are available for synthesizing cellular proteins. To build proteins, cells use peptide bonds to link amino acids.

Protein Synthesis

Genetic material in the nucleus of every cell provides the blueprint for the thousands of proteins needed to perform life functions. To synthesize a protein, cells assemble amino acids in a specific sequence.

Just as one missing part of a car can stop an entire auto assembly line, so can one missing amino acid stop synthesis of an entire protein in the cell. If a nonessential amino acid is missing during protein synthesis, the cell will either make that amino acid or obtain it from the liver via the bloodstream, and protein synthesis will continue. If an essential amino acid is missing, the body may break its own protein down to supply the missing amino acid. If a missing essential amino acid is unavailable, protein synthesis halts, and the partially completed protein is broken down into individual amino acids for use elsewhere in the body.

Genetic defects can cause problems in protein synthesis. People who have sickle-cell anemia cannot construct the correct sequence to form the protein hemoglobin. A genetic error causes the amino acid valine to be substituted for glutamic acid in two locations in the protein chain. This simple error causes the shape of hemoglobin to change so much that the red blood cell becomes stiff and sickle-shaped instead of soft and disk-shaped. Because this faulty protein cannot carry oxygen efficiently, it causes serious medical problems.

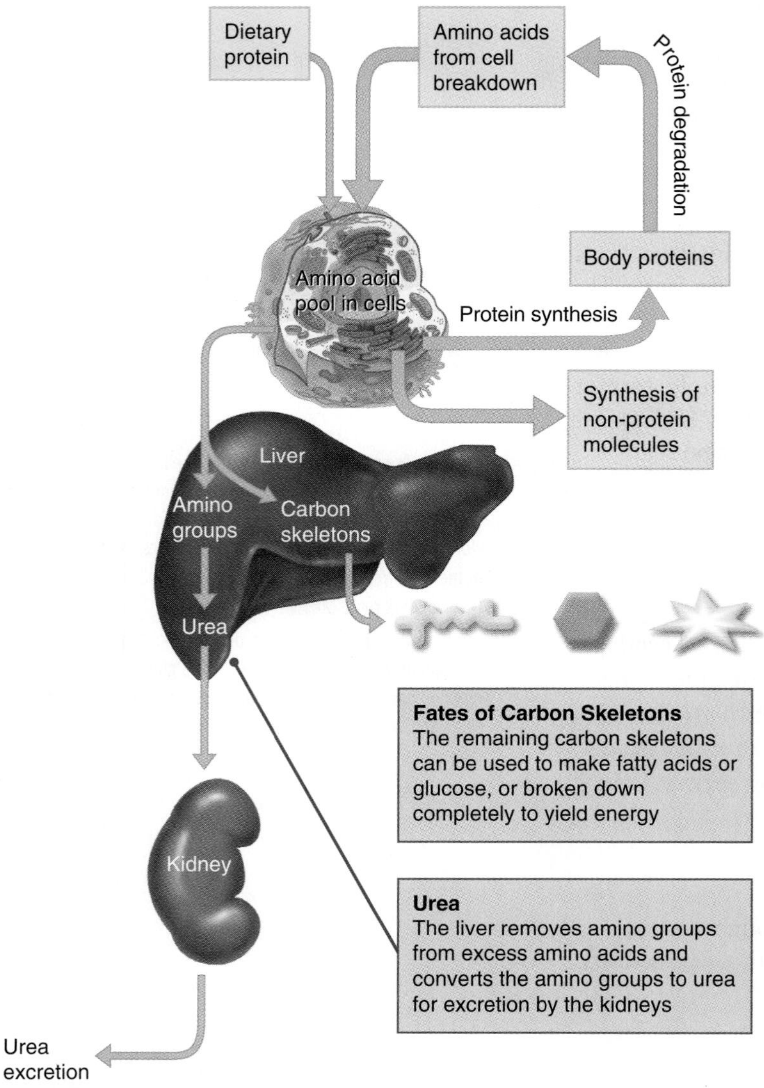
Dietary protein
Amino acids from cell breakdown
Protein degradation
Body proteins
Amino acid pool in cells
Protein synthesis
Synthesis of non-protein molecules
Liver
Amino groups
Carbon skeletons
Urea
Fates of Carbon Skeletons
The remaining carbon skeletons can be used to make fatty acids or glucose, or broken down completely to yield energy
Kidney
Urea
The liver removes amino groups from excess amino acids and converts the amino groups to urea for excretion by the kidneys
Urea excretion

Figure 7.9 **Protein turnover.** Cells draw upon their amino acid pools to synthesize new proteins. These small pools turn over quickly and must be replenished by amino acids from dietary protein and the degradation (breakdown) of body protein. Dietary protein supplies about one-third and the breakdown of body protein supplies about two-thirds of the roughly 300 grams of body protein synthesized daily. When dietary protein is inadequate, increased degradation of body protein replenishes the amino acid pool. This can lead to the breakdown of essential body tissue.

The Amino Acid Pool and Protein Turnover

Cells throughout the body constantly and simultaneously synthesize and break down protein. When cells break down protein, the protein's amino acids return to circulation. (See **Figure 7.9**.) These available amino acids, found throughout body tissues and fluids, are collectively referred to as the **amino acid pool**.[10] Some of these amino acids may be used for protein synthesis; others may have their amino group removed and be used to produce energy or nonprotein substances such as glucose.

The constant recycling of proteins in the body is known as **protein turnover**.[11] Each day, more amino acids in your body are recycled than are supplied in your diet. Of the approximately 300 grams of protein synthesized by the body each day, 200 grams are made from recycled amino acids. This remarkable recycling capacity is the reason we need so little protein in our diet compared with carbohydrate and fat. In a healthful diet, only 10 to 15 percent of our daily calories must come from protein, whereas carbohydrate should supply about 55 to 60 percent and fat no more than 30 percent.

Synthesis of Nonprotein Molecules

Amino acids do more than help build peptides and proteins; they are precursors of many molecules with important biological roles. Your body makes nonprotein molecules from amino acids and the nitrogen they contain. The vitamin niacin, for example, is made from the amino acid tryptophan. Precursors of DNA, RNA, and many coenzymes are formed in part from amino acids. Your body also uses amino acids to make **neurotransmitters**, chemicals that send signals from nerve cells to other parts of the body. Serotonin, which helps regulate mood, is made from tryptophan. Norepinephrine and epinephrine (also called noradrenaline and adrenaline, respectively), which get the body ready for action, are neurotransmitters made from tyrosine. Your body also uses tyrosine to make melanin, a skin pigment, and the hormone thyroxin that helps regulate metabolism. The simple amino acid glycine combines with many toxic substances to make less harmful substances that the body can eliminate. Your body uses the amino acid histidine to make histamine, which dilates blood vessels and is a culprit in allergic reactions.

Protein and Nitrogen Excretion

Cells break down and recycle amino acids. Amino acid breakdown yields amino groups ($-NH_2$). This NH_2 molecule is unstable, and the body quickly converts it to ammonia (NH_3). However, ammonia is toxic to cells, so it is expelled into the bloodstream as a waste product and is carried to the liver. In the liver, an amino group and an ammonia group react with carbon dioxide (through a series of reactions known collectively as the urea cycle) to produce **urea** and water. The nitrogen-rich urea is transported from the liver by way of the bloodstream to the kidneys, where it is filtered from the blood and sent to the bladder for excretion in the urine. Small amounts of other nitrogen-containing compounds, such as ammonia, uric acid, and creatinine, are also excreted in the urine. Some nitrogen is also lost through skin, sloughed-off GI cells, mucus, hair and nail cuttings, and body fluids.

Nitrogen Balance

Because nitrogen is excreted when proteins are recycled or used, we can use the balance of nitrogen in the body to evaluate whether the body is getting enough protein. (See **Figure 7.10**.) We can estimate the balance of nitrogen, and therefore protein, in the body by comparing nitrogen intake to the sum of all sources of nitrogen output (urine, feces, skin, hair, and body fluids).[12]

nitrogen balance = grams of nitrogen intake − grams of nitrogen output

If nitrogen intake equals nitrogen output, **nitrogen balance** is zero and the body is in **nitrogen equilibrium**. If nitrogen intake exceeds nitrogen output, the body is said to be in **positive nitrogen balance**. Positive nitrogen balance means that the body is adding protein; growing children, pregnant women, or people recovering from protein deficiency or illnesses should be in positive nitrogen balance. If nitrogen output exceeds nitrogen intake, the body is in **negative nitrogen balance**. This means that the body is losing protein. People who are starving or on extreme weight-loss diets or who suffer from fever, severe illnesses, or infections are in a state of negative nitrogen balance. Healthy adults are in nitrogen equilibrium, which means that they take in enough protein to maintain and repair tissue. They have no net gain or loss of body protein, and they simply excrete excess dietary protein.

Key Concepts: *Cells throughout the body constantly synthesize and break down protein simultaneously, a process known as protein turnover. Nitrogen-containing end products of protein metabolism are excreted in urine via the kidneys. Comparison*

amino acid pool The amino acids in body tissues and fluids that are available for new protein synthesis.

protein turnover The constant breakdown and synthesis of proteins in the body.

neurotransmitters Substances released at the end of a stimulated nerve cell that diffuse across a small gap and bind to another nerve cell or muscle cell, stimulating or inhibiting it.

urea The main nitrogen-containing waste product in mammals. Formed in liver cells from ammonia and carbon dioxide, urea is carried via the bloodstream to the kidneys, where it is excreted in the urine.

nitrogen balance Nitrogen intake minus the sum of all sources of nitrogen excretion.

nitrogen equilibrium Nitrogen intake equals the sum of all sources of nitrogen excretion; nitrogen balance equals zero.

positive nitrogen balance Nitrogen intake exceeds the sum of all sources of nitrogen excretion.

negative nitrogen balance Nitrogen intake is less than the sum of all sources of nitrogen excretion.

+N balance - intake exceeds output ∴ growth

Figure 7.10 **Nitrogen balance.** Nitrogen balance reflects whether a person is gaining or losing protein.

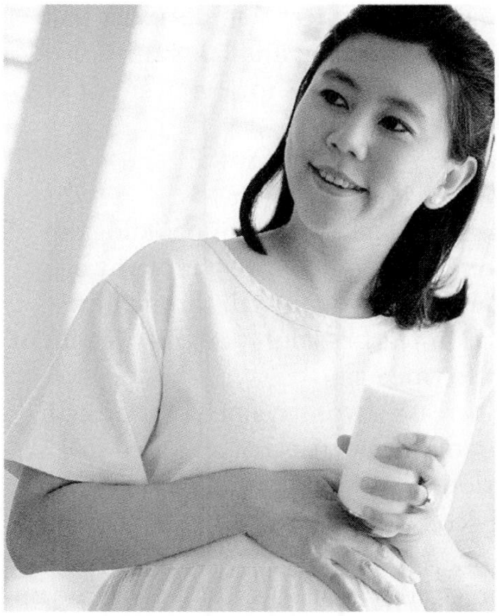

A pregnant woman is adding protein, so she has a positive nitrogen balance.

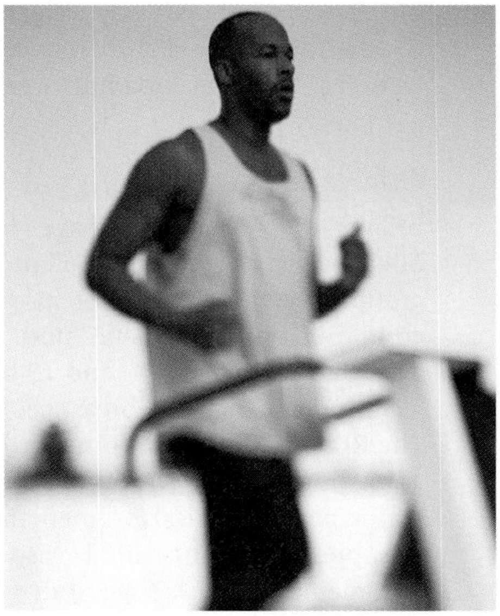

A healthy person who is neither gaining nor losing protein is in nitrogen equilibrium (zero balance).

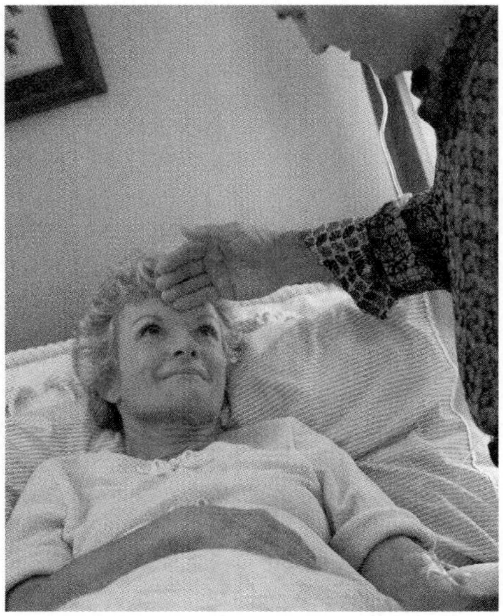

A person who is severely ill and losing protein has a negative nitrogen balance.

of nitrogen intake (from dietary protein) to nitrogen excretion gives a measure of nitrogen balance and indicates protein status in the body.

Proteins in the Diet

Many government and health organizations have made recommendations about the amount of protein in a healthful diet, just as they have for other nutrients. Meat, eggs, milk, legumes, grains, and vegetables are all sources of protein. Fruits contain minimal amounts and, along with fats, are not considered protein sources. **Figure 7.11** shows some good sources of protein.

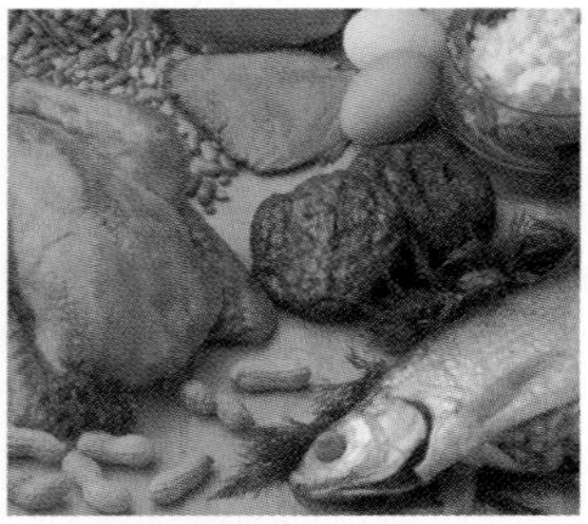

Rich sources of protein include meats, fish, poultry, eggs, dairy products, legumes and nuts.

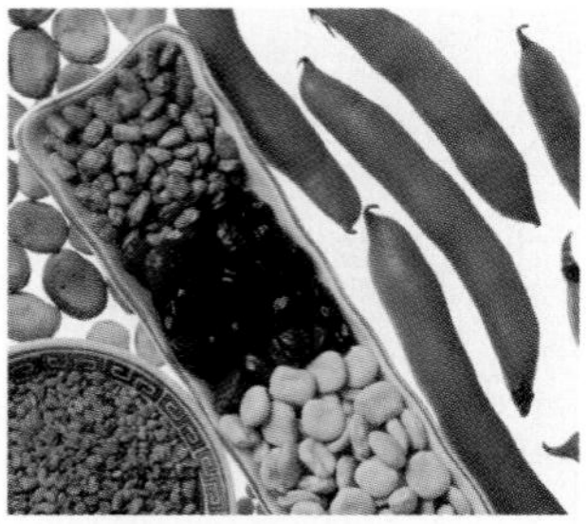

Legumes and nuts are important sources of protein for vegetarians.

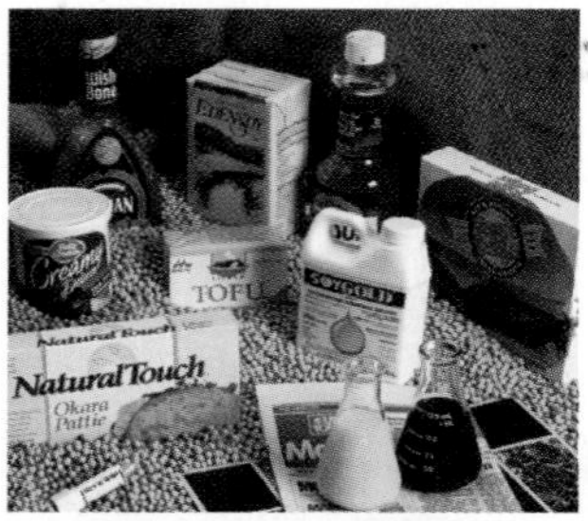

Soybeans and soy products are the only plant sources of complete protein.

Figure 7.11 **Protein sources.** Meat, fish, eggs, dairy products, and soy are excellent protein sources. Legumes, grain products, starchy vegetables, nuts, and seeds also are good sources.

Recommended Intakes of Protein

The World Health Organization (WHO) bases its requirements for essential amino acids on nitrogen balance studies published in the 1950s.[13] These requirements are minimum levels used to develop nutrition and policy interventions around the world. Newer methods of measuring amino acid requirements suggest that some of the WHO values for specific amino acids may be too low.[14] In the United States, the Recommended Dietary Allowance (RDA) is the accepted dietary standard for protein. RDAs are set to meet the nutritional needs of most healthy people, so most of us actually require somewhat less protein than the RDA. RDA values also assume we are consuming adequate energy and other nutrients to allow our bodies to use dietary protein for protein synthesis, rather than for energy. Other countries, such as Canada, make recommendations similar to the RDAs.

People older than 2 years should get about 30 percent or less of their energy intake from fat and about 55 percent or more of their energy intake from carbohydrate.[15] That leaves about 10 to 15 percent of energy to come from protein, an amount that is usually higher than the RDA. Protein currently provides about 15 percent of the average American's energy intake.[16]

Think About It 2

Adults

For adults, the RDA for protein intake is 0.8 grams per kilogram of body weight.[17] This translates into a daily protein recommendation of 58 grams for the average man and 46 grams for the average woman, 19 to 24 years old. Because average body weights are slightly higher in adults older than 25, their RDAs are slightly higher (63 grams for men and 50 grams for women). The RDA for adults works out to be about 8 to 11 percent of average energy intake.

HOW TO CALCULATE PROTEIN RDA

Convert weight to kg
(pounds ÷ 2.2)
Multiply kg by 0.8 = Protein RDA in g

Male, 19–24 years old, 72 kg (158 lb)
72 kg × 0.8 g/kg = 58 g protein

Female, 19–24 years old, 58 kg (128 lb)
58 kg × 0.8 g/kg = 46 g protein

Other Life Stages

Infants under 6 months of age require 2.2 grams of protein per kilogram body weight, the highest protein need relative to body weight of any age group. (See **Table 7.2**.) Protein requirements gradually fall throughout childhood and adolescence until a person reaches adult body size, at about age 15 to 18 for women and 19 to 24 for men.

Both pregnancy and breastfeeding increase a woman's need for protein. The RDA for pregnant women is 60 grams (an increase of about 10 to 15 grams), while the RDA during the period of early milk production is 65 grams. Most American women already consume more than enough protein to support pregnancy and breastfeeding.

Some nutritionists suggest that people older than 50 should consume up to 1.2 grams of protein per kilogram body weight. Although elderly people on average have less lean body mass to maintain than younger people, the body becomes less efficient at digesting, absorbing, and using protein as it ages.[18] (See **Figure 7.12**.) The current RDA for this age group is still 0.8 grams per kilogram, although this may change in upcoming revisions of Dietary Reference Intakes.

Physical Stress

Severe physical stress can increase your body's need for protein. Infections, burns, fevers, and surgery all increase protein losses, and the diet must replace that lost protein. A severe infection can increase protein requirements by one-third. Severe burns can increase requirements two to four times. Less severe physical stressors, such as a viral illness with a mild fever lasting only a few days, rarely increase protein requirements. Muscle-building activities, such as intense weight training, increase protein needs much less than most people think, and the typical American diet supplies an ample amount of protein even for bodybuilders. (See the FYI feature "Do Athletes Need More Protein?")

Protein Consumption in the United States

According to data from the U.S. Department of Agriculture's *1994–1996 Continuing Survey of Food Intake by Individuals*,[19] the average American consumes 75 grams of protein daily. Protein intakes meet or exceed the protein RDA for every age and gender group, except for women aged 70 and older, where average protein intake falls just 3 grams short of the RDA. If you remember that an RDA value is adequate for practically all people in an age and gender group, an average intake slightly below the RDA is not of any real concern. (See Chapter 2, "Nutrition Guidelines," for more on RDAs.)

Key Concepts: *Infants, who are growing rapidly, have the highest protein needs in proportion to body weight. The Recommended Dietary Allowance (RDA) for protein declines from 2.2 grams per kilogram for infants under 6 months old to 0.8 grams per kilogram for adults. Pregnancy, physical changes in old age, and severe physical stress all can alter protein requirements. Americans currently consume about 15 percent of their energy as protein and obtain an average of 75 grams of protein daily—an amount that exceeds the RDA for almost all age and gender categories.*

Protein Quality

Although both animal and plant foods contain protein, the quality of protein in these foods differs. Foods that supply all the essential amino acids in the proportions needed by the body are called high-quality, or **complete proteins**. Foods that lack adequate amounts of one or more essential amino acids are called low-quality, or **incomplete proteins.**

Because we typically eat a variety of foods that provides ample dietary protein, we don't ordinarily worry about protein quality. But for people with marginal protein or energy intake and for people who use only one or a few plant foods as their main dietary protein source, protein quality becomes critical for good health.

Complete Proteins

Animal foods generally provide complete protein; that is, they provide all the essential amino acids in approximately the right proportions. One exception is gelatin, a protein derived from animal collagen that lacks the essential amino acid tryptophan.

Table 7.2 Protein RDA for Infants, Children, and Teens

Age	Protein RDA (g/kg body weight)
0 to 6 months	2.2
6 months to 1 year	1.6
1 to 3 years	1.2
4 to 6 years	1.1
7 to 10 years	1.0
11 to 14 years	1.0
15 to 18 years (males)	0.9
15 to 18 years (females)	0.8

Quick Bites

Mother's Milk

Because it contains less protein, and in particular less casein protein, infants digest human milk more readily than cows' milk. Milks high in casein protein tend to form curds (clumps) in the stomach upon exposure to stomach acid. These tough curds are hard for digestive enzymes to break apart.

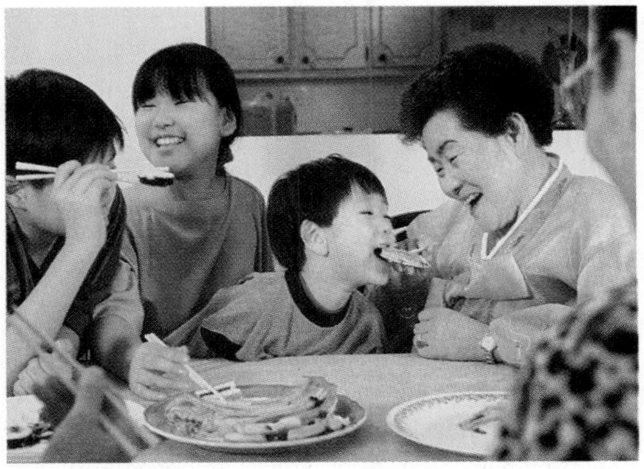

Figure 7.12 Protein needs change as we age. Growing children have higher protein needs (grams per kilogram body weight) than older adults.

complete proteins Proteins that supply all of the essential amino acids in the proportions the body needs. Also known as high-quality proteins.

incomplete proteins Proteins that lack one or more essential amino acids. Also called low-quality proteins.

complementary proteins Two or more incomplete food proteins whose assortment of amino acids make up for, or complement, each other so that the combination provides sufficient amounts of all the essential amino acids.

protein digestibility-corrected amino acid score (PDCAAS) A measure of protein quality that takes into account the amino acid composition of the food and the digestibility of the protein.

Red meats, poultry, fish, eggs, milk, and milk products (all animal foods) contain complete protein. Protein supplies more than 20 percent of the energy content of these foods. In water-packed tuna, protein provides about 80 percent of the energy. The protein isolated from soybeans, unlike protein from other plant foods, is a complete, high-quality protein equal to that of animal protein.[20] Although, compared with animal protein, soy protein contains lower proportions of the amino acids cysteine and methionine, the amount of soy typically consumed provides sufficient quantities. Moreover, soybeans contain no cholesterol or saturated fat.

Americans, on the average, get about 65 percent of their protein intake from animal foods.[21] (See **Table 7.3.**) In other parts of the world, animal proteins play a smaller role. In Africa and East Asia, for example, animal foods provide only 20 percent of protein intake.[22]

Fyi FOR YOUR INFORMATION

Do Athletes Need More Protein?

Athletes not only pump iron these days, they also pump protein supplements in hopes of building muscle and improving performance. Look inside many sports magazines and you'll see ads for protein or amino acid supplements aimed at athletes. You cannot force your body to build muscle by pumping in more protein than you need, any more than you can make your car run faster by adding more gas to a full tank. Extra protein does not build muscles; only regular workouts fueled by a mix of nutrients can do that.

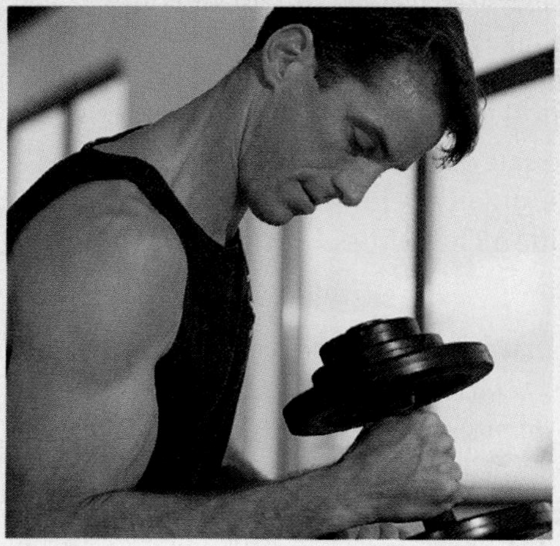

Protein Requirements for Athletes

Many people assume that because muscle fibers are protein, building muscle must require protein. This is only partially true. The heavy resistance-type exercise that is needed to stimulate muscle growth must first be fueled by glucose and fatty acids (glucose will be the predominant fuel). Little protein is used as a fuel source in resistance-type exercise. However, studies show that when men consume the RDA for protein (0.8 g/kg body weight) and engage in heavy resistance exercise, they go into negative nitrogen balance.[1] Further studies estimate the actual protein needs during resistance training as approximately 1.7 to 1.8 grams per kilogram. For endurance athletes, less protein is used for muscle building, but more protein is used as a fuel source. The net effect is that protein needs of endurance athletes are estimated at 1.2 to 1.4 grams per kilogram.

Does this mean the serious athlete has to head for the protein shelves of the local health food store? Since Americans, on average, consume almost twice as much protein as they need, most athletes already get enough protein. An athlete in training (let's make him 70 kg) might consume up to 5,000 kilocalories per day. Even if his diet contained only 10 percent of calories as protein (on the low side in our meat-loving society), he would be getting about 126 grams of protein daily, about 1.8 grams per kilogram. It is unlikely that an athlete would not be able to meet his or her protein needs from a normal, mixed diet, even one that follows the Food Guide Pyramid recommendations.

Risks of Supplements

So, maybe there's no benefit to taking protein or amino acid supplements, but there's no harm either, right? This isn't necessarily true. If excess protein means excess calories, this adds weight as fat, not muscle, and that can slow down your performance. Purified protein supplements can contribute to calcium losses and therefore harm bone health. Excess protein means excess nitrogen that must be excreted, a risk for dehydration if fluid intake is not monitored. Supplements of single amino acids can interfere with absorption of other amino acids and can affect neurotransmitter activity. Contamination of the amino acid L-tryptophan led to devastating illness and ban of this supplement until recently.[2]

So, if you are a weekend athlete, there's no need to increase the protein in your diet, and no reason to expect that doing so will help your performance. If you are a competitive athlete, choosing adequate calories from a wide variety of foods will probably ensure an adequate protein intake, even at levels recommended for strength training. Supplements are unnecessary, expensive, and may disrupt normal protein balance in the body. Play it safe—choose a healthful diet to fuel your exercise.

1 Lemon PWR. Is increased dietary protein necessary or beneficial for individuals with a physically active lifestyle? *Nutr Rev.* 1996;54:S169–S175.

2 Herbert V. L-tryptophan. *Nutr Today.* Mar/Apr 1992;27.

Complementary Proteins

With the exception of soy protein, the protein in plant foods is incomplete; that is, it lacks one or more essential amino acids and does not match the body's amino acid needs as closely as animal foods do. Although the protein in one plant food may lack certain amino acids, the protein in another plant food may be a **complementary protein** that completes the amino acid pattern. So the protein of one plant food can provide the essential amino acid(s) that the other plant food is missing. **Table 7.4** lists some examples of complementary food combinations.

For example, grain products such as pasta are low in the essential amino acid lysine but high in the essential amino acids methionine and cysteine. Legumes such as kidney beans are low in methionine and cysteine but high in lysine. In a dish that combines these foods, such as a pasta–kidney bean salad, the protein from pasta complements the protein from kidney beans, so together they provide a complete protein. Generally, when you combine grains with legumes, or legumes with nuts or seeds, you will get complete, high-quality protein.

Small amounts of animal foods can also complement the protein in plant foods. For example, Asians often flavor rice with small amounts of beef, chicken, or fish, complementing the protein in the rice. Americans eat breakfast cereal with milk, which complements the protein in the cereal.

If you consume little or no animal protein, you should pay attention to complementary proteins. Consuming a wide variety of plant protein sources is the key to obtaining adequate amounts of all the essential amino acids. When protein and energy intakes are adequate, there is no need to plan complementary proteins at each meal.[23] Complementary proteins may still need to be combined in the same meal for infants and very young children.[24]

Boosting your intake of plant protein foods can provide benefits. High-protein plant foods are usually rich in vitamins, minerals, and dietary fiber. Plant foods contain no cholesterol and little fat, and they usually cost less than animal foods high in protein. Lentil loaf, for example, is substantially cheaper to make than meat loaf.

Table 7.3 Top Ten Sources of Protein in the United States

Rank	Food	% of Protein Contributed
1	Beef	18
2	Poultry	14
3	Milk	9
4	Yeast bread	7
5	Cheese	6
6	Fish/shellfish*	4
7	Eggs	3
8	Pork, fresh	3
9	Ham	3
10	Pasta	2

* Does not include tuna.
Source: *1989–1991 Continuing Survey of Food Intake by Individuals.*

Evaluating Protein Quality

A high-quality protein (1) provides all the essential amino acids in the amounts the body needs, (2) provides enough other amino acids to serve as nitrogen sources for making nonessential amino acids, and (3) is easy to digest. If a food protein contains the right proportion of amino acids but cannot be digested and absorbed, it is useless to the body. Protein quality might be assessed to plan a special diet or develop a new product such as infant formula.

A simple way to determine a food's protein quality is to compare its amino acid composition to that of a reference pattern of amino acids. The reference pattern closely reflects the amounts and proportions of amino acids humans need. The **protein digestibility-corrected amino acid score (PDCAAS)** accounts for both the amino acid composition of a food and the digestibility of the protein.

The U.S. Food and Drug Administration (FDA) recognizes the PDCAAS as the official method for determining the protein quality of most food.[25] If the percent Daily Value (%DV) for protein is listed on a food label, it must be based on the food's PDCAAS. It would be misleading to say that, for

Table 7.4 Examples of Complementary Food Combinations

Beans and rice
Beans and corn or wheat tortillas
Rice and lentils
Rice and black-eyed peas
Pea soup with bread or crackers
Hummus: garbanzo beans (chick peas) with sesame paste
Pasta with beans
Peanut butter on bread

example, 8 grams of protein from tuna and 8 grams from kidney beans would contribute equally to amino acid needs, and so even though the amount of protein per serving might be the same, the %DV would be different for these two foods.

Proteins and Amino Acids as Additives and Supplements

Proteins contribute to the structure, texture, and taste of food. They are often added to foods to enhance these properties. The milk protein casein is added to frozen dessert toppings. Gelatin is added to yogurt and fillings. **Protein hydrolysates**—proteins that have been broken down into amino acids and shorter peptides—are added to many foods as thickeners, stabilizers, or flavor enhancers.

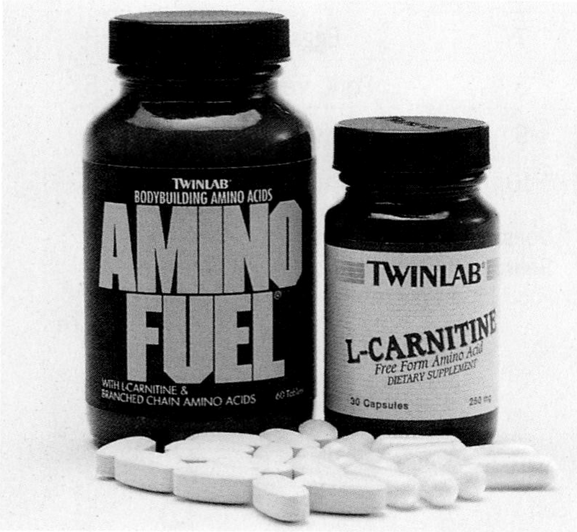

Amino acids are also used as additives. Monosodium glutamate (sodium bound to the amino acid glutamic acid) is a flavor enhancer added to many foods. The artificial sweetener aspartame is a dipeptide composed of aspartic acid and phenylalanine.

Protein and amino acid supplements are sold to dieters, athletes, and people who suffer from certain diseases. Despite a lack of scientific evidence, people buy the amino acid lysine for cold sores and the amino acid tryptophan in hopes that it will relieve pain, depression, and sleep disorders. Some protein powders and amino acid cocktails are marketed with the claims that they enhance muscle building and exercise performance. Although the anecdotal evidence (stories from friends and health food store clerks) for these products may be convincing, few scientific studies back up these claims. Remember, muscle work builds muscle strength and size, and muscles prefer carbohydrate to fuel this type of work.

There is no evidence that consuming large amounts of individual amino acids is beneficial, and the risks are unknown. An excess of a single amino acid in the digestive tract can impair absorption of certain other amino acids. This could cause a deficiency of one or more amino acids and an unhealthy excess of the supplemented amino acid.

Think About It 3

protein hydrolysates Proteins that have been treated with enzymes to break them down into amino acids and shorter peptides.

Key Concepts: *In general, animal foods provide complete protein that contains the right mix of all the essential amino acids. With the exception of soybean protein, plant foods contain incomplete protein—that is, protein lacking in one or more amino acids. Plant foods can be combined to complement each other's amino acid patterns. The FDA uses the PDCAAS as the official method for determining protein quality. Supplements of protein or amino acids are rarely necessary and might be harmful.*

The Pros and Cons of Vegetarian Eating

What did Socrates, Plato, Albert Einstein, Leonardo da Vinci, William Shakespeare, Charles Darwin, and Mahatma Gandhi have in common? They all advocated a vegetarian lifestyle.[26] George Bernard Shaw, vegetarian, famous writer, and political analyst of the early 1900s, wrote, "A man fed on whiskey and dead bodies cannot do the finest work of which he is capable."[27]

Meat-eaters often argue that vegetarian diets don't provide enough protein and other essential nutrients, but this isn't necessarily so. With careful planning, a diet that contains no animal products can be nutritionally complete and also offer many health benefits. Poorly planned vegetarian diets, however, can pose health risks.

Why People Become Vegetarians

In parts of the world where food is scarce, vegetarianism is not a choice but a necessity. Where food is abundant, people choose vegetarianism for many reasons.

People may choose a vegetarian diet because of religious beliefs, concern for the environment, a desire to reduce world hunger and make better use of scarce resources, an aversion to eating another living creature, or concerns about cruelty to animals. Still others become vegetarians because they believe it is healthier for them. The number of vegetarians in the United States has doubled in the last 10 years. Today, more than 12 million Americans consider themselves vegetarian.[28] **Table 7.5** shows three religious groups and their vegetarian practices.

Think About It 4

Table 7.5 Religious Groups with Vegetarian Dietary Practices

Religious Group	Dietary Practices
Buddhism	Some sects lacto-vegetarian, other sects vegan.
Hinduism	Generally lacto-vegetarian, but mutton or pork eaten occasionally.
Seventh-Day Adventists	Lacto-ovo-vegetarian, emphasizing whole-grain foods. Also avoid alcohol, tobacco, and caffeine.

Types of Vegetarians

Although all vegetarians share the common practice of not eating meat and meat products, they differ greatly in specific dietary practices. Lacto-ovo-vegetarians use animal products such as milk, cheese, and eggs, but don't eat the flesh of animals. Vegans eat no animal-based foods and usually avoid products such as cosmetics made with animal-based ingredients. Fruitarians eat only raw fruit, nuts, and green foliage.

Some people eat a semi-vegetarian diet, avoiding red meats but eating small amounts of chicken or fish. The Mediterranean diet, known for reducing the risk of heart disease, is a semi-vegetarian diet rich in grains, pasta, vegetables, cheeses, and olive oil supplemented with small amounts of chicken and fish. **Table 7.6** lists different types of vegetarian diets and the foods typically included and excluded.

Zen macrobiotic diets are mostly vegan and stress whole grains, locally grown vegetables, beans, sea vegetables, and soups. Extreme Zen macrobiotic diets can be very limited, consisting, for example, primarily of brown rice.

Quick Bites

Prophetic Eggs

Can an egg predict the future? In Trinidad and Tobago, people say you can tell the future by the shape an egg white makes when added to warm water on Good Friday.

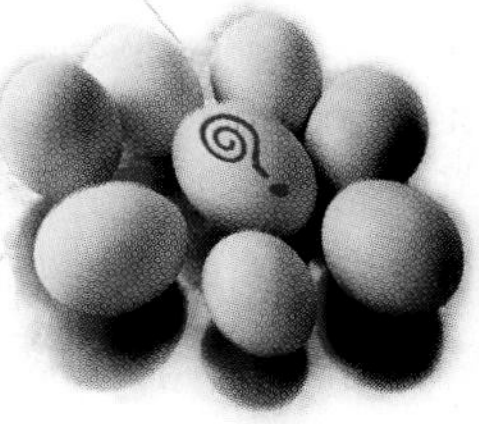

Table 7.6 Types of Vegetarian Diets

Type	Animal Foods Included	Foods Excluded
Semi-vegetarian	Dairy products, eggs, chicken, fish	Red meats (beef, pork)
Pesco-vegetarian	Dairy products, eggs, and fish	Beef, pork, poultry
Lacto-ovo-vegetarian	Dairy products, eggs	Any animal flesh
Lacto-vegetarian	Dairy products	Eggs, all animal flesh
Ovo-vegetarian	Eggs	Dairy products and animal flesh
Vegan	None	All animal products
Fruitarian	None	All foods except raw fruits, nuts, and green foliage

Fyi FOR YOUR INFORMATION — High-Protein Plant Foods

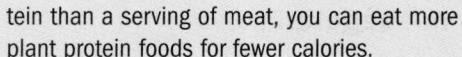

Of the top ten sources of protein in the American diet, only two sources—yeast breads and pasta—are plant-based. (See **Table 7.3**). Lentils, a dense source of plant protein, don't even make the list. Yet look at the comparison between the nutritional profile of lentils and the profile of beef in **Table A**.

Table A How Do Lentils Stack Up Against Beef?

	Cooked Lentils	*Lean Broiled Sirloin*
Amount	1 cup	5 ounces
Energy	230 kcalories	315 kcalories
Protein	18 grams	47 grams
Fat	1 gram	12 grams
Cholesterol	0	139 milligrams
Carbohydrate	40 grams	0
Dietary fiber	9 grams	0
Percent calories from fat	4%	34%

When we consider these two foods in light of the *Dietary Guidelines for Americans* (see Chapter 2, "Nutrition Guidlines"), it's no contest. To reduce fat, saturated fat, and cholesterol and to increase complex carbohydrates and fiber, the lentils win hands down! With all that lentils have going for them, you'd think more Americans would be eating them. Yet dried beans, peas, and lentils combined contribute less than 1 percent of the daily protein intake of Americans, while beef contributes 17.7 percent.

High-protein plant foods also contribute complex carbohydrates, dietary fiber, vitamins, and minerals. Since these plant foods contain little fat, they are nutrient dense; that is, they provide a high amount of protein and nutrients in proportion to their energy contribution.

Sources of Plant Protein

Grains and grain products, legumes (lentils and dried beans and peas such as kidney beans or chickpeas), starchy vegetables, and nuts and seeds all provide protein (**Table B**). A serving of a grain product or starchy vegetable provides an average of 3 grams of protein, a serving of legumes provides about 10 grams of protein, and a serving of vegetables provides about 2 grams of protein. Although a serving of these foods contains less protein than a serving of meat, you can eat more plant protein foods for fewer calories.

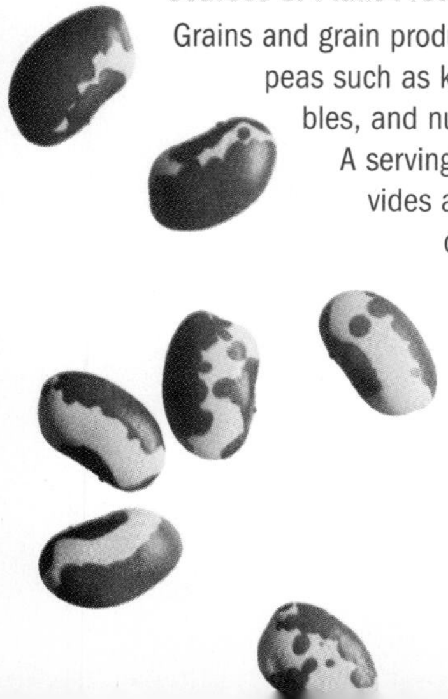

Complementing Plant Proteins

It's important to remember that plant proteins lack one or more of the essential amino acids needed to build body proteins, so individual plant proteins need to complement each other. A simple rule to remember in complementing plant proteins is that combining grains and legumes or combining legumes and nuts or seeds provides complete, high-quality protein.

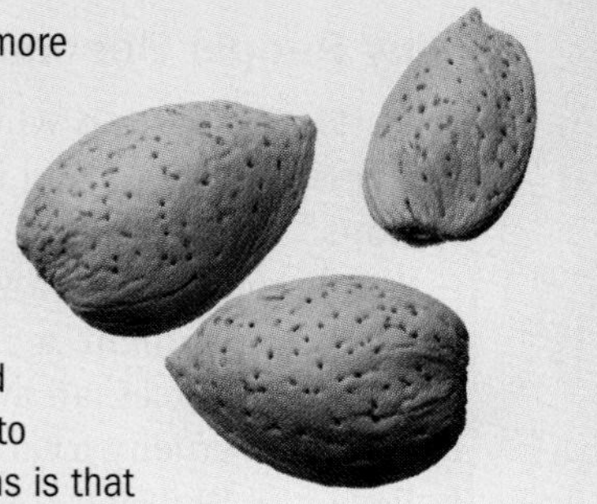

Table B Plant Sources of Protein

Plant Protein Source	*Grams of Protein*	*Kilocalories*
GRAIN PRODUCTS		
1 whole-wheat bagel (3")	6	157
1 whole English muffin, mixed grain	6	155
1 large flour tortilla (10")	6	234
1 cup cooked spaghetti	7	197
1 cup cooked brown rice	5	216
1 cup cooked oatmeal	6	145
2 slices whole-wheat bread	6	138
$^1/_2$ cup low-fat granola	5	213
STARCHY VEGETABLES		
1 cup cooked corn	5	177
1 cup baked hubbard squash	5	103
1 medium baked potato with skin	4	228
LEGUMES		
$^1/_2$ cup tofu	10	97
1 cup lentils	18	230
1 cup cooked kidney beans	15	225
VEGETABLES		
1 cup cooked broccoli	5	44
1 cup cooked cauliflower	2	29
1 cup cooked Brussels spouts	4	61
NUTS AND SEEDS		
2 tablespoons peanut butter	8	190
$^1/_4$ cup peanuts	9	208
$^1/_4$ cup sunflower seeds	7	208

Source: US Department of Agriculture, Agricultural Research Service. *USDA Nutrient Database for Standard Reference,* Release 13; 1999.

Soy Protein

The protein in soybeans is a notable exception to the rule that most plant proteins are not complete. Soy provides complete, high-quality protein comparable to that in animal foods. In addition, soybeans provide no saturated fat or cholesterol, and are rich in isoflavonoids—phytochemicals that help reduce risk of heart disease and cancer and improve bone health.

Isoflavonoids act as antioxidants, protecting cells and tissues from damage. One specific isoflavonoid, genistein, inhibits growth of both breast and prostate cancer cells in the laboratory. Isoflavonoids protect low-density lipoprotein cholesterol (the kind of cholesterol associated with greater risk of heart disease) from oxidation. Oxidized low-density lipoprotein cholesterol contributes to the plaque buildup in arteries. The isoflavonoids in soybeans also act as phytoestrogens, helping to protect older women from cardiovascular disease and osteoporosis. Soy foods that contain most or all of the bean, such as soymilk, sprouts, flour, and tofu, are the best sources of these phytochemicals.

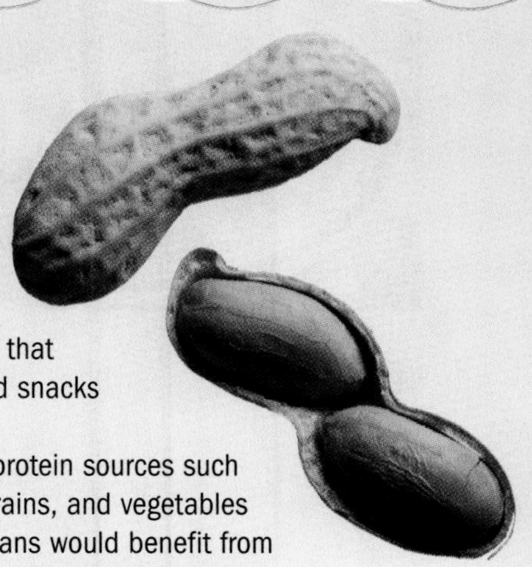

It is easy to incorporate a variety of soy foods into your diet. Tofu, tempeh, ground soy, soymilk, soy flour, and textured soy protein are soy-based products that can be included in many meals and snacks (**Table C**).

The nutritional benefits of plant protein sources such as soy foods and other legumes, grains, and vegetables deserve a closer look. Most Americans would benefit from emphasizing plant protein foods in their diet. Next time you plan to make meat loaf, make lentil loaf instead.

Table C **Soy Food Products and Uses**

Tofu A solid cake of curdled soymilk similar to soft cheese. Tofu comes in hard and soft varieties. It absorbs flavors of the foods it is mixed with. Soft tofu can be substituted for cheese in pasta dishes, stuffed in large shell pasta, blended with fruit, or used to make pie filling. Hard tofu can be used in salads and shish kebabs and can replace meat in stir-fry or mixed dishes.

Tempeh Tempeh is a flat cake made from fermented soybeans. It has a mild flavor and chewy texture. Tempeh can be grilled, included in sandwiches, or combined in casseroles.

Meat analogs Meat analogs are meat alternatives made primarily of soy protein. Flavored and textured to resemble chicken, beef, and pork, they can be substituted for meat in mixed dishes, pizza, tacos, or sloppy joes.

Soymilk Soymilk is the liquid of the soybean. It comes in regular and low-fat versions and in different flavors. Soymilk can be used plain or substituted for regular milk on cereals, in hot cocoa, puddings, or desserts.

Soy flour Soy flour is made from roasted soybeans ground into flour. Soy flour can replace up to one-quarter of the regular flour in a recipe.

Textured soy protein Textured soy protein resembles ground beef. It can be rehydrated and substituted for ground beef in any recipe.

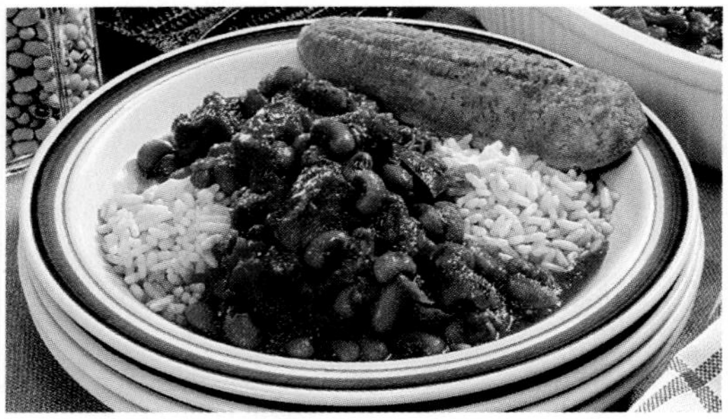

Health Benefits of Vegetarian Diets

Vegetarian diets usually contain less fat, saturated fat, and cholesterol than nonvegetarian diets. Vegetarian diets that emphasize fresh fruits and vegetables contain high amounts of antioxidants such as beta-carotene and vitamins C and E, which protect the body's cells and tissues from damage. Fruits and vegetables also contain dietary fiber and phytochemicals; although these substances are not essential in the diet, they can have important health effects.

On average, vegetarians have lower blood cholesterol levels and are less likely to develop heart disease than nonvegetarians. Vegetarian diets low in fat and saturated fat combined with other healthful lifestyle habits can reverse the clogging of arteries that eventually can lead to heart attack or stroke.[29]

Vegetarians usually weigh less for their height than nonvegetarians, partly because their diets provide less energy and partly because of other healthful lifestyle factors such as regular exercise. High blood pressure occurs less frequently among vegetarians than among nonvegetarians, regardless of body weight or sodium intake.

Certain cancers, such as breast and colon cancers, occur less frequently in vegetarians than nonvegetarians. The high dietary fiber intake typical in vegetarian diets may protect against colon cancer, while the lower estrogen levels of vegetarian women may protect against breast cancer.[30]

Health Risks of Vegetarian Diets

Although vegetarian diets offer many health benefits, certain types of vegetarian diets pose some unique nutritional risks. The more limited the vegetarian diet, the more likely it is to cause nutritional problems. Lacto-ovo-vegetarian diets that contain a variety of foods generally are nutritionally adequate but can be high in fat and cholesterol. However, iron content may be low if the diet contains large amounts of milk products.

Vegan diets tend to be low in iron, zinc, calcium, vitamin D, vitamin B_6, and vitamin B_{12}. The best sources of these nutrients are animal foods—red meat for iron and zinc, fortified milk for calcium and vitamin D, chicken for vitamin B_6, and any animal foods for B_{12}. Plant foods contain a form of iron that is not as well absorbed as the iron in animal foods. (See Chapter 10, "Water and Minerals," for more on iron.) Since vitamin C aids iron absorption into the body, however, the higher vitamin C intakes of vegetarians may offset the lower iron intakes to some degree. Because taking in high amounts of protein increases calcium losses, vegans—who have a lower protein intake—may need less calcium than nonvegetarians.

Vegans tend to have higher intakes of phytates (found in whole grains, bran, and soy products), oxalates (found in spinach, rhubarb, and chocolate), and tannins (found in tea). These compounds can bind minerals, making them less available to the body for absorption.

Very limited vegan diets, such as fruitarian diets or extreme Zen macrobiotic diets, pose the greatest nutritional risks. These diets are likely to be lacking in many essential nutrients.

For most people, vegetarian diets readily provide sufficient nutrients. But for some, especially infants, young children, and pregnant or breastfeeding women, vegetarian diets must be carefully planned to meet the needs of rapid growth.

Quick Bites

Paleolithic Protein

Didn't our ancestors eat a lot of meat too? Researchers estimate that hunter-gatherers had diets that were about one-third meat and two-thirds vegetable. The meat from wild game, however, averages only one-seventh the fat of domesticated beef (about 4 g of fat per 100 g of wild meat, compared with 29 g of fat per 100 g of domestic meat). In addition, compared with the meat at your local supermarket, the fat contained in game animals that graze on the free range has five times as much polyunsaturated fat.

Dietary Recommendations for Vegetarians

Vegetarians can follow a modified version of the Food Guide Pyramid to help plan meals (**Figure 7.13**). Vegetarians who include milk, milk products, and eggs in their diet can easily meet their nutritional needs for protein and other essential nutrients but must take care to choose low-fat milk products and limit eggs to avoid excess saturated fat and cholesterol.

Since grains, vegetables, and legumes (dried beans and peas) all provide protein, vegans who eat a variety of foods also can meet their protein needs easily. Although most plant foods do not contain complete protein, eating complementary plant protein sources during the same day adequately meets the body's needs for protein production.

Vegans who avoid all animal products must supplement their diets with a reliable source of vitamin B_{12}, such as fortified soymilk. Although bacteria in some fermented foods and in the knobby growths of some seaweeds produce vitamin B_{12}, most vegans do not eat enough seaweeds and fermented foods to meet their vitamin B_{12} needs.

The American Dietetic Association gives the following nutritional guidelines for vegetarians:

1. Choose a variety of foods, including whole grains, vegetables, fruits, legumes, nuts, seeds, and, if desired, dairy products and eggs.
2. Choose whole, unrefined foods often and minimize intake of highly sweetened, fatty, and heavily refined foods.
3. Choose a variety of fruits and vegetables.

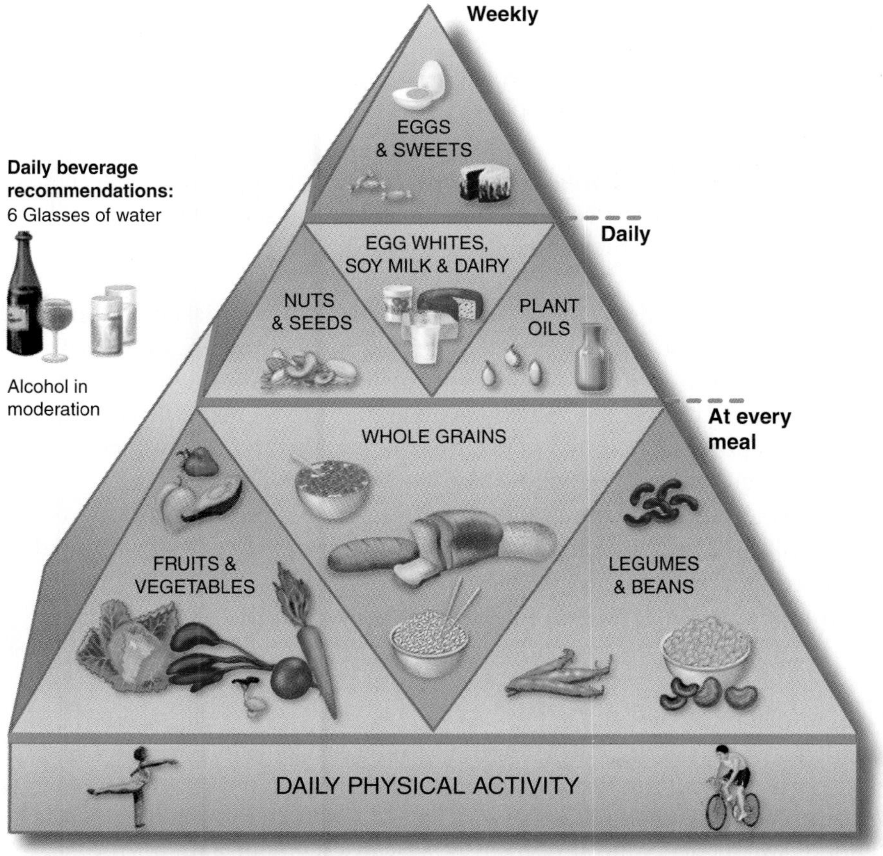

Figure 7.13 **Vegetarian Food Guide Pyramid.** With careful planning, vegetarian diets can be nutritionally complete.
Source: © 2000 Oldways Preservation & Exchange Trust. Reprinted with permission.

4. If animal foods such as dairy products and eggs are used, high-fat dairy foods and eggs should be limited in the diet because of their saturated fat content and because their frequent use displaces plant foods in some vegetarian diets.
5. Vegans should include a regular source of vitamin B_{12} in their diets, along with a source of vitamin D if sun exposure is limited.
6. Infants who receive no food other than breast milk should have supplements of iron after the age of 4 to 6 months and, if sun exposure is limited, a source of vitamin D. Breastfed vegan infants should have vitamin B_{12} supplements if the mother's diet is not fortified.
7. Do not restrict dietary fat in children younger than 2 years. For older children, include some foods higher in fat (eggs, nuts, seeds, nut and seed butters, avocados, and vegetable oils) to help meet nutrient and energy needs.[31]

Key Concepts: *Vegetarian diets eliminate animal products to various degrees. Lacto-ovo-vegetarians include milk and eggs in their diets, while vegans eat no animal foods. Vegetarian diets tend to be low in fat and high in fiber and phytochemicals, which may help reduce chronic disease risks. Careful diet planning is necessary for vegans and growing children to ensure all nutrient needs are met.*

Quick Bites

Protein Makes for Springy Bugs

Resilin is an elastic rubberlike protein in insects, scorpions, and crustaceans. The springiness in the wing hinges of some insects, like locusts and dragonflies, comes from the unique mechanical properties of resilin. The protein also is found in the stingers of bees and ants, the eardrums and sound organs of cicadas, and the little rubber balls in the hips of jumping fleas. The structural properties of resilin are similar to true rubber, which makes it very unusual among structural proteins.

The Health Effects of Too Little or Too Much Protein

Because protein plays such a vital role in so many body processes, protein deficiency can wreak havoc in numerous body systems. If your body doesn't have enough available protein, it will not have the essential amino acids needed to synthesize body proteins.

Protein deficiency occurs when energy and/or protein intake is inadequate. Adequate energy intake spares dietary and body proteins so they can be used for protein synthesis. Without adequate energy intake, the body burns dietary protein for energy rather than using it to make body proteins. Protein deficiency can occur even in people who eat seemingly adequate amounts of protein if the protein they eat is of poor quality or cannot be absorbed.

Although protein deficiency is widespread in poverty-stricken communities and in some nonindustrialized countries, most people in industrialized countries face the opposite problem—protein excess. Although the RDA for a 70-kilogram (154-pound) person is 56 grams, the average American man consumes approximately 105 grams of protein daily and the average woman 65 grams. And many meat-loving Americans eat far more.

Many researchers suggest that high protein intakes pose significant health risks. Links to heart disease, cancer, and osteoporosis have been suggested. However, the independent effects of high protein intake are difficult to determine, since high protein intake often goes hand-in-hand with high intakes of saturated fat and cholesterol.

Protein-Energy Malnutrition

A deficiency of protein, energy, or both in the diet is called **protein-energy malnutrition**, or PEM. Protein and energy intakes are difficult to separate because diets adequate in energy usually are adequate in protein, and diets inadequate in energy inhibit the body's use of dietary protein for protein synthesis.

protein-energy malnutrition (PEM) A condition resulting from long-term inadequate intakes of protein and energy that can lead to wasting of body tissues and increased susceptibility to infection.

Although it can occur at all stages of life, PEM is most common during childhood, when protein is needed to support rapid growth. It is the most common form of malnutrition in the world, affecting an estimated 156 million children under the age of 5 in developing countries.[32] PEM symptoms can be mild or severe and exist in either acute or chronic forms.

Protein-energy malnutrition occurs in all parts of the world but is most common in Africa, South and Central America, East and Southeast Asia, and the Middle East. In industrialized countries, PEM occurs most often among people living in poverty, in the elderly, and in hospitalized patients with other conditions such as anorexia nervosa, AIDS, cancer, or malabsorption syndromes.[33]

Severe PEM takes two forms: kwashiorkor and marasmus. Sometimes people have symptoms of both. Researchers do not understand completely why PEM causes symptoms of kwashiorkor in some people and symptoms of marasmus in others.[34] Historically, kwashiorkor was thought to result from inadequate intake of protein but adequate intake of energy. Marasmus was thought to result from inadequate intake of both protein and energy. Now researchers know that the lines between these two diseases are not so clear and that protein deficiency rarely develops with adequate energy intake.

Researchers believe that kwashiorkor develops from acute PEM, while marasmus develops from chronic PEM. Some researchers also believe that kwashiorkor is an abnormal adaptation to PEM, whereas marasmus is a normal adaptation. Other factors, such as infections or toxins in the diet, may trigger the development of kwashiorkor rather than marasmus.[35] See **Figure 7.14** for signs and symptoms of kwashiorkor and marasmus.

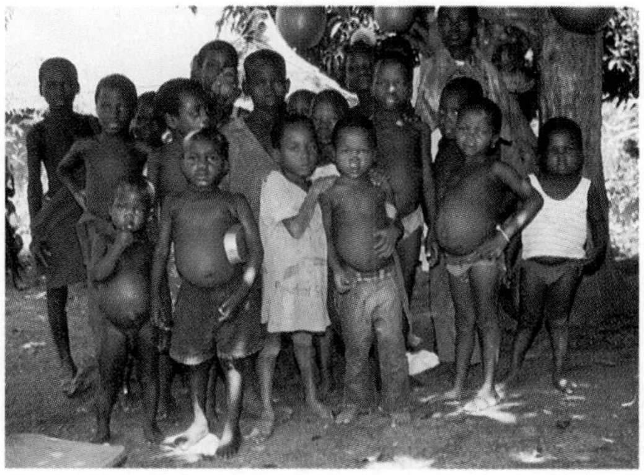

(a)

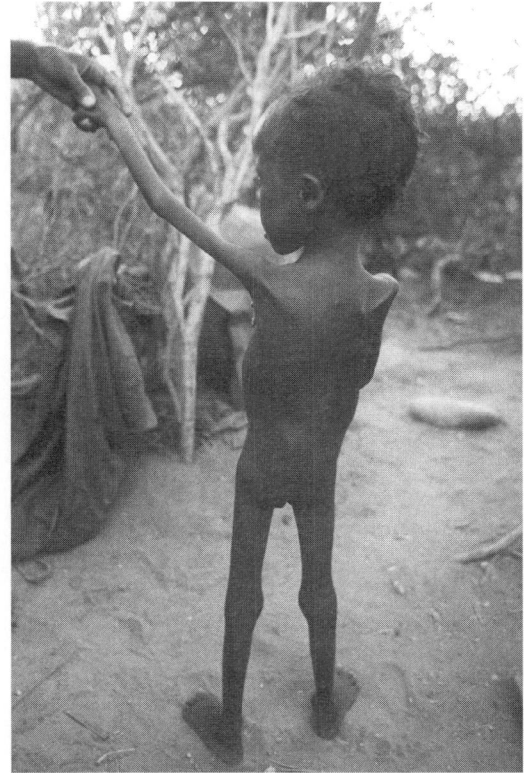

(b)

Figure 7.14 **Kwashiorkor and marasmus.** (a) Edema in the feet and legs and a bloated belly are symptoms of kwashiorkor. (b) Children with marasmus are short and thin for their age and can appear frail and wrinkled.

Kwashiorkor

The term *kwashiorkor* is a Ghanian word that describes the "evil spirit which infects the first child when the second child is born." In many cultures, babies are breastfed until the next baby comes along. When it does, the first baby is weaned from nutritious breast milk and placed on a watered-down version of the family's diet. In areas of poverty, this diet is often low in protein, or the protein is not absorbed easily.

The symptom of kwashiorkor that sets it apart from marasmus is edema, or swelling of body tissue, usually in the feet and legs. Lack of blood proteins reduces the force that keeps fluid in the bloodstream, and, instead, fluid leaks out into the tissues. The belly can also become bloated from both edema and accumulation of fat in the liver, since no proteins are available to transport the fat. Other features of kwashiorkor include stunted weight and height, increased susceptibility to infection, dry and flaky skin, and sometimes skin sores, dry and brittle hair, and changes in skin color. Since the energy deficit is usually not as severe (or as long-standing) in kwashiorkor as in marasmus, people with kwashiorkor may still have some body fat stores left.

Kwashiorkor usually develops in children between 18 and 24 months of age, about the time weaning occurs. Its onset can be rapid and is often triggered by an infection or illness that increases the child's protein needs. In hospital settings, kwashiorkor can develop in situations where protein needs are extremely high (trauma, infection, burns) but dietary intake is poor.

Kwashiorkor is associated with extreme poverty in developing countries and is rare in affluent countries except in people with chronic illness.

Nutritional ignorance and food faddism, however, cause some cases.[36] In one case, for example, well-educated parents primarily fed their child rice-based beverages (incorrectly called rice milk), which are extremely low in protein. When admitted to the hospital, the 22-month-old child had severe kwashiorkor.[37]

Marasmus

Marasmus is derived from the Greek word *marasmos*, which means "withering" or "to waste away." It develops more slowly than kwashiorkor and results from chronic PEM. Protein, energy, and nutrient intakes are all grossly inadequate, depleting body fat reserves and severely wasting muscle tissue, including vital organs like the heart. Growth slows or stops, and children are both short and very thin for their age. Metabolism slows and body temperature drops as the body tries to conserve energy. Children with marasmus are apathetic, often not even crying in an effort to conserve energy. Their hair is sparse and falls out easily. Because muscle and fat are used up, a child with marasmus often looks like a frail, wrinkled, elderly person.

Marasmus occurs most often in infants and children 6 to 18 months of age who are fed diluted or improperly mixed formulas. Because this is a time of rapid brain growth, marasmus can permanently stunt brain development and lead to learning disabilities. Marasmus also occurs in adults who have cancer or are experiencing starvation, including the self-imposed starvation of the eating disorder known as anorexia nervosa.

Nutritional Rehabilitation

To recover, people with PEM need gradual and careful refeeding to correct protein, energy, fluid, and vitamin and mineral imbalances.[38] People with PEM are often dehydrated and have low body potassium stores as a result of diarrhea. These imbalances in fluids and electrolytes are corrected first to raise blood pressure and strengthen the heart. Once that is achieved, the patient receives protein and other nutrients in small amounts that are gradually increased as tolerated.

Quick Bites

The Source of Salisbury Steak

Dr. James Salisbury, a London physician who lived in the late 1800s, believed man to be two-thirds carnivorous and one-third herbivorous. He recommended a diet low in starch and high in lean meat, with lots of hot water to rinse out the products of fermentation. His diet regimen included broiled, lean, minced beef three times a day. Although we call it Salisbury steak as a courtesy to Dr. Salisbury's heritage, minced beef patties are really more like hamburgers.

Excess Dietary Protein

In industrialized countries, an excess of protein and energy is more common than a deficiency. Although not as severe or life-threatening, high protein intake can also cause health problems. (See **Figure 7.15**.) Therefore, the National Research Council recommends that protein intakes not exceed twice the amount recommended in the RDAs.[39]

Kidney Function

Since the kidneys must excrete the products of protein breakdown, high protein intake can strain kidney function and is especially harmful for people with kidney disease or diabetes.

To prevent dehydration, it is important to drink plenty of fluids to dilute the byproducts of protein breakdown for excretion. Human infants should not be fed unmodified cow's milk until they are at least 1 year of age because the high protein concentration in cow's milk combined with an immature kidney system can cause fluid losses and dehydration.

Mineral Losses

If you take in too much protein, your body will excrete more calcium, which can contribute to bone mineral losses and increase the risk of osteo-

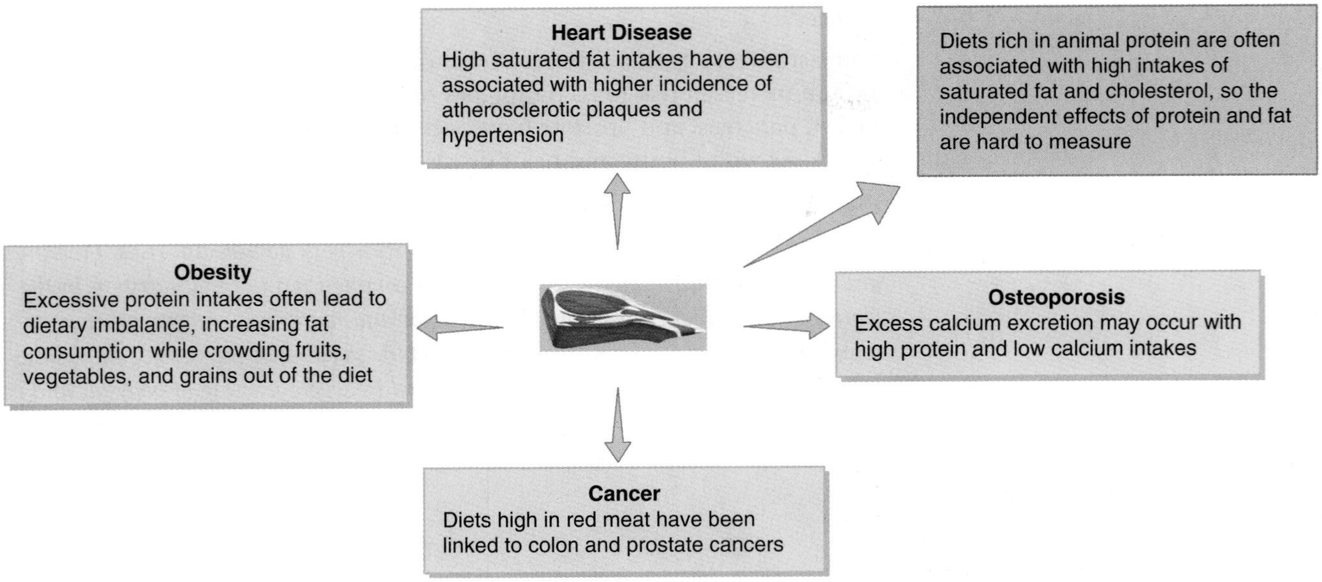
Heart Disease
High saturated fat intakes have been associated with higher incidence of atherosclerotic plaques and hypertension
Diets rich in animal protein are often associated with high intakes of saturated fat and cholesterol, so the independent effects of protein and fat are hard to measure
Obesity
Excessive protein intakes often lead to dietary imbalance, increasing fat consumption while crowding fruits, vegetables, and grains out of the diet
Osteoporosis
Excess calcium excretion may occur with high protein and low calcium intakes
Cancer
Diets high in red meat have been linked to colon and prostate cancers

Figure 7.15 **Excess protein.** In developed countries, excess protein and energy are a greater problem than protein deficiency.

porosis, a disease that causes bones to become porous and brittle. Animal proteins trigger greater calcium losses than plant proteins because animal proteins are especially rich in sulfur-containing amino acids, which are acidic and tend to draw calcium out of the body.[40]

If you meet the Adequate Intake level (AI) for calcium, the calcium losses caused by high protein intake may not be significant. Indeed, the AI for calcium is set high to offset the high protein intake of Americans. However, the calcium intake of many people, especially women, falls short of the AI, while their protein intake typically exceeds the RDA.

Obesity

High-protein foods are also often high in fat. A diet high in fat and protein may provide too much energy, contributing to obesity. Large amounts of high-protein foods will displace fruits, vegetables, and grains—foods that contain fewer calories. Some researchers have recently suggested that high dietary protein intake alters hormones and the body's response to hormones, including leptin, which regulates feeding centers in the brain to reduce food intake.[41] Some studies suggest that because of this effect on hormones, a high protein intake early in life increases the risk of obesity later in life.[42]

Heart Disease

Research has linked high intake of animal protein to high blood cholesterol levels and increased risk of heart disease. Foods high in animal protein, however, are also high in saturated fat and cholesterol. Whether protein alone—independent of fat—plays a role in the development of heart disease is less clear. Soy protein foods, which contain no saturated fat or cholesterol, have been shown to lower blood cholesterol levels and reduce risk for heart disease.[43] The FDA recently approved a health claim saying that soy protein is beneficial in reducing the risk of heart disease. Soy proteins also may have protective effects against obesity, diabetes, irritants in the digestive tract, and bone and kidney diseases.[44]

Cancer

Some studies suggest a link between a diet high in animal protein foods and an increased risk for certain types of cancers.[45] Cancers of the colon, breast, pancreas, and prostate have been linked to high protein and fat intake. As with obesity and heart disease, however, the effects of protein and fat are difficult to separate.

Key Concepts: *Protein deficiency and protein excess both pose health risks. Protein and energy malnutrition (PEM) is the most common form of malnutrition in the world. PEM can take two forms: kwashiorkor and marasmus. Among other symptoms, kwashiorkor is characterized by edema, or swelling of the tissues. Marasmus results from chronic PEM and is characterized by severe wasting of body fat and muscles. Intake of too much protein may contribute to loss of bone calcium, obesity, heart disease, and certain forms of cancer.*

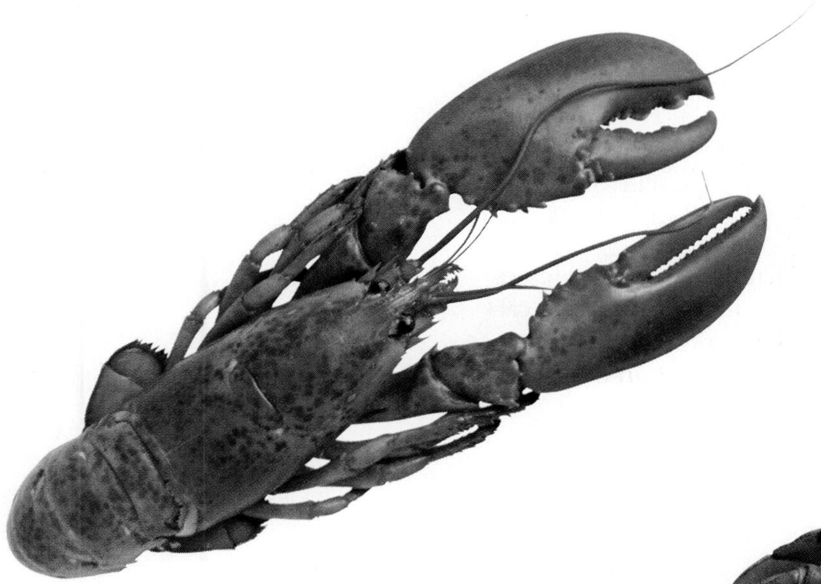

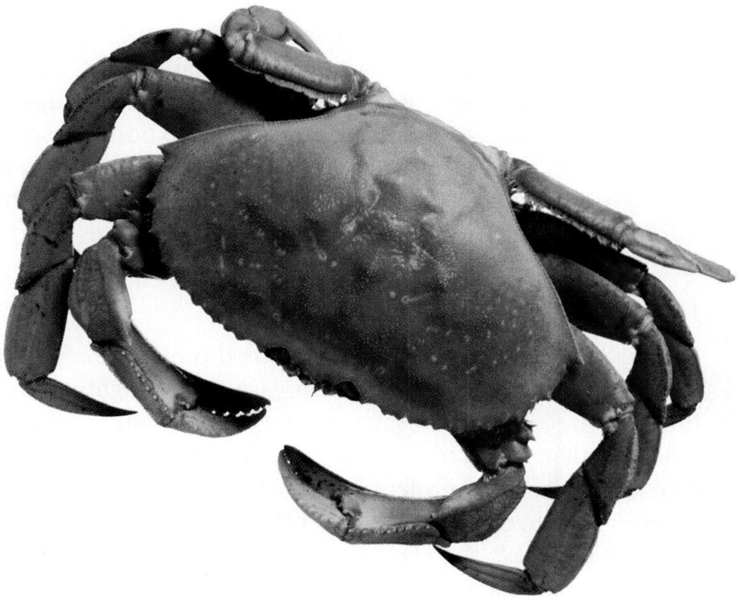

Label [to] Table

Have you ever visited a health food store and noticed all the protein powders, amino acid supplements, and high-protein bars? Do you believe claims like "protein boosts your energy level" or "amino acid X helps you build muscle" or "protein shakes are the best pre-workout fuel"? You know from this chapter that protein is an important nutrient and it's used to build and repair tissue. But do you need one of these supplements? Before reaching into your wallet, check out the Nutrition Facts of this protein powder and determine whether it's a good buy.

Look at this label and note how far down protein is on the list of nutrients. This placement is intentional and attempts to encourage consumers to de-emphasize protein in their diets. You may recall that most Americans eat more protein than they need, and because much of that protein comes from animal foods, they are also getting excess saturated fat. The label doesn't show the %DV for protein—unlike most other nutrients. Manufacturers are not required to give the %DV for protein. Although there is a DV for protein (50 grams), to determine %DV for protein, manufacturers first would have to use the PDCAAS method to determine the food protein's quality.

Do protein and amino acid supplements do what they claim to do? In terms of building muscle, exercise physiologists agree that it takes consistent muscle work (i.e., weight lifting) and a healthful diet that meets the body's calorie needs. Building muscle does not depend on extra protein. In fact, muscles mainly use carbohydrate and fat for fuel, not protein, so these other nutrients are more important for effective workouts.

In terms of protein's ability to boost your energy level, recall that anything with calories (carbohydrates, proteins, and fats) provides the body with "energy." In fact, unlike carbohydrates and fats, only a small amount of protein is used for energy expenditure. Research shows that the best thing to eat before a workout is carbohydrate, not protein, because carbohydrate provides glucose to the muscle cells. Review this label again. What percentage of this protein powder's calories comes from protein?

154 kcalories
11 grams protein × 4 kcalories per gram
= 44 protein kcalories

44 ÷ 154 = 0.28 or 28% protein kcalories

Surprise! Surprise! Only about one-quarter of the powder's calories are protein anyway, so it's OK as a pre-workout fuel not because of its protein content but because of its ample carbohydrate!

Nutrition Facts
Serving Size: 2 scoops
Servings Per Container: 18

Amount Per Serving	
Calories 154 Calories from fat 35	
	% Daily Value*
Total Fat 4g	6%
Saturated Fat 2.5g	12%
Cholesterol 20mg	7%
Sodium 170mg	7%
Total Carbohydrate 17g	6%
Dietary Fiber 0g	0%
Sugars 14g	
Protein 11g	
Vitamin A 4% •	Vitamin C 6%
Calcium 40% •	Iron 0%

* Percent Daily Values are based on a 2,000 calorie diet. Your daily values may be higher or lower depending on your calorie needs:

	Calories:	2,000	2,500
Total Fat	Less Than	65g	80g
Sat Fat	Less Than	20g	25g
Cholesterol	Less Than	300mg	300mg
Sodium	Less Than	2,400mg	2,400mg
Total Carbohydrate		300g	375g
Dietary Fiber		25g	30g

Calories per gram:
Fat 9 • Carbohydrate 4 • Protein 4

LEARNING Portfolio chapter 7

Key Terms

	page
acidosis	203
alkalosis	203
amino acid pool	209
antibodies [AN-tih-bod-eez]	201
buffers	203
celiac disease [SEA-lee-ak]	207
collagen	201
complementary proteins	212
complete proteins	211
conditionally essential amino acids	197
cystic fibrosis	207
deamination	205
denaturation	199
dipeptide	199
edema	204
essential amino acids	197
extracellular fluid	204
hemoglobin [HEEM-oh-glow-bin]	199
immune response	201
incomplete proteins	211
interstitial fluid [in-ter-STISH-ul]	204
intracellular fluid	204
intravascular fluid	204
keratin	201
motor proteins	201
negative nitrogen balance	209
neurotransmitters	209
nitrogen balance	209
nitrogen equilibrium	209
nonessential amino acids	197
oligopeptide	199
peptide bond	199
polypeptide	199
positive nitrogen balance	209
proenzymes	205
proteases	205
protein digestibility-corrected amino acid score (PDCAAS)	212
protein hydrolysates	214
protein turnover	209
protein-energy malnutrition (PEM)	220
tripeptide	199
urea	209
wasting	197

Study Points

- Many vital compounds are proteins, including enzymes, hormones, transport proteins, and regulators of both acid–base and fluid balance.
- Proteins are long chains of amino acids.
- Amino acids are composed of a central carbon atom bonded to hydrogen, carboxyl, amino, and side groups.
- Twenty amino acids are important in human nutrition; nine of these amino acids are considered essential (must come from the diet), while the body can make the other eleven (nonessential) amino acids.
- The amino acid sequence of a protein determines its shape and function.
- Denaturing proteins changes their shape and therefore their functional properties.
- Hydrochloric acid in the stomach denatures proteins so that the enzyme pepsin can begin their digestion.
- Proteins are completely digested in the small intestine and, after absorption, are carried to the liver.
- Dietary protein is found in meats, dairy products, legumes, grains, and vegetables.
- In general, animal foods contain higher-quality protein than is found in plant foods.
- Protein needs are highest when growth is rapid, such as during infancy, childhood, and adolescence.
- The protein intake of most Americans exceeds their RDA.
- Protein deficiency is most common in developing countries and often results in marasmus and kwashiorkor.
- Protein excess is also harmful and may affect risk for osteoporosis, heart disease, and cancer.

Study Questions

Answers can be found at nutrition.jbpub.com/discovering.

1. **List the functions of body proteins.**
2. **Describe the differences among essential, nonessential, and conditionally essential amino acids.**
3. **Why are most plant proteins considered incomplete?**
4. **What are complementary proteins? List three examples of food combinations that contain complementary proteins.**
5. **What health effects occur if you are protein deficient?**
6. **How is protein related to immune function?**
7. **Describe a vegan diet.**
8. **List the potential health benefits of a vegetarian diet.**

[*Try*] This

The Sweetness of NutraSweet

The purpose of this experiment is to see the effect of high temperatures on the dipeptide known as NutraSweet (aspartame). Make a cup of hot tea (or coffee) and add one packet of Equal (one brand of aspartame). Stir and taste the tea; note its sweetness. Reheat the tea (via a microwave or stovetop) so that it boils for 30 to 60 seconds. After the tea cools, taste it. Does it still taste sweet? Why or why not?

The Vegetarian Challenge

The purpose of this activity is to eat a completely vegetarian diet for one day. Begin by making a list of your typical meals and snacks. Once the list is complete, review each food item and determine whether it contains animal products. Cross off items that contain animal products and circle the remaining vegan-friendly options. Double-check the circled list with a friend or roommate. You may have missed something! Create a full day's worth of meals and snacks using your circled foods as well as additional vegan options. Make sure your menu looks complete and nutritionally balanced. Try to stick to this menu for at least one day. Pay attention to deviations you make and determine whether these are vegan food choices.

What About *Bobbie?*

Take a minute to review Bobbie's food intake with a special eye on protein. How do you think she did? Do you think she's lower or higher than her RDA? Let's first calculate her protein RDA. Since Bobbie weighs 155 pounds, her protein RDA is as follows:

155 pounds ÷ 2.2 pounds = 70.5 kilograms
70.5 kilograms × 0.8 grams protein = 56.4 grams

Her protein intake is 97 grams. This is quite high compared to her RDA! Are you surprised to learn she eats nearly twice as much protein as she needs? Her diet doesn't look that high in protein, does it? Here are the foods that contribute the most protein to her diet:

Food	Protein Grams
Turkey breast	*9*
Meatballs	*23*
Bagel	*7*
Spaghetti	*10*
Pizza	*12*

Another way to evaluate Bobbie's protein intake is in terms of calories. If her total protein intake is 97 grams, then 388 kilocalories come from protein. Remember, her total kilocalorie intake is 2,440, which means protein makes up 16 percent of her diet. General guidelines recommend that 10 to 15 percent of energy come from protein.

So what's the deal? Is Bobbie eating way too much protein or just the right amount? Using her RDA as a guide, you'd say she's overconsuming protein, but based on her calories, she's doing just fine. To get to the bottom of this you're going to have to look a little closer. The real issue here is her calorie intake. If you check the RDA table (page i) to see the recommended calorie intake for a 19-year-old woman, you'll see that it's 2,200 kilocalories. So the bigger issue here is that Bobbie may be consuming too many calories. Even though she ate approximately 16 percent as protein, because her calorie intake was high, her total protein intake was high too. Can you calculate what her protein grams should have been if she actually consumed close to the energy RDA?

15% of 2,200 kcalories = 330 protein kcalories
330 protein kcalories ÷ 4 calories per gram = 82 grams

So, Bobbie's protein RDA is 51 grams per day; yet, based on the general protein recommendation of 15 percent of calories, she could consume up to 82 grams. The 51-gram-per-day recommendation based on Bobbie's body weight is more accurate than the 82-gram-per-day recommendation based on the RDA for energy (calories). If you remember the review of Bobbie's diet in the carbohydrate chapter, it should now make sense that she should consume less protein and eat more fruits and vegetables.

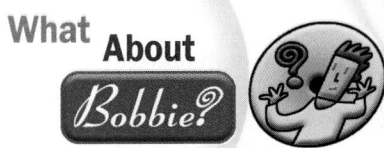

References

1 National Institutes of Health. *Phenylketonuria: Screening and Management.* NIH Consensus Statement. 2000 October 16–18; 17(3):1–27.

2 Griffiths RD, Jones C, Palmer TE. Six-month outcome of critically ill patients given glutamine-supplemented parenteral nutrition. *Nutrition.* 1997;13:295–302.

3 Van der Hulst RR, von Meyenfeldt MR, Soeters PB. Glutamine: an essential amino acid for the gut. *Nutrition.* 1996;12: S78–S81.

4 Alexander JW, Ogle CK, Nelson JL. Diets and infection: composition and consequences. *World J Surg.* 1998;22:209–212.

5 Voet D, Voet JG. *Biochemistry.* 2nd ed. New York: Wiley; 1995.

6 Guyton AC, Hall JE. *Textbook of Medical Physiology.* 10th ed. Philadelphia: W.B. Saunders; 2000.

7 Ibid.

8 Sardesai VM. *Introduction to Clinical Nutrition.* New York: Marcel Dekker; 1998.

9 Ibid.

10 Mathews DE. Proteins and amino acids. In: Shils ME, Olson JA, Shike M, Ross AC, eds. *Modern Nutrition in Health and Disease.* 9th ed. Philadelphia: Lippincott Williams & Wilkins; 1999:11–48.

11 Suryawan A, Hawes JW, Harris RA, et al. A molecular model of human branched-chain amino acid metabolism. *Am J Clin Nutr.* 1998;68:72–81.

12 Mathews DE. Op. cit.

13 Food and Agricultural Organization, World Health Organization, United Nations University. *Energy and Protein Requirements.* Rome: Food and Agricultural Organization; 1985.

14 Basile-Filho A, Beaumier L, El-Khoury E, et al. Twenty-four-hour L-[1-^{13}C] tyrosine and L-[3,3-^{2}H2] phenylalanine oral tracer studies at generous, intermediate, and low phenylalanine intakes to estimate aromatic amino acid requirements in adults. *Am J Clin Nutr.* 1998;67:640–659; and Kurpad AV, El-Khoury E, Beaumier L, et al. An initial assessment, using 24-h [13C] leucine kinetics, of the lysine requirement of healthy adult Indian subjects. *Am J Clin Nutr.* 1998;67:58–66.

15 US Department of Health and Human Services. *Healthy People 2000: National Health Promotion and Disease Prevention Objectives.* Washington, DC: US Government Printing Office; 1991. DHHS Publication No. (PHS) 91-50212.

16 McDowell MA, Briefel RR, Alaimo K, et al. *Energy and Macronutrient Intake of Persons Ages 2 Months and Over in the United States: Third National Health and Examination Survey, Phase 1, 1988–91.* Hyattsville, MD: National Center for Health Statistics; 1994. Advance Data from Vital and Health Statistics, No 255.

17 National Academy of Sciences. *Recommended Dietary Allowances.* 10th ed. Washington, DC: National Academy Press; 1989.

18 Millward DJ, Roberts SB. Protein requirements of older individuals. *Nutr Res Rev.* 1996;9:67–87.

19 US Department of Agriculture, Agricultural Research Service. Data tables: results from USDA's 1994–96 Continuing Survey of Food Intakes by Individuals and 1994–96 Diet and Health Knowledge Survey. On: *1994–96 Continuing Survey of Food Intakes by Individuals and 1994–96 Diet and Health Knowledge Survey,* [CD-ROM]. NTIS Accession Number PB98-500457; 1997.

20 Young VR. Soy protein in relation to human protein and amino acid nutrition. *J Am Diet Assoc.* 1991;91:828–835.

21 Young VR, Pellett PL. Plant proteins in relation to human protein and amino acid nutrition. *Am J Clin Nutr.* 1994;59:1203S–1212S.

22 Ibid.

23 Young VR, Pellett PL. Op. cit.; and American Dietetic Association. Position of the American Dietetic Association: vegetarian diets. *J Am Diet Assoc.* 1997;97:1317–1321.

24 Dwyer JT. Nutritional consequences of vegetarianism. *Ann Rev Nutr.* 1991;11:61–91.

25 Food and Agriculture Organization. *Protein Quality Evaluation: Report of the Joint FAO/WHO Expert Consultation.* Rome: Food and Agriculture Organization; 1991; FAO Food and Nutrition Paper 51; and Sarwar G, McDonough RE. Evaluation of protein digestibility-corrected amino acid score method for assessing protein quality of foods. *J Assoc Official Analytic Chem.* 1990;73:347–356.

26 Ballenntine R. *Transition to Vegetarianism: An Evolutionary Step.* Honesdale, PA: Himalayan International Institute of Yoga Science and Philosophy; 1987; and Null G. *The Vegetarian Handbook: Eating Right for Total Health.* New York: St. Martin's Press; 1987.

27 Null G. Op. cit.

28 Gustafson N. *Vegetarian Nutrition.* 2nd ed. Eureka, CA: Nutrition Dimension; 1997.

29 Gould KL, Ornish D, Scherwitz L, et al. Changes in myocardial perfusion abnormalities by positron emission tomography after long-term intense risk factor modification. *JAMA.* 1995;274:894–901.

30 American Dietetic Association. Op. cit.

31 Ibid. Reprinted with permission.

32 UNICEF. *The state of the World's Children 2001.* www.unicef.org/sow01/tables/table2.htm and www.unicef.org/sow01/tables/table5.htm. Accessed 3/27/02.

33 Swail WS, Samour PQ, Babineau TJ, Bistrian BR. A proposed revision of current ICD-9-CM malnutrition code definitions. *J Am Diet Assoc.* 1996;96:370–373.

34 Manary MJ, Broadhead RL, Yarasheski KE. Whole-body protein kinetics in marasmus and kwashiorkor during acute infection. *Am J Clin Nutr.* 1998;67:1205–1209.

35 Jelliffe DB, Jelliffe EFP. Causation of kwashiorkor: toward a multifactorial consensus. *Pediatrics.* 1992;90:110–112.

36 Liu T, Howard RM, Mancini AJ, et al. Kwashiorkor in the United States: fad diets, perceived and true milk allergy, and nutritional ignorance. *Arch Dermatol.* 2001;137:630–636.

37 Carvalho NF, Kenney RD, Carrington PH, Hall DE. Severe nutritional deficiencies in toddlers resulting from health food milk alternatives. *Pediatrics.* 2001;107:E46.

38 Hoffer JJ. Metabolic consequences of starvation. In: Shils ME, Olson JA, Shike M, Ross AC, eds. *Modern Nutrition in Health and Disease.* 9th ed. Philadelphia: Lippincott Williams & Wilkins; 1999:645–665.

39 Ibid.

40 Itoh R, Nishiyama N, Suyama Y. Dietary protein intake and urinary excretion of calcium: a cross-sectional study in a healthy Japanese population. *Am J Clin Nutr.* 1998;67: 438–444.

41 Rolland-Cachera MR, Deheeger M, Bellisle F. Nutrient balance and body composition. *Reprod Nutr Dev.* 1997;37:727–734; and Schwartz M, Seeley RJ. The new biology of body weight regulation. *J Am Diet Assoc.* 1997;97:54–58.

42 Parizkova J, Rolland-Cachera MF. High proteins early in life as a predisposition for later obesity and further health risks. *Nutrition.* 1997;13:818–819.

43 Sirtori CR, Lovati MR. Soy proteins and cardiovascular disease. *Curr Atheroscler Rep.* 2001;3:47–53.

44 Friedman M, Brandon DL. Nutritional and health benefits of soy proteins. *J Agric Food Chem.* 2001;49:1069–1086.

45 Norat T, Riboli E. Meat consumption and colorectal cancer: a review of epidemiologic evidence. *Nutr Rev.* 2001;59:37–47.

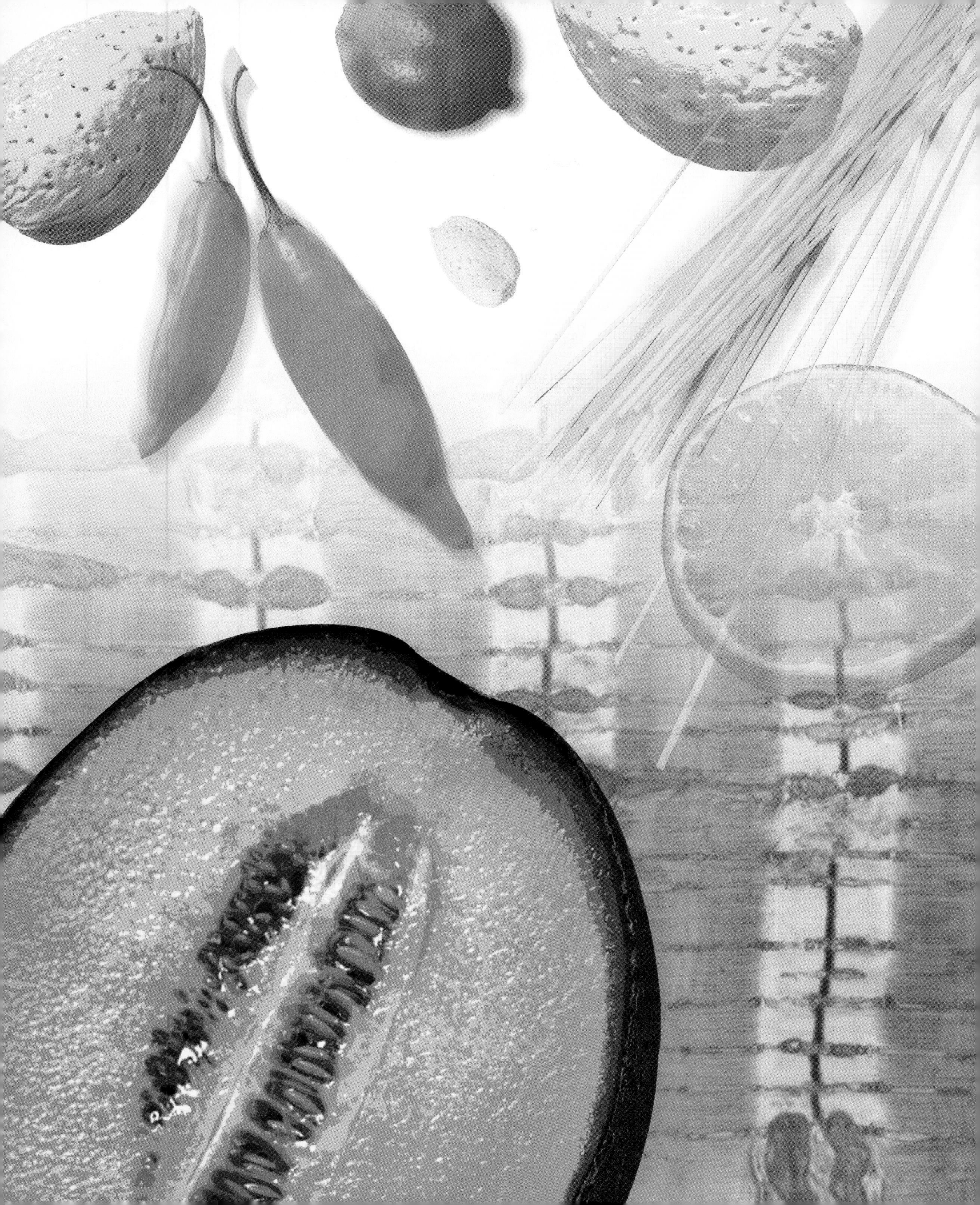

Spotlight on Metabolism

Think About It

1. You are driving on "the energy highway." You stop at the tollbooth. What kind of currency do you need to pay the toll?
2. When you think of "cell power," what comes to mind?
3. What do you think is meant by the saying "Fat burns in a flame of carbohydrate"?
4. When it comes to fasting, what's your body's first priority?

Fyi for your Information

This chapter's FYI box includes practical information on the following topic:
- Do Carbohydrates Turn into Fat?

WWW

The Web site for this book offers many useful tools and is a great source for additional nutrition information for both students and instructors. For information on metabolism, visit the site at **nutrition.jbpub.com/discovering.** You'll find exercises that explore the following topics:
- Mitochondria Malfunctions
- Deadly Dinitrophenol
- The Ketosis Diet
- The Citric Acid Cycle (Krebs Cycle)

Key to Illustrations

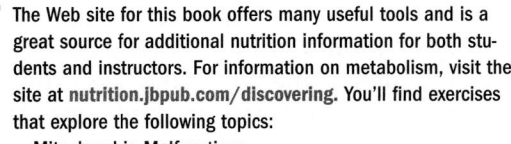

- Amino Acids
- Carbohydrates
- Carbon Dioxide (CO_2)
- Energy
- Fatty Acid
- Fructose
- Galactose
- Glucose
- Glycerol
- Proteins
- Triglyceride

What About Bobbie?

Track the choices Bobbie is making with the EatRight Analysis software.

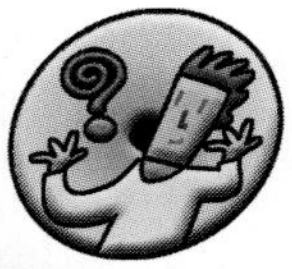

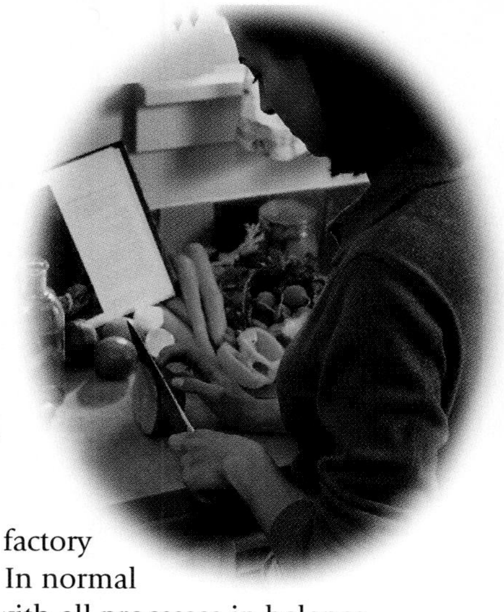

Your body is a wonderfully efficient factory. It accepts raw materials (food), burns some to generate power, uses some to produce finished goods, routes the rest to storage, and discards waste and byproducts. Constant turnover keeps your stored inventory fresh. Your body draws on stored raw materials to produce compounds, and nutrient intake replenishes the supply.

Do you ever wonder how your biological factory responds to changing supply and demand? In normal circumstances, it is humming along nicely with all processes in balance. When supply exceeds demand, your body stores excess raw materials in inventory. When supply fails to meet demand, your body draws on these stored materials to meet its needs. Your biological factory never stops, and even though a storage or energy-production process may dominate, all your factory operations are active at all times.

Collectively, we call these processes **metabolism**. (See **Figure SM.1**.) While some metabolic reactions break down molecules to extract energy, others synthesize building blocks to produce new molecules. To carry out metabolic processes, thousands of chemical reactions occur every moment in cells throughout your body. The most active metabolic sites include your liver and muscle cells.

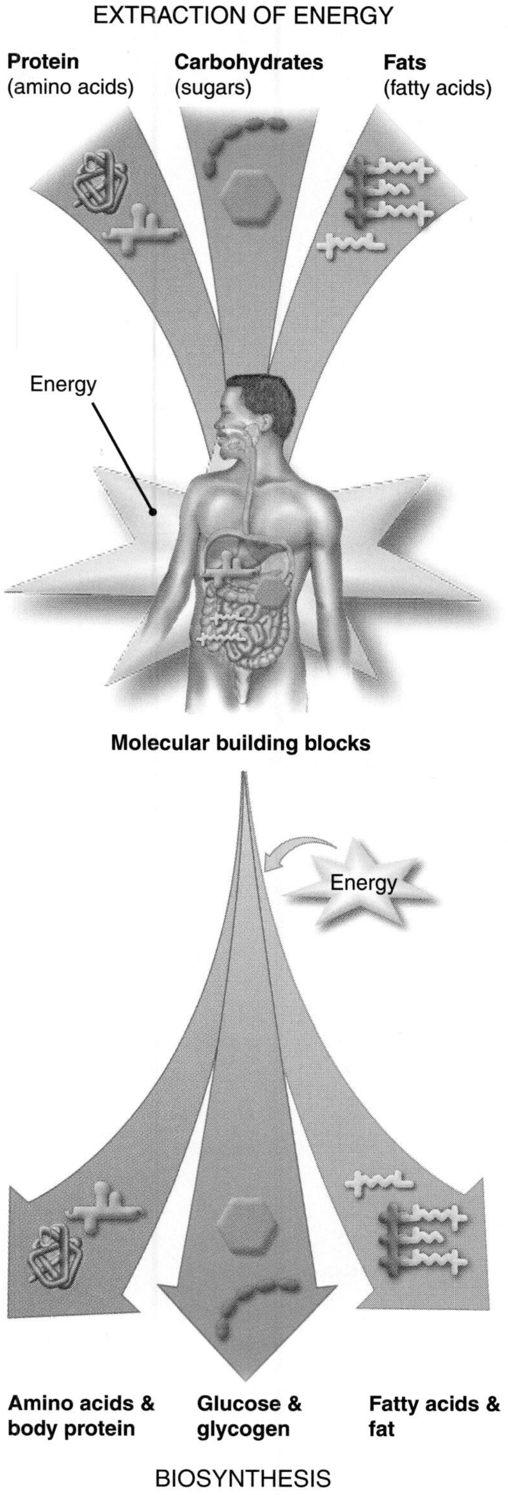

Figure SM.1 **Metabolism.** Cells use metabolic reactions to extract energy from food and to form building blocks for biosynthesis.

Energy: Fuel for Work

To operate, machines need energy. Cars use gasoline for fuel, factory machinery uses electricity, and windmills rely on wind power. So what about you? All cells require energy to sustain life. Even during sleep your body uses energy for breathing, pumping blood, maintaining body temperature, delivering oxygen to tissues, removing waste products, synthesizing new tissue for growth, and repairing damaged or worn-out tissues. When awake, you need additional energy for physical movement (such as standing, walking, talking) and for the digestion and absorption of foods.

Where does the energy come from to power your body's "machinery"? Our cells get their energy from **chemical energy** held in the molecular bonds of carbohydrates, fats, and protein—the energy nutrients—as well as alcohol.[1] This chemical energy originates as light energy from the sun. Green plants use light energy to make carbohydrate in a process called **photosynthesis**. In photosynthesis, carbon dioxide (CO_2) from the air combines with water (H_2O) from the earth to form a carbohydrate, usually glucose ($C_6H_{12}O_6$), and oxygen (O_2). Plants store glucose as starch and release oxygen into the atmosphere. Plants like corn, peas, squash, turnips, potatoes, and rice store especially high amounts of starch in their edible parts. When our bodies extract energy from food and convert it to a form that our cells can use, we lose roughly half of the total food energy as heat.[2]

Transferring Food Energy to Cellular Energy

Our bodies extract energy from food in three stages (see **Figure SM.2**):

Stage 1: Digestion, absorption, and transport. Digestion breaks food down into small subunits—simple sugars, fatty acids, monoglycerides, glycerol, and amino acids—that the small intestine can

absorb. The circulatory system then transports these nutrients to tissues throughout the body.

Stage 2: Breakdown of many small molecules to a few key metabolites. Inside individual cells, chemical reactions convert simple sugars, fatty acids, glycerol, and amino acids to a few key **metabolites** (products of metabolic reactions). This process liberates a small amount of usable energy.

Stage 3: Transfer of energy to a form that cells can use. The complete breakdown of metabolites to carbon dioxide and water liberates large amounts of energy. The reactions during this stage are responsible for converting more than 90 percent of the available food energy to a form of energy our bodies can use.

metabolism All chemical reactions within organisms that enable them to maintain life. The two main categories of metabolism are catabolism and anabolism.

chemical energy Energy contained in the bonds between atoms of a molecule.

photosynthesis The process by which green plants use light energy from the sun to produce carbohydrates from carbon dioxide and water.

metabolites Substances produced during metabolism.

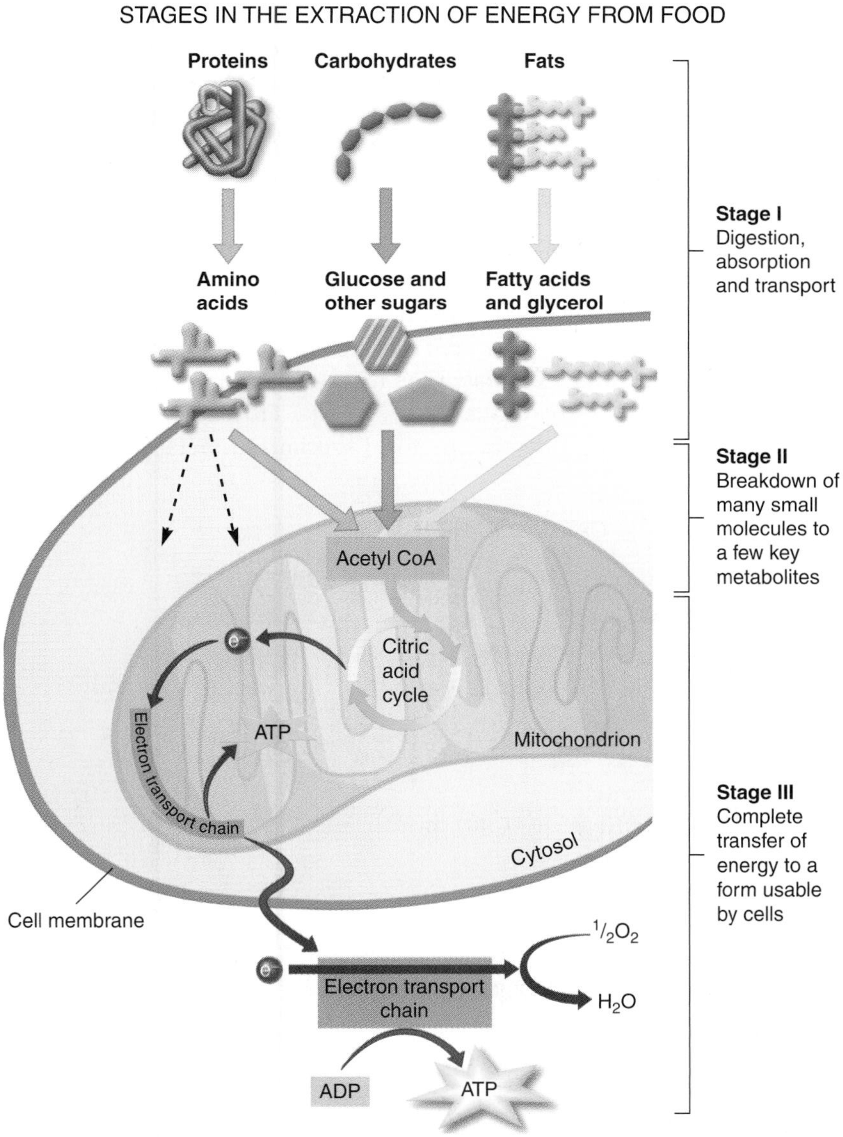

Figure SM.2 **Energy extraction from food.** In the first stage, the body breaks down food into amino acids, sugars, and fatty acids. In the second stage, cells degrade these molecules to a few simple units, such as acetyl CoA, that are widespread in metabolism. In the third stage, the oxygen-dependent reactions of the citric acid cycle and electron transport chain liberate large amounts of energy in the form of ATP.

What Is Metabolism?

Metabolism is a general term that encompasses all chemical changes occurring in living organisms. The term **metabolic pathway** describes a series of chemical reactions that either break down a large compound into smaller units (**catabolism**) or build more complex molecules from smaller ones (**anabolism**).[3] For example, when you eat bread or rice, the GI tract breaks down the starch into glucose units. Cells can further catabolize these glucose units to release energy for activities such as muscle contractions. On the other hand, anabolic reactions take available glucose molecules and assemble them into glycogen for storage. (See **Figure SM.3**.)

Metabolic pathways are never completely inactive. Their activity continually ebbs and flows in response to internal and external events. Imagine, for example, that your instructor keeps you late and you have only five minutes to get to your next class. As you hustle across campus, your body ramps up energy production to fuel the demand created by your rapidly contracting muscles. As you sit in your next class, your body continues to break down and extract glucose from the banana you recently ate. Your body assembles the glucose into branched chains to replenish the glycogen stores you depleted running across campus.

The Cell Is the Metabolic Processing Center

Cells are the "work centers" of metabolism. (See **Figure SM.4**.) Although our bodies are made up of different types of cells (e.g., liver cells, brain cells, kidney cells, muscle cells), most have a similar structure. The basic animal cell has two major parts—the cell **nucleus** and a membrane-enclosed space called the **cytoplasm**. As we zoom in for a closer look, we see that the semifluid **cytosol** fills the cytoplasm. Floating in the cytosol are many **organelles**, small units that perform specialized metabolic functions.

metabolic pathway A series of chemical reactions that either break down a large compound into smaller units (catabolism) or synthesize more complex molecules from smaller ones (anabolism).

catabolism [ca-TA-bol-iz-um] Any metabolic process whereby cells break down complex substances into simpler, smaller ones.

anabolism [an-A-bol-iz-um] Any metabolic process whereby cells build complex substances from simple, smaller units.

cells The basic structural units of all living tissues. Cells have two major parts—the nucleus and cytoplasm.

nucleus The primary site of genetic information in the cell, enclosed in a double-layered membrane.

cytoplasm The cytoplasm is the material of the cell, excluding the cell nucleus and cell membranes. The cytoplasm includes the semifluid cytosol, the organelles, and other particles.

cytosol The semifluid inside the cell membrane, excluding organelles. The cytosol is the site of glycolysis and fatty acid synthesis.

organelles Various membrane-bound structures that form part of the cytoplasm. Organelles perform specialized metabolic functions.

mitochondria (mitochondrion) The sites of aerobic production of ATP, where most of the energy from carbohydrate, protein, and fat is captured. Called the "power plants" of the cell, the mitochondria are where the citric acid cycle and electron transport chain are located. A human cell contains about 2,000 mitochondria.

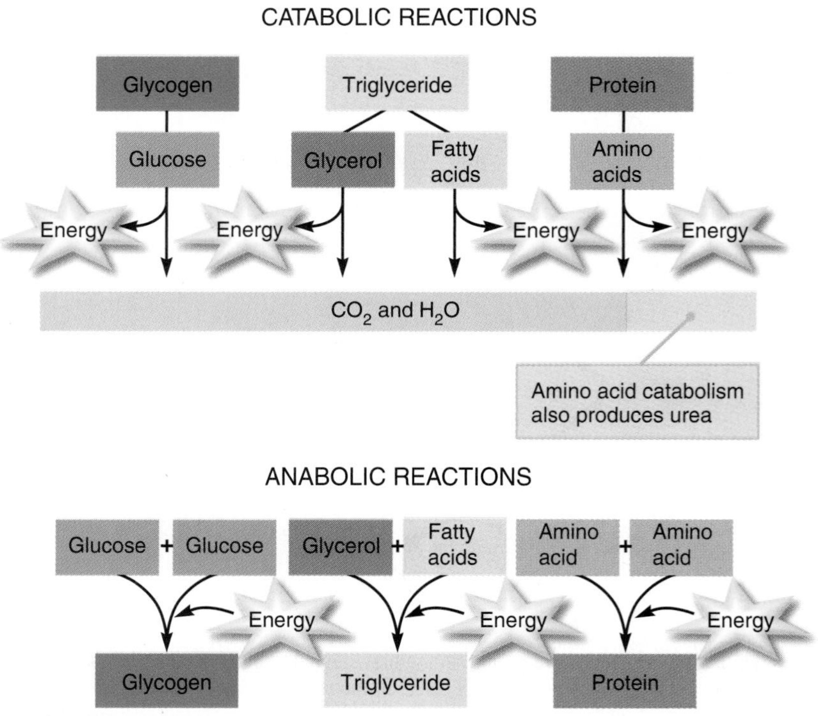

Figure SM.3 **Catabolism and anabolism.** Catabolic reactions break down molecules and release energy. Anabolic reactions consume energy as they assemble complex molecules.

A large number of these—the capsulelike **mitochondria**—are power generators that contain many important energy-producing pathways.

To remember the major parts of a cell, think about a bowl of thick vegetable soup with a single meatball floating in it. For our example, think of the broth as having a runny, jellylike consistency. The bowl surrounds and holds the mixture, similar to the way a cell membrane encloses a cell. The meatball represents the cell nucleus, and the remaining mixture is the cytoplasm. This cytoplasmic soup is made up of a thick, semiliquid fluid (cytosol) and vegetables (organelles). Among the vegetables, think of those kidney beans as mitochondria.

Organelles

Endoplasmic reticulum (ER)
- An extensive membrane system extending from the nuclear membrane.
- Rough ER: The outer membrane surface contains ribosomes. protein synthesis
- Smooth ER: Devoid of ribosomes, the site of lipid synthesis.

Golgi apparatus
- A system of stacked membrane-encased discs.
- The site of extensive modification, sorting, and packaging of compounds for transport.

Lysosome
- Vesicle containing enzymes that digest intracellular materials and recycle the components.

Mitochondrion
- Contains two highly specialized membranes, an outer membrane and a highly folded inner membrane. Membranes are separated by narrow intermembrane space. Inner membrane encloses space called mitochondrial matrix.
- Often called the power plant of the cell. Site where most of the energy from carbohydrate, protein, and fat is captured in ATP (adenosine triphosphate).
- About 2,000 mitochondria in a cell.

Ribosome
- Site of protein synthesis.

Nucleus
- Contains genetic information in the DNA of chromosomes.
- Site of RNA synthesis — RNA needed for protein synthesis.
- Enclosed in a double-layered membrane.

Cytoplasm
- Enclosed in the cell membrane and separated from the nucleus by the nuclear membrane.
- Filled with particles and organelles which are dispersed in a clear semi fluid called cytosol.

Cytosol
- The semifluid inside the cell membrane.
- Site of glycolysis and fatty acid synthesis.

Cell Membrane
- A double-layered sheet, made up of lipid and protein, that encases the cell.
- Controls the passage of substances in and out of the cell.
- Contains receptors for hormones and other regulatory compounds.

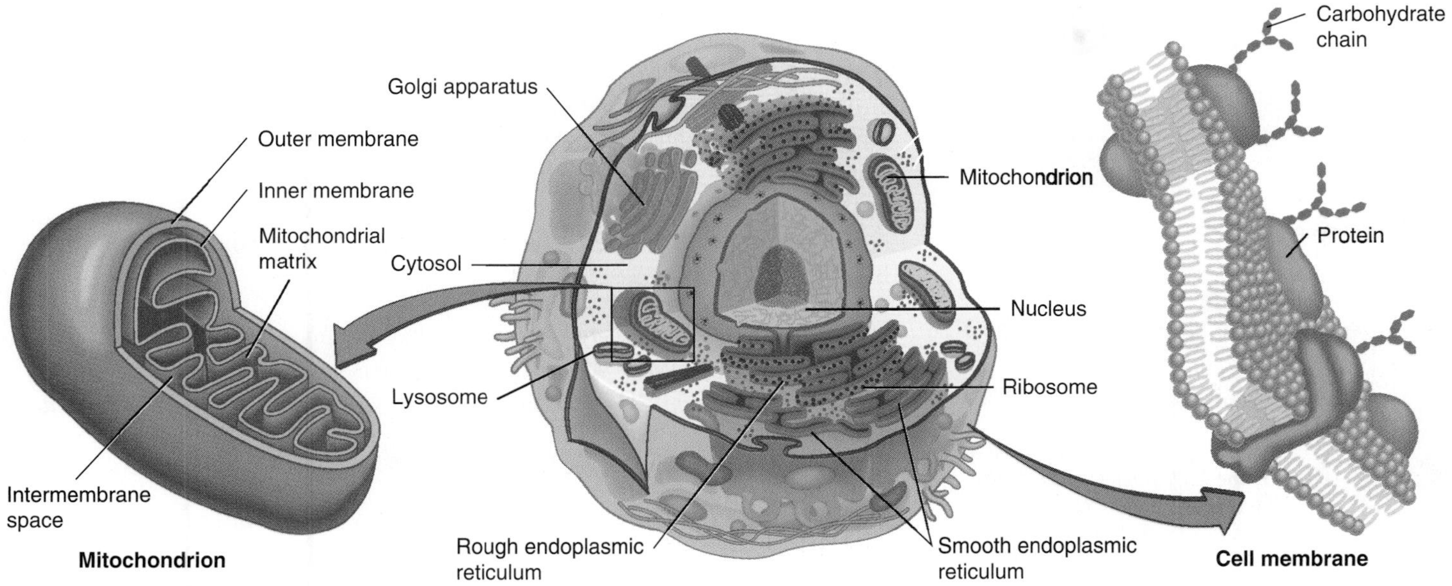

Figure SM.4 **Cell structure.** Liver cells, brain cells, kidney cells, muscle cells, and so forth, all have a similar structure.

cofactors Compounds required for an enzyme to be active. Cofactors include coenzymes and metal ions such as iron, copper, and magnesium.

coenzymes Organic compounds, often derived from B vitamins, that combine with inactive enzymes to form active enzymes.

ATP (adenosine triphosphate) [ah-DEN-oh-seen try-FOS-fate] A high-energy compound composed of adenosine and three phosphate groups. ATP is the main direct fuel that cells use to synthesize molecules, contract muscles, transport substances, and perform other tasks. Breaking down ATP to adenosine diphosphate (ADP) releases energy, and forming ATP from ADP captures energy.

ADP (adenosine diphosphate) [ah-DEN-oh-seen di-FOS-fate] A molecule composed of adenosine and two phosphate groups.

NAD^+/NADH Nicotinamide adenine dinucleotide (NAD^+), a coenzyme derived from the B vitamin niacin, becomes NADH as it accepts a pair of high-energy electrons for transport in cells.

FAD/$FADH_2$ Flavin adenine dinucleotide (FAD), a coenzyme derived from the B vitamin riboflavin, becomes $FADH_2$ as it accepts a pair of high-energy electrons for transport in cells.

Enzymes speed up chemical reactions in metabolic pathways. Many enzymes are inactive unless combined with certain smaller molecules called **cofactors**, which usually are derived from a vitamin or mineral. Vitamin-derived cofactors are also called **coenzymes**. All the B vitamins form coenzymes used in metabolic reactions. (For more on coenzymes see Chapter 9, "Vitamins.")

Key Concepts: *Metabolism refers to the many reactions that take place in cells to build tissue, produce energy, break down compounds, and do other cellular work. Anabolism refers to reactions that build compounds, such as protein or glycogen. Catabolism is the breakdown of compounds to yield energy. Mitochondria, the power plants within cells, contain many of the breakdown pathways that produce energy.*

ATP: The Body's Energy Currency

To power its needs, your body must convert the energy in food to a readily usable form called **adenosine triphosphate (ATP)**. (See **Figure SM.5**.) Cells can break one of the high-energy bonds in an ATP molecule to release usable energy. This converts high-energy ATP to lower-energy **adenosine diphosphate (ADP)**. ATP is the body's universal energy currency that kick-starts many energy-releasing processes, such as the breakdown of glucose and fatty acids, and powers energy-consuming processes, such as the building of glycogen from glucose. Remember that making large molecules from smaller ones (anabolism), like constructing a building from bricks, requires energy.

Think About It 1

Production of ATP is the fundamental goal of metabolism's energy-producing pathways. Just as the ancient Romans could claim that all roads lead to Rome, you can say that, with a few exceptions, your body's energy-producing pathways lead to ATP production.

The body's pool of ATP is a small, immediately accessible energy reservoir rather than a long-term energy reserve. The typical lifetime of an ATP molecule is less than one minute, and ATP production increases or decreases in direct relation to energy needs. At rest, you use about 40 kilograms of ATP in 24 hours (an average rate of about 28 grams per minute). In contrast, if you are exercising strenuously, you can use as much as 500 grams per minute! On average, you turn over your body weight in ATP every day.[4]

NAD^+ and FAD: The Body's Transport Shuttles

During the breakdown of carbohydrate, fat, protein, and alcohol, the body's transport shuttles, **NAD^+** and **FAD**, accept pairs of high-energy electrons and transport them to ATP production sites. (See **Figure SM.6**.) When the empty shuttle molecules (NAD^+ and FAD) pick up their high-energy electron cargo, they also pick up hydrogen and become NADH + H^+ and $FADH_2$. These shuttle molecules highlight the importance of B vitamins. NAD^+ is derived from the B vitamin niacin, and FAD is derived from the B vitamin riboflavin.

Key Concepts: *ATP is the energy currency of the body. Your body extracts energy from food to produce ATP. As energy-yielding compounds break down, the shuttle molecules NAD^+ and FAD transport high-energy electrons to ATP production sites.*

Breakdown and Release of Energy

Bang! The starter's gun echoes in your ears as you leap out of the blocks. With legs pumping, you race to the finish 200 meters away. As you cross the finish line, you congratulate yourself on your best race yet.

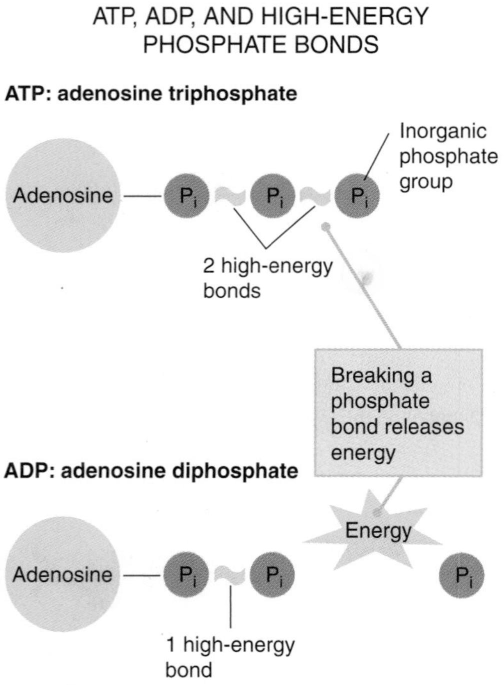

Figure SM.5 **ATP and ADP.** When extracting energy from nutrients, the formation of ATP from ADP + P_i captures energy. Breaking a phosphate bond in ATP to form ADP + P_i releases energy for biosynthesis and work.

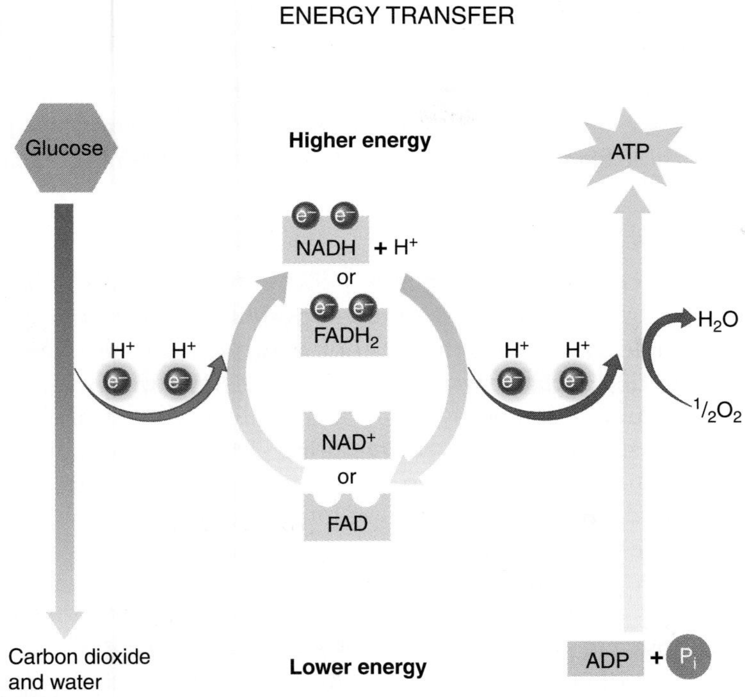

Figure SM.6 **Energy transfer.** As energy moves from glucose to ATP, molecules become high-energy or low-energy as they collect and transfer high-energy electrons and hydrogen ions.

Where did the energy come from to power your muscles at peak effort? Your stores of readily available ATP are used up within the first few seconds. To power the remainder of the race, **anaerobic** reactions (reactions that do not require oxygen) partially break down glucose. Needy cells gobble up glucose and rapidly pour out ATP. Although partial breakdown produces only a small amount of ATP per glucose molecule, it is extremely fast and powers maximal effort for short events.

Bang! The starter's gun signals the beginning of the marathon and you commence running at a moderate pace. For 26 miles, your feet pound the pavement over and over again. Rather than sprinting, you settle into a rhythm. The minutes and hours pass as you maintain your steady pace until reaching the finish.

While anaerobic reactions can power a short, maximal burst of energy for a sprint, they cannot fuel a prolonged event. To sustain muscle contractions during endurance events, **aerobic** reactions (reactions that require oxygen) complete the breakdown of glucose. These aerobic pathways also extract energy from fat and a bit of protein. Compared with anaerobic energy production, aerobic metabolism produces much more energy but at a slower, more easily maintained rate. Anaerobic metabolism may be fast, but for a single glucose molecule, complete aerobic breakdown produces more than 15 times as much ATP.

Although different pathways initiate the breakdown of carbohydrate, fat, and protein, complete breakdown of these nutrients eventually proceeds along two shared catabolic pathways—the citric acid cycle and the electron transport chain. The next section first describes the pathways that catabolize glucose. Then it discusses the breakdown of fat and protein.

anaerobic [AN-ah-ROW-bic] Referring to the absence of oxygen or the ability of a process to occur in the absence of oxygen. Glycolysis is an anaerobic pathway.

aerobic [air-ROW-bic] Referring to the presence of or need for oxygen. The complete breakdown of glucose, fatty acids, and amino acids to carbon dioxide and water occurs only via aerobic metabolism. The citric acid cycle and electron transport chain are aerobic pathways.

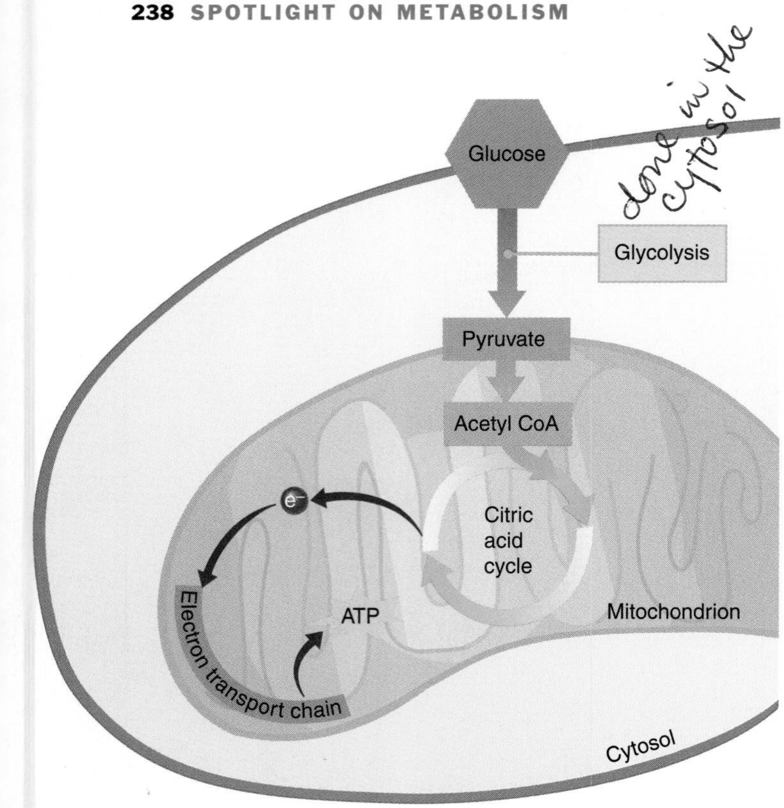

Figure SM.7 **Obtaining energy from carbohydrate.** The complete breakdown of glucose uses four major metabolic pathways: glycolysis, pyruvate to acetyl CoA, the citric acid cycle, and the electron transport chain. Glycolysis takes place in the cytosol of the cell. The remaining reactions take place in the mitochondria.

glycolysis [gligh-COLL-ih-sis] The anaerobic pathway that breaks down a glucose molecule into two molecules of pyruvate and yields two molecules of ATP and two molecules of NADH. Glycolysis occurs in the cytosol of a cell.

pyruvate The three-carbon compound that results from glycolysis. Cells also can make glucose from pyruvate, but this process requires energy and several enzymes not involved in glycolysis. Pyruvate also can be derived from glycerol and some amino acids.

acetyl CoA A key intermediate product in the metabolic breakdown of carbohydrates, fatty acids, and amino acids. It consists of a two-carbon acetate group linked to coenzyme A, which is derived from pantothenic acid.

coenzyme A Coenzyme A is a cofactor derived from the vitamin pantothenic acid.

lactate A three-carbon compound that is produced when insufficient oxygen is present in cells to break down pyruvate to acetyl CoA. Often called lactic acid.

oxaloacetate A four-carbon intermediate compound in the citric acid cycle. Acetyl CoA combines with free oxaloacetate in the mitochondria, forming citric acid and beginning the cycle.

Extracting Energy from Carbohydrate

Cells extract usable energy from carbohydrate via four main pathways: glycolysis, pyruvate to acetyl CoA, the citric acid cycle, and the electron transport chain. (See **Figure SM.7**.) Of these four pathways, the electron transport chain is the major ATP production site.

Glycolysis

Glycolysis (glucose splitting) does not require oxygen. In the cytosol, this sequence of reactions splits one six-carbon glucose molecule into two three-carbon **pyruvate** molecules while producing a relatively small amount of energy. Just as a pump requires priming, glycolysis requires the input of two ATP to get started. Using several reactions, glycolysis then transfers high-energy electrons to NAD^+ shuttle molecules and produces four ATP. Finally, it forms two pyruvate molecules. (See **Figure SM.8**.)

What about the other simple sugars, fructose and galactose? In liver cells, glycolysis also breaks them down.[5] Although fructose and galactose enter glycolysis at intermediate points, the breakdown of each sugar yields the same results as the breakdown of glucose.

Once glycolysis is complete, the two pyruvate molecules easily pass from the cytosol to the interior of mitochondria, the cell's power generators, for further processing.

Pyruvate to Acetyl CoA

When a cell requires energy, and oxygen is readily available, an aerobic reaction in the mitochondria converts each pyruvate molecule to an **acetyl CoA** molecule and transfers a pair of high-energy electrons to an NAD^+ shuttle. (See **Figure SM.9**.) The shuttle carries the electrons to the electron transport chain. To form acetyl CoA, reactions remove one carbon from the three-carbon pyruvate and add **coenzyme A**, a molecule derived from the B vitamin pantothenic acid. After combining with oxygen, the carbon is released as part of carbon dioxide. Remember that glycolysis splits glucose into two pyruvate molecules, so we now have two acetyl CoA molecules.

While many metabolic pathways can proceed forward or backward, the formation of acetyl CoA is a one-way (irreversible) process. Although pyruvate passes easily between the cytosol and the mitochondria, acetyl CoA cannot penetrate the mitochondrial membrane, so it is trapped inside the mitochondria, poised to enter the citric acid cycle.

In rapidly contracting muscle, such as those propelling you to the finish of your 200-meter sprint, oxygen is in short supply, and pyruvate cannot form acetyl CoA. Instead, pyruvate is rerouted to form **lactate**, another three-carbon compound. Lactate is an alternative fuel that muscle cells can use or that liver cells can convert to glucose. When oxygen again becomes readily available, lactate converts back to pyruvate, which irreversibly forms acetyl CoA. You will learn more about lactate production, cycling, and use in Chapter 11, "Sports Nutrition."

Citric Acid Cycle

A series of reactions completes the breakdown of acetyl CoA. In the first reaction, **oxaloacetate** reacts with acetyl CoA to form citric acid. The final reaction forms new oxaloacetate, bringing us back to the starting point.

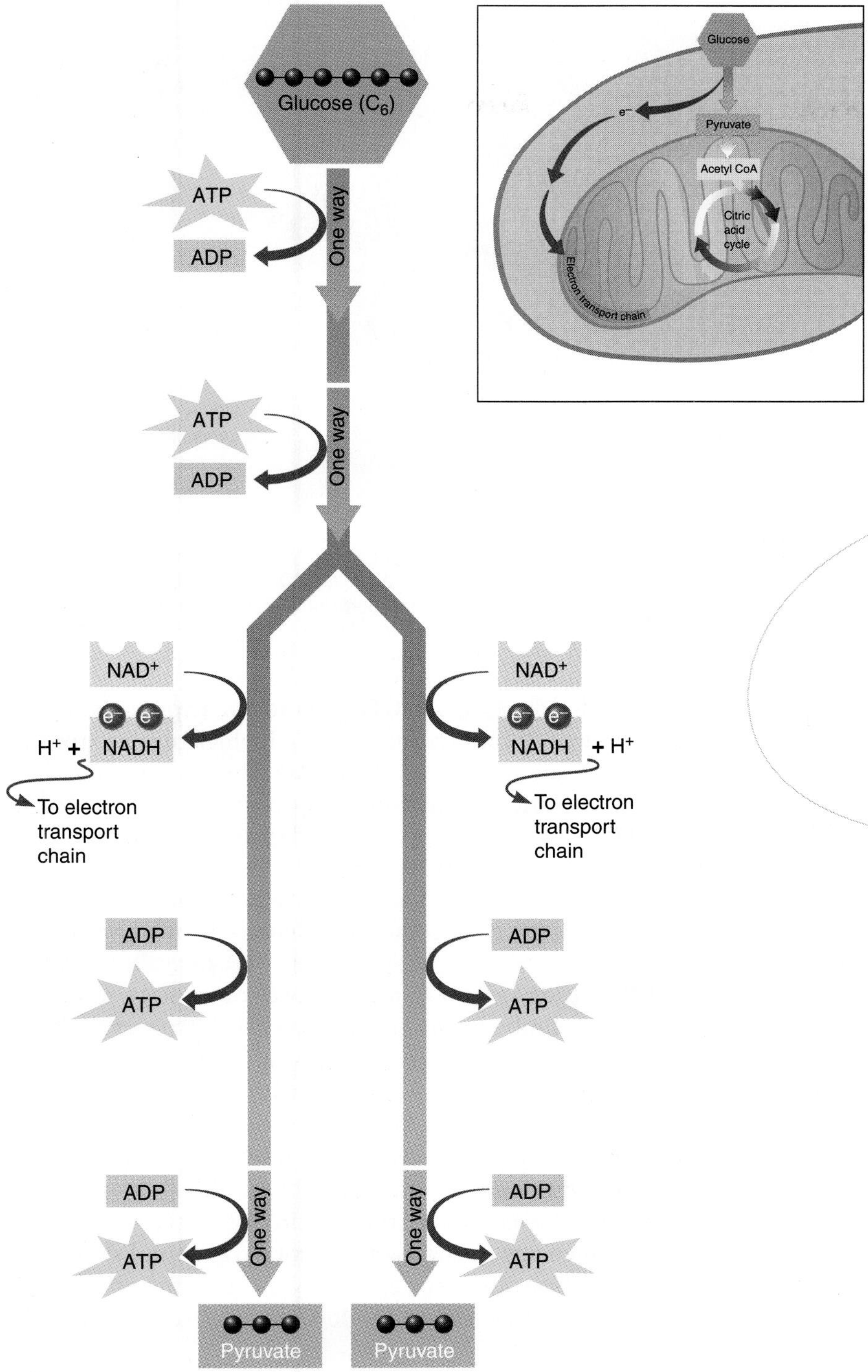

Figure SM.8 **Glycolysis.** The breakdown of one glucose molecule yields two pyruvate molecules, a net of two ATP and two NADH molecules. The two NADH molecules shuttle pairs of high-energy electrons to the electron transport chain for ATP production. Glycolytic reactions do not require oxygen, and some steps are irreversible.

Quick Bites

When Glycolysis Goes Awry

Red blood cells do not have mitochondria, so they rely on glycolysis as their only source of ATP. They use ATP to maintain the integrity and shape of their cell membranes. A defect in red blood cell glycolysis can cause a shortage of ATP, which leads to deformed red blood cells. Destruction of these cells by the spleen leads to a type of anemia called hemolytic anemia.

citric acid cycle The aerobic metabolic pathway in mitochondria that breaks down acetyl CoA to yield two molecules of carbon dioxide, one molecule of GTP, and pairs of high-energy electrons. It transfers the electrons to three molecules of NAD^+ (yielding three NADH) and one molecule of FAD (yielding one $FADH_2$). Also known as the Krebs cycle and tricarboxylic acid cycle.

Since the reactions first form citric acid and eventually come full circle, they are known as the **citric acid cycle**.

To begin the citric acid cycle, acetyl CoA combines with oxaloacetate to form citric acid and release coenzyme A. Subsequent reactions release two carbon atoms that combine with oxygen to form carbon dioxide. Reactions

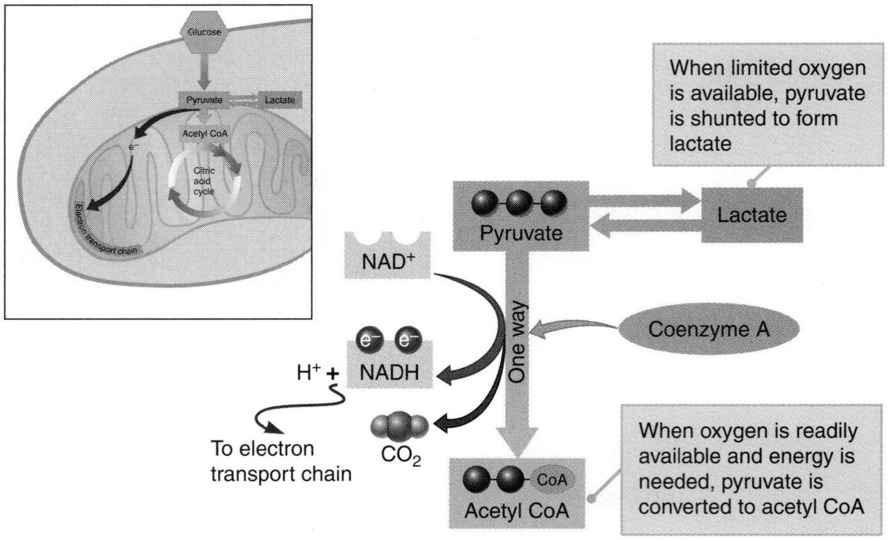

Figure SM.9 **Pyruvate to acetyl CoA.** When oxygen is readily available, each pyruvate formed from glucose yields one acetyl CoA and one NADH. The NADH shuttles high-energy electrons to the electron transport chain for ATP production.

of the citric acid cycle also produce one **GTP (guanosine triphosphate)**, which readily converts to ATP, and transfer pairs of high-energy electrons to three molecules of NAD^+ and one molecule of FAD. The final reaction regenerates oxaloacetate. Since the breakdown of one glucose molecule produces two acetyl CoA molecules, the citric acid cycle will make two complete "turns"—one for each acetyl CoA.

To help visualize the citric acid cycle, think of a merry-go-round at an amusement park. This is a special ride that completes only one revolution per rider and on which the ticket agent rides along. Acetyl CoA is the rider, and oxaloacetate is the ticket agent. Oxaloacetate welcomes acetyl CoA and, hand-in-hand, they climb aboard. Acetyl CoA's ticket (coenzyme A) is dropped into the recycling box. As the merry-go-round whirls by, two NAD^+ shuttles swoop in and grab pairs of high-energy electrons as two carbons combine with oxygen and fly off the ride as carbon dioxide molecules. Who is that jumping off in mid-cycle? Why it's GTP, a molecule similar to ATP. An FAD shuttle swoops in and grabs another pair of high-energy electrons. Nearing the end of the ride, a third NAD^+ shuttle departs with a final pair of high-energy electrons. As the merry-go-round slows to a stop, a new oxaloacetate beckons to the next acetyl CoA waiting in line. The cycle is ready to begin again. **Figure SM.10** shows an overview of the citric acid cycle.

The citric acid cycle also is an important source of building blocks for the **biosynthesis** of amino acids and fatty acids. Many of the cycle's intermediate molecules may be used for biosynthesis rather than the completion of the cycle. For example, oxaloacetate may be converted to glucose or to amino acids for protein synthesis.

Electron Transport Chain

The final step in glucose breakdown is a sequence of linked reactions that take place in the **electron transport chain**, which is located in the inner **mitochondrial membrane**. Most ATP is produced here, and the outpouring of energy can fuel exercise for hours, such as during your marathon

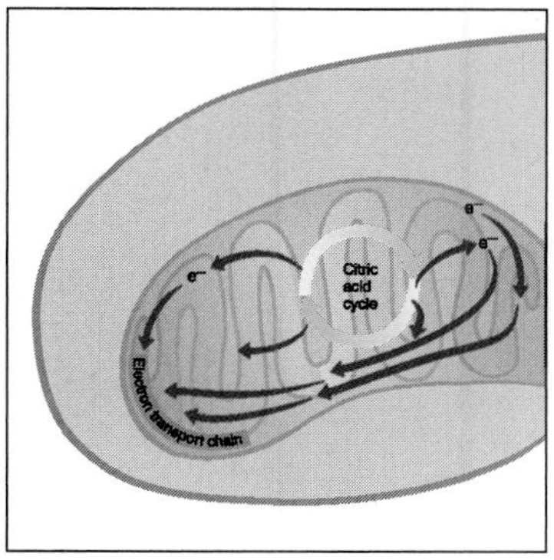

Figure SM.10 **The citric acid cycle.** This circular pathway accepts one acetyl CoA and yields two CO_2, three NADH, one $FADH_2$ and one GTP (readily converted to ATP). The electron shuttles NADH and $FADH_2$ carry high-energy electrons to the electron transport chain for ATP production.

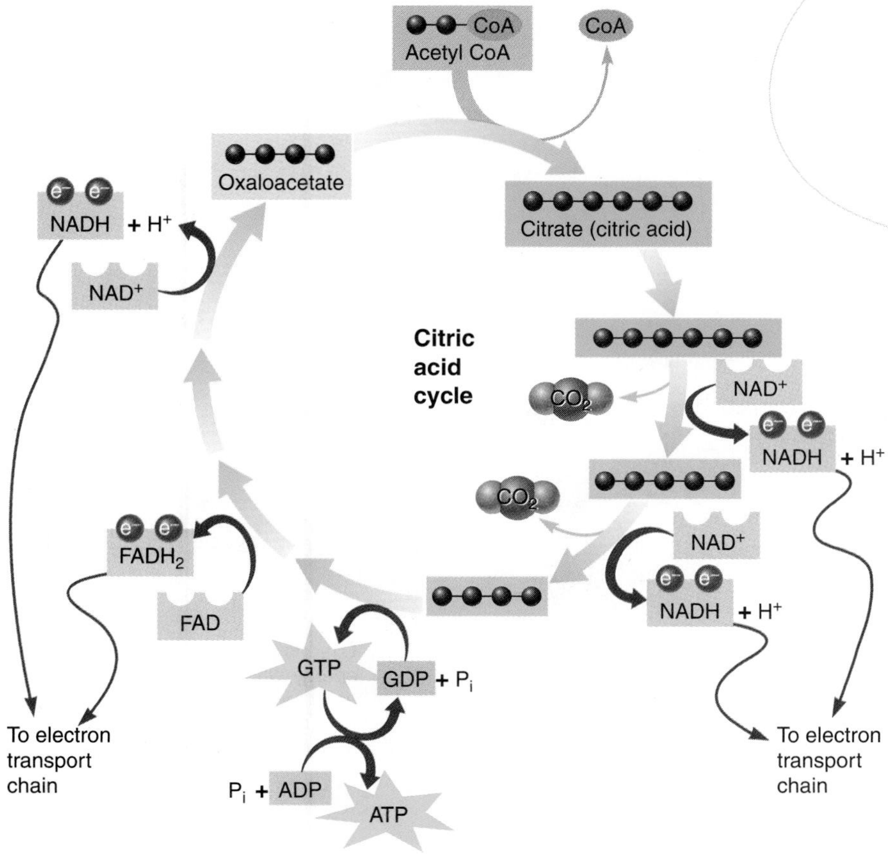

Quick Bites

Cycling Down the Same Pathway

The citric acid cycle goes by many names. It may be called the **Krebs cycle** after Sir Hans Krebs, the first scientist to explain its workings, who was awarded the Nobel Prize in 1953 for his work. It also may be called the **tricarboxylic acid cycle (TCA cycle)** because a tricarboxylic acid (citric acid) is formed in the first step. Most nutritionists use the term *citric acid cycle.*

Think About It 2

race. Because the mitochondrion is the site of both the citric acid cycle and the electron transport chain, it truly is the energy power plant of the cell.

When NAD^+ accepts a pair of electrons, it becomes NADH. Similarly, FAD accepts electrons to become $FADH_2$. These shuttle molecules, NADH and $FADH_2$, deliver their cargo of high-energy electrons to the electron transport chain. As the electrons travel along the electron transport chain, they give up energy to power the production of ATP. At the end of the chain, an oxygen "basket" accepts the energy-depleted electrons and combines with hydrogen to form water (H_2O). (See **Figure SM.11**.) Without oxygen, ATP production would stop, halting the supply of power for our body's essential functions. If our oxygen supply is not restored rapidly, we die.

Because each pair of electrons that traverses the electron transport chain produces slightly fewer ATP than once thought, biochemists have revised

Krebs cycle See *citric acid cycle.*

tricarboxylic acid cycle (TCA cycle) See *citric acid cycle.*

GTP (guanosine triphosphate) A high-energy compound, similiar to ATP, but with three phosphate groups linked to guanosine instead of adenosine.

biosynthesis Chemical reactions in which complex biomolecules, especially carbohydrates, lipids, and proteins, are formed from simple molecules.

electron transport chain An organized series of protein carrier molecules located in mitochondrial membranes. As high-energy electrons delivered by NADH and $FADH_2$ traverse the electron transport chain to oxygen, it produces ATP and water.

mitochondrial membrane The mitochondria are enclosed by a double shell separated by an intermembrane space. The outer membrane acts as a barrier and gatekeeper, selectively allowing some molecules to pass through while blocking others. The inner membrane is where the electron transport chain is located.

Figure SM.11 **Electron transport chain.** This pathway produces most of the ATP available from glucose. NADH deliver pairs of high-energy electrons to the beginning of the chain. The pairs of high-energy electrons from $FADH_2$ enter this pathway farther along, so an electron pair carried by $FADH_2$ produces less ATP than a pair carried by NADH. Water is the final product of the electron transport chain.

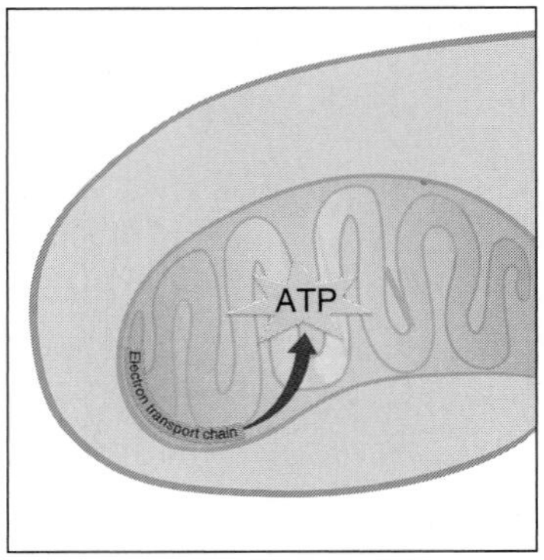

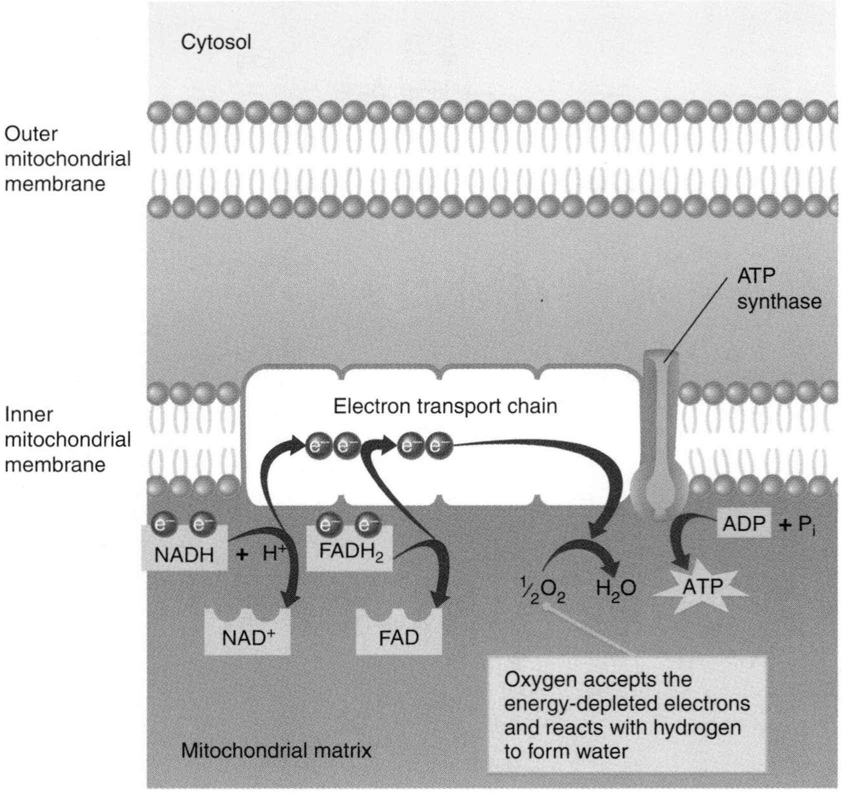

Quick Bites

The Latest ATP Count

The number of ATP (or GTP) formed directly in glycolysis and the citric acid cycle is unequivocally known, but the amount of ATP formed from NADH and $FADH_2$ in the electron transport chain is less certain. Old estimates credited NADH from the citric acid cycle with three ATP and $FADH_2$ with two ATP. The best current estimates are 2.5 and 1.5, respectively. "Hence, about 30 ATP are formed when glucose is completely oxidized to CO_2; this value supersedes the traditional estimate of 36 ATP" (Lubert Stryer, Professor of Biochemistry, Stanford University).

their estimate for the total amount of ATP produced from one glucose molecule. Historically, biologists believed that the complete breakdown of glucose produced 36 to 38 ATP, but the current estimate is 30 to 32 ATP.[6] (See Appendix D to count the number of ATP produced from glucose.)

End Products of Glucose Catabolism

Now you've seen all the steps in glucose breakdown. What has the cell produced from glucose? The end products of complete catabolism are carbon dioxide (CO_2), water (H_2O), and ATP. Both the conversion of pyruvate to acetyl CoA and the citric acid cycle produce CO_2. The electron transport chain produces water. While glycolysis makes small amounts of ATP and the citric acid cycle makes a little GTP, the electron transport chain generates the vast majority of this universal energy currency. **Table SM.1** summarizes the pathways of glucose metabolism.

Table SM.1 Summary of the Major Metabolic Pathways in Glucose Metabolism

Phase	Location	Type	Summary	Starting Materials	End Products
Glycolysis	Cytosol	Anaerobic	A series of reactions that converts one glucose molecule to two pyruvate molecules.	Glucose, ATP	Pyruvate, ATP, NADH
Pyruvate to acetyl CoA	Mitochondria	Aerobic	Pyruvate from glycolysis combines with coenzyme A to form acetyl CoA while releasing carbon dioxide.	Pyruvate, coenzyme A	Acetyl CoA, carbon dioxide, NADH
Citric acid cycle	Mitochondria	Aerobic	This cycle of reactions degrades the acetyl portion of acetyl CoA and releases the coenzyme A portion. This cycle releases carbon dioxide and produces most of the energy-rich molecules, NADH and $FADH_2$, generated by the breakdown of glucose.	Acetyl CoA	Carbon dioxide, NADH, $FADH_2$, GTP
Electron transport chain	Mitochondria (membrane)	Aerobic	As the electrons from NADH and $FADH_2$ pass along this chain of transport proteins, they release energy to power the generation of ATP. Oxygen is the final electron acceptor and combines with hydrogen to form water.	NADH, $FADH_2$	ATP, water

Key Concepts: *Extracting energy from glucose requires several steps. Glycolysis breaks the six-carbon glucose molecule into two pyruvate molecules. After glycolysis the remaining breakdown pathways are traversed twice—once for each pyruvate molecule. Each pyruvate loses a carbon and combines with a coenzyme A to form an acetyl CoA, which then enters the citric acid cycle. Two carbons enter the cycle as part of acetyl CoA, and two carbons leave as part of two carbon dioxide molecules. Finally, the shuttle molecules NADH and $FADH_2$ carry high-energy electrons to the electron transport chain, where ATP and water are produced. When completely oxidized, each glucose molecule yields carbon dioxide, water, and ATP.*

Extracting Energy from Fat

To extract energy from fat, the body first breaks down triglycerides into their component parts, glycerol and fatty acids. Glycerol, a small three-carbon molecule, carries a relatively small amount of energy, and the liver can convert it to pyruvate or glucose. Fatty acids store nearly all the energy found in triglycerides.

The breakdown of fatty acids takes place inside the mitochondria. **Carnitine** has the unique task of ferrying fatty acids across the mitochondrial membrane, from the cytosol to the interior of the mitochondrion. Based on carnitine's role, some people claim carnitine supplements act as "fat burners." Research data show that carnitine supplementation has little or no effect on fatty acid oxidation rates or athletic performance.[7]

carnitine [CAR-nih-teen] A compound that transports fatty acids from the cytosol into the mitochondria, where they undergo beta-oxidation.

beta-oxidation The breakdown of a fatty acid into numerous molecules of the two-carbon compound acetyl coenzyme A (acetyl CoA).

Beta-Oxidation

Once inside a mitochondrion, a process called **beta-oxidation** disassembles the fatty acid chain. Like scissors, enzymes snip the chain into two-carbon "links." Reactions convert each link to acetyl CoA and transfer pairs of high-energy electrons to NAD^+ and FAD shuttles. (See **Figure SM.12.**) These shuttle molecules (now NADH and $FADH_2$) transport their high-energy cargo to the electron transport chain.

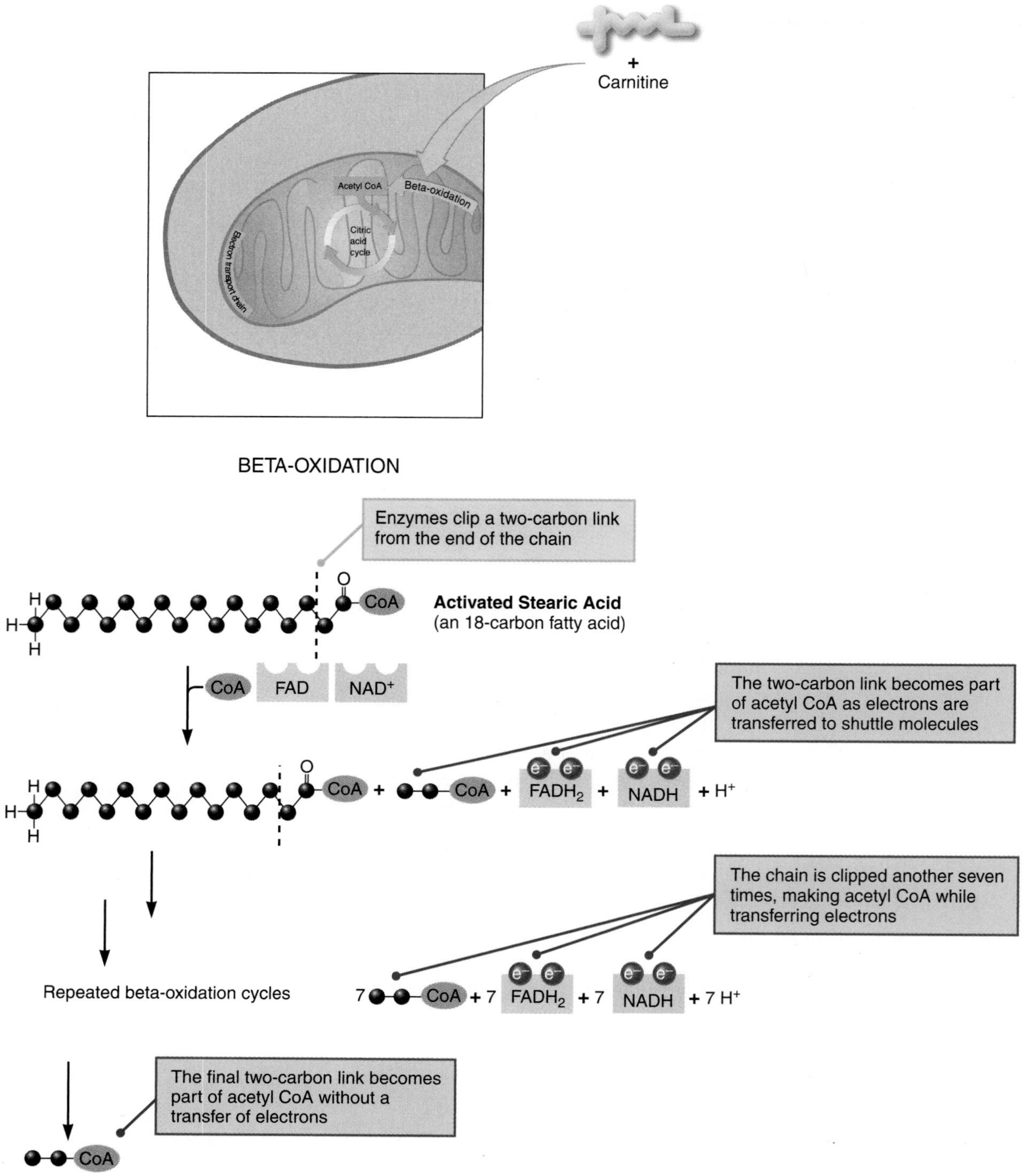
+
Carnitine
Acetyl CoA
Beta-oxidation
Citric acid cycle
Electron transport chain
BETA-OXIDATION
Enzymes clip a two-carbon link from the end of the chain
O
CoA
Activated Stearic Acid
(an 18-carbon fatty acid)
H
CoA
FAD
NAD+
The two-carbon link becomes part of acetyl CoA as electrons are transferred to shuttle molecules
CoA + CoA + FADH2 + NADH + H+
The chain is clipped another seven times, making acetyl CoA while transferring electrons
Repeated beta-oxidation cycles
7 CoA + 7 FADH2 + 7 NADH + 7 H+
The final two-carbon link becomes part of acetyl CoA without a transfer of electrons
CoA

Figure SM.12 **Beta-oxidation.** Beta-oxidation reactions repeatedly clip two carbons from the end of a fatty acid until it is degraded entirely to molecules of acetyl CoA.

Completing Fatty Acid Breakdown

Beta-oxidation of a fatty acid produces a flood of acetyl CoA. The citric acid cycle and electron transport chain complete the extraction of energy from fatty acids. Just as they processed acetyl CoA from glucose, they extract energy from these acetyl CoA molecules and produce ATP.

The end products of fatty acid breakdown are the same as those of glucose breakdown: carbon dioxide, water, and ATP. The exact amount of ATP depends on the length of the fatty acid chain. Longer chains have more carbons. Beta-oxidation of longer chains produces more acetyl CoA and thus more ATP. The complete breakdown of an 18-carbon fatty acid produces 120 ATP. (See Appendix D to count the number of ATP produced from a fatty acid.) Because a fatty acid chain typically contains many more carbon atoms than a molecule of glucose, a single fatty acid produces substantially more ATP. In a single triglyceride with three 18-carbon fatty acids, completely breaking down the fatty acids produces 360 ATP, over 10 times the 30 to 32 ATP from glucose.

Fat Burns in a Flame of Carbohydrate

Acetyl CoA from beta-oxidation can enter the citric acid cycle only when fat and carbohydrate breakdown are synchronized. Without oxaloacetate, acetyl CoA cannot start the citric acid cycle. Conditions like starvation and very-low-carbohydrate diets can deplete oxaloacetate, blocking acetyl CoA from entry. This reroutes the acetyl CoA to form a family of compounds called ketone bodies.

Think About It 3

For fatty acid oxidation to continue efficiently, reactions in the mitochondria help ensure a reliable supply of oxaloacetate. These reactions convert some pyruvate directly to oxaloacetate rather than to acetyl CoA. Since carbohydrate (glucose) is the original source of the pyruvate and, hence, this oxaloacetate, scientists coined the adage "Fat burns in a flame of carbohydrate."

Key Concepts: *Extracting energy from fat involves several steps. First, triglycerides are separated into glycerol and three fatty acids. Glycerol forms pyruvate and can be broken down to yield a small amount of energy. Beta-oxidation breaks down fatty acid chains to two-carbon links that form acetyl CoA, which enters the citric acid cycle. Beta-oxidation and the citric acid cycle transfer electrons to* NAD^+ *and FAD. As NADH and* $FADH_2$*, these shuttle molecules carry high-energy electrons to the electron transport chain, where ATP and water are made. The complete breakdown of a triglyceride yields water, carbon dioxide, and substantially more ATP than one glucose molecule.*

Extracting Energy from Protein

Protein has vital structural and functional roles, so proteins and amino acids are not considered storehouses of energy. However, if energy production falters due to a lack of available carbohydrate and fat, protein comes to the rescue. During starvation, for example, energy needs take priority, so the body breaks down protein and extracts energy from the amino acid building blocks.

Our bodies can't use the nitrogen-containing portion of an amino acid in energy production, so a process called deamination strips down the amino acid to a "carbon skeleton" (see **Figure SM.13**) while producing a nitrogen byproduct that becomes urea. When you eat more protein than you need, your kidneys excrete urea in urine, and your liver uses carbon skeletons to produce energy, glucose, or fat. Much to the dismay of bodybuilders, when they attempt to build muscle by drinking pricey protein drinks, they can end up gaining fat instead!

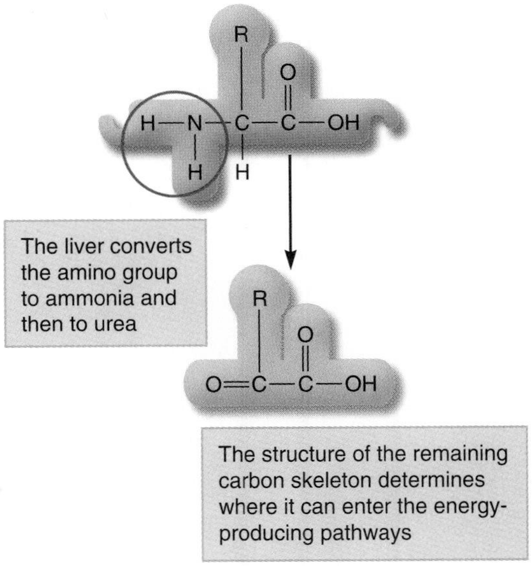
The liver converts the amino group to ammonia and then to urea
The structure of the remaining carbon skeleton determines where it can enter the energy-producing pathways

Figure SM.13 **Deamination.** A deamination reaction strips the amino group from an amino acid.

Carbon Skeletons Enter Pathways at Different Points

Whereas glucose has one main entrance to the breakdown pathways, carbon skeletons from amino acids have several entrance points. Imagine arriving at an amusement park with five entrance gates. The ticket agent hands you a ticket that allows you to enter at your designated gate. Similarly, the structure of an amino acid's carbon skeleton determines which "entrance gate" it uses to enter the breakdown pathways. Some carbon skeletons directly enter the citric acid cycle, others enter at pyruvate, and still others at acetyl CoA.

The complete breakdown of an amino acid yields urea, carbon dioxide, water, and ATP. The carbon skeleton's point of entry to the breakdown pathways determines the amount of ATP it produces. (See **Figure SM.14**.) Whereas the complete breakdown of alanine, for example, produces 12.5 ATP, methionine produces only 5 ATP. Compared with glucose and fatty acids, no amino acid produces much ATP. (See Appendix D to count the number of ATP produced from the amino acids alanine and methionine.)

Key Concepts: *To extract energy from amino acids, cells strip them down to carbon skeletons (deamination). The byproducts become urea, which is removed by the kidneys. The carbon skeleton structure determines where it enters the catabolic pathways. Some carbon skeletons become pyruvate, others become acetyl CoA, and still others become intermediate compounds of the citric acid cycle. Complete breakdown of amino acids yields water, carbon dioxide, urea, and ATP.*

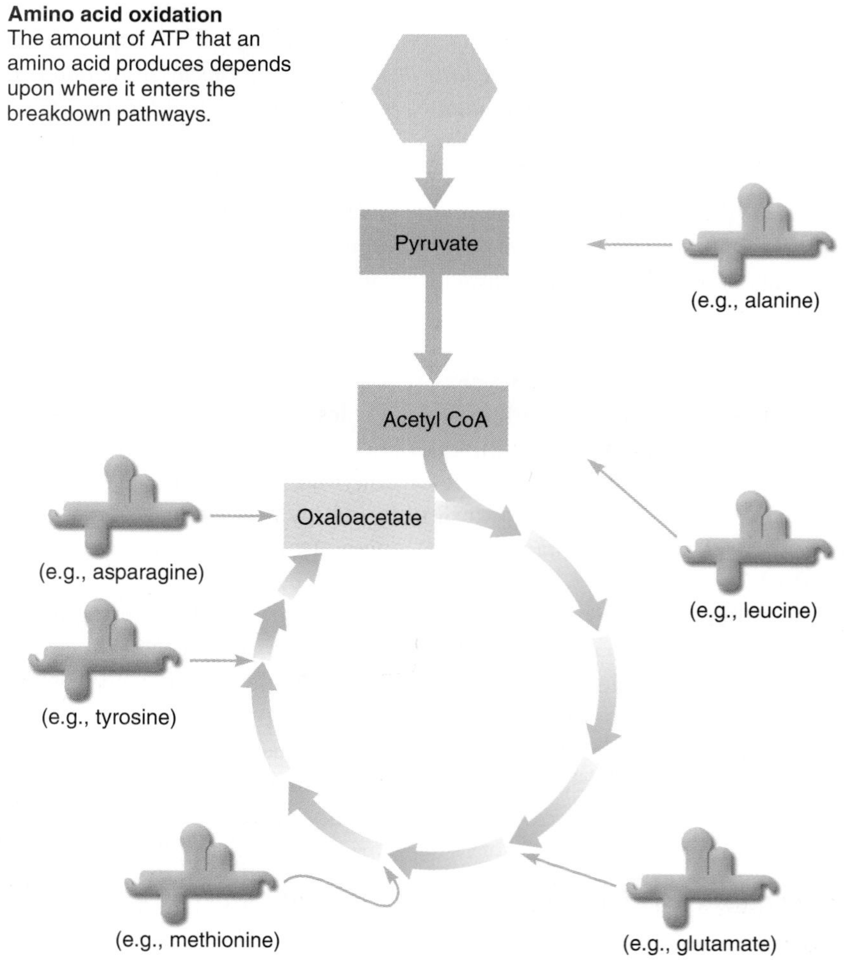

Figure SM.14 **Extracting energy from amino acids.** The carbon skeletons of amino acids have several different entrances to the breakdown pathways. Compared with glucose and fatty acids, amino acids yield much smaller amounts of energy (ATP).

Biosynthesis and Storage

Uh oh! Surveying the results of those holiday dinners and treats, you cringe with regret. Your clothes no longer fit, and you hate the idea of stepping on the scale. Your biosynthetic pathways have been hard at work, building fat stores from your excess intake of energy.

You head for the gym. After sweating through many workouts, your body begins to firm. You drop fat and add muscle. Now any problem with clothes fitting is due to muscle gain, not fat gain. To build muscle protein, different biosynthetic pathways have been busy making amino acids and assembling proteins.

Perhaps you've heard of "carbo loading." (See Chapter 11, "Sports Nutrition.") This strategy uses high-carbohydrate meals to pack carbohydrate into your muscle glycogen stores before a race. Biosynthetic pathways assemble glucose into glycogen chains for storage. When needed, your body also can make glucose from certain amino acids and other precursors.

Both the breakdown and biosynthetic pathways are active at all times. While some cells are breaking down carbohydrate, fat, and protein to extract energy, other cells are busy building glucose, fatty acids, and amino acids. When your body needs energy, the breakdown pathways prevail. When it has an excess of nutrients, the biosynthetic pathways dominate. The activities in these pathways ebb and flow so that they proceed at just the right rate, not too fast and not too slowly. **Figure SM.15** illustrates the interconnections among the metabolic pathways.

gluconeogenesis [gloo-ko-nee-oh-JEN-uh-sis] Synthesis of glucose within the body from noncarbohydrate precursors such as amino acids, lactic acid, and glycerol. Fatty acids cannot be converted to glucose.

Making Carbohydrate (Glucose)

Your body sets a high priority on maintaining an adequate amount of glucose circulating in the bloodstream. Blood glucose is the primary source of energy for your brain, central nervous system, and red blood cells. In fact, while you're at rest, your brain consumes about 60 percent of the energy consumed by your entire body.

Gluconeogenesis: Pathways to Glucose

When you are exercising intensely or when you aren't taking in enough carbohydrate, your body can make glucose through a process called **gluconeogenesis**. Gluconeogenesis and glycolysis share many, but not all, reactions. During gluconeogenesis, reactions flow in the opposite direction as during glycolysis. Because some reactions of glycolysis flow only one way, gluconeogenesis must use energy-consuming detours to bypass them. Thus gluconeogenesis is *not* simply a reversal of glycolysis.

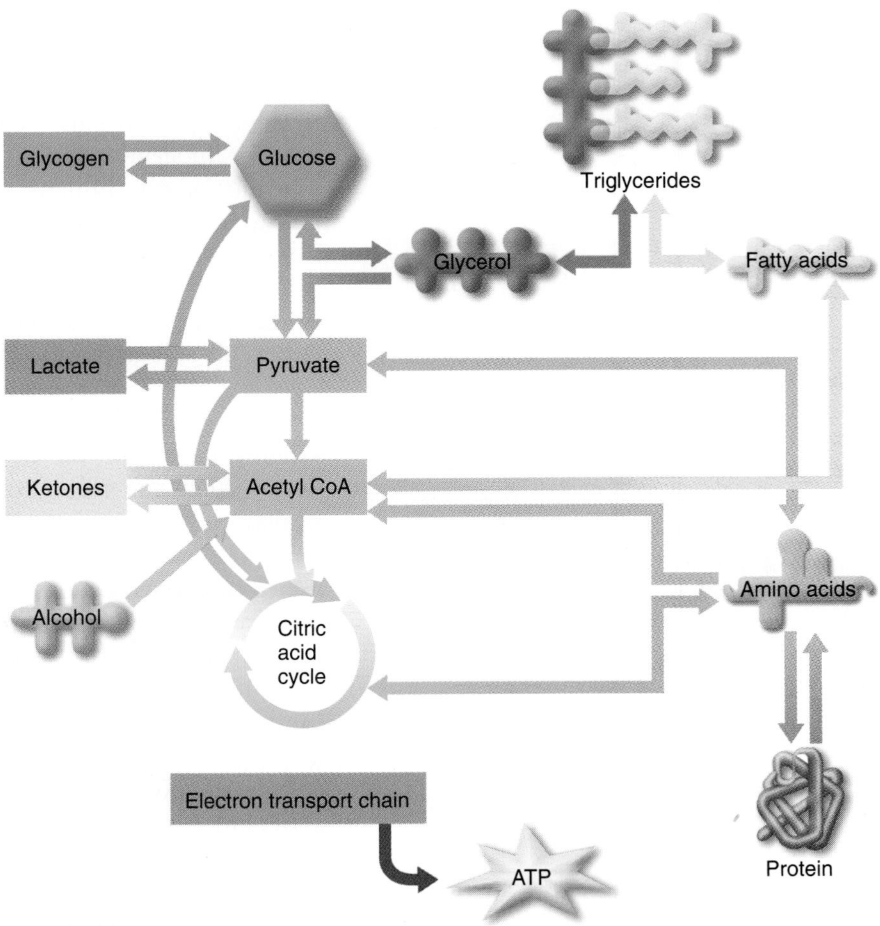

Figure SM.15 **Overview of metabolic pathways.** As if they were traveling a maze of city streets, molecules move through a network of breakdown and biosynthetic pathways. Not all pathways are available to a molecule. Just as traffic lights and one-way streets regulate traffic flow, cellular mechanisms control the flow of molecules in metabolic pathways. These mechanisms include hormones, irreversible reactions, and the location of the reactions in the cell.

Your body can make glucose from pyruvate, lactate, and some noncarbohydrate sources—amino acids and glycerol. Although gluconeogenesis can use the glycerol portion of fat, it cannot make glucose from fatty acids.

Your body cannot make glucose from all amino acids. If the carbon skeleton of an amino acid can be made into glucose, the amino acid is called **glucogenic**. Glucogenic amino acids provide carbon skeletons that become pyruvate or directly enter the citric acid cycle at intermediate points without forming acetyl CoA. If a carbon skeleton of an amino acid directly forms acetyl CoA (which your body can convert to ketone bodies but not glucose), the amino acid is called **ketogenic** (see the section "Ketogenesis").

Quick Bites

Sweet Origins

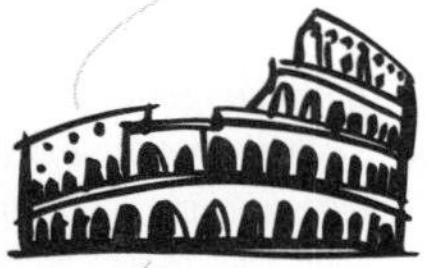

The word *gluconeogenesis* is derived from the Greek words *glyks*, meaning "sweet"; *neo*, meaning "new"; and *genesis*, meaning "origin" or "generation."

Storage: Glucose to Glycogen

Our bodies store glucose as glycogen in the liver and muscles (see Chapter 5, "Carbohydrates"). Liver glycogen serves as a glucose reserve for the blood, and muscle glycogen supplies glucose to exercising muscle tissue. Glycogen stores are limited; fasting or strenuous exercise can deplete them rapidly.

Making Fat (Fatty Acids)

Your body can make long-chain fatty acids using a process called **lipogenesis**. In essence, your body assembles two-carbon acetyl CoA "links" into fatty acid chains. Where do these acetyl CoA building blocks come from? Ketogenic amino acids, alcohol, and fatty acids themselves supply acetyl CoA for lipogenesis.

While you can think of fatty acid synthesis as reassembling the links broken apart by beta-oxidation, lipogenesis is *not* the reversal of beta-oxidation. These processes encompass different sets of reactions that take place in different locations—fatty acid synthesis occurs in the cytosol, and beta-oxidation operates inside the mitochondria. Your body assembles surplus fatty acids and glycerol to form triglycerides for storage as body fat.

glucogenic A term describing an amino acid whose carbon skeleton can be used in gluconeogenesis to form glucose.

ketogenic A term describing an amino acid broken down to acetyl CoA (which can be converted into ketone bodies).

lipogenesis [lye-poh-JEN-eh-sis] Synthesis of fatty acids from acetyl CoA derived from the metabolism of fats, alcohol, and some amino acids.

Storage: From Dietary Energy to Stored Triglyceride

When you overeat, your body uses body fat as a long-term energy storage depot. When you eat an excess of fat, most extra dietary fatty acids head straight to your fat stores. If you eat more protein than your tissues can use, your body converts most of the excess protein to body fat. Interestingly, excess carbohydrate does not readily become fat. In research studies, massive overfeeding of carbohydrate in normal men caused only minimal amounts of fat synthesis. So are carbohydrate calories "free?" Unfortunately not. Although excess carbohydrate does not dramatically increase fat synthesis, it shifts your body's fuel preferences so it burns more carbohydrate and fewer fatty acids.[8] This "fat-sparing" shift in fuel use burns less fat, so a greater proportion of dietary fat accumulates in body fat stores. See **Table SM.2**.

Key Concepts: *Your body can make glucose from pyruvate, lactate, glucogenic amino acids, and glycerol but not from fatty acids. The main storage form of glucose is glycogen. When your diet supplies an excess of energy, your body makes fatty acids and triglycerides. Excess dietary carbohydrate is not readily converted to fat, but instead shifts the body's selection of fuel and encourages the accumulation of dietary fat in body fat stores.*

Table SM.2 Summary of Energy Yield and Interconversions

Dietary Nutrient	Yields Energy?	Convertible to Glucose?	Convertible to Amino Acids and Body Proteins?	Convertible to Fat?
Carbohydrate (glucose, fructose, galactose)	Yes	Yes	Yes, can yield nonessential amino acids when amino groups are available	Insignificant
Fat (triglycerides)				
Fatty acids	Yes, large amounts	No	No	Yes
Glycerol	Yes, small amounts	Small amounts	Yes (see carbohydrate)	Insignificant
Protein (amino acids)	Yes, generally not much (see starvation in text)	Yes, if insufficient carbohydrate is available	Yes	Yes
Alcohol (ethanol)	Yes	No	No	Yes

Fyi FOR YOUR INFORMATION

Do Carbohydrates Turn into Fat? Marc Hellerstein, M.D., Ph.D.

Thirty years ago, Jules Hirsch and his colleagues addressed this question indirectly. They found that the composition of fatty acids in adipose tissue closely resembled the subjects' dietary fat intake. Moreover, when they put these subjects on controlled diets of different fatty acid composition for six months, adipose fatty acids slowly changed to reflect the new dietary fatty acid composition. These studies concluded that "we are what we eat" with regard to body fat and that fatty acid synthesis is minimal at best.

The body's ability to make fat from carbohydrate is called *de novo lipogenesis* (DNL). Numerous studies using a technique called indirect calorimetry have shown that net DNL is absent or very low in humans under most dietary conditions, even after a large carbohydrate meal. But could there be concurrent synthesis *and* use of fat that results in no net change?

Concurrent DNL and burning of fatty acids is called *futile cycling*. About 25 to 28 percent of the carbohydrate energy is lost during the inefficient conversion to fatty acids. Does this costly conversion really happen? New stable isotopic methods have helped answer this question.

Direct Evidence

Direct evidence from stable isotopic methods shows that DNL is minimal in normal (nonobese, nondiabetic, nonoverfed) men. DNL represents less than 1 gram of saturated fat per day, whether the subjects are given large meals, intravenous glucose, or a liquid diet.

Do any circumstances stimulate DNL? Jean-Marc Schwarz gave fructose and glucose orally to lean and obese subjects. The dietary fructose increased DNL up to 20-fold compared with equal calorie loads of glucose. Nevertheless, fat synthesis still represented only a small percentage of the fructose load given (< 5%). Scott Siler has shown that drinking alcohol stimulates DNL. Again, however, only a small percentage (< 5%) of the alcohol was converted to fat; the great majority was released from the liver as acetate.

My laboratory studied the effect of five to seven days of carbohydrate overfeeding or underfeeding in normal men. Fat synthesis by the liver was highly sensitive to the degree of dietary carbohydrate excess. In fact, we could determine exactly which diet a person was eating by measuring DNL. Even so, the absolute amount of fat synthesis remained low, even on massively excessive carbohydrate intakes. DNL may be a sensitive *signal* of excess carbohydrate in the diet, but it is not a quantitatively important route for excess carbohydrate disposal.

Other conditions yield similar findings. Very-low-fat diets (10% of energy as fat; 70% as carbohydrate) stimulate lipogenesis, but, again, not a large amount. In young women, lipogenesis increases during the follicular phase of the menstrual cycle, but the amount is small, representing only 1 to 2 pounds of extra fat per year. A high rate of DNL has been documented in humans only under conditions of massive carbohydrate overfeeding—for example, 5,000 to 6,000 carbohydrate calories per day for more than a week.

Are Carbohydrate Calories "Free"?

Alas, we still become fatter if we overeat carbohydrate. At rest, our bodies normally burn fat as our primary fuel source. An excess of dietary carbohydrate energy causes a fat-sparing shift in fuel selection as it markedly reduces the use of fat to fuel the body. Dietary fat makes a beeline for body fat storage rather than being burned to release energy. Thus, excess dietary carbohydrate is not "free" when the diet also contains fat, because the carbohydrate spares fat use.

Dr. Hellerstein is Professor of Medicine at the University of California, San Francisco, and Professor of Nutritional Sciences at the University of California at Berkeley.

Making Ketone Bodies

Your body makes and uses small amounts of ketone bodies at all times. Although long considered to be just an emergency energy source or the result of an abnormal condition like starvation or uncontrolled diabetes, ketone bodies are normal, everyday fuels. In fact, your heart and kidneys prefer to use the ketone body acetoacetate as their fuel.[9] Some people incorrectly use the term **ketones** to refer to ketone bodies. Although there is some overlap, not all ketones are ketone bodies and not all ketone bodies are ketones.

Ketogenesis: Pathways to Ketone Bodies

During the breakdown of fatty acids, not all acetyl CoA enters the citric acid cycle. Your body converts some acetyl CoA to ketone bodies, a process called **ketogenesis**. (See **Figure SM.16**.) When a person has uncontrolled diabetes or is starving, ketone bodies help provide emergency energy to all body tissues, especially the brain and the rest of the central nervous system. Other than glucose, ketone bodies are your central nervous system's only effective fuel.[10]

To dispose of excess ketone bodies, your kidneys excrete them in urine, and your lungs exhale them. If this removal process cannot keep up, ketone bodies accumulate in the blood—a condition known as ketosis. During ketosis, the blood can become acidic. This condition, known as **ketoacidosis**, can cause brain damage and eventually death.[11] Ketoacidosis is particularly dangerous in uncontrolled type 1 diabetes mellitus. During a short fast, ketoacidosis is rarely a problem.

Given time, your body can adapt to a very-high-fat, low-carbohydrate diet and avoid ketosis. Eskimos, for example, sometimes live almost entirely on fat but do not develop ketosis.[12]

Key Concepts: *While some ketone bodies are made and used for energy all the time, a lack of available carbohydrate accelerates ketone body production. Ketone bodies become an important fuel source during starvation, uncontrolled diabetes mellitus, and high-fat, very-low-carbohydrate diets. In type 1 diabetes mellitus, an accumulation of ketone bodies can acidify the blood and cause ketoacidosis.*

Quick Bites

Will the Smelly Body Please Stand Up?

Ketone bodies (sometimes incorrectly called ketones) include three compounds—acetoacetate, beta-hydroxybutyrate, and acetone. Acetoacetate and beta-hydroxybutyrate are acids, so they may be called keto acids. You may recognize the term *acetone*, which also is a common solvent. In fact, you can smell the strong odor of acetone on the breath of people with high levels of ketone bodies in their blood; their breath smells like nail polish remover!

ketones [KEE-tonez] Organic compounds that contain a chemical group consisting of C=O (a carbon–oxygen double bond) bound to two hydrocarbons. Pyruvate and fructose are examples of ketones. Acetone and acetoacetate are both ketones and ketone bodies. While beta-hydroxybutyrate is not a ketone, it is a ketone body. (See *ketone bodies.*)

ketogenesis The process in which excess acetyl CoA from fatty acid oxidation is converted into ketone bodies.

ketoacidosis Acidification of the blood caused by a buildup of ketone bodies. It is primarily a consequence of uncontrolled type 1 diabetes mellitus and can be life threatening.

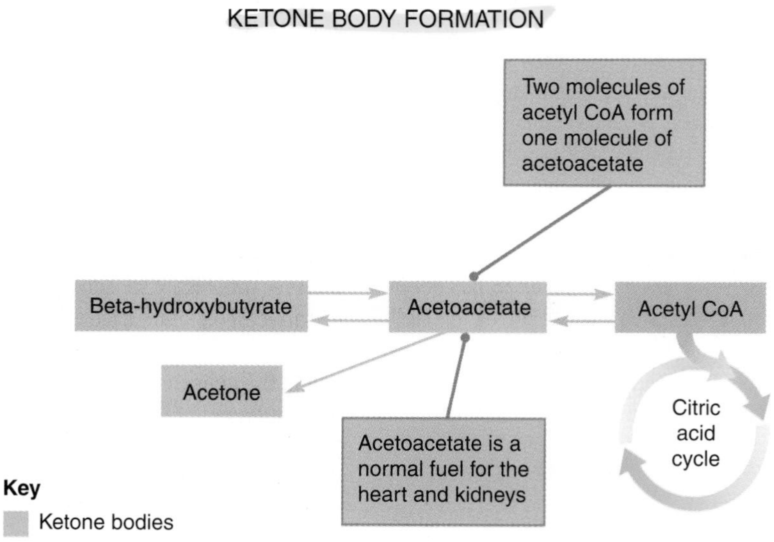
KETONE BODY FORMATION
Two molecules of acetyl CoA form one molecule of acetoacetate
Beta-hydroxybutyrate
Acetoacetate
Acetyl CoA
Acetone
Citric acid cycle
Acetoacetate is a normal fuel for the heart and kidneys
Key
Ketone bodies

Figure SM.16 **Ketogenesis.** For acetyl CoA from fatty acid oxidation to enter the citric acid cycle, fat and carbohydrate metabolism must be synchronized. When acetyl CoA cannot enter the citric acid cycle, it is shunted to form ketone bodies.

Making Protein (Amino Acids)

Your body rebuilds proteins from a pool of amino acids in your cells. But how is that amino acid pool replenished? Your diet supplies some amino acids, the breakdown of body proteins supplies some, and your cells make some. During protein synthesis, your cells can make nonessential amino acids and retrieve essential amino acids from the bloodstream. Your cells cannot make essential amino acids. If a cell lacks one and your diet doesn't supply it, protein synthesis stops. The cell breaks down this incomplete protein into its constituent amino acids, which are returned to the bloodstream. (See Chapter 7, "Proteins and Amino Acids," for more details of protein synthesis.)

Biosynthesis: Making Amino Acids

Your body uses many different pathways to synthesize nonessential amino acids. Each pathway is short, involving just a few steps, and builds amino acids from carbon skeletons. Pyruvate and other compounds involved in glycolysis and the citric acid cycle supply the carbon skeletons.

Key Concepts: *Proteins are made from combinations of essential and nonessential amino acids. The body synthesizes nonessential amino acids from pyruvate, other compounds involved in glycolysis, and compounds from the citric acid cycle.*

Quick Bites

Why Didn't My Cholesterol Levels Drop?

Your body can make cholesterol from acetyl CoA by way of ketones. In fact, all 27 carbons in synthesized cholesterol come from acetyl CoA. The rate of cholesterol formation is highly responsive to cholesterol levels in cells. If levels are low, the liver makes more. If levels are high, synthesis decreases. This is why dietary cholesterol in the absence of dietary fat often has little impact on cholesterol blood levels.

Special States

Now you can put your new knowledge of metabolism to work by evaluating what happens when feasting or fasting. What do you think happens to your metabolism under these situations? Read on to find out which states stimulate breakdown and which stimulate biosynthesis.

Feasting

You're stuffed. You just ate a huge holiday dinner: two servings of turkey with a big ladle of gravy and ample servings of dressing, mashed potatoes, caramelized sweet potatoes, green peas, and two bread rolls. To top it off, you ate a piece of pumpkin pie with whipped cream. You meant to stop there; you loudly proclaimed, "I'm so full I can't eat another bite!" But eventually your grandmother convinced you to taste her special pecan pie. Gosh, that was good! But now you are lying prostrate on the couch, tight and bloated, with your belt loosened. Your feasting may be finished for now, but your body's work has just begun.

Your meal led to a huge influx of carbohydrate, fat, and protein—a plentiful supply for your tissues and far more energy than you need to be a couch potato. The influx of food triggers the command "store, store, store!" Consequently, much of your holiday dinner will wind up stored as fat. The surplus carbohydrate first enters glycogen stores, filling its limited capacity. In the short term, excess carbohydrate primarily readjusts your body's fuel preferences.[13] In a fat-sparing shift, your body maximizes its use of carbohydrate and minimizes its use of fat, thus promoting fat storage.[14] Although your body does not directly make appreciable amounts of fat from carbohydrate, the shift in fuel use triggered by excess carbohydrate still leads to increased fat stores and weight gain.

What happens to the surplus fat and protein? Fat tissue is the perfect energy storage package for both. While a minor amount produces some

Quick Bites

When Men Starve: A Starvation Study

During World War II, researchers at the University of Minnesota conducted a starvation study on 36 male volunteers, all conscientious objectors. Their typical food intake was cut in half and they lost about 25 percent of their body weight. Researchers noted significant psychological changes as well. The subjects began obsessing about food, collecting recipes and cookbooks, and hoarding food-related objects. They became apathetic, chronically exhausted, and lost all interest in sex. Most were afraid to leave the experimental conditions for fear of losing control in the outside world.

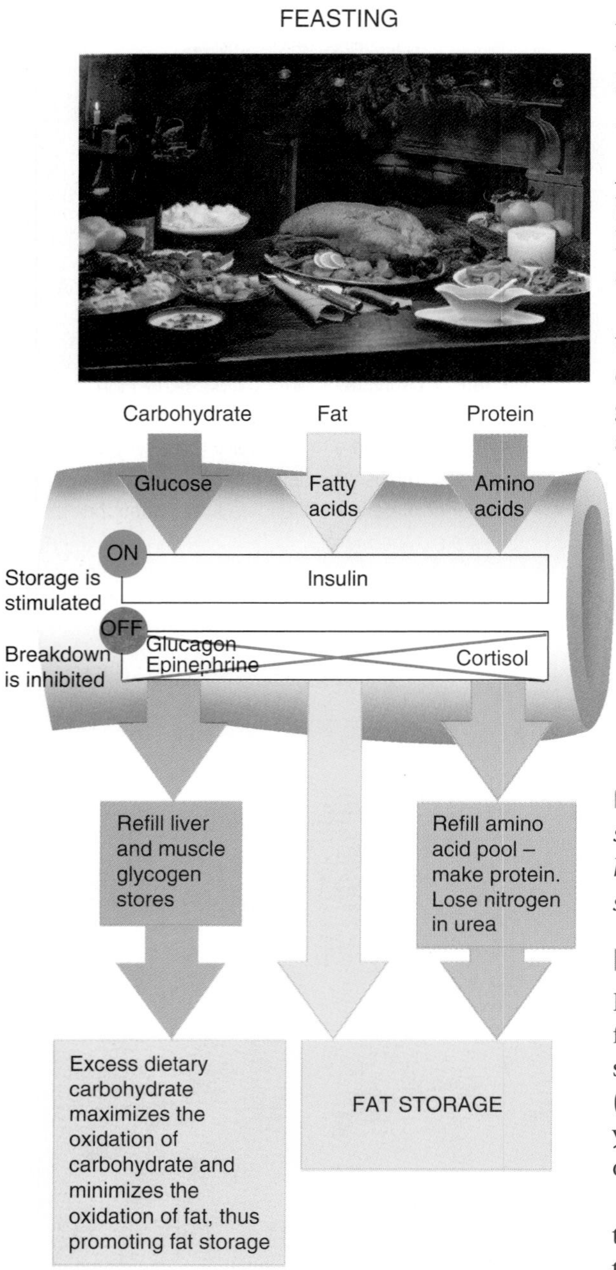

Figure SM.17 **Feasting.** Your body deals with a large influx of nutrients by increasing cellular uptake of glucose and promoting fat storage.

ATP, nearly all excess dietary fat becomes body fat. Excess protein, beyond what's needed to replenish the overall body pool of amino acids, also heads to fat storage. (See **Figure SM.17**.)

The Return to Normal

After this frenzied bout of storage, the amount of glucose circulating in the bloodstream drops to the fasting level. Three to four hours after eating, healthy people have blood glucose levels of 70 to 110 mg/dL. The level of amino acids in the blood also returns to baseline.

Hours later, after a nap, a further decline in blood glucose levels triggers the command "release the glucose!" and your body swings into action to counteract falling blood glucose levels. The body breaks down liver glycogen to glucose, which is released into the bloodstream. Synthesis and storage of glycogen and fatty acids slow. The body breaks down muscle glycogen to form glucose, but this glucose does not enter the bloodstream. If needed, muscles use this glycogen for a "fight-or-flight" response to danger.

If low blood glucose levels persist for hours or days, most cells start shifting their fuel usage from glucose to fatty acids. Gluconeogenesis begins to ramp up and make glucose from circulating amino acids.[15] The body's resources work in concert to maintain blood glucose levels and assure a constant supply of glucose for the central nervous system and red blood cells[16]—until it is time to attack the leftovers!

Key Concepts: *Feasting, or taking in too many calories, stimulates anabolic processes such as glycogen and fat synthesis. Your body resists making fat from excess carbohydrate, but instead shifts its fuel preferences from fat to carbohydrate. This shift still leads to the accumulation of fat stores.*

Fasting

Feasting on a holiday dinner floods your body with excess energy that is stored for future use. On the other hand, fasting and starvation deprive you of energy, so your body must employ an opposing strategy—the mobilization of fuel. (See **Figure SM.18**.) Whether starvation occurs in a child during a famine, a young woman with anorexia nervosa, a patient with AIDS wasting syndrome, or a person intentionally fasting, the body responds in the same way.

Some people deprive themselves of food for a purpose—to lose weight, to stage a political protest, to participate in a religious fast, or to "cleanse" their bodies. The cleansing motivation is ironic, since fasting actually unleashes potentially damaging toxins to circulate throughout the body. Over time, fat stores accumulate environmental toxins, such as DDT, PCBs, and benzene.[17] In the case of PCBs, despite the fact that Congress banned their use decades ago, more than 9 out of 10 Americans still have traces in their body fat.[18] When bound in adipose tissue, toxins are relatively harmless. But fasting breaks down adipose tissue and releases these toxins, giving them a second chance to damage cells. While the liver—the body's detoxification center—and the intestines remove a small portion of these liberated toxins, the balance remain in circulation, where they can wreak havoc.

Survival Priorities and Potential Energy Sources

Starvation confronts your body with several dilemmas. Where is it going to get energy to fuel survival needs? What should it burn first—fat, protein, or carbohydrate? Can it conserve its energy reserves? Which tissues should it sacrifice to ensure survival?

Your body's first priority is to preserve glucose-dependent tissue: red blood cells, brain cells, and the rest of the central nervous system. Your brain will not tolerate even a short interruption in the supply of adequate energy. Once your body depletes its carbohydrate reserves, it begins sacrificing readily available circulating amino acids to make glucose and ATP.

Your body's second priority is to maintain muscle mass. In the face of danger, we rely upon our ability for "fight or flight." This survival mechanism requires a large muscle mass so we can move quickly and effectively. Your body grudgingly uses muscle protein for energy and breaks it down rapidly only in the final stages of starvation.

Although your body stores most of its energy reserve in body fat, triglycerides are a poor source of glucose. Your body can make a small amount of glucose from the glycerol backbone, but it cannot make any glucose from fatty acids. This means your body's primary energy stores—fat—are incompatible with your body's paramount energy priority—glucose for your brain. To meet this metabolic challenge, your body's antistarvation strategies include a glucose-sparing mechanism. Your body shifts to fatty acids and ketone bodies to fuel its needs. In time, even your brain adapts as most, but not all, its cells come to rely on ketone bodies for fuel.

The Prolonged Fast: In the Beginning

What happens during the fasting state? Let's take a metabolic look at Fasting Frank, a political activist determined to make a dramatic statement. Frank begins fasting at sundown, planning to drink nothing but water and to consume no other foods.

The first few hours are no different from your nightly fast between dinner and breakfast. As blood glucose drops to fasting baseline levels, the liver breaks down glycogen to glucose. Gluconeogenesis becomes highly active and begins churning out glucose from circulating amino acids. The liver pours glucose into the bloodstream to supply other organs and altruistically shifts to fatty acids for its own energy needs. Muscle cells also start burning fatty acids. After about 12 hours, the battle to maintain a constant supply of blood glucose exhausts nearly all carbohydrate stores.[19]

During the next few days, fat and protein are the primary fuels. To preserve structural proteins, especially muscle mass, Frank's body first turns to easily metabolized amino acids. It uses some to produce ATP and others to make glucose. Glucogenic amino acids, especially alanine, furnish about 90 percent of the brain's glucose supply. As Frank's body breaks down triglycerides for fuel, the glycerol portion supplies the remaining 10 percent. After a couple of days, production of ketone bodies ramps up, augmenting the fuel supply. (See **Figure SM.19**.)

The Early Weeks

As starvation continues, Frank's body initiates several energy-conservation strategies. It ratchets down its energy use by lowering body temperature, pulse rate, blood pressure, and resting metabolism. He becomes lethargic, reducing the amount of energy expended in activity. Frank may begin to have detectable signs of mild vitamin deficiencies as his body depletes its small reserves of vitamin C and most B vitamins.

If Frank's body continued to rapidly break down protein, he would survive less than three weeks. To avoid such a quick demise, protein breakdown slows drastically and gluconeogenesis drops by two-thirds or more.[20] To pick up the slack, his body doubles the rate of fat breakdown to supply fatty acids for fuel and glycerol for glucose. Ketone bodies pour into the

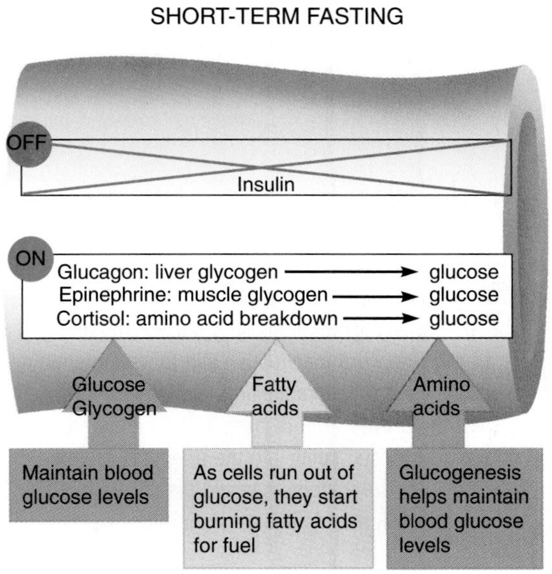

Figure SM.18 **Fasting.** During a short fast, cells first break down liver glycogen to maintain blood glucose levels. They also burn fatty acids and ramp up the production of glucose from amino acids.

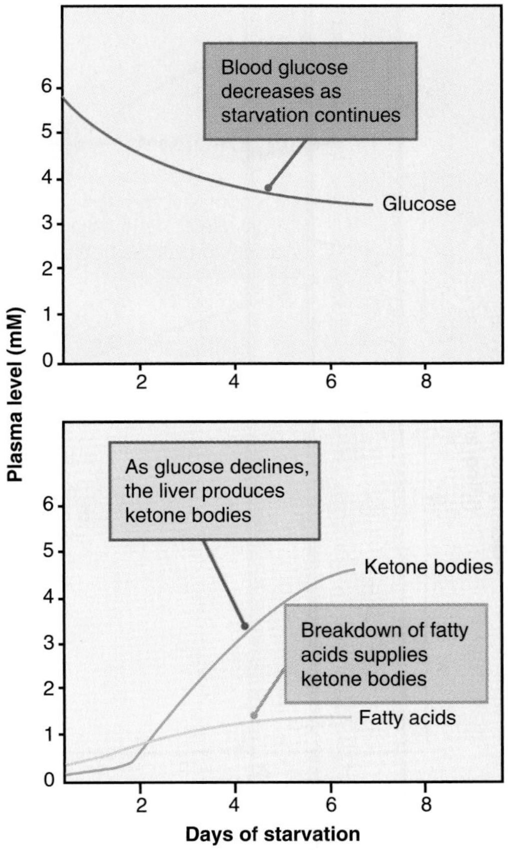

Figure SM.19 **Shifting fuel selection during starvation.** To fuel its needs as blood glucose levels decline, the body shifts from glucose to fatty acids and ketone bodies.

bloodstream. Ketone bodies are an important glucose-sparing energy source for the brain and red blood cells. After about 10 days of fasting, ketone bodies meet most of the nervous system's energy needs. Yet some brain cells can use only glucose. To maintain a small, but essential, supply of blood glucose, protein breakdown crawls along, supplying small amounts of amino acids for gluconeogenesis.

Several Weeks of Fasting

The average person has about three weeks of fat stores, and the rate of fat depletion is fairly constant. As the later stages of starvation exhaust the final fat stores, the body turns again to protein, its sole remaining fuel source. (See **Figure SM.20**.) You can see some of the effects of accelerated protein breakdown in starving children suffering from kwashiorkor. The loss of blood proteins leads to the swollen limbs and bulging stomachs that typify this type of protein-energy malnutrition (PEM). (For more detail on PEM see Chapter 7, "Proteins and Amino Acids.")

The End Is Near

In the final stage of protein depletion, the body deteriorates rapidly. You can see the severe muscle atrophy and emaciation in photos of Holocaust victims. Their bodies sacrificed muscle tissue in attempts to preserve brain tissue. Even organ tissues were not spared. The final stage of starvation attacks the liver and intestines, greatly depleting them. It moderately depletes the heart and kidneys and even mounts a small attack on the nervous system. Amazingly, starving people can cling to life until they lose about half their body proteins, after which death generally occurs.

How long can a person survive total starvation? Several years ago, some Irish prisoners starved themselves to death—the average time was 60 days.[21] Most people survive total starvation for one to three months. Starvation survival factors include:

- *Starting percentage of body fat.* Ample fat tissue prolongs survival.
- *Age.* Middle-aged people survive longer than children and the elderly.
- *Gender.* Women fare better due to a higher proportion of body fat.
- *Energy expenditure levels.* Increased activity leads to an earlier death.

Key Concepts: *Fasting, or underconsumption of energy (calories), favors catabolic pathways. The body first obtains fuel from stored glycogen, then from stored fat and body proteins, such as muscle. Over time, the body adapts to using more and more ketone bodies as fuel because limited carbohydrate is available. Larger stores of fat in adipose tissue extend survival time during starvation. In prolonged starvation, the body catabolizes muscle tissue to continue minimal production of glucose from amino acids.*

Quick Bites

Sweet Urine

The word *diabetes* is Greek for "siphon," from *dia*, meaning "through," and *bainein*, meaning "to go." The word *mellitus* is Latin for "sweetened with honey." *Diabetes mellitus* means the flow of sweetened water. The disease causes a rise in blood sugar that spills into the urine. As early as the 1600s, some doctors would taste a patient's urine to confirm a diagnosis of diabetes mellitus.

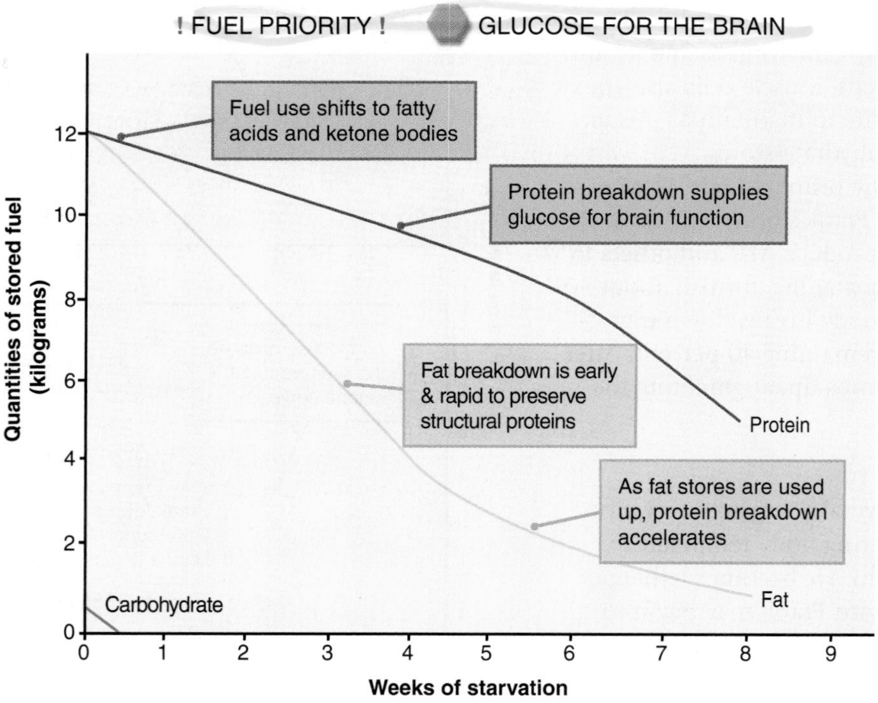

Figure SM.20 **Starvation and Fuel Sources.** During starvation, carbohydrate is exhausted quickly, and fat becomes the primary fuel. Burning fat without available carbohydrate produces ketone bodies, a byproduct that the body can use as fuel. Glucose produced from amino acids and the glycerol portion of fatty acids help fuel the brain. The body conserves protein and breaks it down rapidly only after most fat stores are depleted.

LEARNING *Portfolio* spotlight on metabolism

Key Terms

	page
acetyl CoA	238
ADP (adenosine diphosphate) [ah-DEN-oh-seen di-FOS-fate]	236
aerobic [air-ROW-bic]	237
anabolism [an-A-bol-iz-um]	234
anaerobic [AN-ah-ROW-bic]	237
ATP (adenosine triphosphate) [ah-DEN-oh-seen try-FOS-fate]	236
beta-oxidation	243
biosynthesis	241
carnitine [CAR-nih-teen]	243
catabolism [ca-TA-bol-iz-um]	234
cells	234
chemical energy	233
citric acid cycle	239
coenzymes	236
coenzyme A	238
cofactors	236
cytoplasm	234
cytosol	234
electron transport chain	241
$FAD/FADH_2$	236
glucogenic	248
gluconeogenesis [gloo-ko-nee-oh-JEN-uh-sis]	247
glycolysis [gligh-COLL-ih-sis]	238
GTP (guanosine triphosphate)	241
ketoacidosis	250
ketogenesis	250
ketogenic	248
ketones [KEE-tonez]	250
Krebs cycle	241
lactate	238
lipogenesis [lye-poh-JEN-eh-sis]	248
metabolic pathway	234
metabolism	233
metabolites	233
mitochondria (mitochondrion)	234
mitochondrial membrane	241
$NAD^+/NADH$	236
nucleus	234
organelles	234
oxaloacetate	238
photosynthesis	233
pyruvate	238
tricarboxylic acid cycle (TCA)	241

Study Points

- Energy is necessary to do any kind of work. The body converts chemical energy from food sources—carbohydrates, proteins, and fats—into a form usable by cells.
- Anabolic reactions (anabolism) build compounds. These reactions require energy.
- Catabolic reactions (catabolism) break compounds into smaller units. These reactions produce the energy.
- Adenosine triphosphate, ATP, is the energy currency of the body.
- NAD^+ and FAD accept pairs of high-energy electrons, becoming NADH and $FADH_2$ and shuttling the electrons to the electron transport chain to make ATP.
- Cells extract energy from carbohydrate via four main pathways: glycolysis, pyruvate to acetyl CoA, the citric acid cycle, and the electron transport chain.
- The citric acid cycle and electron transport chain require oxygen. Glycolysis does not.
- The electron transport chain produces more ATP than other catabolic pathways.
- To extract energy from fat, first triglycerides are separated into glycerol and fatty acids. Next, beta-oxidation breaks down the fatty acids to yield acetyl CoA and high-energy electrons that are shuttled to the electron transport chain. The acetyl CoA enters the citric acid cycle, which yields one GTP and more high-energy electrons. In the electron transport chain, the high-energy electrons give up energy to produce ATP.
- To extract energy from an amino acid, first it is deaminated (the amino group is removed). Depending on the structure of the remaining carbon skeleton, it enters the catabolic pathways at pyruvate, acetyl CoA, or the citric acid cycle. The citric acid cycle and the electron transport chain complete the extraction of energy and production of ATP.
- The liver converts the nitrogen portion of amino acids to urea. This product is excreted by the kidney.
- Tissues differ in their preferred source of fuel. The brain, nervous system, and red blood cells rely primarily on glucose, while other tissues use a mix of glucose, fatty acids, and ketone bodies as fuel sources.

- **When carbohydrate is available, glucose can be stored as glycogen in liver and muscle tissue.**
- **Glucose can be produced from the noncarbohydrate precursors glycerol and some (glucogenic) amino acids, but not from fatty acids.**
- **Feasting, or overconsumption of energy, leads to glycogen and triglyceride storage.**
- **Fasting, or underconsumption of energy, leads to the mobilization of liver glycogen and stored triglycerides. Starvation, the state of prolonged fasting, leads to protein breakdown as well and can be fatal.**

Study Questions

Answers can be found at nutrition.jbpub.com/discovering.

1. **What is the "universal energy currency"? Where is most of it produced?**
2. **In the catabolic pathways, what is the primary function of the electron carriers?**
3. **How many pyruvate molecules does glycolysis produce from one glucose molecule? How many acetyl CoA does the oxidative breakdown step after glycolysis produce? The breakdown of one glucose molecule triggers how many "turns" of the citric acid cycle? Why?**
4. **When extracting energy from glucose, which of the four main pathways—glycolysis, pyruvate to acetyl CoA, the citric acid cycle, and the electron transport chain—are anaerobic and which are aerobic?**
5. **What two-carbon molecules does beta-oxidation form as it "clips" the links of a fatty acid chain? What else does beta-oxidation produce that is important to producing ATP?**
6. **What dictates whether an amino acid is considered ketogenic or glucogenic?**
7. **What are ketone bodies, and when are they produced?**
8. **Name the three tissues where energy is stored. Which contains the largest store of energy?**
9. **Define gluconeogenesis and lipogenesis. Under what conditions do they predominantly occur? What are their primary inputs and outputs?**

[Try] This

Comparing Fad Diets

The purpose of this exercise is to have you evaluate two fad diets in regard to their metabolic consequences. The two diets, Cabbage Soup and Super Protein, are described below. Once you've reviewed them, please answer the following questions.

Will these diets result in weight loss? On the seventh day of each of these diets, which of the following metabolic pathways will be highly active?

- Glycogen breakdown
- Fat breakdown
- Gluconeogenesis
- Ketogenesis

Diet 1: The Cabbage Soup Diet

A person following the Cabbage Soup diet only eats a water-based soup made out of cabbage and a few other vegetables. Three to four meals per day of this restricted diet supplies approximately 500 kilocalories per day. The diet is devoid of protein and fat and gets its calories from the small amount of carbohydrate in the vegetables. Think about what happens during starvation.

Diet 2: The Super Protein Diet

In the Super Protein diet a person can eat an unlimited amount of protein-rich foods like meat, poultry, eggs, and seafood. However, no added fats or carbohydrates are allowed. The average person can consume about 1,400 kilocalories if he or she eats three or four small meals a day. Think about what happens when little carbohydrate is available as a person metabolizes fat and protein.

Fasting for Ketones

The purpose of this experiment is to see if a day without eating will cause your body to produce measurable ketones in your urine. Before starting your fast, check with your physician. Go to your local pharmacy and ask the pharmacist for urine ketone strips (often called Ketostix). Bring them home and read the directions. Before you start your one-day fast, test your urine to see if it has a detectable amount of ketones. Start a 24-hour fast (or fast for as long as you can go without food or calorie-containing fluids) and test your urine at 6-hour intervals. Do you detect a color change on the strips as the day goes on? Why? What has happened metabolically as the day progresses?

Remember to drink lots of water!

References

1 Alberts B, Bray D, Lewis J, Raff M, Roberts K, Watson JD, eds. *Molecular Biology of the Cell.* 3rd ed. New York: Garland; 1994.

2 Stipanuk MH. *Biochemical and Physiological Aspects of Human Nutrition.* Philadelphia: WB Saunders; 2000.

3 Murray RK, Granner DK, Mayes PA, Rodwell VW. *Harper's Biochemistry.* 25th ed. Stamford, CT: Appleton & Lange; 1999.

4 Berg J, Tymoczzo J, Stryer L. *Biochemistry*. 5th ed. New York: WH Freeman; 2002.

5 Stipanuk MH. Op. cit.

6 Campbell MK. *Biochemistry*. 3rd ed. Philadelphia: Saunders College Publishing; 1999; and Stryer L. Op. cit.

7 Hawley JA, Brouns F, Jeukendrup A. Strategies to enhance fat utilization during exercise. *Sports Med.* 1998;25:241–257; and Brass EP, Hiatt WR. The role of carnitine and carnitine supplementation during exercise in man and individuals with special needs. *J Am Coll Nutr.* 1998;17:207–215.

8 Hellerstein MK, Schwartz JM, Neese RA. Regulation of hepatic de novo lipogenesis in humans. *Ann Rev Nutr.* 1996;16:527–557.

9 Stryer L. Op. cit.

10 Stein JH. *Internal Medicine.* 4th ed. St. Louis, MO: Mosby-Yearbook; 1994.

11 Anderson JW. Prevention and management of diabetes mellitus. In: Shils ME, Olson JA, Shike M, Ross AC, eds. *Modern Nutrition in Health and Disease.* 9th ed. Philadelphia: Lippincott Williams & Wilkins; 1999:1365–1394.

12 Guyton AC, Hall JE. *Textbook of Medical Physiology.* 10th ed. Philadelphia: WB Saunders; 2000.

13 Shah M, Garg A. High-fat and high-carbohydrate diets and energy balance. *Diabetes Care.* 1996;19:1142–1152.

14 Stubbs RJ, Prentice AM, James WP. Carbohydrates and energy balance. *Ann NY Acad Sci.* 1997;819:44–69.

15 Murray RK, et al. Op. cit.

16 Guyton AC, Hall JE. Op. cit.

17 Scheele JS. A comparison of the concentrations of certain pesticides and polychlorinated hydrocarbons in bone marrow and fat tissue. *Sci Total Environ.* 1998;221:(2–3)201–204.

18 Gower T. The fasting cure. *Health.* April 1999:61–63.

19 Guyton AC, Hall JE. Op. cit.

20 Ibid.

21 Ganong WF. *Review of Medical Physiology.* 20th ed. Stamford, CT: Appleton & Lange; 2001.

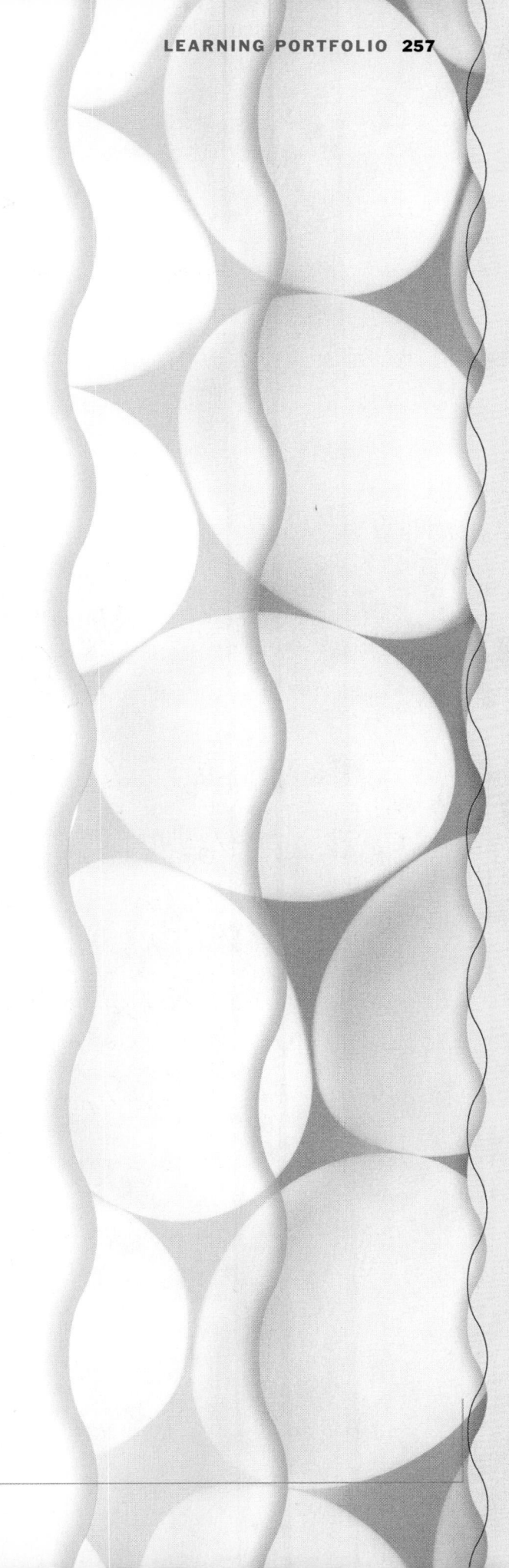

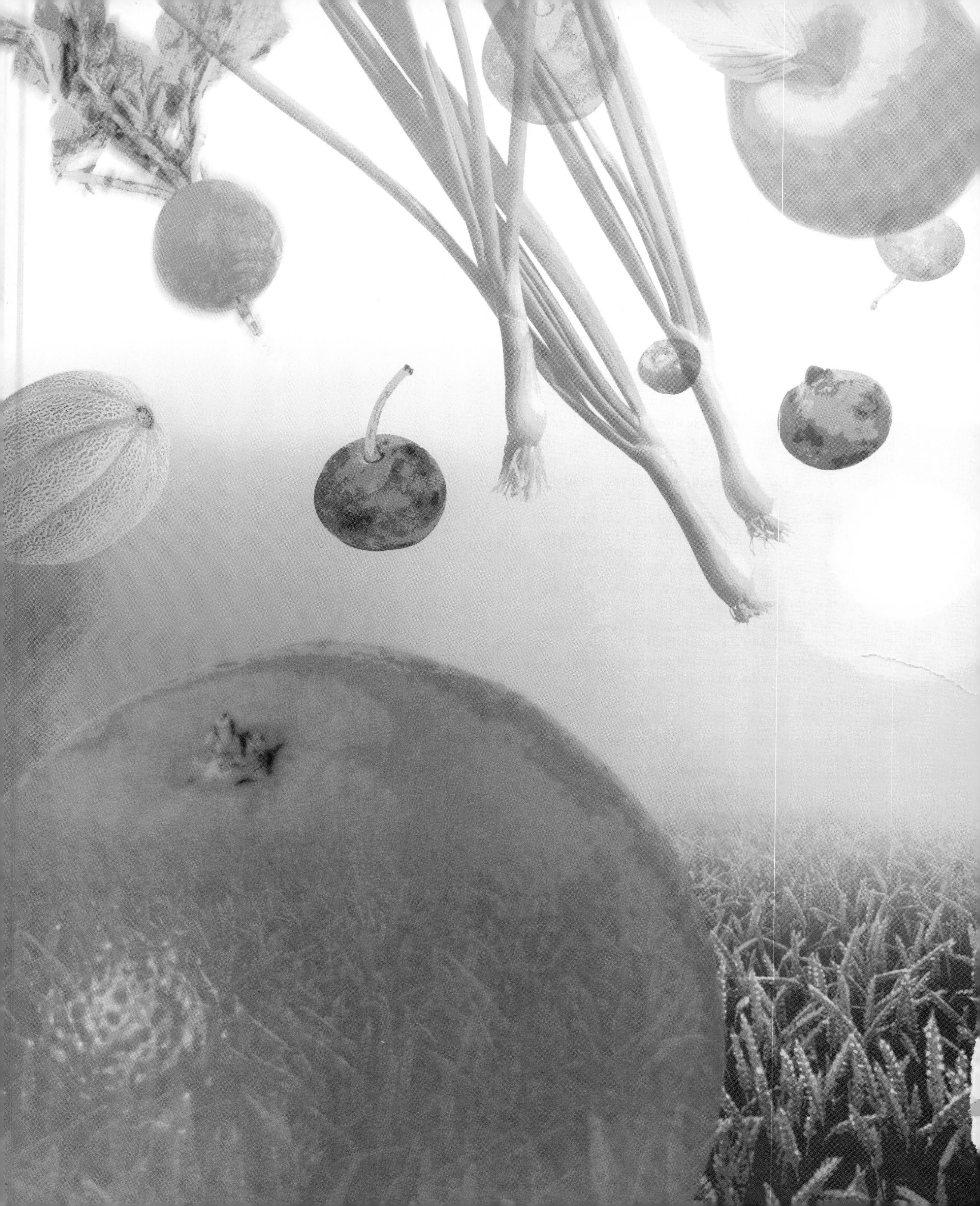

Chapter 8

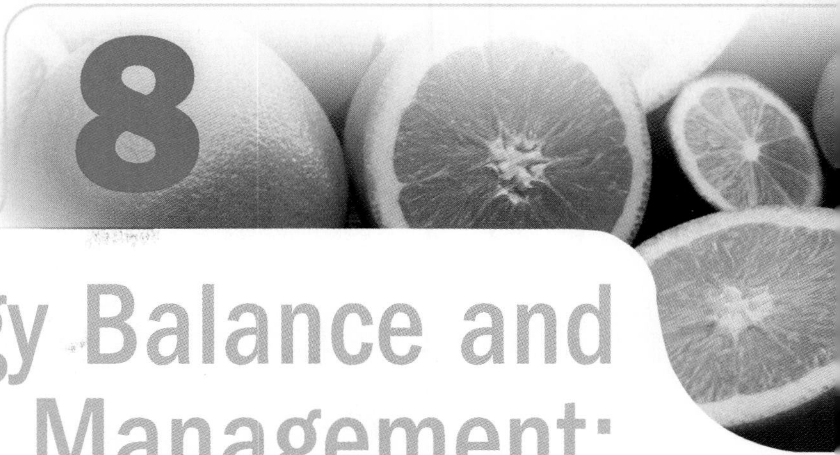

Energy Balance and Weight Management: Finding Your Equilibrium

Think About It

1. How often do you reject dessert after a big meal?
2. When it comes to body fat distribution, are you an apple or a pear?
3. What does it mean to be metabolically fit?
4. How much time do you spend talking with your friends about weight?

Fyi for your Information

This chapter's FYI boxes include practical information on the following topics:

- What's Neat about NEAT?
- How Many Calories Do I Burn?
- High-Protein Diets for Weight Loss: Helpful or Harmful?
- Behaviors That Will Help You Manage Your Weight

www

The Web site for this book offers many useful tools and is a great source for additional nutrition information for both students and instructors. For information on energy balance, body composition, and weight management, visit the site at **nutrition.jbpub.com/discovering.** You'll find exercises that explore the following topics:

- Leptin in Mice and Humans
- Weighing In
- Calculating Your Health
- BMI Calculator
- Childhood Obesity
- Bariatric Surgery

What About Bobbie?

Track the choices Bobbie is making with the EatRight Analysis software.

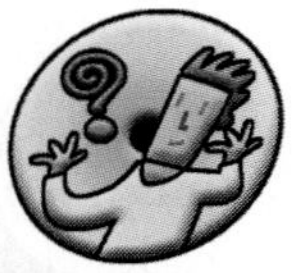

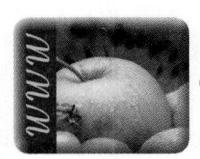

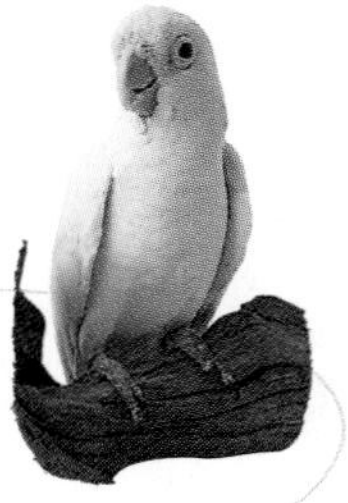

Quick Bites

Early Energy-Balance Experiments

Erasistraus of Chios performed the first recorded experiment on energy balance in 280 B.C.E. Seeking to balance intake with output, he used a jar to fashion a kind of respiration apparatus. He then put two birds in the jar, weighing them and their excreta before and after feeding.

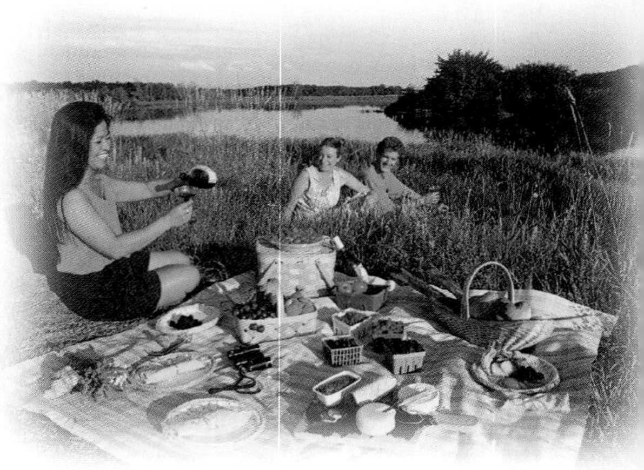

Your body is in the energy exchange business. Here's how it works. You balance the energy you expend with energy from the food in your diet. If you do a fairly good job of equalizing input and output, your body does the rest—maintaining energy equilibrium and keeping your weight steady. But suppose you bring in more energy than your body can handle? It banks the excess energy as fat, and you gain weight. If your "account" grows too big, you become obese. Losing that extra weight—withdrawing the fat from your account—is not always easy.

Energy intake is the amount of calories you take in through consumption of carbohydrate, protein, fat, and alcohol. **Energy output** is the amount of calories you primarily expend on basic body functions, physical activity, and the processing of food. An average adult consumes 2,200 to 3,000 kilocalories per day. In one year, that adds up to 803,000 to 1,095,000 kilocalories! Amazingly, despite such a huge intake of energy over time, most people maintain roughly the same weight during their working lives.

People who maintain a relatively constant weight are in **energy equilibrium**. Within limits, your body automatically regulates your weight, thanks to its ability to balance intake and expenditure. Your body can be in energy equilibrium even if your energy intake is very high, as long as your expenditure also is high. Conversely, your body can be in energy equilibrium when you don't expend much energy, as long as your intake also is low.

When you take in more energy than you need, you have a **positive energy balance**. You store the surplus as fat—the major energy reserve—and as glycogen, the short-term energy/carbohydrate reserve. Pregnant women and growing children need a positive energy balance to increase energy stores. But the positive energy balance that results from overeating and inactivity, a common occurrence around major holidays, leads to unneeded weight gain.

When you take in less energy than you need, you have a **negative energy balance**. Your body uses stores of glycogen and fat for fuel (and body protein, too, if the deficit is extreme), and body weight goes down. Thus, body weight change reflects overall **energy balance**. Starvation reflects an extreme negative energy balance. **Figure 8.1** shows three people with different ratios of energy intake to energy expenditure.

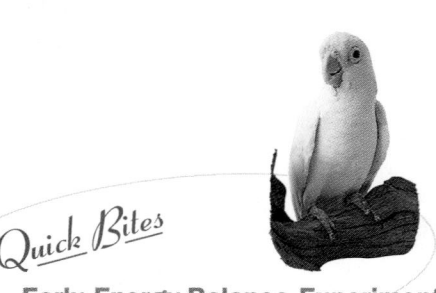

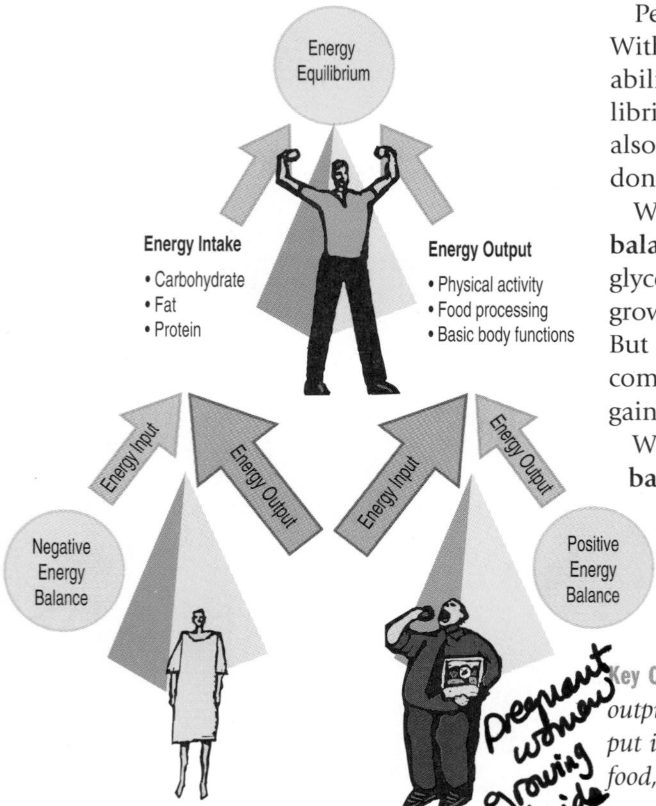

Figure 8.1 **Energy balance.** Most people balance energy intake and output and stay in energy balance. People in negative energy balance lose weight, and those in positive energy balance gain weight.

Key Concepts: *Energy balance is the relationship between energy intake and energy output. Energy intake is the amount of calories contained in the diet. Energy output is the amount of fuel used mainly for basic body functions, the processing of food, and physical activity.*

Energy In

Internal and external cues help the body regulate food consumption and thus maintain energy equilibrium. Internal cues involve interactions and feedback mechanisms among hormones and hormonelike compounds and organ systems. External cues are stimuli in the eating environment and include the sight, smell, and taste of food. Internal and external cues work together to ensure that we eat enough to survive. But the complex interplay of these cues makes it difficult to identify specific factors that cause overeating and obesity or disordered eating.

Hunger, Satiation, and Satiety

We experience internal cues as three different sensations that influence our eating behaviors. (See **Figure 8.2**.) The first, **hunger**, prompts eating ("I'm hungry"). Hunger is a physical sensation that includes the gnawing feeling in your stomach that signals the physiological need to eat. The second, **satiation**, tells you to stop eating ("I'm full"). The third, **satiety**, determines the interval between meals ("I'm not ready to eat again"). Satiety means not being hungry; it is influenced by how many calories you ate at your last meal.

Appetite

External cues can stimulate **appetite**, which complicates the workings of hunger, satiation, and satiety. Hunger and appetite work in tandem to ensure adequate nourishment. Hunger is the physiological need for food. Appetite is the psychological desire to eat and is related to pleasant sensations associated with food. In this sense, hunger is a basic drive, while appetite reflects our eating experiences. When you are truly hungry, any food will do, but your appetite can trigger your desire for a specific food or type of food, even though you may not be hungry. For example, after a big meal of steak, potato, salad, and bread, you probably wouldn't want a second helping. But you might be tempted by the dessert cart! That's appetite. Even when we are hungry, illness and medication can cause loss of appetite and a lack of interest in food.

Think About It 1

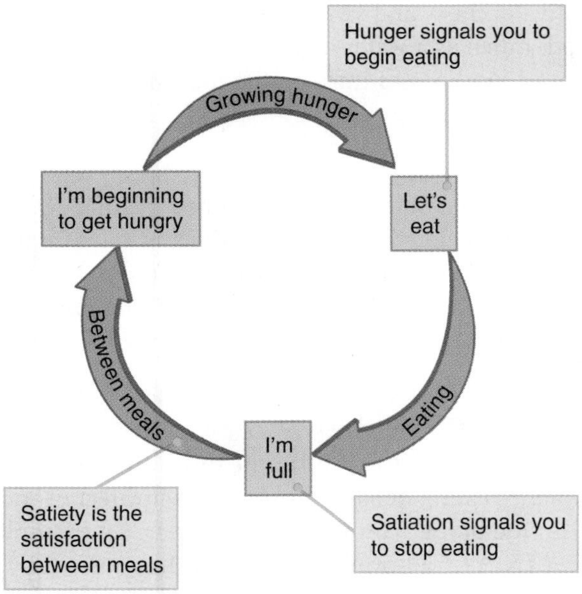

Hunger signals you to begin eating
Growing hunger
I'm beginning to get hungry
Let's eat
Between meals
Eating
I'm full
Satiety is the satisfaction between meals
Satiation signals you to stop eating

Figure 8.2 **Hunger, satiation, and satiety.** Hunger helps initiate eating. Satiation brings eating to a halt. Satiety is the state of nonhunger that determines the amount of time until eating begins again.

energy intake The caloric or energy content of food provided by the sources of dietary energy: carbohydrate (4 kcal/g), protein (4 kcal/g), fat (9 kcal/g), and alcohol (7 kcal/g).

energy output The use of calories or energy for basic body functions, physical activity, and processing of consumed foods.

energy equilibrium A balance of energy intake and output that results in little or no change in weight over time.

positive energy balance Energy intake exceeds energy expenditure, resulting in an increase in body energy stores and weight gain.

negative energy balance Energy intake is lower than energy expenditure, resulting in a depletion of body energy stores and weight loss.

energy balance The balance in the body between amounts of energy consumed and expended.

hunger The internal, physiological drive to find and consume food. Unlike appetite, hunger is often experienced as a negative sensation, often manifesting as an uneasy or painful sensation.

satiation Feeling of satisfaction and fullness that terminates a meal.

satiety The effects of a food or meal that delay subsequent intake. Feeling of satisfaction and fullness following eating that quells the desire for food.

appetite A psychological desire to eat that is related to the pleasant sensations often associated with food.

hypothalamus [high-po-THAL-ah-mus] A region of the brain involved in regulating hunger and satiety, respiration, body temperature, water balance, and other body functions.

neuropeptide Y (NPY) A neurotransmitter widely distributed throughout the brain and peripheral nervous tissue. NPY activity has been linked to eating behavior, depression, anxiety, and cardiovascular function.

leptin A hormone produced by adipose cells that signals the amount of body fat content and influences food intake.

Quick Bites

Why Do We Have Hunger Pangs?

When the stomach has been without food for at least three hours, intense stomach contractions can begin, sometimes lasting two to three minutes. Healthy young people have the strongest contractions, due to good muscle tone in the GI tract. After 12 to 24 hours, contractions of an empty stomach can cause painful hunger pangs.

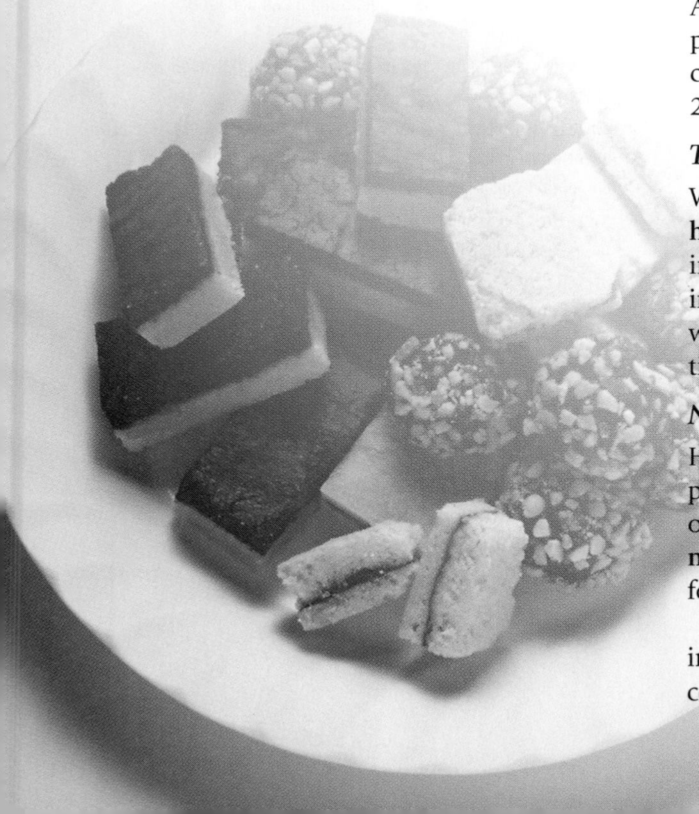

Key Concepts: *Food intake is regulated by sensations of hunger, a physiological drive to eat; satiation, feelings of satisfaction that lead to ending a meal; and satiety, continued feelings of fullness that delay the start of the next meal. Appetite is the psychological urge to eat and often has no relation to hunger.*

Control by Committee

What, then, stimulates hunger, satiation, and appetite? What you eat and responses in the digestive tract, central nervous system, and general circulation influence your eating behavior. Sites throughout the body monitor energy status and send reports to the brain. Even the temperature of our environment affects how much we eat.

Diet Composition

Recent studies suggest that energy density (kcal/g) influences satiation and satiety.[1] People tend to eat a fairly constant amount of food, so diets that are energy dense (typical of high-fat, low-fiber diets) tend to delay satiation and encourage overeating.[2] The amount of energy-dense food that provides satiation has more calories than the same amount of high-fiber, low-fat food. Choosing an energy-dense food means eating more calories before you feel full. Some types of fiber enhance satiation by slowing the rate at which the stomach empties, while others seem to enhance satiation by creating bulk.[3] Protein appears to have a stronger satiating effect than fats or carbohydrates. How varied are your food choices? How tasty are your meals? These factors,[4] as well as the effects of food on blood glucose levels,[5] also influence satiation and satiety.

Gastrointestinal Sensations

As food fills your stomach and small intestine, they stretch and trigger signals to the brain. Your sense of fullness suppresses your urge to eat.[6]

Just passing a reasonable amount of food through the mouth can satisfy hunger temporarily—even if the food never reaches the stomach. When researchers fed large amounts of food to a person with a hole in the esophagus, hunger decreased, even though the food never reached the stomach. As we taste, salivate, chew, and swallow, the brain probably measures the passage of food, much as a water meter measures the flow of water. After a certain amount of food passes through the mouth, hunger diminishes for 20 to 40 minutes.[7]

Temperature

We tend to eat more in cold weather, less in hot weather. Systems in the **hypothalamus** that regulate body temperature and food intake probably interact to link temperature and eating behavior. In cold temperatures, increased food intake helps us survive; it increases the metabolic rate, which helps generate heat, and increases fat stores, which provide insulation to reduce heat loss.[8]

Neurological and Hormonal Factors

Hormones, hormonelike factors, and some drugs (including appetite suppressants) influence eating behavior through their direct or indirect effects on the brain.[9] In the brain, a drop in insulin levels, for example, activates **neuropeptide Y (NPY)**,[10] a hormonelike factor that powerfully stimulates food intake.[11] A rise in insulin levels suppresses NPY.

Animal studies show that the hormone **leptin** suppresses appetite and increases energy output.[12] Fat cells produce this hormone, which tells the central nervous system just how much fat the body is storing.

Administering leptin to experimental obese animals who lack the hormone causes them to attain normal weight. On the other hand, common human obesity is associated with increased, not decreased, leptin levels,[13] and a trial of leptin in obese people resulted in variable amounts of weight loss.[14] Research shows that leptin reverses many of the physiological responses to starvation, and some scientists suggest that leptin's main role may be to respond to food deprivation.[15]

Environmental and Social Factors

The aroma of freshly baked bread or the warmth and chewiness of chocolate chip cookies right out of the oven encourages us to eat more than our hunger dictates! Food's sensory properties—flavor, texture, color, temperature, and presentation—influence its appeal, and such external cues affect food intake.[16] (See **Figure 8.3**.)

Many people use food to cope with stress and negative emotions. Eating can provide a powerful distraction from loneliness, anger, boredom, anxiety, shame, sadness, and inadequacy. To combat low moods, low energy levels, and low self-esteem, people often turn to the refrigerator. When we use food and eating to cope with our emotions, binge eating or other disturbed eating patterns can develop.

Cultural backgrounds and social situations strongly define what we find acceptable or unacceptable as food or as part of a meal (e.g., chips and pretzels for snacks at a party, but not for a formal dinner). While most Americans may find pancakes, bacon, and eggs appealing at breakfast, they might reject a ham sandwich, macaroni and cheese, or chicken stir-fry at a morning meal. For more on cultural influences, see Chapter 1, "Food Choices."

Key Concepts: *Diet composition and factors in the digestive tract and central nervous system influence eating behavior. The brain, especially the hypothalamus,*

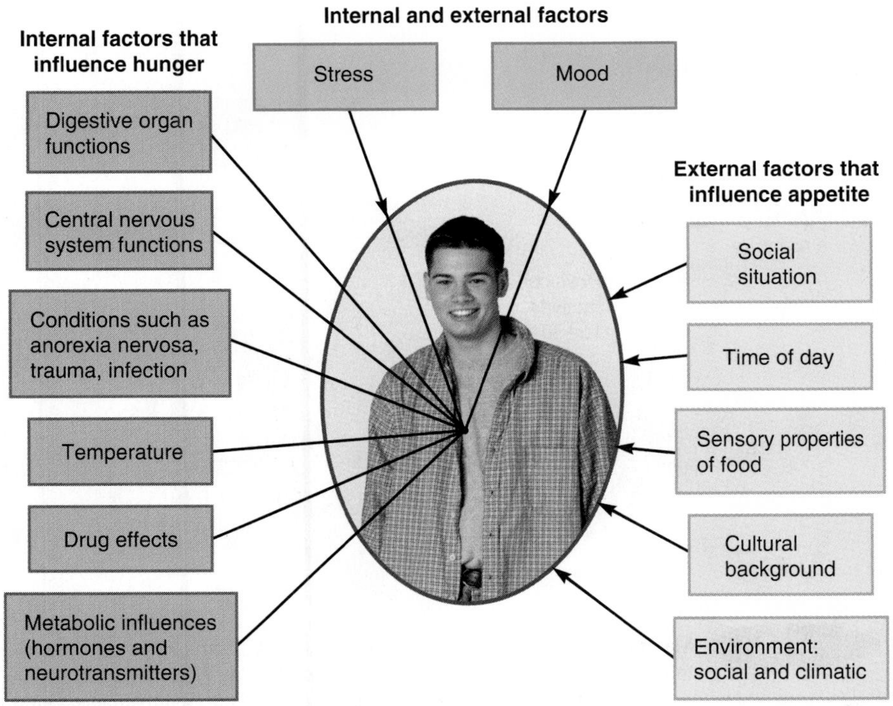

Figure 8.3 **Internal and external influences on hunger and appetite.**

total energy expenditure (TEE) The total of the resting energy expenditure (REE), energy used in physical activity, and energy used in processing food (TEF); usually expressed in kilocalories per day.

resting energy expenditure (REE) The minimum energy needed to maintain basic physiological functions (e.g., heartbeat, muscle function, respiration).

resting metabolic rate (RMR) A clinical measure of resting energy expenditure performed three to four hours after eating or performing significant physical activity. Often used interchangeably with BMR.

basal metabolic rate (BMR) A clinical measure of resting energy expenditure performed upon awakening, 10 to 12 hours after eating, and 12 to 18 hours after significant physical activity. Often used interchangeably with RMR.

receives signals from all over the body about energy status. External factors such as time of day, season of the year, social circumstances, and cultural traditions, as well as the food itself, can enhance or suppress appetite.

Energy Out: Fuel Uses

Your body uses fuel (expends energy) for three primary purposes:

1. to maintain basic physiological functions such as breathing and blood circulation
2. to process the food you eat
3. to power physical activity

We also expend energy to support growth, stay warm in cold environments, metabolize drugs, and deal with physical trauma, fever, and psychological stress. The sum of all energy expended is the **total energy expenditure (TEE)**. **Figure 8.4** illustrates the major components of energy expenditure.

Major Components of Energy Expenditure

Energy Expenditure at Rest

We generally expend most of our energy on the basic body functions needed to sustain life. This **resting energy expenditure (REE)** maintains heartbeat, respiration, nervous function, muscle tone, body temperature, and so on. Resting energy expenditure accounts for 60 to 75 percent of total energy expenditure.[17] The rate of energy expended at rest (as kcal/hr or kcal/day) is measured as either the **resting metabolic rate (RMR)** or the **basal metabolic rate (BMR)**. RMR and BMR are virtually interchangeable; it's just that the ideal conditions for measuring BMR are harder to meet.

Quick Bites

Brrr! Shivering Away Calories

Cold weather increases energy needs. Shivering alone can increase the RMR by 2.5 times. Although shivering bodies use both fat and carbohydrate, carbohydrates are the preferred fuel. In addition, people with less body fat shiver more in the cold.

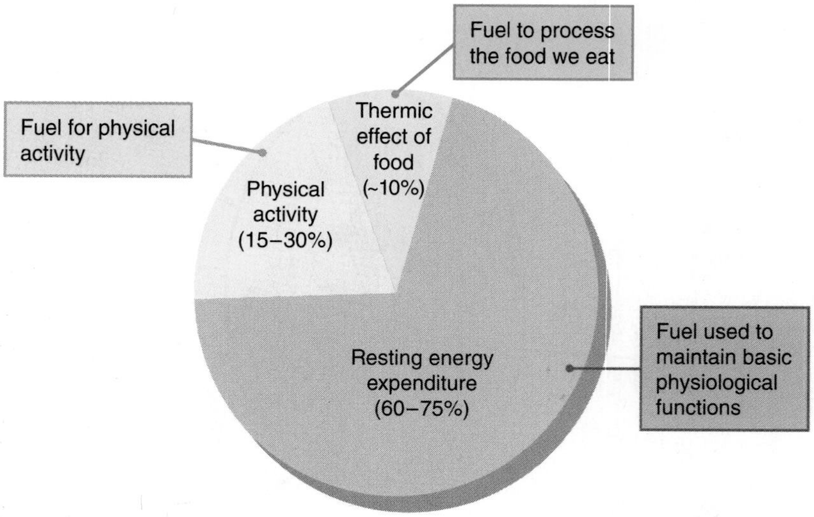

Figure 8.4 **Major components of energy expenditure.** You expend most of your energy to maintain basic body functions. Energy expended in physical activity can be significant and is the most variable component of total energy expenditure. The thermic effect of food is the energy needed to digest, absorb, transport, metabolize, and store ingested food.

Energy expended by organs and resting muscles makes up the greatest proportion of RMR. Other tissues, such as fat, have lower metabolic activity and consume less energy. Muscles, organs, bones, and fluids make up most of what is known as the **lean body mass**—the total mass of the body that isn't fat. An extremely muscular person with a large lean body mass has a higher resting energy expenditure than someone who weighs the same but has a higher proportion of body fat.

Lean body mass tends to decline as we age, and body fatness tends to rise.[18] Keeping physically active helps slow this age-related loss of lean tissue and discourages gain of fat so that we maintain a higher RMR.

Women usually have lower RMRs than men. Women tend to be smaller, and pound for pound they generally have less lean body mass. A woman's RMR also varies during the menstrual cycle, fluctuating from a low point about one week before ovulation to a high point just before the onset of menstruation.[19] **Figure 8.5** shows the factors that affect RMR.

Key Concepts: *We use energy to fuel basic body functions, process the food we eat, and support physical activity. Factors that affect resting energy expenditure include body composition, age, and gender.*

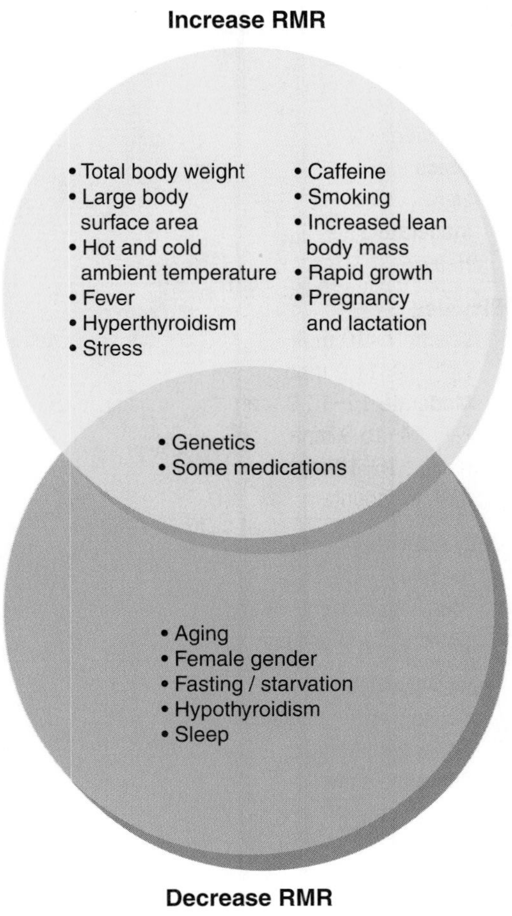

Figure 8.5 **Factors that affect RMR.** Inherited traits determine whether you have a generally high or low RMR. Many environmental and physiological factors may temporarily raise RMR, and other factors may temporarily lower it.

Energy Expenditure for Physical Activity

Physical activity is more than just exercise and sport. It includes work, leisure activities, and other everyday activities, even fidgeting. Depending on whether a person is mostly sedentary or a top athlete in training, energy expended on physical activity is 15 to 30 percent of total energy expenditure.[20] The energy cost of an activity depends on its duration, type (whether it is walking, running, or typing, for example), and intensity. **Table 8.1** shows the amounts of energy expended in specific activities. Body size affects energy cost, too—it takes more energy to move a bigger mass, so a large person expends more calories per minute than a smaller person doing the same activity. Fitness level has an effect as well. Individuals who are fit exercise more efficiently, with lower energy costs. However, they will be able to exercise with greater intensity and duration, burning more calories overall. **Figure 8.6** shows the measurement of energy expended in physical activity.

Mental activity—such as studying for an exam—uses little energy. But if you fidget when you study, you may expend a significant amount of energy. The recently coined term **NEAT** stands for **nonexercise activity thermogenesis**, which is the energy associated with fidgeting, maintenance of posture, and similar contributors to energy expenditure.[21] (See the FYI feature "What's Neat about NEAT?")

Energy Expenditure to Process Food

Our bodies expend energy to digest, absorb, and metabolize the nutrients we take in, and these processes generate heat. This energy output is collectively called the **thermic effect of food (TEF)**. TEF peaks about one hour after eating and normally dissipates within five hours. The TEF is lowest for fat and highest for protein. For a typical mixed diet, TEF accounts for approximately 10 percent of total energy expenditure.[22]

Key Concepts: *An individual's fitness level and weight and the duration, type, and intensity of activity affect the amount of energy expended in physical activity. The thermic effect of food is the energy needed to process the food we eat and is influenced by the amount and mix of nutrients in the diet.*

lean body mass The portion of the body exclusive of stored fat, including muscle, bone, connective tissue, organs, and water.

nonexercise activity thermogenesis (NEAT) The output of energy associated with fidgeting, maintenance of posture, and other minimal physical exertions.

thermic effect of food (TEF) The energy used to digest, absorb, and metabolize energy-yielding foodstuffs. It constitutes about 10 percent of total energy expenditure but is influenced by various factors.

Table 8.1 Amount of Energy Expended in Specific Activities

			Kcal/hr at Different Body Weights				
Description	*kcal/hr/kg*	*kcal/hr/lb*	*50 kg 110 lb*	*57 kg 125 lb*	*68 kg 150 lb*	*80 kg 175 lb*	*91 kg 200 lb*
Aerobics							
Light	3.0	1.36	150	170	205	239	273
Moderate	5.0	2.27	250	284	341	398	455
Heavy	8.0	3.64	400	455	545	636	727
Bicycling							
Leisurely <10 mph	4.0	1.82	200	227	273	318	364
Light 10–11.9 mph	6.0	2.73	300	341	409	477	545
Moderate 12–13.9 mph	8.0	3.64	400	455	545	636	727
Fast 14–15.9 mph	10.0	4.55	500	568	682	795	909
Racing 16–19 mph	12.0	5.45	600	682	818	955	1091
BMX or mountain	8.5	3.86	425	483	580	676	773
Daily Activities							
Sleeping	1.2	0.55	60	68	82	95	109
Studying, reading, writing	1.8	0.82	90	102	123	143	164
Cooking, food preparation	2.5	1.14	125	142	170	199	227
Home Activities							
House painting, outside	4.0	1.82	200	227	273	318	364
General gardening	5.0	2.27	250	284	341	398	455
Shoveling snow	6.0	2.73	300	341	409	477	545
Running							
Jogging	7.0	3.18	350	398	477	557	636
Running 5 mph	8.0	3.64	400	455	545	636	727
Running 6 mph	10.0	4.55	500	568	682	795	909
Running 7 mph	11.5	5.23	575	653	784	915	1045
Running 8 mph	13.5	6.14	675	767	920	1074	1227
Running 9 mph	15.0	6.82	750	852	1023	1193	1364
Running 10 mph	16.0	7.27	800	909	1091	1273	1455
Sports							
Frisbee, ultimate	3.5	1.59	175	199	239	278	318
Hacky sack	4.0	1.82	200	227	273	318	364
Wind surfing	4.2	1.91	210	239	286	334	382
Golf	4.5	2.05	225	256	307	358	409
Skateboarding	5.0	2.27	250	284	341	398	455
Rollerblading	7.0	3.18	350	398	477	557	636
Soccer	7.0	3.18	350	398	477	557	636
Field hockey	8.0	3.64	400	455	545	636	727
Swimming, slow to moderate laps	8.0	3.64	400	455	545	636	727
Skiing downhill, moderate effort	6.0	2.73	300	341	409	477	545
Skiing cross country, moderate effort	8.0	3.64	400	455	545	636	727
Tennis, doubles	6.0	2.73	300	341	409	477	545
Tennis, singles	8.0	3.64	400	455	545	636	727
Walking							
Strolling <2 mph, level	2.0	0.91	100	114	136	159	182
Moderate pace ~3 mph, level	3.5	1.59	175	199	239	278	318
Moderate pace ~3 mph, uphill	6.0	2.73	300	341	409	477	545
Brisk pace ~3.5 mph, level	4.0	1.82	200	227	273	318	364
Very brisk pace ~4.5 mph, level	4.5	2.05	225	256	307	358	409

Source: Adapted from Nieman DC. *Exercise Testing and Prescription.* 4th ed. Mountain View, CA: Mayfield Publishing; 1999.

Table 8.2 Estimating REE from Body Weight, Gender, and Age

Age (yr)	REE Males	REE Females
0–3	(60.9 × wt) − 54	(61.0 × wt) − 51
3–10	(22.7 × wt) + 495	(22.5 × wt) + 499
10–18	(17.5 × wt) + 651	(12.2 × wt) + 746
18–30	(15.3 × wt) + 679	(14.7 × wt) + 496
30–60	(11.6 × wt) + 879	(8.7 × wt) + 829
>60	(13.5 × wt) + 487	(10.5 × wt) + 596

Note: Body weight is in kg and REE is kcal per day.

Estimating Total Energy Expenditure

Nutritionists usually can estimate total energy expenditure from a person's REE and activity level. Recent equations based on large groups of subjects accurately estimate REE from age, gender, and body weight.[23] (See **Table 8.2.**) Because height showed little effect, the equations exclude it. These equations deliver good TEE estimates for a wide range of ages, including children and older people.

For adults, an older abbreviated method provides a quick and easy estimate of REE (see margin). The 1.0 and 0.9 factors for kilocalories per kilogram reflect the differences in body composition between men and women. Men have proportionally more lean body mass and so burn more calories per kilogram of body weight. This abbreviated method dramatically underestimates children's REE, however, and somewhat overestimates older people's REE.

You can estimate your total energy expenditure as a multiple of REE based on your general activity level. (See **Table 8.3.**) The activity level for most of the U.S. population falls in the light or moderate categories. (See the FYI feature "How Many Calories Do I Burn?")

Table 8.3 Estimating Total Energy Expended from REE and Physical Activity

Activity Factor* Men	Activity Factor* Women	Activity Level	Description
1.3	1.3	Sedentary	Mostly resting with little or no activity
1.6	1.5	Light	Occasional unplanned activity, e.g., going for a stroll
1.7	1.6	Moderate	Daily planned activity, such as brisk walks
2.1	1.9	Heavy	Daily workout routine requiring several hours of continuous exercise
2.4	2.2	Exceptional	Daily vigorous workouts for extended hours; training for competition

*The activity factor accounts for the thermic effect of food.

Total energy expenditure (TEE) = REE 3 activity factor

Source: Adapted from Recommended Dietary Allowances, 10th Edition. 1989 National Academy Press.

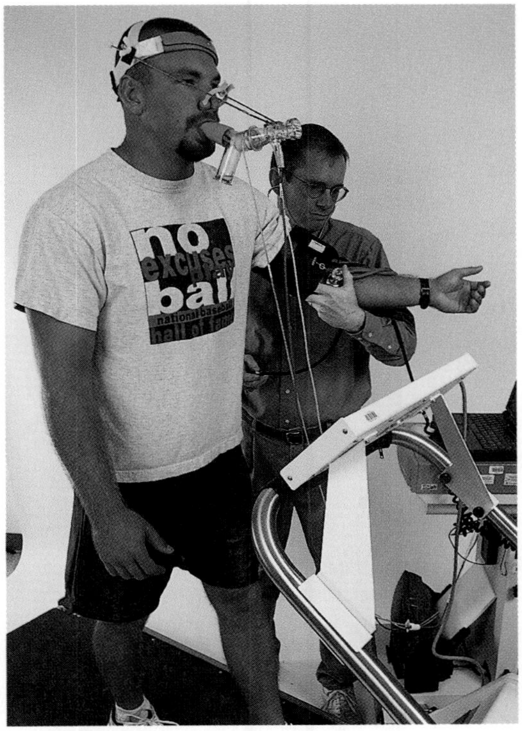

Figure 8.6 **Measuring energy expended in physical activity.** A technician can collect respiratory gases and indirectly calculate energy expenditure during exercise.

Abbreviated Method to Estimate REE

For adult men

$$\text{REE} = \text{weight (kg)} \times 1.0\ \text{kcal/kg} \times 24\ \text{hr}$$
$$\text{REE} = \text{weight (kg)} \times 1.0 \times 24$$

For adult women

$$\text{REE} = \text{weight (kg)} \times 0.9\ \text{kcal/kg} \times 24\ \text{hr}$$
$$\text{REE} = \text{weight (kg)} \times 0.9 \times 24$$

Quick Bites

The Fattest Mammals

Among mammals, humans carry the largest percentage of weight as body fat.

RDA for Energy

The tenth edition of the *Recommended Dietary Allowances* recommends 2,200 kilocalories per day for women aged 19 to 50 years, and 2,900 kilocalories per day for men aged 19 to 50 years.[24] These values assume light to moderate activity levels, and average weights of 55 kilograms (121 lb) for women and 70 kilograms (154 lb) for men. Unlike the RDAs for protein, vitamins, and minerals, energy RDAs represent *average* needs of individuals. If the RDA values for energy were set like the RDAs for other nutrients, they would meet or exceed the needs of 97 to 98 percent of the population, greatly overestimating most people's energy needs.

Body Composition: Understanding Fatness and Weight

body composition The chemical or anatomical composition of the body. Commonly defined as the proportions of fat, muscle, bone, and other tissues in the body.

Stepping onto a scale provides quick and easy feedback about your body weight. Yet many people have a distorted notion of their weight—thinking they're too fat when they are not or thinking their weight is just fine when it isn't. In terms of your health risks, **body composition** is more important than body weight. For example, two people with the same high weight for height may have very different health risks. One may be obese and have many weight-related health risks. The other could be very fit and muscular, with no increased disease risk.

Assessing Body Weight

Height–Weight Tables

Using a height–weight table, you can find a narrow range of body weights (usually by gender) that are associated with good health and "acceptable" appearance. Because bone structure can make a difference, some tables also

Fyi — FOR YOUR INFORMATION

What's Neat about NEAT?

It seems Jan only has to look at food to gain weight. Yet her friend Molly doesn't seem to gain weight no matter what she eats. Both have the same height and frame, eat about the same amount of calories, and get about the same amount of exercise. So what's missing? Recent research suggests that fidgeting and movements such as posture adjustments may be part of the answer.

Studies in the early 1900s first suggested that weight gained in response to overeating wasn't proportional to the extra calories ingested. Following experiments on himself, the German scientist R. O. Neumann coined the term *luxuskonsumption* to describe his observation that excess calories did not result in weight gain and therefore must be lost as heat.[1] Further studies supported this idea, showing wide individual variation in response to overfeeding. Some suggest that the ease of weight gain is genetically based.[2]

A recent study at the Mayo Clinic attributes differences in weight gain in response to overfeeding to a mechanism described as NEAT: nonexercise activity thermogenesis.[3] According to the researchers, NEAT is "the thermogenesis [heat production] that accompanies physical activities other than volitional [intentional] exercise, such as the activities of daily living, fidgeting, spontaneous muscle contraction, and maintaining posture when not recumbent."

In the NEAT study, 16 volunteers (12 men and 4 women) were given an extra 1,000 kilocalories per day—roughly equivalent to two double cheeseburgers—for a period of eight weeks. Before the study began, careful measurements were made over a two-week period to determine each participant's maintenance energy requirements. Physical activity during the study was controlled, and meals were provided only through the Mayo Clinic General Clinical Research Center. Questionnaires and interviews were done to assure compliance.

The average weight gained by the study participants was 4.7 kilograms (10.3 lb), but some gained as much as 7.2 kilograms (15.8 lb), while others added only 1.4 kilograms (3.1 lb). The theoretical expected weight gain from an eight-week excess of 56,000 kilocalories would be 7.3 kilograms (16.0 lb) to 9.1 kilo-

include adjustments for frame size. Weight tables are quick, easy, and cheap, but they ignore body composition, fail to consider other measures of health and fitness, and foster a mentality that there is such a thing as "perfect weight."

Body Mass Index

Body mass index (BMI), also known as the **Quetelet index**, correlates reasonably well with body fatness and health risks.[25] To determine your BMI, accurately measure your height without shoes and your weight with minimal clothing. Then plug these numbers into the equation in the margin.

As **Figure 8.7** shows, correlating BMI with mortality rates produces a J-shaped curve: Low BMI (less than 20 kg/m^2) increases health risks, as does a high BMI (30 to 35 kg/m^2). Mortality rates rise more steeply after BMI exceeds 35 kg/m^2.

Although knowing your BMI will tell you more about your overall health risks than weight tables will, it still doesn't tell you enough about whether you are carrying muscle weight or excess fat. A classic example is the heavy football player or bodybuilder with a large muscle mass who has a BMI greater than 30 kg/m^2 but is not obese. According to NIH guidelines and the *Dietary Guidelines for Americans,* you shouldn't undertake weight loss or other treatments until you evaluate other risk factors associated with obesity, such as high blood pressure, high blood cholesterol, family history of obesity-related disease, or excess abdominal fat (measured by waist circumference).

BMI measurements should be interpreted cautiously when used for children and adolescents who are still growing, pregnant women, people with large body frames, or petite and highly muscular individuals.[26] Revised pediatric growth charts released in 2000 include gender-specific percentile curves for BMI for children 2 to 20 years old.[27] A BMI-for-age at or above

To calculate BMI

$$\text{BMI} = \frac{\text{weight (kg)}}{\text{height (m)}^2}, \text{ or}$$

$$\text{BMI} = \frac{\text{weight (lb)}}{\text{height (in)}^2} \times 704.5$$

body mass index (BMI) Body weight (in kilograms) divided by the square of height (in meters), expressed in units of kg/m^2. Also called Quetelet index.

Quetelet index See *body mass index.*

grams (20.0 lb)—more than the maximum weight gain of any participant!

After accounting for RMR, TEF, and energy used in physical activity, the remaining energy expenditure was attributed to NEAT. The amount of energy expended as NEAT varied among the participants by nearly 800 kilocalories per day. Participants with higher NEAT resisted weight gain, suggesting that people who can effectively activate NEAT tend not to gain weight, even with overeating. Further, this suggests that obese people may not effectively activate NEAT.

Leptin levels do not appear to regulate NEAT. The participants' leptin levels were related to their changes in body fat but not to changes in their energy expenditure as NEAT.[4]

So, is the take-home message "fidget more, stand up straight, and you won't gain weight"? Not exactly. The researchers did not account for factors such as the extra energy needed to move a higher body weight in activity. In addition, they relied on self-reports and pedometers that lacked precision and accuracy.[5] Attributing the entire difference in energy expenditure to NEAT ignores heat production by brown adipose tissue, a type of fat tissue that tends to "waste" energy.[6] Clearly, though, some individuals are able to resist weight gain, and further studies may help to identify and quantify the mechanisms of NEAT.

1 Neumann RO. Experimentalle Beitrage zur Lehre von dem taglichen Nahrungsbedarf der Menschen unter besonder Berucksichtigung der notwendigen Eisewissmenge. *Arch Hyg.* 1902;45:1–2.
2 Bouchard C, Tremblay A, Despres JP, et al. The response to long-term overfeeding in identical twins. *N Engl J Med.* 1990;322:1477–1482.
3 Levine JA, Eberhardt NL, Jensen MD. Role of nonexercise activity thermogenesis in resistance to fat gain in humans. *Science.* 1999;283:212–214.
4 Levine JA, Eberhardt NL, Jensen MD. Leptin responses to overfeeding: relationship with body fat and nonexercise activity thermogenesis. *J Clin Endocrinol Metab.* 1999;84:2751–2754.
5 Ravussin E, Danforth E. Beyond sloth—physical activity and weight gain. *Science.* 1999;283:184–185.
6 Napoli R, Horton ES. Energy requirements. In: Ziegler EE, Filer LJ, eds. *Present Knowledge in Nutrition.* 7th ed. Washington, DC: ILSI Press; 1996; and Levine JA, Eberhardt NL, Jensen MD. Loc. cit.

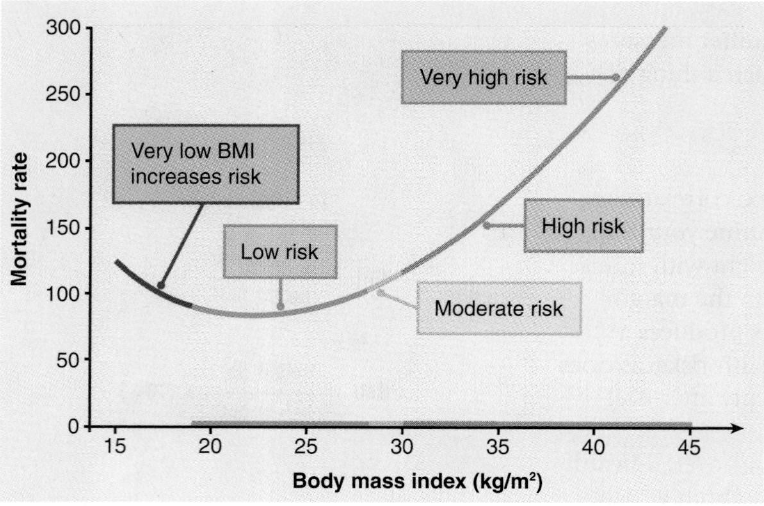

Figure 8.7 **BMI and mortality.** People with a high or very low BMI have a higher relative mortality rate.

the 95th percentile indicates the need for further evaluation and possible treatment. Further evaluation may also be indicated if the child's BMI-for-age is at or above the 85th percentile and is accompanied by other risk factors (mentioned earlier).[28] A BMI-for-age below the 5th percentile suggests the child is underweight.

Key Concepts: *Body composition is a key element in determining energy expenditure and is an important factor in disease risk. Measures of weight and height are used to identify overweight and obesity, but height–weight tables do not address body composition. Weight and height measures can be used to calculate BMI, which is a better assessment tool. Elevated BMI in adults or children can increase health risks.*

Assessing Body Fatness

Body composition is the relative amount of fat and lean body mass. For adult women, body fat is normally 20 to 25 percent of total body weight; for men, the range is 12 to 20 percent. Risk of chronic disease rises dramatically when body fat exceeds 30 percent in women or 25 percent in men.

Body fatness can be assessed by a number of methods. **Underwater weighing**, also called **hydrostatic weighing**, and the **BodPod** use the principle of density to determine relative amounts of fat-free and fat mass. **Figure 8.8** illustrates underwater weighing, and **Figure 8.9** shows the BodPod. **Bioelectrical impedance analysis (BIA)** uses resistance to an electric current to determine amounts of lean tissue. More sophisticated techniques such as **dual energy x-ray absorptiometry (DEXA)**, isotope dilution, **computed tomography (CT)**, and **magnetic resonance imaging (MRI)** more accurately assess body composition; however, their expense limits their usefulness. **Skinfold measurements** assess the thickness of fat deposits directly underneath the skin. Done correctly, body composition estimates from skinfolds correlate well with those from underwater weigh-

Quick Bites

Where's the Fat?

The location of excess abdominal fat may hold information about health risks. Within the abdomen, visceral fat (fat surrounding the organs) may be more harmful than subcutaneous fat (fat under the skin). Only imaging can distinguish between the two.

Fyi — How Many Calories Do I Burn?

FOR YOUR INFORMATION

You can estimate the amount of energy you use each day by using some simple equations. Remember that there will be quite a lot of individual variation in actual energy output, and so these calculated values are just estimates.

1. Convert your weight in pounds to weight in kilograms. For example, a 120-pound weight is 54.5 kilograms.

__________ ÷ 2.2 = __________
weight (lbs) **weight (kg)**

2. From Table 8.2, get the correct REE formula for your age and gender. For example, if you are a 19-year-old woman, the formula is **REE = (14.7 × wt) + 496.**

Using 54.5 kilograms from our example in the last step, REE = 1,298 kilocalories. Calculate your personal REE.

REE = __________ **kilocalories**

3. From Table 8.3, get the correct activity factor for your activity level and gender. A moderately active woman has an activity factor of 1.6, so the total energy expenditure is REE × 1.6 = 2,077 kilocalories. Calculate your personal total energy expenditure.

__________ × __________ = __________
REE **activity factor** **total energy expenditure**

ing, but an inexperienced or careless technician easily can make large errors. Skinfold measurements usually work better for assessing malnutrition than identifying overweight and obesity.

Body Fat Distribution

Measurements of body fatness tell you more about your health risks than your weight does, but still don't tell the whole story. Where the fat is located—**body fat distribution**—can be an independent risk factor.[29] The "pear shape," or **gynoid obesity**, more common in women, has fat distributed predominantly around the hips and thighs. The "apple shape," or **android obesity**, typical of men, has extra fat distributed higher up, around the abdomen. You are at greater health risk with the apple pattern than with the pear pattern of fat distribution. In fact, excess abdominal fat may increase breast cancer risk for women.[30] **Figure 8.10** shows the gynoid and android distributions of body fat.

Think About It 2

Waist Circumference

The *Dietary Guidelines for Americans* suggest that if your **waist circumference** increases, you are probably gaining fat. NIH clinical guidelines suggest that for people with a BMI of 25 kg/m^2 to 34.9 kg/m^2, a waist circumference greater than 40 inches in men or greater than 35 inches in women is a sign of increased health risk. When BMI is 35 kg/m^2 or higher, waist circumference measures cannot predict health risks.

Key Concepts: *Researchers can use a number of different methods to assess body fatness. Expense may limit the usefulness of more sophisticated techniques. Skinfold measurements are better suited for assessing malnutrition than for detecting excess fat. Distribution of body fat is important in evaluating risk of disease. Excess body fat around the abdomen (even with normal to slightly elevated BMI) is associated with higher disease risk than is excess fat around the hips and thighs. Waist circumference can be used to assess body fat distribution.*

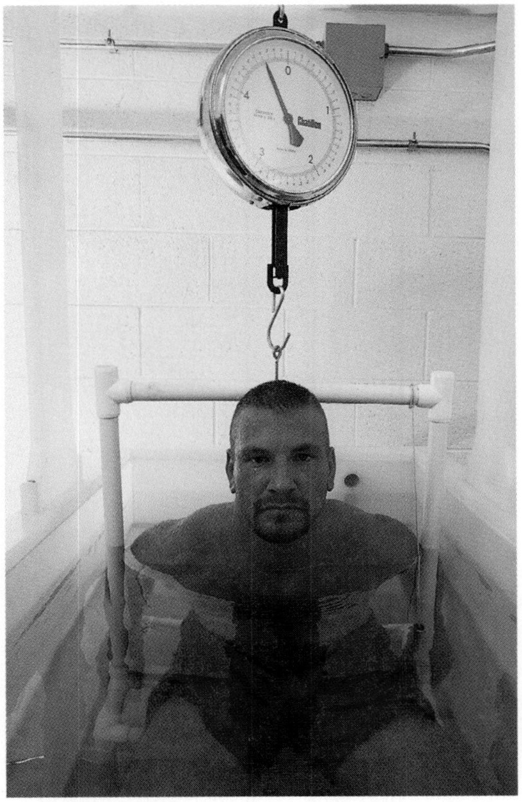

Figure 8.8 **Underwater weighing.** During underwater weighing, the subject must exhale completely, submerge without taking a breath, and remain motionless until the water is still and the scale is steady.

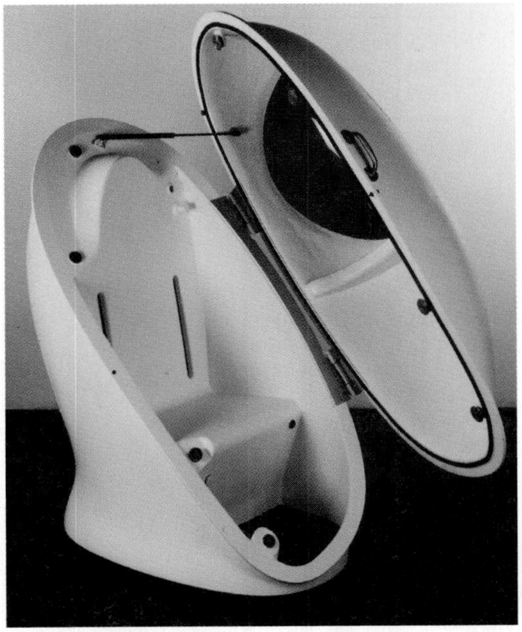

Figure 8.9 **BodPod.** By using air displacement, the BodPod provides an alternative to underwater weighing that is easier, cheaper, and of similar accuracy.

underwater weighing Determining body density by measuring the volume of water displaced when the body is fully submerged in a specialized water tank. Also called hydrostatic weighing.

hydrostatic weighing See *underwater weighing*.

BodPod A device used to measure the density of the body based on the volume of air displaced as a person sits in a sealed chamber of known volume.

bioelectrical impedance analysis (BIA) Technique to estimate amounts of total body water, lean tissue mass, and total body fat. It uses the resistance of tissue to the flow of an alternating electric current.

dual energy x-ray absorptiometry (DEXA) A body composition measurement technique originally developed to measure bone density.

computed tomography (CT) The gathering of anatomical information from cross-sectional images generated by a computer synthesis of x-ray data.

magnetic resonance imaging (MRI) Medical imaging technique that uses a magnetic field and radiofrequency radiation to generate anatomical information.

skinfold measurements A method to estimate body fat by measuring the thickness of a fold of skin and subcutaneous fat.

body fat distribution The pattern of fat distribution on the body.

gynoid obesity Excess storage of fat located primarily in the buttocks and thighs. Also called gynecoid obesity.

android obesity [AN-droyd] Excess storage of fat located primarily in the abdominal area.

waist circumference The waist measurement, as a marker of abdominal fat content, can be used to indicate health risks.

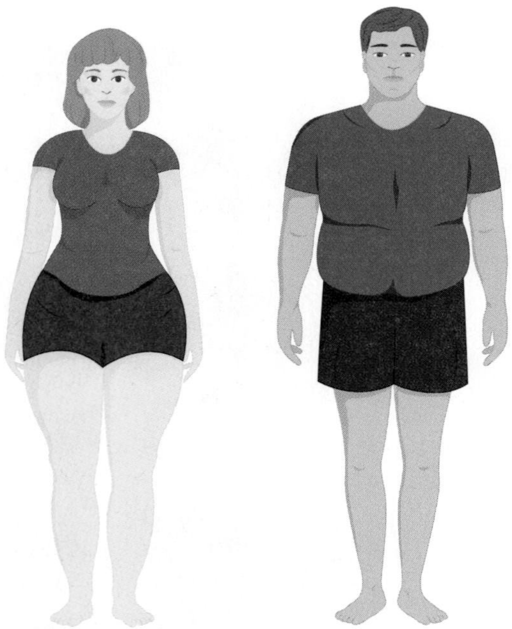

Figure 8.10 **Differences in body fat distribution.** Men tend to carry excess fat around their abdomen (android obesity). Women tend to accumulate excess fat in their hips and thighs (gynoid obesity).

When Energy Balance Goes Awry

Our bodies usually balance energy intake and output closely, but disruptions can cause overweight, obesity, or underweight. **Figure 8.11** can help you determine whether your current weight is a "healthy" weight according to the *Dietary Guidelines for Americans*.

Overweight is generally defined as a BMI greater than 25 but less than 30 or body weight that is 10 to 20 percent above desirable weight or the recommended weight range in a height–weight table. Technically, it is an excess of body weight that includes all body tissues—fat, bone, muscle, water, and so on.

Obesity is generally defined as a BMI greater than or equal to 30 or a body weight that is 20 percent or more above the recommended weight range in a height–weight table. The definition of obesity assumes an excess of body fat.

Underweight is generally defined as body weight 15 to 20 percent or more below desirable weight for height. It is much less common than overweight and obesity and may result from an underlying illness.

Health Risks of Overweight and Obesity

Overweight and obesity are major public health challenges. Obese people are at higher risk for heart disease, the leading cause of death in the United States and Canada, and for stroke, diabetes, hypertension, some forms of cancer, gallbladder and joint diseases, and psychosocial problems. The longer obesity persists, the higher the risks. **Table 8.4** lists the effects that being overweight could have on your health.

Directions: Find your weight on the bottom of the graph. Go straight up from that point until you come to the line that matches your height. Then look to find your weight group.

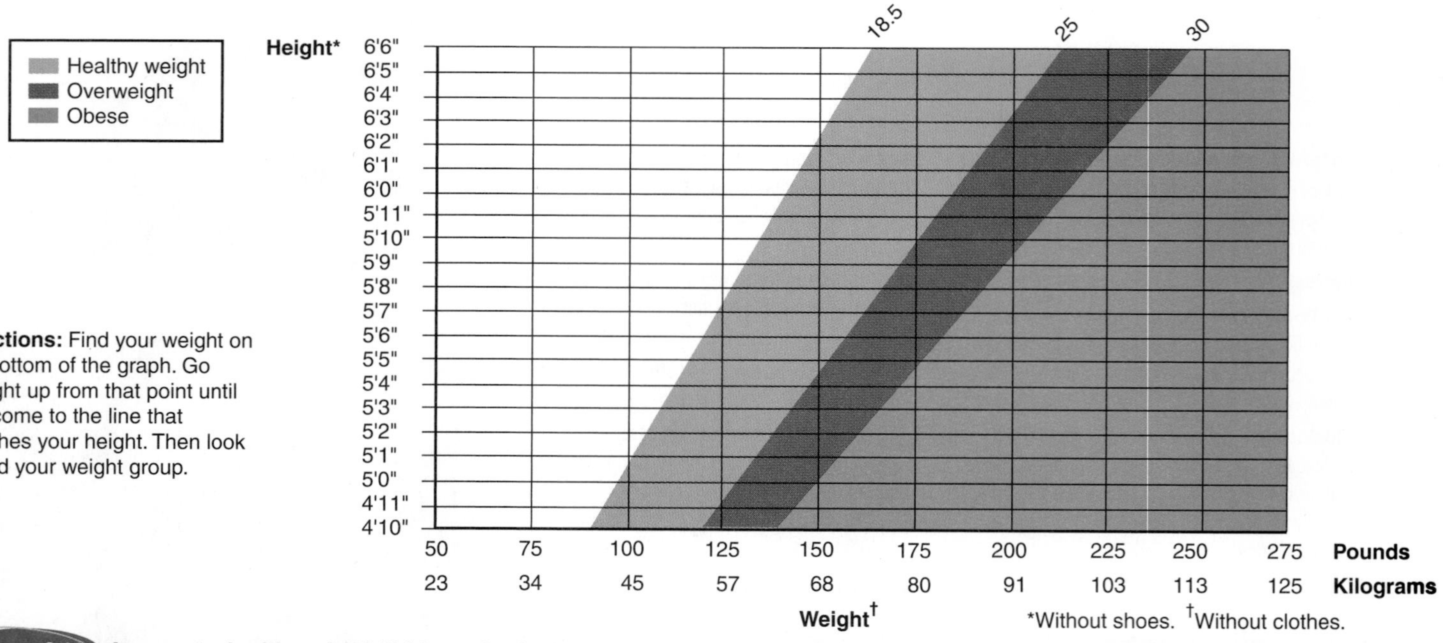

Figure 8.11 **Are you at a healthy weight?** BMI is a ratio of weight in relation to height. The *Dietary Guidelines for Americans* identifies a healthy weight as a BMI between 18.5 and 25. This chart shows weight and height combinations that result in BMI values that are healthy, overweight, or obese.
Source: *Report of the Dietary Guidelines Advisory Committee on the Dietary Guidelines for Americans;* 2000. http://www.usda.gov/cnpp/Pubs/DG2000/Full%20Report.pdf. Accessed 6/14/02.

Table 8.4 What Are the Risks of Being Overweight?

Hypertension

Overweight people are more likely to have high blood pressure, a major risk factor for heart disease and stroke, than people who are not overweight.

Heart Disease and Stroke

Hypertension and very high blood levels of cholesterol and triglycerides (blood fats) can lead to heart disease and often are linked to being overweight. Being overweight also contributes to angina (chest pain caused by decreased oxygen to the heart) and sudden death from heart disease or stroke without any signs or symptoms.

Diabetes

Overweight people are twice as likely to develop type 2 diabetes as people who are not overweight. Type 2 diabetes is a major cause of early death, heart disease, kidney disease, stroke, and blindness.

Cancer

Several types of cancer are associated with being overweight. In women, these include cancer of the uterus, gallbladder, cervix, ovary, breast, and colon. Overweight men are at greater risk for developing cancer of the colon, rectum, and prostate. For some types of cancer, such as colon or breast, it is not clear whether the increased risk is due to the extra weight or a high-fat and high-calorie diet.

Sleep Apnea

Sleep apnea is a serious condition that is closely associated with being overweight. Sleep apnea can cause a person to stop breathing for short periods during sleep and to snore heavily. Sleep apnea may cause daytime sleepiness and even heart failure. The risk for sleep apnea increases with higher body weights. Weight loss usually improves sleep apnea.

Osteoarthritis

Extra weight appears to increase the risk of osteoarthritis by placing extra pressure on weight-bearing joints and wearing away the cartilage (tissue that cushions the joints) that normally protects them. Weight loss can decrease stress on the knees, hips, and lower back and may improve the symptoms of osteoarthritis.

Gout

Gout is a joint disease caused by high levels of uric acid in the blood. Uric acid sometimes forms into solid stone or crystal masses that become deposited in the joints. Gout is more common in overweight people, and the risk of developing the disorder increases with higher body weights.

Note: *Over the short term, some weight-loss diets may lead to an attack of gout in people who have high levels of uric acid or who have had gout before. People who have a history of gout should check with their doctors or other health professionals before trying to lose weight.*

Gallbladder Disease

Gallbladder disease and gallstones are more common if you are overweight. Your risk of disease increases as your weight increases. It is not clear how being overweight may cause gallbladder disease.

Weight loss itself, particularly rapid weight loss or loss of a large amount of weight, can actually increase your chances of developing gallstones. Modest, slow weight loss of about one pound a week is less likely to cause gallstones.

Source: NIH Publication No. 98-4098; May 1998.

The blood lipid levels that typically accompany obesity—high serum triglycerides, low HDL, and a high LDL/HDL ratio—increase the risk for atherosclerosis.[31] Even a person who is only mildly to moderately obese has an elevated risk of coronary heart disease. However, modest weight loss (about 10 percent of body weight) reduces risk.

Type 2 diabetes, the most common form of diabetes in the United States and Canada, is three times more likely to develop in people who are obese, especially if they have abdominal ("apple") obesity. Obesity increases insulin resistance and compromises the ability of body cells to take up glucose. Diabetes in turn is a risk factor for heart disease, kidney disease, and vascular problems. Again, modest levels of weight reduction can improve glucose tolerance.

Weight loss lowers blood pressure in overweight people with hypertension. Overweight people are two to six times more likely to develop hypertension,[32] probably due to increased resistance in the peripheral blood vessels, changes in the way the kidneys handle sodium, and other changes in kidney function.

overweight Body weight in relation to height that is greater than some accepted standard but less than that defined as obesity.

obesity Excessive accumulation of body fat leading to a body weight in relation to height that is substantially greater than some accepted standard.

underweight Body weight in relation to height that is less than some accepted standard.

While the exact reason is unknown, obesity increases the risk of cancer. The same food pattern that contributes to obesity (a diet high in calories and fat, plus low in fiber, fruits, and vegetables) also may be a cancer risk. Inactivity not only encourages obesity, but also increases cancer risk. For example, women who are physically active have a lower risk of breast cancer than sedentary women.[33] People who are obese have increased levels of hormones that influence development of some cancers. Obese women, for example, have more endometrial, gallbladder, cervical, and ovarian cancers.[34]

Obese people are more likely to have obstructive **sleep apnea**, in which the airway collapses during sleep and breathing stops for a short spell. As the body struggles for air, blood pressure spikes upward. Typically, the individual wakes up, gasps for air, begins breathing again, and then falls asleep until the airway collapses again and the cycle repeats; this pattern interrupts sleep and prevents a good night's rest. People with sleep apnea have a higher risk of heart attack and stroke. Modest weight loss alleviates sleep apnea, improves sleep quality, and reduces daytime drowsiness.[35]

Quick Bites

Island Obesity

Some of the most obese people in the world live in the islands of Micronesia. Among these populations, the Naurus are the most obese.

sleep apnea Periods of absence of breathing during sleep.

weight cycling Repeated periods of gaining and losing weight. Also called yo-yo dieting.

Weight Cycling

Weight cycling is a pattern of losing and regaining weight, over and over again. You might expect this behavior to be harmful, perhaps harder on the body than overweight itself. However, research shows that the potential benefits of weight loss for obese individuals outweigh the potential risks of weight cycling.[36]

A recent study reports that women who repeatedly gain and lose weight, especially obese women, have significantly lower levels of HDL, the "good" cholesterol. While low HDL levels are a significant risk factor for coronary artery disease (CAD), the investigators did not observe a direct link between weight cycling and CAD. More research is necessary so that the health and behaviors of these women can be observed over time.[37]

Key Concepts: *Obesity is a risk factor for many chronic diseases, including heart disease, cancer, hypertension, and diabetes. In many cases, a modest amount of weight loss (about 10 percent) can improve symptoms and disease management.*

How Common Is Overweight and Obesity?

The growth in the rate of obesity is alarming. In fact, obesity has become a global problem.[38] Worldwide, obesity is emerging as the most important contributor to ill health—displacing undernutrition and infectious diseases.[39] Not only is obesity prevalent in Europe and the Americas,[40] but it is also on the rise in Southeast Asia. Over the past two decades, Japan and China have seen a marked increase in overweight and obesity. In North Africa, more than half the women in Morocco and Tunisia are overweight or obese.[41] In the Middle East, the United Arab Emirates now recognizes obesity as a major public health problem.[42]

In the United States, overweight and obesity increased dramatically during the 1980s, when the rate jumped from one of every four Americans to one of three.[43] In 1998, 55 percent of adult Americans were overweight or obese (with a BMI of 25 or more). Roughly 22 percent of adults, 11 percent of teens, and 13 percent of children are obese.[44] The escalating problem is blamed on overconsumption of plentiful, tasty, and energy-dense foods, along with decreased physical activity. The goal of *Healthy People 2010* is to cut the prevalence of obesity to no more than 15 percent in adults and 5 percent in children and adolescents.[45]

As overweight and obesity have increased, so have society's emphasis on thinness, and people's efforts at weight management. Every year, the diet industry rakes in about $30 billion to $50 billion from weight-loss programs, diet books, pills, videos, and supplements.

Children and adolescents also are concerned about weight. In studies of grade-school girls from various socioeconomic backgrounds, 28 to 40 percent reported that they sometimes dieted or were very often worried about being fat.[46]

Key Concepts: *Worldwide, the number of overweight or obese people has increased markedly in recent years. At the same time, more people are engaging in weight-control efforts and starting to do so at younger ages.*

fat cell theory The theory that the quantity of fat stored in the body is a result of the number and size of fat cells.

hypercellular obesity Obesity due to an above-average number of fat cells.

hypertrophic obesity Obesity due to an increase in the size of fat cells.

hyperplasia (hyperplastic obesity) Obesity due to an increase in both the size and number of fat cells.

set point theory A theory that a regulatory mechanism operates to keep a certain variable (e.g., body temperature, weight) at a constant value called the set point.

Early Theories of Weight Regulation

What causes obesity? The basics of energy balance tell us that weight gain is a result of positive energy balance: Energy intake is greater than energy output. So what happens when energy regulation goes awry and results in obesity? Several theories have emerged.

Fat Cell Theory

According to the **fat cell theory**, the number and size of fat cells in the body help determine how easily a person gains or loses fat. People with an above-average number of fat cells, **hypercellular obesity**, may have been born with them or may have developed them at certain critical times because of overeating. In **hypertrophic obesity**, fat cells are larger than normal. Fat cells continue to expand as they fill with more fat; when their capacity is reached, the body generates more cells. (See **Figure 8.12**.) Once body fat reaches three to five times the normal amount (by then a person is 40 percent or more overweight), fat tissue is likely to have both bigger fat cells *and* more of them, a condition called **hyperplasia (hyperplastic obesity)**.

Even with weight loss, the number of fat cells does not decline (though presumably some could be removed by liposuction). Fat cells do get smaller, but beyond a certain point, they resist further shrinking and the body strives to refill them with fat. The fat cell theory provides an explanation of why some obese people have difficulty losing weight and regain it easily, but not why they became obese in the first place.

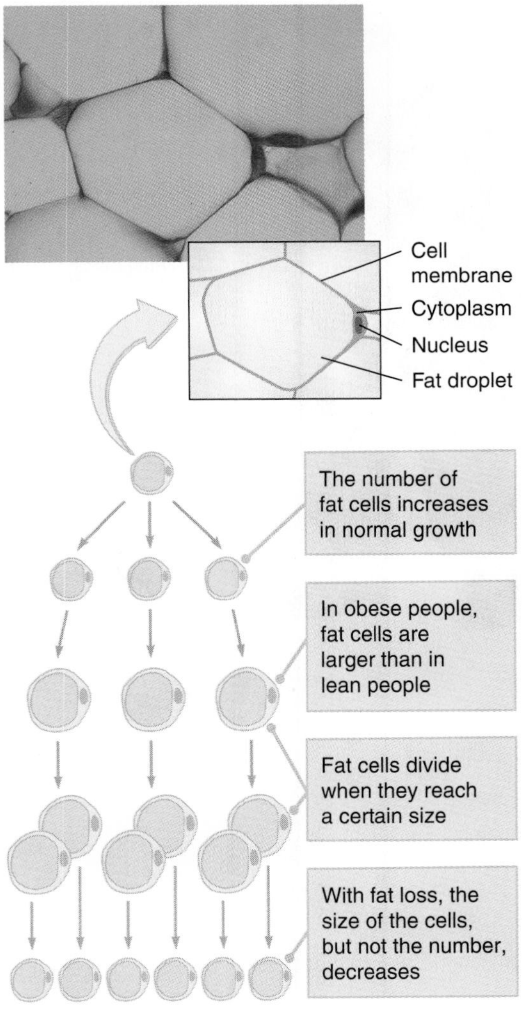

Cell membrane
Cytoplasm
Nucleus
Fat droplet
The number of fat cells increases in normal growth
In obese people, fat cells are larger than in lean people
Fat cells divide when they reach a certain size
With fat loss, the size of the cells, but not the number, decreases

Figure 8.12 **The formation of fat cells.** As body fat accumulates, fat cells enlarge and divide. Fat loss reduces the size of fat cells, but not their number.

Set Point Theory

For most people, body fat and body weight remain constant over long periods despite fluctuations in food intake and activity. Building on this observation, the **set point theory** assumes that the body has internal controls that maintain weight at a set point, even if that weight is unhealthy. During adulthood, however, many people experience significant long-term weight changes, so if set points exist, they vary over a wide range of weights and can be changed. Many researchers have challenged the set point theory as too simplistic, and there is little science to support it.

Additional Early Theories

Although people often have blamed defects in hormonal and metabolic mechanisms for obesity, these rarely occur. To maintain a high body weight, people typically must consume a large number of calories. Yet, obese people often report eating less than what one would expect. Such underreporting is a widely recognized difficulty in dietary intake studies that rely on self-reports.[47]

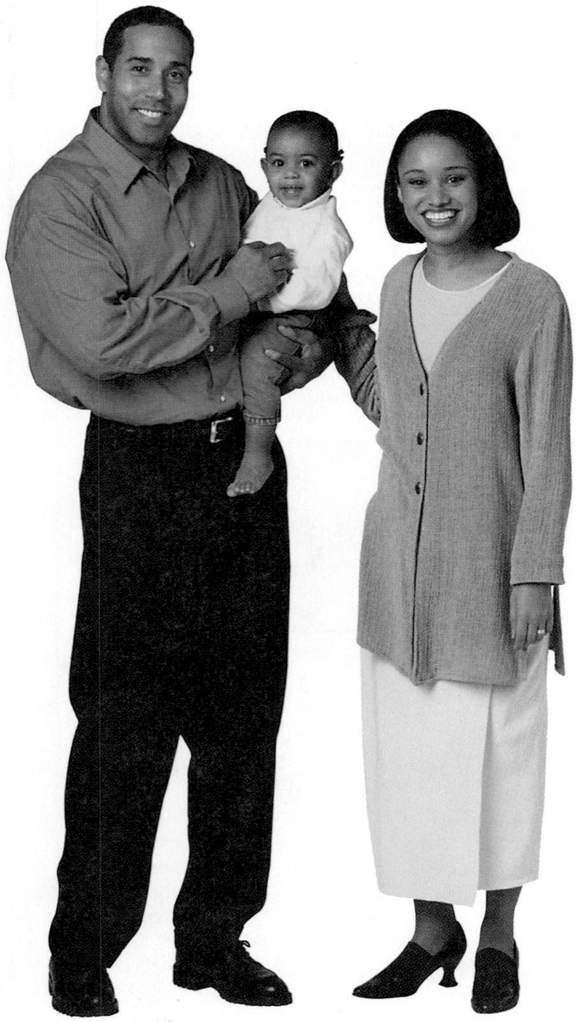

Key Concepts: *Many theories have been proposed to explain obesity. These include the fat cell theory that too many fat cells and enlarged fat cells cause obesity; the set point theory that obese individuals are "programmed" to carry a certain amount of weight; and other theories, all largely discounted today.*

Current Thinking about Obesity

Obesity is a complex disorder that probably involves several regulatory mechanisms and the way they interact and respond to sociocultural and environmental factors, exercise patterns, and biological factors of heredity, age, and gender.

Heredity and Genetic Factors

The search for a genetic role in obesity has barely begun, but the research is promising. So far scientists have identified several genes that when damaged or dysfunctional can cause obesity or increase its likelihood.

Researchers have long recognized hereditary patterns of obesity. When both parents are morbidly obese (body weight 100 percent above normal), the probability that their children will be obese is high (80 percent); when neither parent is obese, the probability that their children will be obese is relatively low (less than 10 percent). However, about 25 to 30 percent of obese individuals have normal-weight parents.[48]

To what extent are family patterns caused by the environment rather than heredity? Because of the interplay between genetics and the environment, the hereditary component is difficult to estimate. Environment and sociocultural influences interact closely with heredity to produce obesity. Researchers estimate that genes alone generally account for 50 to 90 percent of variations in the amount of stored body fat.[49]

Sociocultural Influences

Social factors also influence the development of obesity. Abundant high-calorie, highly palatable foods, pervasive advertising promoting their consumption, and the social enjoyment of eating all create pressures to overeat. At the same time, our culture tells us that we should be thin, and we feel unhealthy pressures to diet. **Table 8.5** summarizes social characteristics that are key predictors of obesity.

Age and Lifestyle

Research links excessive television viewing to obesity in children. For all ages, obesity itself may lead to physical inactivity, though the extent is unclear. As adolescents and young adults, most of us worry about body weight and appearance. A survey of dietetics majors aspiring to become registered dietitians, for example, finds that most dieters in this group wanted to lose weight to improve appearance and increase self-esteem.[50] As we age, we become more concerned with our weight as it relates to health. Both men and women gain the most weight between 25 and 34 years of age. After that, we gain weight more slowly and then start to lose it after we reach age 55.[51] However, it's often important for seniors to maintain weight.

Gender

In general, men and women set different weight standards for themselves. Beginning in grade school, boys are less likely than girls to consider themselves overweight; in fact, males of all ages accept some degree of overweight. Boys typically are more concerned about becoming taller and more

Table 8.5 Sociocultural Influences on Obesity

Social Contexts	
Culture	People in developed societies have more body fat than those in developing societies.
History	Fatness is increasing in the United States, but idealized weights are decreasing.
Social Characteristics	
Age and lifestyle	Fatness increases during adulthood, declines in the elderly.
Gender	Obesity is more prevalent in women than in men.
Race and ethnicity	Obesity is more prevalent in African American, Hispanic, Native American, and Pacific Islander women.
Socioeconomic Status	
Income	Obesity is more prevalent in lower-income women.
Education	Less-educated women have a higher incidence of obesity.
Occupational prestige	Obesity is more prevalent in women (people) in less prestigious jobs.
Employment	Women who are not employed have a higher incidence of obesity.
Household composition	Older people who live with others have a higher incidence of obesity.
Marriage	Married men have a higher incidence of obesity.
Residence	Rural women have a higher incidence of obesity.
Region	People residing in the South have a higher incidence of obesity.

Source: Adapted with permission from Dalton S. Body weight terminology, definitions, and measurements. In: Dalton S, ed. *Overweight and Weight Management: The Health Professional's Guide to Understanding and Practice.* Gaithersburg, MD: Aspen; 1997:314. © Aspen Publishers, Inc.

muscular. By early adulthood, about the same number of men want to lose or gain weight, whereas almost all women want to lose weight. As adults, men tend to see themselves as overweight at higher weights, while women describe themselves as overweight when they are closer to a healthy body weight. (See **Figure 8.13**.) Adult women feel thin only when they weigh less than 90 percent of desirable body weight, whereas men rate themselves as thin even when they weigh as much as 105 percent of healthy body weight.[52]

Although women try harder than men to avoid overweight or to slim down,[53] they frequently become obese after pregnancy and at menopause. In pregnancy, fat stores increase to meet the energy demands of breastfeeding. Many women retain this extra weight after they give birth and become heavier with each child.

Ethnicity

In the United States the prevalence of obesity and attitudes about weight differ among ethnic groups. Black and Latina women are more likely to be

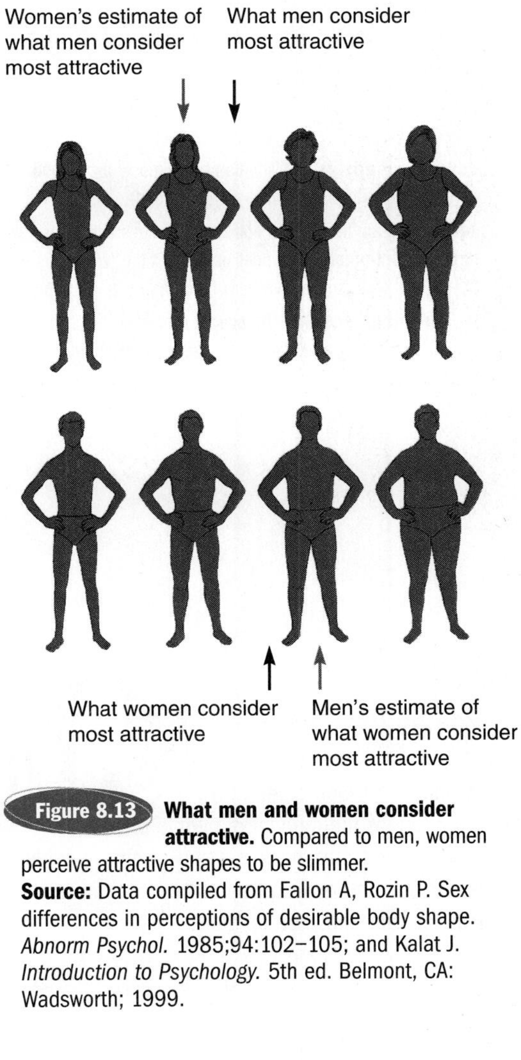

Figure 8.13 What men and women consider attractive. Compared to men, women perceive attractive shapes to be slimmer.
Source: Data compiled from Fallon A, Rozin P. Sex differences in perceptions of desirable body shape. *Abnorm Psychol.* 1985;94:102–105; and Kalat J. *Introduction to Psychology.* 5th ed. Belmont, CA: Wadsworth; 1999.

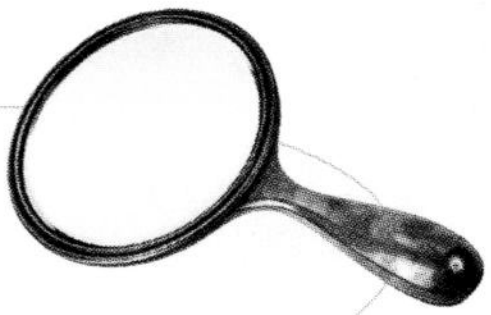

Quick Bites

Mirror, Mirror, on the Wall

A recent study demonstrated that college students and supermarket shoppers ate less in front of a mirror, spreading less full-fat cream cheese on bagelettes and less full-fat margarine on bread than when there was no mirror. The researchers speculated that the mirror decreased food consumption by increasing self-awareness, providing an external reality check on the amount of food being consumed. Mirrors had no effect on the consumption of low-fat or nonfat products, perhaps because people did not perceive these products to be unhealthy.

overweight than white women.[54] As cultures, African Americans, Hispanic Americans, Native Americans, and Pacific Islanders typically value thinness less than white Americans do.[55]

Socioeconomic Status

American women are more likely to be obese if they have low socioeconomic status, and the stigma of obesity can impede their upward mobility. Rural women tend to be heavier than women living in metropolitan areas, and Southern women are the most likely to be overweight.[56]

Employment

Some studies suggest that employed women are thinner than those not in the labor force.[57] Employers tend to hire people of normal weight rather than those who are overweight or obese. Women who work outside the home also have extra income that can be used for healthier food choices, physical activity programs, and health care; on the other hand, they have less time to prepare healthful meals and get routine exercise. Changing jobs, losing a job, or retiring often changes eating patterns and subsequently body weight.

Psychological Factors

Some people adopt eating as a strategy to deal with the stresses and challenges of life. (Others use drugs, alcohol, smoking, shopping, gambling, and so on.) Eating can provide entertainment and alleviate boredom as well; it may be used as a pick-me-up when fatigued. Sometimes people eat to distract themselves from difficult problems or as a means of punishing themselves or others for real or imagined transgressions.

People with a healthy lifestyle have more effective ways to meet their needs. They communicate assertively and manage interpersonal conflict effectively and so don't shrink from problems or overreact. The person with a healthy lifestyle knows how to create and maintain relationships with others and has a solid network of friends and loved ones. Food is used appropriately—to fuel life's activities and gain personal satisfaction, not to manage stress.

Certain obese people may be more prone to emotional eating than others. These subgroups include **restrained eaters** and **binge eaters**.[58]

restrained eaters Individuals who routinely avoid food as long as possible, and then gorge on food.

binge eaters Individuals who routinely consume a very large amount of food in a brief period of time (e.g., two hours) and lose control over how much and what is eaten.

weight management The adoption of healthful and sustainable eating and exercise behaviors that reduce disease risk and improve well-being.

Restrained Eaters Some people try to reduce their calorie intake by fasting or avoiding food as long as possible. They skip meals, delay eating, or severely restrict the types of food they eat. Then, like a dam that bursts, they overeat when environmental or emotional stress triggers a complete release of inhibitions toward eating (disinhibition). Although not all obese binge eaters follow this pattern, the "fast, then binge" behavior is common in obese people who chronically attempt to lose weight.[59] This pattern also occurs in women of "normal" weight who perceive themselves as fat. These restrained eating patterns appear to be passed on from mother to daughter.[60]

Quick Bites

People Persuasion

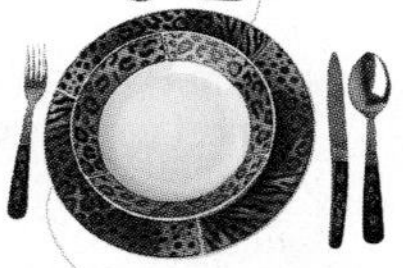

The best predictor of the amount of food eaten at a given time is the amount of people present. Studies show that meals eaten with other people last longer and tend to have 44 percent more calories than those eaten alone.

Binge Eaters A binge eater compulsively overeats, sometimes for days. Some people binge only at night, taking in most of their excess calories between 6 P.M. and the time they go to sleep. Binge eating is common among people enrolled in weight-loss programs—estimates of its prevalence range from 23 to 46 percent.[61] People who binge are more likely to be emotional eaters or to have psychological problems than are those who do not binge. For more information about binge eating, see the "Spotlight on Eating Disorders."

Key Concepts: *Obesity tends to run in families. Gender, age, and sociocultural factors such as socioeconomic status, employment status, marital status, and having children also are related to weight. Overly restrained eating may result in episodes of overeating and weight gain. Binge eating is common among people in weight-loss programs.*

Weight Management

The numerous interrelated factors that lead to obesity are different for every person. Approaches to weight management are just as complex and must be tailored to the individual to be effective. As you continue reading, keep in mind the following definition of **weight management** from the American Dietetic Association; note that there is no mention of weight loss or ideal weight:

Weight management is the adoption of healthful and sustainable eating and exercise behaviors indicated for reduced disease risk and improved feelings of energy and well-being.[62]

The Perception of Weight

The way we view obesity, its causes, and its treatment has changed over time. Until recently many cultures associated obesity with prosperity and good health. In the latter part of the twentieth century, however, Westernized cultures began to see obesity in a different light.

The weights of celebrity models often mold popular notions about desirable weight. In the early 1960s, as today, thin was "in." (At that time, the trendsetter was supermodel Twiggy, who at 5 feet, 7 inches, weighed 98 pounds.) Between 1959 and today, the number of diet and exercise articles in women's magazines escalated, and diet books became bestsellers. Dieting became an institution with its own magazines, television shows, camps and resorts, and weight-loss gurus. The images in **Figure 8.14** show that beauty has not always been associated with thinness.

Despite obesity's link to health risks, a backlash against dieting has emerged. The antidiet advocates' rallying cry is, "Diets don't work!" While acknowledging that severe obesity is dangerous, they argue for size acceptance and challenge the notion that mild obesity is unhealthful.

A new view of obesity evolved in the 1990s: Health professionals now treat it as a complex disorder with multiple contributing factors. (See **Figure 8.15**.) They now emphasize overall health and fitness rather than a number on the bathroom scale. Dietary recommendations emphasize moderation and a balanced diet that is low in fat and high in healthful foods such as fruits, vegetables, and grains. Behavior change is still an important part of weight management, but change is seen as an ongoing process that requires new skills for maintaining a healthy lifestyle over the long run. The requirement for vigorous exercise has been relaxed; experts now stress moderate exercise for improving fitness, regardless of weight.

There are limitations to what each of us can weigh or look like. While we shouldn't abandon efforts to achieve good health, we should balance our desire to lose weight with self-acceptance. If we engage in futile attempts to

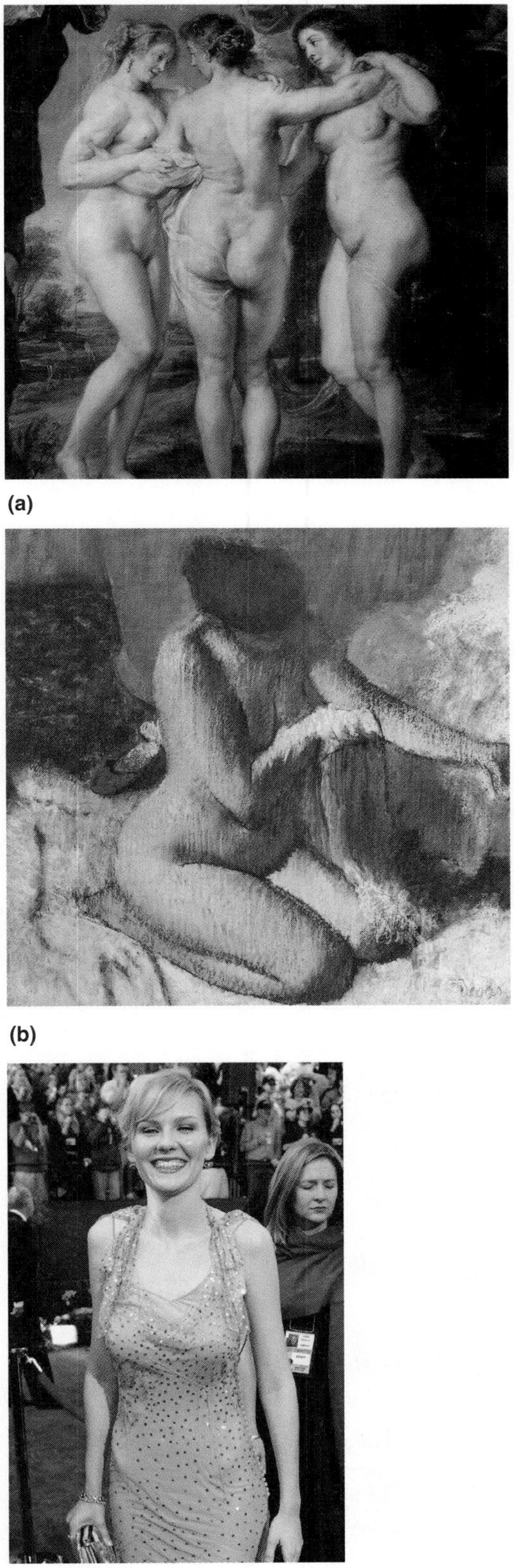

(a)

(b)

(c)

Figure 8.14 **Society's changing standards of beauty.** Over time, society has increasingly valued thinness. (a) Ruben's *The Three Graces*, 1639. (b) Degas's *After the Bath*, 1896. (c) Actress Kirsten Dunst, 2002.

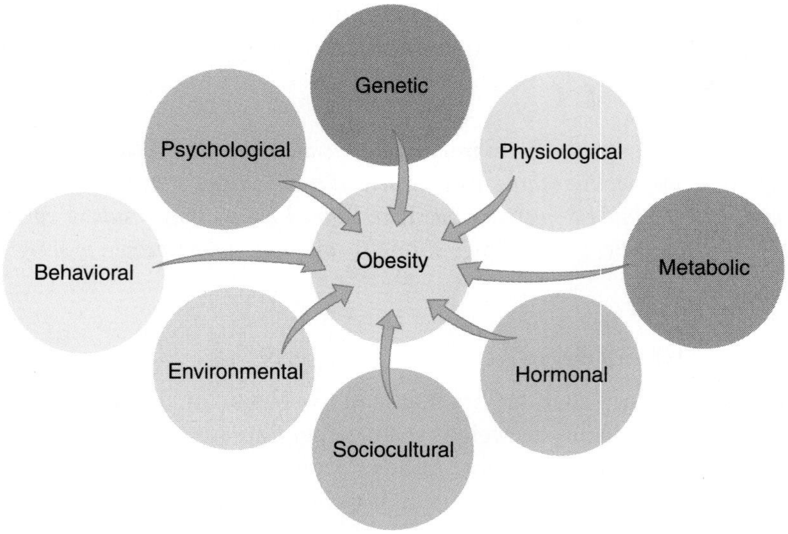

Figure 8.15 **Multiple factors contribute to obesity.** Obesity is a complex disorder that is not easy to treat.

metabolic fitness The absence of all metabolic and biochemical risk factors associated with obesity.

achieve an "ideal" body shape and weight, we may undermine our self-esteem and be harmed emotionally or even physically.

Key Concepts: *Many factors contribute to the complex disorder of obesity. Currently, experts suggest that the best way to manage weight is to improve health by establishing healthful eating and exercise patterns and accepting the limitations of heredity.*

What Goals Should I Set?

What is a reasonable goal for weight management? If you are overweight or obese, a good way to start is with a modest weight-loss goal of roughly 10 percent, enough to produce health benefits and perhaps to encourage continued success. (See **Figure 8.16**.) Another goal might be to restore and maintain a "natural weight," a body weight that is naturally appropriate given the limitations of heredity.

Many health experts suggest that people should aim for **metabolic fitness** rather than a specific weight,[63] especially if they have difficulty achieving or maintaining recommended weight or BMI levels. If you are metabolically fit, you don't have any of the metabolic or biochemical risk factors associated with obesity—such as high cholesterol (especially low HDL cholesterol), high levels of triglycerides, elevated blood glucose levels, insulin resistance, high blood pressure, and elevated fatty acids synthesis. Other risk factors include adult weight gain greater than 18 kilograms (about 40 pounds) and excess abdominal fat.[64] If these risk factors are at normal levels, a person is considered metabolically fit. Abnormal levels increase the risk for coronary heart disease, diabetes, gout, hypertension, and associated conditions. You can reduce these risk factors or even bring them within normal ranges through modest weight loss (5 to 10 percent of initial body weight) achieved by a low-fat, reduced-calorie diet and a moderate increase in physical activity (e.g., walking 30 minutes a day, no fewer than five days a week). You can improve metabolic fitness just by increasing physical activity levels.[65]

Think About It 3

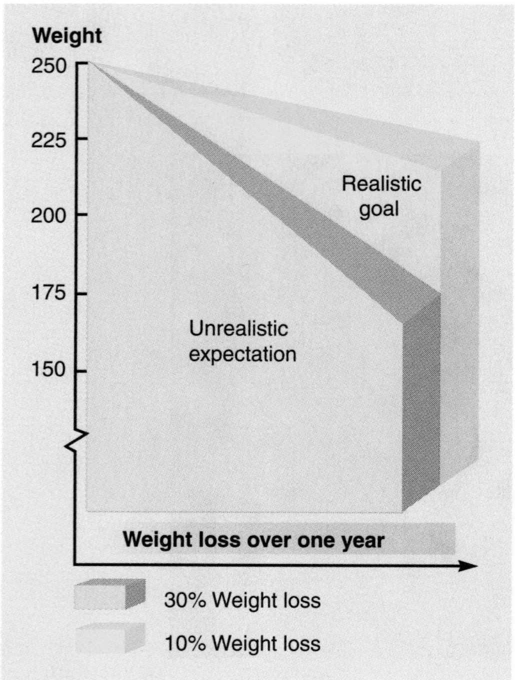

Figure 8.16 **Expectations and reasonable weight goals.** People who establish moderate rather than aggressive goals are more likely to succeed in their weight-loss program.

Think About It 4

Don't focus on a particular weight as your goal. Instead, focus on living a lifestyle that includes eating moderate amounts of healthful foods, getting plenty of exercise, thinking positively, and learning to cope with stress. Learn to use your body's hunger and satiation signals to regulate eating and then let the pounds fall where they may. Most people who follow this advice will approach the recommended weight ranges discussed earlier. Some will still weigh more than societal standards call for—but their weight will be right for them. By letting a healthy lifestyle determine your weight, you can avoid developing unhealthy patterns of eating and a negative body image.

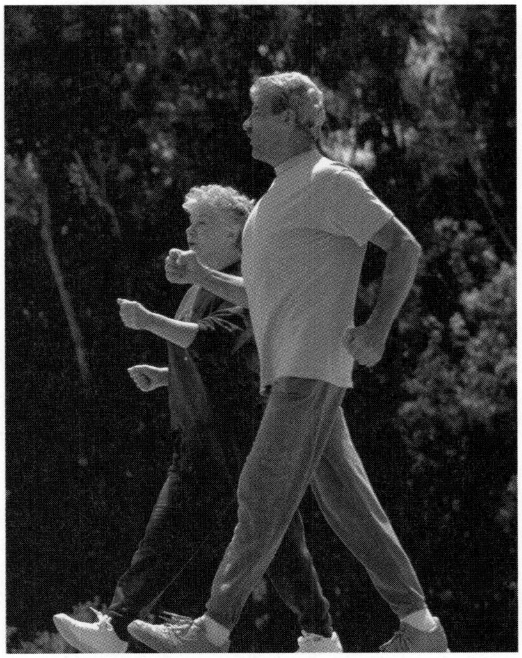

Adopting a Healthy Weight-Management Lifestyle

Most weight problems are lifestyle problems. Even though more and more young people are developing weight problems, most arrive at early adulthood with the advantage of having a "normal" body weight—neither too fat nor too thin. In fact, many young adults get away with terrible eating and exercise habits and don't develop a weight problem. But as the rapid growth of adolescence slows and family and career obligations increase, maintaining a healthy weight becomes a greater challenge. If you develop a lifestyle for successful weight management during early adulthood, healthy behavior patterns have a better chance of taking firm hold.

Permanent weight management is not something you start and stop. You need to adopt health behaviors that you can maintain throughout your life. People who have long-term success share common behavioral strategies that include eating a diet low in fat, frequent self-monitoring of body weight and food intake, and high levels of regular physical activity.[66] To maintain your weight over the long term, focus on healthy behaviors and develop coping strategies to deal with the stresses and challenges in your life.

Key Concepts: *Healthy weight management means focusing on metabolic fitness—healthy levels of blood lipids and blood pressure—rather than on achieving a specific weight. Permanent healthy behaviors are necessary for a long-term weight-management lifestyle.*

Diet and Eating Habits

In contrast to "dieting," which involves some form of food restriction, "diet" refers to your daily food choices. Everyone has a diet, but not everyone is dieting. You need to develop a balanced diet of moderate caloric intake that includes foods you enjoy and that enables you to maintain a healthy body composition. **Figure 8.17** shows the necessary components of an effective weight-management program.

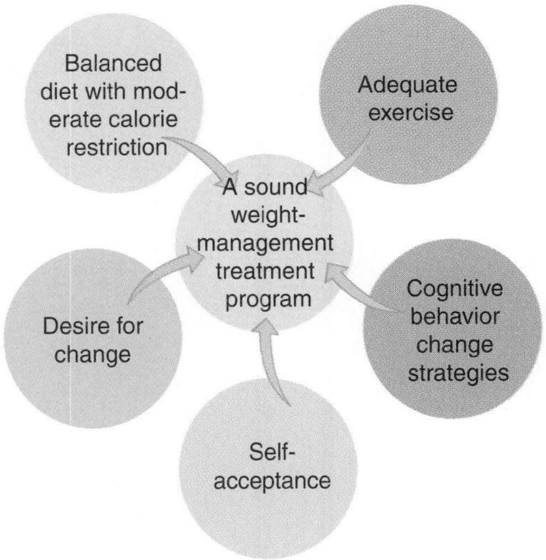

Figure 8.17 Components of a sound weight-management treatment program. Recognizing the need for change, establishing reasonable goals, adopting goal-directed activities and self-monitoring them, and rewarding goal attainment can help successfully implement the components of a sound weight-management program.

Total Calories

If you want to lose weight, you must take in fewer calories than you expend. You are more likely to successfully control your weight over the long term if you work on cutting your intake by 200 to 300 kilocalories a day than by undertaking a drastic diet of only 1,000 to 1,200 kilocalories per day. Eliminating one can of regular soda from your daily routine would reduce your energy intake by about 150 kilocalories. Eating half a serving of fries instead of a whole serving would save another 100 kilocalories. You don't need to make major diet changes; just make small, sustainable changes and focus on the balance of food groups suggested by the Food Guide Pyramid.

Quick Bites

The Beverly Hills Diet

The Beverly Hills Diet, introduced in 1980, begins with ten days of fruit and water only. Many dieters reported an unpleasant side effect—diarrhea.

Quick Bites

Double-Checking Your Recall

When researchers checked the validity of food diaries and self-reports, they found that obese people underreport their energy intake by 20 to 50 percent and lean people underreport by 10 to 30 percent. Energy expenditure in the obese subjects was normal relative to their body size.

Overconsumption of total calories is closely tied with portion sizes. Most of us significantly underestimate the amount of food we eat. Limiting portion sizes to those recommended in the Food Guide Pyramid is critical for weight management. You'll probably find it easier to monitor and manage your total food intake if you concentrate on portion sizes rather than counting calories.

Crash Diets Don't Work

Don't go on a "crash diet" that contains only minimal calories. You need to consume enough food to meet your need for essential nutrients. Once you lose weight, you probably won't maintain it unless you continue to adhere to some degree of the calorie restriction you used to lose weight. So it is important that you adopt a level of food intake that you can live with. A highly restricted diet just won't work long term.

Fat Calories

Although we all need some dietary fat, you should avoid overeating fatty foods. Research evidence suggests that fat calories are more easily converted to body fat than calories from protein or carbohydrate.[67] Limiting fat in the diet also can help you limit your total calories. Fat should supply no more than 30 percent of your average total daily calories, which translates into no more than 65 grams of fat each day in a 2,000-kilocalorie diet.

Some people are better fat burners than others; that is, they burn more of the fat they take in and therefore have less fat to store. People who burn fat at a low rate convert more dietary fat to stored body fat. For these people, the tendency to hoard fat may be an important part of the genetic tendency toward obesity, and so restricting fat calories to a level below 30 percent may help them manage their weight.

Several large surveys of the relationship between what we eat and how much we weigh have found that eating more fat and fewer complex carbohydrates is associated with excess body fat.[68] High-fat, low-fiber diets tend to delay satiation and encourage overeating. If you eat a diet with lots of complex carbohydrates and fresh fruits and vegetables and reduce your reliance on meats and processed foods, you will reduce fat consumption and increase dietary fiber. Watch out for processed foods labeled "fat-free" or "reduced fat"; they can be high in calories despite their lower fat content.

Complex Carbohydrates

To lose weight, dieters often cut back on bread, pasta, and potatoes. But these foods, along with vegetables, legumes, and whole grains, are rich in complex carbohydrates that can help you achieve and maintain a healthy body weight. Complex carbohydrates help provide a feeling of satiation, or fullness, that can keep you from overeating. Carbohydrates should make up about 55 to 60 percent of your total daily calories. Avoid mixing your carbohydrate sources with high-fat toppings and sauces, however. Experiment with lower-fat alternatives. Instead of sour cream on your baked potato, try plain yogurt. Rather than cream sauces on your pasta, use tomato-based sauces.

Simple Sugars and Refined Carbohydrates

High-sugar foods usually provide calories but few nutrients. You should consume them sparingly, so choose fresh fruits and whole grains instead of candy and sugary cereals.

Protein

Periodically, new diet books hit the market proclaiming a "scientific breakthrough"—usually involving a high-protein, low-carbohydrate diet. Even though they promise "all you can eat," such diets typically involve significant calorie restriction. This lower energy intake is what actually causes any weight loss that occurs. A high-protein, low-carbohydrate, low-calorie diet does not conform to the *Dietary Guidelines for Americans* and is difficult to maintain. Most authorities recommend diets high in complex carbohydrates and moderate in protein consumption. (See the FYI feature "High-Protein Diets for Weight Loss: Helpful or Harmful?")

While protein promotes a sense of fullness, foods high in protein often are high in fat. Including small amounts of protein in each meal is a good idea, but stick to the recommended intake of 10 to 15 percent of total daily calories.

Quick Bites

The Fletcherism Fad: Chew Until You...

At the turn of the twentieth century, a retired businessman named Horace Fletcher started a dietary craze known as "Fletcherism." Calling the mouth "Nature's Food Filter," he believed that the sense of taste and the urge to swallow are perfect guides to nutrition. Although he recommended chewing food at least 50 times before swallowing, preferably until tasteless, he far exceeded this by once chewing a piece of onion 722 times. His philosophy did lead to some weight loss; people adhering to Fletcherism cut back on energy intake due to the additional mechanical effort of chewing.

Eating Habits

Equally important to weight management is eating small, frequent meals—three or more a day plus snacks—on a dependable, regular schedule. If you skip meals, you are apt to feel excessively hungry and deprived, and you will be more likely to snack or binge on high-calorie, high-fat, or sugary foods. If you follow a regular pattern of eating and set up some "decision rules" that govern your food choices, you will be able to handle the many details that go into a healthful, low-fat diet. Decision rules governing breakfast, for example, might be

- Most of the time, choose a sugar-free, high-fiber cereal with nonfat milk.
- Once in a while (no more than once or twice a week), have an egg that's hard boiled or scrambled without added fat in the microwave.
- Save pancakes and waffles for special occasions.

When you proclaim some foods "off limits," you are setting up a rule to be broken. Instead, adopt the principle "everything in moderation." Troublesome foods might be placed off limits temporarily until you regain control. If you can learn to eat in moderation, you can achieve a healthful diet and manage your weight successfully; no foods need to be entirely off limits, though some should be eaten prudently. Making the healthier choice more often than not is the essence of moderation.

Key Concepts: *Controlling portion sizes and limiting fat in your diet can help reduce overall energy consumption. Complex carbohydrates provide a feeling of fullness that can help prevent overeating. When planning a diet, aim for caloric intake of 30 percent or less fat, 10 to 15 percent protein, and 55 to 60 percent carbohydrate.*

Physical Activity

Regular physical activity is a vital component of weight management. Physical activity promotes fitness and good health. At the same time, it discourages overeating by reducing stress; it produces positive feelings that reinforce self-worth and a sense of accomplishment; and it often includes pleasant socialization.

You can become more active by incorporating more physical activity into your daily life. (See **Figure 8.18.**) Try to accumulate 30 minutes or more of

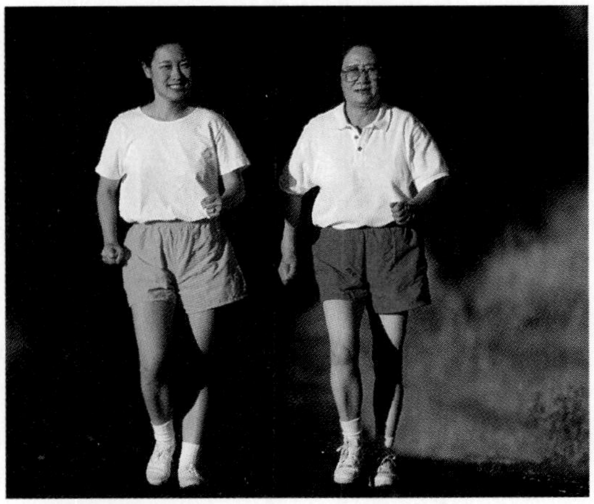

Figure 8.18 **Weight management through lifetime habits.** To achieve long-term weight management, healthy habits must become part of one's daily routine.

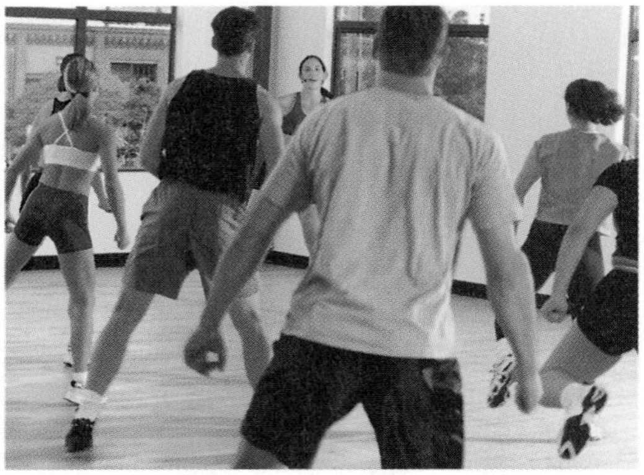

moderate-intensity physical activity each day. Take advantage of routine opportunities to be more active. Walk the dog for an extra half hour daily, for example. Use a stairway instead of an elevator. Walk instead of using transportation. Take up an active hobby like bicycling.

Increasing your activity level by just a small amount can help you maintain your current weight or lose a moderate amount of weight. "Going for the burn" and "no pain, no gain" were the mottoes of the aerobics movement during the 1970s and 1980s, but such intense activity is neither necessary nor desirable. Instead, regular exercise of moderate intensity—any activity that expends 4 to 7 kilocalories per minute (240 to 420 kilocalories per hour, see Table 8.1)—provides substantial health benefits.

Once you have increased your everyday activity level, consider beginning a formal exercise program that includes cardiorespiratory endurance exercise, resistance training, and stretching exercises. Regular, moderate cardiorespiratory endurance exercise, sustained for 45 minutes to 1 hour, can help trim body fat permanently. Strength training helps increase fat-free mass, which results in more calorie burning even outside of exercise periods.

One thing is clear: Regular exercise, maintained throughout life, makes weight management easier. The sooner you establish good habits, the better. You will succeed in maintaining your weight if you make exercise an integral part of the lifestyle you enjoy now and will enjoy in the future.

Key Concepts: *Successful weight management involves regular physical activity as well as healthful food choices. Small increases in activity have significant health benefits and help weight loss and maintenance. You should have at least 30 minutes of moderate exercise in your daily routine.*

Fyi FOR YOUR INFORMATION

High-Protein Diets for Weight Loss: Helpful or Harmful?

High-protein weight-loss diets are in style again. Browse through the weight-loss section of any major bookstore and you will find books like *Protein Power, Dr. Atkins' New Diet Revolution, Sugar Busters,* and *Enter the Zone.* All these books promote various high-protein diets for weight loss.

These diets revisit the idea, popular in the 1970s (and with historical roots dating back nearly 200 years), that carbohydrates (starches and sugars) make us fat. Proponents of high-protein diets point to the fact that throughout the high-carb, low-fat 1980s and early 1990s and with the explosion of fat-free foods, Americans got fatter. They fail to note that although the percentage of calories from fat decreased, Americans ate more total calories and exercised less—a recipe for weight gain.

Common Myths about High-Protein Intake for Weight Loss

1. *Myth:* Early humans existed on a diet that was high in protein, and our bodies are still tuned to eat this way.
   Fact: Early humans were gatherers more than hunters. Most of the time they ate nuts, seeds, fruits, and vegetables; meat was only an occasional part of the diet. Early humans also had a life expectancy about half that of ours today.[1]
2. *Myth:* Dietary protein cannot be converted into body fat.
   Fact: Excess energy from anything—carbohydrate, fat, alcohol, and protein—promotes fat storage.
3. *Myth:* High-protein diets result in quick and permanent weight loss.
   Fact: High-protein diets may result in quick weight loss, but it is seldom permanent. On high-protein diets, initial weight loss comes from loss of body fluids. Later weight loss comes from both fat and muscle tissue. Because unsupervised high-protein diets don't teach lifestyle change or reflect people's usual eating patterns, weight is usually quickly regained when the diet is stopped.
4. *Myth:* You can eat all you want on a high-protein diet and still lose weight.

Thinking and Emotions

What goes on in your head is another factor in a healthy lifestyle and successful weight management. The way you think about yourself and your world influences, and is influenced by, how you feel and how you act. Certain kinds of thinking produce negative emotions, which can undermine a healthy lifestyle.

When we compare ourselves to an internally held picture of an "ideal self," we are more likely to feel low self-esteem and negative emotions. The "ideal self" we envision is often the result of having adopted perfectionistic goals and beliefs about how we and others "should" be. You might know someone who believes "If I don't do things perfectly, I'm a failure" or "It's terrible if I'm not thin." When we accept these irrational beliefs, we may actually cause ourselves stress and emotional conflict. The remedy is to challenge such beliefs and replace them with more realistic ones.

The beliefs and attitudes you hold give rise to self-talk, an internal dialogue you carry on with yourself about events that happen to and around you. When you talk yourself through the steps of a job and then praise yourself when it's successfully completed, you are engaging in **positive self-talk.** When you make self-deprecating remarks or angry and guilt-producing comments and when you blame yourself unnecessarily, you are engaging in **negative self-talk.** Negative self-talk can undermine efforts at self-control and lead to feelings of anxiety and depression.

Your beliefs and attitudes influence how you interpret what happens to you and what you can expect in the future, as well as how you feel and react. Realistic beliefs and goals as well as positive self-talk and problem-solving efforts support a healthy lifestyle.

positive self-talk Constructive mental or verbal statements made to one's self to change a belief or behavior.

negative self-talk Mental or verbal statements made to one's self that reinforce negative or destructive self perceptions.

Fact: Anyone who "goes on a diet" becomes more conscious of what he or she eats and generally eats less. High-protein, low-carbohydrate diets can also induce a state of ketosis that tends to reduce appetite. Look at sample diet plans from high-protein books, and you'll see that they are generally low in calories.

But Do They Work?

People who have tried high-protein weight-loss diets report dramatic weight loss even with abundant amounts of steak, bacon, and eggs. However, rapid initial weight loss from the depletion of glycogen stores may come at a price: Constipation, nausea, weakness, dehydration, and fatigue are common side effects. While ketosis may suppress appetite, it also gives the breath a fruity odor. And a diet that ignores much of the USDA Food Guide Pyramid limits the intake of many vitamins and minerals—so that the plans often recommend supplements. But supplements don't provide fiber or the many phytochemicals found in fruits and vegetables. Diets that contain 60 percent or more of calories from fat may contain more cholesterol and saturated fat than is recommended for heart health.

The Best Diet to Follow

Is there a "best" diet? If there were, we wouldn't have so many diet books vying for our attention and money! What we know about our nutrient needs still points to the Pyramid for guidance; the best diet emphasizes fruits, vegetables, and grains, not high-protein foods. And although weight loss may be the goal of many, weight maintenance is the key to reducing the health risks of obesity. Weight maintenance requires permanent changes to eating habits and, more important, increased physical activity. So, instead of a walk through the diet book aisle, save your money and improve your health with a fitness walk through the mall.

1 Eaton SB, Shostak M, Konner M. *The Paleolithic Prescription.* New York: Harper & Row; 1988.

Antecedents

Her mouth starts watering as she passes by a bakery with delicious sights and aromas.

Behavior

She purchases many pastries, intending some for later. Despite this resolve, she succumbs to the need for instant gratification, immediately eating them all.

Consequences

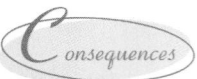

She regrets her behavior and feels guilty. Overeating may leave her feeling ill and nauseated.

Figure 8.19 The ABC model of eating behavior. Conquering overeating often requires a psychological strategy for changing ingrained habits and other behaviors.

Stress Management

Stress management can be an important part of weight management.[69] You can use the **ABC model of behavior** (**Figure 8.19**) to help you cope with daily stresses and their impact on eating behavior.

The ABC model helps you manage events that trigger behaviors and factors that reinforce them. *Antecedents*, the "A" part of the model, are the events that precede the behavior and trigger it. Overeating is a possible *behavior*, the "B" part of the model. The *consequences*, or "C," follow and reinforce the "B." The "C" may be desirable, such as relief from stress, or undesirable, such as guilt or weight gain. The "C" may be immediate or, like weight gain, occur in the future; the consequences that occur immediately have the greatest influence.

Identifying the cues (A) that trigger overeating is the first step to changing or avoiding these triggers. You might remove problem foods from the house or avoid the grocery store's candy aisle. You can sometimes manipulate antecedents to trigger positive behaviors (for example, putting exercise clothes by the door to prompt exercise).

You can affect the behavior of overeating (B) by using positive self-talk to encourage a new behavior and by avoiding excuses and rationalizations to eat something inappropriate.

Positive consequences (C) help to reinforce new behaviors. You could sign a contract with a friend that rewards you for deciding not to overeat. Rewards such as time for physical activity not only reinforce behavior but also develop fitness. **Table 8.6** summarizes cognitive-behavioral tools for changing habits and behavior patterns.

ABC model of behavior A behavioral model that includes the external and internal events that precede and follow the behavior. The "A" stands for antecedents, the events that precede the behavior ("B"), which is followed by consequences ("C") that positively or negatively reinforce the behavior.

Balancing Acceptance and Change

It's not enough to change your behavior to manage obesity. Self-acceptance is equally necessary. (See **Table 8.7**.) Accepting yourself as you are will help your self-esteem and will improve your general satisfaction with life. It is destructive to be overly concerned with the importance of body weight and shape or to have unattainable goals of idealized physical appearance. But don't confuse self-acceptance with complacency or a do-nothing approach that ignores health risks.

If you must diet, do so in combination with exercise, and avoid very-low-calorie diets. Don't try to lose more than ½ to 1 pound per week. Realize that most low-calorie diets cause a rapid loss of body water at first. When this phase passes, weight loss declines. As a result, dieters often are misled into believing that their efforts are not working. They then give up, not realizing that smaller losses later in the diet actually are better than the initial big losses. In fact, the later loss is mostly fat loss, whereas the initial loss was primarily fluid loss.

Key Concepts: *Identifying cues that precede overeating can help a person make behavior changes. Long-term weight management should include self-acceptance and enhanced self-esteem. Goals of idealized body size and shape should be replaced with goals that promote good health and a lifetime of fitness.*

Weight-Management Approaches

Do certain weight-loss diets have adverse health consequences? Is it unhealthy to lose weight quickly? Will the weight stay off? What motivates people to lose weight and to maintain weight? What are the barriers to losing weight and/or to maintaining weight? At the May 2000 National

Table 8.6 Cognitive-Behavioral Tools for Changing Behavior

Tool	Description
Self-monitoring	Prospectively recording information about behavior to identify the antecedents (what precedes and elicits a particular action), the behaviors of interest (usually eating behavior), and the consequences (the thoughts, feelings, and reactions that accompany the behavior of interest).
Environmental management	Avoiding or changing cues that trigger undesirable behavior (e.g., not driving by the doughnut shop, putting the cookie jar out of sight), or instituting new cues to elicit new behaviors (e.g., putting your walking shoes by the door as a reminder to exercise); also called "stimulus control."
Alternate behaviors	Learning new ways of responding to old cues or circumstances that can't be changed or avoided (e.g., taking a walk when you get upset instead of getting something to eat).
Reward	Giving yourself, or arranging to be given, rewards for engaging in desired behaviors.
Negative reinforcement	Arranging to give up something desirable (e.g., money) or to endure something undesirable (e.g., wash your friend's car) for engaging in unwanted behaviors.
Social support	Getting others to participate in or otherwise provide emotional and physical support of your weight-management efforts.
Cognitive coping	Reducing negative self-talk, increasing positive self-talk, and challenging beliefs that undermine your resolve and contribute to negative emotions; setting reasonable goals and avoiding "thinking traps."
Managing emotions	Using reframing, disengagement, imagery, and self-soothing to reduce or manage negative emotions.
Relapse prevention and recovery	Identifying high-risk situations that pose a hazard for relapsing, and learning to recover from small indiscretions before they become major relapses.

Source: Adapted from Nash JD. *The New Maximize Your Body Potential.* Palo Alto, CA: Bull Publishing Company; 1997. Used with permission.

Nutrition Summit, the USDA announced plans for a coordinated nutrition research program to look at questions such as these. The largest part of this research effort is devoted to a series of prospective studies on both the long- and short-term health and nutrition effects of the various types of popular weight-loss diets.[70] Meanwhile, current research provides clues to finding an approach suited to your personal needs.

Self-Help Books and Manuals

Some people respond well to simple information provided in an easy-to-understand format. They are able to change their behavior with good, well-researched self-help manuals and books.[71] The proliferation of diet books is

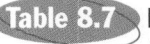

Table 8.7 Basic Tenets of Size Acceptance

- Human beings come in a variety of sizes and shapes. We celebrate this diversity as a positive characteristic of the human race.
- There is no ideal body size, shape, or weight that every individual should strive to achieve.
- Every body is a good body, whatever its size or shape.
- Self-esteem and body image are strongly linked. Helping people feel good about their bodies and about who they are can help motivate and maintain healthy behaviors.
- Appearance stereotyping is inherently unfair to the individual because it is based on superficial factors which the individual has little or no control over.
- We respect the bodies of others even though they might be quite different from our own.
- Each person is responsible for taking care of his/her body.
- Good health is not defined by body size; it is a state of physical, mental, and social well-being.

People of all sizes and shapes can reduce their risk of poor health by adopting a healthy lifestyle.

Source: Excerpted from *Basic Tenets of Health at Every Size,* developed by dietitians and nutritionists who are advocates of size acceptance; their efforts coordinated by Joanne P. Ikeda, MA, RD, Nutrition Education Specialist, Department of Nutritional Sciences, University of California, Berkeley.

Quick Bites

Diet Revolution?

The *Diet Revolution* first promoted by Dr. Atkins in 1972 centered on putting dieters into a state of ketosis by consuming few carbohydrates. In 1973 the American Medical Association called the diet dangerous and required Atkins to testify before the U.S. Senate Select Committee on Nutrition.

Quick Bites

Letter on Corpulence

Published in the early 1800s, *Bantry's Letter on Corpulence* was the first popular diet book in the United States. The book advocated restricting intake of carbohydrates.

very-low-calorie diets (VLCD) Diets supplying 400 to 800 kilocalories per day, which include adequate high-quality protein, little or no fat, and little carbohydrate.

nothing short of phenomenal, however, and each year dozens of dubious weight-loss diet books reach the market. When evaluating a diet book, be alert to the following warning flags:

1. Unbalanced diet patterns. The recommended pattern should not stray too far from the USDA Food Pyramid (see Chapter 2, "Nutrition Guidelines").
2. Claims of a "scientific breakthrough" or promises of "quick and easy" weight loss. There is no quick fix when it comes to weight management.
3. Irrational food instructions: food restrictions (e.g., no fruits), illogical overemphasis of some foods (e.g., five grapefruits daily), and irrational food patterns (e.g., don't mix red and green foods). Such restrictions set the stage for feelings of deprivation and binge eating.
4. The promise of a cure for some disease along with weight loss. That's not only a waste of money, but also potentially dangerous.

Should you decide on the do-it-yourself route, develop specific goals for your diet, exercise, and maintenance plans. (See the FYI feature "Behaviors That Will Help You Manage Your Weight.") Keep tabs on your habits and become more involved in activities other than eating, especially physical activities. Long-term success depends on maintaining the lifestyle changes that helped you lose the weight in the first place.

Self-Help Groups

Self-help groups, often led by laypeople, help many people cope with their weight. Such groups reduce the isolation and alienation some obese people experience and can provide a community in which there is understanding and acceptance of shared experiences.

Commercial Programs

Commercial weight-loss programs provide group or individual counseling and group support. Some sell prepackaged foods or nutritional supplements. Some companies employ dietitians, health educators, psychologists, or physicians to develop and guide the program at the corporate level. In early 1999, the Federal Trade Commission (FTC) issued guidelines encouraging commercial programs to release the following information to potential clients:

- staff training and education
- risks of overweight and obesity
- risks of their products or program
- cost
- program outcomes: success and failure rates

Be sure to obtain this information before you register for a weight-loss program, and think twice about any program that does not willingly provide it.

Several commercial programs, such as Optifast, Medifast, New Directions, and Health Management Resources (HMR), use **very-low-calorie diets (VLCD)** containing only 400 to 800 kilocalories per day as the initial phase of treatment. When such diets were first introduced in the 1970s, several deaths resulted from cardiac abnormalities. As a result, VLCD should be undertaken only with close medical supervision.

Fyi FOR YOUR INFORMATION — Behaviors That Will Help You Manage Your Weight

Set the Right Goals
Setting the right goals is an important first step. Most people trying to lose weight focus just on weight loss. However, you'll be more successful if you focus on dietary and exercise changes that lead to long-term weight change. Successful weight managers select no more than two or three goals at a time.

Effective goals are (1) specific, (2) attainable, and (3) forgiving. "Exercise more" is a commendable ideal, but it's not specific. "Walk five miles every day" is specific and measurable, but is it attainable if you're just starting out? "Walk 30 minutes every day" is more attainable, but what happens if you're held up at work or there's a thunderstorm? "Walk 30 minutes, five days each week" is specific, attainable, and forgiving. In short, a great goal!

Nothing Succeeds Like Success
Select a series of short-term goals that get you closer and closer to the ultimate goal (for example, consider reducing fat intake from 40 percent of calories to 35 percent and later to 30 percent). Nothing succeeds like success. This strategy employs two important behavioral principles: (1) consecutive goals that move you ahead in small steps are the best way to reach a distant point, and (2) consecutive rewards keep the overall effort invigorated.

Reward Success (But Not with Food)
You're more likely to keep working toward your goal if you are rewarded—especially when goals are difficult to reach. An effective reward is something that is desirable, timely, and contingent on meeting your goal. Your rewards may be tangible (e.g., a movie or music CD or a payment toward buying a more costly item) or intangible (e.g., an afternoon off from studying or just an hour of quiet time away from the daily demands of school). Give yourself numerous small rewards as you meet small goals; don't wait to meet your ultimate goal and a large reward. The long, difficult effort might lead you to give up.

Balance Your (Food) Checkbook
Keeping track of your behavior—observing and recording calorie intake, servings of fruits and vegetables, exercise frequency and duration, or any other wellness behavior—can help alter that behavior. Self-monitoring usually changes a behavior in the desired direction and can produce "real-time" records for you and your health care provider. For example, you can track your exercise progress. A record of increasing exercise encourages you to keep up the good work. If the record shows little or no progress, you know that a change of strategy is needed. Some people find that specific self-monitoring forms make it easier, while others prefer to use their own recording system.

Although you don't need to step on the scale every day, monitoring your weight regularly (once a week) can help you maintain your lower weight. Use a graph rather than a list or calendar notations so that you have a picture of cumulative progress. Changes in your body's water content, rather than fat content, are responsible for most of the up and down fluctuations from day to day. A long-term downward trend reflects fat losses.

Avoid a Chain Reaction
Identify the social or environmental cues that seem to encourage undesirable eating, and then change those cues. For example, you may learn from reflection or self-monitoring that you're more likely to overeat while watching television, when treats are on display at the campus cafe, or when you're around a certain friend. You might then try to break the association between eating and the cue (don't eat while watching television), avoid or eliminate the cue (avoid sitting near the display counter), or change the circumstances surrounding the cue (plan to meet with your friend in nonfood settings). In general, visible and accessible food items often are cues for unplanned eating.

Get the (Fullness) Message
Changing the way you go about eating can make it easier to eat less without feeling deprived. It takes 15 or more minutes for your brain to get the message you've been fed. Slowing the rate of eating can allow satiation (fullness) signals to begin by the end of the meal. Eating lots of vegetables also can make you feel fuller. Another trick is to use smaller plates so that moderate portions do not appear meager. Changing your eating schedule, or setting one, can be helpful, especially if you tend to skip or delay meals and overeat later.

The Backsliding Phenomenon
You've just signed a contract with yourself to avoid high-fat desserts for one month when you're presented with an array of your favorite "to die for" desserts. You say to yourself, "just this once" and satisfy your craving. Most of us have experienced the "backsliding phenomenon" in which we have lost our resolve and slipped back into a former bad habit. When it happens, be prepared for it and move on with your resolve. You're most apt to backslide when you're tempted by something unexpected and your self-control is threatened. You can remove high-fat snacks from your home, but not from other places you eat. Imagine tempting situations in your mind's eye and practice coping with them successfully. If you do slip, don't waste time with self-blame. Learn from the experience and get back on track.

Source: Adapted from National Heart, Lung, and Blood Institute. *Guide to behavior change.* http://www.nhlbi.nih.gov/health/public/heart/obesity/lose_wt/behavior.htm. Accessed 3/30/02.

Professional Private Counselors

Private counselors can be physicians, psychotherapists, nutritionists, or dietitians. They provide individualized weight management and the support and attention that some obese people may need. Physicians can also prescribe medication and monitor its safety and effectiveness. Carefully scrutinize the training and credentials of private counselors before committing to any program.

Anti-Obesity Prescription Drugs

The pharmaceutical industry has long been searching for a "magic bullet" to cure obesity. Now that it's clear that obesity involves multiple factors, the focus is moving to drugs with multiple mechanisms and drugs to be used in conjunction with proper diet and exercise.[72]

One of the newest prescription drugs for obesity is Xenical (orlistat), approved in April 1999. Because Xenical blocks fat absorption by up to 30 percent, it must be accompanied by a low-fat diet, or the unabsorbed fat can produce diarrhea and flatulence. It also blocks fat-soluble nutrient absorption, so it's necessary to take a vitamin supplement as well.[73]

In 1998, Meridia (sibutramine), a prescription appetite suppressant, was brought to market. Meridia is believed to be safer than earlier anti-obesity drugs, but like all prescription drugs, it can have side effects—in this case increased blood pressure and heart rate.[74] Other approved anti-obesity prescription drugs include Dexedrine, other amphetamines, and amphetamine derivatives.

The FDA approved these drugs only for use with calorie-restricted diets. Also, aside from Xenical, they are addictive and have the potential for abuse. They shouldn't be used in combination with each other or with other drugs for appetite control because such combinations have not been evaluated for safety. The drugs should be used only in people who are obese—not people looking to lose just a few pounds.

Until September 1997, two other drugs, fenfluramine (one component of a combination called fen-phen) and dexfenfluramine (Redux), were available for treating obesity. But, at the FDA's request, the manufacturers of these drugs voluntarily withdrew them from the market after newer research found that they were the likely cause of life-threatening lung disease and heart valve problems.[75]

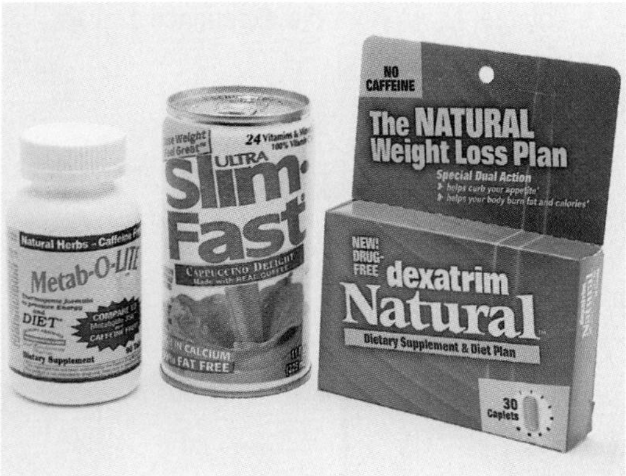

Over-the-Counter Drugs and Dietary Supplements

Nonprescription (over-the-counter, or OTC) weight-loss pills may contain caffeine, benzocaine, or fiber. Caffeine is a stimulant and diuretic. Benzocaine numbs the tongue, reducing taste sensations, thus discouraging eating. Pills with fiber are designed to fill the stomach and provide a feeling of fullness. Although moderately effective, fiber pills can lead to dehydration; much of the lost weight is water, which is easily regained when the pills are stopped.

Numerous dietary supplements are marketed for weight loss, with names like "Weight Away." Common ingredients include chromium picolinate, chitosan, hydroxycitric acid (HCA), ephedra, and St. John's wort. In fact, the combination of ephedra and St. John's wort has been marketed as an "herbal fen-phen." Few studies have been done on the efficacy of these products for weight loss, and what little evidence exists does not support the claims. In addition, ephedra (also known as ma huang) is dangerous to people with hypertension, heart disease, or diabetes. Over-the-counter medicines and dietary supplements are no substitute for exercise and healthful eating. There is no quick, easy way to effectively lose weight.

Surgery

Sometimes, surgery can successfully treat **morbid obesity**—body weight exceeding 100 percent of normal. Surgery should be a last-ditch effort, when all legitimate, less-invasive methods have failed. The most common procedures reduce stomach size by creating a smaller upper stomach, or "pouch." As a result, the patient can eat very few calories at one time.[76] Gastric bypass is another surgical procedure that limits food intake. (See **Figure 8.20**.) Bypassing most of the stomach, however, inhibits not only the digestion and absorption of caloric foods, but also the absorption of some micronutrients—an obvious drawback.

morbid obesity Obesity characterized by body weight exceeding 100 percent of normal; a condition so severe it often requires surgery.

The long-term effectiveness of gastric surgery depends on how patients manage eating. They can defeat the procedure by consuming high-calorie drinks or semisolid foods that overcome stomach size. With time the pouch stretches, allowing more solid foods, but by then, doctors hope that the patient has established healthy eating habits. Also, RMR can decline significantly after gastric surgery, making weight loss more difficult, so exercise is important along with diet modifications.[77] These patients are likely to need lifelong medical supervision.

Liposuction is a cosmetic surgical procedure that reshapes the body by removing fat. Although the procedure removes some fat cells, the body still has billions of other fat cells ready to store extra fat. Thus, liposuction is not effective for significant or long-term weight loss. Liposuction should not be used casually. Risks include blood clots, perforation injuries, skin and nerve damage, and unfavorable drug reactions.

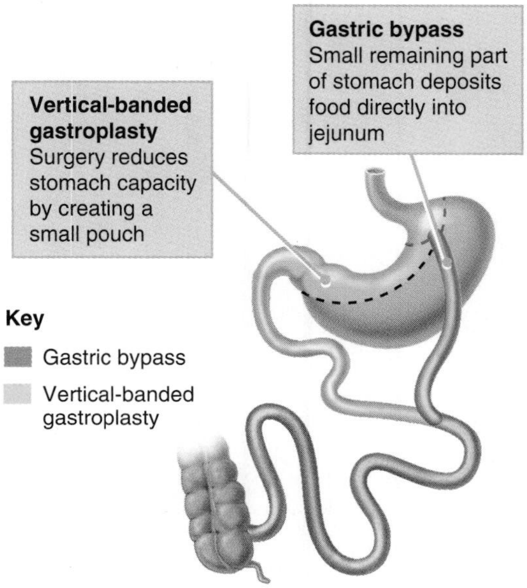
Gastric bypass
Small remaining part of stomach deposits food directly into jejunum
Vertical-banded gastroplasty
Surgery reduces stomach capacity by creating a small pouch
Key
Gastric bypass
Vertical-banded gastroplasty

Figure 8.20 **Gastric surgery in obesity treatment.** In vertical-banded gastroplasty, surgery reduces the size of the stomach. A gastric bypass routes food to the jejunum, bypassing the duodenum and most of the stomach.

Key Concepts: *Books and commercial programs can help some individuals lose weight. However, consumers should always proceed with caution before spending money. Prescription and over-the-counter drugs to lose weight have varying effectiveness. Drugs have potential side effects and must be used with caution and medical supervision. For those who are morbidly obese, surgical intervention is an aggressive, last-resort approach to weight management. Liposuction removes fat cells from specific parts of the body but is not considered an effective approach to weight control.*

Underweight

From a public health standpoint, underweight is much less of a problem than obesity, but those who are underweight can find it troublesome and frustrating. When body weight is 15 to 20 percent or more below desired weight for height, a person is considered underweight. The *Dietary Guidelines for Americans* defines underweight as a BMI under 18.5 kg/m^2.

When underweight is simply an inherited pattern, there is no need to worry about health risks as long as diet and other health behaviors are appropriate. But your health is at risk if your underweight is the result of undernutrition; deficits in protein, vitamins, and minerals, as well as energy, can cause health problems ranging from fatigue to compromised immune function.

Causes and Assessment

The causes of underweight are as diverse as those of overweight. They include

- altered response to hunger, appetite, satiation, satiety, and external cues, described earlier in this chapter

- factors in eating disorders such as distorted body image, compulsive dieting, and compulsive overexercising
- metabolic and hereditary factors
- prolonged psychological and emotional stress
- addiction to alcohol and street drugs
- bizarre diet patterns or diets that are inadequate

Underweight can be a sign of underlying disease, such as cancer. Illness can speed up metabolic rate, spoil the appetite, or interfere with digestion. Correcting underweight helps improve the quality of life.

Weight-Gain Strategies

The way to gain weight is to create positive energy balance. Here are some strategies:

- Have small, frequent meals with nutrient-dense and energy-dense foods and beverages.
- Drink fluids at the end of the meal or, better yet, between meals.
- Use high-calorie weight-gain beverages and foods.
- Use timers or other cues (similar to the ABC model on page 286, but with a different goal) to prompt eating.
- Use a balanced vitamin/mineral supplement to ensure that poor appetite isn't a result of nutritional deficiency.

Sometimes prescription drugs, such as appetite stimulants, are helpful. Medication also can speed stomach emptying, improving appetite for the next meal. Digestive enzyme replacements help people who are underweight due to poor digestion or absorption.

Exercise has a role in weight gain as well. Simple anaerobic or isometric exercise encourages weight gain as lean body mass rather than fat.

Key Concepts: *Underweight is not as common as overweight. Gaining weight can be difficult, but the basic concepts of energy balance apply.*

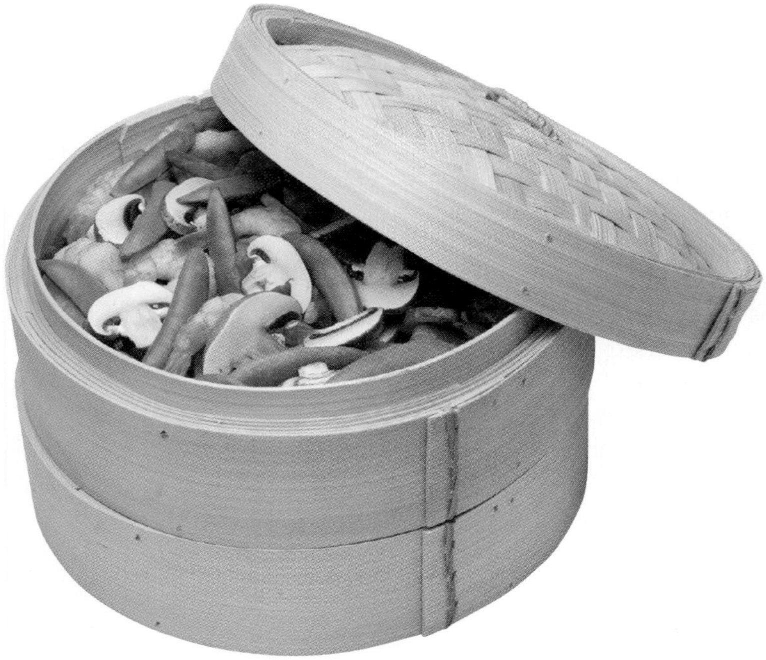

Label [to] Table

Do you believe that by choosing cookies or chips labeled "low-fat" or sticking with certain brand names associated with "diet foods" you are automatically making the right decisions? It may surprise you to know that many low-fat or fat-free products have nearly the same amount of calories as the full-fat versions! After reading this chapter you now know that when it comes to weight loss, total calories are just as important as calories from fat. If you eat a fat-free food, but eat so much of it that your calories are excessive, you will still gain weight. To illustrate this point, let's compare the nutrient labels from some leading cookie manufacturers. The lower-fat cookies (on right) claim they are "better for you" and have "50% less fat" compared with regular cookies. Here are the labels:

Regular Cookie	Lower-Fat Cookie
Serving, 2 cookies (29 g)	*Serving, 2 cookies (26 g)*
Calories, 140	*Calories, 110*
Calories from fat, 50	*Calories from fat, 25*
Total fat, 6 g	*Total fat, 3 g*

True, there is a 50 percent reduction in fat content (6 g vs. 3 g), which is an important part of the picture. However, take a look at the total calories. The lower-fat cookies only have 30 fewer kilocalories than the regular cookies, which may be a surprise to those who think they are saving more.

There is another interesting piece of information on these labels—the serving size. At first glance, you may think the serving sizes of the cookies are the same, two cookies. However, after further inspection you can see that the lower-fat cookies are slightly smaller. A 10 percent reduction in size/weight is certainly worth noting when you are trying to explain how a product can have fewer calories.

The next time you are in the cookie aisle debating whether you should settle a craving with a low-fat product or its full-fat version, be a smart consumer and read the label before you buy!

Nutrition Facts
Serving Size: 2 cookies (26g)
Servings Per Container: 18

Amount Per Serving	
Calories 110 Calories from fat 25	
	% Daily Value*
Total Fat 3g	5%
Saturated Fat 0.5g	3%
Polyunsaturated Fat 0g	
Monounsaturated Fat 1g	
Cholesterol 0mg	0%
Sodium 130mg	5%
Total Carbohydrate 20g	7%
Dietary Fiber 0g	0%
Sugars 10g	
Protein 1g	
Vitamin A 0% • Vitamin C 0%	
Calcium 0% • Iron 2%	

* Percent Daily Values are based on a 2,000 calorie diet. Your daily values may be higher or lower depending on your calorie needs:

		2,000	2,500
Calories:		2,000	2,500
Total Fat	Less Than	65g	80g
Sat Fat	Less Than	20g	25g
Cholesterol	Less Than	300mg	300mg
Sodium	Less Than	2,400mg	2,400mg
Total Carbohydrate		300g	375g
Dietary Fiber		25g	30g

Lower-fat cookie

Nutrition Facts
Serving Size: 2 cookies (29g)
Servings Per Container about 16

Amount Per Serving	
Calories 140 Calories from fat 50	
	% Daily Value*
Total Fat 6g	9%
Saturated Fat 1.5g	8%
Cholesterol 0mg	0%
Sodium 105mg	4%
Total Carbohydrate 21g	7%
Dietary Fiber less than 1g	3%
Sugars 8g	
Protein 2g	
Vitamin A 0% • Vitamin C 0%	
Calcium 0% • Iron 4%	

* Percent Daily Values are based on a 2,000 calorie diet. Your daily values may be higher or lower depending on your calorie needs:

	Calories:	2,000	2,500
Total Fat	Less Than	65g	80g
Sat Fat	Less Than	20g	25g
Cholesterol	Less Than	300mg	300mg
Sodium	Less Than	2,400mg	2,400mg
Total Carbohydrate		300g	375g
Dietary Fiber		25g	30g

Regular cookie

LEARNING *Portfolio* chapter 8

Key Terms

Term	page
ABC model of behavior	286
android obesity [AN-droyd]	271
appetite	261
basal metabolic rate (BMR)	264
binge eaters	278
bioelectrical impedance analysis (BIA)	271
BodPod	271
body composition	268
body fat distribution	271
body mass index (BMI)	269
computed tomography (CT)	271
dual energy x-ray absorptiometry (DEXA)	271
energy balance	261
energy equilibrium	261
energy intake	261
energy output	261
fat cell theory	275
gynoid obesity	271
hunger	261
hydrostatic weighing	271
hypercellular obesity	275
hyperplasia (hyperplastic obesity)	275
hypertrophic obesity	275
hypothalamus [high-po-THAL-ah-mus]	262
lean body mass	265
leptin	262
magnetic resonance imaging (MRI)	271
metabolic fitness	280
morbid obesity	291
negative energy balance	261
negative self-talk	285
neuropeptide Y (NPY)	262
nonexercise activity thermogenesis (NEAT)	265
obesity	273
overweight	273
positive energy balance	261
positive self-talk	285
Quetelet index	269
resting energy expenditure (REE)	264
resting metabolic rate (RMR)	264
restrained eaters	278
satiation	261
satiety	261
set point theory	275
skinfold measurements	271
sleep apnea	274
thermic effect of food (TEF)	265
total energy expenditure (TEE)	264
underwater weighing	271
underweight	273
very-low-calorie diets (VLCD)	288
waist circumference	271
weight cycling	274
weight management	278

Study Points

- Energy balance is the relationship between energy intake and energy output.
- Food intake is regulated by hunger, satiation, satiety, and appetite, which are influenced by complex factors. Hunger is the physiological need to eat. Satiation is the feeling of fullness that leads to termination of a meal. Satiety is the feeling of satisfaction and lack of hunger that determines the interval until the next meal. Appetite is a desire to eat that is influenced by external factors such as flavors and smells, and environmental and cultural factors.
- Gastrointestinal stimulation, circulating nutrients, neurotransmitters, and hormones signal the brain to regulate food intake.
- The major components of energy expenditure are resting energy expenditure, the thermic effect of food, and energy for physical activity.
- Body composition, age, gender, genetics, and hormonal activity affect the amount of energy used for resting metabolism.
- The energy cost of physical activity is affected by a person's size and the intensity and duration of the activity.
- Body composition, the relative amounts of fat and lean body mass, has a major influence on energy expenditure and risk of chronic disease.
- Body mass index, a ratio related to total body fatness and risk of chronic disease, is calculated with height and weight measurements.
- The prevalence of obesity and overweight is escalating worldwide, contributing to chronic disease.

- Health risks associated with obesity are more pronounced when excess body fat is in the abdominal region of the body.
- The factors that cause obesity are not completely understood, but a complex interaction of hormonal and metabolic factors is believed to play a role, along with genetic, sociocultural, and psychological factors.
- Rather than focus on ideal body weight, many professionals now promote health and fitness.
- Physical activity improves fitness and helps achieve the negative energy balance needed for weight reduction.
- Abandoning unrealistic ideas of thinness and accepting body weight and shape are important elements in weight management.
- Long-term weight management includes a balanced diet of moderately restricted calorie intake, adequate exercise, cognitive-behavioral strategies for changing habits and behavior patterns, and attention to balancing self-acceptance and the desire for change.
- Surgical approaches to weight control should be considered only as a last resort for the morbidly obese.
- If the cause is not hereditary, being underweight can pose health problems.
- Gaining weight can be difficult for individuals who are underweight.

Study Questions

Answers can be found at nutrition.jbpub.com/discovering.

1. Explain the concept of energy balance.
2. List and describe the three main components of energy expenditure.
3. Explain the three main factors that determine energy expenditure in activity.
4. Obesity is seen as a complex disorder with multiple contributing factors. List the types of factors involved in the development and maintenance of obesity.
5. What body mass index (BMI) values are associated with being underweight, overweight, and obese? Do these vary for men and women?
6. Describe the concept of metabolic fitness.
7. What is the difference between hyperplastic and hypertrophic obesity?
8. What are the components of a sound approach to weight management?
9. Explain how the ABCs of behavior modification can assist with weight control.
10. Define “underweight.”

[Try] This

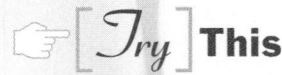

A One-Week Energy Balance Check

The purpose of this exercise is to see if you're in energy balance by monitoring your body weight for one week. Measure your weight on a Monday morning soon after you wake up. Record your weight. Don't change your normal routine of exercise and food intake. One week later weigh yourself again (on a Monday morning just after waking). Did your weight change? If not, your energy intake closely matched your energy output. If so, did you gain or lose weight? What factors do you think contributed to your body weight change? Try repeating this exercise over a longer period of time. Measure and record your weight every Monday morning for six months. What happens?

Increasing Your Energy Output

Physical activity is the part of your energy output that varies the most. The purpose of this exercise is to increase your energy expenditure by committing to daily exercise for one week. Make each exercise session about 30 minutes long, and remember that the longer the duration, the harder the intensity, and the larger the muscle groups involved, the greater the energy expenditure. Choose an exercise you enjoy—such as walking, jogging, cycling, swimming, or rollerblading. Once your week is complete, ask yourself these questions: How did this week's daily exercise affect my energy balance? Have I gained or lost weight during the week? Did I compensate for the extra energy expenditure by increasing my calorie intake?

Changing Your Energy Input

Would you like to change your weight by a pound or two? The purpose of this exercise is to increase or decrease your energy input (calorie intake) so that you gain or lose 1 pound by the end of a week. How? Make only minor adjustments in your usual diet but try to change the energy content for each of your meals by a small amount. Keep a food log and use Appendix A or EatRight Analysis Software to estimate your calorie total for each of the days. Your goal is to change your calorie total by approximately 500 kilocalories per day. You should not consume fewer than 1,500 kilocalories (for women) or 1,800 kilocalories (for men) per day. Weigh yourself at the start of your week and at the end. What change, if any, do you see?

What About Bobbie?

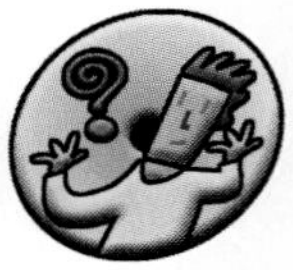

Remember, Bobbie is a 20-year-old college sophomore who weighs 155 pounds and is 5′4″. She gained 10 pounds her freshman year and would like to lose it because she feels healthier when her weight is closer to 145 pounds. She exercises infrequently but likes to walk with her friends and occasionally goes to an aerobics class. How would you suggest she lose the extra 10 pounds? First, let's start by reducing her calorie intake slightly. Here is Bobbie's typical day of eating and a suggested alternative that will save her some calories.

Typical Day	Alternative	Kcalories
BREAKFAST		
1 cinnamon-raisin bagel		
3 Tbsp. light cream cheese	*1 Tbsp. light cream cheese*	*70 saved*
Coffee, 2 Tbsp. 2% milk, 2 tsp. sugar		
SNACK		
1 banana		
LUNCH		
2 slices sourdough bread		
2 ounces turkey lunch meat 2 tsp. regular mayo, 2 tsp. mustard, 1 slice tomato, dill pickle, lettuce leaf		
12 oz. diet coke		
Salad 2 C iceberg lettuce with 2 Tbsp. each: shredded carrot, chopped egg, croutons, kidney beans, Italian dressing	*1 Tbsp. Italian dressing*	*70 saved*
1 chocolate chip cookie		
SNACK		
1 1/2 oz. tortilla chips, 1/2 C salsa	*1 oz. tortilla chips*	*70 saved*
2 C water		
DINNER		
1 1/2 C pasta 3 oz. meatballs, 3 oz. spaghetti sauce, 2 Tbsp. parmesan cheese	*1 C pasta*	*100 saved*
1 slice garlic bread	*delete garlic bread*	*185 saved*
1/2 C green beans	*1 C green beans*	*25 added*
1 tsp. butter	*delete butter*	*30 saved*
SNACK		
1 slice cheese pizza		
	Total	***500 saved***

As you can see, small changes in Bobbie's diet can result in a 500-kilocalorie deficit, which will translate to approximately 1 pound per week of weight loss. This doesn't take into account any extra exercise she might do. So if she starts to work out more regularly, she can make fewer changes in her calorie intake and still lose 1 pound per week.

References

1 McCrory MA, Fuss PJ, Saltzman E, Roberts SB. Dietary determinants of energy intake and weight regulation in healthy adults. *J Nutr.* 2000;130:276S–279S; and Westerterp-Plantenga MS. Analysis of energy density of food in relation to energy intake regulation in human subjects. *Br J Nutr.* 2001;85:351–361.

2 Rolls BJ. The role of energy density in the overconsumption of fat. *J Nutr.* 2000;130(suppl):268S–271S.

3 Burton-Freeman B. Dietary fiber and energy regulation. *J Nutr.* 2000;130:272S–275S.

4 McCrory MA, et al. Op. cit.

5 Ludwig DS. Dietary glycemic index and obesity. *J Nutr.* 2000;130:280S–283S.

6 Guyton AC, Hall JE. *Textbook of Medical Physiology.* 10th ed. Philadelphia: WB Saunders; 2000.

7 Ibid.

8 Ibid.

9 Schwartz MW, Woods SC, Porter D Jr, et al. Central nervous system control of food intake. *Nature.* 2000;404(6):661–671.

10 Schwartz MW, Seeley RJ. *Seminars in medicine of the Beth Israel Deaconess Medical Center: neuroendocrine responses to starvation and weight loss. N Engl J Med.* 1997; 336(25): 1802–1811.

11 Flood JF, Morley JE. Increased food intake by neuropeptide Y is due to an increased motivation to eat. *Peptides.* 1991;12: 1329–1332.

12 Schwartz MW, Baskin DG, Kaiyala KJ, Woods SC. Model for the regulation of energy balance and adiposity by the central nervous system. *Am J Clin Nutr.* 1999;69:584–596.

13 Das SK, Roberts SB. Energy Metabolism. In: Bowman BA, Russell RM, eds. *Present Knowledge in Nutrition.* 8th ed. Washington, DC: ILSI Press; 2001.

14 Bowles L, Kopelman P. Leptin: of mice and men? *J Clin Pathol.* 2001;54:1–3.

15 Ibid.

16 Stubbs RJ, Johnstone AM, Mazalan N, et al. Effect of altering the variety of sensorially distinct foods, of the same macronutrient content, on food intake and body weight in men. *Eur J Clin Nutr.* 2001;55:19–28.

17 Wilmore JH, Costill DL. *Physiology of Sport and Exercise.* 2nd ed. Champaign, IL: Human Kinetics; 1999.

18 Mahan LK, Escott-Stump S. *Krause's Food, Nutrition & Diet Therapy.* 10th ed. Philadelphia: WB Saunders; 2000.

19 Ibid.

20 Wilmore JH, Costill DL. Op. cit.

21 Levine JA, Eberhardt NL, Jensen MD. Role of nonexercise activity thermogenesis in resistance to fat gain in humans. *Science.* 1999;283:212–214.

22 Wilmore JH, Costill DL. Op. cit.

23 National Academy of Sciences: Energy. *Recommended Dietary Allowances.* 10th ed. Washington, DC: National Academy Press; 1989.

24 Ibid.

25 Rippe JM, Crossley S, Ringer R. Obesity as a chronic disease: modern medical and lifestyle management. *J Am Diet Assoc.* October 1998(suppl):S9–S15. Theme issue.

26 USDA Center for Nutrition Policy and Promotion. *Body Mass Index and Health.* Nutrition Insights series, No. 16. March 2000; updated March 2001.

27 National Center for Health Statistics. CDC growth charts: United States. http://www.cdc.gov/growthcharts. Accessed 3/31/02.

28 Barlow, SE, Dietz WH. Obesity evaluation and treatment: expert committee recommendations. *Pediatrics* [online]. 1998;102, E29. http://www.pediatrics.org/cgi/content/full/102/3/e29. Accessed 3/31/02.

29 Despres JP, Allard C, Tremblay A, et al. Evidence for a regional component of body fatness in the association with serum lipids in men and women. *Metabolism.* 1985;34:967–973.

30 Ziegler RG. Anthropometry and breast cancer. *J Nutr.* 1997;127(suppl 5):924S–928S.

31 Blackburn GL. Effects of weight loss on weight-related risk factors. In: Brownell KD, Fairburn CG, eds. *Eating Disorders and Obesity.* New York: Guilford; 1995:406–410.

32 National High Blood Pressure Education Program (NHBPEP) Working Group. Report on primary prevention of hypertension. *Arch Intern Med.* 1993;153:186.

33 Rockhill B, Willett WC, Hunter DJ, et al. A prospective study of recreational physical activity and breast cancer. *Arch Intern Med.* 1999;59(19):2290–2296.

34 Pi-Sunyer XF. Medical complications of obesity. In: Brownell KD, Fairburn CG, eds. *Eating Disorders and Obesity.* New York: Guilford; 1995:401–405.

35 Blackburn GL. Op. cit.

36 Kirschenbaum DS, Fitzgibbon ML. Controversy about the treatment of obesity: criticisms or challenges? *Behav Ther.* 1995;26:43–68.

37 Olson MB, Kelsey SF, Bittner V, et al. Weight cycling and high-density lipoprotein cholesterol in women: evidence of an adverse effect. A report from the NHLBI-sponsored WISE study. *J Am Coll Cardiol,* 2000;36(5):1565–1571.

38 Friedman JM. Obesity in the new millennium. *Nature.* 2000;404:632–634.

39 Kopelman PG. Obesity as a medical problem. *Nature.* 2000;404:635–643.

40 Uauy R, Albala C, Kain J. Obesity trends in Latin America: transitioning from under- to overweight. *J Nutr.* 2001;131: 893S–899S.

41 Mokhatar N, Elati J, Chabir R, et al. Diet culture and obesity in northern Africa. *J Nutr.* 2001;131:887S–892S.

42 Kopelman PG. Op. cit.

43 Dalton S. Trends in prevalence of overweight in the United States and other countries. In: Dalton S, ed. *Overweight and Weight Management: The Health Professional's Guide to Understanding and Practice.* Gaithersburg, MD: Aspen; 1997:142–160.

44 Kuczmarski RJ, Carrol MD, Flegal KM, Troiano RP. Varying body mass index cut-off points to describe overweight prevalence among U.S. adults: NHANES III (1988 to 1994). *Obes Res.* 1997;5:542–548.

45 US Department of Health and Human Services. Leading health indicators. *Healthy People 2010: Understanding and Improving Health.* 2nd ed. Washington, DC: US Government Printing Office; 2000.

46 Gustafson-Larson AM, Terry RD. Weight-related behaviors and concerns of fourth-grade children. *J Am Diet Assoc.* 1992;92: 818–822.

47 Johansson L, Solvoll K, Bjorneboe G-EA, Drevon CA. Under- and overreporting of energy intake related to weight status and lifestyle in a nationwide sample. *Am J Clin Nutr.* 1998;68: 266–274.

48 Bouchard C. Genetic factors and body weight regulation. In: Dalton S, ed. Op. cit., 161–186.

49 Barsh GS, Faroogi S, O'Rahilly S. Genetics of body-weight regulation. *Nature.* 2000;404:644–651.

50 McArthur LH, Howard AB. Dietetics majors' weight-reduction beliefs, behaviors, and information sources. *J Am Coll Health.* 2001;49:175–181.

51 Williamson DF, Kahn HS, Remington PL, Anda RF. The 10-year incidence of overweight and major weight gain in US adults. *Arch Intern Med.* 1990;150:665–672.

52 Anderson AE. Eating disorders in males. In: Brownell KD, Fairburn CG, eds. *Eating Disorders and Obesity.* New York: Guilford; 1995:177–182.

53 Pliner P, Chaiken S, Flett GL. Gender differences in concern with body weight and physical appearance over the life span. *Personal Soc Psychol Bull.* 1990;16:262–273.

54 Kopelman PG. Op. cit.

55 James W. The epidemiology of obesity. In: Chadwick D, Cardew G, eds. *The Origins and Consequences of Obesity.* Chichester: Wiley; 1996:1–16.

56 Sobal J, Troiano R, Frongillo E. Rural-urban differences in obesity. *Rural Sociol.* 1996;61:289–305.

57 Sobal J, Rauschenbach B, Frongillo E. Marital status, fatness, and obesity. *Social Sci Med.* 1992;35:915–923.

58 Faith MS, Allison DB, Geliebter A. Emotional eating and obesity. In: Dalton S, ed. Op. cit., 439–465.

59 Arnow B, Kenardy J, Agras WS. The emotional eating scale: the development of a measure to assess coping with negative affect by eating. *Int J Eating Dis.* 1995;18:79–90.

60 Cutting TM, Fisher JO, Grimm-Thomas K, Birch LL. Like mother, like daughter: familial patterns of overweight are mediated by mothers' dietary disinhibition. *Am J Clin Nutr.* 1999;69: 608–613.

61 Marcus MD. Binge eating in obesity. In: Fairburn CG, Wilson GT, eds. *Binge Eating: Nature, Assessment, and Treatment.* New York: Guilford; 1993:77–96.

62 Position of the American Dietetic Association on weight management. *J Am Diet Assoc.* 1997;97(1):71–74.

63 Campfield LA. Treatment options and the maintenance of weight loss. In: Allison DB, Pi-Sunyer FX, eds. *Obesity Treatment: Establishing Goals, Improving Outcomes, and Reviewing the Research Agenda.* New York: Plenum; 1995:93–95.

64 Blackburn GL. Obesity and the metabolic syndrome. 1999. http://www.obesity.org/obmetabolic.htm. Accessed 3/31/02.

65 Irwin ML, Mayer-Davis EJ, Addy CL, et al. Moderate-intensity physical activity and fasting insulin levels in women: the Cross-Cultural Activity Participation Study. *Diabetes Care* 2000;23(4):449.

66 Wing RR, Hill JO. Successful weight loss maintenance. *Ann Rev Nutr.* 2001;21:323–341.

67 Stubbs RJ, Prentice AM, James WP. Carbohydrates and energy balance. *Ann NY Acad Sci* 1997;819:44–69.

68 Miller WC, Niederpruem MG, Wallace JP, Lindeman AK. Dietary fat, sugar, and fiber predict body fat content. *J Am Diet Assoc.* 1994;94:612–615.

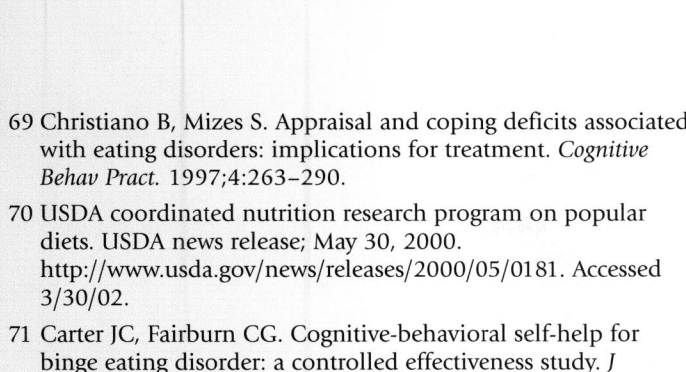

69 Christiano B, Mizes S. Appraisal and coping deficits associated with eating disorders: implications for treatment. *Cognitive Behav Pract.* 1997;4:263–290.

70 USDA coordinated nutrition research program on popular diets. USDA news release; May 30, 2000. http://www.usda.gov/news/releases/2000/05/0181. Accessed 3/30/02.

71 Carter JC, Fairburn CG. Cognitive-behavioral self-help for binge eating disorder: a controlled effectiveness study. *J Consult Clin Psychol.* 1998;66:616–623.

72 Campfield LA. The role of pharmacological agents in the treatment of obesity. In: Dalton S, ed. Op. cit., 466–485.

73 Lucas KH, Kaplan-Machlis B. Orlistat—a novel weight loss therapy. *Ann Pharmacother*. 2001;35:314–328.

74 Aronne LJ. Modern medical management of obesity: the role of pharmaceutical intervention. *J Am Diet Assoc.* 1998;98:10 (suppl 2):S23–S26.

75 Weissman NJ. Appetite suppressants and valvular heart disease. *Am J Med Sci.* 2001;32:285–291.

76 Pi-Sunyer FX. Obesity. In: Shils ME, Olson JA, Shike M, Ross AC, eds. *Modern Nutrition in Health and Disease.* 9th ed. Philadelphia: Lippincott-Williams & Wilkins; 1999.

77 Followup. *HealthNews.* February 2001;7:8.

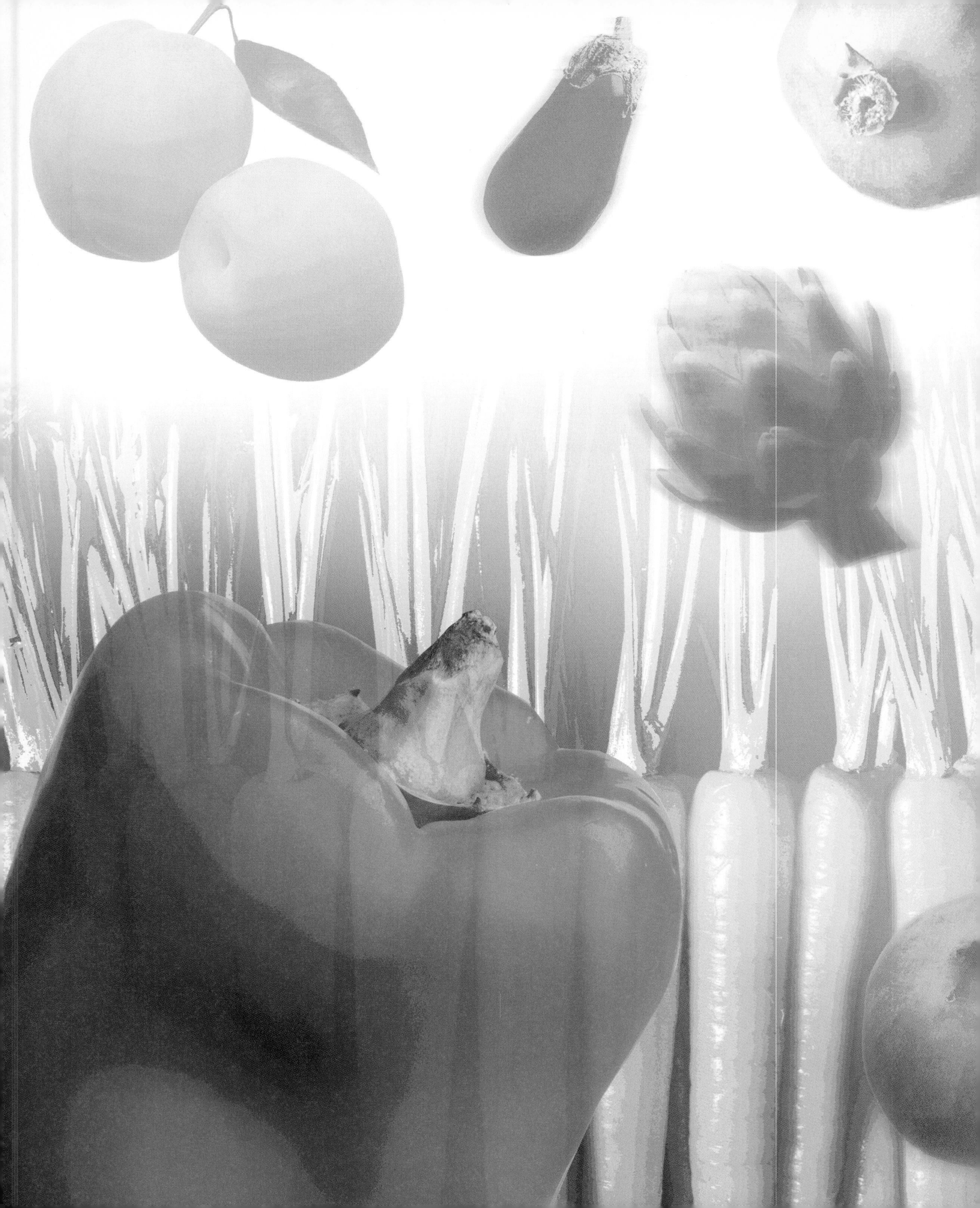

Chapter 9

Vitamins: Vital Keys to Health

Think About It

1 Do you prefer vegetables or meat? What food group, if any, supplies most of your vitamin needs?

2 From a well-lighted area, you step into a dark room. Over time, you see details. What's going on?

3 You decide to follow a strict vegetarian lifestyle. What vitamin deficiencies should you watch out for?

4 Do you know anyone who takes vitamin C to prevent colds? What do you think of this strategy?

Fyi for your Information

This chapter's FYI boxes include practical information on the following topics:

- Fresh, Frozen, or Canned? Raw or Cooked?
- Antioxidants and Free Radicals
- The B Vitamins and Heart Disease

WWW

The Web site for this book offers many useful tools and is a great source for additional nutrition information for both students and instructors. For information on fat-soluble vitamins, visit the site at nutrition.jbpub.com/discovering. You'll find exercises that explore the following topics:

- New Roles for Vitamin A?
- Vitamin D
- Vitamin E in 3-D
- "K" Is for Clotting
- Exercise and Water-Soluble Vitamins

Key to Illustrations

- Chylomicron
- Enzymes
- Fat-Soluble Vitamins
- Free Radical
- Proteins
- Water-Soluble Vitamins

What About Bobbie?

Track the choices Bobbie is making with the EatRight Analysis software.

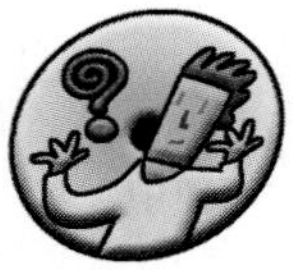

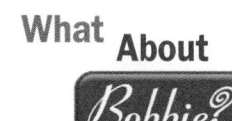

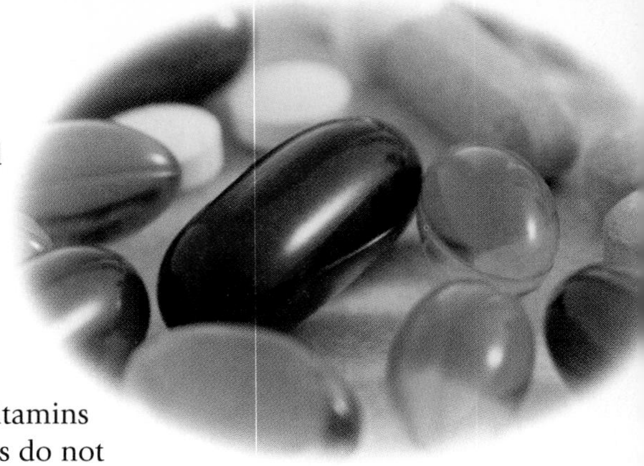

Feeling tired, run down, stressed out? You must need a vitamin, right? Surely you've heard that vitamins give you energy, so a lack of energy must be a signal that you need more vitamins, right? Well, probably not.

Although many people think of vitamins as energy boosters, in truth, vitamins do not supply the body with energy in the form of calories—a fact that distinguishes them from fat, carbohydrate, and protein. However, you do need certain vitamins to obtain energy from those nutrients.

In times of stress, you need more energy, so a supplement is in order, right? Well, yes and no. Certainly physical stresses, such as injury or illness, increase your body's need for energy, protein, vitamins, and minerals to aid healing. But emotional stress, such as that caused by anxiety or fear, does not. It may seem that you expend a lot of energy worrying about finals, but worrying requires no more energy than sitting and chatting with friends.

But surely if you do more physical exercise, you should take a vitamin, right? Again, not necessarily. Physical activity requires energy and the vitamins to metabolize it. But the extra food you eat to meet your greater energy needs contains vitamins too—unless your diet consists mostly of chips, sodas, and the like. In most cases, adding fruits, vegetables, and grains as energy sources provides all the vitamins you need. So, check out your diet before you check out the vitamin supplements!

Quick Bites

What Do You Believe about Vitamins?

Thirty-five percent of Americans surveyed in 1997 said that they believed vitamin supplements were necessary to ensure good health. Women were more likely than men to believe they needed supplements.

Understanding Vitamins

Vitamins differ from fat, protein, and carbohydrate in many important ways. For one, the body requires large amounts of carbohydrates, proteins, and fats—amounts measured in grams. By comparison, the daily needs for vitamins are infinitesimal—a mere microgram or two in some cases. In addition, unlike fat, protein, and carbohydrate, vitamins are not an energy source. However, many vitamins play crucial roles in extracting energy from those nutrients. Another difference is structural: Vitamins are individual units rather than long chains of smaller units.

Like fat, carbohydrate, and protein, however, vitamins are organic (carbon-containing) compounds essential for normal functioning, growth, and maintenance of the body. Vitamins often work together to get their jobs done (see **Figure 9.1**), so a deficiency of just one can cause profound health problems.

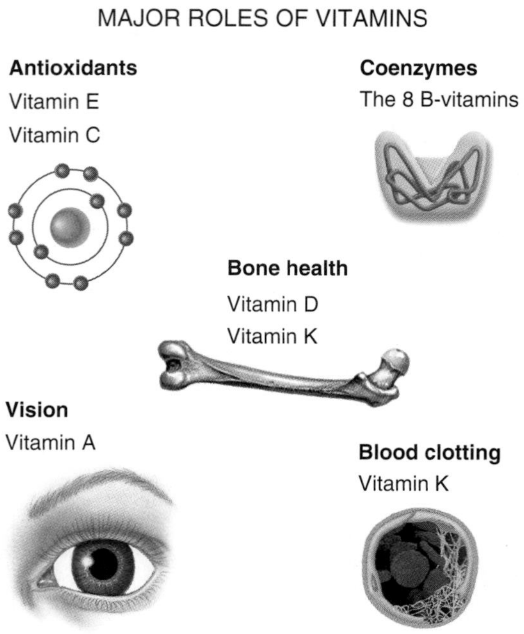

Figure 9.1 **Major roles of vitamins.** Compared with carbohydrate, fat, and protein, the body needs tiny amounts of vitamins. Vitamins, however, are crucial for normal functioning, growth, and maintenance of body tissues.

Fat-Soluble versus Water-Soluble Vitamins

Scientists classify vitamins as "fat-soluble" and "water-soluble." Vitamins A, D, E, and K are fat-soluble vitamins. The B vitamins and vitamin C, on the other hand, are water-soluble vitamins. This difference in solubility affects the way our body absorbs, transports, and stores vitamins. (See **Figure 9.2**.)

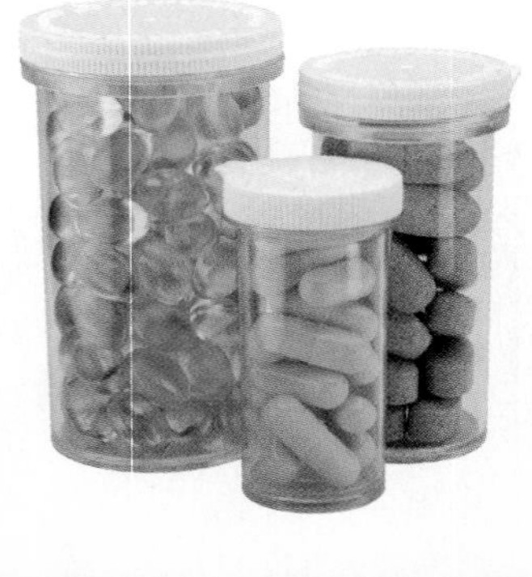

Intestinal cells absorb fat-soluble vitamins along with dietary fat and package them in lipoproteins, which are released to the lymph system. Fat-soluble vitamins travel through the lymph system, and eventually the bloodstream, until they reach the liver.

Suppose you eat and absorb more fat-soluble vitamins than you need. As vitamin intake rises above the body's needs, the amount absorbed generally falls. Excess fat-soluble vitamins accumulate in your liver and fatty tissues, building up reserves that can tide you over for weeks or months.

Water-soluble vitamins are dissolved in the watery compartments of foods. Intestinal cells absorb water-soluble vitamins directly into the bloodstream. Because your body does not store most water-soluble vitamins in appreciable amounts, they should be a part of your daily diet. An exception is vitamin B_{12}, which the liver stores in large amounts. Small variations in daily intake typically do not cause problems, however. For example, symptoms of vitamin C deficiency do not emerge until after 20 to 40 days of a diet deficient in this water-soluble vitamin.

In general, excess fat-soluble vitamins, which tend to be stored in the body, are more likely to cause adverse effects than water-soluble vitamins. The kidneys filter out most excess water-soluble vitamins and excrete them in urine. But there are exceptions. Fat-soluble vitamins E and K are unlikely to be toxic. And large amounts of some water-soluble vitamins—vitamin B_6, folate, niacin—can be problematic, often seriously so.

Vitamin toxicity is rarely linked to high vitamin intakes from food or to the use of supplements that contain 100 to 150 percent of the recommended amounts. However, people who take megadoses of one or more vitamins risk consuming toxic amounts.

Figure 9.2 **Absorption of vitamins.** Water-soluble vitamins are absorbed by intestinal cells and delivered directly to the bloodstream. Fat-soluble vitamins are absorbed with fat into the lymphatic system.

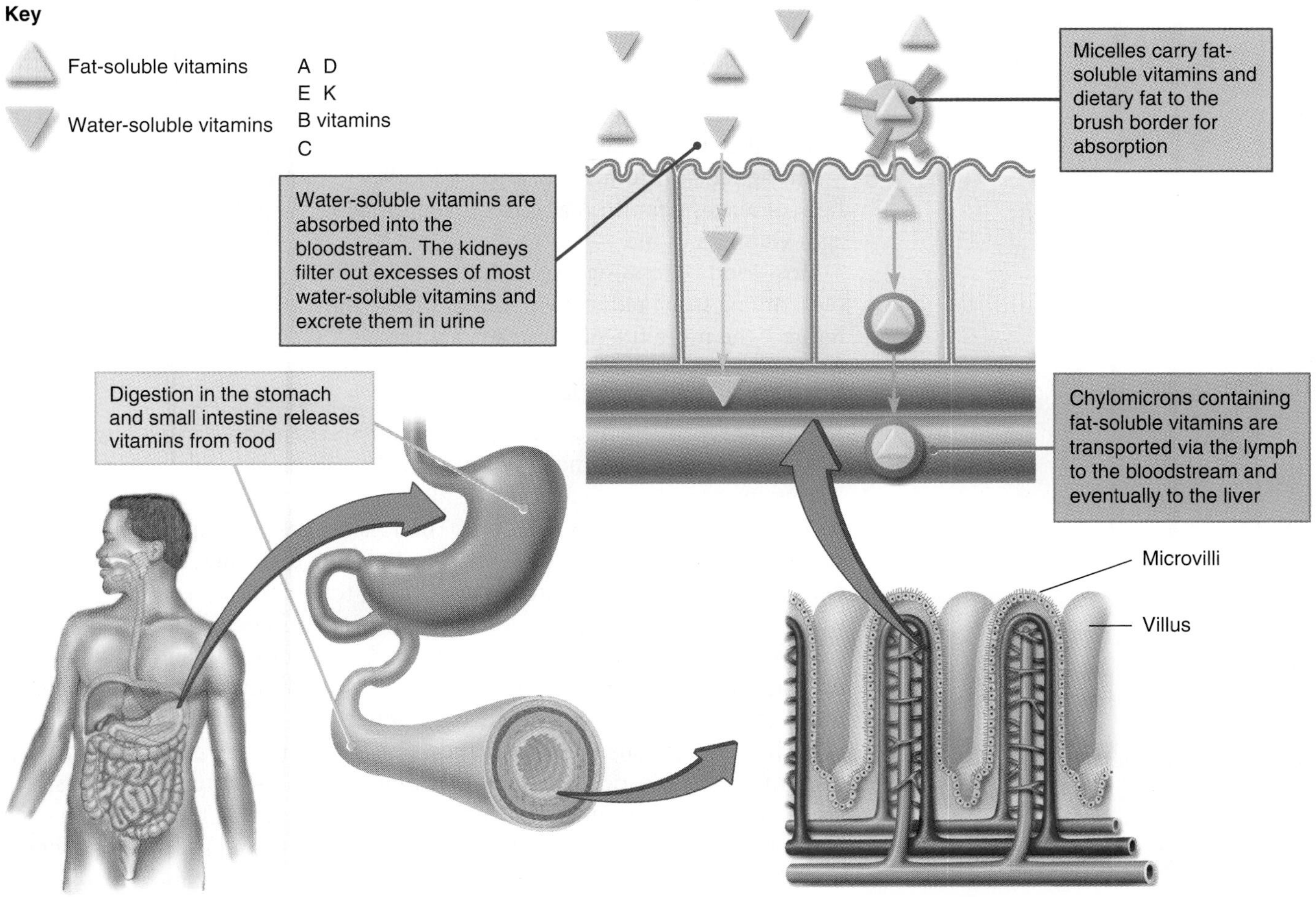
Key
Fat-soluble vitamins
A D
E K
Water-soluble vitamins
B vitamins
C
Water-soluble vitamins are absorbed into the bloodstream. The kidneys filter out excesses of most water-soluble vitamins and excrete them in urine
Micelles carry fat-soluble vitamins and dietary fat to the brush border for absorption
Digestion in the stomach and small intestine releases vitamins from food
Chylomicrons containing fat-soluble vitamins are transported via the lymph to the bloodstream and eventually to the liver
Microvilli
Villus

Key Concepts: *Vitamins are organic substances needed in minuscule amounts to help regulate body processes. Vitamins can be classified as fat-soluble (vitamins A, D, E, and K) or water-soluble (the B vitamins and vitamin C). Fat-soluble vitamins, which are stored in the liver and fatty tissues of the body, are excreted more slowly than water-soluble vitamins, and reserves last longer. Fat-soluble vitamins, when consumed in excess, generally pose a greater risk of toxicity than water-soluble vitamins.*

Vitamins in Foods

Vitamins are found in every food group, including the fats and oils that many of us are trying to reduce in our diets. This is one more reason to eat a variety of foods. No single food group or single choice within a food group is a good source of all vitamins. Think About It 1

Several factors determine the amounts of specific vitamins in a food. Because animals store and concentrate vitamins in their tissues, animal products tend to have fairly constant vitamin levels. Fruits and vegetables can be a different story. Soil composition, sunlight, moisture, growing conditions, and the plant's maturity at harvest all affect vitamin content. Fortunately, our foods are grown in diverse locales, so eating a varied diet supplies plenty of vitamins.

In general, water-soluble vitamins are more fragile than fat-soluble vitamins, and some cooking practices are particularly harmful. Many cooks add baking soda, which is alkaline, to cooking water to reduce cooking time and intensify a vegetable's color. Both alkalinity and heat destroy vitamin C and the B vitamins thiamin and riboflavin. When vegetables are boiled, cooking water easily leaches water-soluble vitamins. Yet cooking only partially destroys a food's vitamin content, and some cooking methods are less destructive than others. The best cooking methods—steaming, stir-frying, and microwaving—use minimal amounts of water. (See the FYI feature "Fresh, Frozen, or Canned? Raw or Cooked?")

Packaging and storage can affect a food's vitamin content. Exposure to light damages vitamin A and the B vitamin riboflavin. Exposure to air damages vitamins C and E.

Most food processing (e.g., refining oils, milling grain, canning vegetables, drying fruit) reduces vitamin content. The more a food is processed or refined, the more it tends to lose vitamins.

Enrichment and Fortification

Milling or refining grains removes the bran and germ to make white flour, white rice, refined cornmeal, flour for pasta, and most breakfast cereals. Processing grains also removes most B vitamins, vitamin E, and minerals such as iron, magnesium, and zinc. The loss of these nutrients from such staple foods could be devastating. In fact, during the nineteenth and early twentieth centuries, widespread adoption of these milling techniques left a wake of vitamin deficiency diseases like beriberi and pellagra.

To prevent overt deficiencies, processors now return iron and three B vitamins to the grains they process. Replacing lost nutrients is called "enrichment." Most countries now require enriching staple grain products.

Food processors also "fortify" foods. Fortification is the process of adding extra nutrients to foods where they wouldn't be found naturally in consistently significant amounts. Iodized table salt is a fortified food. Read the labels on some breakfast cereals—the ones with the long list of added vitamins and minerals are fortified foods. Fortification is sometimes required

Quick Bites

Is It a Fruit or Vegetable?

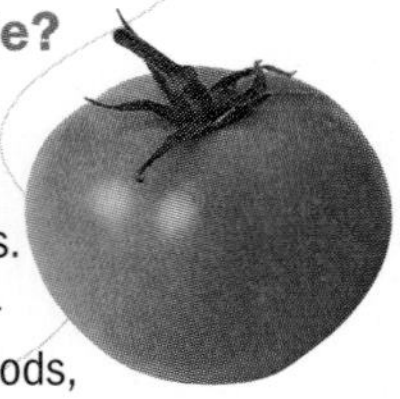

In the eighteenth century, botanists defined fruits as the organ surrounding the seeds. This definition considers cucumbers, eggplants, peppers, pea pods, and corn kernels as fruits. Legally though, these are all vegetables. In the late 1800s, the U.S. Supreme Court, while trying the case of a tomato importer, established a definition based on linguistic custom and usage. The importer had to pay the vegetable tax.

provitamins Inactive forms of vitamins that the body can convert into active usable forms. Also referred to as vitamin precursors.

vitamin precursors See *provitamins.*

by law, as in the addition of vitamins A and D to milk and, most recently, the addition of folic acid to enriched cereal and grain products.

Enrichment and mandatory fortification programs helped eliminate most overt deficiency diseases in the United States and many other countries. However, mandatory enrichment replaces only some of the many nutrients lost in milling. Moreover, the American diet contains lots of highly refined foods that are not fortified or enriched, foods that have calories but almost no micronutrients.

Provitamins

Some vitamins in foods are in inactive forms, called **provitamins** or **vitamin precursors.** The body must change them to an active form. One familiar provitamin is beta-carotene, found in many fruits and vegetables. Your body converts much of the beta-carotene you eat to its active form, vitamin A. (See **Figure 9.3**.) When experts calculate vitamin requirements or monitor consumption, they must take provitamins into account.

Key Concepts: *Growing conditions, storage, processing, and cooking affect the amounts of vitamins in foods. Enrichment and fortification programs replace some vitamins and minerals lost in processing and add other nutrients to foods. Provitamins are vitamin precursors that can be converted to an active vitamin form.*

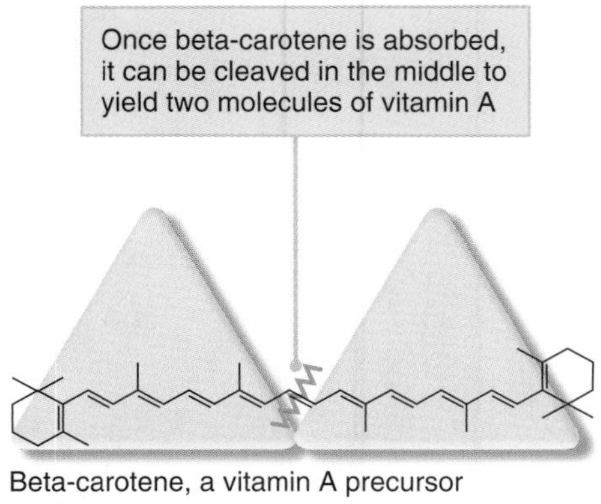
Once beta-carotene is absorbed, it can be cleaved in the middle to yield two molecules of vitamin A
Beta-carotene, a vitamin A precursor

Figure 9.3 **Beta-carotene.** Beta-carotene may be cleaved at different locations, so it may yield less than two molecules of vitamin A. Other provitamin A carotenoids yield less vitamin A than beta-carotene.

Fyi FOR YOUR INFORMATION — Fresh, Frozen, or Canned? Raw or Cooked?

Selecting and Preparing Foods to Maximize Vitamin Content

Wouldn't it be great if we could all shop daily for fresh fruits and vegetables? When picked at their peak ripeness, fresh fruits and vegetables are packed with many different vitamins. Remember that light, heat, air, acid, and alkali can destroy many vitamins, and cooking liquids can leach them out. Even if you can't buy fresh foods daily, you can still minimize nutrient loss after purchase. Start by choosing clean, undamaged produce at each of your regular shopping trips. Then store foods with minimal exposure to light and air. Many fruits, most vegetables, and all animal products require refrigeration. Get them cold right away, and keep them cold. Because vitamin content can decrease with time, plan on using fruits and vegetables soon after purchase. The vitamin C of fresh green beans, for example, drops by half after six days at home.

What about frozen and canned foods? Their vitamin content is much better than you might guess. True, the heat used in canning is destructive. But the processor typically uses fresh-picked produce, which is higher in vitamins than food transported to faraway markets. The vitamin levels in canned foods remain relatively constant, even after two years. Often, vitamins end up in the liquid in which the food is packed.[1] Use the liquids from canned vegetables in soups and stews to get the benefit.

Carotenoids are stable during the canning process. In fact, current research suggests the lycopene in processed tomato products is better absorbed into the body than that from raw tomatoes.[2] Unfortunately, vitamin C is lost from fruits and vegetables during canning, but much of the lost vitamin remains in the canning liquid or juice.

What is the best way to cook vegetables? To maximize vitamin content, think minimal—minimal heat, minimal cooking water, and minimal exposure to air. A good rule of thumb: "minimize to maximize." Try to minimize handling the food before and during cooking. Dicing a food such as a potato reduces cooking time, but also exposes more surface area to vitamin destruction. So, cut if you must, but not too small.

Because steaming, stir-frying, and microwaving minimize cooking time and water use, they are the best cooking methods for preserving vitamin content. If you boil foods, use the cooking water for sauces, stews, or soups to salvage lost water-soluble vitamins. And do not add baking soda to beans or vegetables (some folks do that to intensify color and tenderize). Baking soda destroys some vitamins.

Remember, to retain the most vitamins in your food, be gentle with storage, kind with cooking, and "minimize to maximize"!

1 University of Illinois, Department of Food Science and Human Nutrition. *Nutrient Conservation in Canned, Frozen, and Fresh Foods.* Urbana University of Illinois; 1997.
2 Tonucci LH, Holden JM, Beecher GR, et al. Carotenoid content of thermally processed tomato-based food products. *J Agr Food Chem.* 1995;43:579–583.

Fat-Soluble Vitamins A, D, E, K, and the Carotenoids

Despite their common property of fat-solubility, the fat-soluble vitamins have diverse roles. Vitamin A is crucial for vision and renewing cells. Vitamin D helps regulate blood levels of calcium and is essential for bone health. Vitamin E and the carotenoids are antioxidants that help protect cells from damage. Vitamin K is known for its role in blood clotting, but it also is crucial for bone health along with vitamin D. Unlike the water-soluble B vitamins, none of the fat-soluble vitamins are coenzymes.

Vitamin A: The Retinoids

Vitamin A's most dramatic effects are in the eye. You need vitamin A to change light images to sight and to keep the eye's surface healthy. Vitamin A also helps direct development of the body's cells—how and when they grow and divide and what form they take. As such, this vitamin is essential to proper growth and reproduction. It plays a role in immune function, both as a cell regulator and by helping maintain the skin and mucous membranes. In fact, vitamin A plays a crucial role in maintaining or regulating many tissues throughout the body.

The liver holds over 90 percent of the body's vitamin A reserves, with the rest deposited in fat tissue, lungs, and kidneys.[1] A healthy liver can store up to a year's supply of vitamin A, releasing it in just the right amounts to maintain normal vitamin A blood levels—a nice benefit, but one with a drawback: Large doses of vitamin A can exceed storage capacity and cause toxicity.

retinol The alcohol form of vitamin A; one of the retinoids; the main physiologically active form of vitamin A; interconvertible with retinal.

retinal The aldehyde form of vitamin A; one of the retinoids; the active form of vitamin A in the retina; interconvertible with retinol.

retinoic acid The acid form of vitamin A; one of the retinoids; formed from retinal but not interconvertible; helps growth, cell differentiation, and the immune system; does not have a role in vision or reproduction.

retinoids Compounds in foods that have chemical structures similar to vitamin A. Retinoids include the active forms of vitamin A (retinol, retinal, and retinoic acid) and the main storage forms of retinol (retinyl esters).

carotenoids A group of yellow, orange, and red pigments in plants. Some of these compounds are precursors of vitamin A.

Forms of Vitamin A

The body uses three active forms of vitamin A—**retinol**, **retinal**, and **retinoic acid**—known collectively as the **retinoids**. (See **Figure 9.4**.) While all three forms are essential, retinol is the key player in the vitamin A family.[2]

Colorful plant pigments called **carotenoids** are precursors of vitamin A. There are several hundred carotenoids found in nature, but your body converts only a handful of them to vitamin A. Of the carotenoids, beta-carotene supplies the most vitamin A.

Functions of Vitamin A

Vitamin A is crucial for vision, for maintaining healthy cells—particularly skin cells—for fighting infections and bolstering immune function, and for promoting growth and development. (See **Figure 9.5**.)

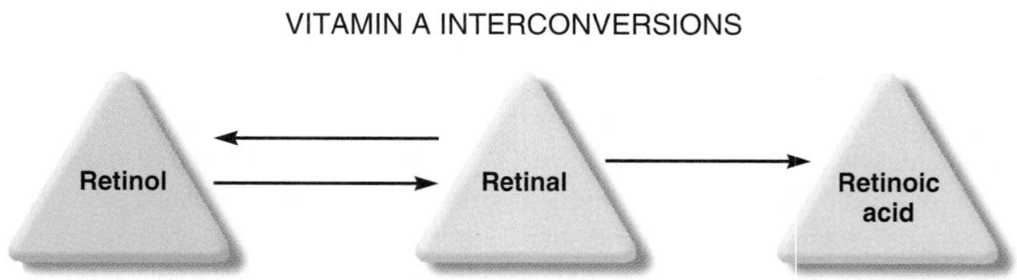

Figure 9.4 **Forms of vitamin A.** Whereas retinol and retinal are interconvertible, the reaction that forms retinoic acid is irreversible.

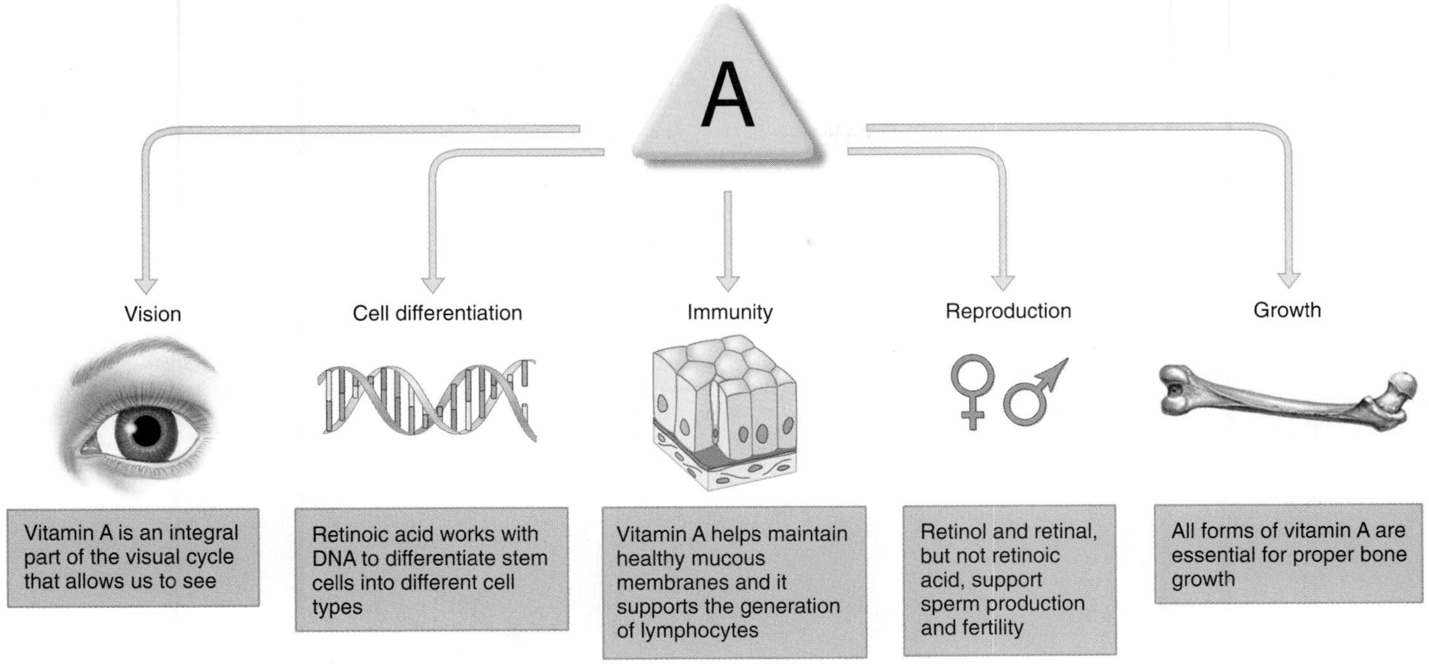
A
Vision
Cell differentiation
Immunity
Reproduction
Growth
Vitamin A is an integral part of the visual cycle that allows us to see
Retinoic acid works with DNA to differentiate stem cells into different cell types
Vitamin A helps maintain healthy mucous membranes and it supports the generation of lymphocytes
Retinol and retinal, but not retinoic acid, support sperm production and fertility
All forms of vitamin A are essential for proper bone growth

Figure 9.5 **Major functions of vitamin A.** Vitamin A plays a crucial role in vision and is essential for proper cell synthesis, reproduction, and bone growth.

Vision: Night and Day

Vitamin A allows night and color vision, by actually becoming a functioning part of the retina. The **retina** is the paper-thin tissue lining the back of the eye, where light images are received and relayed to the brain, resulting in vision. (See **Figure 9.6**.) **Rod cells**, the cells in the retina that react to dim light, are rich in a purple pigment called **rhodopsin**, or "visual purple." Rhodopsin is composed of a protein, **opsin**, plus vitamin A.

Light entering the eye and striking the retina splits rhodopsin, causing it to lose color as it releases opsin and vitamin A. This **bleaching process** triggers electric impulses that the brain interprets as black-and-white visual images. In well-nourished people, vitamin A recombines with opsin, forming new rhodopsin that again can respond to light. If vitamin A levels are low, the body cannot re-form rhodopsin, and **night blindness** results. Although the eyes contain only 0.01 percent of the body's vitamin A, they are so sensitive to vitamin A levels that one injection of the vitamin can relieve this type of night blindness within minutes.[3]

If you awaken in the middle of the night and turn on a bright light, the light level is blinding until your eyes adjust. Rhodopsin breaks down quickly in bright light, and the reduced supply makes the rod cells less light sensitive. Conversely, when you enter a dark room, not only do your eyes dilate, but they also produce rhodopsin to increase their sensitivity to light. Known as **dark adaptation**, the speed of adjustment to dim light is related directly to the amount of vitamin A available to regenerate rhodopsin. People with night blindness cannot adjust to dim light or regain vision quickly after exposure to a flash of bright light.

Think About It 2

Color vision also requires vitamin A. **Cone cells**, which are responsible for color vision, are rich in the pigment **iodopsin**. The iodopsin cycle is

retina A paper-thin tissue that lines the back of the eye and contains cells called rods and cones.

rod cells Light-sensitive cells in the retina that react to dim light and transmit black-and-white images.

rhodopsin Found in rod cells, this light-sensitive pigment molecule consists of a protein called opsin combined with retinal.

opsin A protein that combines with retinal to form rhodopsin in rod cells.

bleaching process A complex light-stimulated reaction in which rod cells lose color as rhodopsin is split into vitamin A (retinal) and opsin.

night blindness The inability of the eyes to adjust to dim light or to regain vision quickly after exposure to a flash of bright light.

dark adaptation The process that increases the rhodopsin concentration in your eyes, allowing them to detect images in the dark better.

cone cells Cells in the retina that are sensitive to bright light and translate it into color images.

iodopsin Color-sensitive pigment molecules in cone cells that consist of opsinlike proteins combined with retinal.

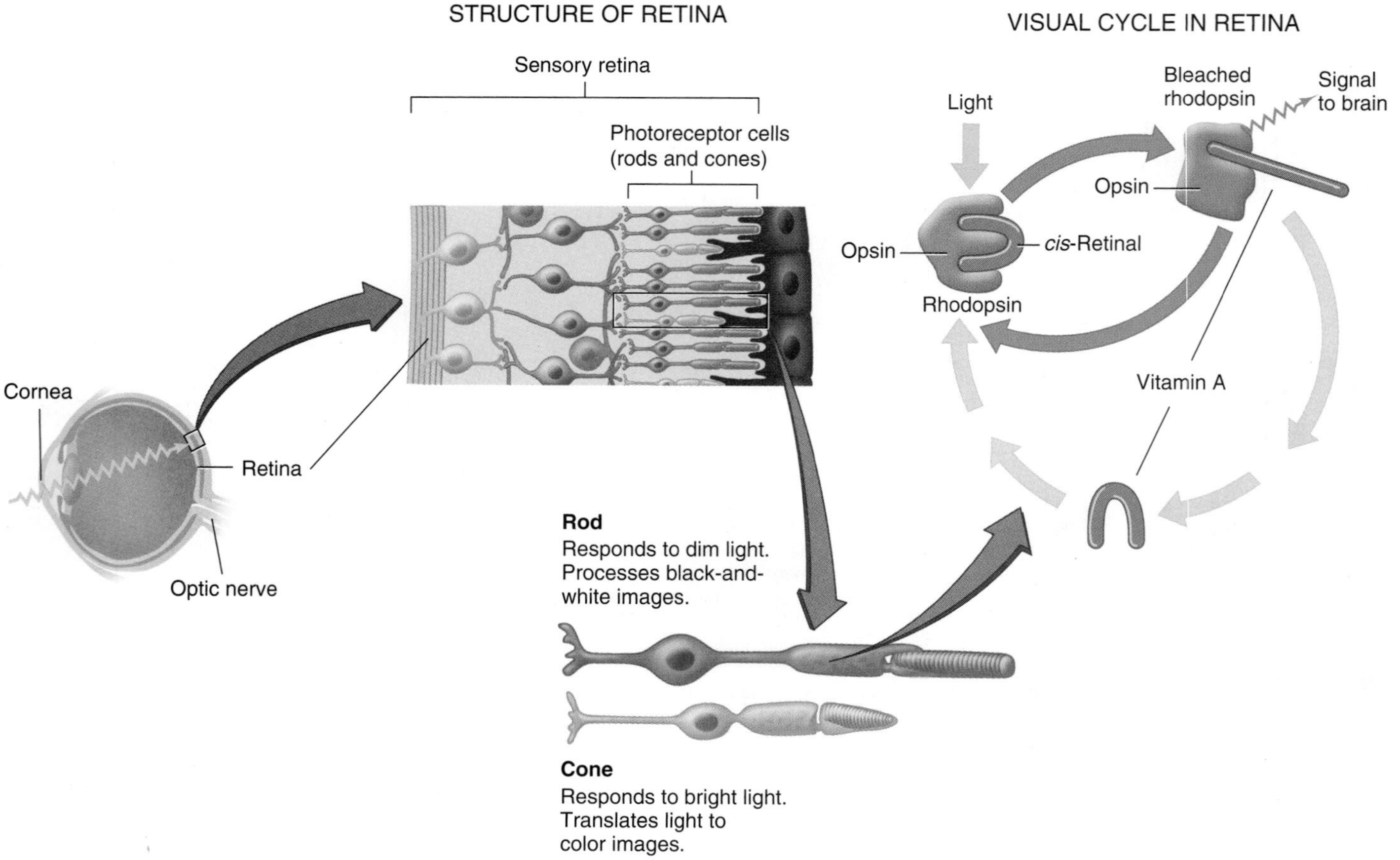

Figure 9.6 **Vitamin A and the visual cycle.** Rhodopsin is the combination of the protein opsin and vitamin A (retinal). When stimulated by light, both opsin and vitamin A change shape. This sends a signal to the brain, and you see an image in black and white. A similar process using a different protein called iodopsin provides color.

similar to the rhodopsin cycle, with vitamin A playing a crucial role. A prolonged lack of vitamin A impairs color vision, but because it affects rod cells before cone cells, night blindness emerges first.

Vitamin A in Cell Production and Differentiation

When your body needs to make the proteins that form new cells or other protein compounds, vitamin A plays a role in directing protein production. It helps regulate production of enzymes, blood carrier proteins, structural proteins such as those in skin, and more.

Vitamin A works in cell differentiation, the process that causes immature, characterless cells (undifferentiated cells called **stem cells**) to mature into specific kinds of cells. For example, if you cut your hand, the new cells produced to repair the cut are specifically suited to the job; stomach cells or lung cells would not do.

With these very basic, crucially important biological functions, vitamin A plays a role in building and maintaining tissues throughout the body.

stem cells Formative cells whose daughter cells may differentiate into other cell types.

epithelial tissues Closely packed layers of epithelial cells that cover the body and line its cavities.

epithelial cells The millions of cells that line and protect the external and internal surfaces of the body. Epithelial cells form epithelial tissues such as skin and mucous membranes.

Vitamin A and Skin

Skin, mucous membranes, and other lining materials in the body are all **epithelial tissues**. Together they cover us on the outside, act as a lining or covering on the inside, and provide lubrication where it's needed—for example, along bronchial tubes and the digestive tract. **Epithelial cells** are on the front line protecting your body, and they are destroyed and replaced relatively quickly. This requires vitamin A. Because the turnover of skin cells is rapid, signs of vitamin A deficiency show up early in the skin and mucous membranes.[4]

Vitamin A and Immune Function

Epithelial tissue is your body's first line of defense against bacterial, parasitic, and viral attack. But if dangerous microorganisms successfully breach these barriers, your body's defense system mobilizes immune cells to attack the invaders. To produce these immune cells, your body needs vitamin A.[5]

Vitamin A and Reproduction

Vitamin A aids reproduction, probably by keeping the secretion-producing linings of the reproductive tract healthy. In women, vitamin A helps maintain fertility. In men, it is needed for sperm production. Vitamin A's role in cell production and differentiation also makes it crucial to the proper development of an embryo.

Vitamin A and Bones

Vitamin A helps produce bone cells needed for growth and is required for bone "remodeling." As children grow, their bones get longer. But simply adding length would produce some strange-looking bones. Therefore during normal growth, the bone ends are actually broken down and then lengthened; that is, they are remodeled. A lack of vitamin A in the growing child disrupts bone remodeling and interferes with the development of immature bone cells. The result is weak, poorly formed bones.

Dietary Recommendations for Vitamin A

Remember, vitamin A includes retinoids—retinol, retinoic acid, and retinal—and is formed from precursor carotenoids. Similar amounts of dietary retinoids and carotenoids do not provide the same amount of vitamin A. To reconcile the differences, scientists use a measure called **retinol activity equivalent (RAE)**. One retinol activity equivalent equals the activity of 1 microgram (1/1,000,000 of a gram) of retinol. On average, 12 micrograms of beta-carotene from food produce 1 microgram of retinol. Other provitamin carotenoids like alpha-carotene are converted even less efficiently: 24 micrograms produce 1 microgram of retinol.[6] (See **Figure 9.7**.)

Because the term RAE and its definition have been adopted only recently, you may read about the outdated measure "retinol equivalents," or RE, in older texts. You also may see another outdated measure, **International Units (IU)**, on vitamin labels. One IU equals about 0.3 microgram of retinol from animal foods and 3.6 micrograms of beta-carotene from plant foods.

Most Americans take in adequate amounts of vitamin A and have large stores of the vitamin in their livers. The RDA for vitamin A for males aged 14 years and older is 900 micrograms RAE per day. For females aged 14 years and older, the vitamin A RDA is 700 micrograms RAE per day. Pregnant women should consume slightly more vitamin A (770 micrograms), and women who are breastfeeding their children are advised to consume 1,300 micrograms RAE.[7]

Sources of Vitamin A

Only foods of animal origin contain retinoids. Plant foods, especially yellow-orange vegetables and fruits, contain **provitamin A** carotenoids such as

Quick Bites

Vitamin A Isn't Just for Eyes

A recent study conducted in Nepal showed that women who took vitamin A supplements during pregnancy had a much lower risk of maternal mortality than those who took a placebo. The researchers concluded that regular and adequate intake of vitamin A or beta-carotene can reduce the risk of pregnancy-related death in areas where vitamin A deficiency is common.

retinol activity equivalent (RAE) A unit of measurement of the vitamin A content of a food. One RAE equals 1 microgram of retinol.

International Units (IU) An outdated system to measure vitamin activity, this measurement does not consider differences in bioavailability.

provitamin A Carotenoid precursors of vitamin A in foods of plant origin, primarily deeply colored fruits and vegetables.

1 retinol activity equivalent (RAE) = 1 μg retinol
= 2 μg supplemental beta-carotene
= 12 μg dietary beta-carotene
= 24 μg dietary carotenoids

Figure 9.7 **Retinol activity equivalents conversion.**

beta-carotene. (Read more under "The Carotenoids" later in this chapter.) On average, we get about a third of our vitamin A as carotenoids, mainly beta-carotene, but that figure varies widely.[8]

Liver is the richest source of vitamin A, just as you would expect, knowing that the liver stores vitamin A. Historically, people consumed fish oils, such as cod liver oil, for their vitamin A (and vitamin D) content, and cod liver oil remains a popular supplement today. Other good sources include butter, butterfat-containing dairy foods, and egg yolk. (See **Figure 9.8**.)

Because low-fat milk is fortified, it is a good vitamin A source, despite having little or no butterfat. Producers also fortify some foods of plant origin, including margarine, some breakfast cereals, and some special dietary foods like "nutrition bars."

Key Concepts: *Vitamin A occurs in three forms in the body: retinol, retinal, and retinoic acid. Retinol is found in a few animal-derived foods. Vitamin A is also formed from precursors called carotenoids. Intake recommendations for vitamin A are expressed in RAEs (retinol activity equivalents) to account for differences between retinoids and carotenoids. Most vitamin A is processed and stored in the liver and is released as needed. Vitamin A in the cells of the retina plays a crucial role in vision. It is also involved in cell differentiation, reproduction, maintaining epithelial tissue, supporting other immune functions, and bone health.*

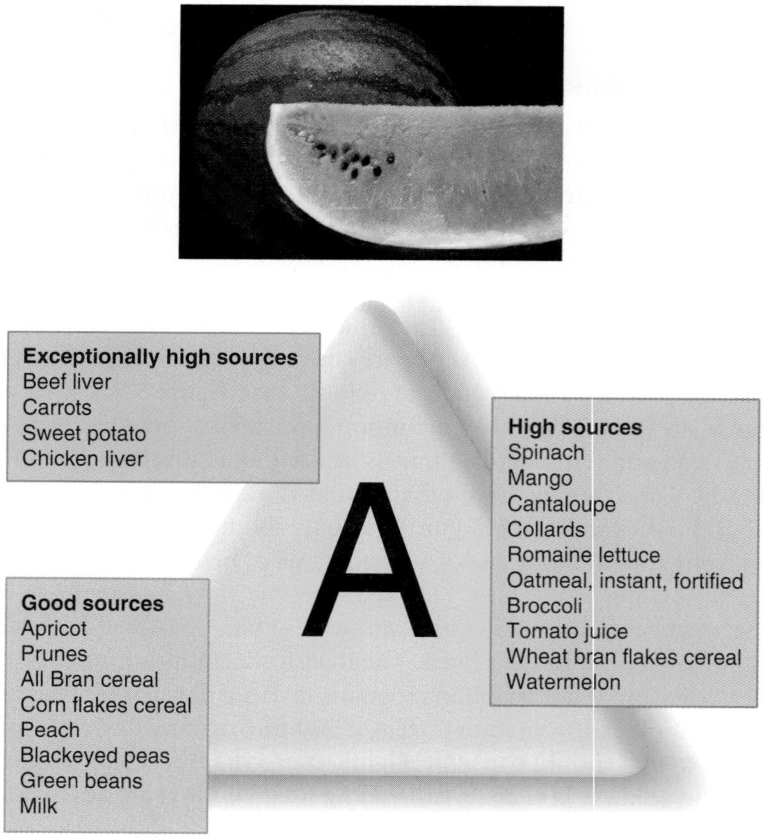

Figure 9.8 **Food sources of vitamin A.** Vitamin A is found as retinol in animal foods and as beta-carotene and other carotenoids in plant foods. Some of the best sources are liver, orange and deep-yellow vegetables, and dark-green leafy vegetables.

Vitamin A Deficiency

Although dietary deficiency of vitamin A is rare in North America and Western Europe, it is the leading cause of childhood blindness worldwide, especially in Southeast Asia, parts of Africa, and Central and South America. In these regions, vitamin A deficiency typically results from general protein-energy malnutrition in infants and young children. Protein deficiency reduces levels of retinol-binding protein, the blood carrier protein that transports vitamin A in the blood. Vitamin A deficiency interacts with other nutrient deficiencies and with infection, worsening respiratory infections or diarrhea and causing countless deaths. (See **Figure 9.9**.)

Certain North American groups are at risk for vitamin A deficiency. Premature infants do not have vitamin A reserves in their livers. People with alcoholism or liver disease may have damaged livers that cannot store much vitamin A. Fat malabsorption diseases and medicines that inhibit fat absorption also impair vitamin A absorption. Because the body needs zinc to use vitamin A efficiently, inadequate zinc intake can cause vitamin A deficiency symptoms.

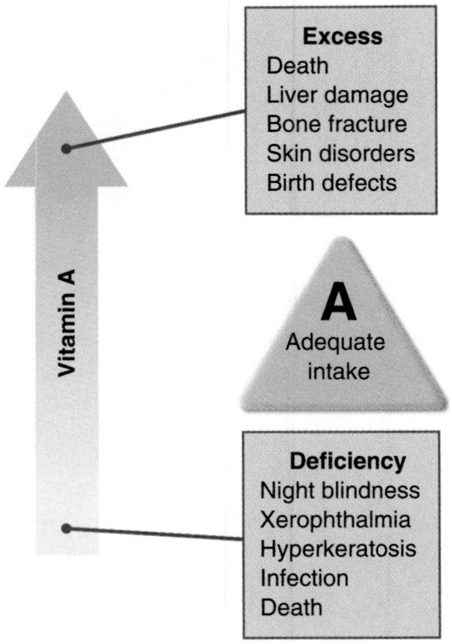

Figure 9.9 **Vitamin A toxicity and deficiency.** A broad range of vitamin A intake is adequate and provides for normal function. Too much or too little vitamin A can have serious consequences.

The Eyes

Early treatment can rapidly correct night blindness, an early symptom of vitamin A deficiency. But a worsening and prolonged deficiency threatens eyesight. Cells in the **cornea** (part of the eye's covering) stop reproducing, and the deficiency damages mucous membranes that provide lubrication. Without adequate moisture, dirt and bacteria accumulate as the eye dries out. As the cornea deteriorates, foamy white patches called Bitot's spots appear on the eye. In extreme cases, the cornea eventually develops sores and scars and may even liquefy, causing total blindness. Collectively, these are the symptoms of **xerophthalmia**, an irreversible condition.

The Skin and Other Epithelial Cells

Hard, bumpy, scaly skin—"goose flesh" that doesn't go away—is an early symptom of vitamin A deficiency. The deficiency disrupts epithelial cell production, and tough **keratin** protein plugs the skin's hair follicles.[9] Vitamin A deficiency also impairs normal secretions, blocking perspiration and mucus. The lack of mucus damages the linings of the mouth, respiratory tract, and urinary and genital tracts. Sperm production slows, and female fertility declines.

Immune Function

Vitamin A deficiency leaves a person especially vulnerable to infection.[10] Damaged epithelium allows microorganisms to breach this first line of defense. Under ordinary circumstances, entry of these enemy invaders would then trigger protective immune cells to quickly multiply. But immune cells need vitamin A to multiply. With too few immune cells to mount an effective attack, the invading microorganisms can cause severe, even fatal diarrhea or respiratory infection. When a child is deficient in vitamin A, a relatively harmless infection like measles becomes a killer.[11]

Other Effects

Because vitamin A is essential to cell growth and differentiation, a deficiency causes a variety of problems that include growth retardation, bone deformities, defective teeth, and kidney stones.

cornea The transparent outer surface of the eye.

xerophthalmia A condition caused by vitamin A deficiency that dries the cornea and mucous membranes of the eye.

keratin A sulfur-containing protein normally present in the outermost surface of the skin as well as in hair, nails, and tooth enamel.

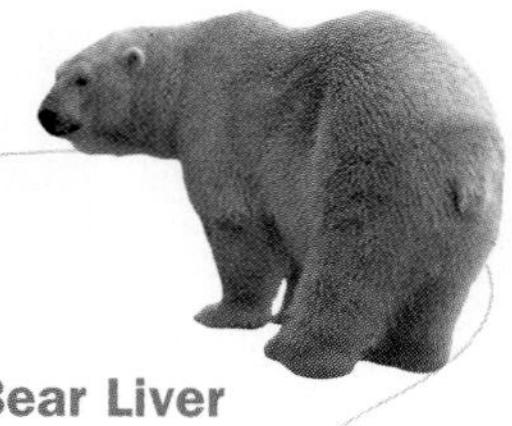

Quick Bites

Avoid Polar Bear Liver

Liver and onions may be your favorite meal, but do not use polar bear liver. Polar bear liver is so rich in vitamin A that a single serving can be toxic for humans.

Vitamin A Toxicity

Although it is difficult to overdo vitamin A from natural foods, the enthusiasm for megadose vitamin supplements has increased the potential for toxic dosing. Vitamin A toxicity has a wide range of symptoms, both subtle and overt, including fatigue, vomiting, abdominal pain, bone and joint pain, loss of appetite, skin disorders, headache, blurred or double vision, and liver damage. (See Figure 9.9.) Vitamin A toxicity can be acute, but more often it develops gradually over months or years. A recent analysis from the long-term Nurses' Health Study suggests that high intake of vitamin A (≥2000 micrograms of retinol) is related to increased risk of hip fractures in older women.[12]

Excess retinol is a known **teratogen** (causes birth defects). The birth defects it causes include cleft palate, heart abnormalities, and brain malfunction.[13] It is most dangerous during the first three months of pregnancy, when cell differentiation is most intense. Pregnant women should take retinol-containing supplements only with the approval of their doctor.

teratogen Any substance that causes birth defects.

The Tolerable Upper Intake Level (UL) for vitamin A for men and women, including women who are pregnant or breastfeeding, is 3,000 micrograms of retinol per day. Check out some vitamin A supplement labels. Those that contain 10,000 IU of retinol (not from carotenoids) are providing the UL of vitamin A. You may be surprised to see supplements with 25,000 IU—far above safe levels.

You may know people who consumed so much carrot juice that their skin acquired a yellowish-orange cast. Dark-skinned people may notice a yellowing of the palms and soles of their feet. Accumulation of excess beta-carotene in the blood is responsible for this harmless condition. But are beta-carotene supplements harmless? Large trials of adult smokers suggest megadose supplementation with beta-carotene increased the long-term risk of lung cancer.[14]

Acne Treatment

Some "close cousins" (or analogs) of vitamin A are given in therapeutic doses to treat skin problems. Two, Retin-A and Accutane, are widely used for acne. But, like vitamin A, these retinoids cause birth defects. Any woman who may become pregnant should not use these medicines.[15] In fact, because these medications accumulate in fat stores, even when applied on the skin, women should discontinue them at least two years before pregnancy.

Key Concepts: *Vitamin A deficiency causes blindness; damages skin, bone, and other tissues; and limits immune function, leaving a person vulnerable to infection. Excessive vitamin A supplementation can cause toxicity, even with doses just a few times higher than the RDA. Vitamin A toxicity during pregnancy could be devastating; pregnant women should be wary of retinol-containing supplements and avoid retinoid-containing medicines.*

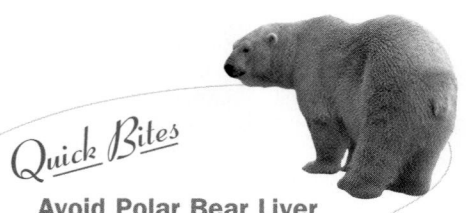

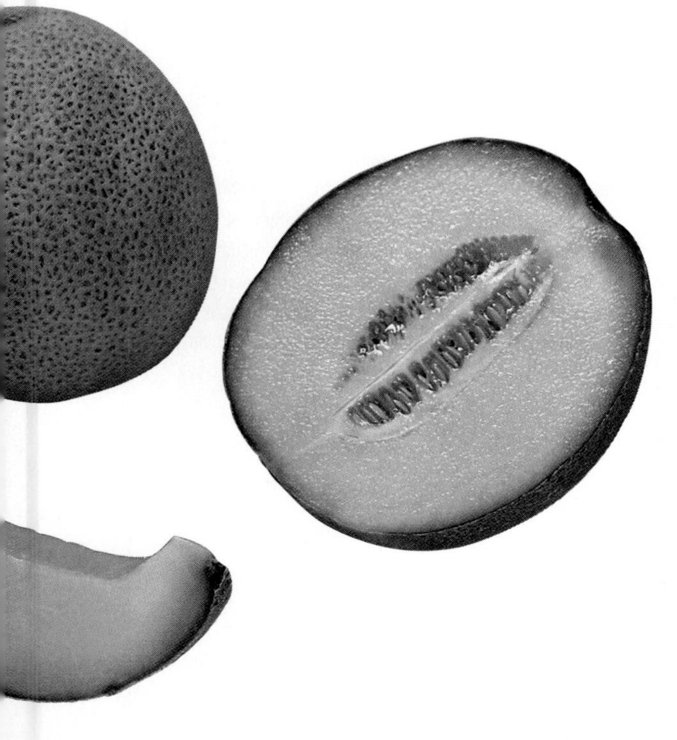

The Carotenoids

Carotenoids are plant pigments that give the deep yellow, orange, and red colors to fruits and vegetables such as apricots, carrots, and tomatoes. The major carotenoids are alpha-carotene, beta-carotene, lutein, zeaxanthin, cryptoxanthin, and lycopene. Among them, beta-carotene, the yellow-orange pigment in cantaloupe, carrots, and squash, is the most common. Alpha-carotene, beta-carotene, and beta-cryptoxanthin can be converted to vitamin A. Lycopene, lutein, and zeaxanthin cannot be converted, so they have no vitamin A activity.

Functions of Carotenoids

Aside from conversion to vitamin A, the carotenoids do not appear essential in the technical sense; a carotenoid-free diet does not cause deficiency disease. Therefore, the Food and Nutrition Board has not established DRIs for them.[16] Yet people who eat generous amounts of the foods that are rich in the carotenoids reduce their risk of the major degenerative diseases. Although the exact role that carotenoids play in risk reduction is still unclear, they may act as antioxidants. (See **Figure 9.10**.) Antioxidants can prevent damage that may lead to premature aging, cancer, atherosclerosis, cataracts, age-related macular degeneration, and an array of degenerative diseases.[17] (For more information on antioxidants, see the FYI feature "Antioxidants and Free Radicals.")

Carotenoids and Vision

Lutein and zeaxanthin are found in the macula of the eye, the central portion of the retina responsible for sharp, detailed vision. Scientists believe these carotenoids protect the macula by filtering harmful light rays and by antioxidant activity.[18] Epidemiological studies have found lower rates of macular degeneration and cataracts—major causes of blindness in the elderly—among people who eat the most lutein- and zeaxanthin-containing foods.[19]

Carotenoids and Cancer

Scientists believe the carotenoids may inhibit some cancers by preventing damaged cells from multiplying.[20] People with the highest intakes of carotenoid-rich fruits and vegetables and/or high levels of specific carotenoids tend to have the lowest risk for certain cancers. Eating tomato products like tomato sauce (yes, even ketchup), for example, is associated with reduced risk of prostate cancer.[21] Tomato products are excellent sources of the carotenoid lycopene.

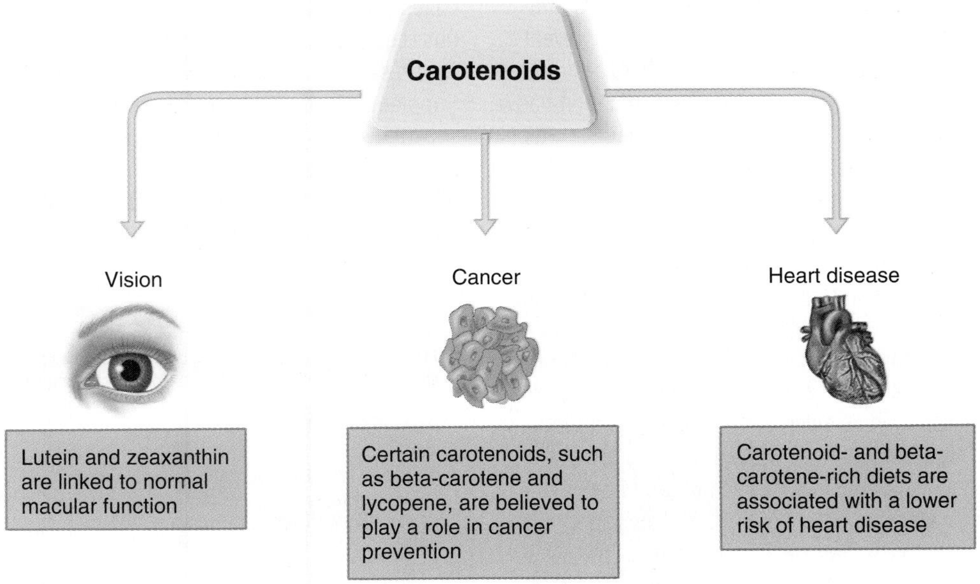

Figure 9.10 **Major functions of carotenoids.** Independent of vitamin A activity, carotenoids may be involved in normal macular function and reduced risk of heart disease and cancer.

These studies reflect food intake, not supplement use. To date, trials of beta-carotene supplements for cancer prevention have been disappointing, and paradoxically megadose supplements are associated with increased lung cancer among smokers or those exposed to asbestos.[22]

Beta-Carotene and Skin

One of the few proven effective uses of beta-carotene supplements is for people who are missing natural protection to ultraviolet (UV) light, due to a hereditary illness. Large doses of beta-carotene help protect their skin.[23]

[Fyi] Antioxidants and Free Radicals

FOR YOUR INFORMATION

An antioxidant prevents the damaging effects of oxygen. Say, wait a minute. Oxygen's a good thing, isn't it? Certainly, you couldn't live long without it!

But some forms of oxygen are very unstable. We call these unstable molecules "free radicals." They are extremely active and, when out of control, can attack or react with healthy body cells, damaging fragile cell membranes and genetic material and changing the character of fats and proteins.[1] Antioxidants "neutralize" or "quench" free radicals, keeping them from becoming excessive or getting out of control. Several vitamins act as antioxidants.

Free radicals are generated during normal metabolism and they are normal substances. We put their destructive capabilities to good use. Their oxidizing action kills harmful microorganisms. They even destroy our body's own damaged cells, thus preventing cancerous growth.

Household bleach, a familiar oxidizing agent, is a good example of the "good guy–bad guy" nature of free radicals. Add it to dirty clothes, and it cleans them well, even killing germs. But add too much, and your clothes get holes. The sun's oxidizing rays are also bleaching agents, very helpful for white fabrics, but damaging to colors. Other examples of oxidative damage are the rusting of iron and the rancidity of fats.

Outside agents, such as tobacco smoke, toxic chemicals, excessive sunshine, and even some medical treatments, form free radicals in our bodies. In the presence of these agents, our antioxidants are depleted more quickly.

Excessive oxidation in the body is problematic.[2] Chronic, excessive exposure to sunshine, for example, is associated with age-related macular degeneration and cataracts, two conditions that cause blindness. Researchers believe oxidative damage plays a role in these conditions; there's preliminary evidence that the carotenoids lutein and zeaxanthin help protect us from that damage.[3] The oxidizing rays of the sun also accelerate skin wrinkling and, worse, cause skin cancer, due in part to oxidative damage of skin cells. Other cancers may originate when cellular DNA is damaged by free radicals; foods rich in antioxidants may prevent this damage.[4]

There is good evidence that oxidation has a pivotal role in initiating atherosclerosis. Free radicals oxidize blood lipids such as cholesterol; the damaged lipids are then deposited on the inside surface of artery walls, the beginning of atherosclerotic plaques. Vitamin E, our major fat-soluble antioxidant, may help block this process.[5]

Vitamin C and, under some circumstances, riboflavin are other antioxidants. Some minerals such as selenium function in antioxidant systems as well. The antioxidants often work in cooperation with each other. Vitamin C, a water-soluble antioxidant, restores vitamin E that is altered by its antioxidant activity. Selenium also works with vitamin E. In fact, to a certain extent, a selenium-rich diet can help treat a vitamin E deficiency.

Vitamins and minerals are only part of your antioxidant defense. Your body makes many of its own antioxidants. Examples are glutathione, coenzyme Q_{10} (ubiquinone), and superoxide dismutase. Several of these have now been put into supplements. To have an effect, however, they must survive digestion, be absorbed, and reach their site of activity in the body. Their value in supplement form remains largely unproved.

In addition to vitamins, fruits and vegetables contain many other antioxidants, which protect the plants from sunshine and other oxidants. These substances, along with other plant-produced chemicals, are sometimes called phytonutrients, phytochemicals, or nutraceuticals. Ingesting them probably gives us the same protection they give the plant. Supplement manufacturers also put these substances—examples are the bioflavonoids—in pills and add them to beverages marketed as "health-promoting." In these forms, neither their value nor their safety have been proved.

1 Jacob RA, Burri BJ. Oxidative damage and defense. *Am J Clin Nutr.* 1996;63:985S–990S.

2 Rock CL, Jacob RA, Bowen PE. Update on the biological characteristics of the antioxidant micronutrients: vitamin C, vitamin E, and the carotenoids. *J Am Diet Assoc.* 1996;96:693–702.

3 Ibid.

4 Institute of Medicine, Food and Nutrition Board. *Dietary Reference Intakes for Vitamin C, Vitamin E, Selenium, and Carotenoids.* Washington, DC: National Academy Press; 2000.

5 Ibid.

Carotenoids and Immunity

There is some evidence that carotenoids play a role in immune system function. Beta-carotene supplements have improved measures of immune function in elderly men and nonsmoking men.[24] It remains unclear whether this translates into better health.

Food Sources, Absorption, and Storage of Carotenoids

Orange and yellow fruits and vegetables generally contain beta-carotene, alpha-carotene, and cryptoxanthin. Good sources of beta-carotene include carrots, winter squash, sweet potatoes, and some orange-colored fruits like cantaloupe, peaches, apricots, and mango. Dark-green vegetables also contain abundant carotenoids, although plentiful green chlorophyll pigment masks the carotenoid colors. Carotenoids from dark-green leafy vegetables, however, produce less vitamin A than those from ripe orange-colored fruit.[25]

Surprisingly oranges and tangerines have little beta-carotene, but they are rich in cryptoxanthin. Lycopene has a more reddish color; you will see it in tomatoes, pink grapefruit, guava, and watermelon. Lutein and zeaxanthin are in leafy green vegetables, pumpkin, and red pepper. Since it's hard to identify carotenoids in food just by looking, and because we know all of the major carotenoids are important, eating a wide variety of fruits and vegetables, and plenty of them, assures a good intake of all.

Your body absorbs only 20 to 40 percent of the carotenoids you eat, even less if your intake is high. Dietary fat increases absorption. Factors that limit fat absorption limit carotenoid absorption as well. That includes olestra, the fat substitute in some snack foods. Although manufacturers fortify olestra with retinol, they do not add carotenoids—a reason for concern among some nutritionists.

It's now known that cell walls of carotenoid-rich plants inhibit absorption. Cooking vegetables a few minutes breaks the cell walls, releasing the carotenoids and improving their absorption.

Carotenoid Supplementation

Carotenoid supplements have become popular in recent years. However, the Food and Nutrition Board advises against them for the general population, recommending carotenoid-rich fruits and vegetables instead. A UL has not been set for the carotenoids.

Vitamin D

This fat-soluble nutrient is called the sunshine vitamin. When the ultraviolet rays of the sun strike your skin, they convert a precursor to vitamin D. Vitamin D is unique because, given sufficient sunlight, your body can make all that it needs—dietary vitamin D is unnecessary. However, when coupled with too little sun exposure, a lack of dietary vitamin D does cause a vitamin deficiency.

Vitamin D is essential for bone health. In children, it promotes bone development and growth. In adults, it is necessary for bone maintenance. In the elderly, vitamin D helps prevent bone loss and fractures.

Forms and Formation of Vitamin D

Vitamin D is a group of about ten related compounds. The most important of these are vitamin D_2 (ergocalciferol), found in a few plant foods, and vitamin D_3 (cholecalciferol), found naturally only in a few animal-derived

Quick Bites

And They Called It Cantaloupe

The word *cantaloupe* comes from a papal garden in a small town near Rome named Cantaloupo. One-half of a cantaloupe has 444 RAE as beta-carotene.

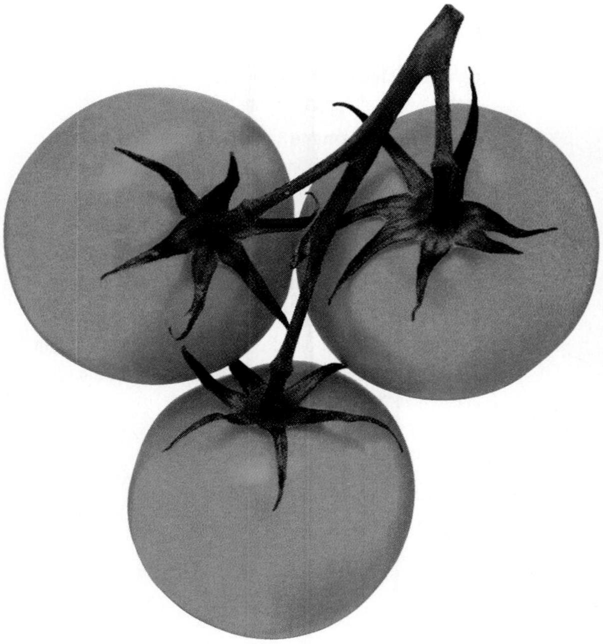

Quick Bites

Pizza versus Tomato Juice

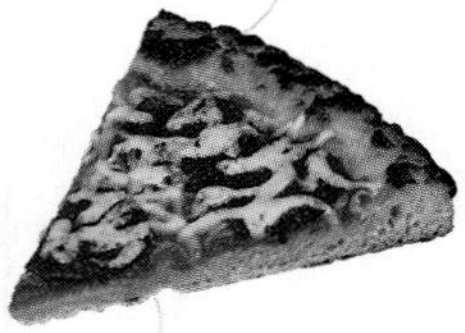

One U.S. study linked intake of tomato sauce, tomatoes, and pizza to lowered risk of prostate cancer. Tomato juice, however, was not protective. That's not surprising. According to John Erdman, Ph.D., of the University of Illinois in Urbana, the cancer-fighting carotenoid found in tomatoes (lycopene) is a fat-soluble substance, so it needs some fat like that found in pizza and most pasta sauces to be absorbed. The lycopene in tomato juice, however, seems to be especially poorly absorbed.

foods. Our skin makes vitamin D_3 and supplies about 90 percent of our vitamin D.[26]

In the skin, UV radiation converts a form of cholesterol to cholecalciferol, which travels to the liver. The liver converts both synthesized and dietary vitamin D to an intermediate form, which it sends to the kidneys. The kidneys perform the final step—conversion to **calcitriol**, the predominant, active form of vitamin D.

Quick Bites

Do You Know Vitamin D When You See It?

The general terms *vitamin D* and *calciferol* are used to refer to both vitamin D_2 (ergocalciferol) and vitamin D_3 (cholecalciferol), and to any combination of these two compounds.

calcitriol The active form of vitamin D, it is an important regulator of blood calcium levels.

parathyroid hormone (PTH) A hormone secreted by the parathyroid glands in response to low blood calcium. It stimulates calcium release from bone and calcium absorption by the intestines, while decreasing calcium excretion by the kidneys. It acts in conjunction with calcitriol to raise blood calcium. Also called parathormone.

calcitonin A hormone secreted by the thyroid gland in response to elevated blood calcium. It stimulates calcium deposition in bone and calcium excretion by the kidneys, thus reducing blood calcium.

Functions of Vitamin D

Many simply regard vitamin D as a vitamin that keeps bones healthy. But it is first and foremost a regulator. (See **Figure 9.11**.) Because vitamin D made in one part of the body regulates activities in other parts, scientists consider it a hormone. As such, it may play a role in cancer prevention, an area of considerable research activity. Investigators also are looking for ways vitamin D and its derivatives might treat other conditions of abnormal cell growth, such as psoriasis.

Regulation of Blood Calcium Levels

Calcitriol's primary regulatory role involves keeping blood calcium and phosphorus levels within a normal range. Calcitriol acts in concert with two other hormones: **parathyroid hormone (PTH)** from the parathyroid glands and **calcitonin** from the thyroid gland. Together, levels of these three hormones continually rise and fall, adjusting blood calcium levels by changing urinary calcium excretion, intestinal calcium absorption, and the flow of calcium in and out of bone.

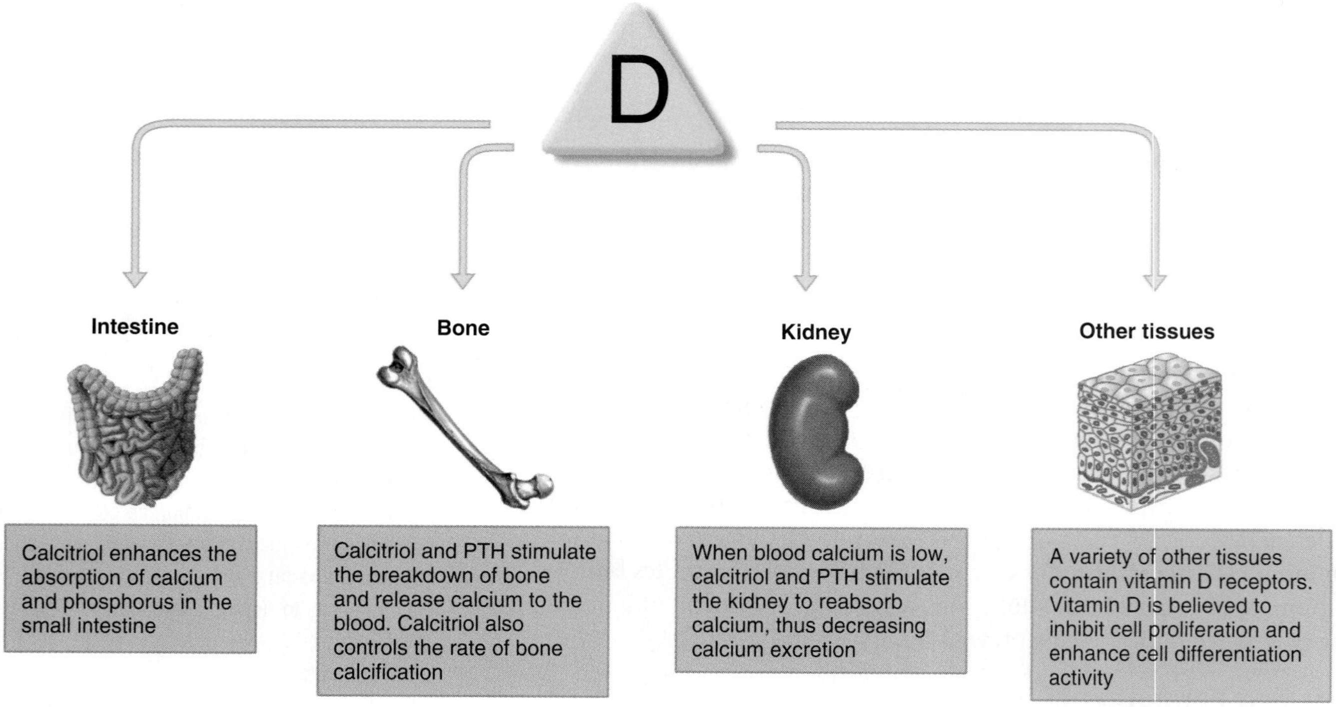

D
Intestine
Bone
Kidney
Other tissues
Calcitriol enhances the absorption of calcium and phosphorus in the small intestine
Calcitriol and PTH stimulate the breakdown of bone and release calcium to the blood. Calcitriol also controls the rate of bone calcification
When blood calcium is low, calcitriol and PTH stimulate the kidney to reabsorb calcium, thus decreasing calcium excretion
A variety of other tissues contain vitamin D receptors. Vitamin D is believed to inhibit cell proliferation and enhance cell differentiation activity

Figure 9.11 **Major functions of vitamin D.** Vitamin D and calcium are essential to bone health. To regulate blood calcium levels, vitamin D works with parathyroid hormone (PTH) to stimulate the body to move calcium back and forth between the blood and the reservoir of calcium in bone.

Here's how it works. Much like a thermostat monitoring temperature, the parathyroid glands monitor blood calcium levels, releasing PTH when calcium levels drop. PTH signals specific bone cells to break down bone tissue and release calcium into the bloodstream. PTH also signals the kidneys to slow calcium excretion and increase calcitriol production. In turn, calcitriol stimulates the small intestine to absorb more calcium from food, thereby raising blood calcium levels further.

When blood calcium levels become too high, the thyroid gland releases calcitonin and the parathyroid glands slow their release of PTH. Calcitonin inhibits factors causing bone breakdown, allowing bone-forming activities to prevail. Bone-forming cells remove calcium from the blood and deposit it in bone. Lower PTH levels allow the kidneys to continue excreting calcium and decrease calcitriol production. In turn, low calcitriol levels cause the small intestine to reduce calcium absorption from food, thereby lowering blood calcium levels further. (For more on blood calcium regulation, see Chapter 10, "Water and Minerals.")

Dietary Recommendations for Vitamin D

Despite our ability to synthesize vitamin D, it is an essential nutrient, and the Food and Nutrition Board has set dietary intake recommendations. Because sunlight varies throughout the year and some people have limited sun exposure, the Board assumed no vitamin D synthesis when setting the Adequate Intake (AI) amounts.[27] Still, the AI is small, only 5 micrograms daily for infancy through 50 years.

Newborns have vitamin D stores that last about nine months. Because breast milk contains little vitamin D, breastfed babies who receive little exposure to sunlight need supplemental vitamin D. (Infant formula is fortified with vitamin D.) Because vitamin D skin synthesis decreases markedly with age, AI recommendations increase in later adulthood.[28] For men and women aged 51 through 70, the AI increases to 10 micrograms per day; and for people older than 70, the AI rises to 15 micrograms per day.

On food and supplement labels, vitamin D is often stated in International Units (IU) rather than micrograms. One microgram of vitamin D equals 40 IU. Therefore, 200 IU is the equivalent of the AI for those 50 years and younger.

Quick Bites

A Fishy Cure

Cod liver oil was well known in the early nineteenth century as a treatment for rickets, a bone disease common in children. It wasn't until the early 1900s, however, that vitamin D was identified as the "antirachitic" (antirickets) substance in cod liver oil.

Sources of Vitamin D

How much exposure to the sun is needed for an adequate supply of vitamin D? Most adults under 50 need about 10 or 15 minutes of daily sunlight on the hands for adequate vitamin synthesis. Adults over 50 need more.[29] The exact amount of sun exposure depends on several factors, including time of day, season, location, sunscreen use, and skin type. The sun's rays are more intense at latitudes closer to the equator and during midday and summertime. Topical sunscreens (those with sun protection factor [SPF] of 8 or greater) block UV light. People with dark skin do not absorb UV rays as well as light-skinned people do. Pollution and smog can reduce UV rays.

The major dietary sources of vitamin D are fortified foods, mainly fortified milk and fortified breakfast cereals. The few foods that naturally contain vitamin D include oily fish (e.g., salmon and sardines), egg yolk, butter, and liver, with amounts dependent on the animal's diet. (See

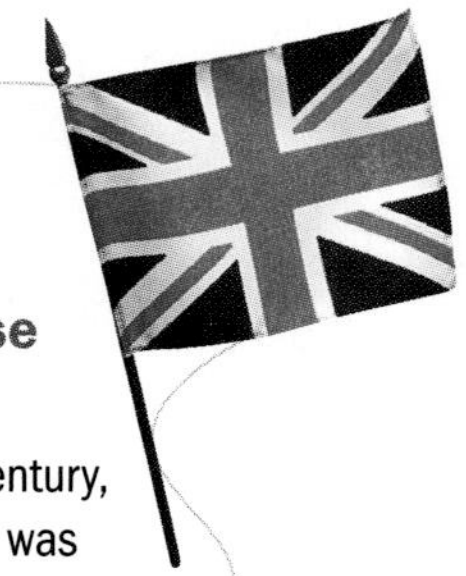

Quick Bites

"Children's Disease of the English"

In the seventeenth century, vitamin D deficiency was so common in British children that rickets was called the "children's disease of the English." Diets provided little vitamin D, and the lack of sun during many months of the year inhibited vitamin D synthesis in the skin.

Figure 9.12.) More concentrated vitamin D is available in cod liver or other fish liver oils. Plants are poor sources, so strict vegetarians must get their vitamin D through exposure to sunlight, fortified foods, or supplements.

Vitamin D Deficiency

Vitamin D deficiency damages bones. Babies with vitamin D deficiency have soft, weak bones, which bend and bow under their weight as they start to walk. The condition is called **rickets** and is characterized by "bow legs," "knock-knees," and other skeletal deformities. In the United States and Canada, nutritional rickets has been all but eliminated by vitamin D fortified milk, infant vitamin supplements, and vitamin supplements for children with fat malabsorption conditions. Recently, however, scattered cases of rickets have been seen in dark-skinned infants who were breastfed, drank nonfortified soymilk, or in some cases had metabolic disorders.[30] Although severe vitamin D deficiency in children and adults is rare, deficiency does exist among sick people and the elderly.[31]

In adults, vitamin D deficiency causes **osteomalacia**, or "soft bones." The condition reduces calcium absorption and increases calcium loss from bone, increasing the risk of bone fractures. People with diseases that affect organs responsible for absorption or activation of vitamin D have a high risk of osteomalacia.

Osteoporosis is closely related to osteomalacia, with similar symptoms of bone loss and increased risk of fractures.[32] In seniors, supplemental

rickets A bone disease in children that results from vitamin D deficiency.

osteomalacia A disease in adults that results from vitamin D deficiency; it is marked by softening of the bones, leading to bending of the spine, bowing of the legs, and increased risk for fractures.

osteoporosis A bone disease characterized by a decrease in bone mineral density and the appearance of small holes in bones due to loss of minerals.

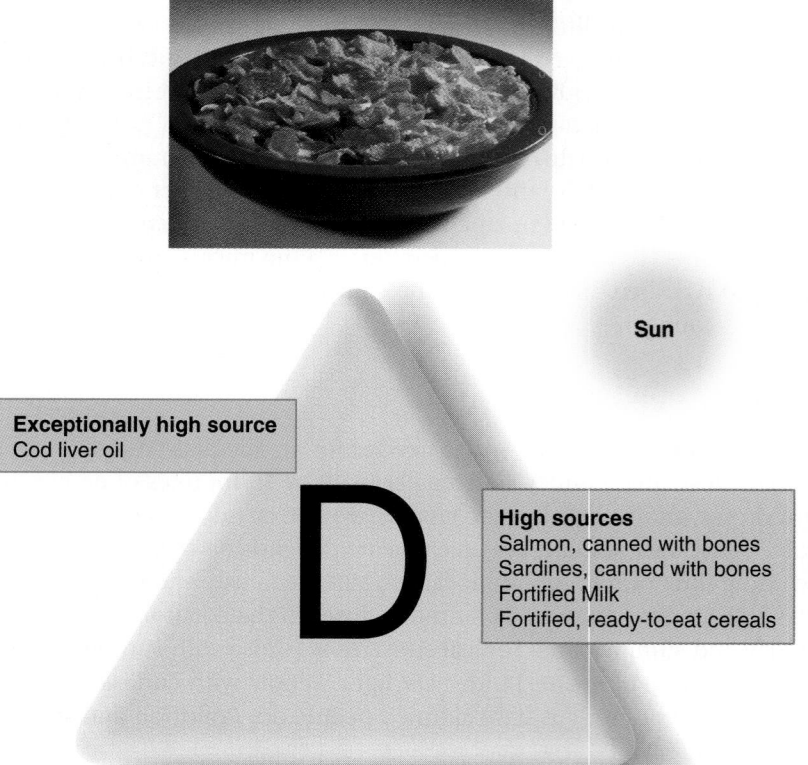

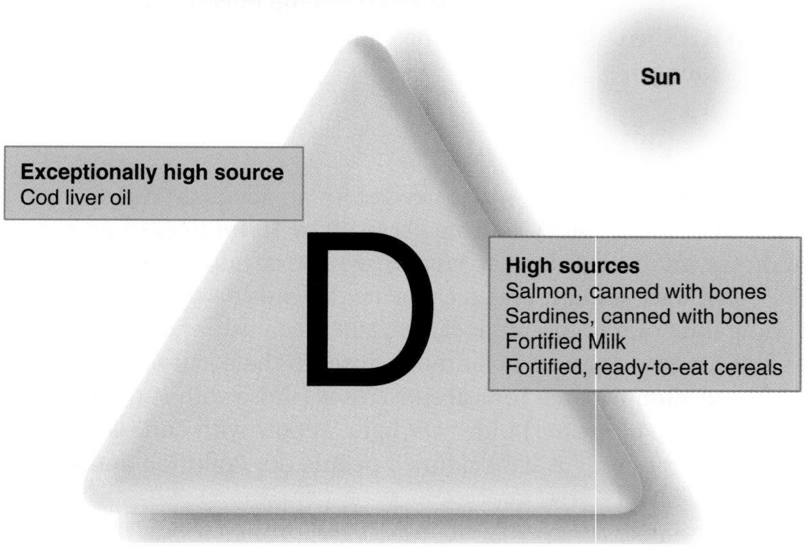

Figure 9.12 **Sources of vitamin D.** Given sufficient sunlight, your body can make all the vitamin D it needs. Only a few foods are naturally good sources of vitamin D. Therefore, fortified foods such as milk and some cereals are important dietary sources, especially for people with limited exposure to the sun.

vitamin D can slow bone turnover, increase bone density, and, in people with low vitamin D blood levels, substantially reduce the risk of osteoporotic fractures, especially hip fractures.[33] (For more information on osteoporosis, see Chapter 10, "Water and Minerals.")

Do we get optimal amounts of vitamin D? Enough to protect us from bone loss? A 1998 study investigated this question in about 300 Boston hospital patients. Surprisingly, in almost three of five people, vitamin D levels were too low to maintain optimal bone calcium.[34] The reasons may be increased use of sunscreen, the northern climate (see **Figure 9.13**), the age of the patients, or diets that exclude milk or other fortified foods. For such people, vitamin D supplements may be warranted.

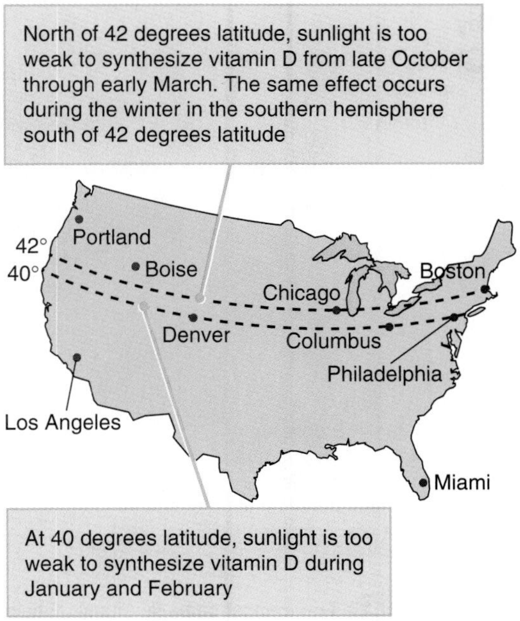
North of 42 degrees latitude, sunlight is too weak to synthesize vitamin D from late October through early March. The same effect occurs during the winter in the southern hemisphere south of 42 degrees latitude
42°
40°
Portland
Boise
Chicago
Boston
Denver
Columbus
Philadelphia
Los Angeles
Miami
At 40 degrees latitude, sunlight is too weak to synthesize vitamin D during January and February

Figure 9.13 **Mapping vitamin D synthesis.** Vitamin D synthesis halts for part of the winter if sunlight is too weak. In Los Angeles and Miami, the sunlight is strong enough to synthesize vitamin D year round, even in January.

Vitamin D Toxicity

Although sun exposure does not cause vitamin D toxicity, supplement megadoses are highly toxic. The daily UL for adults over 19 years of age is 50 micrograms per day (2,000 IU). (A physician may prescribe higher doses for some diseases.)

The hallmark of vitamin D toxicity is a high concentration of calcium in the blood. Initially, this increases urination and thirst. If prolonged, the body deposits excess calcium in soft tissues, causing pain and organ damage. Other symptoms include severe depression, nausea, vomiting, and loss of appetite. Ironically, excess vitamin D also causes loss of bone mass.

Key Concepts: *The active form of vitamin D is calcitriol. Its best-understood function is regulation of blood calcium levels. Along with two other hormones, it regulates urinary calcium excretion, intestinal calcium absorption, and the amount of calcium in bone. Dietary needs increase with age, as the ability of skin to synthesize vitamin D declines. Most dietary vitamin D is from fortified milk and other fortified foods. Vitamin D deficiency in children causes rickets; in adults it leads to osteomalacia and contributes to osteoporosis. In excess, vitamin D causes loss of bone and deposits of calcium in soft tissue.*

Vitamin E

Consumers have long embraced the practice of taking large amounts of vitamin E. Since its discovery in 1922 and the finding that its deficiency made laboratory rats sterile, vitamin E has been a reputed aphrodisiac. Vitamin E supplements have also been promoted for "anti-aging," with the ability to prevent everything from gray hair and wrinkles to cancer and heart disease. Although science does not support most rumored benefits, a growing body of research suggests vitamin E may be important in defending against chronic diseases associated with aging.

Quick Bites

Too Much Cover

Many Arab women are clothed so that only their eyes are exposed to sunlight. Even though these women live in sunny climates near the equator, many suffer from osteomalacia.

Forms of Vitamin E

Vitamin E is actually a family of eight similar compounds: alpha-, beta-, gamma-, and delta-**tocopherol** and alpha-, beta-, gamma-, and delta-**tocotrienol**. All are absorbed, but alpha-tocopherol is considered to be the only one with significant vitamin E activity. Alpha-tocopherol is the most common form of vitamin E in food, and milligrams of alpha-tocopherol are the standard measure of vitamin E.

Unlike the fat-soluble vitamins A and D, vitamin E is not stored primarily in the liver. Body fat holds about 90 percent of the vitamin E reserves. Virtually every tissue has some vitamin E providing protection within every cell membrane.

tocopherol The chemical name for vitamin E. There are four tocopherols (alpha, beta, gamma, delta), but only alpha-tocopherol is active in the body.

tocotrienol Four compounds (alpha, beta, gamma, delta) chemically related to tocopherols. The tocotrienols and tocopherols are collectively known as vitamin E.

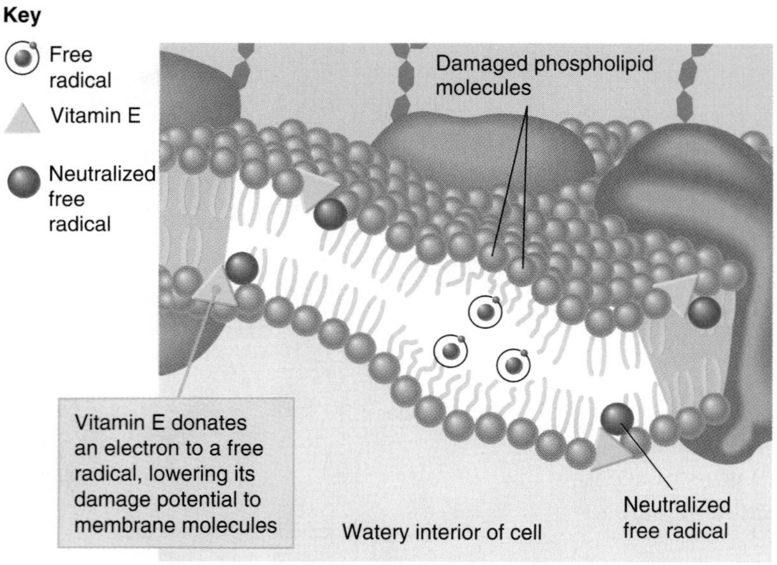
Key
Free radical
Vitamin E
Neutralized free radical
Damaged phospholipid molecules
Vitamin E donates an electron to a free radical, lowering its damage potential to membrane molecules
Watery interior of cell
Neutralized free radical

Figure 9.14 **Free radical damage.** Vitamin E helps prevent free radical damage to polyunsaturated fatty acids in cell membranes.

Functions of Vitamin E

Vitamin E is our body's major fat-soluble antioxidant. It protects vulnerable polyunsaturated lipids in cell membranes, in the blood, and elsewhere throughout the body. (See **Figure 9.14**.) Like carotenoids, it works by countering, or "scavenging," free radicals. (For more on antioxidants, see the FYI feature "Antioxidants and Free Radicals.")

A large and growing body of evidence suggests that high intakes of vitamin E may lower the risk of some chronic diseases, especially heart disease.[35] However, only four published, large-scale, randomized, double-blind clinical intervention studies have tested the ability of vitamin E to prevent heart attack. One was strongly positive, but the other three had neutral results. Currently, there are insufficient data to recommend supplemental vitamin E for heart disease prevention in the general population.[36]

What about other age-related diseases? In some people, supplemental vitamin E appears to reverse age-related declines in immune function. Promising preliminary results suggest vitamin E may slow the progression of Alzheimer's disease, but it still is too early to draw any conclusions. Some evidence suggests vitamin E may protect against prostate cancer, but overall evidence supporting a role against cancer is weak.[37] See **Figure 9.15** for the major functions of vitamin E.

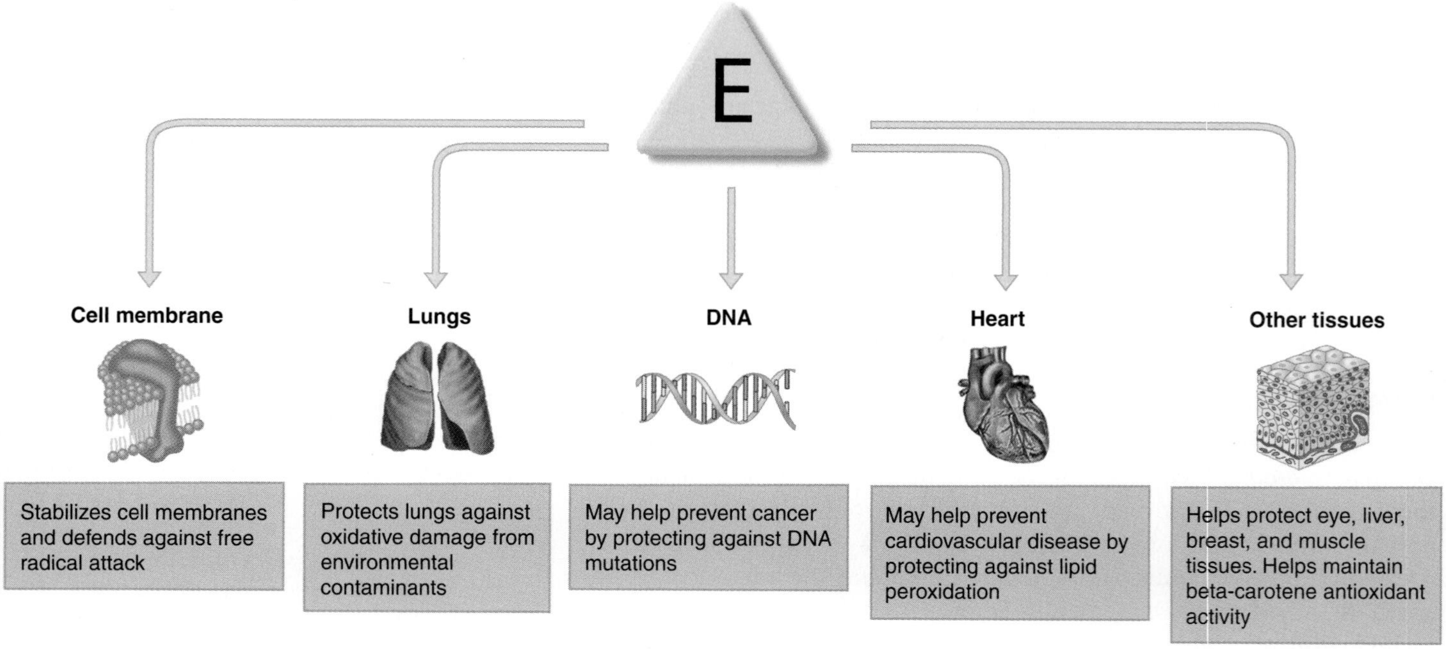
E
Cell membrane
Lungs
DNA
Heart
Other tissues
Stabilizes cell membranes and defends against free radical attack
Protects lungs against oxidative damage from environmental contaminants
May help prevent cancer by protecting against DNA mutations
May help prevent cardiovascular disease by protecting against lipid peroxidation
Helps protect eye, liver, breast, and muscle tissues. Helps maintain beta-carotene antioxidant activity

Figure 9.15 **Major functions of vitamin E.** The antioxidant activity of vitamin E helps stabilize cell membranes, protects tissues from oxidative damage, and may reduce the risk of cancer and heart disease.

Dietary Recommendations for Vitamin E

Vitamin E needs are related to the intake of polyunsaturated fatty acids (PUFA), which are especially vulnerable to destructive oxidation. When you eat minimal amounts of PUFA, you need smaller amounts of protective vitamin E. When you eat more vegetable oils, the major PUFA source, you need more vitamin E. Since the vitamin E in vegetable oils tends to be proportional to their PUFA content, to some extent these oils help provide extra vitamin E as needed.

The RDA for vitamin E accommodates generous PUFA intake. It is set at 15 milligrams per day of alpha-tocopherol for adults (including pregnant women) and 19 milligrams per day for women who are breastfeeding. Supplement labels may list vitamin E content in International Units, but these can be converted to milligrams of alpha-tocopherol. A supplement with 30 IU of natural vitamin E would equate to 20 milligrams of alpha-tocopherol (30×0.67). If the supplement contained synthetic vitamin E, the equivalent alpha-tocopherol would be 13.5 milligrams (30×0.47).

Sources of Vitamin E

For most people, small amounts of vitamin E from several sources, rather than a large amount from a single source, meet dietary requirements. Nuts and seeds, such as sunflower seeds, are among the best food sources. Because vitamin E is found naturally in the germ of grains, whole-grain products provide vitamin E. Wheat germ oil has one of the highest vitamin E concentrations. Most fruits and vegetables contribute only small amounts, and animal-derived products are inconsistent sources, depending on the animal's diet. (See **Figure 9.16**.)

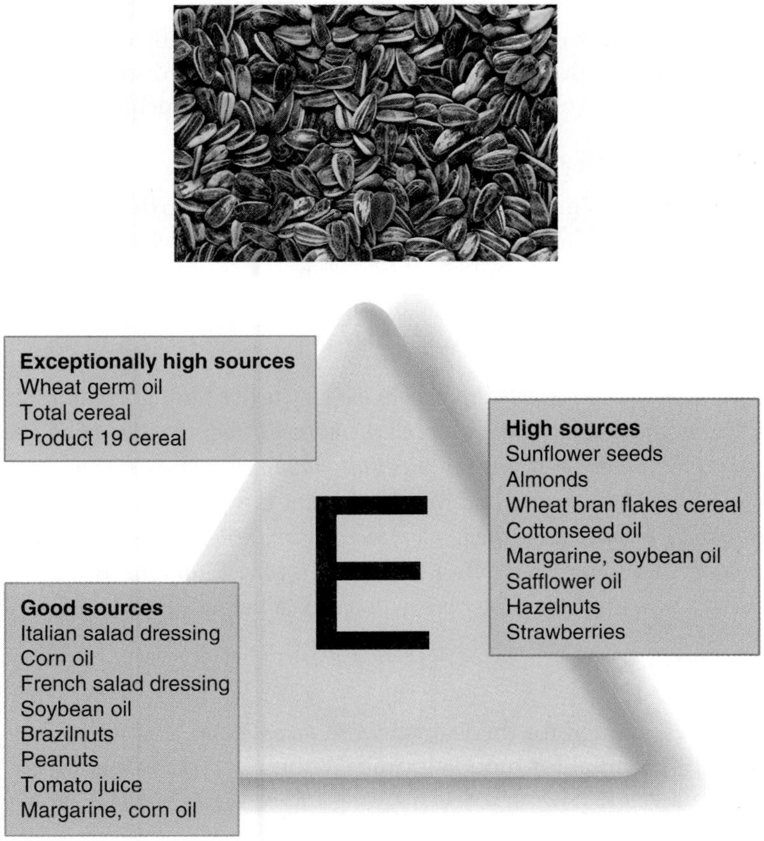

Figure 9.16 **Food sources of vitamin E.** Nuts and seeds, vegetable oil, and products made from vegetable oil, such as margarine, are among the best sources of vitamin E.

Table 9.1 **Reported Storage and Processing Losses of Vitamin E**

Food	Test Conditions	Vitamin E Loss
Peanut oil	Frying at 347°F (175°C), 30 minutes	32%
Safflower oil	Storing at room temperature, 3 months	55%
Tortillas	Storing at room temperature, 12 months	95%
Almonds	Roasting	80%
Wheat germ	Storing at 39°F (4°C), 6 months	10%
Wheat	Processing to white flour	92%
Bread	Baking	5–50%

Source: *Vitamin E Factbook.* LaGrange, IL: VERIS; 1999. Reprinted by permission of Veris Research Information Services.

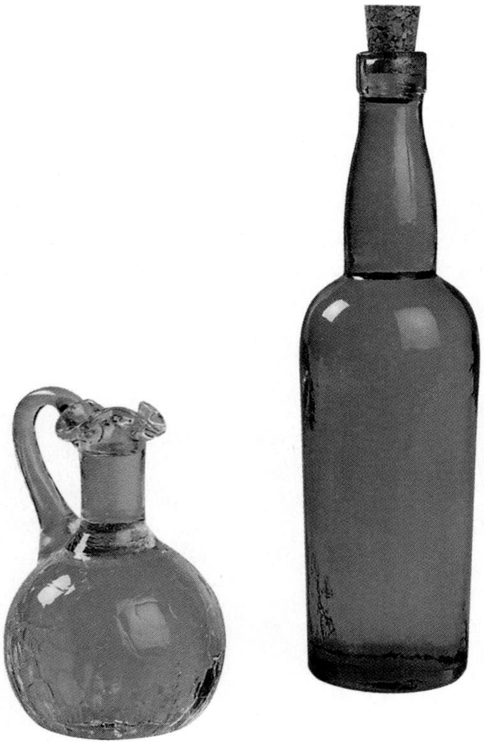

Vegetable oils such as sunflower and safflower, and foods made with them, such as margarine or salad dressing, are good sources. Although soybean and corn oils contain much vitamin E, only about 10 percent is alpha-tocopherol, the active form of vitamin E.[38] Cooking, processing, and storage can reduce the vitamin E content of foods substantially. (See **Table 9.1.**) Light and heat accelerate vitamin E's destruction. Safflower oils stored at room temperature for three months lose more than half of their vitamin E. Roasting destroys 80 percent of the vitamin E in almonds.

Vitamin E Deficiency

Overt vitamin E deficiency is so rare in humans that the Food and Nutrition Board could not use signs of deficiency (e.g., neurological abnormalities) as a basis for estimating dietary requirements. Vitamin E deficiency occurs mostly in people with fat malabsorption or rare genetic disorders. In adults, it takes 5 to 10 years of a deficiency before symptoms emerge.

Vitamin E Toxicity

For a fat-soluble vitamin, vitamin E is surprisingly nontoxic. However, it is not totally safe, and large amounts interfere with blood clotting, especially if taken along with anticoagulant medication or with aspirin.[39] For adults, the UL is 1,000 milligrams per day of supplemental alpha-tocopherol. Amounts greater than that can cause bleeding.[40]

Key Concepts: *Alpha-tocopherol is probably the only active form of vitamin E in the body. It is an antioxidant, protecting cell membranes from the damaging effects of oxidation. Preliminary evidence suggests that vitamin E might delay degenerative diseases such as heart disease and cancer. Vitamin E is found mainly in vegetable oils and products made from them. Considerable vitamin E is lost in food processing, cooking, and storage. Vitamin E deficiency is rare. Vitamin E is relatively nontoxic, though large doses interfere with blood clotting.*

phylloquinone The form of vitamin K that comes from plant sources. Also known as vitamin K_1.

menaquinones The form of vitamin K that comes from animal sources or is produced by intestinal bacteria. Also known as vitamin K_2.

menadione A medicinal form of vitamin K. Also known as vitamin K_3.

Vitamin K

Vitamin K was named for the Danish word *koagulation*. The name says it all. Vitamin K is essential for blood clotting. Without it, you would bleed to death from a single cut.

Vitamin K is a family of compounds known as quinones. It includes **phylloquinone** from plant sources, **menaquinones** from animal sources and synthesized by our intestinal bacteria, and **menadione**, a synthetic form. The liver holds most of the body's vitamin K reserve. Unlike other fat-soluble vitamins, the liver rapidly breaks down vitamin K and eliminates it, and thus reserves can be depleted quickly.

Quick Bites

Does Blocking Vitamin K Cure or Kill?

The medication warfarin (Coumadin) prevents undesired blood clotting by blocking vitamin K. Warfarin in very large amounts is also used in common rat poison to cause internal hemorrhage and death.

Functions of Vitamin K

When you bleed from a cut, your body starts a chain of reactions that forms a clot and stops the flow of blood. Many reactions in this coagulation cascade require vitamin K and calcium. Megadoses of vitamin E interfere with vitamin K's clotting activities.

Vitamin K also helps form bone. (See **Figure 9.17**.) Low blood levels of vitamin K are associated with increased fractures.[41]

Dietary Recommendations for Vitamin K

Typical diets easily meet the dietary recommendations for vitamin K. The AI for vitamin K for adult men is 120 micrograms daily, and for women, including those pregnant or breastfeeding, it is 90 micrograms.[42]

Sources of Vitamin K

Plant foods, especially green vegetables like spinach, turnip greens, broccoli, and Brussels sprouts, are our primary vitamin K source. Although many vegetable oils also contain vitamin K, they are not reliable sources.[43] Light exposure degrades vitamin K, so the vitamin content of oil in transparent containers diminishes with storage, causing variability from one bot-

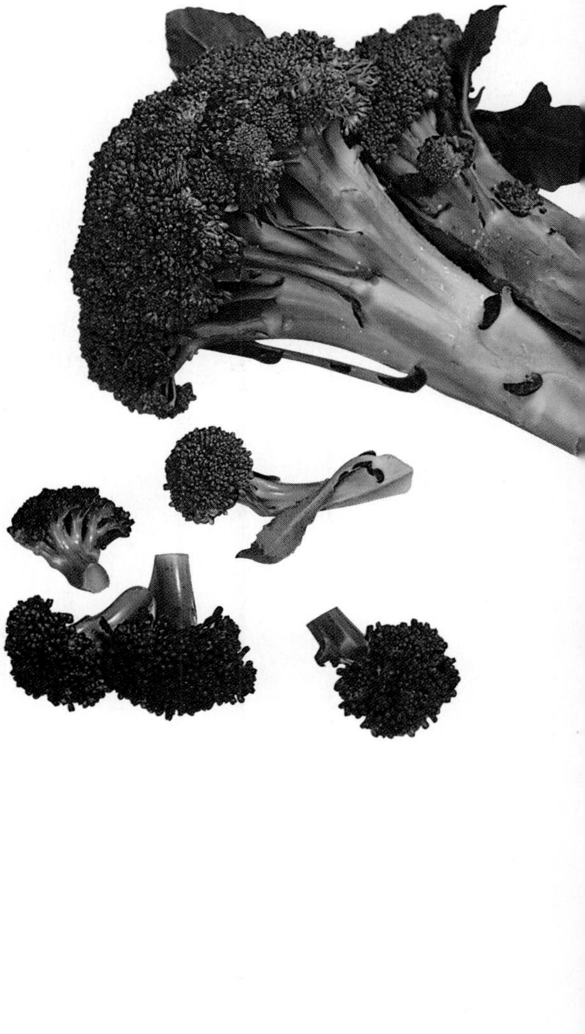

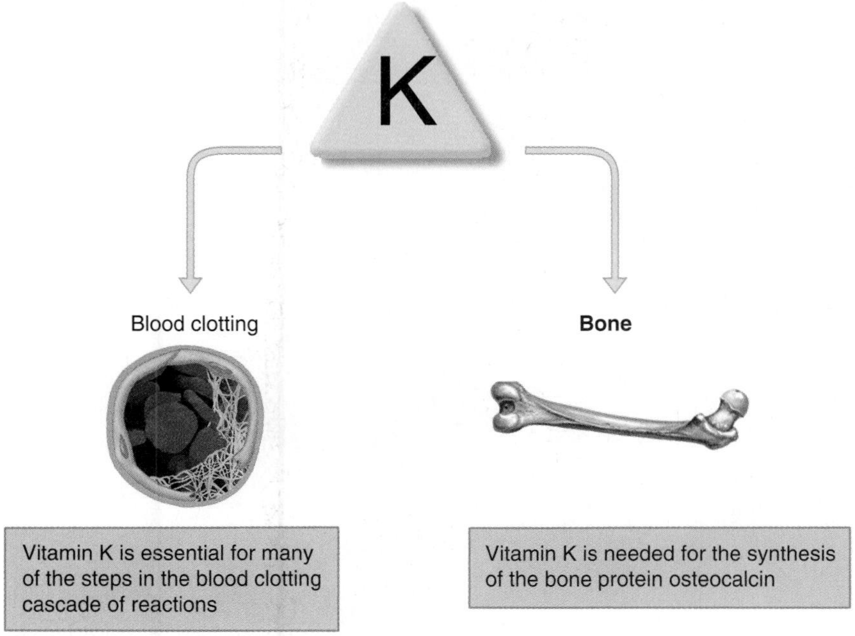
K
Blood clotting
Bone
Vitamin K is essential for many of the steps in the blood clotting cascade of reactions
Vitamin K is needed for the synthesis of the bone protein osteocalcin

Figure 9.17 **Major functions of vitamin K.** Without vitamin K, our blood would not clot and our bones would become weak.

tle of oil to another. Liver and some cheeses, egg yolk, and butter are fair sources.[44] (See **Figure 9.18**.)

Intestinal bacteria in the lower bowel also produce vitamin K, but the amount actually absorbed by the body is difficult to measure. Although intestinal bacteria were once thought to supply about half of the body's vitamin K, research suggests they supply only 10 to 15 percent.[45]

Vitamin K Deficiency

In adults, vitamin K deficiency is extremely rare and usually occurs in people with fat malabsorption problems. However, newborn babies lack vitamin K-producing intestinal bacteria, so they are at risk of vitamin K deficiency. Because breast milk has little vitamin K, breastfed babies are especially vulnerable. Physicians routinely give infants a vitamin K injection at birth. This usually meets the infant's needs for several weeks, until vitamin K-producing bacteria become established in the intestine.

Because large fluctuations in vitamin K intake could interfere with medicines that prevent blood clots, people who take these medications may need to keep their vitamin K intake low or at least fairly constant.[46]

Vitamin K Toxicity

Because the body excretes vitamin K much more rapidly than other fat-soluble vitamins, toxicity from food is rare. The Food and Nutrition Board has not set a UL for vitamin K.

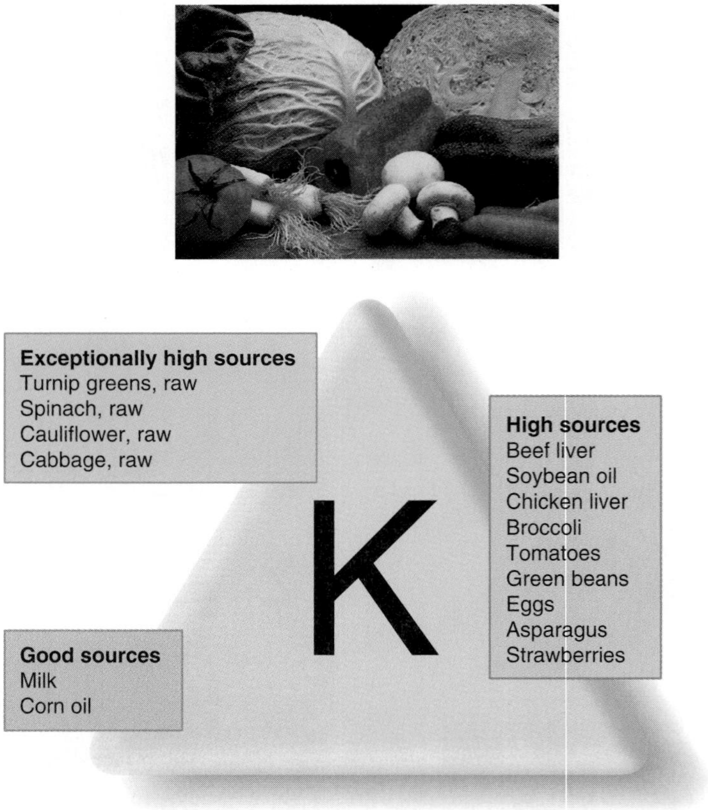

Figure 9.18 **Food sources of vitamin K.** The best sources of vitamin K are vegetables, especially those in the cabbage family. Liver, eggs, and milk are good sources as well.

Key Concepts: *Vitamin K is required for blood clotting and bone health. It is found primarily in green vegetables and in some vegetable oils. Newborns are routinely given injections of vitamin K at birth. Deficiencies are very rare. Because vitamin K is readily excreted, especially compared with other fat-soluble vitamins, toxicity also is rare.*

The Water-Soluble Vitamins: Eight Bs and a C

The scientists who first discovered vitamin B believed "it" was a single compound. As they learned more, they realized "it" was actually several vitamins. In fact there are eight B vitamins. Initially, to differentiate them, numbers were added to the letter B—vitamins B_6 and B_{12}, for example. Today, with the exception of B_6 and B_{12}, we usually refer to the B vitamins by their names: thiamin (B_1), riboflavin (B_2), niacin (B_3), pantothenic acid, biotin, and folate.

B vitamins act primarily as coenzymes (or parts of coenzymes)—the keys that unlock the action of enzymes. Enzymes regulate countless life-sustaining chemical reactions. They hurry reactions along or slow them down, as needed, even allowing them to proceed when it would otherwise be impossible. But many enzymes cannot work until the body supplies a missing component—a coenzyme. B vitamins primarily act as coenzymes or parts of coenzymes.

Let's use an analogy to clarify how vitamins function as coenzymes. Suppose you had an appointment in 15 minutes and 10 miles away. You could walk there, but you would be too late. You could drive your car, but you cannot find your key. Now you find your key (the coenzyme), turn on your car (the enzyme), and quickly drive to your destination (the reaction taking place in your body). (See **Figure 9.19**.)

Vitamin C is an antioxidant, but unlike the antioxidant vitamin E, it is water-soluble. Despite differences in solubility, vitamin C and vitamin E work together. When vitamin E quenches a free radical, vitamin E in turn becomes a free radical, although a less reactive one. Vitamin C can stabilize it, restoring vitamin E's antioxidant abilities.

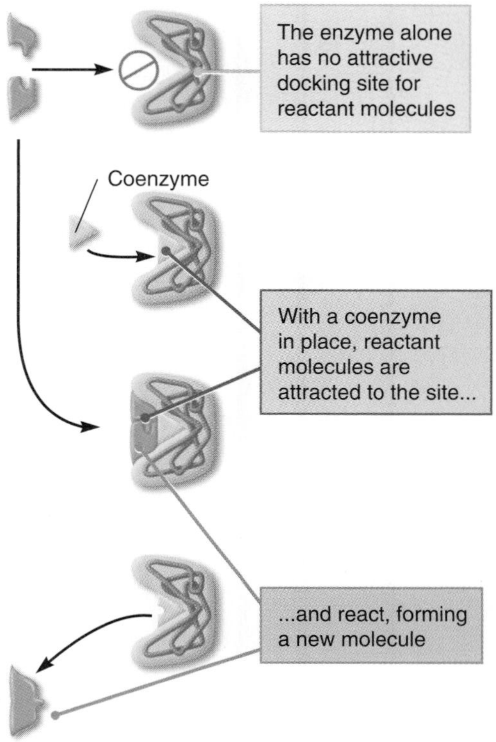
The enzyme alone has no attractive docking site for reactant molecules
Coenzyme
With a coenzyme in place, reactant molecules are attracted to the site...
...and react, forming a new molecule

Figure 9.19 **The coenzyme–enzyme partnership.** The B vitamins form coenzymes that enable specific enzymes to catalyze reactions.

Thiamin

The thiamin-deficiency disease **beriberi** was first described in Chinese writings over 4,000 years ago. But it was not widespread until the nineteenth century, when highly milled or "polished" white rice became popular. In 1855 Dr. K. Takaki of the Japanese Naval Medical Services first demonstrated beriberi's dietary origins. He cured sailors sick with beriberi by adding meat, milk, and whole grains to their diets. Years later, Christian Eijkman, a Dutch medical officer, fed birds only white rice until they had beriberi and then cured them by adding bran to their diet. This led to the discovery of an "anti-beriberi" factor—thiamin.

Functions of Thiamin

Thiamin works as a coenzyme in reactions that produce energy. Deprive your body of thiamin, and you deprive every cell of its ability to use energy. As the vitamin component of the coenzyme **thiamin pyrophosphate (TPP)**, thiamin helps reactions break down glucose, make RNA and DNA, or produce energy-rich molecules that power protein synthesis. TPP also helps synthesize and regulate neurotransmitters—chemicals that act as messengers between nerve cells.

beriberi Thiamin-deficiency disease. Symptoms include muscle weakness, loss of appetite, nerve degeneration, and edema in some cases.

thiamin pyrophosphate (TPP) A coenzyme of which the vitamin thiamin is a part. It plays a key role in removing carboxyl groups and helps drive the reaction that forms acetyl CoA from pyruvate during metabolism.

Dietary Recommendations and Sources of Thiamin

Because thiamin needs are related to energy requirements and carbohydrate intake, they are slightly greater for men than women. The RDA for adult men aged 19 years and older is 1.2 milligrams per day; for adult women, it is 1.1 milligrams. Pregnancy and breastfeeding increase energy requirements, so thiamin RDAs rise to 1.4 milligrams per day during pregnancy and 1.5 when a woman is breastfeeding. If a person's diet supplies adequate energy and includes thiamin-rich foods, it generally contains enough thiamin.

Because thiamin is found in small amounts throughout the food supply, eating a wide variety of foods is the best way to ensure a good intake. Pork and wheat germ are the richest sources. Seeds (e.g., sunflower seeds), legumes (mature beans and peas), nuts, and organ meats (e.g., liver) are good sources. (See **Figure 9.20**.) Other meats, dairy products, seafood, and most fruits contain little thiamin. Most thiamin in the American diet comes from enriched grain products: bread, pasta, rice, and ready-to-eat cereals.[47] Heat and alkaline cooking water easily destroy thiamin, so cooking reduces a food's thiamin content.

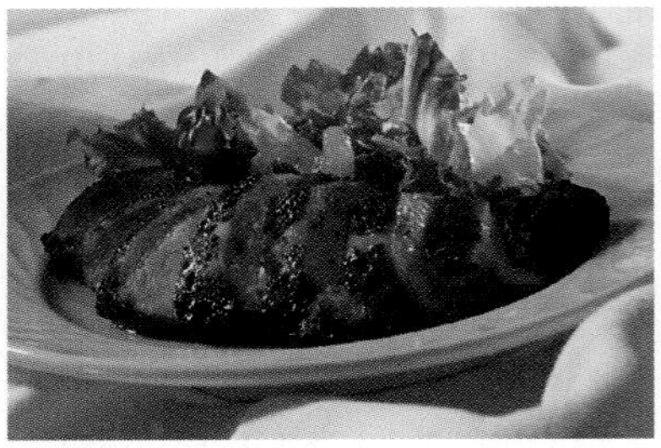

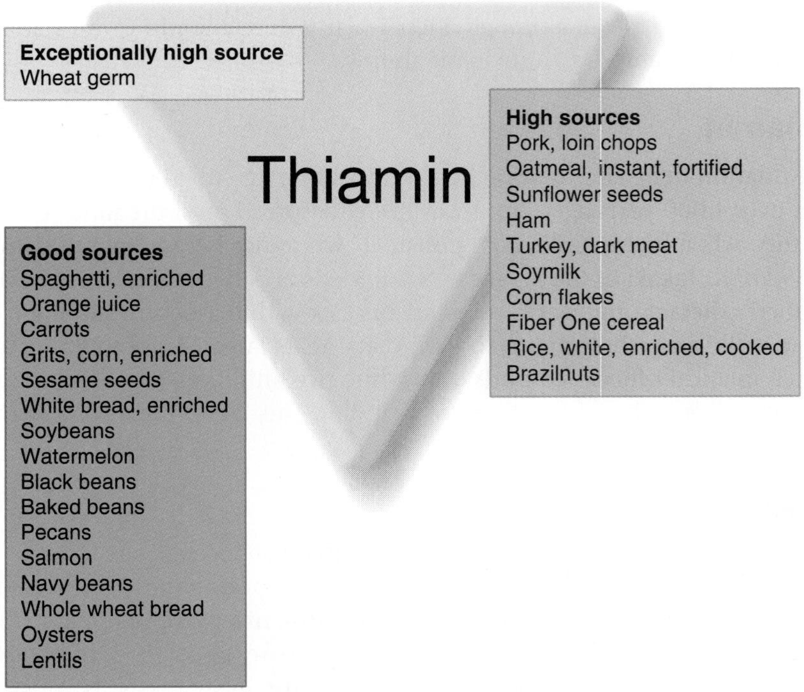

Figure 9.20 **Food sources of thiamin.** Pork, whole and enriched grains, and fortified cereals are rich in thiamin. Most animal foods contain little thiamin.

Thiamin Deficiency

Beriberi means "I can't, I can't," in one of the languages of Southeast Asia. The phrase describes how doctors long ago diagnosed the disease: Their patients were unable to rise from a squatting position. In fact, overall profound muscle weakness combined with nerve destruction ultimately leaves the victim of beriberi almost unable to move.

Milder symptoms of thiamin deficiency can appear after only 10 days on a thiamin-free diet. These include headache, irritability, depression, and loss of appetite—signs of nervous system disturbance—and contribute to a worsening food intake, causing further muscle weakness and nerve degeneration.

Those body systems with high energy needs deteriorate first. Digestive damage causes diarrhea, muscle damage causes muscle wasting and pain, and nerve damage disrupts coordination and causes "pins and needles" sensations in hands and feet. Death, however, most often comes from damage to the heart. As the heart muscle fails, feet and legs fill with fluid (edema), the so-called wet beriberi. (See **Figure 9.21**.) Outbreaks of beriberi commonly occur in refugee and displaced populations dependent on international food aid. They often must subsist on milled white cereals, including polished rice and white flour, all poor sources of thiamin when not enriched.[48]

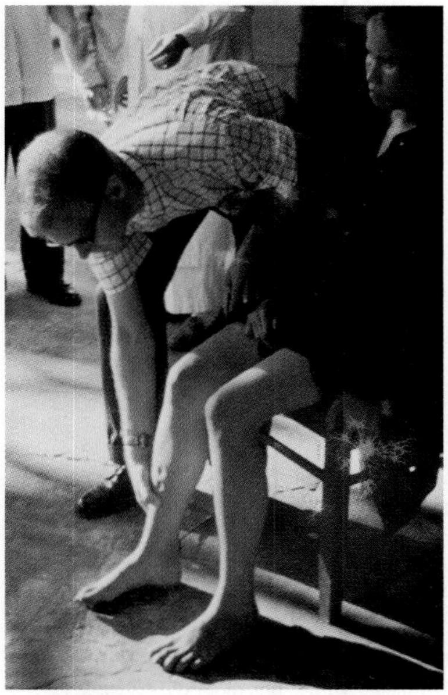

Figure 9.21 Edema is a symptom of wet beriberi.

In industrialized countries, thiamin deficiency usually is related to chronic alcoholism coupled with a poor diet. Alcohol interferes with B vitamin absorption. Alcohol-induced thiamin deficiency produces Wernicke-Korsakoff syndrome—symptoms include mental confusion and memory loss, staggered gait, and constant rapid eye movement. Although the syndrome most often is associated with the stereotypical "Skid Row" alcoholic, it can occur in any heavy drinker, especially the aging alcoholic.

Thiamin Toxicity

Thiamin supplements, which are cheap to produce, often include up to 200 times the Daily Value for thiamin, but to date, there have been no reports of thiamin toxicity. Following doses of 5 milligrams or more, thiamin absorption declines rapidly, and the kidneys quickly excrete excess.[49] The Food and Nutrition Board has not set a thiamin UL.

Riboflavin

At first, riboflavin and thiamin were considered the same vitamin. When riboflavin was finally isolated from the "anti-beriberi factor" it was dubbed vitamin B_2, and later "riboflavin" for its yellowish-green color (*flavin* means "yellow" in Latin). In foods, though, it may give a green or bluish cast. You'll notice the color in uncooked egg whites and some brands of fat-free milk.

Functions of Riboflavin

Riboflavin is a part of two coenzymes (flavin mononucleotide and flavin adenine dinucleotide). Both coenzymes are required in reactions that extract energy from glucose, fatty acids, and amino acids.[50] Riboflavin also supports the antioxidant activity of **glutathione peroxidase.**

glutathione peroxidase A selenium-containing enzyme that reduces toxic hydrogen peroxide formed within cells; works with vitamin E to reduce free radical damage.

Dietary Recommendations and Sources of Riboflavin

As with thiamin, riboflavin requirements increase along with increasing energy needs. For adults aged 19 and older, the RDA is 1.3 milligrams per

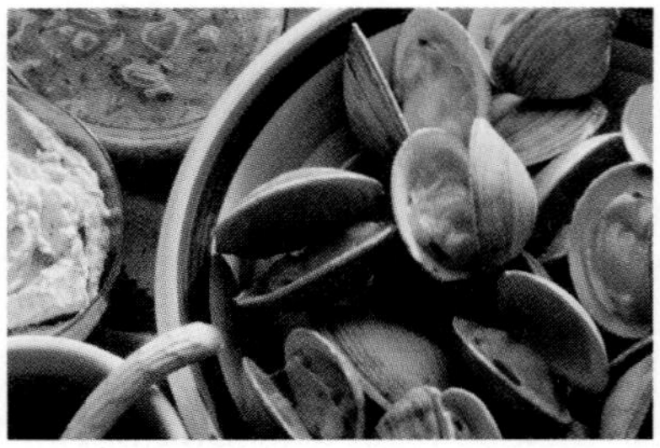

ariboflavinosis Riboflavin deficiency.

glossitis Inflammation of the tongue; a symptom of riboflavin deficiency.

stomatitis Inflammation of the mouth; a symptom of riboflavin deficiency.

cheilosis Cracking of the skin at the corners of the mouth and inflammation of the lips.

seborrheic dermatitis Disease of the oil-producing glands of the skin; a symptom of riboflavin deficiency.

anemia Abnormally low concentration of hemoglobin in the bloodstream; can be caused by impaired synthesis of red blood cells, increased destruction of red blood cells, or significant loss of blood.

tryptophan An amino acid that serves as a niacin precursor in the body. In the body, 60 milligrams of tryptophan yield about one milligram of niacin, or 1 niacin equivalent (NE).

niacin equivalents (NE) A measure that includes preformed dietary niacin as well as niacin derived from tryptophan; 60 milligrams of tryptophan yield about 1 milligram of niacin.

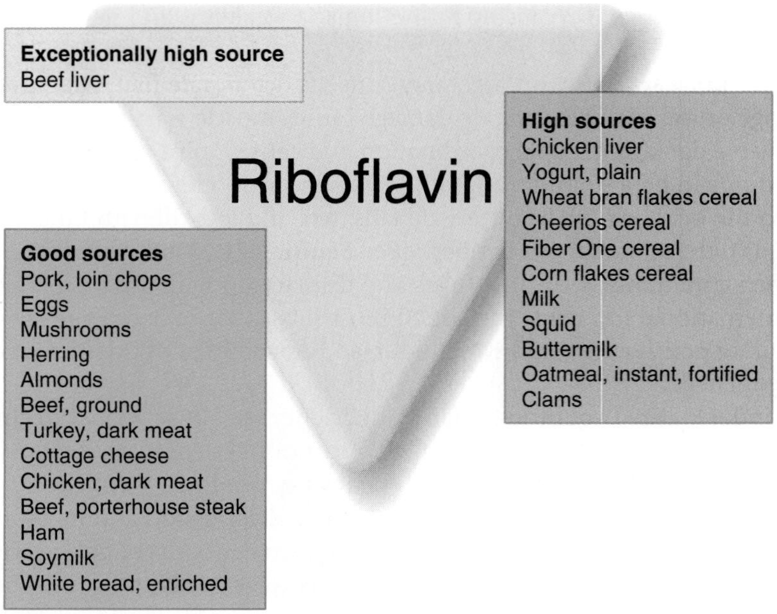

Figure 9.22 **Food sources of riboflavin.** The best sources of riboflavin include milk, liver, whole and enriched grains, and fortified cereals.

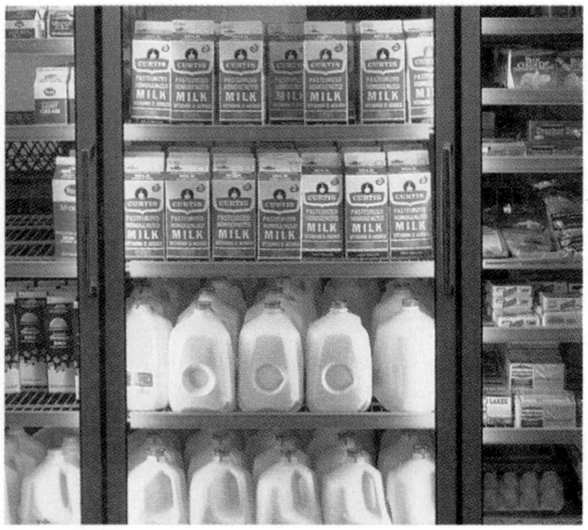

Figure 9.23 **Packaging affects riboflavin content in milk.** Light breaks down riboflavin easily, so foods high in riboflavin (e.g., milk) are best stored in opaque containers.

day for men, and 1.1 milligrams for women, reflecting higher energy needs of men. Pregnancy increases the riboflavin RDA to 1.4 milligrams per day; breastfeeding increases it to 1.6 milligrams.

Milk and milk-containing beverages, cottage cheese, and yogurt are excellent riboflavin sources. Enriched grain products, eggs, and organ meats also are good sources. (See **Figure 9.22**.) In general riboflavin is more stable than thiamin, but light can destroy it. Riboflavin-rich foods should be stored in opaque packages. For example, packaging milk in paper or plastic cartons rather than clear glass better protects milk's riboflavin content. (See **Figure 9.23**.)

Riboflavin Deficiency

Overt riboflavin deficiency (**ariboflavinosis**) is now rare, and like thiamin deficiency, occurs most often in chronic alcoholism. Long-term use of sedatives and other barbiturates accelerates liver breakdown of riboflavin and contributes to deficiency.

Riboflavin deficiency shows up first around the mouth. The tongue gets shiny, smooth, and inflamed (**glossitis**); the mouth becomes painful and sore (**stomatitis**); the lips also become sore, and fissures develop at the corners of the mouth (**cheilosis**). The oil-producing glands of the skin become clogged (**seborrheic dermatitis**); and as the deficiency becomes severe, a characteristic **anemia** develops. Riboflavin deficiency usually exists along with other nutrient deficiencies. In fact, it may even make other deficiencies worse; for example, riboflavin deficiency disrupts vitamin B_6 metabolism and can precipitate a B_6 deficiency.[51]

Riboflavin Toxicity

Excess riboflavin is readily excreted, and even large doses don't appear harmful. There are no reported cases of toxicity. A UL has not been set for riboflavin.

Quick Bites

Are You Smoking That Bread?

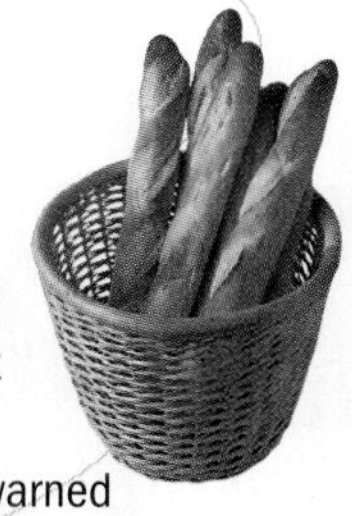

In the 1940s, antitobacco forces were confused about the differences between niacin and nicotine. They mistakenly warned that niacin-enriched bread could cause an addiction to cigarettes!

Niacin

Niacin is the name for two similar compounds: nicotinic acid and nicotinamide (also known as niacinamide). Ironically, this healthful substance got its name from a singularly unhealthful substance. In 1867, nicotinic acid was produced from nicotine in tobacco. Understand clearly, though, that nicotinic acid is not the same as or even closely related to nicotine. In the early 1940s, with its role as a vitamin established, it was renamed "niacin" so people wouldn't confuse it with nicotine.

Functions of Niacin

Niacin forms a part of crucially important coenzymes that participate in at least 200 metabolic pathways. As such, it plays a key role in energy metabolism, both under normal conditions and during times of vigorous activity when energy use swings into high gear. The body also needs niacin to synthesize fatty acids.

Dietary Recommendations and Sources of Niacin

Niacin is unique among the B vitamins—your body can make it from the amino acid **tryptophan** as well as obtain it from foods. Intake recommendations are expressed as **niacin equivalents (NE)**, a measure that includes both niacin and tryptophan. The RDA is 16 milligrams of NE per day for adult men and 14 milligrams per day for adult women, increasing to 18 milligrams during pregnancy and 17 milligrams during breastfeeding.

Most niacin in the American diet comes from meat, poultry, fish, nuts and peanuts, and enriched and whole-grain products.[52] (See **Figure 9.24**.) Niacin is stable when heated, so little is lost during cooking.

The niacin precursor tryptophan supplies about half of our niacin intake. Tryptophan is an essential amino acid and is an integral part of dietary protein. It is in almost all protein foods, but is notably low in the protein of corn. Sixty milligrams of tryptophan yield about 1 milligram of niacin, or 1 niacin equivalent (NE). Because the body needs other

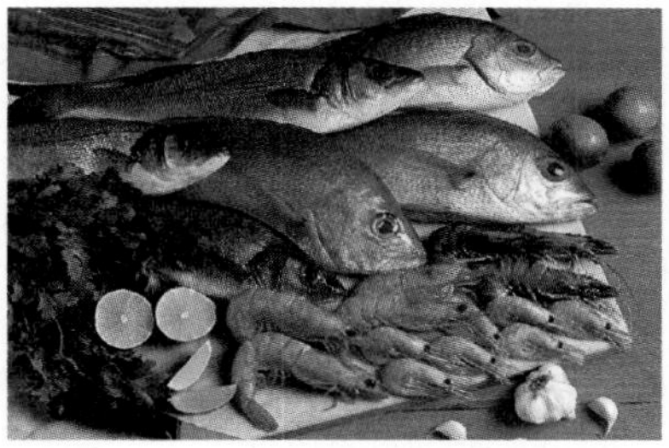

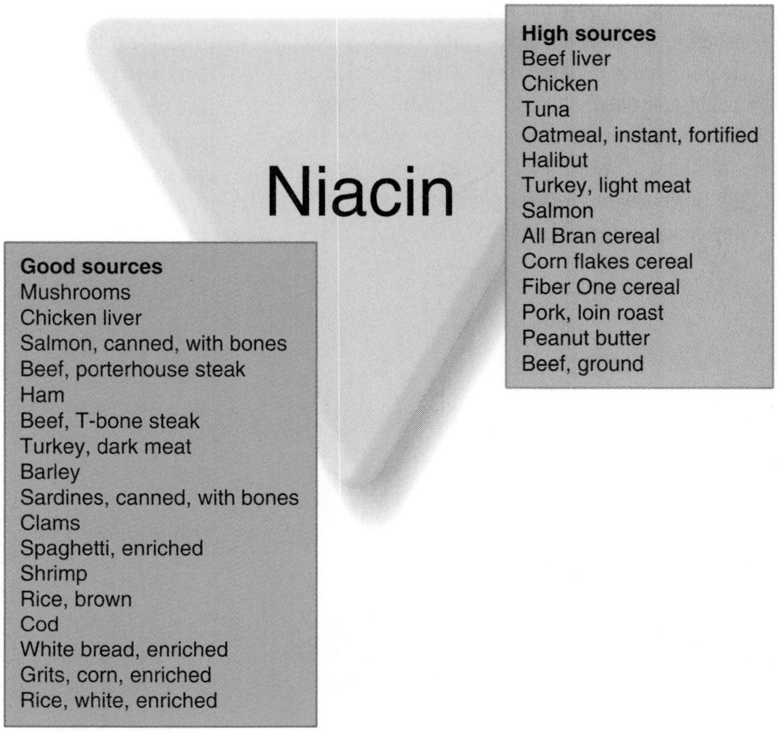

Figure 9.24 **Food sources of niacin.** Niacin is found mainly in meats and grains. Enrichment adds niacin as well as thiamin, riboflavin, folic acid, and iron to processed grains.

nutrients (riboflavin, vitamin B_6, and iron) to convert tryptophan to niacin, a deficit of any of them can worsen a niacin deficiency.

Niacin Deficiency

Pellagra is the disease of severe niacin deficiency. The word *pellagra* means "rough skin" in Italian and describes the dermatitis—a rough, darkened rash—that occurs where the victim's skin is exposed to sunlight. However, because niacin coenzymes are involved in just about every metabolic pathway, deficiency devastates the entire body. The hallmarks of pellagra are "the four Ds": dermatitis, diarrhea, dementia, and, ultimately, death. Deficiencies of other nutrients such as iron, riboflavin, and vitamin B_6 can contribute to the damage.

Descriptions of pellagra were first recorded in 1735. But the great pellagra epidemic in America's South did not emerge until the early twentieth century. The rural poor began subsisting on a diet of corn (maize), molasses, and fatty salt pork, all poor sources of niacin and tryptophan. Although corn contains niacin, the niacin is bound to a protein, which impairs absorption.[53] We now know that soaking corn in lime water helps release niacin, which much improves absorption. (See **Figure 9.25**.)

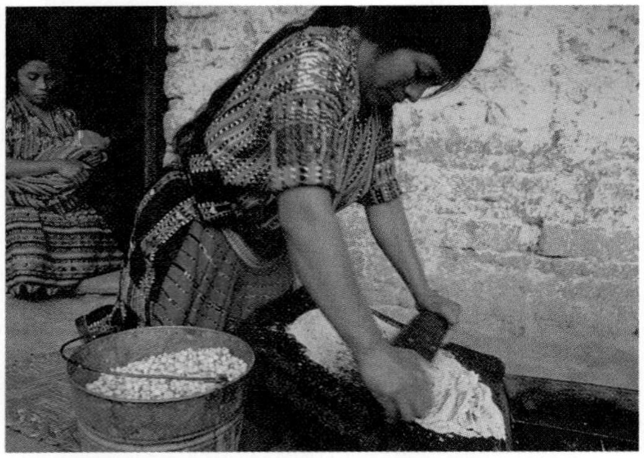

Figure 9.25 Soaking corn in lime water releases bound niacin.

Widespread pellagra began to decline during World War II after the federal government mandated enrichment of bread flour and other cereal grains with niacin. Today, pellagra has virtually disappeared in industrialized countries, except in some people with chronic alcoholism or disorders that disrupt synthesis from tryptophan. Pellagra continues to plague people living in Southeast Asia and Africa, however, whose diets lack sufficient niacin and protein.

Quick Bites

Disputing Conventional Wisdom

Early 1900s medical theory wrongly held that bacterial infection due to poor sanitation caused pellagra. Dr. Joseph Goldberg of the U.S. Public Health Service suffered much social criticism as he fought conventional wisdom to prove the crucial link between poor nutrition and the scourge pellagra. About 10 years later Conrad A. Elvehjem at the University of Wisconsin identified the "pellagra-preventive factor" as niacin.

Niacin Toxicity and Medicinal Uses of Niacin

The UL for niacin is 35 milligrams per day for adults. Because megadoses of niacin lower LDL cholesterol and raise HDL cholesterol, physicians may prescribe it. Even at one-fourth the medicinal dose, niacin can cause an uncomfortable flushing reaction with a hot, red rash on the face and arms, nausea, headache, and blurred vision.[54] While sustained-release supplements may alleviate these symptoms, chronic use over months or years can cause liver damage.[55] In some people, high-dose supplements can cause liver abnormalities within a week.

Key Concepts: *Thiamin, riboflavin, and niacin are all incorporated into coenzymes that metabolize carbohydrate, protein, and fat. Enriched grains are a major source of these B vitamins, with pork ranking as a good source of thiamin, milk as a major source of riboflavin, and high-protein foods as sources of niacin. Overt deficiencies of these vitamins are rare in North America. High doses of thiamin and riboflavin appear to be harmless, but megadoses of niacin should be taken only under medical supervision.*

Vitamin B_6

Vitamin B_6 (also known as pyridoxine) is a group of six compounds, three with a phosphate group and three without. Digestion strips the phosphate group and sends the remaining compounds to the liver, which converts them to pyridoxal phosphate (PLP), the primary active coenzyme form.[56]

microcytic hypochromic anemia Anemia characterized by small, pale red blood cells that lack adequate hemoglobin to carry oxygen; can be caused by deficiency of iron or vitamin B_6.

Functions of Vitamin B_6

PLP is a coenzyme for more than 100 different enzymes. Its better-known roles involve protein and amino acid metabolism. Enzymes that require PLP help change one amino acid into another and enable us to make the nonessential amino acids. Without adequate vitamin B_6, all amino acids become essential—the body cannot make them and must get them from food. (See the discussion of amino acids in Chapter 7, "Proteins and Amino Acids.") Vitamin B_6 also helps make glucose from amino acids (gluconeogenesis) and helps release energy from glycogen.

PLP supports white blood cell synthesis and a healthy immune system. Healthy red blood cells also need PLP. The coenzyme helps synthesize their oxygen-carrying hemoglobin and helps bind oxygen. PLP also helps produce a number of major neurotransmitters.

Vitamin B_6, folate, and vitamin B_{12} work in concert to lower blood levels of the amino acid homocysteine. Each vitamin forms a coenzyme that helps convert homocysteine to other amino acids—cysteine and methionine. (See **Figure 9.26**.) Low intake of B_6 or folate can increase homocysteine levels, and moderately high homocysteine levels are associated with fatal heart attacks. Because the body has large vitamin B_{12} stores, variations in B_{12} intake seldom affect homocysteine levels. A recent study found that women with the highest intakes of B_6 and folate have about half the risk of a heart attack as women with the lowest intakes. Furthermore, when intakes were considered separately, B_6 and folate had similar disease-reduction effects.[57]

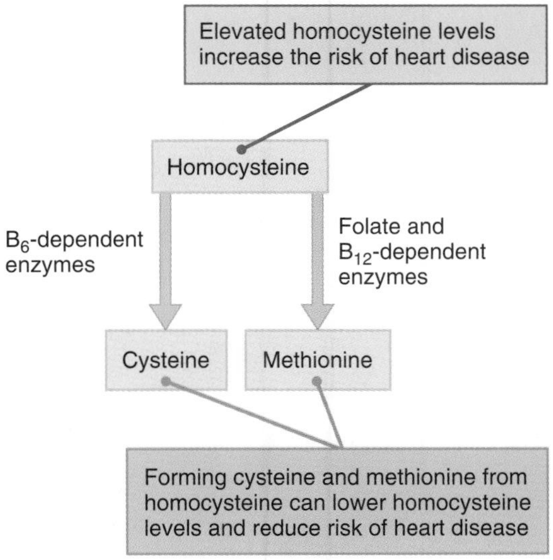

Figure 9.26 **Homocysteine and heart disease.** Elevated homocysteine levels are linked to an increased risk of heart disease. Enzymes dependent on B_6, B_{12}, and folate help lower the amount of homocysteine by converting it to cysteine and methionine.

Dietary Recommendations and Sources of Vitamin B_6

The vitamin B_6 RDA for men and women 19 to 50 years old is 1.3 milligrams per day. Because requirements appear to increase with age, the RDA is set at 1.7 milligrams for older men and 1.5 milligrams for older women.[58]

Good sources of vitamin B_6 include meat (especially organ meats like liver), fish, or poultry; potatoes and other starchy vegetables; and fortified soy-based meat substitutes.[59] Whole grains contain vitamin B_6, but it is lost in refining and is not replaced by enrichment. However, it is added to some fortified breakfast cereals. Vitamin B_6 also pops up in unexpected places: bananas, watermelon, and sunflower seeds, for example. (See **Figure 9.27**.)

Vitamin B_6 is not particularly stable and is especially sensitive to temperature. Heat can destroy up to half of a food's vitamin B_6.

Vitamin B_6 Deficiency

Overt vitamin B_6 deficiency is rare, although some medications can cause deficiency. Excessive alcohol interferes with the vitamin's absorption and its coenzyme activities, worsening B_6 deficits created by the alcoholic's typically poor diet.

Overt vitamin B_6 deficiency produces a skin rash and anemia and also disrupts nervous system activity. Inadequate vitamin B_6 disrupts the synthesis of red blood cells and their oxygen-binding ability, causing an anemia in which red blood cells are small and pale (**microcytic hypochromic anemia**). The pale color reflects their lack of adequate hemoglobin to carry sufficient oxygen. Vitamin B_6

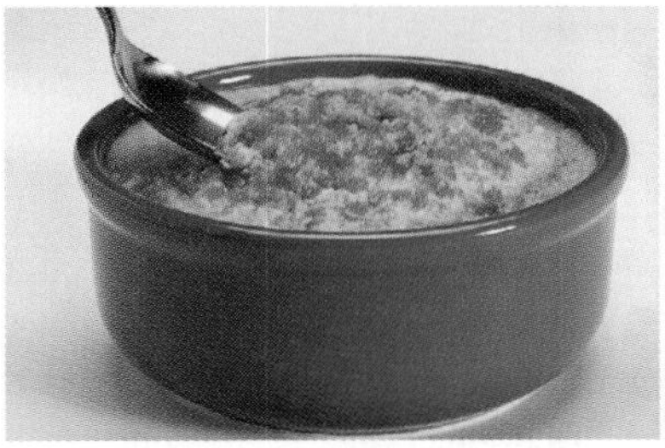

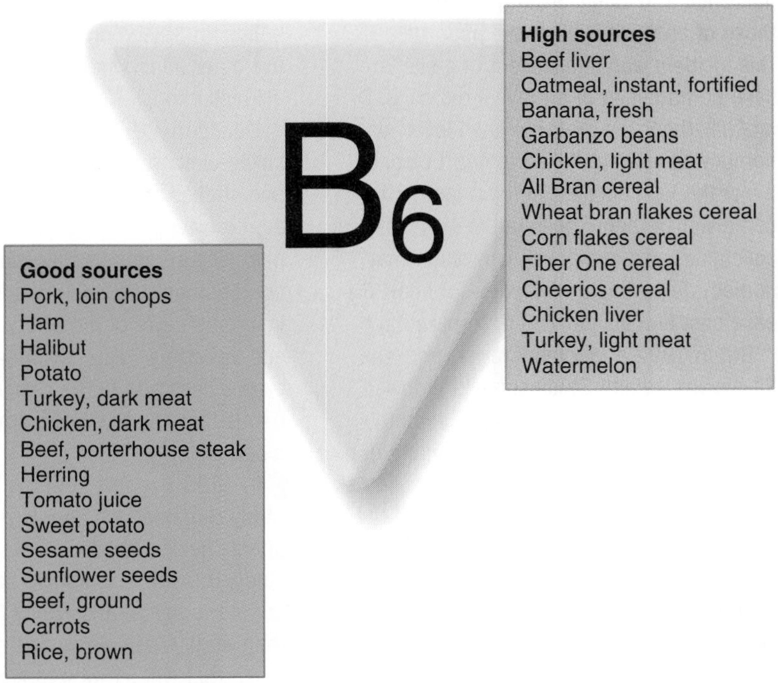

Figure 9.27 **Food sources of vitamin B_6.** Meats are generally good sources of vitamin B_6, along with certain fruits (e.g., bananas, watermelon) and vegetables (e.g., potatoes, carrots).

deficiency also damages the nervous system, causing depression, headaches, confusion, and convulsions.

More subtle deficits of vitamin B_6 disrupt homocysteine metabolism, leading to increased levels that are a risk factor for heart disease. (See the FYI feature "The B Vitamins and Heart Disease.")

Vitamin B_6 Toxicity and Medicinal Uses of Vitamin B_6

Some women take large doses of vitamin B_6 to treat premenstrual syndrome (PMS)—a set of symptoms that may occur before the onset of menstruation. Doses as low as 50 milligrams appear helpful, but more research is needed to establish its effectiveness for PMS.[60]

High-dose vitamin B_6 has also been used for carpal tunnel syndrome—a wrist injury that causes painful tingling in hands and fingers. Most well-designed scientific studies have found no evidence that vitamin B_6 improves carpal tunnel syndrome, however.[61]

Fyi — FOR YOUR INFORMATION: The B Vitamins and Heart Disease

In 1968 a young pathologist named Kilmer McCully examined the body of a 2-month-old boy who had died of the rare genetic disease homocystinuria—a condition with sky-high levels of the amino acid homocysteine in the urine. The child's arteries were so hardened and clogged that they resembled those of an adult with severe heart disease. This incident was reminiscent of a similar case he had seen of an 8-year-old child. Dr. McCully theorized that their high levels of homocysteine were linked to heart disease.

For the next decade, he held fast to his controversial theory despite the skepticism of colleagues. His outspoken conviction that homocysteine was a risk factor for heart disease cost him his job and his reputation.[1]

But in 1992 a landmark report from the Physicians' Health Study sparked renewed interest in Dr. McCully's theory. The study, which monitored the health of a large group of physicians, showed that heart disease risk more than tripled in those doctors with the highest blood levels of homocysteine.[2] Homocysteine appeared to be on a par with high blood cholesterol and smoking as an independent risk factor for cardiovascular disease.

In 1993 a research team from the Jean Mayer USDA Human Nutrition Research Center on Aging at Tufts University showed that high homocysteine levels go hand in hand with low blood levels of vitamins B_6, B_{12}, and especially folate.[3] Because these three nutrients interact in the body's metabolism of homocysteine, this association makes sense. When one or more is lacking, homocysteine builds up. Based on the Tufts study, one in five older adults may have homocysteine levels high enough to put them at risk.

During the 1990s scores of studies clearly linked elevated homocysteine to heart attacks and strokes, blood clots in the legs, and damage to arteries.[4] Homocysteine appears to help clog arteries by triggering the proliferation of smooth muscle cells just beneath the innermost layer of the artery wall. This thickens the artery wall, narrowing the artery. The excess cells add to the plaque and other debris that line the arteries and promote blood clots.

In 1998 a report from the Nurses' Health Study examined whether B vitamin intake affects heart disease risk. In this ongoing study, Harvard researchers have been monitoring the health and eating habits of more than 80,000 female nurses since 1980. They found that women who took in the most folate—from either food or supplements—were 31 percent less likely to suffer a heart attack than the women who consumed the least folate. The same held true for vitamin B_6.[5] More research is under way to determine whether the results hold up in different populations, such as men, and under different circumstances.

Do we need B vitamin supplements to reduce heart disease risk? Most research suggests that consuming the RDA for folate, vitamin B_6, and vitamin B_{12} is sufficient. Should we have our homocysteine levels tested? At this time, no major health organization recommends across-the-board testing for homocysteine. Some physicians, however, do advise testing for people with a strong family history of heart disease and those who have suffered a heart attack or other coronary event in the absence of high blood cholesterol or other risk factors.

1 McCully KS. *The Homocysteine Revolution.* New Canaan, CT: Keats Publishing; 1997.
2 Stampfer MJ, Malinow MR, Willett WC, et al. A prospective study of plasma homocyst(e)ine and risk of myocardial infarction in US physicians. *JAMA.* 1992;268:877–881.
3 Selhub J, Jacques PF, Wilson PW, et al. Vitamin status and intake as primary determinants of homocysteinemia in an elderly population. *JAMA.* 1993;270:2693–2698.
4 McCully KS. Homocysteine, folate, vitamin B6, and cardiovascular disease. *JAMA.* 1998;279:392–393.
5 Rimm E, Willett WC, Hu FB, et al. Folate and vitamin B6 from diet and supplements in relation to risk of coronary heart disease among women. *JAMA.* 1998;279:359–364.

Vitamin B_6 megadoses are not without risk. Over time, daily supplements of 1,000 milligrams or more can cause painful, partly irreversible nerve damage that causes numbness in the extremities and interferes with walking.[62]

The UL for vitamin B_6 intake is 100 milligrams per day. Unfortunately, over-the-counter supplements often contain this amount or more. Doses above the UL should be taken only under medical supervision.

neural tube defects (NTD) Birth defects resulting from failure of the neural tube to develop properly during early fetal development.

dietary folate equivalents (DFE) A measure of folate intake used to account for the high bioavailability of folic acid taken as a supplement compared with the lower bioavailability of the folate found in foods.

Folate

Folate is named for its best natural source: green leafy vegetables (foliage). The term *folate* actually refers to a group of several closely related folate forms. Folic acid is the most stable form and is used for supplementation and fortification.

Functions of Folate

As a coenzyme, folate is crucial to DNA synthesis and cell division, amino acid metabolism, and the maturation of red blood cells and other cells. This involvement in basic cell reproduction and growth makes folate essential for healthy embryonic development. Good folate status in early pregnancy greatly reduces the risk of a type of birth defect called **neural tube defects (NTD)**.[63] However, many women do not realize they have become pregnant or don't seek prenatal care until it's too late. That is why experts recommend folic acid supplements before pregnancy to all women who may become pregnant. And it is why the government mandated folic acid fortification.

Dietary Folate Equivalents

1 μg DFE = 1 μg food folate

= 0.5 μg folic acid taken on an empty stomach

= 0.6 μg folic acid consumed with meals

Folate functions in close cooperation with vitamins B_6 and B_{12}. All three support red blood cell synthesis and help control homocysteine levels. By lowering homocysteine blood levels, folate cuts the risk of heart attack.[64] (See the section "Vitamin B_6" and the FYI feature "The B Vitamins and Heart Disease.")

Folate also lowers cancer risk. When women took multivitamins containing folate for at least 15 years, they had a 75 percent reduction in colon cancer risk, according to the Harvard Nurses' Health Study. Folate intakes of more than 600 micrograms per day reduced breast cancer risk by 50 percent.[65]

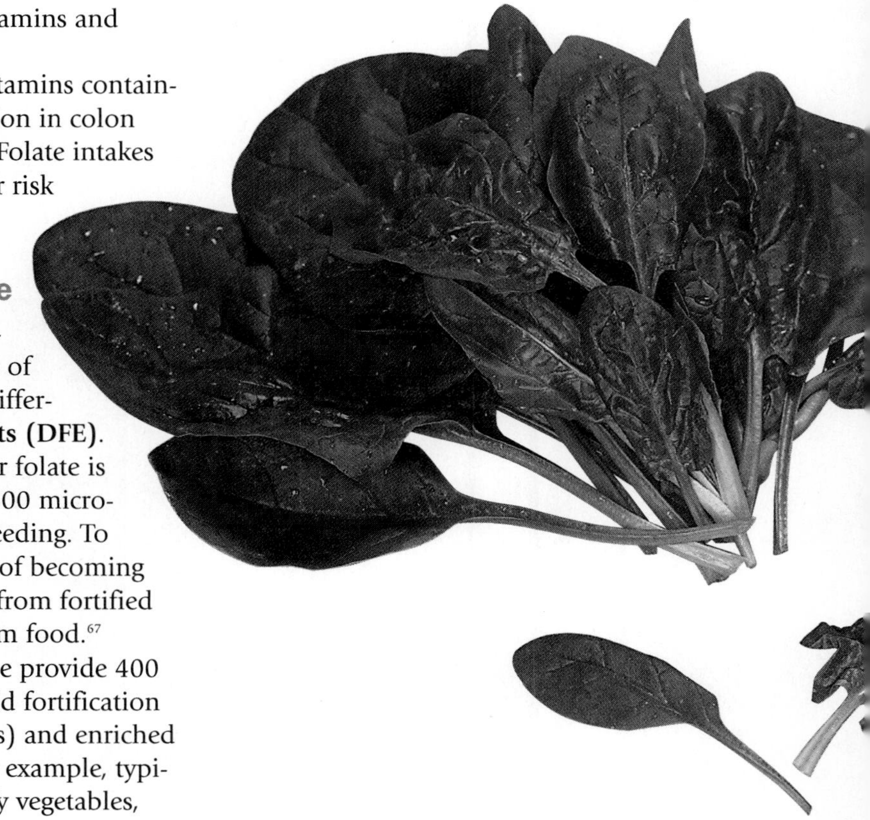

Dietary Recommendations and Sources of Folate

The body absorbs nearly 100 percent of folic acid in supplements and fortified foods, but only about half to two-thirds of the folate naturally present in food.[66] To account for these differences, RDA values are expressed as **dietary folate equivalents (DFE)**.

For men and women aged 19 years and older, the RDA for folate is 400 micrograms of DFE per day. Requirements increase to 600 micrograms during pregnancy and 500 micrograms while breastfeeding. To reduce the risk of birth defects, all women who are capable of becoming pregnant should get 400 micrograms of folic acid each day from fortified foods or supplements, in addition to any folate they get from food.[67]

Fortified breakfast cereals supply most dietary folate. Some provide 400 micrograms in a moderate-size serving. Since 1998, folic acid fortification of enriched flour (including that used by commercial bakers) and enriched grain products has been mandatory.[68] A serving of pasta, for example, typically provides 30 percent of the folate RDA. Dark-green leafy vegetables, asparagus, broccoli, orange juice, wheat germ, liver, sunflower seeds, and legumes are other good sources. (See **Figure 9.28**.)

Folate is extremely vulnerable to heat, ultraviolet light, and oxygen. Cooking and other food-processing and preparation techniques can destroy up to 90 percent of a food's folate. Experts recommend eating folate-rich fruits and vegetables raw or cooking them quickly in minimal amounts of water via steaming, stir-frying, or microwaving. Vitamin C in foods also helps protect folate from oxidation.

megaloblastic anemia Excess amounts of megaloblasts (immature red blood cells) in the blood caused by deficiency of folate or vitamin B_{12}.

spina bifida A type of neural tube birth defect.

microencephaly A type of neural tube birth defect in which the brain is abnormally small.

anencephaly A type of neural tube birth defect in which part or all of the brain is missing.

Folate Deficiency

Until recently, folate deficiency was probably the most prevalent of all vitamin deficiencies in the United States. This dubious honor may disappear with mandatory folic acid fortification—our levels of blood folate have started to improve.[69]

Other factors along with diet affect folate status. A significant number of people have a genetic variation in an enzyme that limits their ability to process folate effectively.[70] Many prescription medicines interfere with folate metabolism, and some medical conditions increase folate needs. Plus, low vitamin B_6 levels worsen folate absorption.

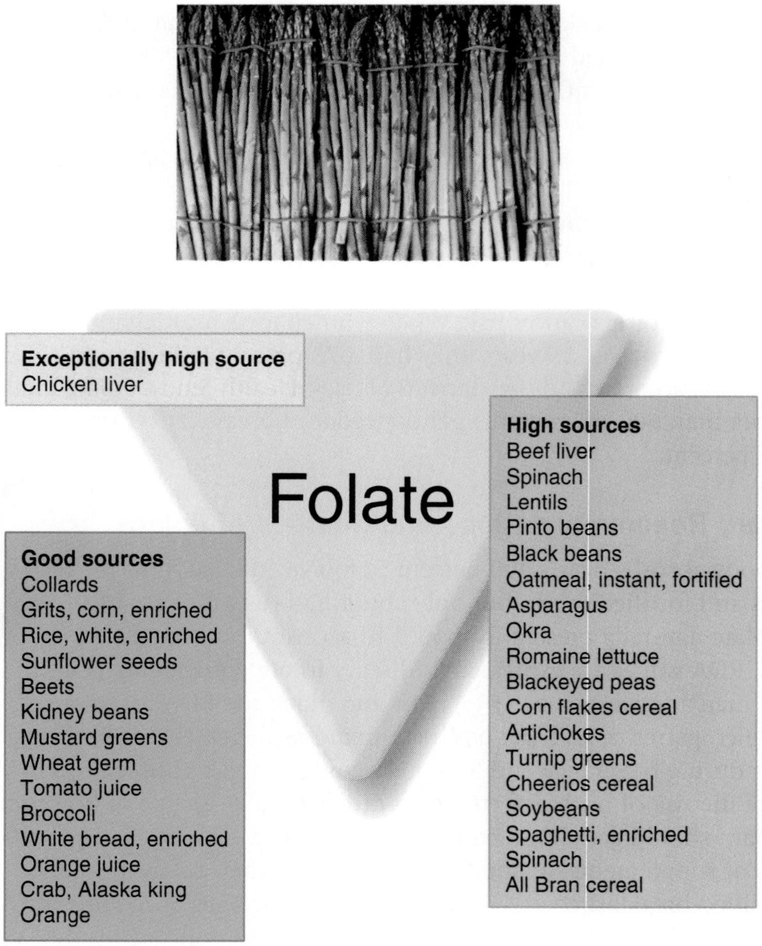

Figure 9.28 **Food sources of folate.** Good sources of folate are a diverse collection of foods: liver, legumes, leafy greens, and orange juice. Enriched grains and fortified cereals are other ways to include folic acid in the diet.

When your folate reserves are good, your body normally can store enough folate to last two to four months without additional intake. Abnormal cell reproduction due to folate deficiency can be corrected within 24 hours by vitamin replacement.

Anemia and Diarrhea

Both folate and vitamin B_{12} are required for DNA synthesis and normal cell growth. A deficiency shows up soonest in cells that are reproducing the fastest. Red blood cells are rapidly dividing cells that must be replaced about every 120 days; they are among the first cells to be damaged by deficiency. The immature red blood cells cannot grow normally and cannot mature normally. Instead, these fragile blood cells grow into large bizarre shapes and have greatly shortened life spans. These abnormal cells displace normal red blood cells, leading to a type of anemia called **megaloblastic anemia**. (See **Figure 9.29**.) A lack of folate also impairs the synthesis of white blood cells, which are vital to the immune response.

Like blood cells, cells lining the gastrointestinal tract also divide rapidly and need frequent replacement. And like blood cells, impaired DNA synthesis prevents gastrointestinal cells from maturing normally. Large, immature cells accumulate along the digestive tract. In the intestine, they interfere with absorption, causing diarrhea. In the mouth, the defective cells make the tongue sore and "beefy red."

Birth Defects

Low folate levels during the early stages of pregnancy dramatically increase risk of neural tube defects. These central nervous system defects occur within the first 30 days after conception.[71] Most common is **spina bifida**, in which a protective covering fails to form over part or all of the fragile spinal cord. (See **Figure 9.30**.) Other neural tube defects include abnormally small brain (**microencephaly**) or no brain at all (**anencephaly**). Worldwide, between 1 and 9 of every 1,000 infants are born with these conditions.

Heart Disease

Poor folate status can lead to elevated homocysteine levels, an important risk factor for heart disease. Homocysteine levels were a primary factor in setting the folate RDA, and recommended folate intakes help maintain homocysteine at reduced levels.

Folate Toxicity

Deficiency of either folate or vitamin B_{12} produces the same type of anemia, but B_{12} deficiency also causes nerve damage. Taking folate supplements can mask the symptoms of B_{12} deficiency anemia until nerve damage becomes irreversible. (See the section "Vitamin B_{12} Deficiency.")

Although rare, hypersensitive people who take folic acid supplements may suffer hives or respiratory distress. The UL for adults is 1,000 micrograms per day of folic acid from supplements and fortified foods.

Vitamin B_{12}

Vitamin B_{12} is unlike other B vitamins. Plants do not provide it, and your body stores large reserves. Vitamin B_{12} is a group of cobalt-containing compounds, known collectively as cobalamin. In the United States, cyanocobalamin is the only form of vitamin B_{12} commercially available in supplements.

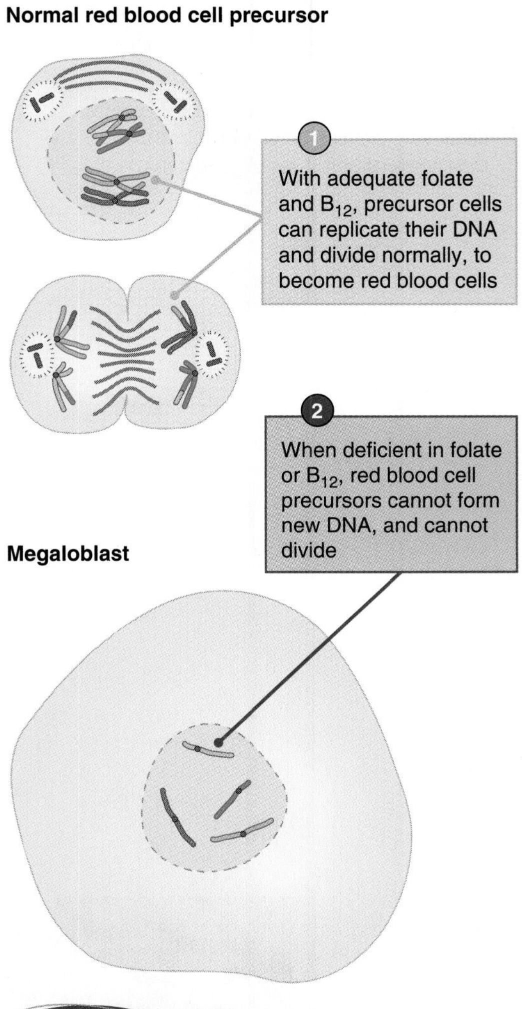
Normal red blood cell precursor
1
With adequate folate and B_{12}, precursor cells can replicate their DNA and divide normally, to become red blood cells
2
When deficient in folate or B_{12}, red blood cell precursors cannot form new DNA, and cannot divide
Megaloblast

Figure 9.29 **Megaloblastic anemia.** When red blood cell precursors in the bone marrow cannot form new DNA, they cannot divide normally. These precursor cells continue to grow and become large, fragile, immature cells called megaloblasts. Megaloblasts displace red blood cells, resulting in megaloblastic anemia.

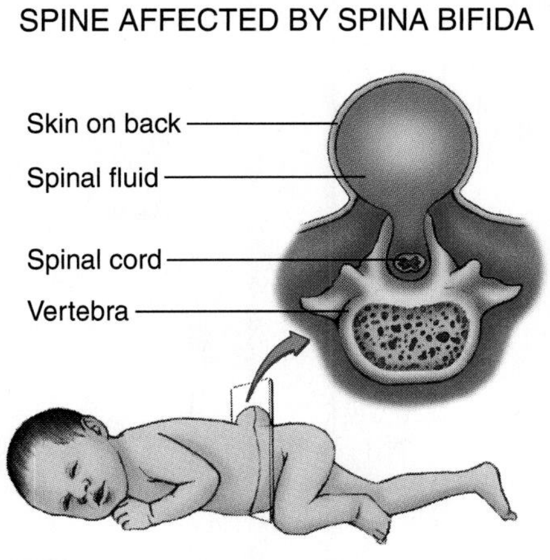
SPINE AFFECTED BY SPINA BIFIDA
Skin on back
Spinal fluid
Spinal cord
Vertebra

Figure 9.30 **Neural tube defects.** Poor folate status during the early stages of pregnancy, even before a woman may realize she is pregnant, increases the risk of a neural tube defect.

myelin sheath The protective coating that surrounds nerve fibers.

pernicious anemia Result of vitamin B_{12} deficiency. Hallmarks of the condition are megaloblastic anemia and nerve degeneration that can result in paralysis and death.

Functions of Vitamin B_{12}

Vitamin B_{12} transforms folate into an activated form. Without vitamin B_{12}, folate cannot function in DNA synthesis or blood cell synthesis, nor can it metabolize homocysteine. All folate functions are blocked. Thus, a deficiency of vitamin B_{12} will produce folate deficiency symptoms, even though folate levels might be adequate.

Vitamin B_{12} has another essential job. It helps maintain the **myelin sheath**, a protective coating that surrounds nerve fibers. A vitamin B_{12} deficiency ultimately destroys nerve cells.

Dietary Recommendations and Sources of Vitamin B_{12}

For healthy adults, the RDA for vitamin B_{12} is 2.4 micrograms per day. Because up to 30 percent of people older than 50 may malabsorb vitamin B_{12} from food, experts advise them to consume B_{12}-fortified foods or supplements. Our bodies more efficiently absorb vitamin B_{12} from these sources.[72]

All naturally occurring vitamin B_{12} originates with bacteria. Bacteria produce it, and animals obtain it from bacteria on their food or from their intestinal bacteria. Animals concentrate and store B_{12}, mainly in the liver. Consequently animal-derived foods are our only good natural source of vitamin B_{12}, and liver is the richest source.

Plants do not make vitamin B_{12}, but contaminating traces do exist on plant foods. Blue-green algae (cyanobacteria) are sometimes promoted as a B_{12} plant source, but their cobalamin is an inactive form. For vegans (vegetarians who avoid eggs and dairy, as well as meats), the most reliable food sources are fortified breakfast cereals, fortified soy products, and other foods fortified with B_{12}. (See **Figure 9.31**.)

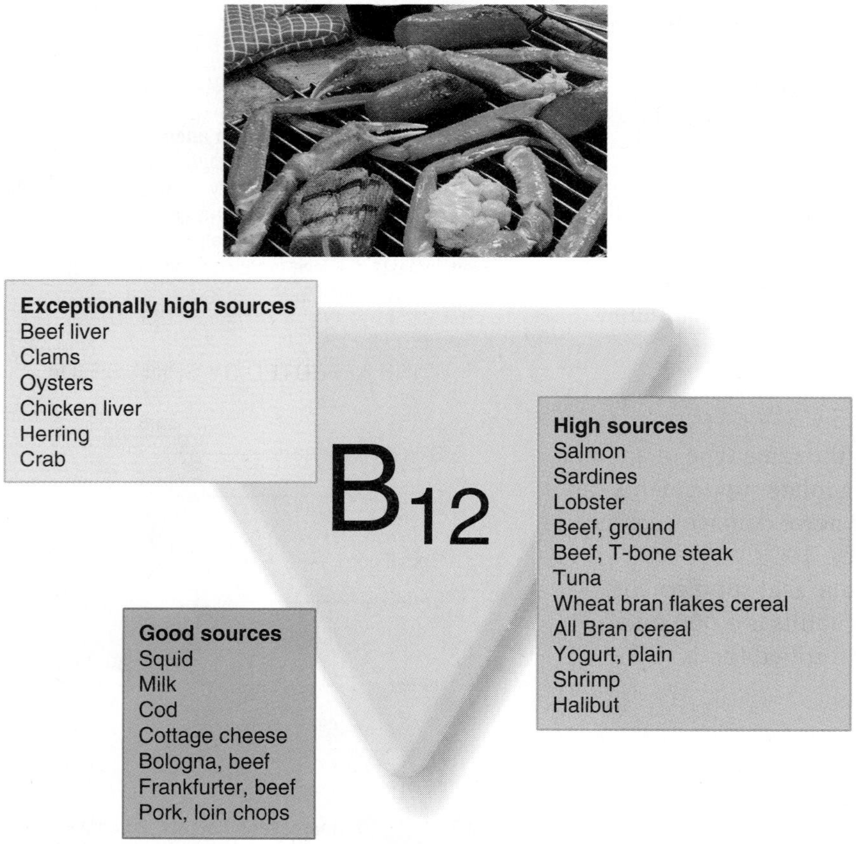

Figure 9.31 **Food sources of vitamin B_{12}.** Vitamin B_{12} is found naturally only in foods of animal origin, such as liver, meats, and milk. Some cereals are fortified with vitamin B_{12}.

Absorption of Vitamin B_{12}

Unless you're a vegan, it's easy to get enough vitamin B_{12} from your diet. But absorbing it is another matter. Readying B_{12} for absorption is a complex multistep digestive process, starting in the mouth and ending with absorption in the small intestine. The process requires production of adequate stomach acid and a substance called intrinsic factor. (See **Figure 9.32**.) A defect in any step can cause B_{12} deficiency.

Vitamin B_{12} Deficiency

We can store enough vitamin B_{12} in the liver to last more than 2 years, and symptoms of deficiency may not appear for up to 12 years. A vitamin B_{12} deficiency is almost always due to impaired absorption. Deficiency is treated with B_{12} injections or oral doses that are high enough to overcome impaired absorption.[73] Vegans who do not eat fortified cereals regularly or do not take vitamin B_{12} supplements also risk

Think About It 3

Think About It 3

vitamin B_{12} deficiency. Vegan mothers who breastfeed but do not take supplemental vitamin B_{12} may put their infants at risk of long-term neurologic problems.

Vitamin B_{12} deficiency causes **pernicious anemia**. In this type of anemia, red blood cells are large, fragile, and strangely shaped, just like in folate-deficiency anemia. But when a B_{12} deficiency causes the anemia, nerve cells are irreversibly destroyed. This is the crucial difference between B_{12} deficiency anemia and folate deficiency anemia—folate deficiency does not destroy nerves. If pernicious anemia is incorrectly treated with folic acid, anemia symptoms may disappear as nerve degeneration continues. The mistake may not become apparent until the damage is irreversible. Proper treatment of pernicious anemia includes B_{12} injections or megadose supplements.

Vitamin B_{12} Toxicity

Large vitamin B_{12} doses have no apparent ill effect. Doses of 1,000 micrograms are used routinely in medical situations. A UL for vitamin B_{12} has not been determined.

Key Concepts: *Vitamin B_6, folate, and vitamin B_{12} work closely together. Deficiency of folate increases risk for birth defects. Deficiency of B_{12} causes irreversible nerve damage. All three deficiencies cause anemia. All three deficiencies compromise homocysteine metabolism, a risk factor for heart disease. Fortified grains have become an important folate source. Only animal-derived or fortified foods contain significant amount of vitamin B_{12}. Megadoses of vitamin B_6 can cause nerve damage.*

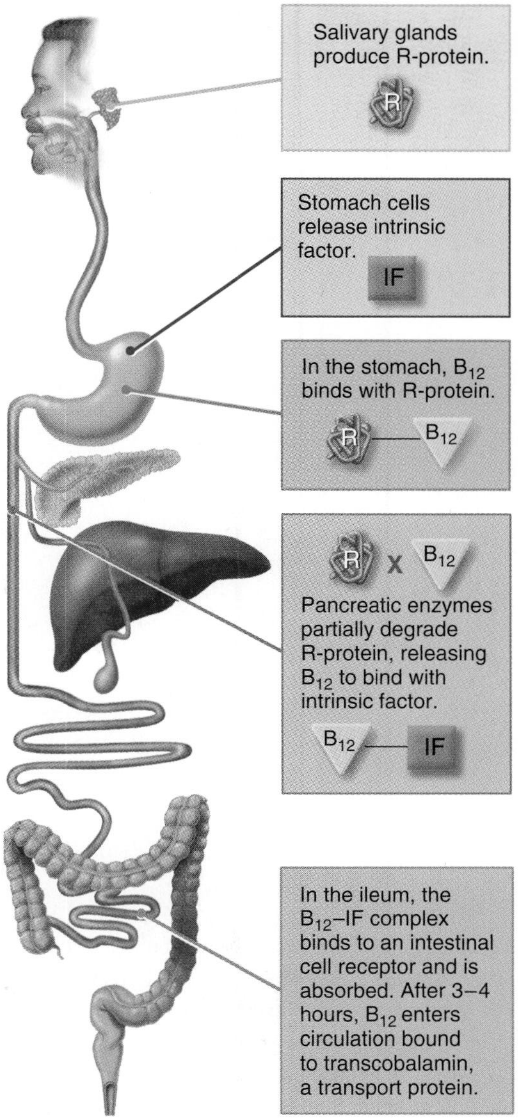

Figure 9.32 **Absorption of vitamin B_{12}.** Absorption of B_{12} is a complex process that involves many factors and sites in the GI tract. Defects in this process, especially a lack of intrinsic factor, impair B_{12} absorption and can result in pernicious anemia.

Pantothenic Acid

Pantothenic acid is widespread in the food supply; in fact, its name comes from the Greek word *pantothen*, meaning "from every side." Although marketers have promoted pantothenic acid supplements as an "antistress" vitamin, there is no evidence from controlled studies to suggest it reduces feelings of anxiety or stress.[74]

Functions of Pantothenic Acid

Pantothenic acid is a component of coenzyme A (CoA), which in turn is part of acetyl CoA, a compound that sits at the crossroads of energy-generating and biosynthetic pathways. (See **Figure 9.33**.) It is critical to the extraction of energy from nutrients and for building new fatty acids. (For more on coenzyme A, acetyl CoA, and metabolic pathways, see the "Spotlight on Metabolism.")

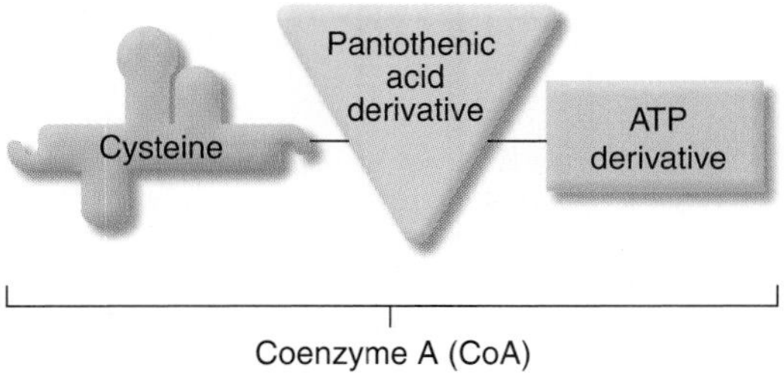

Figure 9.33 **Pantothenic acid and coenzyme A.** Pantothenic acid forms part of coenzyme A, which in turn is a component of acetyl CoA. Through coenzyme A, pantothenic acid is involved in many metabolic reactions that extract energy from nutrients and other reactions that build fatty acids.

Dietary Recommendations and Sources of Pantothenic Acid

There are few data upon which to base dietary recommendations for pantothenic acid, so an Adequate Intake level has been set instead. For adults aged 19 to 50, the AI is 5 milligrams per day.

Mother Nature must have known the importance of this vitamin, because it is found throughout the food supply. Pantothenic acid is in foods as diverse as meat, mushrooms, and oats.[75] Pantothenic acid is damaged easily. Freezing and canning appear to decrease the pantothenic acid content, and refining grains destroys nearly 75 percent.[76]

Pantothenic Acid Deficiency

Pantothenic acid deficiencies are virtually nonexistent. In research settings, deficiency-induced symptoms include irritability and restlessness, fatigue, digestive disturbance, sleep disturbance, numbness and tingling, muscle cramps, staggered gait, and low blood glucose levels.

Pantothenic Acid Toxicity

High intakes of pantothenic acid have no apparent adverse effects. Therefore a UL has not been established.

Biotin

In 1924 researchers thought they had identified three growth factors—"bios II," "vitamin H," and "coenzyme R." But it soon became clear that there was only one substance at work—the B vitamin biotin.

Functions of Biotin

Like the other B vitamins, biotin acts as a coenzyme in dozens of reactions. Among these reactions are amino acid metabolism, including the conversion of amino acids to glucose (gluconeogenesis); fatty acid synthesis and release of energy from fatty acids; and DNA synthesis.

Dietary Recommendations and Sources of Biotin

We know so little about biotin requirements that the AI for adults is mathematically determined from the infant AI, which in turn is based on the biotin levels of human milk.[77] The AI for biotin for adults is 30 micrograms daily.

We also have little information on the biotin content of foods. We do know that some good sources are cauliflower, liver, peanuts, and cheese, while most fruits and meats are poor sources.

In raw egg white, a protein called **avidin** binds biotin and prevents its absorption. Cooking denatures avidin, preventing it from binding to biotin. Egg yolks are a good biotin source, as long as eggs are cooked.

Quick Bites

Busy Bacteria

You may be aware that bacteria in the colon synthesize vitamin K, but did you know that these bacteria also make some biotin? However, in synthesizing this B vitamin these busy microbes may be undertaking a futile effort. Since the colon is downstream from the small intestine, the site of most biotin absorption, the bacteria's biotin may not be absorbed efficiently. Bacterial synthesis of biotin probably does not make an important contribution to your body's supply of biotin.

Biotin Deficiency

Deficiency is rare, but it can occur. Eating raw egg whites—about a dozen or more daily over months or years—could produce biotin deficiency, but this scenario is unlikely. Some anticonvulsant drugs break down biotin, increasing risk of deficiency.

A rare genetic defect can lead to biotin depletion in infants. Symptoms progress from initial hair loss, rash, and delayed growth and development to convulsions and other neurological problems. Early diagnosis and daily biotin supplements usually clear up symptoms. If untreated, biotin deficiency can lead to coma and death.

avidin A protein in raw egg whites that binds biotin, preventing its absorption. Avidin is denatured by heat.

Biotin Toxicity

High doses of biotin do not appear toxic, and no UL for biotin has been established.

Key Concepts: *Pantothenic acid and biotin are widespread in the food supply, and deficiencies are rare. Like the other B vitamins, they are parts of coenzymes involved in the metabolism of fat, carbohydrate, and protein.*

Vitamin C

For centuries, the treacherous disease scurvy dogged mankind. Explorers and seafaring men especially feared this mysterious ailment that inflicted aching pain and made each journey a gamble with death. Writings dating back as far as 1500 B.C.E. describe their suffering in detail.

In 1747 James Lind, a Scottish physician, proved that eating lemons and oranges cured the disease. (See Figure 1.11 in Chapter 1.) But not until 1930 did scientists isolate the substance responsible for curing scurvy and name it vitamin C.

Vitamin C has two forms: ascorbic acid and dehydroascorbic acid. Most animals manufacture their own vitamin C, but humans cannot, sharing this dubious distinction with fruit-eating bats, guinea pigs, pigs, and a few other isolated species.

Functions of Vitamin C

Unlike the B vitamins, vitamin C does not act as a coenzyme. Yet it is an important participant in many reactions and is known for its antioxidant activities.

Antioxidant Activity

Like vitamin E, vitamin C is an antioxidant and helps protect cells from oxidative damage.[78] But unlike vitamin E, vitamin C is water-soluble rather than fat-soluble. (See the FYI feature "Antioxidants and Free Radicals.") Vitamin C may reduce the risk of chronic diseases such as heart disease, certain forms of cancer, and cataracts. In fact, studies consistently show that people who eat more foods rich in vitamin C have a lower risk of these diseases.[79] But study results are contradictory for vitamin C supplements.

Collagen Synthesis

We need vitamin C to form collagen, a fibrous protein that helps reinforce the **connective tissues** that hold together the structures of the body. Collagen is the most abundant protein in our bodies and the main fibrous component of skin, bone, tendons, cartilage, and teeth.

connective tissues Tissues composed primarily of fibrous proteins such as collagen and containing few cells. Their primary function is to bind together and support various body structures.

Other Vital Roles

Your body needs vitamin C to make many other essential compounds, among them thyroid hormone, steroid hormones, bile acids, the neurotransmitter serotonin, and parts of the DNA molecule. Also, vitamin C enhances the absorption of iron from plant foods.

Vitamin C enables lymphocytes and other cells in our immune system to function effectively. Based in part on the vitamin's importance to immunity, vitamin C has been reputed to prevent or cure the common cold. However, studies show that, at best, vitamin C may reduce the severity and duration of a cold somewhat.[80]

Think About It 4

Dietary Recommendations and Sources of Vitamin C

For adults the RDA for vitamin C is 90 milligrams per day for men and 75 milligrams per day for women, increasing to 85 milligrams per day during pregnancy and 120 milligrams during breastfeeding (levels far above the 5 or 10 milligrams required daily to prevent scurvy). Cigarette smoking increases the need for vitamin C by 35 milligrams per day.[81]

Many, but not all, fruits and vegetables are high in vitamin C. Good sources include citrus fruits, tomatoes, fortified juice drinks, broccoli,

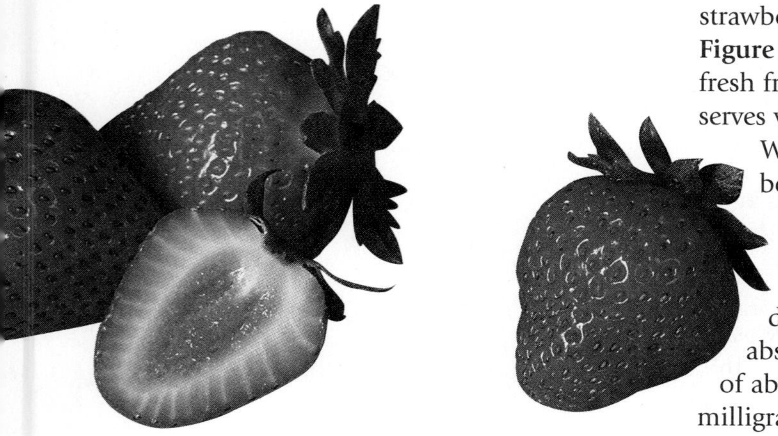

strawberries, kiwi fruit, cabbage, leafy greens, peppers, and potatoes. (See **Figure 9.34**.) Because vitamin C is highly vulnerable to heat and oxygen, fresh fruits and vegetables are best. Frozen orange juice concentrate preserves vitamin C content better than cartons of ready-to-drink orange juice. When choosing ready-to-drink juices, purchase them 3 to 4 weeks before the expiration date and consume them within 1 week of opening.[82]

The more vitamin C you consume, the less efficiently your intestines absorb the vitamin. If your intake is under 30 milligrams daily, you absorb nearly all of it. Between 30 and 120 milligrams, you absorb about 80 to 90 percent. As intake increases further, the efficiency of absorption continues to decline, falling to about 20 percent at 6,000 milligrams. Any excess vitamin C that is absorbed is excreted in urine.

Vitamin C Deficiency

After about a month on a diet without vitamin C, symptoms of scurvy start to surface. As the body loses its ability to synthesize collagen, connective tissue starts breaking down. Gums and joints begin to bleed. Small blood

Quick Bites

Chili Peppers Are Hot Stuff

An estimated one-quarter of the world's adults eat chili peppers every day. By weight, chili peppers are one of the richest sources of vitamins A and C. In addition, capsaicin, the substance that causes your mouth to burn, jump-starts the digestive process by stimulating salivation, gastric secretions, and gut motility.

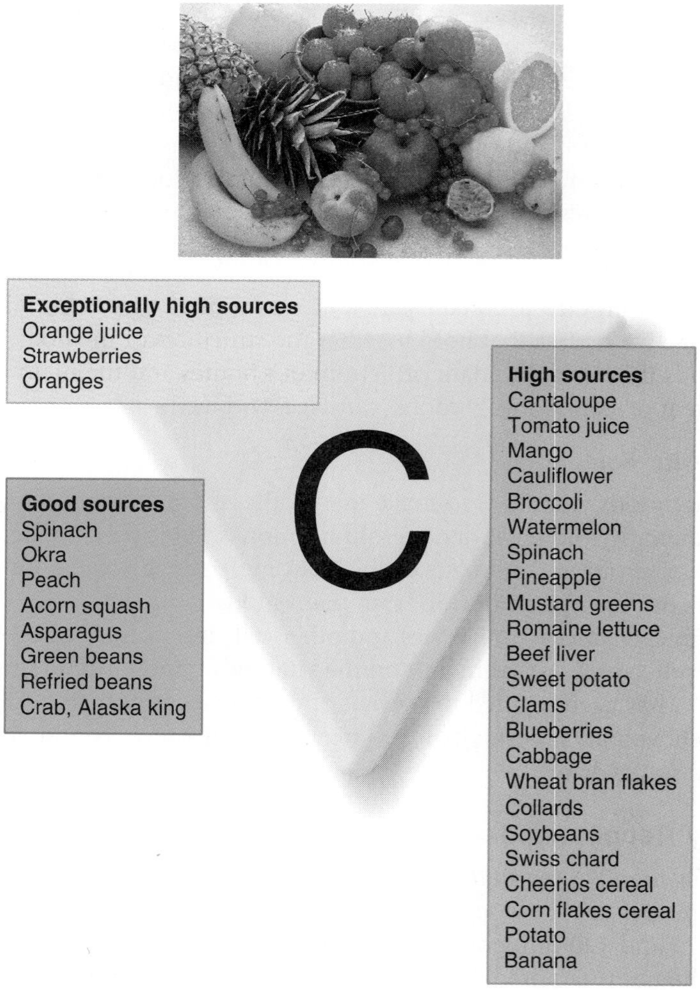

Figure 9.34 **Food sources of vitamin C.** Vitamin C is found mainly in fruits and vegetables. Although citrus fruits are notoriously good sources, many other popular fruits and vegetables are rich in vitamin C.

vessels break, and tiny hemorrhages appear just under the skin. Mild bruising produces exaggerated "black and blue marks." As the disease progresses, previously healed wounds reopen. Teeth are lost. Bone pain, fractures, diarrhea, and psychological problems such as depression appear. Left untreated, scurvy is fatal.

Scurvy is rare in developed countries, except among alcoholics or those on severely restricted diets.[83] Marginal deficiency is more common; its symptoms include sore, inflamed gums and fatigue.

Vitamin C Toxicity

Megadoses greater than 2,000 milligrams daily may cause abdominal cramps and diarrhea. In certain kidney conditions, excess vitamin C may cause kidney stones.[84] High vitamin C increases iron absorption—useful for some people, but problematic for those who already have too much body iron. (See the section on iron and hemochromatosis in Chapter 10, "Water and Minerals.") At megadose levels, some laboratory research suggests vitamin C may switch from its antioxidant role to encouraging oxidation.[85] The UL for vitamin C is 2,000 milligrams per day.

Key Concepts: *Vitamin C is found in many fruits and vegetables. It functions in collagen synthesis, acts as an antioxidant, helps boost iron absorption, plays a role in immunity, and helps synthesize many essential substances. Deficiency causes scurvy. Megadoses can cause digestive disturbance.*

Choline: A Vitamin-Like Substance

Choline is a vitamin-like substance, but differs from a true vitamin. You can synthesize most, but probably not all, of the choline you need. Men who stay on a choline-free diet develop a deficiency over time. For this reason dietary recommendations are now made for choline.

Along with vitamins B_{12}, B_6, and folate, choline helps metabolize homocysteine. But unlike most vitamins, choline is more than a catalyst or coenzyme. Most choline in your body is actually a component of other substances, such as the neurotransmitter acetylcholine. It is also a component of phospholipids. You may recall from Chapter 6, "Lipids," that a phospholipid has two fatty acids (responsible for solubility in fat) and choline (responsible for solubility in water). In cell membranes phospholipids help protect the cell, allowing only certain substances to enter and leave, and they help maintain the cell's shape. Throughout the body, phospholipids act as emulsifiers, enabling fatty substances to mix with water-soluble ones.

The AI for choline is 550 milligrams per day for adult men and 425 milligrams for women.[86] Milk, liver, egg yolk, and peanuts are good sources, but overall it is abundant in the food supply. Deficiency in healthy people is unlikely. A deficiency produces fat accumulation in the liver, then liver damage.

High doses of choline can cause diarrhea, falling blood pressure, and a disconcerting fishy body odor. The UL for choline is 3,500 milligrams per day.

Conditional Nutrients and Bogus Vitamins

Relatively speaking, there are few substances we need for life that our bodies cannot make. These substances are nutrients like vitamins that we must get from food. Our bodies routinely make countless other essential substances. However, under some circumstances—illnesses or inherited metabolic errors—we cannot make enough, so we must obtain them from our diets. These substances are "conditional nutrients." Inositol, carnitine, taurine, and lipoic acid are examples of nutrients that probably are conditional. Inositol helps form cell membrane phospholipids and precursors of eicosanoids, substances that work like hormones. Carnitine transports fatty acids to sites in the cell where your body can break them down. Taurine, derived from the amino acids methionine and cysteine, seems to play a role in such diverse functions as vision, insulin activity, and cell growth. Lipoic acid is a potent antioxidant and a necessary cofactor in many energy-releasing reactions. You may see conditional nutrients in dietary supplements, and they may be prescribed medically.

Bogus Vitamins

Some supplements contain clearly unnecessary substances. Yet hucksters often call them "vitamins" and tout their supposed benefits: "health boosters," "youth-enhancers," "physical performance enhancers," and the like. Other products are subtly and unethically promoted to cure disease. Despite ample scientific evidence to the contrary, quacks still hawk laetrile ("vitamin B_{17}") as a cancer cure. Some supplements contain hesperidin, para-aminobenzoic acid (PABA), pangamic acid, or rutin, even though these substances are not essential for human health. Think twice before you buy them.

Key Concepts: *The vitamin-like substance choline is a component of phospholipids and neurotransmitters. A conditional nutrient is not ordinarily required from our diet. People with certain medical conditions may benefit from supplements of some conditional nutrients.*

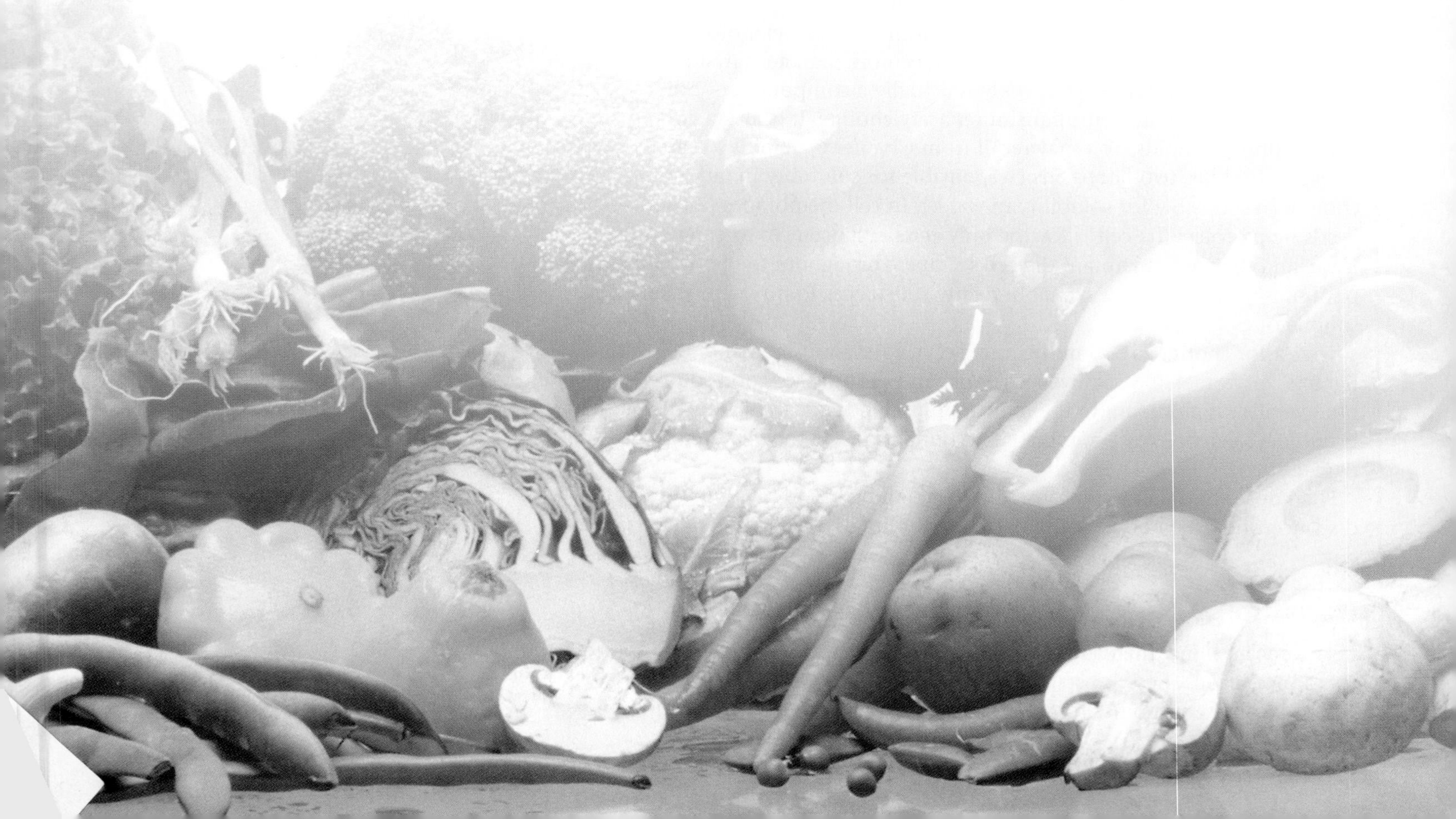

Label [to] Table

You've probably heard that milk is an excellent source of calcium, but did you know that milk also contains three of the four fat-soluble vitamins and contains a significant amount of some of the water-soluble vitamins? Let's take a look at the Nutrition Facts from a carton of nonfat milk.

Skim milk

Calories	*90*
Total Fat	*0*
Cholesterol	*less than 5 mg*
Sodium	*130 mg*
Total Carbohydrate	*13 g*
Dietary Fiber	*0 g*
Sugars	*12 g*
Protein	*9 g*
Vitamin A	*10% DV*
Vitamin C	*4% DV*
Calcium	*30% DV*
Iron	*0% DV*
Vitamin D	*25% DV*
Vitamin B_6	*5% DV*
Vitamin B_{12}	*15% DV*
Riboflavin	*18% DV*

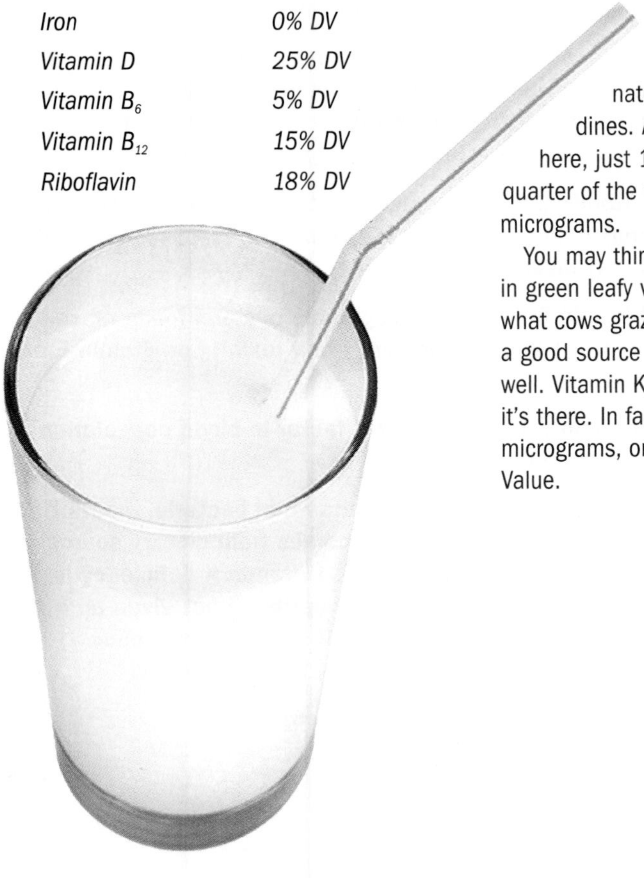

Milk contains the fat-soluble vitamins A, D, and K. Vitamin A is found naturally in whole milk, but all milk is fortified with this vitamin. That includes whole, reduced-fat, evaporated, powdered, lactose-free, and fat-free milks. (But yogurt, cheese, and ice cream are not generally fortified.) Fortification provides 10 percent of the Daily Value for vitamin A in 1 cup. Drink 3 cups in a day, and you'll get about a third of your recommended vitamin A. That's good news because dietary vitamin A is not always easy to obtain.

Keep in mind when selecting milk that nonfat (skim) milk contains vitamins A and D just like whole milk. Don't let the large banner "Vitamin A and D" printed on containers of whole milk trick you into thinking it contains more. It doesn't!

Vitamin D is important for bone health, because it helps with absorption of calcium and phosphorus. Fortifying milk with vitamin D assures that growing children will have the vitamin D they need, even if they don't get much sunlight or eat foods naturally rich in vitamin D like sardines. As shown on the nutrition label here, just 1 cup of milk gives you one-quarter of the vitamin D Daily Value, or 2.5 micrograms.

You may think of vitamin K as being mainly in green leafy vegetables. But just think about what cows graze. So it's not surprising milk is a good source of this fat-soluble vitamin as well. Vitamin K is not listed on the label, but it's there. In fact, 1 cup of milk provides 10 micrograms, or 13 percent of your Daily Value.

Let's take a look at a few of the water-soluble vitamins now since milk is a good source of those too. The vitamin C Daily Value is always required on food labels, but riboflavin and vitamins B_6 and B_{12} are not. They've been added here to emphasize that 1 cup of milk contributes 15 percent of your vitamin B_{12} and 18 percent of your riboflavin needs for the day. Notice that Vitamins C and B_6 are also found in milk at 4 percent and 5 percent of their Daily Value, respectively. This means drinking milk not only helps you grow and maintain a healthy skeleton but also provides B vitamins for other key body functions.

Nutrition Facts
Serving Size: 1 cup (240mL)
Servings Per Container about 8

Amount Per Serving	
Calories 90 Calories from fat 0	
	% Daily Value*
Total Fat 0g	0%
Saturated Fat 0g	0%
Cholesterol less than 5mg	1%
Sodium 130mg	5%
Total Carbohydrate 13g	4%
Dietary Fiber 0g	0%
Sugars 12g	
Protein 9g	18%
Vitamin A 10% •	Vitamin C 4%
Calcium 30% •	Iron 0%
Vitamin D 25%	

* Percent Daily Values are based on a 2,000 calorie diet. Your daily values may be higher or lower depending on your calorie needs:

	Calories:	2,000	2,500
Total Fat	Less Than	65g	80g
Sat Fat	Less Than	20g	25g
Cholesterol	Less Than	300mg	300mg
Sodium	Less Than	2,400mg	2,400mg
Total Carbohydrate		300g	375g
Dietary Fiber		25g	30g
Protein		50g	65g

Calories per gram:
Fat 9 • Carbohydrate 4 • Protein 4

AMOUNTS PER 1 CUP SERVING:	FAT
WHOLE MILK	8g
FAT FREE MILK	0g

INGREDIENTS: GRADE A FAT FREE MILK, VITAMIN A PALMITATE, VITAMIN D_3.

LEARNING Portfolio chapter 9

Key Terms

	page
anemia	328
anencephaly	334
ariboflavinosis	328
avidin	338
beriberi	325
bleaching process	307
calcitonin	316
calcitriol	316
carotenoids	306
cheilosis	328
cone cells	307
connective tissues	339
cornea	311
dark adaptation	307
dietary folate equivalents (DFE)	333
epithelial cells	308
epithelial tissues	308
glossitis	328
glutathione peroxidase	327
International Units (IU)	309
iodopsin	307
keratin	311
megaloblastic anemia	334
menadiones	322
menaquinones	322
microcytic hypochromic anemia	330
microencephaly	334
myelin sheath	336
neural tube defects (NTD)	333
niacin equivalents (NE)	328
night blindness	307
opsin	307
osteomalacia	318
osteoporosis	318
parathyroid hormone (PTH)	316
pernicious anemia	336
phylloquinone	322
provitamin A	309
provitamins	304
retina	307
retinal	306
retinoic acid	306
retinoids	306
retinol	306
retinol activity equivalent (RAE)	309
rhodopsin	307
rickets	318
rod cells	307
seborrheic dermatitis	328
spina bifida	334
stem cells	308
stomatitis	328
teratogen	312
thiamin pyrophosphate (TPP)	325
tocopherol	319
tocotrienol	319
tryptophan	328
vitamin precursors	304
xerophthalmia	311

Study Points

- There are two classes of vitamins: fat-soluble vitamins (A, D, E, and K) and water-soluble vitamins (eight B vitamins and vitamin C).
- Vitamin A comes from preformed retinoids and the precursor carotenoids. Sources include butterfat, liver, green leafy and yellow-orange vegetables, and yellow-orange fruits.
- Vitamin A is essential to vision, cell differentiation, growth and development, and immune function. Night blindness is an early symptom of vitamin A deficiency that, if not treated, can result in permanent blindness.
- In large doses, vitamin A is toxic. When taken during pregnancy, excess vitamin A may cause birth defects.
- Because UV light hitting the skin converts a cholesterol precursor to vitamin D, vitamin D is known as the "sunshine vitamin." Ultimately, the kidney converts this to the active form of vitamin D—calcitriol.
- Vitamin D in foods is available mainly from fortified milk and other fortified products.
- The primary function of vitamin D is the regulation of blood levels of calcium. Vitamin D deficiency contributes to skeletal problems. Vitamin D can be toxic at doses just a few times larger than the AI level.
- Vitamin E is an important antioxidant in the body and may help reduce the risk of chronic diseases such as heart disease and cancer.
- Vitamin E is found in vegetable oils and foods made from those oils. Deficiency and toxicity of vitamin E are relatively rare.
- Vitamin K is an important factor in blood coagulation and bone health.
- Although synthesized by intestinal bacteria, most of the vitamin K in the body comes from dietary sources, especially green vegetables. Vitamin K deficiency is rare, but newborns are susceptible if not given an injection of vitamin K at birth. Because the body excretes vitamin K easily, toxicity is unlikely.
- All B vitamins function as coenzymes.

- **Thiamin deficiency results in the classic disease beriberi. In industrialized countries, thiamin deficiency most often is associated with alcoholism. High doses of thiamin do not appear to be toxic.**
- **Milk is a good source of riboflavin, but light can destroy the vitamin. Packaging milk in paper or plastic cartons rather than clear glass better protects milk's riboflavin content.**
- **Niacin deficiency results in pellagra, a disease characterized by diarrhea, dermatitis, dementia, and death. High doses of niacin, such as in the treatment of high blood cholesterol, can have toxic side effects, including liver damage.**
- **Vitamin B_6, folate, and vitamin B_{12} work together to control blood levels of homocysteine. Increased intake of vitamin B_6 and folate is more important than vitamin B_{12} intake for lowering homocysteine levels.**
- **A deficiency of vitamin B_6 can lead to microcytic anemia—small, pale red blood cells.**
- **Poor folate status is associated with development of neural tube defects during pregnancy. Therefore, women of childbearing age need folic acid from foods or supplements in addition to other dietary folate.**
- **Deficiency of either folate or vitamin B_{12} can lead to megaloblastic anemia, but vitamin B_{12} deficiency (pernicious anemia) also causes irreversible nerve damage.**
- **Pantothenic acid is widespread in the food supply, and deficiency is virtually nonexistent. In the body, pantothenic acid is part of coenzyme A.**
- **Biotin deficiency is rare, but may be induced by regularly consuming large quantities of raw egg whites.**
- **Vitamin C (ascorbic acid) functions in the synthesis of collagen and other vital compounds and also works as an antioxidant. Vitamin C deficiency causes scurvy.**
- **Choline is a vitamin-like substance that the body makes but which, under some circumstances, must be supplied by diet.**

Study Questions

Answers can be found at nutrition.jbpub.com/discovering.

1. **List at least three characteristics of fat-soluble vitamins.**
2. **List at least three characteristics of water-soluble vitamins.**
3. **What are the main roles of vitamin A in the body? What is an early sign of vitamin A deficiency?**
4. **What is vitamin D's nickname? Why? Why is vitamin D also considered a hormone?**
5. **What is vitamin E's primary function and what are the best sources of vitamin E?**
6. **What is the best-known function of vitamin K?**
7. **Which two fat-soluble vitamins potentially are the most toxic? Which two are the least toxic?**
8. **List the nine water-soluble vitamins and one main function for each.**
9. **Name the diseases and/or characteristic symptoms of deficiencies of each water-soluble vitamin.**
10. **A lack of which three B vitamins can cause anemia? Describe the differences among these anemias.**
11. **List the water-soluble vitamins demonstrated to be toxic in large doses. What signs indicate toxic levels of each vitamin?**

Try This

The PUFA Protection Challenge: Vitamin E vs. Oxygen

The object of this experiment is to see if vitamin E protects polyunsaturated fats (PUFA) from oxidation. You'll need two glasses, one bottle of either safflower or corn oil, and some liquid vitamin E gel caps (can be purchased at any pharmacy). Pour equal amounts of oil in each of the glasses. Bite a hole in 10 of the vitamin E gel caps, squeeze their contents into *one* of the glasses, and stir. Mark this glass with tape and write the letter E on it. Let the glasses sit uncovered on a countertop for several days or weeks. Check the freshness or rancidity of the oils by smelling them and noting whether they look clear or cloudy. Over time, one will become more rancid than the other. Which glass container won the challenge—the one with or without vitamin E? Why?

Supplemental Income

The object of this exercise is to critically review vitamin supplements. Go to the drug store and look at a few multivitamin supplements and "stress" formulas. Look at the %DV for the water-soluble vitamins. Do you see any that have more than 1000% of the DV? Compare prices. Is it more expensive to buy supplements with more of these vitamins? Considering what you learned in this chapter, would it benefit you to take supplements that contain such a high amount of these vitamins? Why do you think supplements contain such large quantities of these vitamins?

What About Bobbie?

Let's take a look at Bobbie's intake of fat-soluble vitamin A and five water-soluble vitamins: thiamin, riboflavin, niacin, vitamin B_{12}, and vitamin C. Let's examine her day of eating (see Chapter 1) using the guidelines you've learned in this chapter. How did Bobbie do in terms of these vitamins?

She did well; she consumed ample amounts of most due to her varied food choices. Here is a summary of each of the vitamins.

Vitamin A

Bobbie's intake of 680 RAE is quite close to the RDA of 700 RAE, so Bobbie is likely meeting her needs for vitamin A. Her best sources of vitamin A were both preformed vitamin A sources (foods of animal origin such as cream cheese and pizza cheese) and foods with vitamin A precursors (e.g., beta-carotene from carrots).

Although Bobbie's intake of vitamin A was on target with her RDA, if this day's intake is typical of her usual eating pattern, she may want to try some of the following ideas to keep her vitamin A intake adequate:

- Use spinach greens as the base of her salad instead of iceberg lettuce.
- Continue adding shredded carrots to her salad and consider adding them to her sandwich too.
- Add a slice or two of tomato on top of the bagel with cream cheese.
- Alternate bagels (not high in vitamin A) and fortified cereals (high in vitamin A) for breakfast. This change also would add some milk to her diet, which would further increase her vitamin A intake (130 RAE per cup).

Thiamin

Bobbie consumed 1.8 milligrams of thiamin, which is 164 percent of the RDA of 1.1 milligrams. Most of the foods Bobbie ate this day contributed to her thiamin intake, but the ones that contributed the most were the enriched grains from the bread, bagel, and spaghetti.

Riboflavin

Bobbie consumed 1.9 milligrams of riboflavin on this day, or 171 percent of the RDA of 1.1 milligrams. As with thiamin, a variety of foods contributed to her riboflavin intake, but the enriched grains (bread, bagel, and pasta) were among the best contributors. The meatballs Bobbie ate at dinner also contributed riboflavin.

Niacin

Bobbie's intake of niacin also was above her RDA. She consumed 21.7 milligrams this day compared to her RDA of 14 milligrams. If you remember from the protein chapter that Bobbie's intake of protein was quite high, it shouldn't surprise you that her niacin intake is high, too. Meat, poultry, fish, and other protein-containing foods are some of the best sources of niacin. In this case, Bobbie's turkey sandwich, meatballs, and cheese pizza contributed niacin.

Vitamin B_{12}

Bobbie's intake of vitamin B_{12} (3.6 micrograms), like her intake of the other B vitamins, was above the RDA (2.4 micrograms). The foods that contributed to Bobbie's vitamin B_{12} intake were the animal products (turkey, egg, meatballs, parmesan cheese, and cheese pizza).

Vitamin C

Although Bobbie enjoys tomato products like salsa, spaghetti sauce, and pizza sauce, her intake of vitamin C (61 milligrams) was less than the RDA of 75 milligrams. Here are some other ways Bobbie could include more vitamin C in her diet:

- Have some orange or grapefruit juice with breakfast.
- Choose spinach, broccoli, or Brussels sprouts instead of green beans for dinner.
- Use spinach as the base of her salad instead of iceberg lettuce.
- Add some sliced red pepper to her salad at lunch.
- Have an orange as a snack instead of the tortilla chips.

References

1 Mahan KL, Escott-Stump S, eds. *Krause's Food, Nutrition & Diet Therapy*. Philadelphia: W.B. Saunders; 2000.
2 Institute of Medicine, Food and Nutrition Board. *Dietary Reference Intakes for Vitamin A, Vitamin K, Arsenic, Boron, Chromium, Copper, Iron, Manganese, Molybdenum, Nickel, Silicon, Vanadium, and Zinc*. Washington, DC: National Academy Press; 2001.
3 Guyton AC, Hall JE. *Textbook of Medical Physiology*. 10th ed. Philadelphia: W.B. Saunders; 2000.
4 McCollough FS, Northrop-Clewes CA, Thurnham DI. The effect of vitamin A on epithelial integrity. *Proc Nutr Soc*. 1999;58:289–293.
5 Semba RD. The role of vitamin A and related retinoids in immune function. *Nutr Rev*. 1998;56(1 pt 2):S38–48.
6 Institute of Medicine, Food and Nutrition Board. 2001. Op. cit.
7 Ibid.
8 Wood M. New clues about carotenes revealed. *Agricultural Res*. March 2001:12–13.
9 McCollough FS, Northrop-Clewes CA, Thurnham DI. Op. cit.
10 Stephensen CB. Vitamin A, infection, and immune function. *Annu Rev Nutr*. 2001;21:167–192.
11 Semba RD. Op. cit.
12 Feskanich D, Singh V, Willett WC, Colditz GA. Vitamin A intake and hip fractures among postmenopausal women. *JAMA*. 2002;287:47–54.
13 Rothman KJ, Moore LL, Singer MR, et al. Teratogenicity of high vitamin A intake. *N Engl J Med*. 1995;333(21):1360–1373; and Oakley GP, Erickson JD. Vitamin A and birth defects. *N Engl J Med*. 1995;333(21):1414–1415.
14 The Alpha-Tocopherol, Beta Carotene Cancer Prevention Study Group. The effect of vitamin E and beta carotene on the incidence of lung cancer and other cancers in male smokers. *N Engl J Med*. 1994;330:1029–1035; and Omenn GS, Goodman GE, Thornquist MD, et al. Effects of a combination of beta carotene and vitamin A on lung cancer and cardiovascular disease. *N Engl J Med*. 1996;334:1150–1155.
15 Koo J. Acne: psychological effects are more than skin deep. *Skin Care Today*. 1998;4:4–5.
16 Institute of Medicine, Food and Nutrition Board. *Dietary Reference Intakes for Vitamin C, Vitamin E, Selenium, and Carotenoids*. Washington, DC: National Academy Press; 2000.
17 Rock CL, Jacob RA, Bowen PE. Update on the biological characteristics of the antioxidant micronutrients: vitamin C, vitamin E, and the carotenoids. *J Am Diet Assoc*. 1996;96:693–702.
18 Ibid.
19 Institute of Medicine, Food and Nutrition Board. 2000. Op. cit.
20 Rock CL, Jacob RA, Bowen PE. Op. cit.; and Zhang LX, Cooney RV, Bertram JS. Carotenoids up-regulate connexin43 gene expression independent of their provitamin A or antioxidant properties. *Cancer Res*. 1992;52:5707–5712.
21 Giovannucci E. Tomatoes, tomato-based products, lycopene, and cancer: review of the epidemiologic literature. *J Natl Cancer Inst*. 1991;91:317–331.
22 Institute of Medicine, Food and Nutrition Board. 2000. Op. cit.
23 Mathews-Roth MM. Carotenoids in erythropoietic protoporphyria and other photosensitivity diseases. *Ann NY Acad Sci*. 1993;691:127–138.
24 Santos MS, Meydani SN, Leka L, et al. Natural killer cell activity in elderly men is enhanced by beta-carotene supplementation. *Am J Clin Nutr*. 1996;64:772–777; and Hughes DA, Wright AJ, Finglas PM, et al. The effect of beta-carotene supplementation on the immune function of blood monocytes from healthy male nonsmokers. *J Lab Clin Med*. 1997;129:309–317.
25 Institute of Medicine, Food and Nutrition Board. 2001. Op. cit.
26 Eastell R, Riggs BL. Vitamin D and osteoporosis. In: Feldman D, Glorieux FH, Piek JW, eds. *Vitamin D*. San Diego: Academic Press; 1997:695–711.
27 Institute of Medicine, Food and Nutrition Board. *Dietary Reference Intakes for Calcium, Phosphorus, Magnesium, Vitamin D, and Fluoride*. Washington, DC: National Academy Press; 1997.
28 Ibid.
29 Need AG, Morris HA, Horowitz M, Nordin C. Effects of skin thickness, age, body fat, and sunlight on serum 25-hydroxyvitamin D. *Am J Clin Nutr*. 1993;58:882–885; and Holick MF, Matsuoka LY, Wortsman J. Age, vitamin D, and solar ultraviolet [letter]. *Lancet*. 1989;2(8671):1104–1105.
30 Gessner BD, de Schweinitz E, Petersen KM, Lewandowski C. Nutritional rickets among breast-fed black and Alaska Native children. *Alaska Med*. 1997;39:72–74, 87; Severe malnutrition among young children—Georgia, January 1997–June 1999. *MMWR*. 2001;50:224–227; and Rowe P. Why is rickets resurgent in the USA? *Lancet* 2001;357:1100.
31 Utiger RD. The need for more vitamin D. *N Engl J Med*. 1998;328:828–829.
32 Eastell R, Riggs BL. Vitamin D and osteoporosis. In: Feldman D, Glorieux FH, Piek JW, eds. Op. cit., 695–711; and Chapuy M-C, Meunier PJ. Vitamin D insufficiency in adults and the elderly. In: Feldman D, Glorieux FH, Piek JW, eds. Op. cit., 679–693.
33 Chapuy MC, Arlot ME, Duboeuf F, et al. Vitamin D3 and calcium to prevent hip fractures in elderly women. *N Engl J Med*. 1992;327:1637–1642; Chapuy MC, Arlot ME, Delmas PD, Meunier PJ. Effect of calcium and cholecalciferol treatment for three years on hip fractures in elderly women. *BMJ*. 1994;308:1081–1082.
34 Thomas MK, Lloyd-Jones DM, Thadhani RF, et al. Hypovitaminosis D in medical inpatients. *N Engl J Med*. 1998;338:777–783.
35 Jialal I, Traber M, Devaraj S. Is there a vitamin E paradox? *Curr Opin Lipidol*. 2001;12:49–53; and Kaul N, Devaraj S, Jialal I. Alpha-tocopherol and atherosclerosis. *Exp Biol Med*. 2001;226:5–12.
36 Institute of Medicine, Food and Nutrition Board. 2000. Op. cit.
37 Ibid.
38 Ibid.
39 Horwitt MK. Critique of the requirement for vitamin E. *Am J Clin Nutr*. 2001;73:1003–1005.
40 Ibid.
41 Sokoll LJ, Booth SL, O'Brien ME, et al. Changes in serum osteocalcin, plasma phylloquinone, and urinary g-carboxyglutamic acid in response to altered intakes of dietary phylloquinone in human subjects. *Am J Clin Nutr*. 1997;65:779–784.
42 Institute of Medicine, Food and Nutrition Board. 2001. Op. cit.

43 Booth SL, Davidson KW, Lichtenstein AH, Sadowski JA. Plasma concentrations of dihydro-vitamin K1 following dietary intake of a hydrogenated vitamin K1-rich vegetable oil. *Lipids.* 1996;31:709–713; and Fenton ST, Price RJ, Bolton-Smith C, Harrington D, Shearer MJ. Nutrient sources of phylloquinone (vitamin K1) in Scottish men and women [abstract]. *Proc Nutr Soc.* 1997;56:301.
44 Shearer MJ, Bach A, Kohlmeier M. Chemistry, nutritional sources, tissue distribution and metabolism of vitamin K with special reference to bone health. *J Nutr.* 1996;126(suppl): 1181S–1186S.
45 "Special K" takes on new meaning. *Tufts University Health & Nutrition Letter.* 1997;15(5):1, 7.
46 Booth SL, Charnley JM, Sadowski JA, et al. Dietary vitamin K1 and stability of oral anticoagulation: proposal of a diet with constant vitamin K1 content. *Thromb Haemost.* 1997;77:504–509.
47 Institute of Medicine, Food and Nutrition Board. *Dietary Reference Intakes for Thiamin, Riboflavin, Niacin, Vitamin B6, Folate, Vitamin B12, Pantothenic Acid, Biotin, and Choline.* Washington, DC: National Academy Press; 1998.
48 Prinzo ZW. Thiamine deficiency and its prevention and control in major emergencies. WHO. 1999;1–5. http://www.who.int/nut/documents/thiamine_in_emergencies_eng.pdf. Accessed 4-27-02.
49 Institute of Medicine, Food and Nutrition Board. 1998. Op. cit.
50 Ibid.
51 McCormick DB. Two interconnected B vitamins: riboflavin and pyridoxine. *Physiol Rev.* 1989;69:1170–1198.
52 Institute of Medicine, Food and Nutrition Board. 1998. Op. cit.
53 Carpenter KJ, Lewin WJ. A reexamination of the composition of diets associated with pellagra. *J Nutr.* 1985;115:543–552.
54 McKenney JM, Proctor JD, Harris S, Chinchili VM. A comparison of the efficacy and toxic effects of sustained- vs. immediate-release niacin in hypercholesterolemic patients. *JAMA.* 1994;271:672–677.
55 Ibid; and Gibbons LW, Gonzalez V, Gordon N, Grundy S. The prevalence of side effects with regular and sustained-release nicotinic acid. *Am J Med.* 1995;99:378–385.
56 Institute of Medicine, Food and Nutrition Board. 1998. Op. cit.
57 Rimm EB, Willett WC, Hu FB, et al. Folate and vitamin B6 from diet and supplements in relation to risk of coronary heart disease among women. *JAMA.* 1998;279:359–364.
58 Institute of Medicine, Food and Nutrition Board. 1998. Op. cit.
59 Ibid.
60 Wyatt KM, Dimmock PW, Jones PW, Shaughn O'Brien PM. Efficacy of vitamin B-6 in the treatment of premenstrual syndrome: systematic review. *BMJ.* 1999;318(7195):1375–1381.
61 Franzblau A. The relationship of vitamin B6 status to median nerve function and carpal tunnel syndrome among active industrial workers. *J Occup Environ Med.* 1996;38:485–491.
62 Schaumberg H, Kaplan J, Windebank A, et al. Sensory neuropathy from pyridoxine abuse. *N Engl J Med.* 1983;309: 445–448.
63 Brent RL, Oakley GP Jr, Mattison DR. The unnecessary epidemic of folic acid-preventable spina bifida and anencephaly. *Pediatrics.* 2000;106:825–827.
64 Institute of Medicine, Food and Nutrition Board. 1998. Op. cit.
65 Giovannucci E, Stampfer MJ, Colditz GA, et al. Multivitamin use, folate, and colon cancer in women in the Nurses' Health Study. *Ann Intern Med* 1998;129:517–524.
66 Institute of Medicine, Food and Nutrition Board. 1998. Op. cit.; and Suitor CW, Bailey LB. Dietary folate equivalents: interpretation and application. *J Am Diet Assoc.* 2000;100:88–94.
67 Institute of Medicine, Food and Nutrition Board. 1998. Op. cit.; and Mills JL. Fortification of foods with folic acid: how much is enough? *N Engl J Med.* 2000;342:1442–1445.
68 US Department of Health and Human Services. FDA announces name changes for lower-fat milks and folic acid fortification for bakery products. *HHS News;* December 31, 1997.
69 Lawrence JM, Petitti DB, Watkins M, et al. Trends in serum folate after food fortification. *Lancet.* 1999;354:915–916; and Caudill MA, Le T, Moonie SA, et al. Folate status in women of childbearing age residing in Southern California after folic acid fortification. *J Am Coll Nutr.* 2001;20(suppl2):129–134.
70 Molloy AM, Daly S, Mills JL, et al. Thermolabile variant of 5,10-methylenetetrahydrofolate reductase associated with low red-cell folates: implications for folate intake recommendations. *Lancet.* 1997;349:1591–1593.
71 Knowledge and use of folic acid among women of reproductive age—Michigan 1998. *MMWR.* 2001;50:185–190.
72 Hurwitz A, Brady DA, Schaal SE, et al. Gastric acidity in older adults. *JAMA.* 1997;278:659–662.
73 Kuzminski AM, Del Giacco EJ, Allen RH, et al. Effective treatment of cobalamin deficiency with oral cobalamin. *Blood.* 1998;92:1191–1198.
74 Sarubin A. *The Health Professional's Guide to Popular Dietary Supplements.* Chicago, IL: The American Dietetic Association; 2000.
75 Institute of Medicine, Food and Nutrition Board. 1998. Op. cit.
76 Ibid.
77 Ibid.
78 Sauberlich HE. Pharmacology of vitamin C. *Ann Rev Nutr.* 1994;14:371.
79 Khaw KT, Bingham S, Luben R, et al. Relation between plasma ascorbic acid and mortality in men and women in EPIC-Norfolk prospective study: a prospective population study. *Lancet.* 2001;357:657–663.
80 Ibid.
81 Institute of Medicine, Food and Nutrition Board. Op. cit. 2000.
82 Johnston CS, Bowling DL. Stability of ascorbic acid in commercially available orange juices. *J Am Diet Assoc.* 2002;102: 525–529.
83 Institute of Medicine, Food and Nutrition Board. 2000. Op. cit.
84 Ibid.
85 Halliwell B. Antioxidants: sense or speculation? *Nutr Today.* 1994;29:15–19.
86 Institute of Medicine, Food and Nutrition Board. 1998. Op. cit.

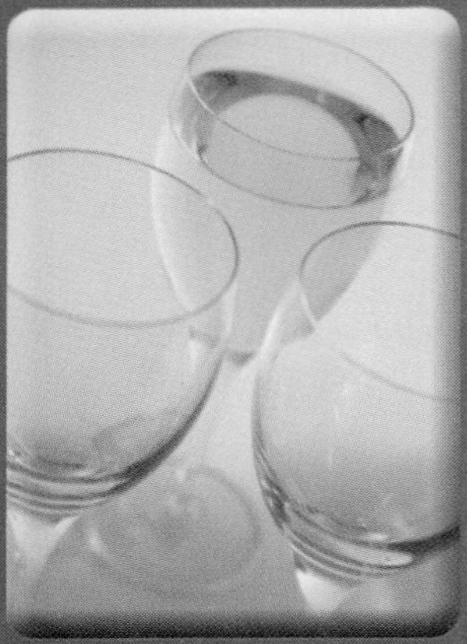
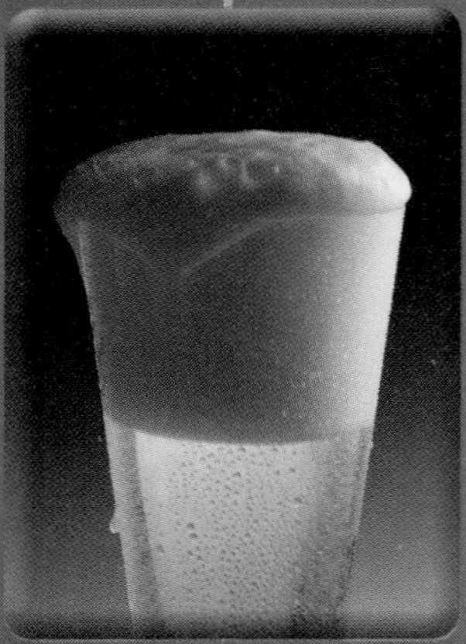
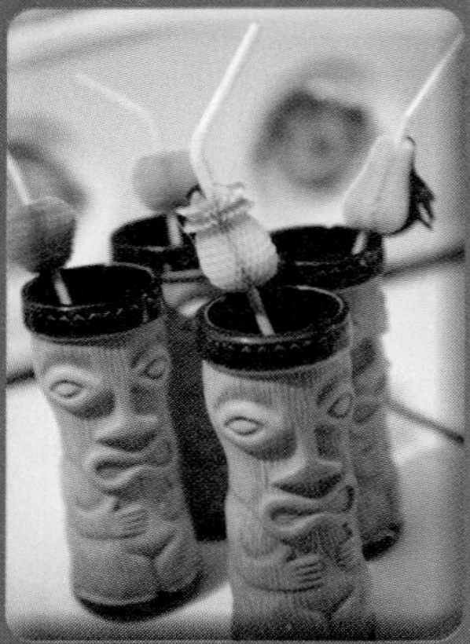
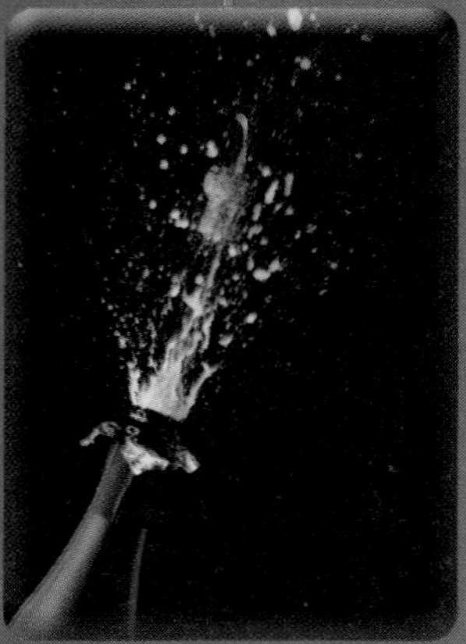
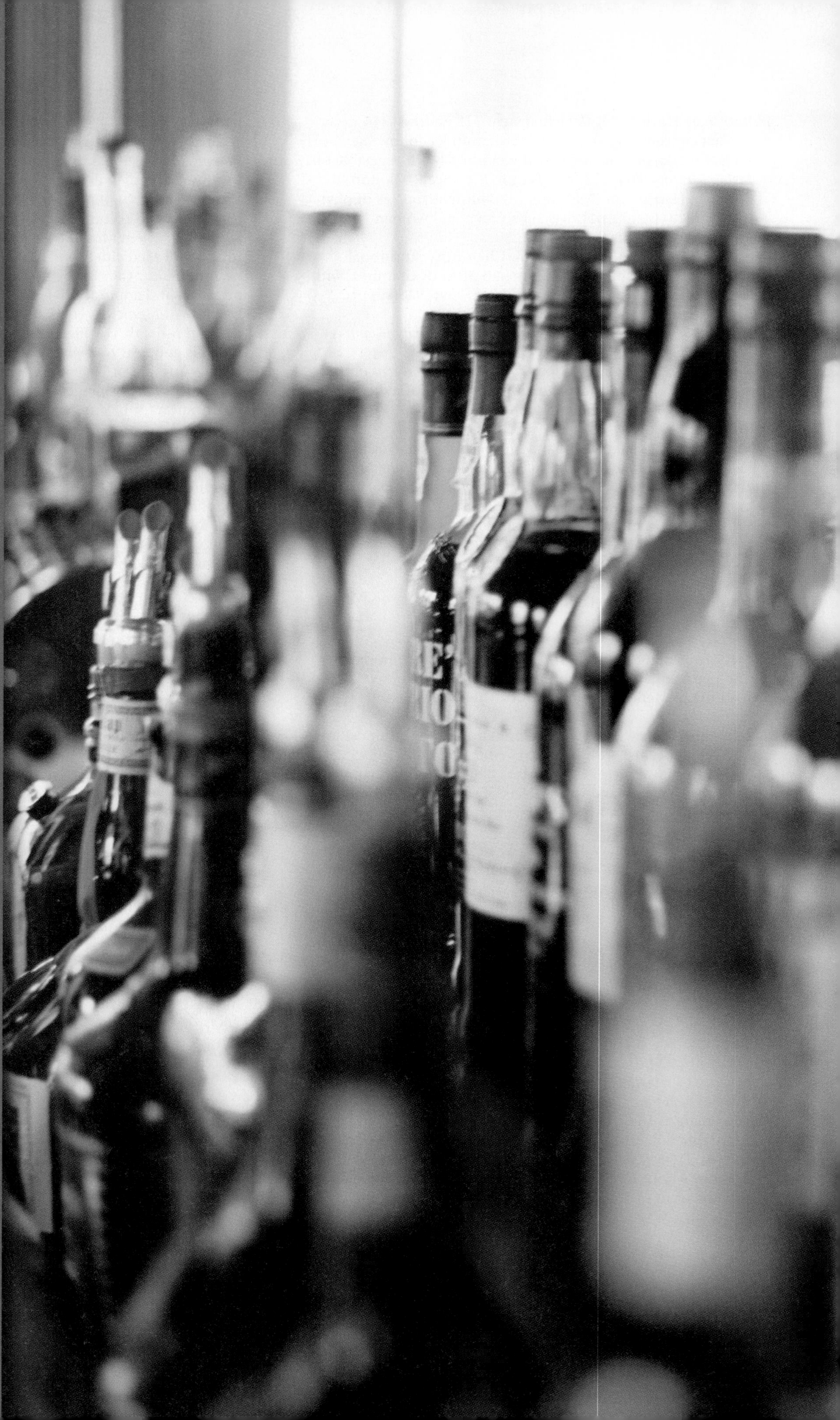

Spotlight on Alcohol

Think About It

1 In a word or two, how would you describe alcohol? Is it a nutrient?

2 What's your impression of the alcohol content of wine compared with that of beer? How about compared with vodka?

3 Have you ever thought of alcohol as a poison?

4 After a night of drinking and carousing, your friend awakens with a splitting headache and asks you for a pain reliever. What would you recommend?

Fyi for your Information

This chapter's FYI boxes include practical information on the following topics:

- College Drinking Culture
- Myths about Alcohol

WWW

The Web site for this book offers many useful tools and is a great source for additional nutrition information for both students and instructors. For information on alcohol, visit the site at **nutrition.jbpub.com/discovering.** You'll find exercises that explore the following topics:

- The Legal Age Around the World
- Time to Hand Over the Car Keys?
- Diabetics and Alcohol
- The Culture of Alcohol

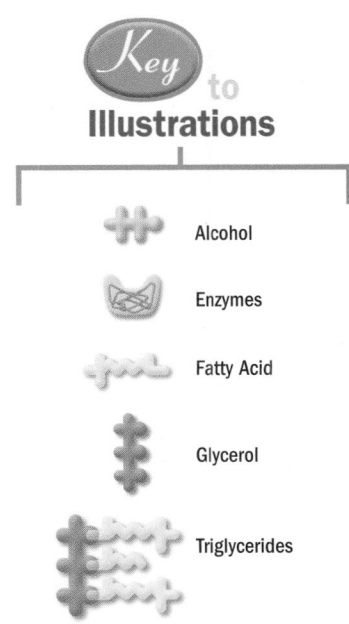

Key to Illustrations

- Alcohol
- Enzymes
- Fatty Acid
- Glycerol
- Triglycerides

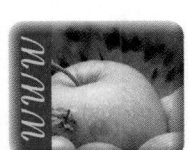

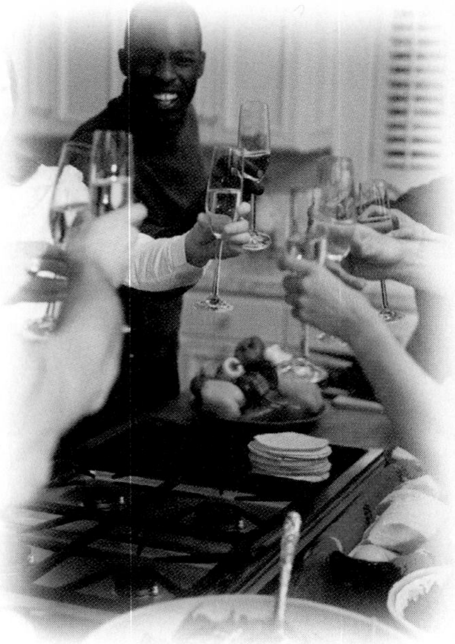

Think about alcohol. What image comes to mind: Champagne toasts? Elegant gourmet dining? Hearty family meals in the European countryside? Or do you think of wild parties? Or sick, out-of-control drunks? Violence? Car accidents? Broken homes? No other food or beverage has the power to elicit such strong, disparate images—images that reflect both the healthfulness of alcohol in moderation, the devastation of excess, and the political, social, and moral issues surrounding alcohol.

Alcohol has a long and somewhat checkered history. More drug than food, alcoholic beverages produce druglike effects in the body while providing little, if any, nutrient value other than energy. Yet there are several reasons why it still is important to consider alcohol in the study of nutrition. Alcohol is common to the diets of many people. In moderation, it may have significant health benefits, yet even small quantities can raise risks for birth defects and breast cancer. In large amounts, it interferes with our intake of nutrients as well as the body's ability to use them, and it causes significant damage to every organ system in the body. The *Dietary Guidelines for Americans* advise us, "If you drink alcoholic beverages, do so in moderation."

Quick Bites

Preferred Beverages

Beer is the national beverage of Germany and Britain. Wine is the national beverage of Greece and Italy.

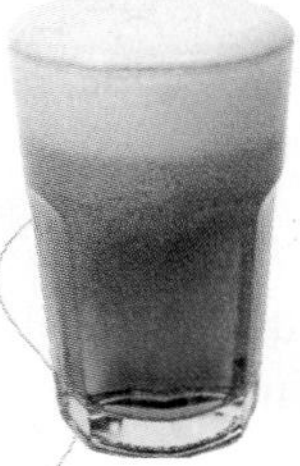

For most people, alcohol consumption is a pleasant social activity. Moderate alcohol use is not harmful for most adults. Nonetheless, many people have serious trouble with drinking. Heavy drinking can increase the risk for certain cancers. It can also cause liver cirrhosis, brain damage, and harm to the fetus during pregnancy. In addition, drinking increases the risk of death from automobile crashes, recreational accidents, and on-the-job accidents and also increases the likelihood of homicide and suicide.

History of Alcohol Use

Alcohol has had a prominent role throughout history. Old religious and medical writings frequently recommend its use, although with warnings for moderation. Thanks to alcohol's antiseptic properties, fermented drinks were safer than water during the centuries before modern sanitation, especially as people moved to towns and villages where water supplies were contaminated. Even mixing alcohol with dirty water afforded some protection from bacteria.[1]

At a time when life was filled with physical and emotional hardships, people valued alcohol for its analgesic and euphoric qualities. People relied on it to lift spirits, ease boredom, numb hunger, and dull the discomfort, even pain, of daily routine. Before the twentieth century, it was one of the few painkillers available in the Western world.

In sharp contrast to what is allowed today, drinking was often encouraged at the work site. Workers might be given alcohol as an inducement to do boring, painful, or dangerous jobs. Distilled spirits, beer, and wine accompanied sailors and passengers on all long voyages, supplying relatively pathogen-free fluid and calories. Legend has it that even the Puritans, a group known for rigid morality, disembarked at Plymouth Rock because their beer supply was depleted.[2]

The Character of Alcohol

Although there are many types of alcohol, the term **alcohol** commonly refers to the specific alcohol compound in beer, wine, and spirits. (See **Figure SA.1**.) Its technical name is **ethanol**, or **ethyl alcohol**. Ethanol is commonly abbreviated to "EtOH," shorthand often preferred by health professionals. In this chapter, when we use the term *alcohol*, we are referring to ethanol.

Other types of alcohol are unsafe to drink. The simplest alcohol is **methanol**, also called **methyl alcohol** or **wood alcohol**, a solvent used in paints and for woodworking. Some years ago, down-on-their-luck alcoholics thought they had discovered a way to save money—wood alcohol used at that time to heat chafing dishes was intoxicating but considerably cheaper than beer or wine. Unfortunately, methanol caused blindness and death. Methanol is no longer used in these products, but methanol poisoning from other sources still occurs.[3] Today, methanol is used in a number of consumer products, including paint strippers, duplicator fluid, model airplane fuel, and dry gas. Most windshield washer fluids are 50 percent methanol.

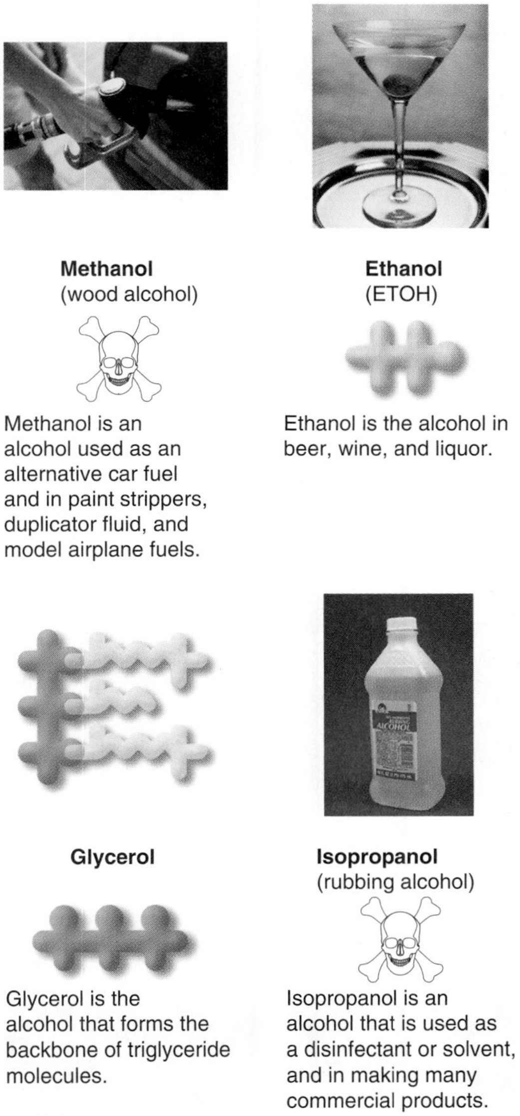

Methanol
(wood alcohol)
Methanol is an alcohol used as an alternative car fuel and in paint strippers, duplicator fluid, and model airplane fuels.
Ethanol
(ETOH)
Ethanol is the alcohol in beer, wine, and liquor.
Glycerol
Glycerol is the alcohol that forms the backbone of triglyceride molecules.
Isopropanol
(rubbing alcohol)
Isopropanol is an alcohol that is used as a disinfectant or solvent, and in making many commercial products.

Figure SA.1 **Alcohols.** Ethanol is not the only alcohol people consume. When people eat fat, they consume the alcohol glycerol. Consuming the alcohol methanol or isopropanol can be deadly.

Alcohol: Is It a Nutrient?

Alcohol eludes easy classification. Like fat, protein, and carbohydrate, it provides energy when metabolized. Laboratory experiments in the nineteenth century demonstrated that upon oxidation pure alcohol releases 7 kilocalories per gram, but many people doubted it actually produced energy in the body. These doubts were the basis of the controversial conclusion that alcohol was not food—a conclusion used by early Prohibitionists in their fight against alcohol. (See **Figure SA.2**.) However, energy researchers Francis Atwater and Wilbur Benedict did a series of experiments which showed that alcohol did indeed produce 7 kilocalories per gram in the body—findings that were a great disappointment to the Temperance Movement because it showed alcohol was a food.[4]

But alcohol's status as a nutrient is more questionable. It is certainly different from any other substance in the diet. It provides energy but is not essential, performing no necessary function in the body. Unlike the nutrients, alcohol is not stored in the body. It provides calories, but chronic overconsumption does not usually lead to obesity. And for no nutrient are the dangers of overconsumption so dramatic and the window of safety so narrow. In the small amounts most people usually consume, alcohol acts as a drug, producing a pleasant euphoria. For some people, it is addictive, with the characteristics of tolerance, dependence, and withdrawal symptoms. Certainly alcohol is a substance available in the diet, but it does *not* meet the definition of a nutrient.

Think About It 1

Key Concepts: *Alcohol, or more specifically, the compound ethyl alcohol, has been part of people's diets for thousands of years. Although it provides calories, alcohol performs no essential function in the body and, therefore, is not a nutrient.*

alcohol Common name for ethanol or ethyl alcohol. As a general term, it refers to any organic compound with one or more hydroxyl (–OH) groups.

ethanol Chemical name for drinking alcohol. Also known as ethyl alcohol.

ethyl alcohol See *ethanol.*

methanol The simplest alcohol. Also known as methyl alcohol and wood alcohol.

methyl alcohol See *methanol.*

wood alcohol Common name for methanol.

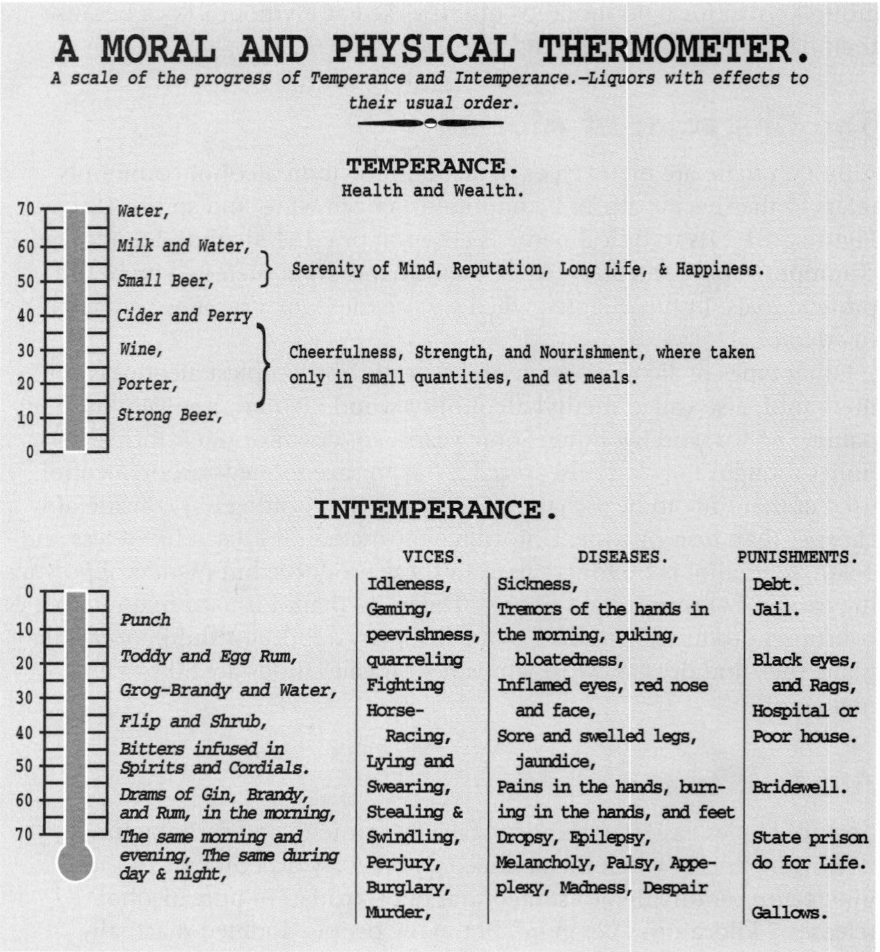

A MORAL AND PHYSICAL THERMOMETER.

A scale of the progress of Temperance and Intemperance.–Liquors with effects to their usual order.

TEMPERANCE.

Health and Wealth.

Scale	Liquors	Effects
70	*Water,*	
60	*Milk and Water,*	Serenity of Mind, Reputation, Long Life, & Happiness.
50	*Small Beer,*	
40	*Cider and Perry*	Cheerfulness, Strength, and Nourishment, where taken only in small quantities, and at meals.
30	*Wine,*	
20	*Porter,*	
10	*Strong Beer,*	
0		

INTEMPERANCE.

Scale	Liquors	VICES.	DISEASES.	PUNISHMENTS.
0		Idleness,	Sickness,	Debt.
10	*Punch*	Gaming, peevishness,	Tremors of the hands in the morning, puking,	Jail.
20	*Toddy and Egg Rum,*	quarreling	bloatedness,	Black eyes,
30	*Grog-Brandy and Water,*	Fighting	Inflamed eyes, red nose and face,	and Rags,
40	*Flip and Shrub,*	Horse-Racing,	Sore and swelled legs,	Hospital or Poor house.
50	*Bitters infused in Spirits and Cordials.*	Lying and Swearing,	jaundice,	
60	*Drams of Gin, Brandy, and Rum, in the morning,*	Stealing & Swindling,	Pains in the hands, burning in the hands, and feet	Bridewell.
70	*The same morning and evening, The same during day & night,*	Perjury, Burglary, Murder,	Dropsy, Epilepsy, Melancholy, Palsy, Appeplexy, Madness, Despair	State prison do for Life. Gallows.

Figure SA.2 **A moral and physical thermometer of temperance and intemperance.** As part of a late eighteenth century temperance movement, Philadelphian Dr. Benjamin Rush (1745–1813) created the *Moral and Physical Thermometer* and distributed it to the clergy in a campaign against heavy drinking.

Source: Reprinted with permission from *Quarterly Journal of Studies on Alcohol*, vol 4, pp. 321–341, 1943 (presently *Journal of Studies on Alcohol*). Copyright Journal of Studies on Alcohol, Inc., Rutgers Center of Alcohol Studies, Piscataway, NJ 08854.

fermentation The anaerobic conversion of various carbohydrates to carbon dioxide and an alcohol or organic acid.

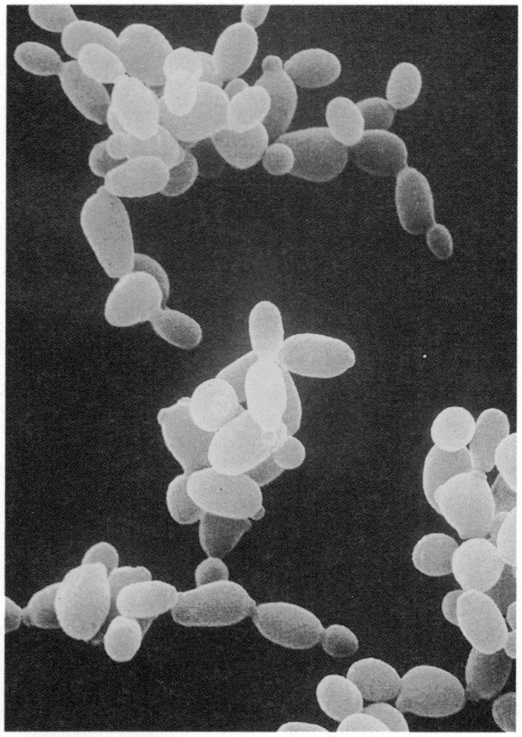

Figure SA.3 A micrograph of a yeast plant.

Formation or Production of Alcohol and Its Sources

When yeast cells metabolize sugar, they produce alcohol and carbon dioxide by a process called **fermentation**. If little oxygen is present, these cells produce more alcohol and less carbon dioxide. **Figure SA.3** shows living yeast cells.

Fermentation can occur spontaneously in nature—all that's needed is sugar, water, a warm environment, and yeast (whose spores are present in air and soil). Human experience with alcohol probably began at least 10,000 years ago with spontaneously fermented fruits or honey. It's reasonable to assume that humans have always had small quantities of alcohol in their diets, since all humans possess the enzymes to metabolize at least minimal amounts of alcohol.[5] Very small amounts of alcohol are even produced by the microorganisms in our intestines.

Humans probably learned to make wine from fruits, mead from honey, and beer from grain about 5,000 years ago. In some areas, people made alcohol-containing dairy products. Using simple yeast fermentation, they could not produce beverages with alcohol levels above 16 percent—the point at which alcohol kills off the yeast, halting alcohol production. Later, seventh-century Egyptian chemists discovered how to use distillation to capture concentrated alcohol, which could be added to drinks to boost alcohol content. Distilled alcoholic beverages (such as rum, gin, and whiskey) are called spirits, liquor, or hard liquor.

Think About It 2

Beer, wine, and liquor have different alcohol levels: Most beer is up to 5 percent alcohol, although some beers exceed 6 percent; wine is 8 to 14 percent alcohol; and hard liquor is typically 35 to 45 percent alcohol. Beer and wine are labeled with the percentage of alcohol, but hard liquor is labeled by "proof," which is twice the alcohol percentage (an 80 proof whiskey is 40 percent alcohol).

Pure alcohol, a clear, colorless liquid used in chemistry labs, is 95 percent alcohol. (Even "pure" alcohol contains some water.) The beverage closest to pure alcohol is vodka, which is alcohol and water and almost nothing else; gin is similar but flavored with juniper berries. Scotch, rum, rye, whiskeys, and other liquors have residual flavor traces of the grain from which they were fermented or flavors introduced during storage. All liquors, however, contain little of nutritional value besides energy. Beer and wine do contain unfermented carbohydrates and a trace of protein but, like liquor, have negligible minerals. With the exception of niacin in beer, alcoholic beverages have negligible vitamins as well. **Table SA.1** shows the number of calories in various alcoholic beverages.

Quick Bites

Nutrients in Beer?

Most of the carbohydrate used in the production of alcohol is converted to ethanol. In beer, however, some carbohydrate remains, along with a little protein and some vitamins. So while it is technically correct to say there are nutrients in beer, the amounts are small when beer is consumed at recommended low levels.

Table SA.1 Calories and Alcohol in Selected Beverages

Beverage	Serving Size	Kcalories	Alcohol (g)
Light beer	12 fl oz	99	11.3
Beer	12 fl oz	146	12.8
White table wine	4.5 fl oz	90	12.3
Red table wine	4.5 fl oz	95	12.3
Dessert wine	4.5 fl oz	203	20.2
Distilled beverages (gin, rum, vodka, whiskey)			
80 proof	1.5 fl oz	97	14.0
86 proof	1.5 fl oz	105	15.1
90 proof	1.5 fl oz	110	15.9
94 proof	1.5 fl oz	116	16.7
100 proof	1.5 fl oz	124	17.9
Coffee liqueur, 53 proof	1.5 fl oz	175	11.9
Bloody Mary cocktail	4 fl oz	92	11.1
Daiquiri cocktail	4 fl oz	224	27.8
Whiskey sour cocktail	4 fl oz	163	20.1
Tequila sunrise cocktail	4 fl oz	137	11.6
Piña colada cocktail	4 fl oz	233	12.4

Sources: US Department of Agriculture, Agricultural Research Service. 2001. *USDA Nutrient Database for Standard Reference*, Release 14. Nutrient Data Laboratory Home Page, http://www.nal.usda.gov/fnic/foodcomp. Accessed 4/27/02; and Pennington JAT. *Bowes and Church's Food Values of Portions Commonly Used.* 17th ed. Philadelphia: Lippincott-Raven; 1998.

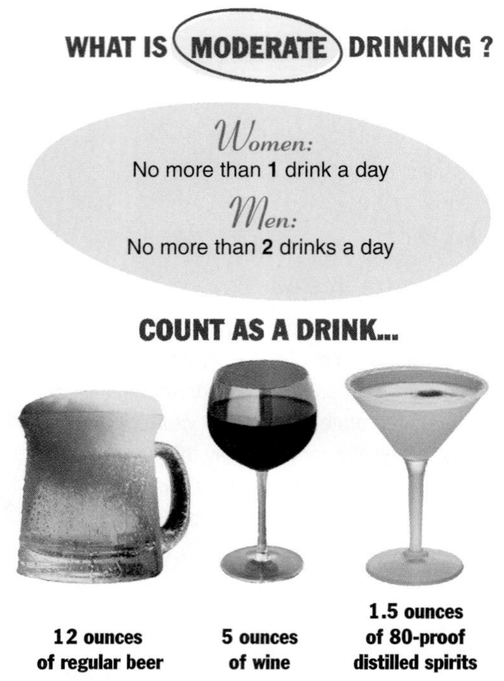
WHAT IS MODERATE DRINKING ?
Women:
No more than 1 drink a day
Men:
No more than 2 drinks a day
COUNT AS A DRINK...
12 ounces of regular beer
5 ounces of wine
1.5 ounces of 80-proof distilled spirits

Figure SA.4 **Moderate drinking.**
Source: USDA Center for Nutrition Policy and Promotion.

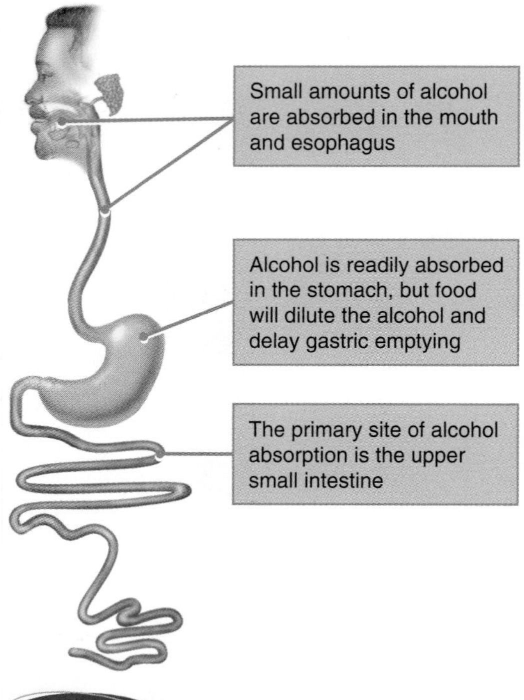
Small amounts of alcohol are absorbed in the mouth and esophagus
Alcohol is readily absorbed in the stomach, but food will dilute the alcohol and delay gastric emptying
The primary site of alcohol absorption is the upper small intestine

Figure SA.5 **Alcohol absorption.** Alcohol easily diffuses in and out of cells, so most alcohol is absorbed unchanged.

Distillation can yield more than just ethanol. Traces of other compounds, such as methanol, evaporate and then condense in the distilled product. These are called **congeners**. These biologically active compounds help to create the distinctive taste, smell, and appearance of alcoholic beverages like whiskey, brandy, and red wine. But congeners are also suspected of causing or contributing to hangovers and may play a role in alcohol's relationship to cancer.[6]

One serving of alcohol, or a **standard drink**, is generally defined as 12 ounces of beer, 4 to 5 ounces of wine, or 1½ ounces (a "jigger") of liquor. All contain roughly 15 grams (1 measuring tablespoon) of pure alcohol. Most health professionals who speak of "moderate alcohol intake" usually mean no more than one (for women) or two (for men) servings in a day.[7] (See **Figure SA.4**.) Moderate intake is not an average of seven drinks per week, when there are six days of abstinence followed by seven drinks in one night! That's **binge drinking**, and it's dangerous.

Key Concepts: *Alcohol is formed when yeast ferments sugars to yield energy. Distillation methods produce concentrated solutions, with up to 95 percent alcohol. A typical serving of beer, wine, or distilled spirits contains about 15 grams of alcohol.*

Alcohol Absorption

Absorption begins immediately in the mouth and esophagus, where small quantities enter the bloodstream. Although alcohol absorption continues in the stomach, the small intestine efficiently absorbs most of the alcohol a person consumes.[8] (See **Figure SA.5**.)

You've heard it before: "Don't drink on an empty stomach." Eating before or with a drink slows down the rush of alcohol into the bloodstream in several ways. Food, especially if it contains fat, delays emptying of the stomach into the small intestine. The delay also provides a longer opportunity for oxidizing stomach enzymes to work. And food dilutes the stomach contents, lowering the concentration of alcohol and its rate of absorption.

About 80 to 95 percent of alcohol is absorbed unchanged. However, some oxidation does take place in the digestive tract, mainly in the stomach, and products of this metabolism join alcohol as it diffuses into the gut cells.[9] These products travel via the portal vein directly to the liver, where most alcohol metabolism takes place. When all goes well, metabolism achieves two goals: energy production and protection from the damaging effects of alcohol and its even more toxic metabolite **acetaldehyde**.

Alcohol Metabolism

The body cannot store potentially harmful alcohol and so works extra hard to get rid of it. To prevent alcohol from accumulating and destroying cells and organs, the body quickly metabolizes it and removes it from the blood. The liver selectively metabolizes alcohol before other compounds and has alternative pathways to handle excess consumption.

Metabolizing Small Amounts of Alcohol

Alcohol dehydrogenase (ADH) is a zinc-containing enzyme that catalyzes the conversion of small to moderate amounts of alcohol to acetaldehyde, a toxic substance. To avoid toxic buildup, another enzyme, **aldehyde dehydrogenase (ALDH)**, quickly and effectively converts acetaldehyde to acetate. (See **Figure SA.6**.) People differ in their ability to eliminate toxic acetaldehyde, and small amounts of it are found in the blood of intoxicated people.[10]

Dehydrogenases in the gastrointestinal tract and the liver are responsible for almost all alcohol metabolism. Probably about 4 to 9 percent, possibly as much as 20 percent, of alcohol is changed to acetaldehyde in the digestive tract.[11] Gastrointestinal aldehyde dehydrogenase does not completely convert acetaldehyde to acetate. The remaining acetaldehyde is more destructive than alcohol itself and can damage the mucous membranes lining the gut.[12]

Alcohol breakdown always takes priority over the breakdown of carbohydrates, proteins, and fats. Liver cells detoxify alcohol and use the products to synthesize fatty acids, which are assembled into fats. Fat accumulation in the liver can be seen after a single bout of heavy drinking, and fatty acid synthesis accelerates with chronic alcohol consumption. **Fatty liver** is the first stage of liver destruction in alcoholics.

Metabolizing Large Amounts of Alcohol

Large amounts of alcohol can overwhelm the alcohol dehydrogenase system, the usual metabolic path. As alcohol builds up, the body identifies it as foreign and routes it into the primary overflow pathway, the **microsomal ethanol-oxidizing system (MEOS)**. (See **Figure SA.7**.) The liver ordinarily uses the MEOS bypass pathway to metabolize drugs and detoxify "foreign" substances. Chronic heavy drinking appears to activate MEOS enzymes, which may be responsible for transforming the pain reliever acetaminophen into chemicals that can damage the liver.

To transform alcohol into acetaldehyde, the MEOS pathway uses different enzymes than the alcohol dehydrogenase system. When repeatedly exposed to large doses of alcohol, the MEOS pathway increases its capacity and processing speed. Whether alcoholics metabolize alcohol differently from nonalcoholics is unknown. Clearly, chronic ingestion of alcohol leads to changes in the liver, and the alcohol abuser acquires an increased tolerance to alcohol and to drugs such as sedatives, tranquilizers, and antibiotics.

Quick Bites

Alcohol Aversion Therapy

In alcohol aversion therapy, the medication disulfiram (Antabuse) deliberately blocks the conversion of toxic acetaldehyde to acetate (acetic acid). Even small amounts of alcohol trigger the highly unpleasant Antabuse–alcohol reaction, which includes a throbbing headache, breathing difficulties, nausea, copious vomiting, flushing, vertigo, confusion, and a drop in blood pressure.

METABOLIZING SMALL TO MODERATE AMOUNTS OF ALCOHOL

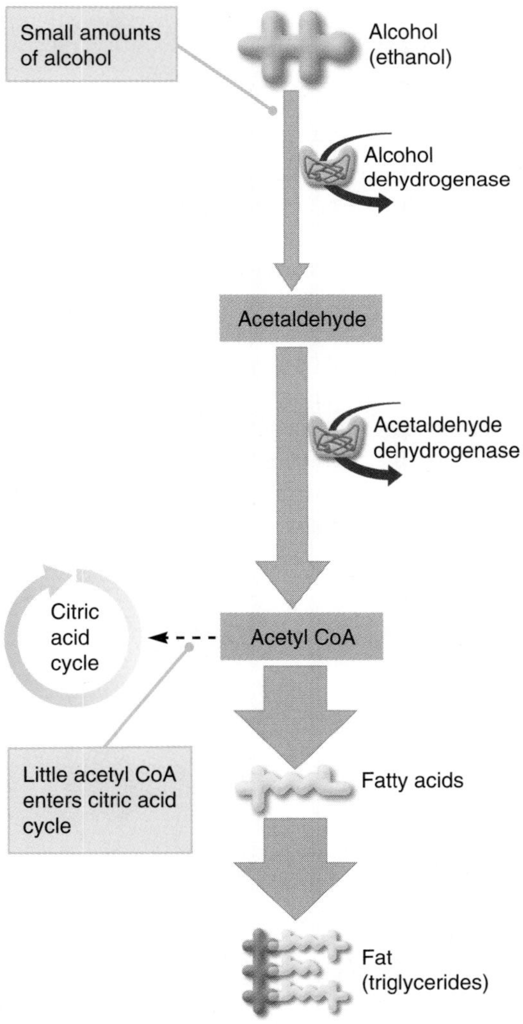

Figure SA.6 **Metabolizing alcohol.** The metabolism of alcohol inhibits the citric acid cycle and primarily forms fat.

congeners Biologically active compounds in alcoholic beverages that include nonalcoholic ingredients as well as other alcohols such as methanol. Congeners contribute to the distinctive taste and smell of the beverage and may increase intoxicating effects and subsequent hangover.

standard drink One serving of alcohol (about 15 grams), defined as 12 ounces of beer, 4 to 5 ounces of wine, or 1.5 ounces of liquor.

binge drinking Consuming excessive amounts of alcohol in short periods of time.

acetaldehyde A toxic intermediate compound formed by the action of alcohol dehydrogenase enzyme during the metabolism of alcohol.

alcohol dehydrogenase (ADH) The enzyme that catalyzes the oxidation of ethanol and other alcohols.

aldehyde dehydrogenase (ALDH) The enzyme that catalyzes the conversion of acetaldehyde to acetate, which forms acetyl CoA.

fatty liver Accumulation of fat in the liver, a sign of increased fatty acid synthesis.

microsomal ethanol-oxidizing system (MEOS) An energy-requiring enzyme system in the liver that normally metabolizes drugs and other foreign substances. When the blood alcohol level is high, alcohol dehydrogenase cannot metabolize it fast enough, and the excess alcohol is metabolized by MEOS.

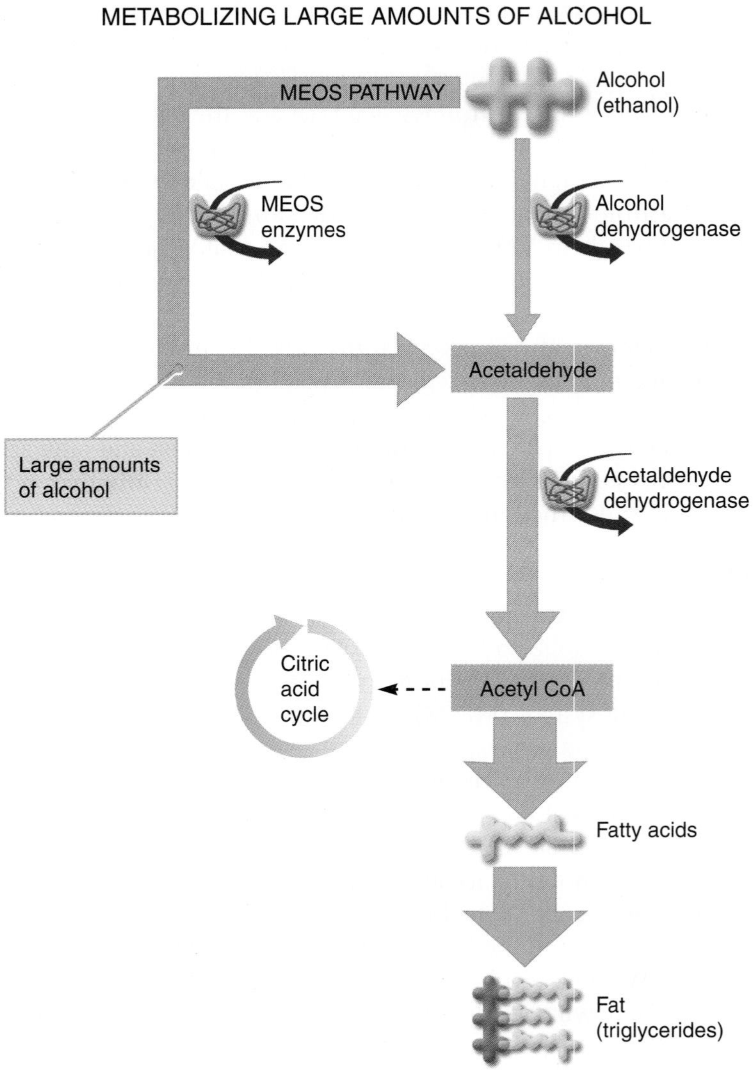

Figure SA.7 **The MEOS overflow pathway.** Large amounts of alcohol can overwhelm its typical metabolic route, so excess alcohol enters an overflow pathway called the microsomal ethanol-oxidizing system (MEOS).

Quick Bites

How to Shock Your Surgeon

If a former alcoholic neglects to disclose past alcohol use before undergoing surgery, the surgeon could be in for a big surprise. Even if the patient is now a teetotaler, his MEOS could still act like that of an alcoholic—operating at the faster speed it once needed to process alcohol quickly. The overactive MEOS would deplete anesthesia much quicker than expected. Theoretically, the patient could wake up in the middle of surgery, much to the shock of the surgeon. That's why anesthesiologists and surgeons ask their patients about alcohol use, past and present.

Removing Alcohol from Circulation

Despite its multiple alcohol-processing pathways, the liver can metabolize only a certain amount of alcohol per hour, regardless of the amount in the bloodstream. The rate of alcohol metabolism depends on several factors, including the amount of metabolizing enzymes in the liver, and varies greatly between individuals. In general, after one standard drink, the amount of alcohol in the drinker's blood (blood alcohol concentration, or BAC) peaks in 30 to 45 minutes. (See **Figure SA.8**.) When absorption exceeds the liver's capacity, a bottleneck is created, and alcohol enters the systemic circulation. Alcohol diffuses rapidly, dispersing equally into all body fluids, including cerebrospinal fluid and the brain and, during pregnancy, into the placenta and fetus. About 10 percent of circulating alcohol is lost in urine, through the lungs, and through skin. Consequently, urine tests and breathalyzer tests both reflect concentrations of blood alcohol as well as alcohol levels in the brain and can indicate how much a person's mental and motor functions may be impaired.

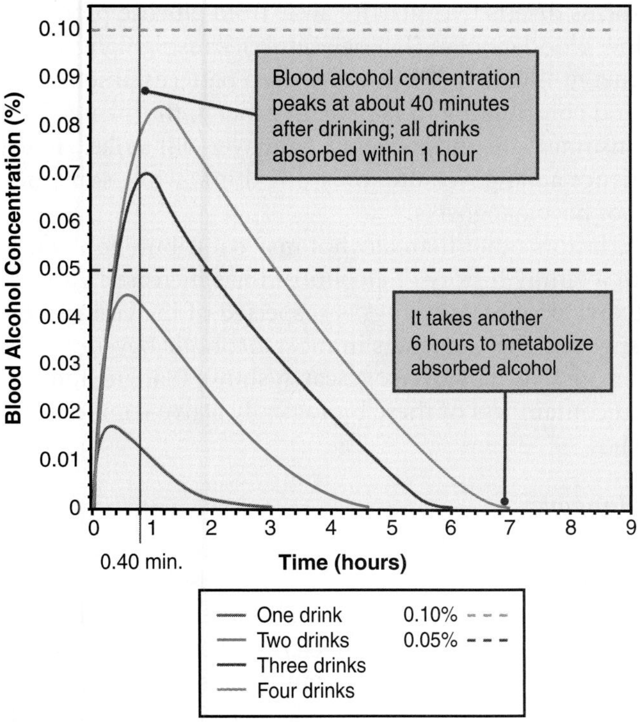

Figure SA.8 **Blood alcohol concentration over time.** Because the body metabolizes alcohol at a relatively constant rate, it clears small amounts faster than large amounts. **Source:** National Institute on Alcohol Abuse and Alcoholism. Alcohol Alert No. 35. PH371; January 1997. http://www.niaaa.nih.gov/publications/aa35.htm. Accessed 4/27/02.

alcohol poisoning An overdose of alcohol. The body is overwhelmed by the amount of alcohol in the system and cannot metabolize it fast enough.

hangover The collection of symptoms experienced by someone who has consumed a large quantity of alcohol. Symptoms can include pounding headache, fatigue, muscle aches, nausea, stomach pain, heightened sensitivity to light and sound, dizziness, and possibly depression, anxiety, and irritability.

Think About It 3

Excessive alcohol consumption deprives the brain of oxygen. The struggle to deal with an overdose of alcohol and lack of oxygen eventually causes the brain to shut down functions that regulate breathing and heart rate. This shutdown leads to a loss of consciousness and, in some cases, coma and death. When a drinker passes out, the body is actually protecting itself: When you lose consciousness, you can't add more alcohol to your system. When you hear of an **alcohol poisoning** death, it usually is the result of consuming such a large quantity of alcohol in such a short period of time that the brain of the victim is overwhelmed. Heart and lung functions shut down, and the person dies.

The Morning After

After a night of drinking, the drinker may suffer from a pounding headache, fatigue, muscle aches, nausea, and stomach pain as well as a heightened sensitivity to light and noise—a **hangover** in full force. The sufferer may be dizzy, have a sense that the room is spinning, and be depressed, anxious, and irritable. Usually a hangover begins within several hours after the last drink, when the blood alcohol level is dropping. Symptoms normally peak about the time the alcohol level reaches zero, and they may continue for an entire day.[13]

What causes a hangover? Scientists have identified several causes of the painful symptoms of a hangover. (See **Figure SA.9**.) Alcohol causes dehydration, which leads to headache and dry mouth. Alcohol directly irritates the stomach and intestines, contributing to stomach pain and vomiting. The sweating, vomiting, and diarrhea that can accompany a hangover cause additional fluid loss and electrolyte imbalance. Alcohol's hijack of the

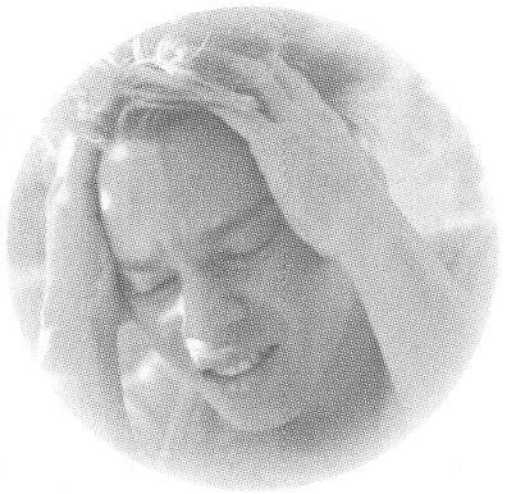

Hangover Symptoms

Constitutional—fatigue, weakness, and thirst
Pain—headache and muscle aches
Gastrointestinal—nausea, vomiting, and stomach pains
Sleep and biological rhythms—decreased sleep, decreased dreaming when asleep
Sensory—vertigo and sensitivity to light and sound
Cognitive—decreased attention and concentration
Mood—depression, anxiety, and irritability
Sympathetic hyperactivity—tremor, sweating, increased pulse, and blood pressure

Possible Contributing Factors

Direct effects of alcohol
- Dehydration
- Electrolyte imbalance
- Gastrointestinal disturbances
- Low blood glucose levels
- Sleep and biological rhythm disturbances

Alcohol withdrawal
Alcohol metabolism (i.e., acetaldehyde toxicity)
Nonalcohol factors
- Compounds other than alcohol in beverages, especially the congener methanol
- Use of other drugs, especially nicotine
- Personality traits such as neuroticism, anger, and defensiveness
- Negative life events and feelings of guilt about drinking
- Family history for alcoholism

Figure SA.9 **Hangovers.** Factors other than just alcohol contribute to the misery of a hangover.

metabolic process diverts liver activity away from glucose production and can lead to low blood glucose (hypoglycemia), causing light-headedness and lack of energy. Alcohol also disrupts sleep patterns, interfering with the dream state and contributing to fatigue. In general, the greater the amount of alcohol consumed, the more likely a hangover will strike. However, some people experience a hangover after only one drink, while some heavy drinkers do not have hangovers.[14]

In addition, factors other than alcohol may contribute to the hangover. A person with a family history of alcoholism has increased vulnerability to hangover. Mixing alcohol and drugs is suspected of increasing the likelihood of a hangover. The congeners in most alcoholic beverages can contribute to more vicious hangovers. Research shows that gin and vodka, beverages that contain less of these biologically active compounds, cause fewer headaches.[15]

Treating a Hangover

So what can you do about a hangover? Few treatments have undergone rigorous, scientific investigation. Time is the most effective treatment—symptoms usually disappear in 8 to 24 hours. Consuming fruits, fruit juices, or other fructose-containing foods may decrease a hangover's intensity, but this has not been well studied. Eating bland foods that contain complex carbohydrates, such as toast or crackers, can combat low blood glucose and possibly nausea. Sleep can ease fatigue, and drinking nonalcoholic, noncaffeinated beverages can alleviate dehydration (caffeine is a diuretic and increases urine production). Taking vitamin B_6 before drinking may reduce the severity of hangover symptoms.[16] Certain medications can relieve symptoms. Antacids may relieve nausea and stomach pains. Aspirin may reduce headache and muscle aches but could increase stomach irritation. Avoid acetaminophen because alcohol metabolism enhances its toxicity to the liver.[17] People who drink three or more alcoholic beverages a day should avoid all over-the-counter pain relievers and fever reducers. These heavy drinkers may have an increased risk of liver damage and stomach bleeding from medicines that contain aspirin, other salicylates, acetaminophen (Tylenol), ibuprofen (Advil), naproxen sodium (Aleve), or ketoprofen (Orudis KT and Actron).[18]

Think About It 4

People with hangovers should avoid "the hair of the dog that bit you," a remedy that calls for drinking more alcohol. Additional drinking only enhances the toxicity of the alcohol previously consumed and extends the recovery time.

Quick Bites

Ancient Hangover Helpers

According to the ancient Persians, eating five almonds could prevent a hangover. The Romans and Greeks had a different solution: celery.

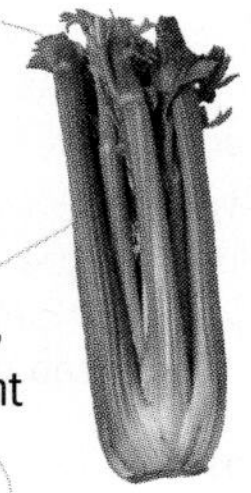

Individual Differences in Alcohol Metabolism

Individuals vary in their ability to metabolize alcohol and acetaldehyde and thus differ in their susceptibility to inebriation, hangover, and, in the long term, addiction and organ damage.

The result of individual differences is easiest to see in acute responses to alcohol. For example, when people of Asian descent drink alcohol, about half experience flushing around the face and neck, probably as a result of high blood acetaldehyde levels.[19] These individuals lack gastric alcohol dehydrogenase, and their livers have an inefficient form of aldehyde dehydrogenase. This may explain why their ancestors depended on boiled water (for teas) as a source of safe fluid. In contrast, Europeans are able to metabolize larger quantities of alcohol and historically have relied on fermentation to produce fluids that were safer to drink.[20]

Elderly people often find their tolerance for alcohol is less than it used to be. Due to decreased tolerance, the effects of alcohol, such as impaired coordination, occur at lower intakes in the elderly than in younger people, whose tolerance *increases* with increased consumption. This reduced tolerance is compounded by an age-related decrease in body water, so that blood alcohol concentrations in older people are likely to rise higher after drinking.[21]

Women and Alcohol

Men and women respond differently to alcohol. (See **Figure SA.10**.) Blood alcohol rises faster in women, so they become more intoxicated than men with an equivalent dose of alcohol.[22] Accordingly, moderate drinking is usually defined as "two standard drinks for men and one for women."[23] Women also metabolize alcohol more slowly than men. Several factors are responsible for alcohol's greater effect on women.

Body Size and Composition Women on average are smaller than men and have smaller livers, and therefore they have less capacity for metabolizing alcohol. Women also have lower total body water and higher body fat than men of comparable size. After alcohol is consumed, it diffuses uniformly into all body water, both inside and outside cells. Because of their smaller quantity of body water, after drinking equivalent amounts of alcohol, women have higher concentrations of alcohol in their blood than men.

Less Enzyme Activity For nonalcoholics, alcohol dehydrogenase (the primary enzyme involved in the metabolism of alcohol) is 40 percent less active in the stomachs of women than of men.[24] This contributes to higher blood alcohol concentrations and lengthens the time needed to metabolize and eliminate alcohol. The gender difference in alcohol levels is due mainly to the significantly lower activity of gastric enzymes in women.[25]

Chronic Alcohol Abuse Alcoholism and other abuses exact a greater physical toll on women than men. Female alcoholics have death rates 50 to 100 percent higher than those of male alcoholics. Further, a greater percentage of female alcoholics die from suicides, alcohol-related accidents, circulatory disorders, and cirrhosis of the liver.

Key Concepts: *Alcohol does not need to be digested prior to absorption and moves easily across the GI tract lining into the bloodstream. Once absorbed, the liver metabolizes alcohol. The primary metabolic enzymes are alcohol dehydrogenase and aldehyde dehydrogenase. When large amounts of alcohol are consumed, some is metabolized by the MEOS pathway. There are a number of genetic and gender differences in the amount and activity levels of alcohol-metabolizing enzymes.*

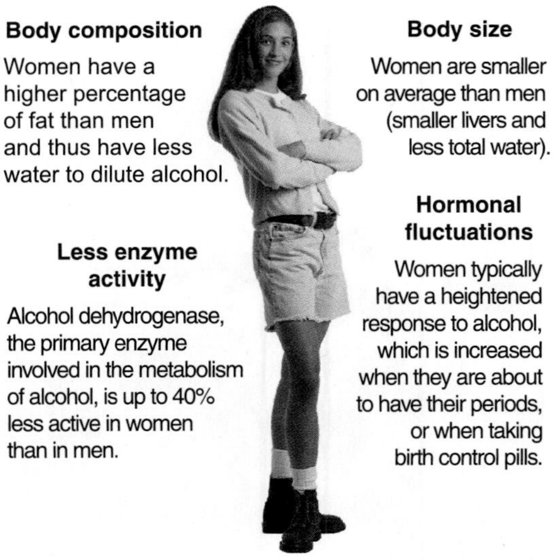

Body composition
Women have a higher percentage of fat than men and thus have less water to dilute alcohol.
Body size
Women are smaller on average than men (smaller livers and less total water).
Less enzyme activity
Alcohol dehydrogenase, the primary enzyme involved in the metabolism of alcohol, is up to 40% less active in women than in men.
Hormonal fluctuations
Women typically have a heightened response to alcohol, which is increased when they are about to have their periods, or when taking birth control pills.

Figure SA.10 **Women and men respond differently to alcohol.** Women tend to have a lower capacity for alcohol than men.

When Alcohol Becomes a Problem

Alcohol affects every organ system in the body. In the short term, small amounts of alcohol change the levels of neurotransmitters in the brain, reducing inhibitions and physical coordination. In the long term, chronic intake of large amounts of alcohol damages the heart, liver, GI tract, and brain. When a pregnant woman drinks, alcohol can have a devastating effect on the development of her baby.

Alcohol in the Brain and the Nervous System

Alcohol diffuses readily into the brain, and because a small amount is absorbed from the mouth directly into circulating blood, its effects can be almost immediate, reaching the brain in as little as one minute after consumption. **Figure SA.11** shows the effects alcohol has on the brain.

Because alcohol is soluble in fat, it can easily cross the protective fatty membrane of nerve cells. There, it disrupts the brain's complex system for communicating between nerve cells. Neurotransmitters that excite nerve cells and those that inhibit nerve cells are thrown out of balance. Excess of some neurotransmitters produces sleepiness; high levels of others cause a loss of coordination; an imbalance of others impairs judgment and mental ability; and still other neurotransmitters perpetuate the desire to keep drinking, even when it's clearly time to stop. Changes in these messengers are suspected of leading to addiction and symptoms of alcohol withdrawal.[26] In the short run, they probably contribute to a hangover.

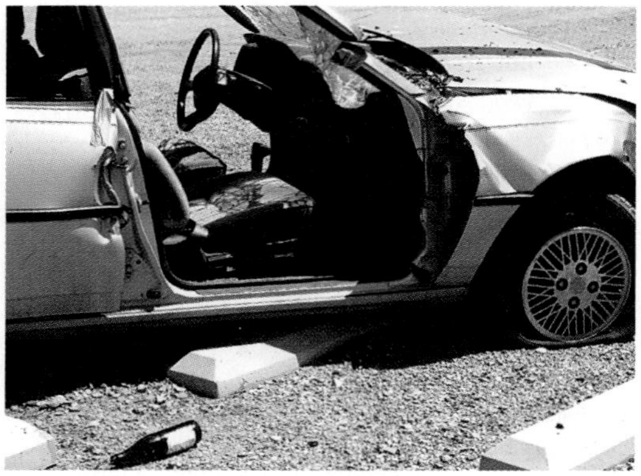

Alcohol's short-term effects are related to how much a person drinks. One or two drinks typically bring alcohol blood levels to 0.04 percent and usually cause only mild, pleasant changes in mood and release of inhibitions. With more drinks and rising blood alcohol levels, coordination, judgment, reaction time, and vision are increasingly impaired. In many states and Canada, it is illegal for a person whose blood level of alcohol has reached or exceeds 0.08 percent to drive a motor vehicle. A recent review of 112 studies concludes that certain skills required to drive a motor vehicle can become significantly impaired at a BAC as low as 0.05 percent.[27] **Table SA.2** shows the effects various amounts of alcohol have on mood and behavior.

The acute effect of a large alcohol intake—swallowed accidentally by children, for example—is hypoglycemia (low blood glucose) severe enough to kill.[28] Binge drinking, especially following several days of little food, also can be deadly. The lack of food depletes glycogen stores, and heavy drinking suppresses gluconeogenesis. The resulting severe hypoglycemia is a medical emergency with the potential for coma and death.

Chronic alcoholism produces many different mental disorders. Malnutrition is a probable factor in most of these, even when diet appears adequate. After years of drinking, brain cells become permanently damaged and unable to metabolize nutrients properly.

Alcohol's Effect on the Gastrointestinal System

Years of heavy drinking and ongoing contact with alcohol and acetaldehyde eventually damage the gastrointestinal system, which in turn discourages

Figure SA.11 **Effects of alcohol on the brain.** As blood alcohol concentration rises, different parts of the brain are affected.

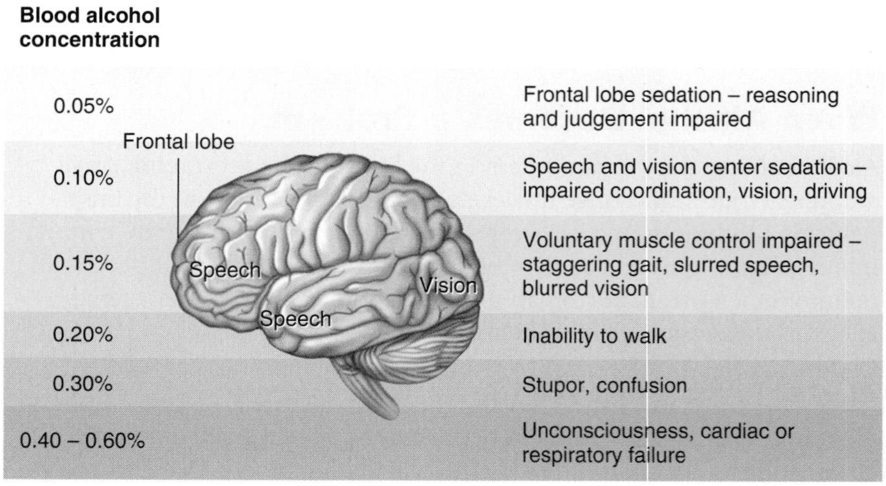

eating, affects absorption of protective nutrients, and leaves the digestive lining even more vulnerable to damage as the vicious cycle continues.

Chronic irritation from alcohol and acetaldehyde erodes protective mucosal linings, causing inflammation and release of destructive free radicals. **Esophagitis** (inflammation of the esophagus), esophageal stricture (closing), and swallowing difficulties are common among alcoholics. When the stomach is repeatedly exposed to alcohol at high concentrations, **gastritis** (inflammation of the stomach) often develops. Alcoholics frequently have diarrhea and malabsorption, evidence of intestinal damage. The

esophagitis Inflammation of the esophagus.
gastritis Inflammation of the stomach.

Table SA.2 Alcohol Impairment Chart

This chart is intended as a guide, not a guarantee.
IMPAIRMENT BEGINS WITH YOUR FIRST DRINK.
FOR SAFETY'S SAKE, NEVER DRIVE AFTER DRINKING!

Men

Drinks	Body Weight in Pounds: 100	120	140	160	180	200	220	240	
	Approximate Blood Alcohol Percentage								
1	.04	.03	.03	.02	.02	.02	.02	.02	Impairment Begins
2	.08	.06	.05	.05	.04	.04	.03	.03	Driving Skills Significantly Affected
3	.11	.09	.08	.07	.06	.06	.05	.05	
4	.15	.12	.11	.09	.08	.08	.07	.06	
5	.19	.16	.13	.12	.11	.09	.09	.08	Possible Criminal Penalties
6	.23	.19	.16	.14	.13	.11	.10	.09	
7	.26	.22	.19	.16	.15	.13	.12	.11	Legally Intoxicated
8	.30	.25	.21	.19	.17	.15	.14	.13	
9	.34	.28	.24	.21	.19	.17	.15	.14	Criminal Penalties
10	.38	.31	.27	.23	.21	.19	.17	.16	

Subtract .01% for each 40 minutes of drinking.
One drink is 1.25 oz. of 80 proof liquor, 12 oz. of beer, or 5 oz. of table wine.

Women

Drinks	Body Weight in Pounds: 90	100	120	140	160	180	200	220	240	
	Approximate Blood Alcohol Percentage									
1	.05	.05	.04	.03	.03	.03	.02	.02	.02	Impairment Begins
2	.10	.09	.08	.07	.06	.05	.05	.04	.04	Driving Skills Significantly Affected
3	.15	.14	.11	.10	.09	.08	.07	.06	.06	
4	.20	.18	.15	.13	.11	.10	.09	.08	.08	Possible Criminal Penalties
5	.25	.23	.19	.16	.14	.13	.11	.10	.09	
6	.30	.27	.23	.19	.17	.15	.14	.12	.11	Legally Intoxicated
7	.35	.32	.27	.23	.20	.18	.16	.14	.13	
8	.40	.36	.30	.26	.23	.20	.18	.17	.15	
9	.45	.41	.34	.29	.26	.23	.20	.19	.17	Criminal Penalties
10	.51	.45	.38	.32	.28	.25	.23	.21	.19	

Note: Data supplied by the Pennsylvania Liquor Control Board.

Source: The National Clearinghouse for Alcohol and Drug Information, Substance Abuse and Mental Health Services Administration. http://www.health.org/nongovpubs/bac-chart/. Accessed 4/27/02.

Fyi College Drinking Culture

FOR YOUR INFORMATION

From car crashes to alcohol poisonings—the culture of drinking on many college campuses puts students at grave risk. An overwhelming number of college students, many of whom are younger than the legal drinking age, use alcohol. The findings of a recent nationwide survey are typical of studies on campus drinking: More than 80 percent of college students had had at least one drink of alcohol during the 30 days preceding the survey, and nearly half (47 percent) of student drinkers say they drink to get drunk.[1] Such figures are averages for all campuses, however, and mask variability among schools. There is little drinking in some schools, a troubling level in many others.[2]

Binge Drinking

Binge drinking is especially worrisome, and it is widespread on college campuses. What is binge drinking? Binge drinking is defined as the consumption of at least five drinks in a row for men or four drinks in a row for women. Just over two in five (44 percent) students report binge drinking behaviors, and about one in four (23 percent) report bingeing frequently, three or more times in a two-week period. Frequent binge drinkers average more than 14 drinks per week and account for more than two-thirds of the alcohol consumed by college students.[3] College binge drinkers may drink not for sociability, but solely and purposefully to get drunk.

Binge drinkers often do something they later regret—argue with friends, make fools of themselves, get sick, engage in unplanned (and often unprotected) sexual activity, or drive drunk. Afterward they may forget where they were or what they did, but the consequences of the binge remain. These consequences may include alienated friends, a hangover, and embarrassment. Or the consequences could be much more serious, such as sexually transmitted disease, hospitalization, permanent injury, rape, pregnancy, and death.

Abstaining

There is a polarizing trend in college drinking, with binge drinkers at one end and abstainers at the other. The number of college students who drink no alcohol is rising and now is nearly equal to the number who frequently binge. About one in five (19 percent) students report consuming no alcohol within the past year.[4]

The Campus Drinker

Researchers have looked closely at the students who are binge drinkers. The findings tend to agree on the following characteristics:

- *Ethnicity.* Studies suggest that college students who are members of racial and/or ethnic minorities drink less than white students.[5]
- *Age.* Younger students are more likely than older students to binge-drink and to have alcohol-related problems.[6]
- *Past alcohol use.* Binge drinking during high school, especially among men, is a strong predictor of binge drinking in college.[7]
- *Athletic participation.* Although competitive athletes are viewed as being health-conscious, athletes may be more likely than other students to binge-drink.[8]
- *Personality characteristics.* Heavy drinking and alcohol-related problems during college are associated with psychological factors such as impulsiveness, depression, anxiety, or early deviant behavior. A family history of alcohol abuse is another risk factor.[9]
- *Group and peer influence on drinking behavior.* "But my friends drink more than I do" is a common refrain. Students often believe that they drink less than others and generally overestimate how much their peers drink. This exaggerated perception leads to greater personal consumption.
- *Drinking in groups.* Group influence can exaggerate any behavior, and drinking is no exception.[10]
- *Serving oneself.* The convenience of self-serve at college parties also boosts alcohol consumption.[11]
- *Fraternities and sororities.* Fraternity and sorority members drink greater amounts of alcohol and drink more frequently than other groups on campus.[12]

Some students have a romanticized notion of heavy drinking. The image of the macho drinker, the sophisticated drinker, or the creative artistic drinker may hold special appeal for the student with a poor self-image.

Binge Drinkers and Problem Behaviors

Interestingly, students who are frequent binge drinkers or who report specific alcohol-related problems do not see themselves as problem drinkers.[13] Yet these students are more likely than their classmates to:

- damage property
- have unprotected sex
- drink and drive
- have trouble with authorities
- perform poorly in classes
- miss classes
- have hangovers
- get injured[14]

Heavy drinking on campus creates problems for all students. In 1998, approximately 600,000 students were assaulted by drinking students.[15] In colleges where significant binge drinking goes on, classmates are more often insulted or humiliated; their property is damaged more often; and they receive more unwanted sexual advances—all as a result of their peers' drinking. Classmates of binge drinkers are more likely to have their studies disturbed or to have to take care of a drunken student.[16]

The most serious consequence of high-risk college drinking is death. The U.S. Department of Education has evidence that at least 84 college students have died since 1996 because of alcohol poisoning, or related injury—and they believe the actual total is higher because of incomplete reporting.

When alcohol-related traffic crashes and off-campus injuries are taken into consideration, it is estimated that over 1,400 college students die each year from alcohol-related unintentional injuries.[17]

Interventions

Many campuses have programs for both prevention and treatment of alcohol abuse. Treatment must often start with helping students recognize that their drinking is a problem. Group programs are very helpful for students, just as they are for other populations. However, other innovative treatments are also helping students. The Alcohol Skills Training Program focuses on monitoring and moderating one's own drinking. The goal is reduction of alcohol use, not necessarily abstinence. Heavy-drinking students who took the course said one year later they were drinking less, compared with similar students who took a more traditional alcohol education course. A single individual motivational session for heavy-drinking freshmen has also helped reduce alcohol-related problems during the first two years of college.[18]

The National Advisory Council Task Force on College Drinking recommends that colleges and universities:

- Pay careful attention to environmental factors on campus and in the community. They are extremely important in influencing college drinking behaviors both positively and negatively.
- Actively enforce existing drinking age laws on campus; they help decrease alcohol consumption.
- Use social norms interventions to correct misperceptions and change drinking practices. When discussing college drinking problems, do not inadvertently reinforce the notion that hazardous drinking is the norm. Help students understand that they have the right not to drink and to have negative feelings about the consequences they experience due to other students' excessive drinking.
- Communicate the institution's, the community's, and the state's alcohol policies to students and parents before and after students arrive on campus.
- Be cautious about making alcohol available on campus. In the general population, increased availability is associated with increased consumption.[19]

Many questions remain about college binge drinking: What is the best way to keep students from heavy drinking and to intervene effectively when they do binge-drink? How can we prevent students from harming themselves and others, from squandering the opportunities of a college education, from becoming addicted to alcohol? Questions on social policy must be explored, too, and answered honestly. For example, does prohibiting alcohol on campus cause students to drive in search of a drink? How effective are restrictions on alcohol advertising? Do restrictions interfere with the rights of students who are 21 and older? To what degree must schools act as surrogate parents? The questions are difficult, but the answers are crucial.

1 Wechsler H, Lee JE, Kuo M, Lee H. College binge drinking in the 1990s: a continuing problem. *J Am Coll Health.* 2000;48(10):199–210.

2 Wechsler H, Dowdall GW, Davenport A, Rimm EB. A gender-specific measure of binge drinking among college students. *Am J Public Health.* 1995;85:982–985.

3 Wechsler H, Lee JE, Kuo M, et al. Trends in college binge drinking during a period of increased prevention efforts: Findings from 4 Harvard School of Public Health College Alcohol Study Surveys: 1993–2001. *J Am Coll Health.* 2002;50(5):203–217.

4 Ibid.

5 Ibid.

6 Ibid.

7 Ibid.

8 Nelson TF, Wechsler H. Alcohol and college athletes. *Med Sci Sports Exerc.* 2001;33:43–47.

9 Baer JS, Kivlahan DR, Marlatt GA. High-risk drinking across the transition from high school to college. *Alcohol: Clin Exp Res.* 1995;19(1):54–61.

10 Marlatt GA, Baer JS, Larimer M. Preventing alcohol abuse in college students: a harm-reduction approach. In: Boyd GM, Howard J, Zucker RA, eds. *Alcohol Problems Among Adolescents: Current Directions in Prevention Research.* Hillsdale, NJ: Lawrence Erlbaum; 1995:147–172.

11 Geller ES, Russ NW, Altomari MG. Naturalistic observations of beer drinking among college students. *J Appl Behav Anal.* 1986;19(4):391–396; and Geller ES, Kalsher MJ. Environmental determinants of party drinking: bartenders versus self-service. *Environ Behav.* 1990;22(1):74–90.

12 Wechsler H, Dowdall GW, Davenport A, Rimm EB. Op. cit.; Marlatt GA, Baer JS, Larimer M. Op. cit.; and Baer JS, Kivlahan DR, Marlatt GA. Op. cit.

13 Presley CA, Meilman PW, Cashin JR, Lyerla R. *Alcohol and Drugs on American College Campuses: Use, Consequences, and Perceptions of the Campus Environment.* Vol 3, *1991–1993.* Carbondale, IL: Core Institute; 1996.

14 Wechsler H, Lee JE, Kuo M, Lee H. Op. cit.

15 Hingson R, Heeren T, Zakocs R, Kopstein A and Wechsler H. Magnitude of alcohol-related morbidity, mortality, and alcohol dependence among U.S. college students age 18–24. *J Studies Alcohol.* 2002;63(2):136–144.

16 Ibid.

17 NIAAA National Advisory Council Task Force on College Drinking. *How to reduce high-risk college drinking: use proven strategies, fill research gaps. Final report of the panel on prevention and treatment.* April 2002. http://www.collegedrinkingprevention.gov/Reports/Panel02/Panel02_TOC.aspx. Accessed 4/27/02.

18 Marlatt GA, Baer JS, Larimer M. Op. cit.

19 NIAAA National Advisory Council Task Force on College Drinking. Op. cit.

mouth, throat, esophagus, stomach, and small and large intestines are all at greatly increased risk of cancer. Smoking dramatically multiplies this risk.

Alcohol and the Liver

Metabolizing and detoxifying alcohol is almost entirely the responsibility of the liver. So it's not surprising that too much drinking hurts the liver more than any other site in the body. In the United States, heavy alcohol use is considered the most important risk factor for chronic liver disease. During the 1980s, alcoholic fatty liver, acute alcoholic hepatitis, and alcoholic cirrhosis together accounted for 46 percent of deaths from chronic liver disease and 49 percent of hospitalizations for liver disease.[29]

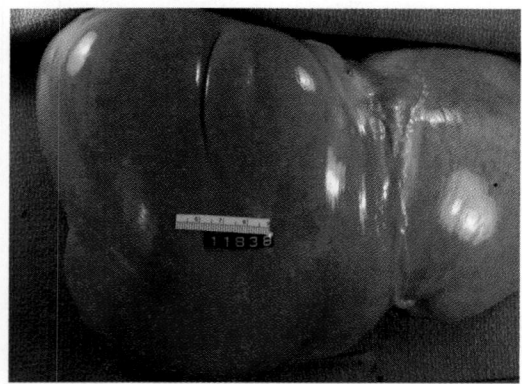

Figure SA.12 **Fatty liver.**

The earliest evidence of liver damage is fat accumulation, which can appear after only a few days of heavy drinking. Fatty liver (see **Figure SA.12**) recedes with abstinence but persists with continued drinking. Is fatty liver in and of itself harmful? The answer is controversial among liver researchers, with some experts suggesting it's a benign condition. However, studies show 5 to 15 percent of people with alcoholic fatty liver who continue to drink develop liver fibrosis (excessive fibrous tissue) or cirrhosis (scarring) in only 5 to 10 years.[30]

Fat accumulation is one of several factors resulting in alcoholic liver disease. With regular, high intakes of alcohol, alcohol and acetaldehyde continually irritate and inflame the liver, producing alcoholic hepatitis (persistent inflammation of the liver) in 10 to 35 percent of heavy drinkers. The inflammatory process also generates free radicals that batter away at liver cells. The destruction of liver cells becomes self-perpetuating, especially if antioxidant nutrients are unavailable to help break the cycle. If the intestines also have been damaged, toxins, including those produced by the gut's microorganisms, may be able to cross the intestinal barrier into circulation and worsen inflammation.[31]

Quick Bites

Are Alcoholics More Likely to Get Food Poisoning?

When alcohol inhibits the breakdown of another toxin, the effect can be dramatic. Consider seafood toxins, for example. The alcoholic who sits down for a good fish dinner should be extra careful about seafood because alcoholic liver disease makes him or her 200 times more likely to die from *Vibrio vulnificus*, a bacterium found in raw oysters. Alcohol also accentuates the symptoms of *ciguatera*, or "fish poisoning," a relatively common food poisoning in tropical areas where people eat large fish from infected waters.

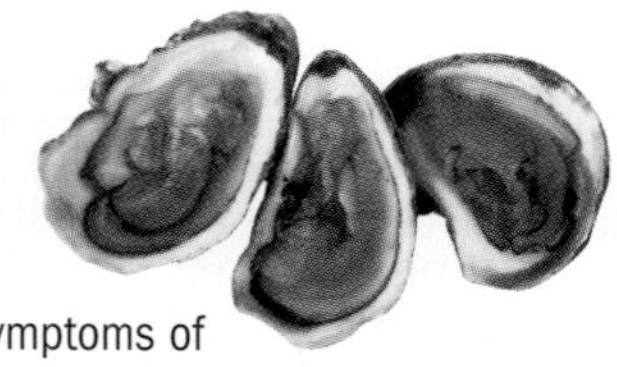

Alcoholic hepatitis may be treatable, but it's often fatal. Alcoholic hepatitis also predisposes a person to liver cancer and cirrhosis, conditions that are usually fatal. With continued inflammation, the liver makes excessive collagen and becomes fibrous (fibrotic liver disease) and scarred (cirrhosis). This ultimately kills liver cells by choking off tiny blood vessels that nourish them. About 10 to 20 percent of heavy drinkers develop cirrhosis.[32]

Dietary changes may be helpful in liver disease, but abstinence from alcohol is essential to treatment. Reducing dietary fats somewhat reduces fat accumulation in the liver. Adequate micronutrients and a healthful balance of macronutrients probably speed recuperation from liver diseases in their earlier stages.[33] In late-stage liver disease, dietary restrictions, often of proteins, may slow disease progression or improve symptoms.

Fetal Alcohol Syndrome

Fetal alcohol syndrome is perhaps alcohol's saddest result. The severely affected victims of the syndrome have a variety of congenital defects: mental retardation, coordination problems, and heart, eye, and genitourinary malformations, as well as low birth weight and slowed growth rate. Most apparent are characteristic facial abnormalities. Severe cases of fetal alcohol syndrome are rare, but subtle damage with one or two abnormalities, sometimes called "fetal alcohol effects," is probably much more widespread. Symptoms of the syndrome may not emerge until months after birth and are apt to go undiagnosed.[34] This disorder, a major cause of mental retardation in the United States, is preventable.

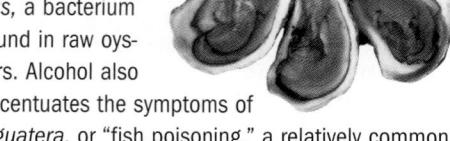

fetal alcohol syndrome A set of physical and mental abnormalities observed in infants born to women who abuse alcohol during pregnancy. Affected infants exhibit poor growth, characteristic abnormal facial features, limited hand-eye coordination, and mental retardation.

Alcohol is especially damaging in the early weeks of pregnancy, before a woman may know she's pregnant. It crosses the placenta into the tiny body of the fetus, where its effects are grossly magnified. Both the congeners in alcoholic beverages and the associated disturbed metabolism of vitamin A and folic acid, nutrients clearly required for fetal growth and development, can interfere with embryonic development.[35]

Relatively small amounts of alcohol may cause fetal alcohol syndrome. A safe level during pregnancy is not known; therefore, pregnant women should abstain from alcohol consumption. Unlike most other alcohol-related diseases, fetal alcohol damage does not require chronic intake. A binge, even several drinks at a party, at the wrong moment of pregnancy can cause problems. However, population studies show that babies with neurodevelopmental problems are more common among women who drink more frequently during pregnancy.[36]

Official health advisories issued in 1981, 1990, and 1995 warn women against drinking alcohol if they are pregnant or considering becoming pregnant. Labels on alcoholic beverages must carry a warning for pregnant women. Yet government surveys estimate that consumption increased between 1991 and 1995. In 1995, 16 percent of pregnant women consumed alcohol, and 3.5 percent did so frequently.[37] **Figure SA.13** shows the prevalence of alcohol consumption by women of childbearing age.

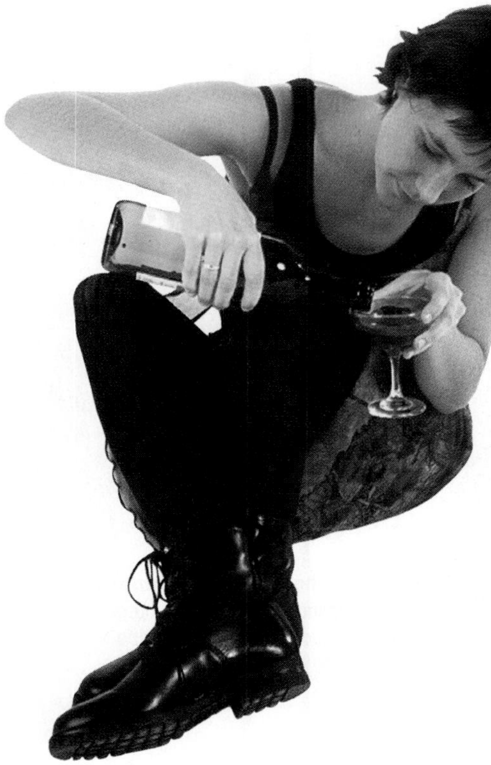

Key Concepts: *Alcohol affects every organ system of the body. In the brain and nervous system, alcohol is a depressant. In the GI tract, alcohol damages cells of the esophagus and stomach and increases the risk for GI cancers. The liver is most affected by alcohol consumption, culminating in alcoholic hepatitis and cirrhosis after years of alcohol abuse. Alcohol intake during pregnancy can have devastating effects on fetal development.*

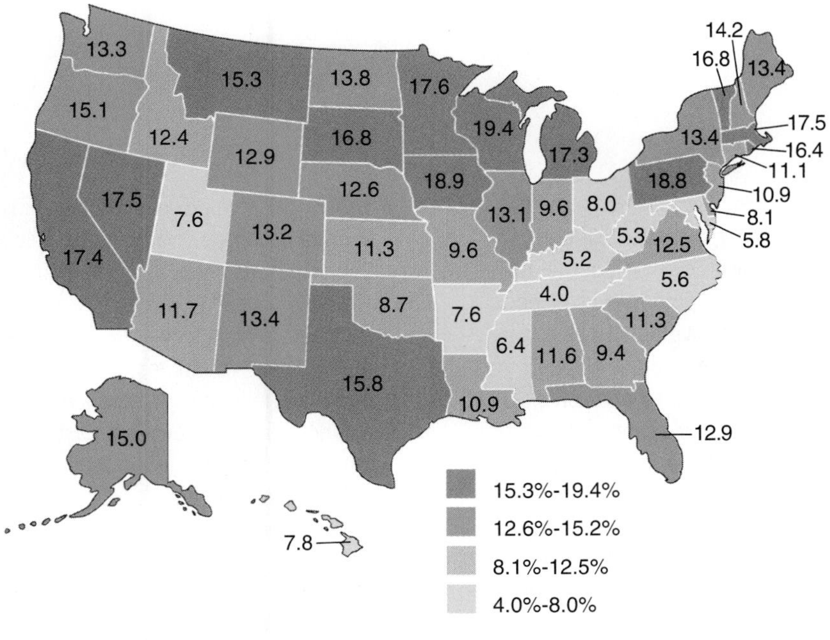

* Consumption of an average of seven or more drinks per week or five or more drinks on at least one occasion during the preceding month.

Figure SA.13 **Prevalence of frequent alcohol consumption among women of childbearing age (18–44 years).** Alcohol is especially damaging to the fetus during the early weeks of pregnancy—before a woman may know she is pregnant. **Source:** Alcohol consumption among pregnant and childbearing-aged women. *MMWR.* 1997;46:346–350.

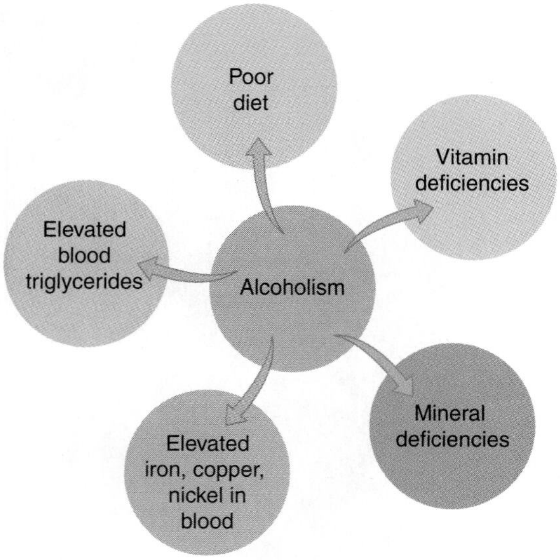

Figure SA.14 **Alcoholism and malnutrition.** Alcoholics' poor diets interact with alcohol's toxicity to worsen their malnutrition.

Alcoholics and Malnutrition

In the United States and Canada, where food is plentiful and fortification of foods with vitamins and minerals is common, overt nutrient deficiencies are rare—except among alcoholics. The results of their poor diet interact with the results of alcohol's toxicity—which include diarrhea, malabsorption, liver malfunction, bleeding, bone marrow changes, and hormonal changes—to worsen malnutrition. (See **Figure SA.14**.) In general, the more a person drinks, the worse the malnutrition.

Poor Diet

Disordered eating is common among heavy drinkers, especially among alcoholic women.[38] Factors responsible for the poor diet of alcoholics are much easier to identify than to correct. Economic factors include poverty, lack of cooking facilities, and homelessness. Anxiety, depression, loneliness, and isolation are all characteristic of alcoholism, and all contribute to loss of appetite. So can physical pain. Lack of interest in food is common. There may be an aversion to many specific foods or to eating in general, especially after the experience of diarrhea, painful indigestion, or difficulty swallowing.

Heavy drinkers who get about half their calories from alcohol cannot eat enough to obtain adequate vitamins and minerals. Severely malnourished alcoholics often have multiple deficiencies.

Vitamin Deficiencies

Inadequate intake, poor absorption, increased vitamin destruction in the body, and urinary losses all contribute to vitamin deficiencies in the alco-

[Fyi] Myths about Alcohol

FOR YOUR INFORMATION

Poor alcohol, so misunderstood. Myths and misunderstandings just keep circulating about alcohol. Some of these statements are partly true, but most are completely false. You may have heard some of the following:

- *Alcohol is a stimulant.* No. It's actually a depressant, but its initial depressing effect on inhibitions and judgment may make it seem stimulating.
- *Alcohol keeps you warm.* Partly true. It dilates blood vessels near the body's surface, giving a feeling of warmth. But as body heat escapes, alcohol cools the inner body.
- *Alcohol is an aphrodisiac.* Partly true. By suppressing inhibitions, it may loosen behavior. However, sexual function is often compromised by alcohol.
- *Most alcoholics live on skid row.* No. The highly visible skid-row alcoholic represents only a minority of alcoholics.
- *Beer is a source of vitamins.* Partly true. Beer does contain a fair amount of niacin. But you'd need about 1 liter to fulfill daily niacin requirements. Levels of other vitamins are much lower.
- *Alcohol helps you sleep.* No. Alcohol disrupts sleep patterns, leading to a restless, unsatisfying sleep.
- *Laboratory animals love to drink.* No. Alcohol is usually given by tube feeding because most animals refuse to drink it willingly.
- *It's good to have a beer before breastfeeding.* No. Alcohol may be relaxing and allow milk to flow more readily, but alcohol concentrations in breast milk are similar to those in the mother's blood. Alcohol in breast milk reduces milk production by reducing the intensity of the infant's suckling.

holic. Alcohol also interferes with the conversions of vitamin precursors to active forms.

Folate, thiamin, and vitamin A are most often affected by alcoholism. Folate deficiency contributes to malabsorption, anemia, and nerve damage—all of which worsen malnutrition. Vitamin A deficiency also creates a vicious cycle by damaging gastrointestinal epithelium and by impairing immunity, leaving the victim susceptible to infections. Thiamin deficiency contributes to classic diseases of alcoholism: the brain damage of Wernicke-Korsakoff syndrome, polyneuropathy (nerve inflammation), and cardiomyopathy (heart inflammation). Alcoholics can have overt scurvy from vitamin C deficiency. Vitamin B_6 and vitamin B_{12} deficiencies are less common.

Alcohol metabolism interferes with the normal metabolism of vitamins and other nutrients. For example, metabolism of ethanol uses up the dehydrogenase enzyme that is also used for metabolism of retinol.[39] Retinol (vitamin A) uses that enzyme for its conversion to other active forms of vitamin A, and the disruption of its metabolism is probably one way alcohol increases cancer risk. The same disruption may produce fetal birth defects when pregnant women drink.

Alcohol-induced fat malabsorption and metabolic abnormalities contribute to depletion of fat-soluble vitamins A, D, E, and K. Blood-clotting factors drop with depleted vitamin K, increasing risk of bleeding and anemia. Vitamin E deficiency is not generally recognized as a complication of alcoholism, but its depletion due to fat malabsorption is possible. Optimal vitamin E status is necessary to quench free radicals generated during alcohol metabolism.[40]

Mineral Deficiencies

Alcoholics are commonly deficient in minerals such as calcium, magnesium, iron, and zinc. Alcohol itself does not seem to affect their absorption. Rather, fluid losses and an inadequate diet are the primary culprits. Magnesium deficiency causes "shakes" similar to that seen in alcohol withdrawal. Chronic diarrhea and loss of epithelial tissue (caused by skin rashes or sloughing off of the digestive lining) may seriously deplete zinc, a mineral needed for immune function. In cases of bleeding, especially gastrointestinal blood loss, iron levels fall.

But not all minerals are lower in heavy drinkers than in nondrinkers. If there is no bleeding, a heavy drinker's iron levels tend to be higher than normal in the blood and liver, potentially contributing to harmful oxidation. Copper and nickel may also be elevated in advancing disease, but the reason and the effects are unclear.[41]

Macronutrients

Animal experiments can demonstrate a number of ways alcohol alters digestion and metabolism of carbohydrate, fat, and protein, but the relevance to humans at usual levels of intake is not certain. Alcohol interferes with amino acid absorption, but its direct overall effect on protein balance appears minimal. It inhibits gluconeogenesis and lowers blood glucose levels, probably contributing to hangovers and, at the most extreme, causing acute, potentially lethal hypoglycemia if a person who drinks heavily neglects to eat.[42]

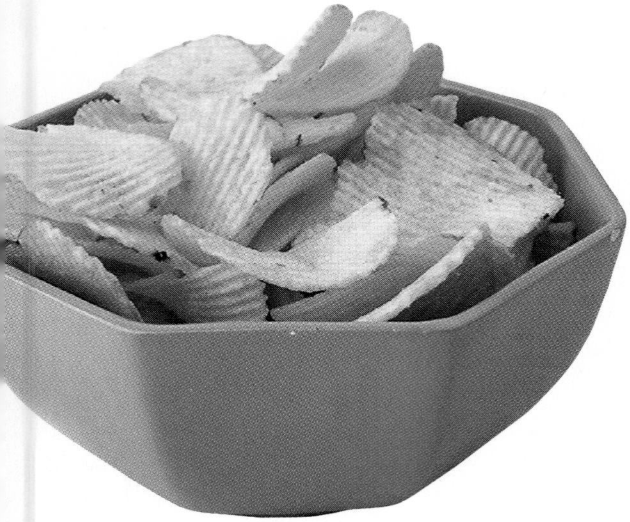

Alcohol's most dramatic effect is on fats. You have seen that alcohol causes fatty liver. In the blood, excess alcohol has the undesirable effect of raising triglyceride levels, often significantly. Hyperlipidemia (high blood fats) is common among heavy drinkers. Abstinence and a balanced diet can usually return blood lipids to normal.[43] On the other hand, moderate alcohol use increases protective high-density lipoproteins (HDL, or "good cholesterol"), an important factor in alcohol's relationship to the reduced risk for coronary artery disease.

Body Weight

Although alcohol is relatively high in calories, alcohol consumption does not necessarily result in increased body weight. While some studies report weight gain,[44] other studies show that when chronic heavy drinkers substitute alcohol for carbohydrates in their diets, they lose weight and weigh less than their nondrinking counterparts. Furthermore, when chronic heavy drinkers eat an otherwise normal diet, they do not gain weight.[45] Some possible explanations for this seeming paradox are (1) the high levels of alcohol consumed by alcoholics are metabolized mainly by the MEOS backup pathway, which is less efficient and loses more energy as heat than other alcohol-metabolizing pathways;[46] (2) with so much alcohol to handle, the liver is unable to efficiently process fats; (3) energy-producing mitochondria are permanently damaged;[47] and (4) energy is lost from malabsorbed nutrients, especially fat.

Key Concepts: *Alcohol interferes with normal nutrition by reducing the intake of nutrient-dense foods and by affecting the absorption, metabolism, and excretion of many vitamins and minerals. Although alcohol contains a significant number of calories (7 kilocalories per gram), during alcohol metabolism excess intake often is wasted as heat, and the weight gain that accompanies high intakes is less than might be expected from the calorie content.*

Does Alcohol Have Benefits?

Can a potentially harmful drink like alcohol play a role in a healthful diet? The consensus of health experts is that it can—but not for everyone. The question continues to arouse much debate, however, and even those supporting alcohol's usefulness often have reservations. Public health statements on alcohol are typically accompanied by plenty of "ifs" and "buts."

Consistent epidemiological evidence suggests that low to moderate drinking reduces mortality among some groups.[48] (**Table SA.3** gives definitions of different levels of drinking.) Tracked against alcohol intake, death rates typically follow what statisticians describe as a "U-shaped curve." Compared with people who rarely or never drink, people who drink slightly or moderately have lower total mortality rates. The lowest rate is seen in people who consume one drink per week. Increasing the number of drinks confers no additional benefit. As the number of drinks increases, the mortality rate rises. People who consume two drinks per day have about the same mortality rate as nondrinkers.[49] Beyond three drinks per day, the death rate rises dramatically.[50] Alcohol's primary benefit is to raise protective HDL cholesterol levels. It may also inhibit formation of blood clots, but this connection is less clear.[51] In addition, alcohol may have subjective benefits like stress relief and relaxation.

In most studies, wine, beer, and spirits appear equal in offering protection against heart disease. Recent findings of reduced rates of nonfatal heart

Table SA.3 How Much Is Too Much?

Term	Criterion
Moderate drinking (NIAAA)	Men: ≤ 2 drinks per day Women: ≤ 1 drink per day Over 65: ≤ 1 drink per day
At-risk drinking (NIAAA)	Men: > 14 drinks per week or > 4 drinks per occasion Women: > 7 drinks per week or > 3 drinks per occasion
Alcohol abuse (APA)	Maladaptive pattern of alcohol use leading to clinically significant impairment or distress, manifested within a 12-month period by one or more of the following: • Failure to fulfill role obligations at work, school, or home • Recurrent use in hazardous situations • Legal problems related to alcohol • Continued use despite alcohol-related social or interpersonal problems • Symptoms have never met criteria for alcohol dependence
Alcohol dependence (APA)	Maladaptive pattern of alcohol use leading to clinically significant impairment or distress, manifested within a 12-month period by three or more of the following: • Tolerance (either increasing amounts used or diminished effects with the same amount) • Withdrawal (withdrawal symptoms or use to relieve or avoid symptoms) • Use of larger amounts over a longer period than intended • Persistent desire or unsuccessful attempts to cut down or control use • Great deal of time spent obtaining or using or recovering from use • Important social, occupational, or recreational activities given up or reduced • Use despite knowledge of alcohol-related physical or psychological problems
Hazardous use (WHO)	Person at risk for adverse consequences
Harmful use (WHO)	Use resulting in physical or psychological harm

Note: NIAAA = National Institute on Alcohol Abuse and Alcoholism; APA = American Psychiatric Association; WHO = World Health Organization.
Source: O'Connor PG, Schottenfeld RS. Patients with alcohol problems. *N Engl J Med.* 1998;338(9):593. Copyright © 1998 Massachusetts Medical Society. All rights reserved. Adapted with permission.

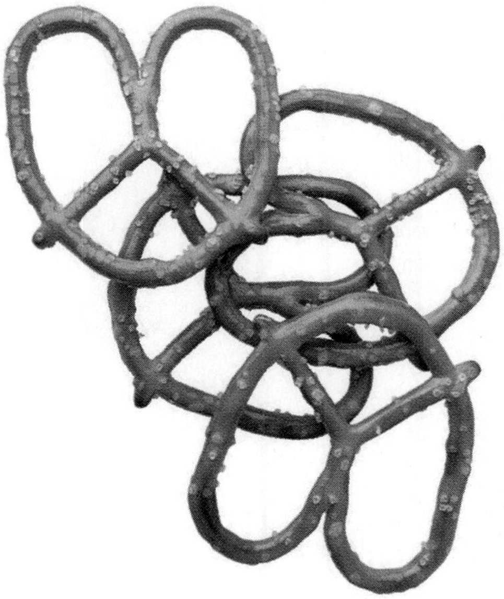

attacks among exclusive beer drinkers support the view that protective benefits of moderate drinking are due to alcohol itself rather than other substances in alcoholic beverages.[52] However, international comparisons that highlight unexpectedly low rates of heart disease in France, despite a high-fat diet (the **French paradox**), suggest red wine may have a unique protective effect. The apparent benefits of red wine may result from overall healthier behavior of people who drink red wine. As yet, a direct connec-

French paradox The phenomenon observed in the French, who have a lower incidence of heart disease than people whose diets contain comparable amounts of fat. Part of the difference has been attributed to the regular and moderate drinking of red wine.

Quick Bites

A What?

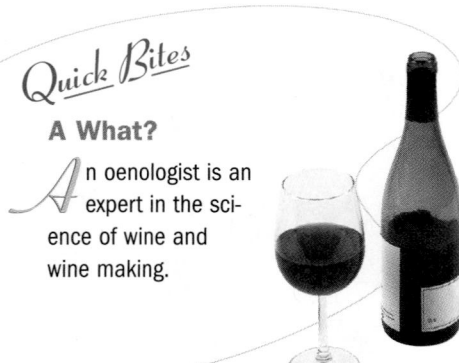

An oenologist is an expert in the science of wine and wine making.

tion between red wine and health benefits remains unproved.[53] Nevertheless, recognizing that alcohol generally confers moderate protection and the possibility that wine has a particular benefit, the Bureau of Alcohol, Tobacco and Firearms recently granted permission for wine labels to include one of the following statements:

> *"The proud people who made this wine encourage you to consult your family doctor about the health effects of wine consumption."*
>
> *"To learn the health effects of wine consumption, send for the Federal Government's Dietary Guidelines for Americans ..."*[54]

Because of the many harmful effects of alcohol (see **Figure SA.15**), public health agencies and organizations caution against inappropriate drinking. While low to moderate alcohol use may have some benefit, these groups advise people to discuss their alcohol intake with their doctors, and they urge moderation. Public health officials also point out that numerous groups should not drink any alcohol:

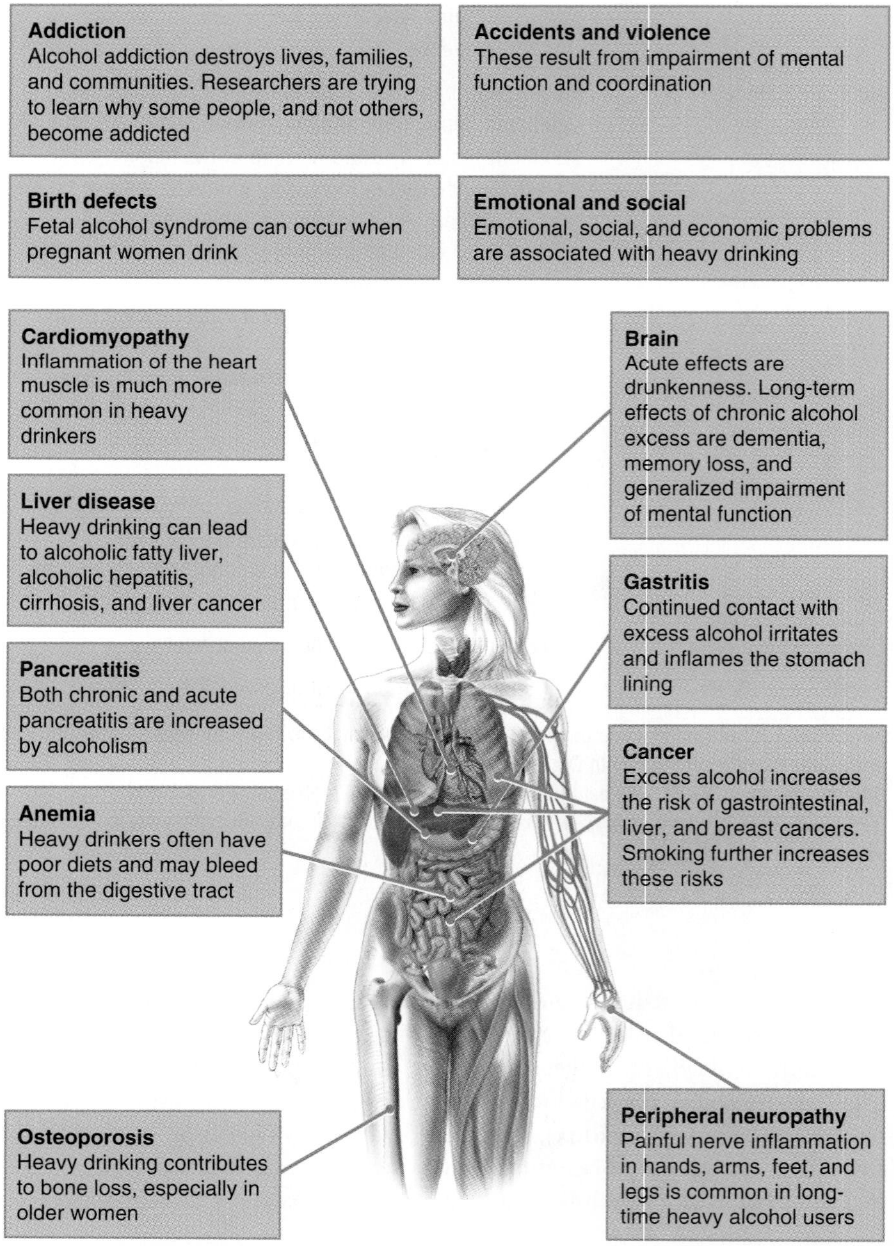

Addiction
Alcohol addiction destroys lives, families, and communities. Researchers are trying to learn why some people, and not others, become addicted
Accidents and violence
These result from impairment of mental function and coordination
Birth defects
Fetal alcohol syndrome can occur when pregnant women drink
Emotional and social
Emotional, social, and economic problems are associated with heavy drinking
Cardiomyopathy
Inflammation of the heart muscle is much more common in heavy drinkers
Liver disease
Heavy drinking can lead to alcoholic fatty liver, alcoholic hepatitis, cirrhosis, and liver cancer
Pancreatitis
Both chronic and acute pancreatitis are increased by alcoholism
Anemia
Heavy drinkers often have poor diets and may bleed from the digestive tract
Osteoporosis
Heavy drinking contributes to bone loss, especially in older women
Brain
Acute effects are drunkenness. Long-term effects of chronic alcohol excess are dementia, memory loss, and generalized impairment of mental function
Gastritis
Continued contact with excess alcohol irritates and inflames the stomach lining
Cancer
Excess alcohol increases the risk of gastrointestinal, liver, and breast cancers. Smoking further increases these risks
Peripheral neuropathy
Painful nerve inflammation in hands, arms, feet, and legs is common in long-time heavy alcohol users

Figure SA.15 **Harmful effects of alcohol.** Because excess alcohol reaches all parts of the body, it causes a wide array of physical problems. Here are some of the ways alcohol can harm.

- children and adolescents
- people on certain medications
- people who have an alcohol-related illness or another illness that will be worsened by alcohol
- people who will be driving or operating machinery
- pregnant women or women who may be in the early weeks of pregnancy and don't know they are pregnant
- people with a personal or strong family history of alcoholism[55]

Key Concepts: *Although alcohol has the potential to reduce risk for heart disease, most health organizations recommend moderate to no drinking. It is too early in the scientific investigation of alcohol's benefits to recommend alcohol intake for all adults. Some people, such as pregnant women, should not drink alcohol at all.*

Label [to] Table

Have you ever wondered how much protein, carbohydrate, and fat are in a can of beer? If you've ever looked at a beer label, you know it's quite different from a food label. Look at the following information from a can of light beer and see if you can calculate the calories from carbohydrate, fat, and protein.

Serving size = 12 fl oz

Calories = 105 (kcal)

Carbohydrate = 5 g

Protein = 0.7 g

Fat = 0 g

First, to figure out how many calories come from the three macronutrients, multiply the number of grams by their respective calorie contribution per gram:

5 g carbohydrate × 4 kcal/g =
20 kcal from carbohydrates

0.7 g protein × 4 kcal/g =
2.8 kcal from protein

0 g fat × 9 kcal/g = 0 kcal from fat

Uh oh. Is this adding up correctly? So far we have accounted for only 23 of the 105 kilocalories in this beer. Where are the other 82 kilocalories? Don't forget that many of the calories in beer come from alcohol, and it's easy to calculate just how many grams are in this can of light beer. Remember, alcohol has 7 kcalories per gram, so the remaining 82 kilocalories come from 12 grams of alcohol (82 ÷ 7 = 11.7).

So, for the 105 kilocalories this beer provides, you get very little (if any) protein, carbohydrate, or fat. Instead, a majority of the calories come from alcohol. This holds true for the micronutrients as well—beer contains negligible amounts of vitamins or minerals.

This is why people say alcoholic beverages have only "empty calories." They provide calories, but almost no nutrient value!

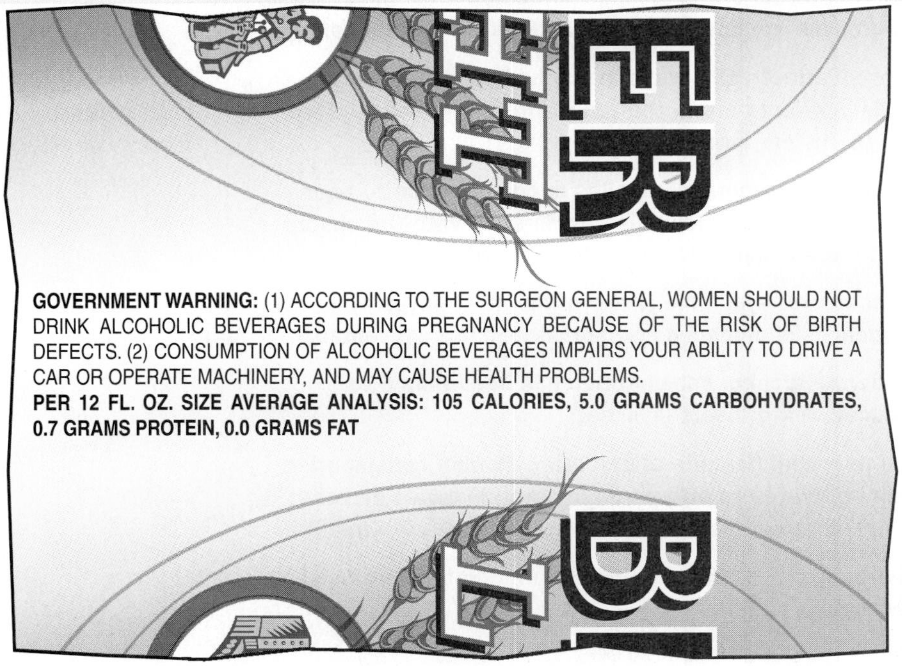
GOVERNMENT WARNING: (1) ACCORDING TO THE SURGEON GENERAL, WOMEN SHOULD NOT DRINK ALCOHOLIC BEVERAGES DURING PREGNANCY BECAUSE OF THE RISK OF BIRTH DEFECTS. (2) CONSUMPTION OF ALCOHOLIC BEVERAGES IMPAIRS YOUR ABILITY TO DRIVE A CAR OR OPERATE MACHINERY, AND MAY CAUSE HEALTH PROBLEMS.
PER 12 FL. OZ. SIZE AVERAGE ANALYSIS: 105 CALORIES, 5.0 GRAMS CARBOHYDRATES, 0.7 GRAMS PROTEIN, 0.0 GRAMS FAT

LEARNING Portfolio

spotlight on alcohol

Key Terms

	page
acetaldehyde	357
alcohol	353
alcohol dehydrogenase (ADH)	357
alcohol poisoning	359
aldehyde dehydrogenase (ALDH)	357
binge drinking	357
congeners	357
esophagitis	363
ethanol	353
ethyl alcohol	353
fatty liver	357
fermentation	354
fetal alcohol syndrome	366
French paradox	371
gastritis	363
hangover	359
methanol	353
methyl alcohol	353
microsomal ethanol-oxidizing system (MEOS)	357
standard drink	357
wood alcohol	353

Study Points

- Alcohol provides 7 kilocalories per gram but no essential function for the body; therefore, alcohol is not a nutrient.
- Alcohol requires no digestion and is absorbed easily all along the gastrointestinal tract.
- Fatty liver is apparent even after one night of binge drinking.
- Different rates of alcohol metabolism can be attributed to different levels of the alcohol-metabolizing enzymes; these differences are due to genetic and gender variations.
- Alcohol affects all organs in the body, but the most obvious effects are in the brain and the nervous system, the GI system, and the liver.
- Malnutrition among alcoholics is common due to poor food choices and alcohol's interference with the absorption, metabolism, and excretion of nutrients.
- Fetal alcohol syndrome is one of the most devastating consequences of alcohol consumption, and it is preventable.
- Moderate alcohol consumption has been linked to reduced risk of heart disease.
- The potential benefits of moderate alcohol consumption may be related to effects on lipoprotein levels and the antioxidant components of beverages such as wine.
- Health organizations recommend moderate to no alcohol consumption.

Study Questions

Answers can be found at nutrition.jbpub.com/discovering.

1. How much alcohol is in a standard drink of beer, of wine, and of liquor?
2. List the ways food helps to delay or avoid inebriation.
3. Where does alcohol metabolism take place?
4. What causes a hangover? Is there any way to relieve one?
5. Among health authorities, what is the consensus about drinking alcohol?
6. List some factors that affect our ability to metabolize alcohol.
7. Why do health care professionals advise pregnant women not to drink alcohol?
8. List the positive and the negative effects of alcohol.

Try This

Cruising through the Medicine Cabinet

This exercise will increase your awareness of the amounts of alcohol in over-the-counter medications. Look through your medicine cabinet and check the ingredient lists of all the products there. In particular, take a close look at any mouthwash or cough syrup. Which products contain alcohol? How much? What do you think its purpose is in these medicines?

References

1 Roe DA. *Alcohol and the Diet.* Westport, CT: AVI Publishing; 1979.

2 Ibid.

3 Mittal BV, Desai AP, Khade KR. Methyl alcohol poisoning: an autopsy study of 28 cases. *J Postgrad Med.* 1991;37:9–13.

4 Roe DA. Op. cit.

5 Vallee BL. Alcohol in the Western world. *Scientific American.* June 1998;80–85.

6 Swift R, Davidson D. Alcohol hangover: mechanisms and mediators. *Alcohol Health Res World.* 1998;22:54–60.

7 USDA Center for Nutrition Policy and Promotion. Does alcohol have a place in a healthy diet? *Nutr Insights.* August 1997;4.

8 Seitz HK, Oneta CM. Gastrointestinal alcohol dehydrogenase. *Nutr Rev.* 1998;56:52–60.

9 Ibid.

10 Swift R, Davidson D. Op. cit.

11 Seitz HK, Oneta CM. Op. cit.

12 Ibid.

13 Swift R, Davidson D. Op. cit.

14 Ibid.

15 Ibid.

16 Wiese JG, Slipak MG, Browner WS. The alcohol hangover. *Ann Intern Med.* 2000;132:897–902.

17 Swift R, Davidson D. Op. cit.

18 Nordenberg T. "An aspirin a day..." just another cliché? *FDA Consumer.* March–April 1999;15–17.

19 Steinmetz CG, Xie P, Weiner H, et al. Structure of mitochondrial aldehyde dehydrogenase: the genetic component of ethanol aversion. *Br J Psych.* 1996;168:762–767.

20 Vallee BL. Op.cit.

21 National Institute on Alcohol Abuse and Alcoholism (NIAAA). *Alcohol Alert: Alcohol and Aging.* April 1998;40.

22 NIAAA. *Alcohol Alert: Moderate Drinking.* April 1992;16.

23 USDA Center for Nutrition Policy and Promotion. Op. cit.

24 Swift R, Davidson D. Op. cit.

25 Baraona E, Abbittan CS, Dohmen K, et al. Gender differences in pharmacokinetics of alcohol. *Alcohol Clin Exp Res.* 2001;25:502–507.

26 Valenzuela CF. Alcohol and neurotransmitter interactions. *Alcohol Health Res World.* 1997;21:108–148.

27 NIAAA. *Alcohol Alert: Alcohol and Transportation Safety.* April 2001;52.

28 Bradford DE. Alcohol and the young child. *Alcohol Alcohol.* 1984;19:173–175.

29 Deaths and hospitalizations from chronic liver disease and cirrhosis—United States, 1980–1989. *MMWR.* 1993;41:969–973.

30 Teli MR, Day CP, Burt AD, et al. Determinants of progression to cirrhosis or fibrosis in pure alcoholic fatty liver. *Lancet.* 1995;346:987–990.

31 NIAAA. *Alcohol Alert: Alcohol and the Liver: Research Update.* 1998;42.

32 Ibid.

33 Teli MR, Day CP, Burt AD, et al. Op. cit.

34 Identification of children with fetal alcohol syndrome and opportunity for referral of their mother for primary prevention, Washington, 1993–1997. *MMWR.* 1998;47:861–864.

35 Roe DA. Op. cit.

36 Alcohol consumption among pregnant and childbearing-aged women—United States, 1991 and 1995. *MMWR.* 1997;46:346–350.

37 Ibid.

38 Lilenfeld LR, Kaye WH. The link between alcoholism and eating disorders. *Alcohol Health Res World.* 1996;20:94–99.

39 Seitz HK, Oneta CM. Op. cit.; and Wang XD. Chronic alcohol intake interferes with retinoid metabolism and signaling. *Nutr Rev.* 1999;57:51–59.

40 Feinman L, Lieber CS. Nutrition and diet in alcoholism. In: Shils ME, Olson JA, Shike M, eds. *Modern Nutrition in Health and Disease.* 8th ed. Philadelphia: Lippincott Williams & Wilkins; 1999:1523–1542.

41 Ibid.

42 Ibid.

43 Ibid.

44 NIAAA. *Alcohol Alert: Alcohol Metabolism.* 1997;35.

45 Ibid.

46 Suter PM, Hassler E, Vetter MD. Effects of alcohol on energy metabolism and body weight regulation: is alcohol a risk factor for obesity? *Nutr Rev.* 1997;55:157–171.

47 Lands EM. Alcohol and energy intake. *Am J Clin Nutr.* 1995;62(suppl 5):1101S–1106S.

48 Klatsky AL. Should patients with heart disease drink alcohol? *JAMA.* 2001;285:2004–2006.

49 Gazino JM, Gaziano TA, Glynn RJ, et al. Light-to-moderate alcohol consumption and mortality in the Physicians' Health Study enrollment cohort. *J Am Coll Cardiol.* 2000;35:96–105.

50 Pearson TA. Alcohol and heart disease. *Circulation.* 1996;94:3023–3025.

51 Klatsky AL. Op. cit.

52 Bobak M, Skodova Z, Marmot M. Effect of beer drinking on risk of myocardial infarction: population based case-control study. *BMJ.* 2000;320:1378–1379.

53 Tjonneland A, Gronbaek M, Stripp C, Overvad K. Wine intake and diet in a random sample of 48763 Danish men and women. *Am J Clin Nutr.* 1999;69:49–54.

54 Treasury announces actions concerning labeling of alcoholic beverages. Treasury Department, Bureau of Alcohol Tobacco and Firearms press release; February 5, 1999.

55 Pearson TA. Op. cit.

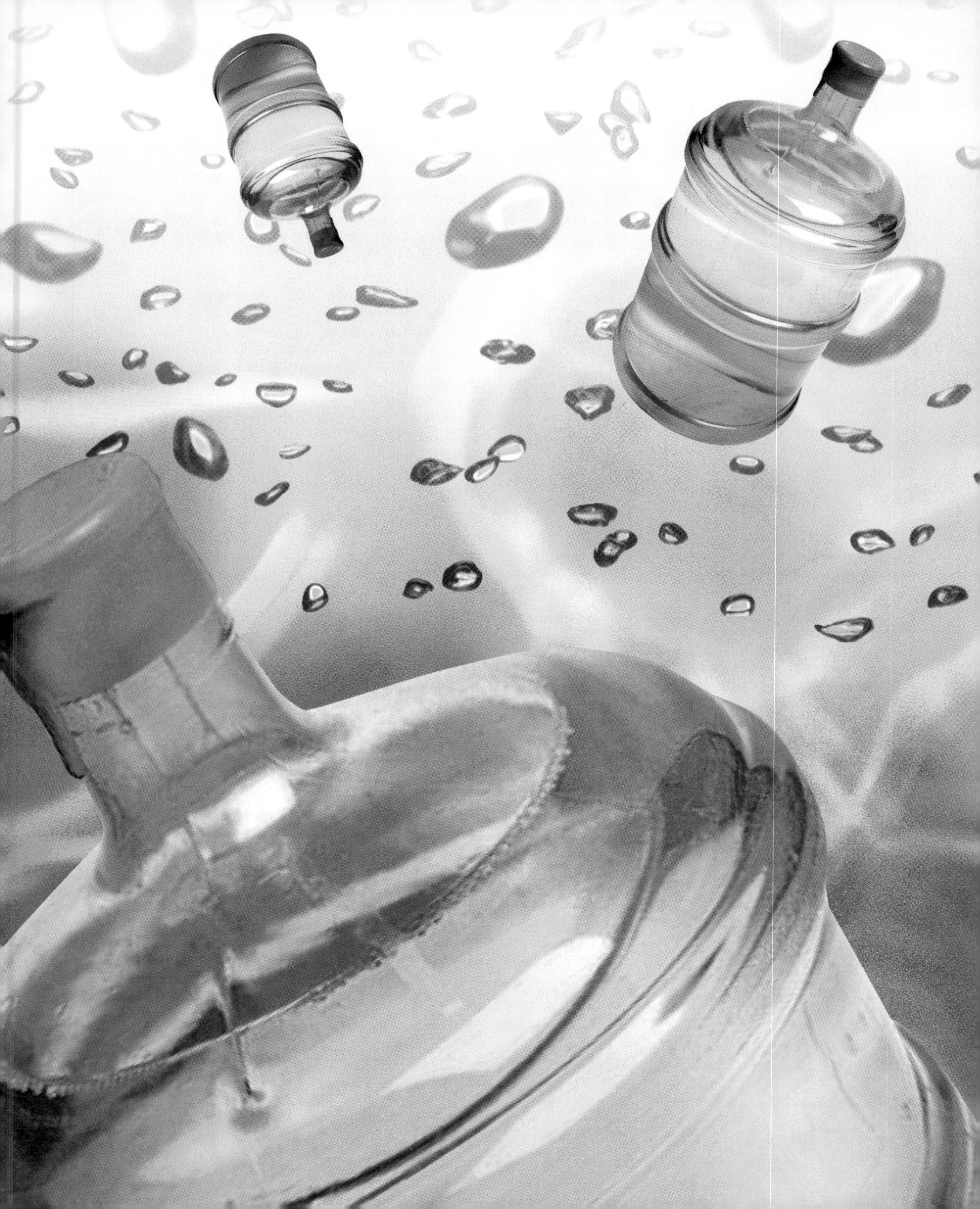

Chapter 10

Water and Minerals: The Ocean Within

Think About It

1 Do you ever feel dehydrated?

2 How often do you salt your food before tasting it?

3 You disclose to a friend that you tend to be low in iron. She knows you are a vegetarian and suggests you drink milk. What false assumption might she be making?

4 Some people argue that fluoridation is overdone. What is your position? Would you vote for fluoridating all water supplies?

Fyi for your Information

This chapter's FYI boxes include practical information on the following topics:

- Tap, Filtered, or Bottled: Which Water Is Best?
- Calcium Supplements: Are They Right for You?
- Zinc and the Common Cold

www

The Web site for this book offers many useful tools and is a great source for additional nutrition information for both students and instructors. For information on water and major minerals, visit the site at **nutrition.jbpub.com/discovering.** You'll find exercises that explore the following topics:

- The Water in Your State
- The DASH Diet
- Calcium
- Making Hard Water Soft
- Highlighting Heme
- The ADA's Stand on Supplements
- What Food Labels Can Claim
- Glowing Thyroids!

Key to Illustrations

Minerals

Water

What About Bobbie?

Track the choices Bobbie is making with the EatRight Analysis software.

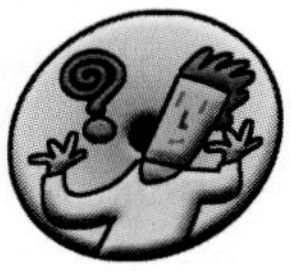

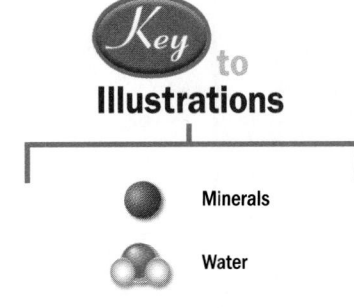

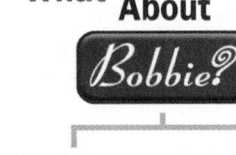

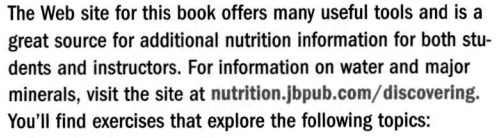

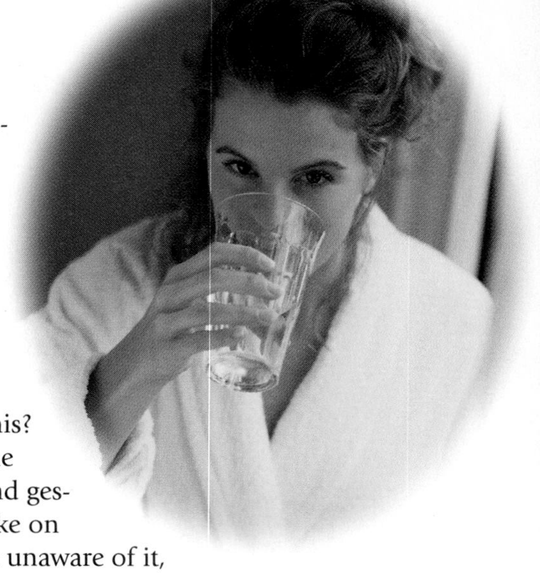

You take a coast-to-coast flight with your father and your brother. You watch as your father drinks water frequently throughout the flight, while your brother alternates between Coke and beer. When you arrive at your destination, your brother complains of feeling utterly exhausted. In contrast, your father is lively and ready for a "night on the town"! How do you explain this?

First, it's important to know that the familiar beverage cart is not just a kind gesture by the airlines; regular fluid intake on flights is necessary! Although you are unaware of it, water evaporates from the skin at an accelerated rate in the low-humidity, high-altitude, pressurized cabin of an airplane. And so drinking fluids during the flight helps prevent dehydration. But you must choose fluids carefully. Alcohol and caffeine are diuretics. This means that beverages containing them increase fluid loss as urine and therefore do not replace fluid losses as effectively as water, juice, and caffeine-free beverages.

Your brother's lack of energy may be a symptom of mild dehydration. Although he has been drinking fluids, the diuretic effect of alcohol and caffeine limits replacement of fluid. Dad, however, had the right idea—plenty of water along the way.

plasma The fluid portion of the blood that contains blood cells and other components.

salts Compounds that result when the hydrogen of an acid is replaced with a metal or a group that acts like a metal.

ions Atoms or groups of atoms with an electrical charge resulting from the loss or gain of one or more electrons.

electrolytes [ih-LEK-tro-lites] Substances that separate into charged particles (ions) when dissolved in water or other solvents and thus become capable of conducting an electrical current. The terms *electrolyte* and *ion* often are used interchangeably.

cations Ions that carry a positive charge

anions Ions that carry a negative charge.

osmosis The movement of a solvent, such as water, through a semipermeable membrane from the dilute to the concentrated side until the concentrations on both sides of the membrane are equal.

Water: Crucial to Life

Water is absolutely essential. You could probably survive weeks without food. But you can live only a few days without water. Humans have no capacity to store "spare" water, so we must quickly replace any that's lost.

Overall, water makes up between 50 and 75 percent of a person's weight. (See **Figure 10.1**.) About two-thirds of body water is intracellular fluid, the fluid inside cells. The remaining one-third is extracellular fluid, which is mainly between cells (interstitial) and in blood (the **plasma** portion). (See **Figure 10.2**.)

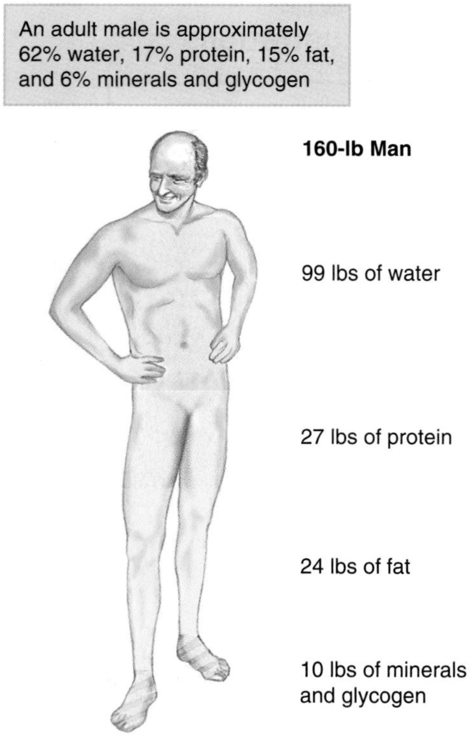

Figure 10.1 **Body composition.** The main constituent of the body is water. Adult males have more lean tissue (and therefore more water) and less fat than adult females.

Electrolytes and Water: A Delicate Balance

When minerals or **salts** dissolve in water, they form **ions (electrolytes)**. Sodium and potassium, for example, form **cations** (positively charged ions), whereas chloride and phosphate form **anions** (negatively charged ions).

Your body precisely controls and balances the concentration of electrolytes dissolved in its watery fluids—there must be just the right mix of water and electrolytes, both within and outside of each cell. Cells use pumps embedded in their membranes to move electrolytes in and out. In concert with the movement of electrolytes, water flows back and forth through the cell membrane, a process called **osmosis**. When electrolytes are more concentrated on one side of the membrane, osmosis moves water from the dilute side to the concentrated side to equalize the concentrations. (See **Figure 10.3**.)

Cells must contain just the right amount of water. Too little and the cell will shrink and die. Too much and the cell will burst. Too much water in spaces surrounding cells causes swelling (edema).

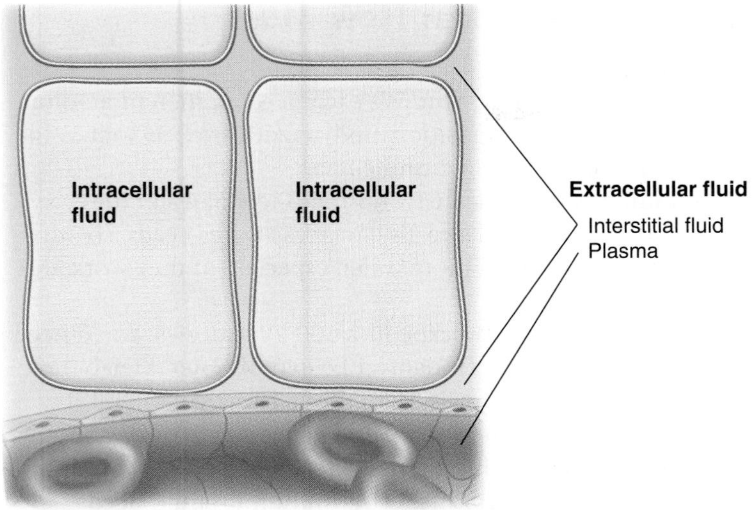

Figure 10.2 **Intracellular and extracellular fluid.** Extracellular fluids and their dissolved substances (except for proteins) move across capillary membranes easily. Plasma (the fluid portion of the blood) has a higher concentration of proteins than interstitial fluid. Excluding protein, their compositions are roughly the same.

heat capacity The amount of energy required to raise the temperature of a substance 1°C.

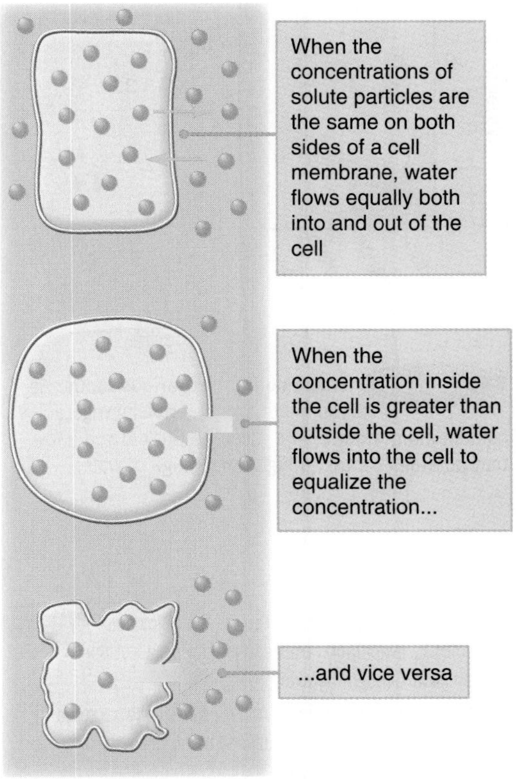

When the concentrations of solute particles are the same on both sides of a cell membrane, water flows equally both into and out of the cell
When the concentration inside the cell is greater than outside the cell, water flows into the cell to equalize the concentration...
...and vice versa

Figure 10.3 **Osmosis.** Water moves across cell membranes to equalize concentrations of dissolved particles.

Functions of Water

Water is the highway that moves nutrients and wastes between cells and organs. It carries food through your digestive system, transports nutrients to your cells and tissues, and carries waste out of your body in urine. (See **Figure 10.4**.) What about nutrients and wastes that are not water-soluble? Your body either modifies them chemically so they dissolve in water or packages them with proteins (e.g., lipoproteins). Your body's watery fluids, such as the bloodstream, can easily transport these protein packages throughout the body.

Watery fluids also have mechanical functions. They act as shock absorbers, lubricators, and cleansing agents. For example, amniotic fluid cushions and protects the fetus, synovial fluid allows joints to move smoothly, tears lubricate and cleanse the eyes, and saliva moistens food and makes swallowing possible.

Water is an essential part of your body's chemistry. It helps break apart substances and is a byproduct in many anabolic reactions (reactions that combine substances). Reactions involving water also help maintain the body's acid–base (pH) balance in the narrow range required for life.

Water has a high **heat capacity**, meaning a large amount of energy must be added or removed to raise or lower its temperature. When microwaving food, for example, you may have noticed that watery foods like soup heat much more slowly than foods like pizza that contain little water. Since your body is nearly two-thirds water, your body temperature remains relatively stable. Plus, water is the prime component of your body's cooling system. If you get too warm, blood vessels dilate and you begin to sweat. The perspiration on your skin evaporates and cools you off.

Key Concepts: *Water is so essential that we cannot survive without it for more than a few days. We need water for temperature regulation, acid–base balance, lubrication, and protection. Water dissolves or carries vital substances throughout the body and participates in chemical reactions.*

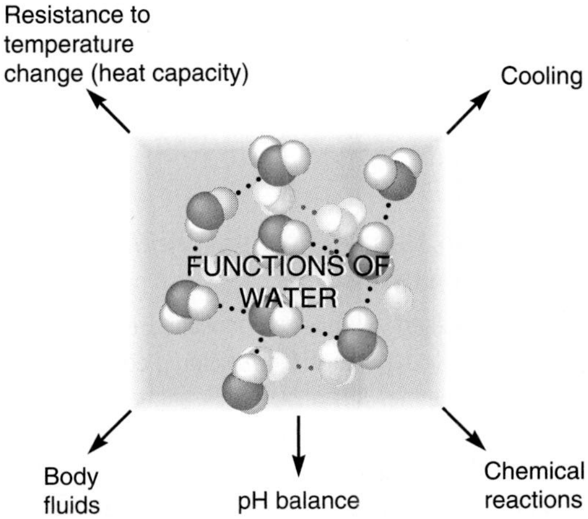

Figure 10.4 **Functions of water.** Water is so critical that we can live only a few days without it.

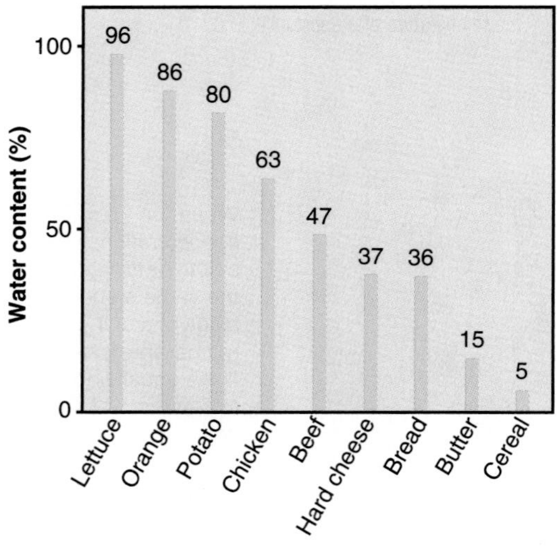

Figure 10.5 **Water content of various foods.** As you might expect, crunchy vegetables contain more water than dry cereal. But did you know that potatoes contain a high percentage of water?

insensible water loss The continual loss of body water by evaporation from the respiratory tract and diffusion through the skin.

antidiuretic hormone (ADH) A hormone secreted by the pituitary gland that increases blood pressure and prevents fluid excretion by the kidneys. Also called vasopressin.

aldosterone [al-DOS-ter-own] A hormone secreted from the adrenal glands that acts on the kidneys to regulate electrolyte and water balance. It raises blood pressure by promoting retention of sodium (and thus water) and excretion of potassium.

Quick Bites

How Do Desert-Dwelling Animals Avoid Dehydration?

Some desert animals can concentrate their urine to nearly 100 times the maximum concentration of human urine. This allows such animals to survive on water obtained from food and their own metabolic reactions. Aquatic animals, on the other hand, minimally concentrate their urine. Beavers concentrate their urine to only about half that of humans.

Intake Recommendations: How Much Water Is Enough?

There is no one answer to this question. We each need a different amount, depending on our size, body composition, and activity level, as well as the temperature and humidity of the environment.

A good rule of thumb is to replace 1 to 1.5 milliliters of water for every kilocalorie expended.[1] Activity and sweating increase water needs, so athletes and active people need much more water, especially if they work and train in warm, humid climates.

On an "average" day, suppose you expend 2,400 kilocalories. You'd need to replace at least 2,400 milliliters (roughly 10 cups) of water. Metabolic reactions in your body produce some water (about 1 to 2 cups), but the rest must come from beverages and food. Food generally supplies about 1,000 milliliters (about 4 cups) of water daily. (See **Figure 10.5**.) So drinking another 4 or 5 cups of fluid will meet your minimum fluid needs. Remember, if you are highly active or sweating, these needs can double easily.

Water Excretion: Where Does the Water Go?

We continuously lose water through various routes—exhaled air, perspiration, feces, and urine. (See water sources and water output in **Figure 10.6**.) **Insensible water loss**—the continuous evaporation of water from the lungs and skin—typically accounts for about one-quarter to one-half of daily fluid loss. These losses increase at high altitudes and during low humidity. During a coast-to-coast airplane flight, the low cabin humidity can cause fluid losses of 4 to 6 cups (about 1,000 to 1,500 milliliters)![2]

Each day we typically lose about 1 to 2 liters of water in urine. If we eat the typical American diet containing excess protein and salt, our urine production increases to eliminate surplus urea (a breakdown product from protein) and sodium. Fever, coughing, rapid breathing, and watery nasal secretions all increase water loss significantly. This is one reason why doctors recommend increasing your fluid intake when you are sick.

Key Concepts: *A typical adult needs 1.0 to 1.5 milliliters of fluid per kilocalorie expended. Water intake comes from a combination of foods, fluids, and water produced in normal metabolism. Fluid is lost mainly by urination. Additional losses occur through the skin and lungs and in feces. Water is critical in eliminating the body's waste products.*

Water Balance

Our bodies carefully maintain water balance by manipulating water intake and output. When water intake is low, the kidneys conserve water and only excrete a small volume of concentrated urine. When the body has an excess of water, the kidneys excrete a large volume of dilute urine.

How do the kidneys know when to conserve water? Special cells in the brain sense the need to dilute rising sodium levels in the body. They signal the pituitary gland to release **antidiuretic hormone (ADH)**, which in turn signals the kidneys to conserve water. Sensors in the kidneys themselves can detect a rapid loss of fluid through a drop in blood pressure. They trigger a complex process that includes the release of the hormone **aldosterone** by the adrenal glands. Aldosterone signals the kidneys to retain sodium. To avoid an increased concentration of sodium, osmosis drives the simultaneous reabsorption of water.

Thirst

While taste, availability, cultural patterns, and personal habits influence our consumption of fluids, thirst remains our most important stimulus for drinking fluids. Yet thirst is not always a reliable guide to avoiding dehydration. By the time dehydration triggers thirst, you will have lost 1 to 2 percent of your body weight in water.[3] Hot weather or heavy exercise can cause fluid losses of up to 1 to 2 liters per hour.[4] And after you drink water, your body can take 30 to 60 minutes to absorb and distribute it throughout the body. For example, imagine you are rollerblading in the hot sun and after an hour you pause momentarily to quench your thirst with a ½-liter bottle of water. That's not enough! You still have a deficit of ½ to 1½ liters of water, and you'll continue to lose water while your body absorbs and distributes the water you just drank. To avoid dehydration in hot weather or when exercising, you need to drink fluids early and often. (See the FYI feature "Tap, Filtered, or Bottled: Which Water Is Best?")

Think About It 1

Key Concepts: *The body uses complex mechanisms to precisely regulate water balance. Antidiuretic hormone (ADH) stimulates water reabsorption in the kidneys, while aldosterone stimulates the kidneys to reabsorb sodium and water. Although our sense of thirst usually reminds us to drink enough so that we don't become dehydrated, it is an unreliable signal during hot weather or heavy exercise, when fluid losses are high.*

Alcohol, Caffeine, and Common Medications Affect Fluid Balance

Anyone who regularly consumes alcohol probably realizes that it is a diuretic—a substance that increases fluid loss through increased urination. Alcohol suppresses ADH production, and excessive alcohol consumption can cause dehydration with symptoms of thirst, weakness, dryness of mucous membranes, dizziness, and light-headedness—all common effects of a hangover.

A cup of coffee can provide a morning pick-me-up, but the caffeine is a diuretic. A typical pattern of many busy Americans is a few cups of coffee in the morning, a caffeinated soda with lunch, another in the afternoon, and maybe a glass of wine or a beer with dinner. Although some suggest that a fondness for caffeinated beverages can cause chronic mild dehydration, most Americans seem to consume a sufficient quantity and variety of beverages to maintain fluid balance.[5]

Doctors often prescribe diuretic medications to help lower blood pressure or decrease swelling caused by fluid retention. Since these medications can disrupt sodium and potassium balance, doctors typically monitor the patient's blood electrolyte levels and may prescribe potassium supplements to maintain a proper balance.

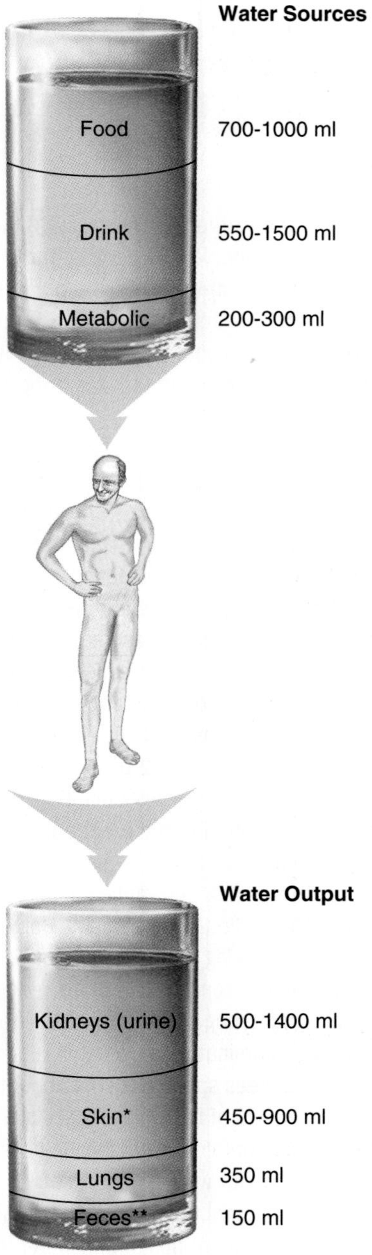

* (Insensible and perspiration)
The volume of perspiration is normally about 100 ml per day. In very hot weather or during heavy exercise, a person may lose 10 to 20 times this amount (1 to 2 liters) per hour.

** People with severe diarrhea can lose several liters of water per day in feces.

Figure 10.6 **Typical daily water intake and output.** To maintain water balance, your body regulates its fluid intake and output.

Dehydration

Any condition causing rapid water loss is dangerous: burns in which damaged skin cannot control water evaporation, the heat of fever, extreme environmental heat, or exertion without replenishing water. Early signs of dehydration include fatigue, dry mucous membranes, headache, and dark urine with a strong odor. Physical and mental performance slip. A

Fyi FOR YOUR INFORMATION Tap, Filtered, or Bottled: Which Water Is Best?

Everywhere you look, it seems as if more and more people are carrying and sipping from bottles of water. Theme parks even sell shoulder holsters for you to carry your bottle around with you. What's with the water craze? And what's wrong with the good old water fountain?

The popularity of bottled water exploded in the 1980s. Initially, bottled mineral waters, like Perrier, were associated with wealth and glamour. But like many trends adopted by the wealthy (white bread, for instance), bottled water soon became desirable to a wider range of people. It is now estimated that Americans drink 2.5 billion gallons of bottled water each year![1] Worldwide, bottled water is a $35 billion industry. In 1999, U.S. bottled water sales exceeded $5.2 billion.[2] Even the major soft drink companies Coca-Cola and PepsiCo have gotten into the act and now sell their own brands of bottled water.

There are probably several factors fueling the growth of the bottled-water industry. Baby boomers are seeking natural, low-calorie beverages, and fitness consciousness has reemphasized the importance of hydration. Media reports of contaminated tap water in major metropolitan areas spark concerns about the safety and quality of tap water. Most Americans choose bottled water for what they think is not in it, rather than for what it contains.

From a nutritional perspective, it's important to drink plenty of fluids, and water is one of the best ways to replace lost fluids. And so, at the simplest level, the source of water doesn't really matter. Standards for municipal water systems are enforced by the Environmental Protection Agency (EPA), which requires regular testing and monitoring. Tap water can be considered a safe, clean source of water. Many municipal water systems add fluoride to tap water, an important weapon in the prevention of tooth decay. However, home-installed filtration systems for removing chlorine also may remove added fluoride, and most bottled waters do not contain fluoride.

Some people don't like the taste of their local water supply and don't want to bother with maintaining a filtration system. In this case, or if you want your water "to go," bottled water may be the choice. The bottled-water industry offers

- high-volume, returnable containers from suppliers who stock the water coolers for offices or supermarkets
- the familiar brands (e.g., Evian, Zephyrhills, Dannon, Nala) that are sold as alternatives to soft drinks
- bottled water in vending machines

The bottled-water industry is regulated by the Food and Drug Administration (FDA), which, in 1995, published Standards of Identity for bottled water, set maximum allowable standards for contaminants, and established Current Good Manufacturing Practices (CGMP) for bottling plants. Keep in mind that the FDA regulates bottled waters that are sold interstate and not those sold only in a particular area or state. Individual states may have their own quality standards for locally distributed waters.

Look beyond the terms like *artesian, mineral, spring,* or *purified* (see Table A). The labels on most bottled water list the source of the water. Some consumers may be surprised to find that their favorite brand of water is really from a municipal source, not an underground spring! Nutrition Facts labels are required if the manufacturer makes a claim (e.g., sodium-free) or adds minerals. These labels often do not show the natural mineral content of the water, which is really the only other nutritional aspect that could be expected.

Once again, the choice is up to the consumer—for water, no choice is clearly best. Cost, taste, convenience, and safety are all issues to consider.

1 American Dietetic Association. Tip of the Day! Water to tap. http://www.eatright.org/erm/erm070797.html. Accessed 4/27/02.

2 BottledWaterWeb. www.bottledwaterweb.com/indus.html. Accessed 4/27/02.

Table A Definitions of Bottled Water Terms

- *Mineral water* must contain at least 250 parts per million (ppm) of dissolved minerals and come from a geologically and physically protected underground water source.
- *Purified water* is tap or ground water that has been treated by distillation, deionization, or reverse osmosis. This may be labeled "distilled water" if produced by steam distillation and condensation.
- *Spring water* comes from an underground formation from which water flows naturally to the surface; it is collected either at the spring or from a bore hole to the underground formation.
- *Artesian water* comes from tapping a confined underground aquifer that is below the natural water table. Generally the artesian well is located in a depression where the water table of the surrounding hills is higher. The "head" of pressure from the water table forces the water up through the tap line.
- *Ground water* comes from a subsurface saturated zone and is not under the direct influence of surface water.
- *Well water* comes from a drilled hole that taps the water of an aquifer, and is pumped to the surface.

Source: Bottled Water Industry Facts. http://www.bottledwaterweb.com/regulations.html. Accessed 4/27/02; and FDA regulations 21CFR165.110. http://vm.cfsan.fda.gov/~lrd/n095-323.txt. Accessed 4/27/02.

water loss of 20 percent of body weight can cause coma and death. (See **Figure 10.7**.)

Seniors and infants are particularly vulnerable to dehydration. The sense of thirst often diminishes with age, and seniors commonly take diuretic medications. For a variety of reasons, seniors may eat and drink less. The resulting physical and mental deterioration creates a vicious cycle, with food and fluid intake continuing to worsen.

Because infants can lose water rapidly through their skin, they need ample fluid relative to their size. Breast milk or infant formula generally provides all the fluid a baby needs. Severe diarrhea can cause swift and deadly dehydration, especially in seniors and infants. Normally, the intestines reabsorb nearly all the fluid secreted by digestive organs. But when intestinal disease causes diarrhea or prolonged vomiting, dehydration can occur. Worldwide, dehydration is a major killer of babies and young children, with infection the underlying culprit.

Water consumption, of course, is the primary treatment for dehydration. Often electrolytes also must be replaced, particularly in cases of diarrhea and vomiting. For moderate to severe dehydration, intravenous fluids and hospitalization may be necessary. In remote areas or developing countries, "rehydration packets"—a mix of potassium and sodium salts and sugar—dissolved in boiled water have saved countless lives.

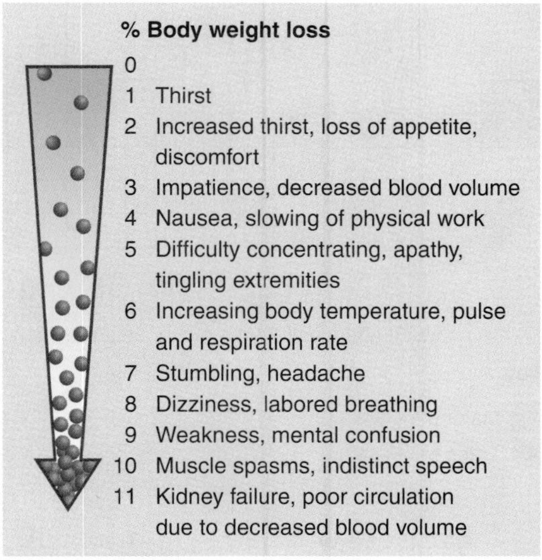

Figure 10.7 **Effects of progressive dehydration.** Dehydration quickly diminishes physical and mental performance. Severe dehydration can be fatal.

Water Intoxication

Because drinking fluids temporarily alleviates thirst, we rarely drink to the point of overhydration and dilution of body fluids. Overhydration can occur in people with untreated glandular disorders that cause excessive water retention. Some mentally ill people have a compulsion to drink more water than their kidneys can handle (over 15 to 20 liters daily). Overhydration first causes headaches and then seizures. Several years ago, some dieters overenthusiastically followed a fad weight reduction diet calling for massive water intake and suffered seizures from overhydration.

Key Concepts: *Alcohol, caffeine, and diuretic medications increase urinary fluid losses. Dehydration is a potential consequence of gastrointestinal disease, burns, and heavy sweating. Treatment involves replacing fluids, along with electrolytes if the condition is severe. Although unlikely, water intoxication is possible.*

Quick Bites

Water, Water Everywhere and Not a Drop to Drink!

When shipwrecked sailors drink seawater, they quickly become severely dehydrated. This is because the concentration of salt in seawater is about double the maximum concentration of salt in urine. Thus, it takes 2 liters of urine to rid the body of the solutes ingested by drinking 1 liter of seawater.

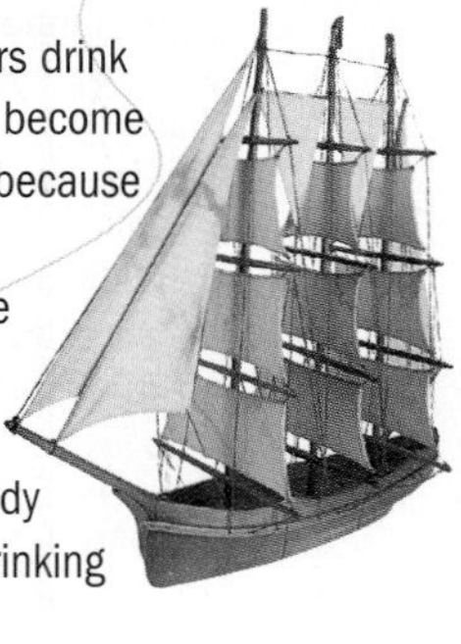

Minerals

What distinguishes minerals from vitamins, carbohydrates, proteins, and fats? Minerals are elemental atoms or ions rather than organic compounds. Unlike vitamins, minerals are not destroyed by heat, light, acidity, or alkalinity. Calcium, for example, remains calcium, be it in seashells, milk, or bones. Iron remains iron, whether it is part of a cast-iron skillet or part of hemoglobin.

Like vitamins, however, minerals are "micronutrients." Compared with carbohydrates, proteins, and fats, they are needed in relatively small amounts—at most a gram or two per day.

Minerals often are grouped as **major minerals** and **trace minerals**. The classification is arbitrarily based on the amount you need in your diet and the amount present in your body. You need more than 100 milligrams per

major minerals Major minerals are required in the diet and present in the body in large amounts compared with trace minerals.

trace minerals Minerals required in the diet and present in the body in very small quantities.

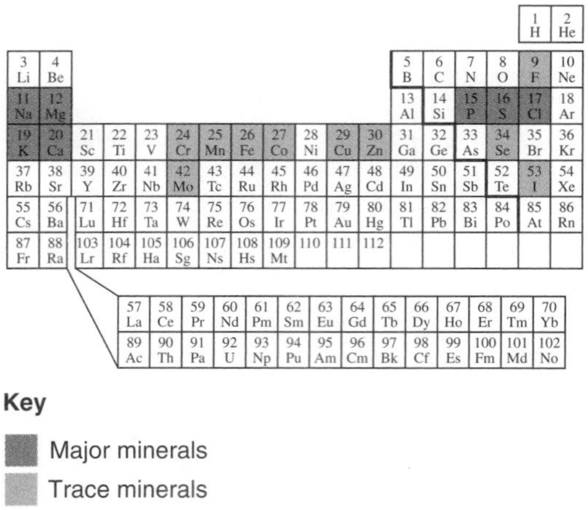

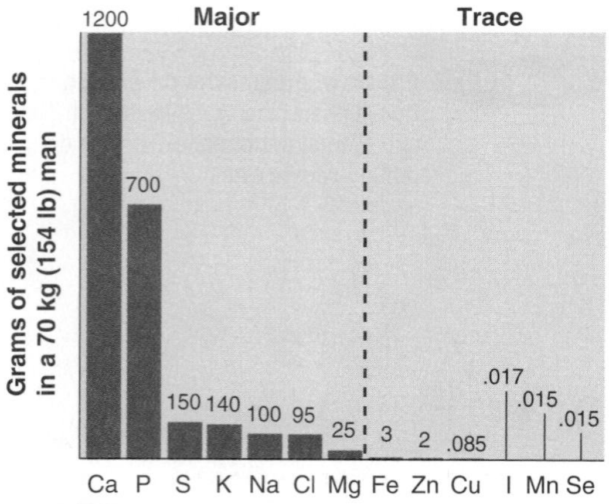

Figure 10.8 **Minerals in the human body.** Dietary minerals also are elements in the periodic table. Based on the amount of a mineral needed in the diet and the amount in the body, nutritionists categorize a mineral as major or trace. Other minerals are found in minute quantities in the body, and may or may not be essential nutrients.
Source: Groff JL, Gropper SS. *Advanced Nutrition and Human Metabolism.* 3rd ed. Belmont, CA: Wadsworth/Thomson Learning; 2000; and Stipanuk MH. *Biochemical and Physiological Aspects of Human Nutrition.* Philadelphia: WB Saunders; 2000.

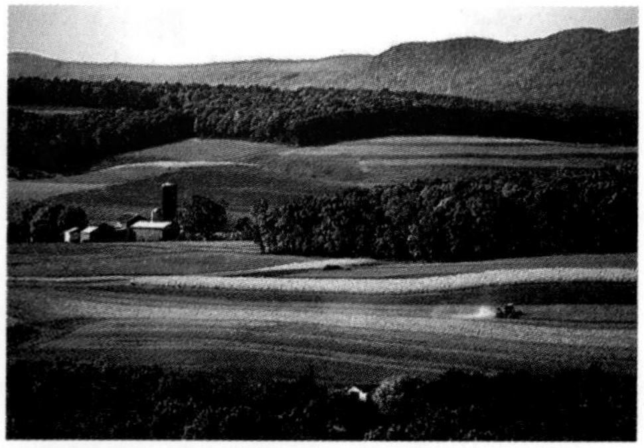

Figure 10.9 **Growing conditions influence mineral content.** The mineral content of plants reflects the mineral content of the soil in which they are grown.

day of each major mineral and less than 100 milligrams daily of each trace mineral. (See **Figure 10.8**.)

Compared with the major minerals, the total amount of each trace mineral present in your body is small. For example, your total body iron, a trace mineral, is 2 to 4 grams, or about the amount of iron in a small nail. Contrast that with your total body calcium, a major mineral. Most adult bodies contain over 1,000 grams.[6]

Despite the amounts found in the body or required from diet, both major and trace minerals are crucially important. Often a single mineral has several quite diverse functions. Some, like iodine, are components of hormones. Many are components of enzymes or enzyme cofactors. Others serve a structural function; for example, calcium and phosphorus are among the minerals that make bones hard.

Minerals in Foods

Foods from both plants and animals are sources of minerals. Generally speaking, animal tissue contains minerals in the proportion that the animal needs, so animal-derived foods are more reliable mineral sources.

Plant foods can be excellent sources of several minerals, but the mineral content of plants can vary dramatically depending on the minerals in the soil where the plants are found. (See **Figure 10.9**.) Even the maturity of a vegetable, fruit, or grain can influence its mineral content. Since actual mineral content varies so much, the values published in food composition tables can be misleading. Often these values are omitted. Like plant foods, drinking water has variable mineral content. But it sometimes can be a significant source of minerals such as sodium, magnesium, and fluoride.

Bioavailability

Our GI tracts absorb a much smaller proportion of minerals than vitamins—and probably for good reason. Once absorbed, excess minerals often are difficult for the body to flush out. In many cases, the body adjusts mineral absorption in relation to needs. For example, a calcium-deficient person absorbs calcium more readily than does a person with normal calcium levels.

Megadosing with single-mineral supplements can hamper the absorption of other minerals. Minerals like calcium, iron, zinc, and magnesium, for example, all have similar chemical properties and compete for absorption.

Fiber and other components of food also affect mineral bioavailability. (See **Figure 10.10**.) High-fiber diets reduce absorption of iron, calcium, zinc, and magnesium. **Phytate** (a component of whole grains) binds minerals and carries them out of the intestine unabsorbed. **Oxalate** (found in spinach and rhubarb) binds calcium, markedly reducing calcium absorption.

Key Concepts: *Minerals are essential inorganic elements. They are in a wide variety of foods, but absorption is limited by several factors, among them our physiological need, presence of competing minerals, and presence of fiber.*

Major Minerals and Health

The seven major minerals—sodium, potassium, chloride, calcium, phosphorus, magnesium, and sulfur—have significant roles, and when mineral status goes awry, your health can suffer. Two disorders in which major minerals play critical parts are hypertension and osteoporosis.

Hypertension

Hypertension is persistent high blood pressure. It affects nearly one quarter of American adults and more than half of people over 65. Most cases are **essential hypertension**, in which the cause is unknown.

Left untreated, the excessive pressure of blood on the arteries eventually scars and narrows them, reducing their elasticity. This increases the likelihood of atherosclerosis, because fatty plaque accumulates where arteries are damaged. (See Chapter 6, "Lipids," for more on atherosclerosis.) The heart, forced to work much harder pumping blood through the narrowed arteries, becomes enlarged and inefficient. Eventually the heart is unable to supply enough nutrients and oxygen to organs and tissues. The kidneys, the brain, and the heart are especially vulnerable to the damaging effects of high blood pressure.

Blood clots also tend to form at sites of artery damage, further limiting blood flow. The clots can break loose and travel to the brain, causing a stroke, or to the heart, causing heart attack.

Blood pressure is expressed as two numbers. The **systolic** is the higher number and represents pressure during the heart's contraction. **Diastolic** is the lower number, measured during the heart's rest phase. Normal blood pressure is generally defined as 120/80 mm Hg (millimeters of mercury) or lower. Persistent systolic pressure of 140 or higher or diastolic pressure of 90 or higher, or both, usually requires treatment.

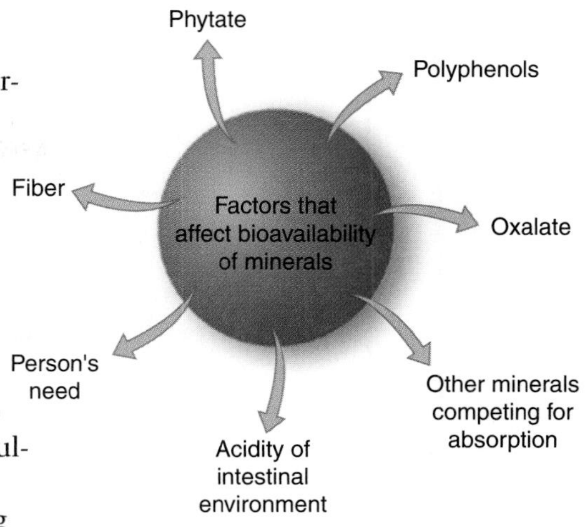

Figure 10.10 **Factors that affect the bioavailability of minerals.** A person's need and the dietary components of a meal can enhance or inhibit the absorption of a mineral.

Sodium and Hypertension

Clearly, there is a genetic predisposition to essential hypertension. For example, African Americans are more likely to develop hypertension and at an earlier age than Caucasians.[7] If both parents have high blood pressure, then the probability their children also will have it rises dramatically.

But does diet also play a role? Could changing our diets prevent or delay high blood pressure? And for people who have hypertension, can changing their diet help control their blood pressure?

Think About It 2

Excessive sodium can hold excessive fluid in the body, at least temporarily. These excesses can be burdensome on the kidneys, heart, and blood vessels. The consensus among heart disease experts is that too much sodium, ingested routinely over the years, plays a role in the underlying causes of hypertension in genetically predisposed or "salt-sensitive" people. The more salt they eat, the higher their blood pressure.

Population studies appear to bear this out. Rates of hypertension are greater in countries with high sodium intakes. On the other hand, primitive people, whose diets contain very little sodium, seldom have hypertension. Their blood pressure does not rise with age if they continue to eat their traditional diet. But if they adopt a "modern" (higher-sodium) diet, blood pressure tends to rise, and they are more likely to become hypertensive.[8]

The relation of dietary sodium to hypertension is one of the most heavily researched issues in nutrition. Unfortunately, study conclusions often differ. Among the most influential studies are the DASH (Dietary Approaches to Stop Hypertension) studies, two large, carefully controlled trials sponsored by the National Heart, Lung and Blood Institute (NHLBI). The most recent study found that strictly reducing sodium for four weeks, along with eating generous amounts of fruits, vegetables, and low-fat dairy foods, lowered systolic blood pressure an average 7.1 mm Hg in nonhypertensive people and 11.5 mm Hg in hypertensive people.[9] Limiting sodium, but not eating the extra fruits, vegetables, and dairy foods, lowered systolic blood pressure by an average 6.7 mm Hg.

phytate (phytic acid) A phosphorus-containing compound in the outer husks of cereal grains that binds with minerals and inhibits their absorption.

oxalate (oxalic acid) An organic acid in some leafy green vegetables, such as spinach, that binds to calcium to form calcium oxalate, an insoluble compound the body cannot absorb.

hypertension Condition in which resting blood pressure persistently exceeds 140 mm Hg systolic or 90 mm Hg diastolic.

essential hypertension Hypertension for which no specific cause can be identified; 90 to 95 percent of people with hypertension have essential hypertension.

systolic Pertaining to a heart contraction. Systolic blood pressure is measured during a heart contraction, a time period known as systole.

diastolic Pertaining to the time between heart contractions. Diastolic blood pressure is measured at the point of maximum cardiac relaxation.

Other Dietary Factors

Sodium is not the only dietary factor associated with hypertension. The carefully controlled DASH study also showed that foods low in fat and rich in calcium, magnesium, and potassium reduce blood pressure as well. Eating 10 servings of fruit and vegetables and 2 to 3 servings of low-fat dairy products daily, while limiting fat and saturated fat, brought systolic blood pressure down by 5.9 mm Hg, even at the highest sodium intake of 3,450 milligrams.[10] In an earlier eight-week study, a similar diet reduced systolic blood pressure by 3.5 mm Hg in nonhypertensive people and 11.3 mm Hg in people with hypertension.[11]

The DASH studies show that limiting sodium, fat, and cholesterol, as well as increasing fruits, vegetables, and low-fat dairy foods, can lower blood pressure. The NHLBI recommends that all Americans follow the DASH combination diet. Controlling weight, getting regular exercise, and reducing alcohol consumption also help reduce blood pressure.

Key Concepts: *Hypertension is a risk factor for atherosclerosis, kidney disease, and stroke. Excess sodium intake raises blood pressure in those who are salt-sensitive. Inadequate levels of potassium, calcium, and possibly magnesium may also contribute to hypertension. Limiting sodium intake, along with eating lots of low-sodium vegetables, fruits, and low-fat dairy products, will probably help reduce hypertension and its side effects.*

Osteoporosis

Osteoporosis means "porous bone." It's a good description. In osteoporosis, bone mass or density declines, and bone quality deteriorates, leaving the bones fragile and vulnerable to fracture. (See **Figure 10.11**.) The hip, spine, and wrist bones are especially vulnerable. Often called a "silent disease," osteoporosis develops over several years without outward symptoms or diagnosis. Eventually bone loss makes bones so weak, they break with a mild strain, bump, or gentle fall. In fact, the break may occur first and cause the fall! Osteoporosis is the major cause of bone fracture in older adults, primarily postmenopausal women.[12]

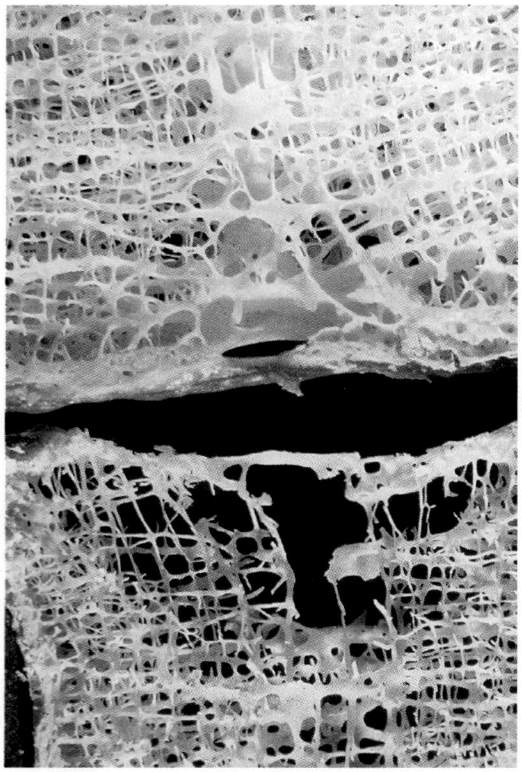

Figure 10.11 **Osteoporosis.** Normal bone (top) and osteoporotic bone (bottom). The osteoporotic bone is noticeably less dense.

Osteoporosis affects more than 25 million Americans, making it a major public health problem. Although 80 percent of those with osteoporosis are women, by age 75 one-third of all men have osteoporosis. During their lifetimes, one in two women and one in five men will break a bone weakened by osteoporosis.[13] **Table 10.1** lists the risk factors for osteoporosis.

Development of Osteoporosis

Bone mass typically peaks sometime around age 30. Starting in midlife, bone breakdown begins to exceed bone formation, and the progressive loss of bone begins. If earlier calcium and vitamin D intakes maximized bone mass, when bone loss begins you are likely to be a long way from low bone density and fractures.

Because declining estrogen levels accelerate bone loss, postmenopausal women have the highest risk for osteoporosis. By age 65, some women have lost half their skeletal mass. Women who reach menopause with low bone mass have a greatly increased risk of fractures.

Calcium and Osteoporosis

Adequate calcium intake throughout life helps prevent osteoporosis. Good calcium intake during childhood and adolescence helps maximize peak bone mass. Even in adulthood, adequate calcium slows bone loss, and it reduces fracture rates in postmenopausal women.

Calcium is clearly an important nutrient in bone health, but it's not the only one. Normal mineralization and maintenance of bone also require vitamins D, A, and K; phosphorus, fluoride, and magnesium; and protein.

Other Dietary and Lifestyle Factors

You need vitamin D for calcium absorption and bone maintenance. Since aging limits the ability to manufacture active vitamin D, older people should use vitamin D-fortified foods such as milk or consider vitamin D supplements. Phytate and oxalate, caffeine, and smoking can reduce calcium absorption or increase excretion rates. Regular weight-bearing exercise enhances bone remodeling and strength. Exercise helps maximize bone mass when you're young and will slow bone loss during your later years. To promote bone health and slow the development of osteoporosis, exercise experts suggest:

1. Exercise should be weight-bearing and put stress on bones. Examples include walking and running.
2. For continued improvement, exercise intensity should increase progressively.
3. People with small total bone mass have the greatest potential for improvement.
4. There is a maximum achievable bone density. As this is approached, greater efforts are needed to achieve smaller gains.
5. Discontinuing an exercise program reverses the benefits.[14]

In summary, these steps help reduce the risk of osteoporosis: Maintain adequate calcium and vitamin D intake throughout life; eat a healthful diet rich in other bone-building nutrients; perform weight-bearing exercise; and in the case of postmenopausal women, consider estrogen supplements.[15]

Key Concepts: *Osteoporosis is the progressive loss of bone mass, resulting in fragile bones that break easily. Osteoporosis primarily affects postmenopausal women who have lower estrogen levels and accelerated rates of bone loss. Adequate calcium intake early in life helps maximize peak bone mass and reduces the risk of osteoporosis. Adequate amounts of vitamin D and regular exercise also are important for bone health.*

Table 10.1 Risk Factors for Osteoporosis

Advanced age
Female
Thin and/or small frame
Family history of osteoporosis
Early menopause, whether natural or surgically induced
Low testosterone levels in men
Abnormal absence of menstrual periods (amenorrhea)
Anorexia nervosa or bulimia nervosa
Medical conditions such as thyroid disease, rheumatoid arthritis, and problems that block intestinal absorption of calcium
Use of certain medications, such as corticosteroids and anticonvulsants
Insufficient dietary calcium
Lack of weight-bearing exercise
Cigarette smoking
Excessive use of alcohol or caffeine

Sodium

You probably know sodium best as a component of table salt. Table salt, or sodium chloride, is 40 percent sodium. And you've probably heard that we eat too much sodium. The *Dietary Guidelines* tell us to "choose and prepare foods with less salt."[16]

But excess sodium is a relatively recent problem. For centuries in many regions, salt was highly prized and hard to come by. Our language reflects that: "He's worth his salt" means he's a valuable person; the word *salary* is derived from the Latin word for salt. Sodium is, in fact, an essential nutrient of great importance.

Sodium is critical for regulating both cellular fluid and total body fluid. Although most sodium is in extracellular fluid, it acts in concert with other electrolytes both within and outside of cells to regulate fluid levels, blood

Quick Bites

Why Do Salty Foods Make You Thirsty?

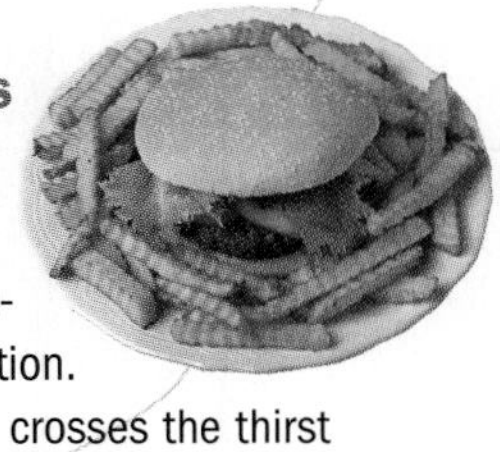

The thirst mechanism is highly sensitive to extracellular sodium concentration. Even a tiny rise in sodium crosses the thirst threshold and triggers the desire to drink.

pressure, and pH (acidity and alkalinity). The movement of sodium back and forth across cell membranes helps regulate the transit of other substances that tag along or travel in the opposite direction. Sodium, as well as other electrolytes, also helps transmit nerve impulses and other electrical messages.

Dietary Recommendations and Sources of Sodium

There is no RDA for sodium. We rarely eat too little; in fact most of us eat substantially more than we need. The Food and Nutrition Board estimates that healthy adults require a minimum of 500 milligrams daily.[17] The American Heart Association recommends limiting sodium to 2,400 milligrams per day (the amount in about 1 teaspoon of table salt); this level is used for the Daily Value on food labels.

The typical American diet contains 3,000 to 6,000 milligrams of sodium daily. Not only do Americans consume more than the recommended amounts of sodium, but they also are poor judges of the amount of sodium in their diets.[18] Surprisingly, processed foods—not table salt—contribute the most sodium. (See **Table 10.2**.)

A breakdown of the sources of sodium in our diets shows

75 percent	Added during food processing
10 percent	Occurring naturally in foods
15 percent	Used in cooking and at the table

Soy sauce and other sauces; pickled foods; salty or smoked meats, cheese, and fish; salted snack foods; bouillon cubes; and canned and instant soups are all high-sodium foods. Seasonings based on salt (such as "lemon salt" and "seasoning salt") and those containing the flavor enhancer monosodium glutamate (MSG) also are high in sodium. If your diet is based on Asian foods that contain liberal amounts of soy sauce and MSG, you could be taking in 12,000 to 16,000 milligrams of sodium per day.

Quick Bites

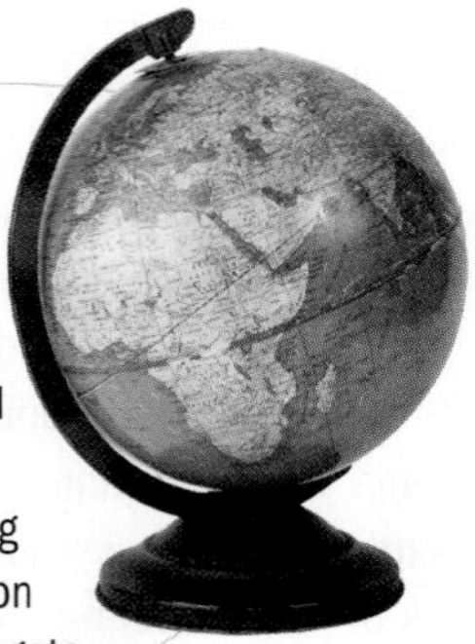

Sacred Salt

The physiological need for salt played an important role in shaping human history. Population groups tended to congregate where salt could be found, and civilizations in Africa, India, the Middle East, and China developed around rich salt deposits. At times, salt was traded at a value twice that of gold.

Table 10.2 Sodium Content of Various Foods

Food	Serving Size	Sodium (mg)
Cucumber, fresh	1 large (8 1/4")	6
Dill pickle	1 large (4")	1,730
Roast pork	3 oz (85 g)	50
Ham, cured	3 oz (85 g)	1,180
Whole-wheat bread	1 slice	150
Biscuit from mix	1	540
Fresh tomato	1 medium	10
Spaghetti sauce, jar	1/2 C	520
Two-percent milk	1 C (240 mL)	120
American cheese	1 oz	400
Baked potato	1 medium	8
Potato chips	1 oz	170

As food becomes more processed, the sodium content increases

Source: US Department of Agriculture, Agricultural Research Service. 2001. *USDA Nutrient Database for Standard Reference*, Release 14. Nutrient Data Laboratory Home Page. http://www.nal.usda.gov/fnic/foodcomp. Accessed 4/27/02.

Dealing with Excess Sodium

While some illnesses can drive down blood sodium to dangerously low levels, our bodies usually must deal with an excess of sodium. In some people, eating too much sodium over a long period of time can contribute to hypertension. (See the section "Hypertension" in this chapter.) Your intestinal tract absorbs nearly all dietary sodium, which travels throughout the body in the bloodstream. Your kidneys, those remarkable organs, retain the exact amount of sodium the body needs and excrete the excess sodium in the urine along with water.

Because excreting excess sodium wastes water, taking in too much sodium and not enough water can worsen dehydration. The old practice of giving athletes salt tablets before or after exercise is unnecessary and possibly harmful. On the other hand, radical sodium restriction is not a good idea, either. Even though most Americans consume too much sodium, severe sodium restriction can limit the availability of other essential nutrients like vitamin B_6, calcium, iron, and magnesium.[19]

Key Concepts: *Sodium in the extracellular fluid plays a critical role in regulating water distribution and blood pressure. There is no RDA for sodium, and the American diet contains an overabundance—3,000 to 6,000 milligrams daily, versus recommended limits of 2,400 milligrams. Processed foods supply most of the sodium in our diets. Extreme sodium restriction is unwise and may reduce the availability of some vitamins and minerals.*

Potassium

Nearly all the body's potassium resides within cells, with the highest amount in muscle cells. The flow of potassium in and out of cells is coupled to the flow of sodium. Together, they help contract muscles, transmit nerve impulses, and regulate blood pressure and heartbeat. The central nervous system zealously protects its potassium, maintaining constant levels even when muscle and blood levels drop.

Like sodium, potassium affects blood pressure, but in a different way. When people with hypertension eat a diet low in sodium and rich in high-potassium foods (like fruits and vegetables), their blood pressure often improves.[20]

Dietary Recommendations and Sources of Potassium

For potassium, the Daily Value on food labels is 3,500 milligrams, and experts estimate that healthy adults should average no less than 2,000 milligrams per day. Vegetables and fruits, especially potatoes, spinach, melons, and bananas, are important dietary potassium sources. Meat, fish, poultry, and dairy products are also good sources. (See **Figure 10.12**.) Many but not all salt substitutes contain potassium chloride. A balanced healthy diet generally contains between 2,000 and 4,000 milligrams per day.

Although food manufacturers often add sodium to processed foods, they do not routinely add potassium. So if a person's diet includes a lot of processed foods, it may fail to meet the minimum potassium recommendations.

When Potassium Balance Goes Awry

Dietary deficiency of potassium is uncommon. The most common cause of potassium deficiency is excessive losses. Prolonged

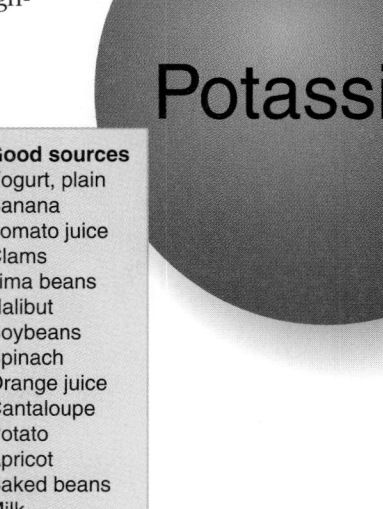

Quick Bites

Banana Facts

You may know that bananas are high in potassium, but did you also know that they have an unusually high carbohydrate content? Before ripening, a banana is almost entirely starch. After ripening, the dessert varieties are almost entirely sugar—as much as 20 percent by weight.

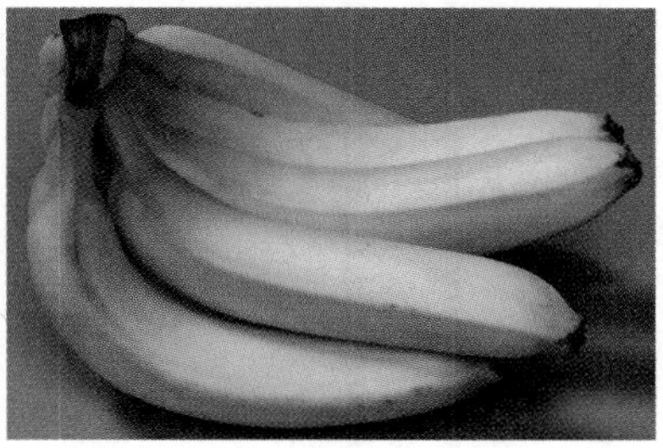

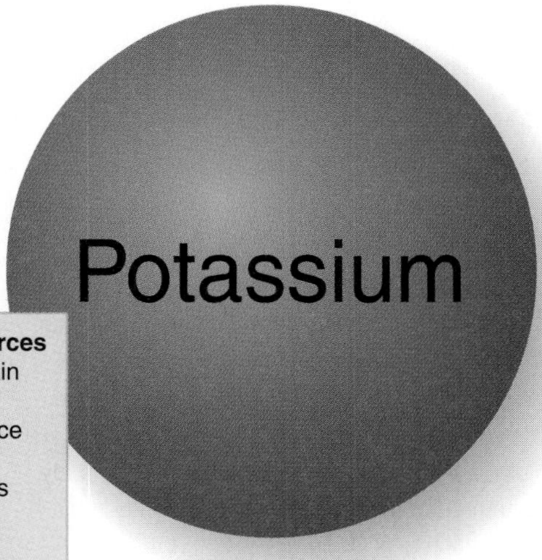

Good sources
Yogurt, plain
Banana
Tomato juice
Clams
Lima beans
Halibut
Soybeans
Spinach
Orange juice
Cantaloupe
Potato
Apricot
Baked beans
Milk
Acorn squash

Figure 10.12 Food sources of potassium. The best food sources of potassium are fresh fruits and vegetables, certain dairy products, and fish.

vomiting, chronic diarrhea, laxative abuse, and use of diuretics are the most common causes of low blood potassium. Physicians monitor electrolyte blood levels of patients taking diuretics and recommend potassium supplements if needed. Symptoms of low blood potassium include muscle weakness, loss of appetite, and confusion. If potassium depletion is severe or rapid, heart rhythms may be disrupted—a potentially fatal problem.

Because the kidneys effectively remove excess potassium, in healthy people the risk of toxicity from dietary intake is low. Potassium supplements, available over the counter and sold in health food stores, should be taken only when recommended by a physician. Extremely high blood potassium levels can slow and eventually stop the heart.

Key Concepts: *Potassium is found mainly in intracellular fluid. Along with sodium, it regulates muscle contractions and nerve impulse transmissions. For healthy adults, the minimum potassium requirement is 2,000 milligrams per day. Vegetables and fruits are low in sodium, but many are good potassium sources. Extremely high or low blood potassium can cause heartbeat irregularities and death.*

Quick Bites

Versatile Potassium

During the Middle Ages, saltpeter (potassium nitrate) was discovered to be a useful substance. It was used as a means of extracting other minerals from rock, as a fertilizer, and as an ingredient in gunpowder. It wasn't used to cure meat until the sixteenth or seventeenth century. Saltpeter was a major ingredient in the curing mixture until 1940, about the time that refrigeration emerged. Today, food manufacturers use small amounts of nitrites rather than saltpeter to preserve foods such as bacon, ham, and some sausages.

Chloride

Chloride is a component of table salt and other salts. (Do not confuse chloride with chlorine. Chlorine is a highly reactive gas used in water treatment plants to kill germs.)

Both sodium and chloride help maintain the body's fluid balance. You have probably noticed the salty taste that sodium chloride (NaCl) imparts to blood, sweat, and tears. While chloride readily moves in and out of cells, it resides mainly in extracellular fluid. Chloride is crucial to transmitting nerve impulses and to maintaining acid–base balance. It also is a component of hydrochloric acid produced by the stomach. Hydrochloric acid is required for digestion; it also kills disease-causing bacteria ingested in food. White blood cells also use chloride ions to kill invading bacteria.[21]

Quick Bites

Low-Calorie Chlorine?

Sucralose is a low-calorie sweetener made from sugar. During manufacture, a multistep process substitutes three chlorine atoms for three hydrogen–oxygen groups on the sugar molecule. This creates an exceptionally stable molecular structure that is 600 times sweeter than sugar. The sucralose molecule is chemically and biologically inert, so it passes through the body without being digested and is eliminated after consumption.

Dietary Recommendations and Sources of Chloride

Most of us consume much more chloride than the 750 milligrams per day that is the adult minimum requirement estimated by the Food and Nutrition Board. The Daily Value for chloride is 3,400 milligrams. Most of our chloride intake comes from salt (for dietary sources, see the "Sodium" section earlier in this chapter). You usually can estimate the chloride content of processed foods from the sodium content with this simple formula:

$$\text{chloride content} = 1.5 \times \text{sodium content}$$

The average intake of chloride from salt alone is 4,500 milligrams per day (7.5 grams of salt), which is much more than adequate. The kidneys excrete excess chloride, and some chloride also is lost in sweat. Severe dehydration is the only known cause of high blood chloride levels.

Who Risks Chloride Deficiency?

Excessive chloride loss is the most common cause of chloride deficiency. Vomiting expels stomach acid (hydrochloric acid), which contains a lot of chloride. People with bulimia nervosa compulsively gorge and purge, so they often have low chloride levels. Low blood chloride slows blood flow to the brain and oxygen delivery to tissues. It also disrupts the body's acid–base balance and causes heartbeat irregularities. Untreated low blood chloride levels can be life threatening.[22]

Key Concepts: *In addition to its role as an electrolyte, chloride is a component of hydrochloric acid. The minimum chloride requirement for healthy adults is 750 milligrams per day, far below average intakes. People who frequently induce vomiting risk chloride deficiency.*

Quick Bites

Discouraging Discoloration

Cutting or bruising causes discoloration of many fruits and vegetables such as apples, bananas, pears, eggplants, avocados, and raw potatoes. Chloride ions inhibit the responsible enzyme, so salt will retard discoloration although it changes the flavor.

Calcium

Although only 1.5 to 2 percent of our body weight, calcium is the most abundant mineral in our bodies. It's important to have adequate calcium throughout life, so bones and teeth can remain strong into old age. Recently, calcium-containing foods have been shown to help reduce hypertension.

Functions of Calcium

Over 99 percent of your body's calcium is found in bones and teeth, making them hard and strong. Although less than 1 percent of body calcium is in blood and soft tissue, that tiny amount has vitally important roles in muscle contraction, nerve impulse transmission, blood clotting, and cell metabolism. (See **Figure 10.13**.)

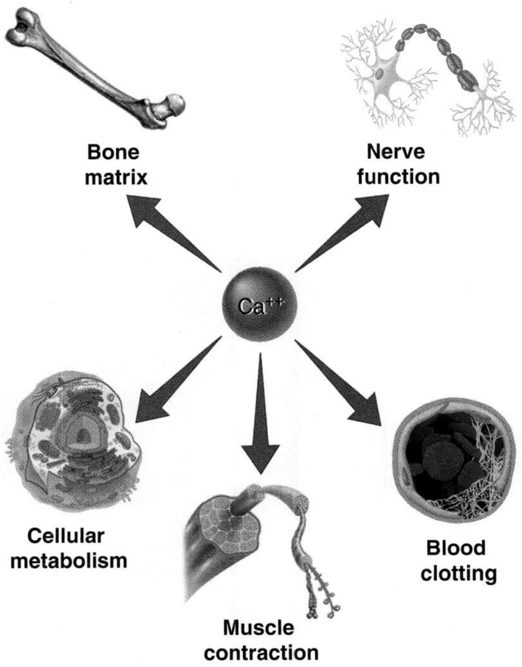

Figure 10.13 **Functions of calcium.** In addition to its key role in bone health, calcium in blood and soft tissues is essential for such diverse functions as blood clotting, muscle contractions, and nerve impulse transmission.

Bone Structure

Think of bone as living tissue that responds to physical stresses. Most of the time, bone is able to withstand tremendous force without breaking. In fact, healthy bone has about the same strength as reinforced concrete.[23] By weight, bone is two-thirds mineral and one-third water and protein, primarily collagen. Most bone calcium is part of **hydroxyapatite**—a hard, crystalline complex of calcium and phosphorus that surrounds collagen fibers.

Our bones undergo constant remodeling by two types of bone cells—**osteoblasts** and **osteoclasts**. Osteoblasts are the construction team, and osteoclasts are the demolition team. Together they determine how bones grow and change over time. Bone **mineralization** is greatest while children are growing taller and for 5 to 10 years thereafter. Although we usually achieve our peak bone mass at around age 30, bone responds to physical activities throughout our lives. In areas under repeated stress, bone thickens and becomes denser. Even elderly adults can strengthen and rebuild their bones through weight-bearing exercise such as walking or weight lifting.[24]

Bone also is a reservoir of calcium and phosphorus. When needed, blood and soft tissues can draw upon this calcium reserve. Blood calcium levels must be kept constant at all costs, even at the expense of bone strength, so that calcium's roles in nerve function, blood clotting, muscle contraction, and cellular metabolism can proceed without a hitch.

Calcium, Blood Clots, and Nerve Transmission

Blood cannot clot without calcium, but blood calcium levels seldom fall this low. Calcium participates in nearly every step in the production of **fibrin**, the protein that gives structure to blood clots. Nerve cells need calcium to transmit signals. In fact, the strength of a nerve signal is in direct proportion to the number of calcium ions crossing the nerve cell membrane.

Calcium, Muscles, and Metabolism

Calcium has a central role in muscle contractions, as the flow of calcium ions inside muscle cells causes muscles to contract or relax. During exercise,

hydroxyapatite A crystalline mineral compound of calcium and phosphorus that makes up bone.

osteoblasts Bone cells that synthesize and excrete the extracellular matrix that forms the structure of bone.

osteoclasts Bone cells that break down bone structure and release calcium and phosphate into the blood.

mineralization The addition of minerals, such as calcium and phosphate, to bones and teeth.

fibrin A stringy, insoluble protein that is the final product of the blood-clotting process.

one cause of muscle fatigue is the impaired activity of calcium in muscle cells.

Calmodulin is a calcium-sensing protein found throughout the body. When it binds calcium, calmodulin helps regulate a number of cellular processes, including cell division, cell proliferation, **ciliary action**, and cell secretions.

calmodulin A calcium-binding protein that regulates a variety of chemical reactions and physiological activities, such as muscle contractions and norepinephrine release.

ciliary action Wavelike motion of small hairlike projections on some cells.

Regulation of Blood Calcium Levels

To prevent even minor dips in blood calcium levels, your body will demineralize bone. Even if calcium intake is very low, blood calcium levels remain steady. Three hormones, calcitriol (the active form of vitamin D), parathyroid hormone (PTH), and calcitonin, regulate calcium status.

When blood calcium levels are low, calcitriol increases intestinal absorption of calcium. PTH from the parathyroid glands activates osteoclasts that release bone calcium. PTH also signals the kidneys to conserve more calcium and to produce more calcitriol. When calcium levels become too high, the thyroid gland secretes calcitonin, which acts in opposition to PTH.

Dietary Recommendations for Calcium

During every life stage, optimal calcium intake is critical. If children and young adults fail to take in enough calcium, they are more likely to develop osteoporosis later in life. As we age, optimal calcium intake slows bone loss, helping preserve bone density.

Adequate Intake (AI) recommendations are aimed at minimizing osteoporosis risk. AIs are 1,000 milligrams calcium per day for adults aged 19 to 50 years, increasing to 1,200 milligrams for people 51 years and older. The AI for those 9 to 18 years is 1,300 milligrams per day, a level meant to maximize peak bone mass.

Unfortunately, many of us fall far short of recommended calcium intakes. In fact, calcium intake by adolescent girls—probably the group for whom calcium is most important—is well below recommendations, leaving them vulnerable to osteoporosis as they age.[25] Excessive caffeine, alcohol, and sodium intake and misuse of diuretics—factors that increase urinary calcium—make bone loss worse.[26]

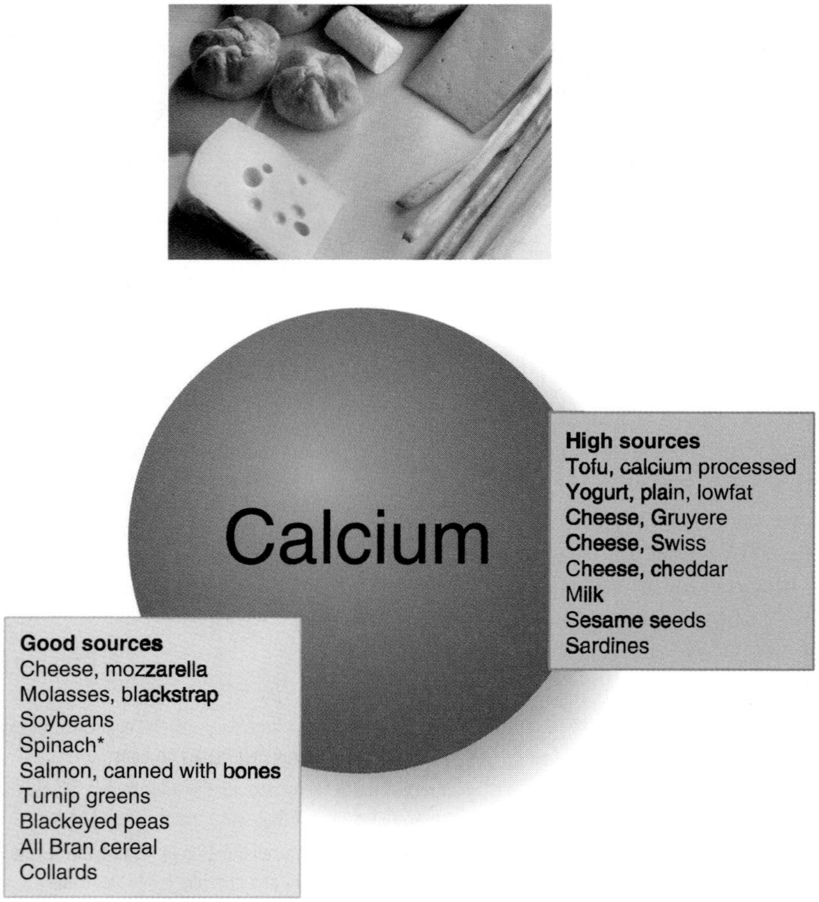

* In spinach, oxalate binds calcium and prevents absorption of all but about 5 percent of the plant's calcium.

Figure 10.14 Food sources of calcium. Calcium is found in milk and dairy products, certain green leafy vegetables, and canned fish with bones.

Sources of Calcium

Dairy products are the best source of calcium in the American diet.[27] (See **Figure 10.14**.) Nonfat milk and yogurt are especially good, providing high calcium with minimal calories and little or no fat. Although ice cream and cheese are good sources, they are high in fat. Among dairy foods, cottage cheese and cream cheese contain the least calcium.

Other significant sources are green vegetables such as broccoli, Chinese cabbage, turnip greens and other "greens," and tofu processed with calcium. However, leafy vegetables in the spinach family are high in the mineral oxalate, which binds to calcium, thus preventing intestinal absorption. (See **Figure 10.15**.) If you eat the bones, canned fish with bones, such as sardines, provide lots of calcium.

Certain brands of soy milk, fruit juice, breakfast cereal, and bread are now fortified with calcium. These are convenient calcium sources for people who don't eat dairy foods. Check labels carefully because only a few products are fortified with calcium. Some dairies also add extra calcium or calcium-containing milk solids to their products.

People with limited dairy intake may need calcium supplements to ensure adequate intake. Flavored, chewable, calcium-containing antacids are an inexpensive and easy-to-take source of extra calcium. (See the FYI feature "Calcium Supplements: Are They Right for You?")

Calcium Absorption

We usually absorb 25 to 75 percent of the calcium we eat, and absorption efficiency is inversely related to calcium intake—the more calcium you eat, the less you absorb.[28] Other dietary factors also affect absorption. Wheat bran, phytate (in whole grains, nuts, and seeds), and oxalate (in foods like spinach) reduce calcium absorption. High supplement doses of phosphorus and magnesium may also interfere with calcium absorption. Because calcium depends on vitamin D to enter intestinal cells, calcium absorption drops dramatically if vitamin D status is poor.

Calcium absorption is particularly efficient during pregnancy and infancy and is least efficient in old age. If both a healthy child and a healthy adult eat exactly the same meal, all other things being equal, the growing child will absorb a much greater proportion of the dietary calcium than the

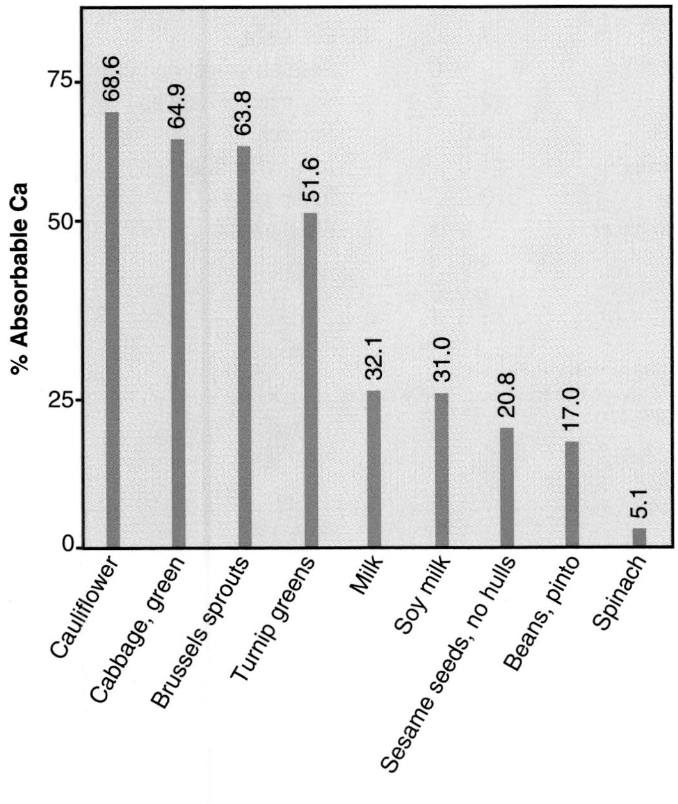

Figure 10.15 Bioavailability of calcium from different sources. Your body can absorb more than two-thirds of the calcium in cauliflower, but only about 5 percent of the calcium in spinach. Oxalate in spinach binds calcium and inhibits its bioavailability.

Source: Adapted from Weaver CM, Plawecki KL. Dietary calcium: adequacy of a vegetarian diet. *Am J Clin Nutr.* 1994;59(suppl):1238S–1241S.

[*Fyi*] Calcium Supplements: Are They Right for You?

FOR YOUR INFORMATION

After reading the section on calcium, you may be wondering whether you need a calcium supplement. After all, calcium is critical for so many bodily functions, and getting enough calcium reduces the risk of osteoporosis later in life.

Before you head to the supplement aisle at the grocery store, take a critical look at your diet, especially your intake of milk and other dairy products. In the United States and Canada, dairy foods are the major sources of dietary calcium; without them, it may be difficult to reach the AI for calcium. People who exclude dairy products, such as vegans and those with milk allergy, must choose foods carefully to find rich calcium sources.

Calcium sources vary widely in their bioavailability. While labels are required to list the %DV for calcium, they don't indicate how much of that calcium the body will absorb. For example, ½ cup of spinach contains about 120 milligrams of calcium, but the body will absorb only 5 percent of that calcium! Intake recommendations are based on the mix of sources in the typical American diet. Other cultures manage on much lower intakes in part because they do not consume the many food constituents that deplete calcium or reduce its absorption. Vegetarians may, in fact, need less calcium than meat eaters. If you are considering spinach as your sole source of calcium, however, check out Table A. It shows the amount of certain foods needed to equal the calcium available from 1 cup of milk (about 30 percent of the 300 milligrams of calcium in 1 cup of milk is bioavailable).

You can see from Table A that the amount of bioavailable calcium varies quite a bit among green leafy vegetables! If your diet is low in calcium, try adding some of the foods that are higher in calcium. Incorporating calcium-rich foods into the diet adds other important vitamins and minerals.

Even armed with more information about calcium in the diet, you may still decide to investigate the supplement market. Again, you have a variety of choices: calcium carbonate, calcium citrate, calcium lactate, calcium phosphate . . . how to decide? First, it's important to know that the absorption of calcium from most supplements is about equal—roughly 30 percent. The calcium citrate malate that is used in some brands of fortified juice and a limited number of supplements is absorbed better, 35 percent. However, a typical calcium citrate malate tablet has less calcium than a tablet of another type such as calcium carbonate. Calcium carbonate is usually the most concentrated per tablet, so taking fewer pills per day will supply enough; also, this type of supplement tends to be less expensive. Chelated calcium supplements can improve absorption a bit, but the extra expense probably is not worth it.

Other factors to consider are that calcium supplements may be absorbed better if taken between meals. Also, you need to get plenty of vitamin D, either through casual exposure to the sun, in fortified milk, or as part of a supplement (many calcium supplements have added vitamin D). Vitamin D is important for the absorption of calcium. In addition, bones get stronger with regular, weight-bearing exercise, so make sure to include that in your healthful lifestyle.

Table A **Foods That Provide the Calcium Equivalent of 1 Cup (8 fl oz) of Milk**

Almonds, dry roasted	6 oz	Mustard greens	1 1/3 C
Beans, pinto	6 1/3 C	Radish	4 1/2 C
Beans, red	7 C	Rutabaga	2 1/4 C
Beans, white	2 1/2 C	Sesame seeds, no hulls	12 oz
Broccoli	2 1/2 C	Soy milk, unfortified	30 C
Brussels sprouts	4 C	Spinach	7 3/4 C
Cabbage, Chinese	1 C	Tofu, calcium set	1/2 C
Cabbage, green	3 C	Turnip greens	1 C
Calcium-fortified juices*	5 fl oz	Watercress	3 1/2 C
Cauliflower	4 C		
Kale	1 3/4 C		
Kohlrabi	3 1/2 C		

*Fortified with calcium as calcium citrate malate.

Source: Adapted from Weaver CM, Plawecki KL. Dietary calcium: adequacy of a vegetarian diet. *Am J Clin Nutr.* 1994;59(suppl):1238S–1241S.

adult. Low estrogen levels in postmenopausal women can lower calcium absorption to about 20 percent. Older women may take estrogen supplements, as well as calcium supplements, to maintain calcium absorption.

When Calcium Balance Goes Awry

Because the body uses bone calcium to maintain normal blood calcium levels, low blood calcium is relatively uncommon in the absence of illness or vitamin D deficiency. Chronically low calcium intake can overtax this reserve and lead to suboptimal bone growth in childhood and adolescence or increased rate of bone loss after menopause. (See the section "Osteoporosis" in this chapter.) Studies also link low calcium intake to an increased risk of hypertension, colon cancer, and preeclampsia (a complication of pregnancy marked by hypertension, fluid retention, and protein in the urine).[29]

Although certain illnesses can cause high blood calcium, dietary calcium intake does not. Of greater dietary concern is the interaction of calcium supplements with the absorption of iron, zinc, magnesium, and phosphorus. Although calcium supplements can dramatically affect absorption of other minerals, dietary calcium intake has not been shown to cause a deficiency for any of these minerals. Thus calcium interactions with other minerals represent a potential risk rather than an adverse effect.[30] Calcium from food or supplements can interfere with absorption of some medications, such as tetracycline.[31] The Food and Nutrition Board has established a Tolerable Upper Intake Level (UL) for calcium of 2,500 milligrams per day.

Key Concepts: *Calcium is a major component of bones and teeth. It is also required for muscle contraction, nerve impulse transmission, blood clotting, and regulation of cell metabolism. The body assures adequate blood calcium levels by withdrawing it from bone if needed. Dairy foods and fortified foods are major dietary sources of calcium. Optimal calcium intake throughout life reduces chances of osteoporosis.*

Quick Bites

Paleolithic Calcium Intake

Hunter-gatherer populations during the late Paleolithic period did not drink milk or consume dairy products. Nonetheless, they do not appear to have suffered from calcium deficiency. Researchers estimate that the calcium intake by these populations was almost 1,600 milligrams per day, mostly from wild plants and nectars.

Phosphorus

Phosphorus, along with calcium, is a component of the mineral complex hydroxyapatite in bone. Bones are the major storehouse of phosphorus, holding nearly 85 percent of our supply. The remaining phosphorus is found in cells of soft tissues, with a little bit in extracellular fluid. Most of the body's phosphorus is in the form of phosphate ion (phosphorus joined to oxygen), our most abundant anion.

Phosphorus helps activate and deactivate enzymes during the final steps in the extraction of energy from carbohydrate, fat, and protein. It also is a component of ATP, the universal energy source, and of DNA and RNA. And phosphorus is a component of phospholipids, found in cell membranes and lipoproteins.

Quick Bites

The Double Helix Depends on Phosphorus

The backbone of DNA's twisting ladderlike structure contains alternating molecules of phosphoric acid and deoxyribose.

Dietary Recommendations and Sources of Phosphorus

The phosphorus RDA for adolescents is 1,250 milligrams per day to support growth. While adults need only 700 milligrams per day, the average adult consumes much more, about 1,000 to 1,500 milligrams per day.

Phosphorus is abundant in our food supply. Foods rich in protein (milk, meat, and eggs) generally are rich in phosphorus. (See **Figure 10.16**.) Food additives, especially those in processed meat and soft drinks, supply up to 30 percent of our phosphorus. To improve moisture retention and smoothness, food processors often add phosphate salts to processed foods.

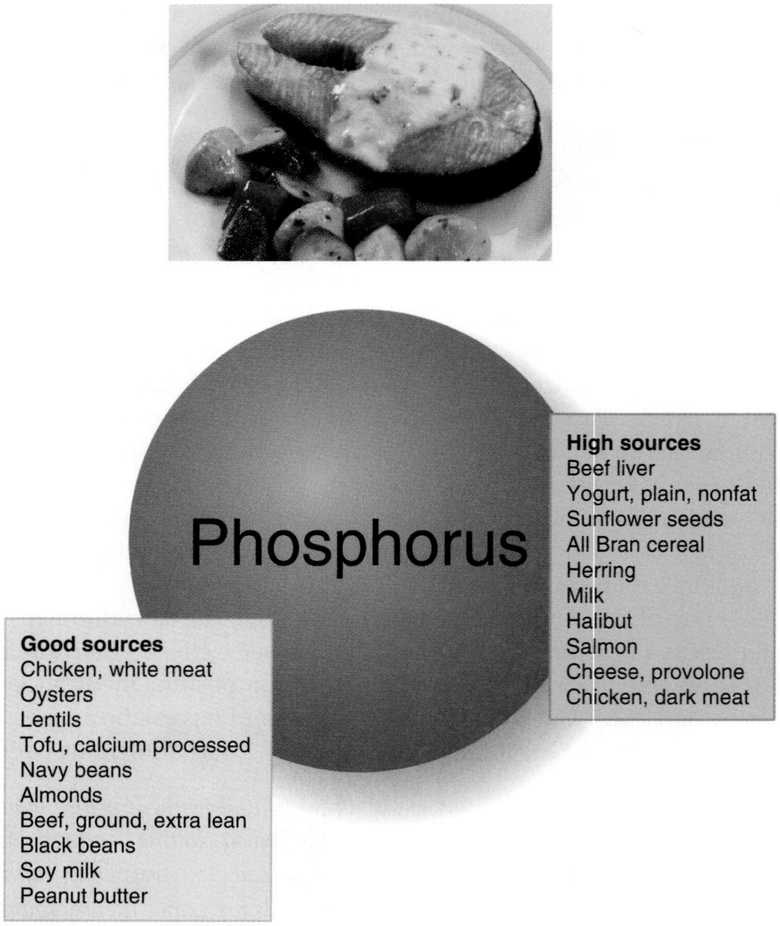

Figure 10.16 **Food sources of phosphorus.** Phosphorus is abundant in the food supply. Meats, legumes, nuts, dairy products, and grains tend to have more phosphorus than fruits and vegetables.

Since cow's milk contains more phosphorus than most foods, people with high dairy-product intakes have high-phosphorus diets. Soft drinks often contain phosphoric acid, although the phosphorus level is not high—about 50 milligrams in a 12-ounce cola. However, among heavy soda drinkers, soda is an important contributor to phosphorus intake.[32] Dairy products have phosphorus plus calcium, whereas sodas have phosphorus but virtually no calcium—an important distinction.

We absorb about 55 to 70 percent of the phosphorus we eat. Although phosphorus is part of phytate in plant seeds (beans, peas, cereals, and nuts), we can still absorb about 50 percent. Two familiar hormones, PTH (parathyroid hormone) and calcitriol (activated vitamin D), regulate intestinal absorption of phosphorus. When phosphorus levels are low, calcitriol enhances intestinal absorption of both calcium and phosphorus. When levels are high, PTH greatly increases urinary excretion of phosphorus.

When Phosphate Balance Goes Awry

Phosphorus is so common in foods that only near total starvation causes deficiency. Some medical disorders, however, can cause low blood phosphate. Kidney disease is the most common cause of high blood phosphate. Other causes include overuse of vitamin D supplements, overuse of phosphate-containing laxatives, and diseases of the parathyroid gland. At the extreme, symptoms include muscle spasms and convulsions.

In the short run, high phosphorus intake is unlikely to produce problems in healthy people.[33] But over the long run, eating too much phosphorus, together with too little calcium, may increase bone loss. People who replace milk with cola increase their ratio of dietary phosphorus to calcium, possibly increasing their risk of osteoporosis later in life. The UL for phosphorus is 4,000 milligrams per day for people aged 9 to 70.

Key Concept: *Phosphorus is a component of bone, ATP, phospholipids, and genetic material. It acts as an electrolyte regulator as well. Milk, meat, and food additives are major sources of dietary phosphorus. Diets high in phosphorus and low in calcium can contribute to bone loss.*

Quick Bites

Magnesium Says: "Let the Competition Begin!"

The pigment chlorophyll, which is responsible for the deep green color of vegetables, contains a magnesium atom at its molecular center. Heat easily displaces this magnesium, and in acidic cooking water, hydrogen ions rush in to replace it. The altered chlorophyll is grayish-green. This replacement of magnesium by hydrogen is the most common cause of the dull, olive-green color of many cooked vegetables. On the other hand, if the acidic cooking water also contains zinc or copper ions, these minerals beat out hydrogen in the race for the central spot in the chlorophyll. This combination makes cooked vegetables bright green.

Magnesium

Magnesium is the fourth most abundant cation in our bodies. Bone holds about half, with the remainder distributed equally between muscle and other soft tissue. Like bone calcium, bone magnesium is a large reservoir that soft tissue can draw upon when needed. Most magnesium resides in cells, with only 1 percent in extracellular fluid.

Magnesium participates in more than 300 types of enzyme-driven reactions, including those in DNA and protein synthesis, blood clotting, muscle contraction, and ATP production. Since ATP is the universal energy source, an absence of magnesium would halt all cellular activity.

Dietary Recommendations and Sources of Magnesium

The magnesium RDA is 400 milligrams per day for men aged 19 to 30 years, and 310 milligrams per day for women. The RDA rises for those 31 and older, to 420 milligrams for men and 320 milligrams for women. The average American gets only about three-fourths this level. Yet, overt symptoms of low magnesium are relatively uncommon in healthy people.[34]

Magnesium is found throughout the food supply. Our main sources are plant foods. Whole grains, many vegetables, legumes, tofu, and some seafood are good sources, and chocolate contains modest amounts. (See **Figure 10.17**.) In some communities, "hard" tap water has significant amounts of magnesium. Unfortunately, processing and refining removes much magnesium—up to 80 percent in refined grains—and enrichment does not replace it. In general, refined foods are low in magnesium.

We absorb about 50 percent of dietary magnesium. High-fiber diets, high phosphorus intake, and overuse of calcium supplements (over 2,600 milligrams of calcium daily) all can interfere with magnesium absorption.

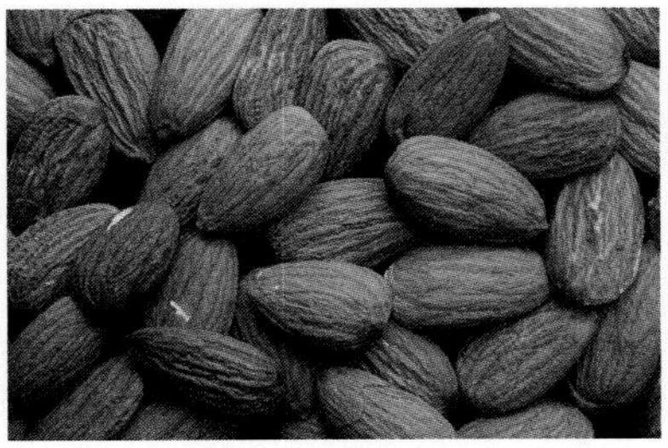

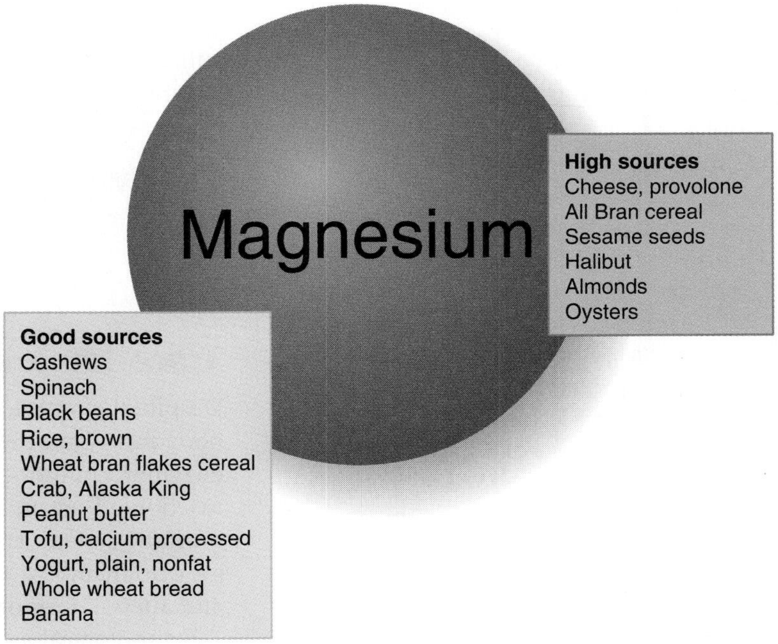

Figure 10.17 **Food sources of magnesium.** Most of the magnesium in the diet comes from plant foods like grains, vegetables, and legumes.

When Magnesium Balance Goes Awry

Magnesium deficiency is often associated with alcoholism. Alcohol increases urinary magnesium excretion. Poor magnesium intake typically goes hand in hand with poor intake of other nutrients, and magnesium deficiency by itself is unusual.[35] Deficiency also occurs with certain diseases and is worsened by diarrhea.

In research studies, healthy people on magnesium-deficient study diets have no symptoms for several weeks. Once bone reserves are depleted, loss of appetite, nausea, and weakness gradually develop. Then muscle cramps, irritability, and confusion occur. Low magnesium disrupts heart rhythm; and if the deficiency becomes extreme, heart abnormalities can lead to death. Studies have shown that people living in areas with high magnesium content in the water have a lower incidence of sudden death from heart attacks.[36]

In the absence of kidney disease, an abnormally high blood level of magnesium is uncommon. The UL for supplemental magnesium is 350 milligrams per day.

Key Concepts: *Magnesium participates in more than 300 reactions, including several in energy metabolism. It's required for cardiac and nerve function. Magnesium reserves are stored in bone. Whole grains and vegetables are good sources. People with chronic diarrhea, poor diet, and heavy alcohol use are at risk of deficiency. Because magnesium ions help regulate heartbeat, heart rhythm irregularities occur if blood levels are too low.*

Quick Bites

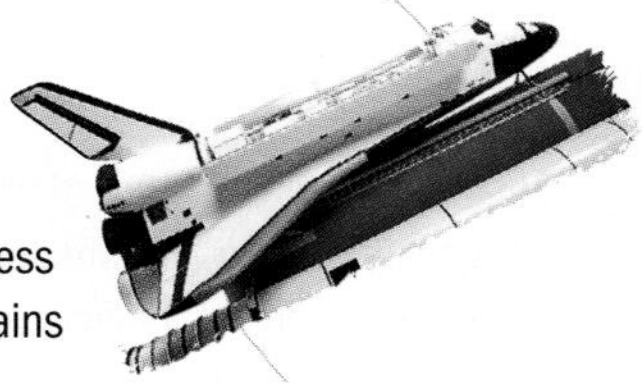

Lost in Space

Knowing that stress on bones maintains their strength, what would you guess happens in the gravity-free environment of outer space? Experience with prolonged space travel has made it clear that extensive bone and mineral loss are one health hazard of living without gravity's constant pull. Interestingly, changes in non-weight-bearing bones were not seen in studies of space travelers. As humans spend longer periods in space, scientists will be challenged to discover how to preserve bone strength without the constant stimulation of gravity on weight-bearing bones.

Sulfur

Unlike the other minerals discussed in this chapter, sulfur does not function alone. In the body, sulfur is primarily a component of organic (carbon-containing) nutrients, such as the vitamins biotin and thiamin, as well as the amino acids methionine and cysteine. The sulfur in amino acids helps stabilize the three-dimensional shapes of proteins such as those in skin, hair, and nails. The liver's detoxification pathways require sulfur, and sulfate (sulfur combined with oxygen) helps maintain acid–base balance.

Typical diets contain ample sulfur, and deficiency is unknown in humans.

Key Concepts: *Sulfur is a component of some amino acids and the vitamins biotin and thiamin. It helps proteins maintain their functional shapes. Sulfur is important in liver function and in maintaining acid–base balance. Human sulfur deficiency is unknown.*

Quick Bites

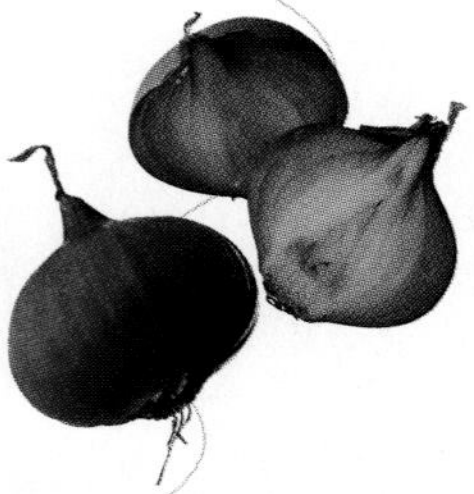

Do Onions Make You Cry?

The cabbage and onion families have sulfur-based compounds that are transformed into odiferous compounds when their tissues are broken. Cutting into a raw onion mixes the contents of its cells, bringing enzymes into contact with an odorless precursor substance apparently derived from the sulfur-containing amino acid cysteine. The volatile result, a powerful sulfur-containing irritant, causes most people's eyes to water, apparently by dissolving in fluids that surround the eye and forming sulfuric acid.

Trace Minerals

Despite the minute amounts in the body, trace minerals are crucial to many body functions. (See **Figure 10.18**.) Trace minerals serve as cofactors for enzymes, components of hormones, and participants in many chemical reactions. They are essential for growth and for normal functioning of the immune system. Deficiencies may cause delayed sexual maturation, poor growth, mediocre work performance, faulty immune function, tooth decay, and altered hormonal function.

Technological advances in recent years have triggered an explosion of exciting new research because scientists can now track trace minerals throughout the body more effectively. Working together, nutritionists,

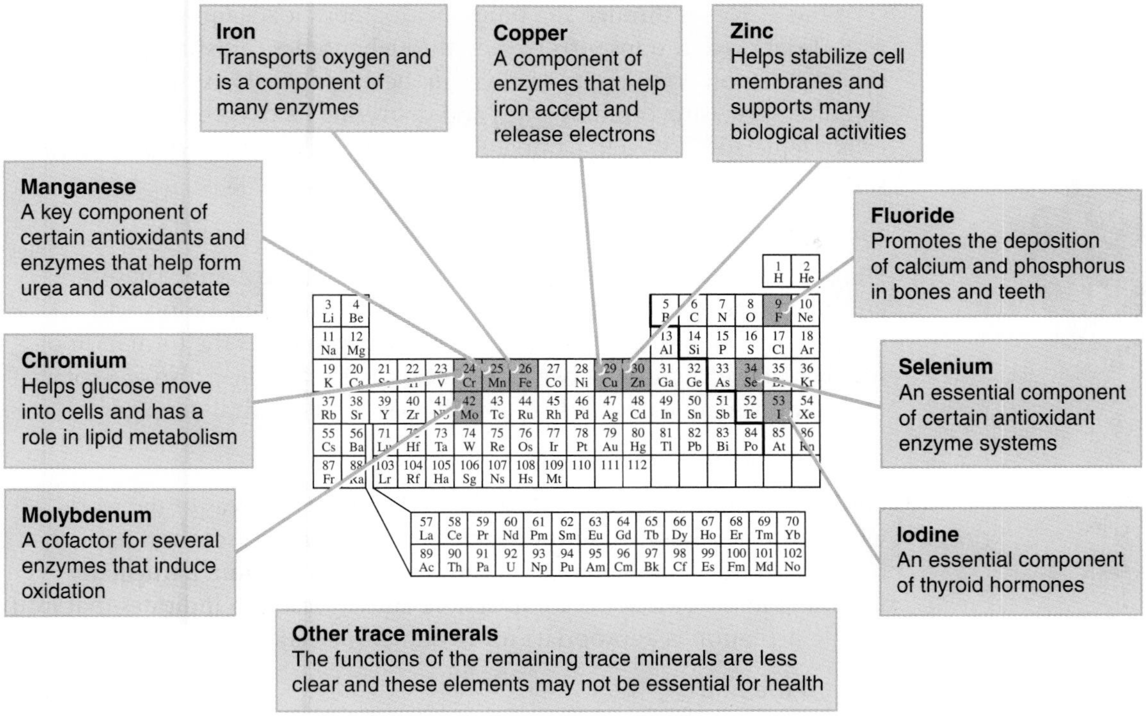
Iron
Transports oxygen and is a component of many enzymes
Copper
A component of enzymes that help iron accept and release electrons
Zinc
Helps stabilize cell membranes and supports many biological activities
Manganese
A key component of certain antioxidants and enzymes that help form urea and oxaloacetate
Fluoride
Promotes the deposition of calcium and phosphorus in bones and teeth
Chromium
Helps glucose move into cells and has a role in lipid metabolism
Selenium
An essential component of certain antioxidant enzyme systems
Molybdenum
A cofactor for several enzymes that induce oxidation
Iodine
An essential component of thyroid hormones
Other trace minerals
The functions of the remaining trace minerals are less clear and these elements may not be essential for health

Figure 10.18 **Trace minerals on the periodic table.** Trace minerals are found in the body and required in the diet in small amounts, but they play important roles in the body.

biochemists, biologists, immunologists, geneticists, and epidemiologists are uncovering the mysteries behind many of these fascinating minerals and finding new links between trace minerals and a variety of diseases and genetic disorders.

heme A chemical complex with a central iron atom that forms the oxygen-binding part of hemoglobin and myoglobin.

myoglobin The oxygen-transporting protein of muscle that resembles blood hemoglobin in function.

Iron

Iron is among the most abundant minerals in the earth's crust. Yet iron deficiency is the most common nutrient deficiency in the world. It's estimated that 500 to 600 million people suffer from iron-deficiency anemia.[37]

Iron has a special property that allows it to easily transfer electrons to and from other atoms. This ability makes iron essential for numerous reactions and allows it to easily bind and release oxygen. Iron's abilities also endow it with a "dark side"—the ability to promote formation of destructive free radicals.

Functions of Iron

Iron is well known for its role in transporting oxygen in the blood. Iron also is an essential component of hundreds of enzymes, many of which are involved in energy metabolism. In addition, iron plays a role in brain development and in the immune system. (**Figure 10.19** shows the functions of iron.)

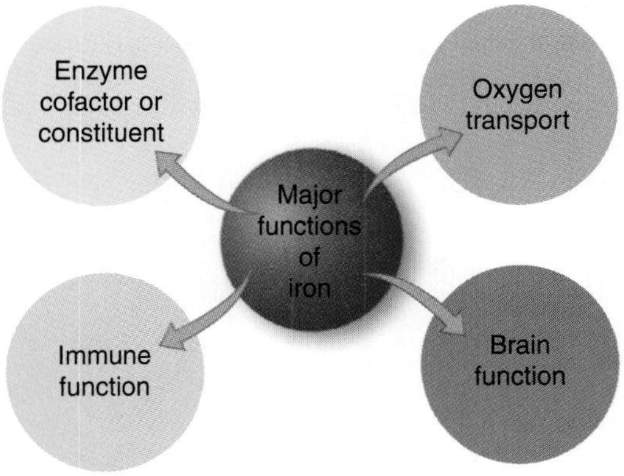

Figure 10.19 **Major functions of iron.** Well known for its role in transporting oxygen in the blood, iron also is essential for optimal immune function and nerve health. In addition, it is a cofactor in numerous reactions.

Oxygen Transport

Iron is vital to oxygen transport and sits at the center of **heme**—the iron-containing portion of hemoglobin and **myoglobin**. (See **Figure 10.20**.) Hemoglobin carries oxygen in the blood; myoglobin resides in muscle and moves oxygen into muscle cells.

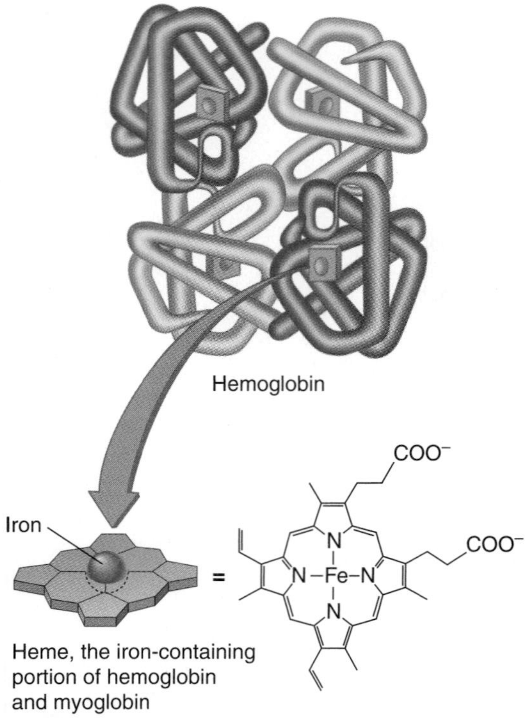

Figure 10.20 **Heme in hemoglobin.** Iron in the heme portion of hemoglobin and myoglobin binds and releases oxygen easily. Hemoglobin in red blood cells transports oxygen in the blood and gives blood its red color.

As blood passes through the lungs, hemoglobin loads up on oxygen and turns bright red. It transports oxygen through arteries to tissues throughout the body. Upon reaching its destination, hemoglobin flows through tiny capillaries, crossing capillary walls and delivering its oxygen cargo to target cells. Depleted of oxygen, hemoglobin turns a dark bluish-red and travels through veins back to the lungs for another load of oxygen.

Enzymes

Hundreds of enzymes contain iron or need iron as a cofactor. These enzymes drive reactions necessary for energy production, amino acid metabolism, and muscle function. Excess iron promotes the formation of highly reactive and destructive free radicals. Ironically, iron also is a cofactor of antioxidant enzymes that protect against free radical damage.

Immune Function

Optimal immune function requires iron. However, in areas of the world with rampant disease and iron deficiency, a dilemma arises. Iron nourishes bacteria, so iron supplementation can worsen an infection, particularly malaria.[38] In the absence of an infection, current research indicates that iron supplementation is appropriate for treating iron deficiency.[39]

Brain Function

Iron is essential for optimal brain and nervous system development and function. Children with iron-deficiency anemia often have learning and behavior problems.[40] Scientists are now studying specific ways that iron affects the brain. We know that iron is involved in producing the protective covering, or myelin sheath, that surrounds nerve cells.[41] Iron is also involved in producing neurotransmitters, chemicals that carry messages between nerve cells.

Regulation of Iron in the Body

Total body iron averages a little less than 4 grams in men and a little more than 2 grams in women. Most of your body's iron is in hemoglobin, with the remainder in myoglobin and enzymes. If you're well nourished, you'll have good iron reserves stored as **ferritin** and **hemosiderin**.[42]

But too much iron is toxic. So your body carefully performs a balancing act, adjusting iron absorption, transport, storage, and loss to optimize the amounts of actively functioning iron and iron reserves without exceeding safe levels.

ferritin A major storage form of iron.

hemosiderin An insoluble form of storage iron.

heme iron The iron found in the hemoglobin and myoglobin of animal foods.

non-heme iron The iron in plants and animal foods that is not part of hemoglobin or myoglobin.

polyphenols Organic compounds may produce bitterness in coffee and tea.

Iron Absorption

Intestinal cells act as gatekeepers, absorbing needed iron but turning away excess (and potentially harmful) iron. The actual amount absorbed depends on the body's iron status and need, normal GI function, the amount and type of iron in the diet, and dietary factors that enhance or inhibit iron absorption. Once intestinal cells admit iron, they can use it immediately, release it to the blood, or store it for later. During normal cell turnover, the GI tract sloughs intestinal cells. When excreted, these dead cells carry their stored iron out of the body.

Effect of Iron Status on Iron Absorption Depending on need, iron absorption can vary from less than 1 percent to greater than 50 percent. On average, adult men absorb about 6 percent of dietary iron, and nonpregnant women of childbearing age absorb about 13 percent. Women absorb a higher proportion to make up for iron losses from menstruation.

Normally, absorption is more efficient when circulating iron and iron reserves are low. Absorption is highest among iron-deficient people, and it slows as iron reserves become filled. An increase in red blood cell production—during pregnancy, for example, or after blood loss—increases the body's need for iron and can trigger a severalfold increase in iron uptake.[43]

Effect of GI Function on Iron Absorption To prepare iron for intestinal absorption, you need adequate stomach acid. Since stomach acid generally declines with aging, iron absorption tends to be less efficient in seniors. Overuse of antacids also can affect iron bioavailability.

Effect of the Amount and Form of Iron in Food All other factors being equal, the less iron in your diet, the greater the proportion you absorb. This ability to conserve dietary iron no doubt helped people survive when iron-rich foods were scarce. But it has its limits—if iron intake is routinely too low, anemia will emerge over time.

Food contains two types of iron: **heme iron** and **non-heme iron**. Most heme iron is a part of hemoglobin and myoglobin, so it is found only in animal tissue. Meat, fish, and poultry contain about 40 percent heme iron and 60 percent non-heme iron. In contrast, plant foods and iron-fortified foods contain only non-heme iron. (See **Figure 10.21**.) Vegan diets, by definition, contain no heme iron.

Heme iron is much more bioavailable than non-heme iron.[44] Therefore, meats, poultry, fish, and seafood have the most efficiently absorbed iron. Vegetarians need more iron than people who eat foods with heme iron.

Dietary Factors That Enhance Iron Absorption You can improve the bioavailability of non-heme iron with vitamin C (ascorbic acid). (See **Table 10.3**.) Eating fruits and vegetables—good sources of ascorbic acid—along with iron-containing foods enhances non-heme iron absorption. Eating heme-iron foods along with non-heme-iron foods also improves non-heme-iron absorption.

Dietary Factors That Inhibit Iron Absorption Whole grains contain phytate, which inhibits iron absorption. However, whole-grain foods are healthy in other respects, so don't avoid them. Instead, include vitamin C-rich fruits and vegetables, which counter the inhibitory effects of phytate.

Polyphenols, found in tea, coffee, other beverages, and many plants, limit non-heme iron absorption. Foods from soybeans, foods containing oxalates, and high-fiber foods in general also tend to inhibit non-heme iron absorption.

Calcium, zinc, and iron compete for absorption, and each can inhibit absorption of another.[45] Many women take calcium supplements to reduce their risk of osteoporosis. To minimize interference with iron absorption, they should take their calcium supplements alone at bedtime rather than with meals.

Table 10.3 Factors That Affect Iron Absorption

Inhibitors	Enhancers
Fiber and phytate	Vitamin C (ascorbic acid)
Calcium and phosphorus (milk/dairy)	Factor in meat, poultry, and fish
Tannins, found in tea	HCl secreted in the stomach
Polyphenols	Citric, malic, and lactic acid
Oxalate	

MEAT

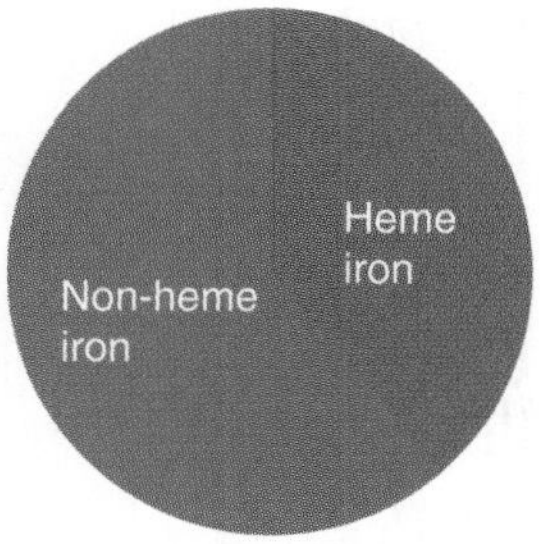

Beef, chicken, and fish contain about 40% heme and 60% non-heme iron. Eggs and dairy products contain no hemoglobin or myoglobin, so they contain only non-heme iron.

LEGUMES AND VEGETABLES

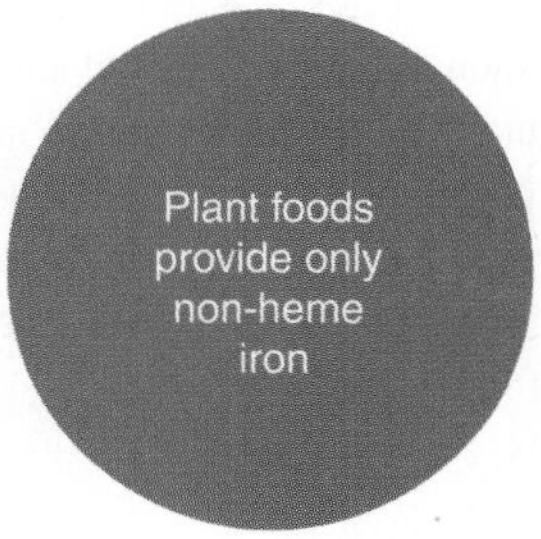

Beans, fortified cereals, soybeans, and green leafy vegetables are sources of non-heme iron.

AVERAGE DAILY DIET

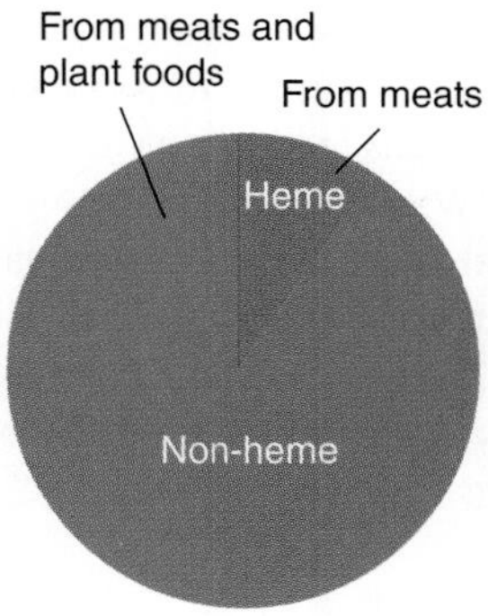

The average diet contains much more non-heme iron than heme iron.

Figure 10.21 Sources of heme and non-heme iron. Heme iron is found only in meats. Non-heme iron is found in both plant and animal foods. Eggs and dairy products contain small amounts of non-heme iron only.

transferrin A protein synthesized in the liver that transports iron in the blood to the red blood cells for use in heme synthesis.

Iron Transport and Storage

Transferrin is the carrier protein that ferries iron through the blood. It delivers iron from the intestines to the bone marrow for manufacture into hemoglobin, and it carries iron to all other body tissues as needed. (See **Figure 10.22**.)

The body stores surplus iron in two forms. Most iron is stored as ferritin, and smaller amounts are stored as hemosiderin. Although small amounts of ferritin circulate in blood, the liver, bone marrow, spleen, and skeletal muscle hold most iron reserves. Over time, a negative iron balance can deplete these reserves and iron deficiency begins.

Iron Turnover and Loss

The body is good at conserving iron, a trait probably acquired in ancient times when availability of high-iron foods was uncertain and irregular. The normal, routine destruction of old red blood cells releases iron, which the body recycles as it builds new red blood cells. A healthy adult man, for example, produces new red blood cells with about 95 percent recycled iron. Diet or iron stores must supply the remaining 5 percent. During periods of rapid growth and blood expansion, iron needs outstrip the supply of recycled and stored iron. Dietary iron makes up the difference. During infancy, for example, dietary iron supplies about 30 percent of iron for new red blood cells.

We lose small amounts of iron every day—a milligram or so in feces, sweat, and sloughed-off mucosal and skin cells. Women lose considerably more during menstruation. Pregnancy, with its high growth demands, and childbirth, with its high blood loss, increase iron needs markedly. Women with repeated pregnancies have very high iron needs.

Digestive disorders can increase blood and iron losses significantly. Any condition in which there is bleeding or accelerated destruction of intestinal cells—ulcer, cancer, inflammatory bowel disease, parasitic infection—can lead to iron-deficiency anemia.

Quick Bites

But It Worked in the Lab...

Carefully conducted clinical trials have shown that supplements reduce iron deficiency during pregnancy. However, public health programs to provide iron supplements in communities often are unsuccessful. Why? Programs in the "real world" have several limiting factors: inadequate supply of iron tablets, limited access to care, poor or nonexistent nutrition counseling, lack of knowledge, and the uncomfortable side effects experienced by some women. These are some reasons pregnant women don't take iron supplements even when programs to supply them are available.

Grandma's Cast-Iron Skillet Helped Her Avoid Iron Deficiency

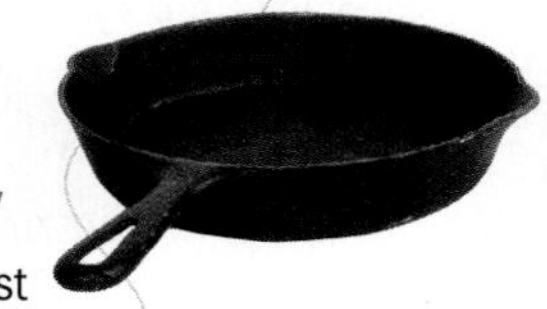

Iron deficiency is the most common form of malnutrition in the United States. However, this is a relatively recent phenomenon. Americans used to cook using cast-iron pots and pans. A study showed that using these utensils to cook acidic foods like spaghetti sauce and apple butter increases the iron content of such foods by 30- to 100-fold. Our preference for stainless steel, aluminum, and enamelware eliminates this fortification.

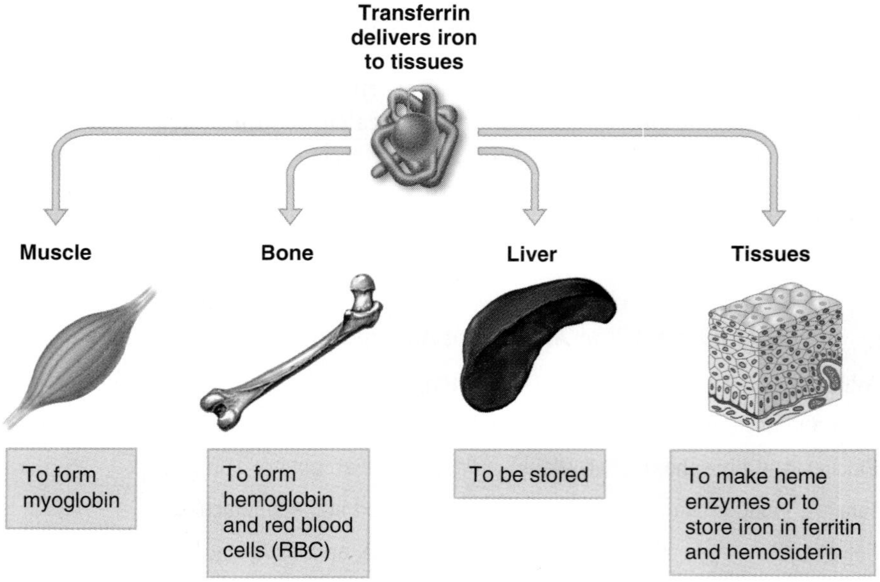

Figure 10.22 **Iron in the body.** Transferrin transports iron to tissues for the synthesis of heme or storage in ferritin and hemosiderin.

Dietary Recommendations for Iron

The RDA for men and postmenopausal women is 8 milligrams per day. The RDA for women of childbearing age is 18 milligrams per day. Most men consume more than their RDA,[46] but many women fall well short of recommended amounts.

The iron needs of infants are a special concern. During the final weeks of pregnancy, babies ideally store enough iron in the liver, bone marrow, spleen, and hemoglobin-rich blood to see them through their first six months of life. However, if the mother's iron nutrition is poor or the baby is born early, the baby's iron stores are smaller and do not last. To help ensure that babies have adequate iron, pregnant women are urged to consume adequate iron. Infant baby cereal and many infant formulas are fortified with iron.

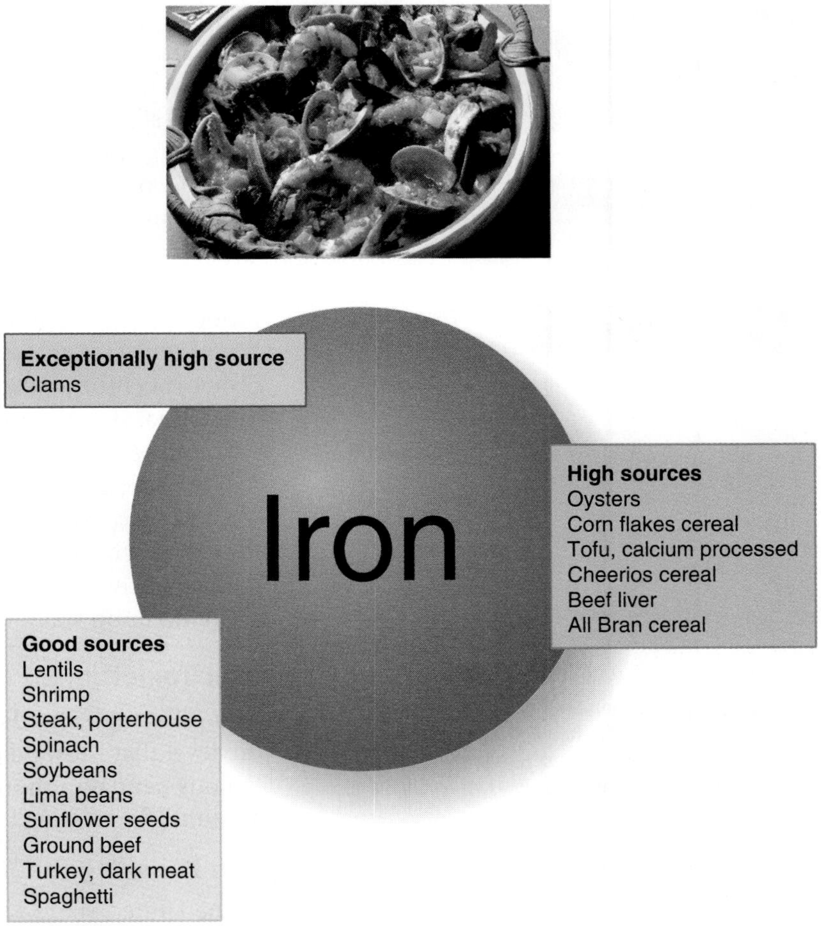

Figure 10.23 **Food sources of iron.** Iron is found in red meats, certain seafood, vegetables, and legumes, and is added to enriched grains and breakfast cereals.

Sources of Iron

In terms of both amount and bioavailability, beef is an excellent dietary source of iron. Other excellent sources include clams, oysters, tofu, and liver. Poultry, fish, pork, lamb, and legumes are also good sources. (See **Figure 10.23**.) Whole-grain and enriched-grain products contain less bioavailable iron than meat, but are significant sources of iron because they make up a major part of our diets. Fortified cereals also make an important contribution to iron intake in the United States and Canada. Dairy products are low in iron.

Think About It 3

A varied diet (adequate in calories, rich in fruits and vegetables, and with small amounts of lean animal flesh) generally provides adequate iron. Vegetarians who consume no animal tissue can maximize iron bioavailability from other sources by consuming vitamin C-rich fruits and vegetables with every meal.

Iron Deficiency

Iron deficiency is the most common nutrient deficiency worldwide, especially in developing countries. Although less prevalent in the United States and Canada, it remains a public health concern. Infants and toddlers, adolescent girls, women of childbearing age, and pregnant women are particularly vulnerable.

Iron deficiency most commonly occurs in young children between 6 and 24 months old. This is the age when cognitive and motor skills develop most rapidly, and inadequate iron during this critical time can cause irreversible developmental and intellectual deficits.

Progression of Iron Deficiency

Iron deficiency is not the same as iron-deficiency anemia. Iron deficiency progresses through three stages. (See **Table 10.4**.)

Table 10.4 Stages of Iron Deficiency

Stage	Functional Implications
Depletion of iron stores	None
Depletion of functional iron	Decreased physical performance
Iron-deficiency anemia	Cognitive impairment, poor growth, decreased performance, and decreased exercise tolerance

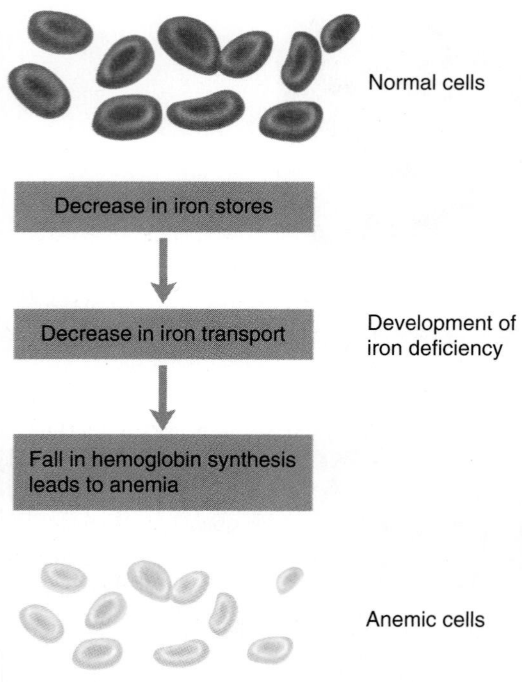

Figure 10.24 Development of iron-deficiency anemia. Iron deficiency can progress to iron-deficiency anemia, a severe form of iron deficiency that is accompanied by low hemoglobin levels.

During the first stage of iron deficiency, the body depletes iron stores, but there are no physiological impairments. During the second stage, the body depletes its supply of iron in circulating transferrin, and heme production starts to slip. Enzymes that need an iron cofactor cannot function properly, and energy production starts to suffer; an iron-deficient person may not be able to work at full capacity. The third and most severe stage is iron-deficiency anemia. (See **Figure 10.24**.)

During iron-deficiency anemia, a lack of iron inhibits production of normal red blood cells, while normal cell turnover continues to deplete the red blood cell population. Red blood cell production falters, producing red blood cells that are small and pale and lack sufficient hemoglobin (microcytic hypochromic anemia). Inadequate vitamin B_6 also can cause this type of anemia. (See Chapter 9, "Vitamins.")

The symptoms of iron-deficiency anemia vary according to its severity and the speed of its development. They include fatigue, pale skin, breathlessness with exertion, poor tolerance to cold temperature, poor immune function, behavioral changes, cognitive impairment, and decreased work performance. In children, iron deficiency causes impaired growth, apathy, short attention span, irritability, and reduced ability to learn.[47]

Iron Toxicity

Iron pills can be hard on your digestive system. The UL for iron is based on the level that causes digestive distress. For adults, the UL for iron is 45 milligrams per day, although physicians may prescribe supplements with larger amounts for treating iron-deficiency anemia.

Iron Poisoning in Children

In the United States accidental iron overdose is a leading cause of poisoning deaths in young children.[48] Even a few iron pills or a relatively moderate adult dose can cause the death of a small child. Parents often fail to appreciate the potential toxicity of iron and don't take precautions they would ordinarily use for other medicines. Symptoms of iron intoxication include nausea, vomiting, diarrhea, rapid heartbeat, dizziness, and confusion. Death can occur within hours of ingestion. If iron poisoning is suspected, the child must receive immediate emergency medical care.

Hereditary Hemochromatosis

In hereditary **hemochromatosis**, a genetic defect causes excessive iron absorption and chronic **iron overload**. Although it was once believed to be rare, scientists now know that mild forms are quite common.[49] Iron buildup over the years leads to severe organ damage, causing diabetes, heart disease, arthritis, liver cirrhosis, and liver cancer.

Men are more vulnerable to hemochromatosis than women, who lose iron through menstruation and pregnancy. Early diagnosis and treatment control the condition and prevent organ damage. Treatment includes minimizing iron intake, avoiding excess vitamin C, and periodically removing some blood.

Key Concepts: *Iron is a key component of the oxygen transporters hemoglobin and myoglobin and of many enzymes involved in energy metabolism. The body carefully regulates iron absorption, based on its iron needs. Heme iron is absorbed more efficiently than non-heme iron. Iron can be bound to transferrin for transport or stored as ferritin or hemosiderin. The best dietary sources of iron are organ meats and red meat. Plant foods contain only non-heme iron. Vitamin C-containing*

Quick Bites

Oceans Can Get Anemia, Too

Stretching from South America to New Zealand is a large region of the South Pacific Ocean that suffers from an iron deficiency. Phytoplankton and plant life are not growing properly in this area. Researchers have identified iron deficiency as the reason.

hemochromatosis A hereditary disorder in which excessive absorption of iron results in abnormal iron deposits in the liver and other tissues.

iron overload Toxicity from excess iron.

foods improve bioavailability of non-heme iron. Iron deficiency develops gradually, and anemia is the most severe manifestation of deficiency. Iron poisoning, whether accidental or due to hemochromatosis, is potentially deadly.

Zinc

It's hard to believe that a nutrient so important to health could go unnoticed for so long. In fact, human zinc deficiency was not recognized until 1961.[50] Some young men in Iran had a peculiar set of symptoms: severe growth retardation, poorly developed testicles (**hypogonadism**), anemia, and, among several, poor night vision. Their diet consisted mainly of wheat bread and was almost devoid of animal protein. They also ate clay (**geophagia**). Could their high-phytate, low-protein diet, along with geophagia, impair absorption of zinc and iron to such an extent? Six years later, a study in Egypt confirmed zinc's role; among a similar group of patients, zinc supplementation improved growth and genital development.[51]

Functions of Zinc

Your body contains a small amount of zinc—1.5 to 2.5 grams, or about the amount of zinc that's in the thin zinc layer on a **galvanized** nail. Yet zinc is found in every body cell.

The functions of zinc fall into three categories: catalytic, structural, and regulatory. Zinc is a cofactor for nearly 100 enzymes representing all the major enzyme types. In its structural role, zinc helps fold proteins into functional shapes. As a regulator, zinc helps control many diverse functions, including gene expression, cell death, and nerve transmission.[52] (See **Figure 10.25**.)

Zinc and Enzymes

In many enzymes, zinc helps provide structural integrity or helps activate catalytic ability. For example, zinc performs a structural role in copper-zinc superoxide dismutase, an enzyme that speeds antioxidant reactions and helps protect cells from free radical damage. In the retina of the eye, the enzyme that activates vitamin A depends on zinc. Consequently, a lack of zinc can create a condition that resembles the night blindness caused by vitamin A deficiency.

Zinc and Gene Regulation

As a component of certain small proteins, zinc enables those proteins to fold into a special form that interacts with DNA. The interaction "turns on" the gene, beginning the steps to protein production and cell multiplication.[53]

In severe zinc deficiency, cells fail to replicate. This may explain zinc's importance for normal growth of children and sexual maturation of adolescents. Furthermore, certain tissues with high turnover rates, such as cells lining the GI tract, skin cells, immune cells, and blood cells, are particularly vulnerable to a zinc deficiency. As a result, zinc-deficient people often have diarrhea, dermatitis, and depressed immunity.

Zinc and the Immune System

Zinc is vital to a vigorous immune response and is essential to the proper development and maintenance of the immune system. Without zinc, your body could not fight off invading viruses, bacteria, and fungi. Even mild deficiency may increase the risk of infection.

Quick Bites

Bizarre Behavior or Nutritional Deficiency?

In all cultures, races, and geographic regions, certain people have strange cravings for nonfood items. These cravings include ice (pagophagia), clay and dirt (geophagia), cornstarch (amylophagia), stone (lithophagia), paper, toilet tissue, soap, and foam. Pica, the compulsive consumption of nonfood items, often is associated with either iron or zinc deficiency, but it may also be the result of cultural beliefs or a response to family stresses. Whatever the cause, the behavior is not benign. It can injure teeth as well as cause constipation, intestinal obstruction or perforation, lead poisoning, pregnancy complications, poor growth in children, and mineral deficiencies.

hypogonadism Decreased functional activity of the gonads (ovaries or testes) with retardation of growth and sexual development.

geophagia Ingestion of clay or dirt.

galvanized Describes iron or steel with a thin layer of zinc plated onto it to protect against corrosion.

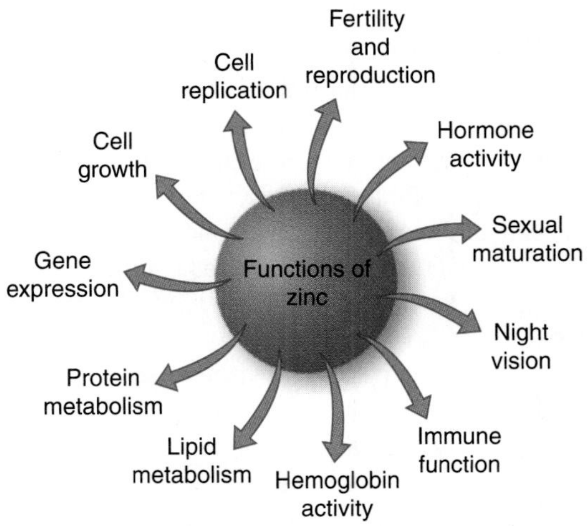

Figure 10.25 **Functions of zinc in the body.** Because zinc is involved in so many different functions, it is fortunate that overt zinc deficiency is rare.

Other Zinc Functions

Among zinc's many other functions, it interacts with hormones like insulin and assists in linking oxygen to hemoglobin. Of special interest to nutritionists is zinc's role in the sense of taste. Zinc deficiency reduces taste perception, and poor appetite generally follows.

Regulation of Zinc in the Body

When dietary zinc is low, our bodies have no long-term storehouse of zinc to draw upon. We maintain zinc balance, even when confronted with varying needs and dietary conditions, by adjusting absorption and excretion.

Zinc Absorption

Much about absorption of dietary zinc is similar to that of iron. We absorb only about 10 to 35 percent of the zinc in our diets. The proportion that's absorbed depends on our zinc status, the zinc content of the meal, and the presence of competing minerals. People with zinc deficiency absorb zinc more efficiently than do people with optimal zinc status. Zinc absorption

Fyi FOR YOUR INFORMATION — Zinc and the Common Cold

The common cold, one of our most common illnesses, affects American adults two to four times per year and children six to eight times per year.[1] Colds are even more frequent in young children in day-care settings and preschools. Because of missed work and decreased productivity, colds can be an economic stressor as well as a physical nuisance. A cure for the common cold would be of great benefit, and scientists have long pursued this goal. Because of zinc's role in immune function, 11 placebo-controlled studies between 1984 and 1998 investigated the effect of zinc lozenges on the common cold. Roughly half of the studies produced positive results and the other half had negative findings.

One study with positive results received considerable attention from the press. As a result, zinc lozenges are on nearly every pharmacy shelf in the United States. This study recruited 100 people during the winter of 1994. Researchers enrolled subjects within 24 hours of the onset of their common cold symptoms. Every two hours while awake, half the subjects took placebo lozenges and half took lozenges containing 13 milligrams of zinc, an average of six lozenges per day. They could take acetaminophen, but they were asked to refrain from taking other cold medicines or antibiotics during the trial. In the zinc group, colds resolved in an average of four days. In comparison, cold symptoms in the placebo group persisted for seven days.[2]

Though scientists have suggested several hypotheses, the mechanism for the effect is unclear. Zinc deficiency is known to impair immune function, but could all these people have been zinc-deficient? This is doubtful. Some speculate that zinc may inhibit viral replication.

During the trial, many of the experimental subjects experienced side effects, including nausea, bad taste, and sore mouths. In addition to the mild side effects and the cost of the lozenges, such high doses of zinc could have harmful effects. Long-term use of high doses of zinc induces copper deficiency. On average, those in the experimental group took close to 480 milligrams of zinc during the week of their cold. If children have eight colds per year and take nearly 500 milligrams of zinc per cold, could that be enough to induce widespread copper deficiency?

The same research group studied 249 randomly selected children in a double-blind, placebo-controlled trial. The experimental group took zinc gluconate lozenges at the first sign of cold symptoms. Depending on age, each child received 50 to 60 milligrams of zinc per day. There was no difference between groups in the time for all cold symptoms to resolve—a median of nine days. Although the researchers noted several limitations of their study, they concluded that we still need additional studies to determine what role, if any, zinc has in treatment of the common cold.[3]

Since only half of the studies produced positive effects, and excess zinc intake can cause deficiencies of other minerals, we should think twice before routinely giving children (and ourselves) zinc lozenges every time a cold strikes.

1 Gwaltney JM, Hendley JO, Simon G, Jordan WS. Rhinovirus infections in an industrial population. *N Engl J Med.* 1966;275:1261–1268.
2 Mossad SB, Macknin ML, Medendorp SV, Mason P. Zinc gluconate lozenges for treating the common cold: a randomized, double-blind placebo-controlled study. *Ann Intern Med.* 1996;125:81–88.
3 Macknin ML, Piedmonte M, Calendine C, et al. Zinc gluconate lozenges for treating the common cold in children: a randomized controlled trial. *JAMA.* 1998;279:1962–1967.

also increases during times of increased need, such as growth spurts, pregnancy, and lactation. As with iron, intestinal cells act as gatekeepers as they adjust their zinc absorption to maintain proper body levels.

Large amounts of phytate from whole grains and fiber inhibit zinc absorption. Some vegetarian diets contain enough phytate and fiber to depress zinc absorption significantly, but most American diets do not.[54] Calcium supplements combined with a high-phytate meal depress zinc absorption much more than phytate alone.

Very-high-dose iron supplements (which are non-heme) also depress zinc absorption, but heme iron (from meat) has no effect.[55] Iron-fortified foods are unlikely to inhibit zinc absorption.[56]

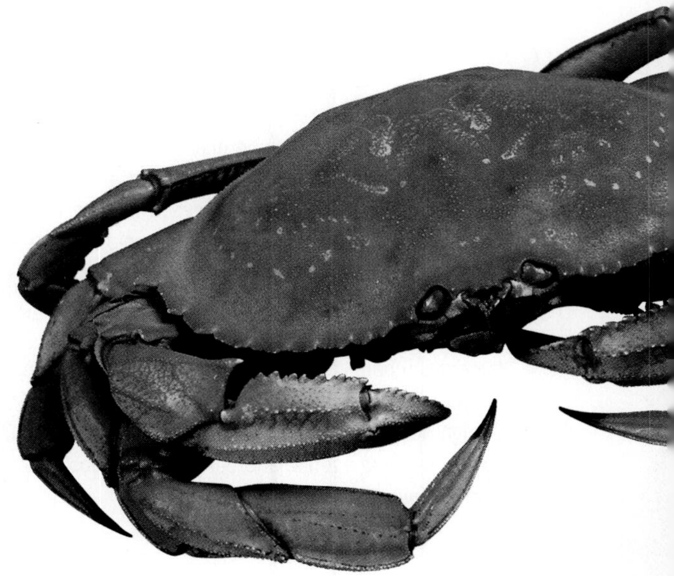

Zinc Transport, Distribution, and Excretion

Zinc circulates in the bloodstream bound to protein, traveling to the liver and tissues where it is most needed. Muscle and bone contain 90 percent of the body's zinc.

During digestion, the pancreas secretes a considerable amount of zinc in pancreatic juice. When needed, intestinal cells reabsorb most of this zinc. Otherwise, it is lost in feces along with unabsorbed dietary zinc. Zinc is also lost from sloughed-off intestinal cells, skin, and hair; and minor amounts are excreted in urine, sweat, and other fluids.

Dietary Recommendations for Zinc

The RDA for men is 11 milligrams per day, and for women over age 18, it is 8 milligrams per day, increasing to 11 milligrams during pregnancy and to 12 milligrams while breastfeeding.[57] Most people in the United States and Canada consume more than the RDA, but a significant number do not.

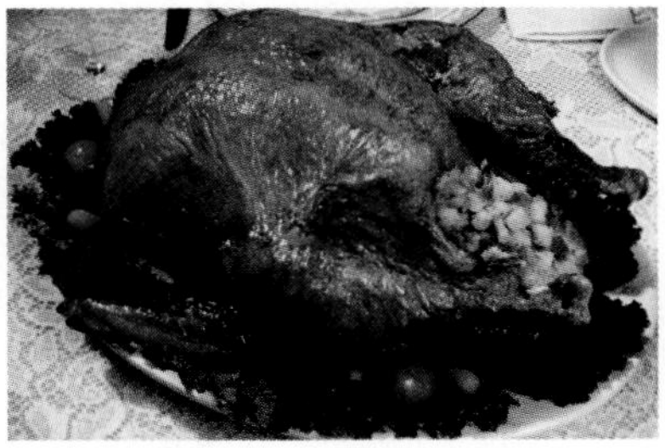

Sources of Zinc

Zinc usually is abundant in foods that are good sources of protein, especially red meat, and seafood such as oysters and clams. (See **Figure 10.26.**) For poultry, dark meat is a richer source than white meat. The zinc in animal foods is generally well absorbed. Conversely, whole grains have a relatively high amount of zinc, but it is poorly absorbed. Fruits and vegetables generally are poor zinc sources. Because diets that exclude meat are excluding the best zinc sources, adequate intake is a special concern for vegetarians.

Zinc Deficiency

Zinc deficiency is uncommon in the United States and Canada. It usually occurs in people with illnesses that impair absorption.

In other parts of the world, zinc deficiency is most prevalent in populations that subsist on cereals and little else. Zinc in cereal grains is poorly absorbed. Among these populations, infections with pneumonia and diarrhea are commonplace

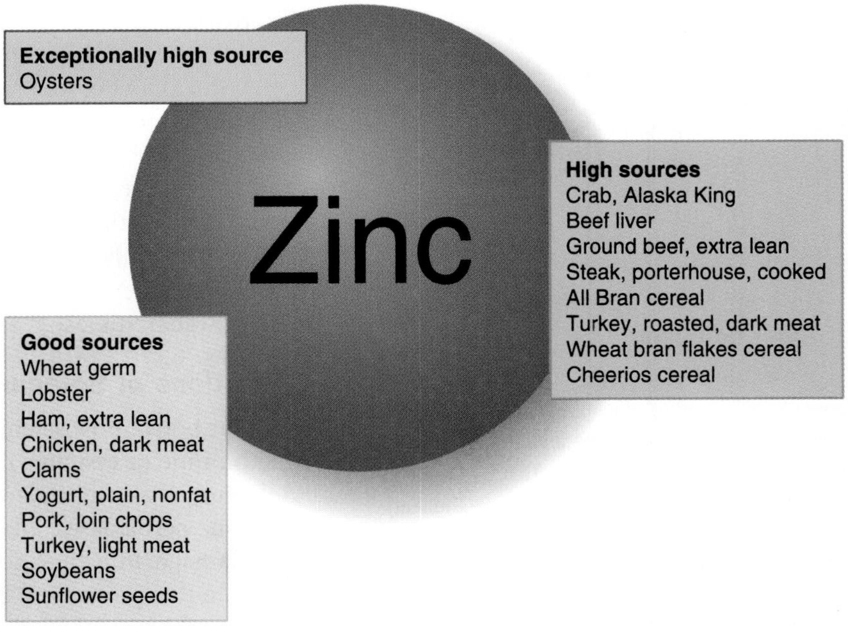

Figure 10.26 **Food sources of zinc.** Meat, organ meats, and seafood are the best sources of zinc.

Quick Bites

Hair Analysis Is a Misguided Measure

Although its use has been discredited, hair analysis is promoted with the claim that it can reveal mineral deficiencies. However, this measure lacks sensitivity and is unreliable. The color, diameter, and rate of growth of a person's hair, the season of the year, the geographic location, and the person's age and gender can affect the levels of minerals in hair. It is possible for hair concentration of an element (zinc, for example) to be high even though deficiency exists in the body. Hair dyes, colors, perming agents, and certain shampoos also alter the mineral content of hair.

Wilson's disease Genetic disorder of increased copper absorption, which leads to toxic levels in the liver and heart.

Keshan disease Selenium deficiency disease that impairs the structure and function of the heart.

hypothyroidism The result of a lowered level of circulating thyroid hormone, with slowing of mental and physical functions.

Quick Bites

On Your Next Moonlit Stroll, Think Selenium!

Selenium takes its name from the Greek word *Selênê*, "moon," because it has a pasty white color. In mythology, Selene is the Greek goddess of the moon. Ancient Greeks often blamed Selene and her brother Helios (god of the sun) for pestilent diseases and death.

and cause significant zinc losses. A downward spiral results: Zinc deficiency lowers immunity, and infection causes zinc loss, more infection, and more zinc loss. In some regions, zinc supplementation programs have cut the incidence of childhood respiratory infections and diarrhea.

Symptoms of moderate to severe zinc deficiency include poor growth, delayed or abnormal sexual development, diarrhea, severe skin rash and hair loss, impaired immune response, and impaired taste acuity. During pregnancy, zinc deficiency may contribute to complications and low birth weight.[58]

Zinc Toxicity

While toxicity from high dietary zinc intake is rare, chronic supplementation with too much zinc has adverse effects. Daily doses of 100 to 150 milligrams of zinc can decrease immune function.[59] Doses greater than 200 milligrams per day typically cause vomiting. The UL for zinc is set at 40 milligrams per day.

Chronic high dosing of zinc relative to copper inhibits copper absorption and with time may induce a copper deficiency. But for people with **Wilson's disease**, there's a benefit. Wilson's disease is a genetic disorder that causes excessive accumulation of copper in the body. Zinc supplements of 100 to 150 milligrams daily help prevent the copper accumulation.[60]

Key Concepts: *Zinc is important for normal growth and development, immune function, and the function of many enzymes. Zinc balance is maintained by regulating intestinal absorption. The best food sources are good protein sources, especially red meats and seafood. Zinc deficiency occurs most often among populations that subsist on cereals and grains.*

Selenium

The story of selenium (Se) is a recent one and becomes more complex as scientists continue to explore its roles. Historically, because animals grazing on selenium-rich soils suffered selenium poisoning, scientists focused on its toxicity. This changed in 1957, when researchers first demonstrated selenium's nutritional benefits in vitamin E-deficient animals. But not until 1979 did evidence emerge that selenium is essential for humans. Chinese scientists reported an association between low selenium status and **Keshan disease**, a heart disorder that strikes children in the Keshan province of China. The Chinese scientists demonstrated that selenium supplements could prevent the disease. Although selenium deficiency does not cause the disease, it predisposes a child to heart damage after a particular type of viral infection. When selenium intake is adequate, the virus apparently does not cause Keshan disease.

Functions of Selenium

In your body, most selenium joins up with one of two amino acids, methionine or cysteine, for storage or for its role as an antioxidant. Selenium is a component of a well-known family of antioxidants, the glutathione peroxidases. Like vitamin E, these enzymes work to prevent oxidative damage. In fact, to some extent selenium and vitamin E "spare" each other in this protection. A generous intake of one reduces the requirement for the other.

Selenium-containing enzymes are also involved in thyroid metabolism, converting thyroid hormone to its most active form. A deficiency of seleni-

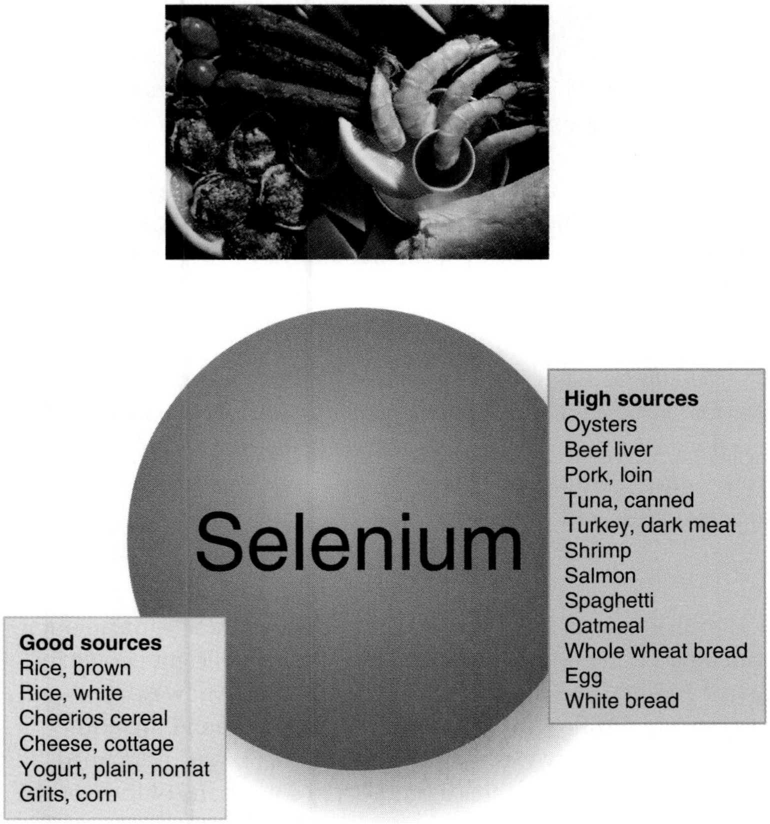

Figure 10.27 **Food sources of selenium.** Selenium is found mainly in meats, organ meats, seafood, and grains.

um worsens the **hypothyroidism** caused by iodine deficiency. (See the discussion of iodine later in this chapter.)

Selenium is important to immune function. As the Keshan studies showed, the body needs selenium to fight infections. Animals with depleted selenium get sicker from viral infections, and low selenium levels are associated with faster progression of viral disease in humans. Selenium may have some anticancer benefits, but more research is needed to clarify the relationship.[61]

Absorption and Excretion of Selenium

Most selenium in food is bound to the amino acids methionine or cysteine, and in this form, about 50 to 90 percent is bioavailable. Vitamins A, C, and E enhance selenium absorption, and phytate inhibits it. Excess selenium leaves the body mainly through feces and urine.

Dietary Recommendations and Sources of Selenium

For both men and women the selenium RDA is 55 micrograms per day.[62] The American diet generally provides these levels.

Selenium is found in both plant and animal-derived foods. Selenium levels are quite variable in plant foods and generally reflect the selenium content of the soil in which the plant was grown. Brazil nuts are particularly high in selenium. The soil in Venezuela, where most Brazil nuts are harvested, is rich in selenium. As a result, a single Brazil nut provides more than the RDA for selenium. The selenium content of animal-derived foods is much more consistent. Organ meats, fish, seafood, and meats are consistently good sources. (See **Figure 10.27**.)

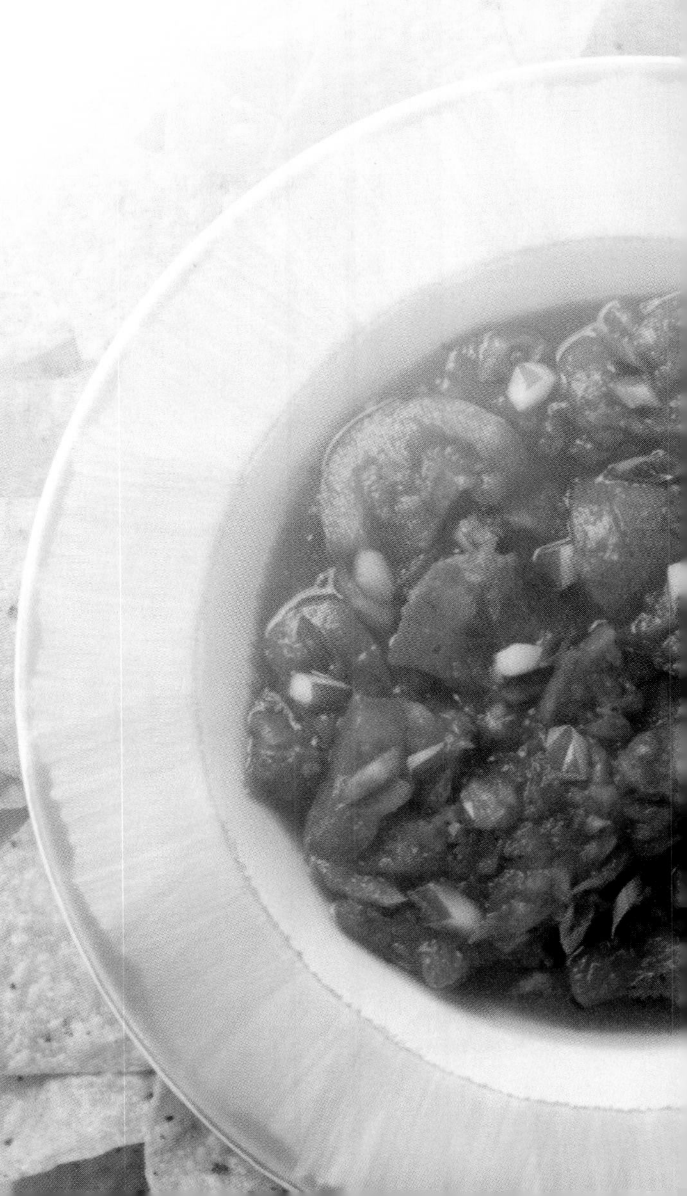

Quick Bites

Iodine or Iodide: What's in a Name?

Although the terms *iodine* and *iodide* often are used interchangeably, chemically they are not identical.

Iodine (I_2) is a bluish-black solid that gives off a purple vapor, which gives the element its name. *Iodine* stems from the Greek word *iôdêdes*, meaning "violet-colored."

Iodide (I^-) is the colorless negative ion of iodine. Iodine circulates in the body either bound to protein or as free iodide ions. Sodium iodide and potassium iodide are iodide salts commonly used in medicines.

goitrogens Compounds that interfere with iodine absorption and can induce goiter.

Selenium Deficiency and Toxicity

Chronic selenium deficiency interferes with immune function and predisposes a person to Keshan disease. Borderline deficiency appears to limit the ability to fight viral infections and may predispose a person to some kinds of cancer.[63]

There are isolated reports of selenium toxicity. Outward signs are brittle hair and nails and a garliclike body odor. Excessive intake may be accidental or the result of overenthusiastic supplementation. Chronic selenium toxicity also exists in isolated regions of the world where soil levels are very high. The UL is set at 400 micrograms per day for adults.

Key Concepts: *Selenium functions in antioxidant systems and spares vitamin E. It is involved in thyroid metabolism and immune function. Good dietary sources are Brazil nuts, organ meats, and seafood. Selenium deficiency is associated with Keshan disease, a rare heart ailment. Marginal deficiency may compromise immune function and increase cancer risk.*

Iodine

Iodine deficiency has existed for centuries. The ancient Chinese wrote about it, and European artists of the Middle Ages included iodine-deficient people in their paintings.[64] Iodine deficiency existed in the American Midwest, too, until supplementation and fortification programs were begun around the mid-1900s. Prior to that, deficiency was so common the region was nicknamed "the goiter belt." Iodine deficiency remains a problem in some parts of the world, and its eradication is an important goal of the World Health Organization.[65]

Iodine is an essential component of thyroid hormones, which help regulate body temperature, basal metabolic rate, reproduction, and growth. Not surprisingly, most of the body's iodine is found in the thyroid gland. Selenium-dependent enzymes activate the major thyroid hormone, so a selenium deficiency can lead to inefficient use of iodine.

In food, iodine is mostly in its ion form—iodide. Your intestines absorb nearly all dietary iodide. Raw vegetables in the cabbage family contain compounds known as **goitrogens**. These interfere with iodine absorption and can worsen deficiency. Cooking inactivates goitrogens. We excrete most excess iodine in urine, but also lose some in sweat, especially in hot, humid climates.

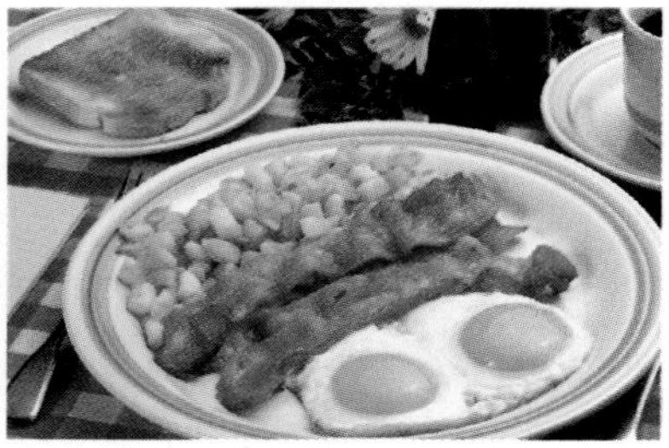

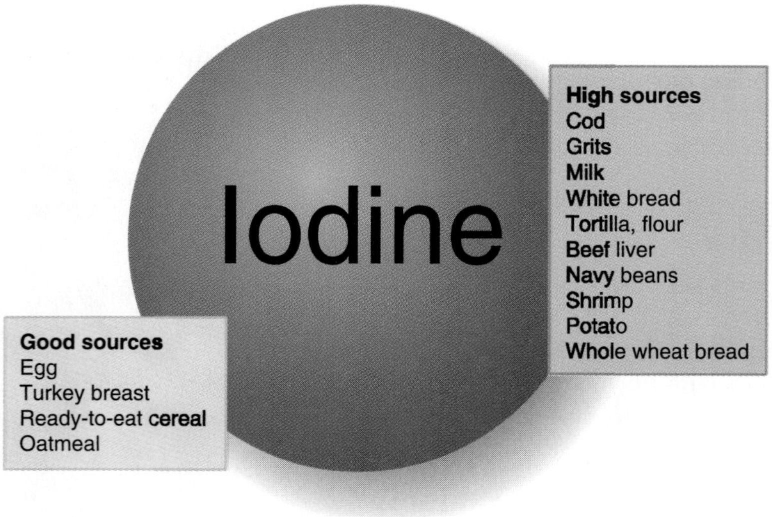

Figure 10.28 **Food sources of iodine.** Few foods are rich in iodine; it is found mainly in milk, seafood, and some grain products.

Dietary Recommendations and Sources of Iodine

The iodine RDA for men and women is 150 micrograms per day, an amount that replaces iodine losses and provides a generous margin of safety.[66]

Because the ocean is the best iodine source, the best food sources are ocean products: fish, seafood, and seaweed. (See **Figure 10.28**.) Saltwater fish have higher concentrations of iodine than freshwater fish. Natural iodine levels in plants reflect soil iodine levels, and foods grown near the ocean are considerably richer in iodine than foods grown far inland.

Because eons ago the midwestern United States and Canada were covered by glaciers rather than the ocean, these regions have iodine-poor soils and produce food with little iodine.

The dairy industry adds iodine to cattle feed and uses sanitizing solutions that contain iodine. This substantially increases the iodine in milk and dairy products, which are now major contributors of iodine to the American diet. For many people, iodized salt is their primary iodine source. In the United States, iodized salt contains an average of 76 micrograms of iodine per gram of salt.

Iodine Deficiency

Iodine deficiency causes hypothyroidism, low levels of thyroid hormones. Its most apparent sign is **goiter**—an enlarged thyroid gland in the neck. (See **Figure 10.29**.) If iodine deficiency occurs during pregnancy, the infant may be born with **cretinism**, a form of mental retardation.

Iodine deficiency inhibits thyroid hormone production. The body senses low levels of thyroid hormones and produces more and more **thyroid-stimulating hormone (TSH)**. The excessive TSH in turn stimulates the thyroid gland to grow, eventually causing a goiter. Other symptoms of hypothyroidism are intolerance to cold temperatures, decreased body temperature, weight gain, and sluggishness. In children, deficiency severe enough to cause goiter also affects intelligence.[67]

Severe iodine deficiency during early pregnancy causes cretinism in the baby. Symptoms are mental retardation, stunted growth, deafness, and muteness.

Iodine deficiency has disappeared from the United States and Canada, but it still exists in the world's poor and isolated areas where the soils are low in iodine and little food from outside enters the local food supply. Deficiency may be worsened by diets low in selenium and high in goitrogenic vegetables.

Iodine Toxicity

Large amounts of iodine inhibit synthesis of thyroid hormone, surprisingly, and stimulate thyroid growth and goiter. In other words, both too much and too little iodine cause goiter. Overzealous supplementation is the most common cause of iodine toxicity. The UL for iodine is 1,100 micrograms per day.

Key Concepts: *Iodine is an essential component of thyroid hormones. Iodine deficiency causes overstimulation of the thyroid gland and eventual goiter. Deficiency during pregnancy can cause cretinism in the offspring. Important food sources include ocean fish and seafood, dairy products, and iodized salt. Worldwide, iodine deficiency continues to exist in some regions. Iodizing salt is a powerful preventive measure.*

Copper

During the 1960s, researchers learned that copper was essential when they uncovered **Menkes' syndrome**, a rare genetic disease of copper deficiency. Dietary copper deficiency is not a significant public health concern, but excessive supplementation of other trace minerals can cause a secondary copper deficiency.

As a part of coenzymes, copper participates in dozens of reactions, among them energy release, skin pigment (melanin) production, and the produc-

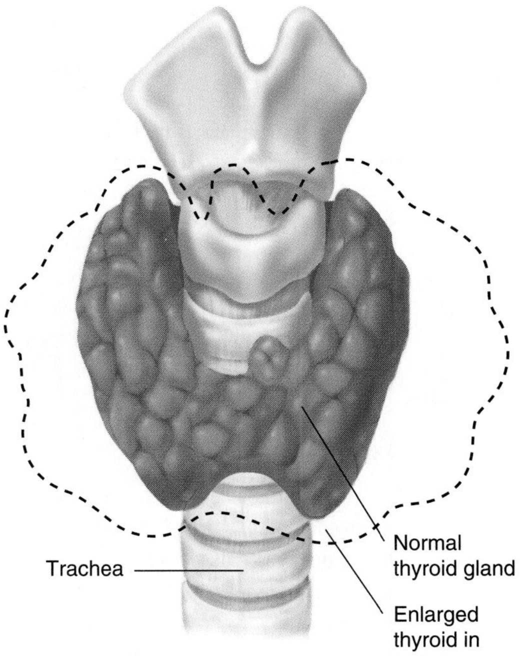

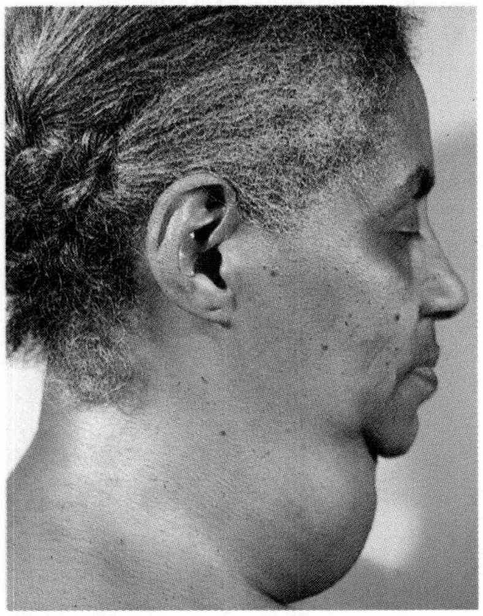

Figure 10.29 Enlargement of the thyroid gland in goiter. Iodine deficiency results in goiter. Use of iodized salt dramatically reduces goiter rates. This finding led to the widespread fortification of table salt with iodine.

goiter A chronic enlargement of the thyroid gland, visible as a swelling at the front of the neck; usually associated with iodine deficiency.

cretinism A congenital condition often caused by severe iodine deficiency during gestation; characterized by arrested physical and mental development.

thyroid-stimulating hormone (TSH) Hormone secreted from the pituitary gland at the base of the brain; regulates synthesis of thyroid hormones.

Menkes' syndrome A genetic disorder that results in copper deficiency.

ceruloplasmin A copper-dependent enzyme that enables iron to bind to transferrin. Also known as ferroxidase I.

albumin A protein that circulates in the blood and helps transport many minerals and some drugs.

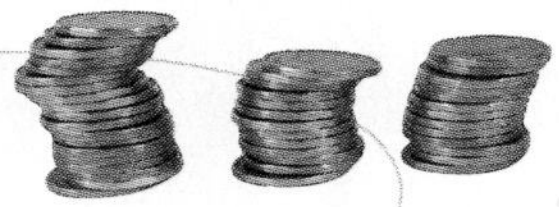

Quick Bites

A Penny for Your ...

How do the amounts of zinc and copper in a U.S. penny compare with the amounts in your body? Today's penny is mostly zinc (2.4 grams), covered with some copper plating (62.5 mg). A penny's zinc is in the upper range of the body's zinc content, but the amount of copper falls short. It takes the copper in about $1^{1}/_{2}$ pennies to equal the amount of copper in your body.

Quick Bites

Egg Whites? Please Stand Up!

Although cooking food in a copper pot is inadvisable, copper mixing bowls can be a plus. Meringues made in ceramic or steel bowls tend to be snowy white and drier than those made in copper bowls. Making meringue in a copper bowl leads to a creamier, yellowish foam that is harder to overbeat into a lumpy liquid. The copper bowl contributes copper ions to conalbumin, a metal-binding protein, thus stabilizing the whipped egg whites.

tion of the connective tissue proteins collagen and elastin. It plays a role in maintaining nerve health, immune function, and heart function. Copper is also a component of the superoxide dismutases, enzymes involved in antioxidant reactions. And copper is a component of **ceruloplasmin**, an enzyme required for iron transport. Without ceruloplasmin, iron accumulates in the liver, creating symptoms similar to hemochromatosis.

Copper Absorption and Storage

Copper absorption varies with dietary intake and can range from 20 to 50 percent. Most absorption takes place in the small intestine, though some occurs in the stomach. Some mineral supplements, most notably iron and zinc, can interfere with copper absorption. So can excessive use of antacids.

Albumin transports copper to the liver, where most is incorporated into ceruloplasmin. Little copper is stored. Unabsorbed copper, copper sloughed off in intestinal cells, and excess copper secreted in bile all leave the body via feces.

Dietary Recommendations and Sources of Copper

The copper RDA for both men and women is 900 micrograms per day. It's not difficult to achieve because copper is widely distributed in foods. The richest food sources for copper include organ meats, shellfish, nuts and seeds, legumes, peanut butter, and chocolate. (See **Figure 10.30**.)

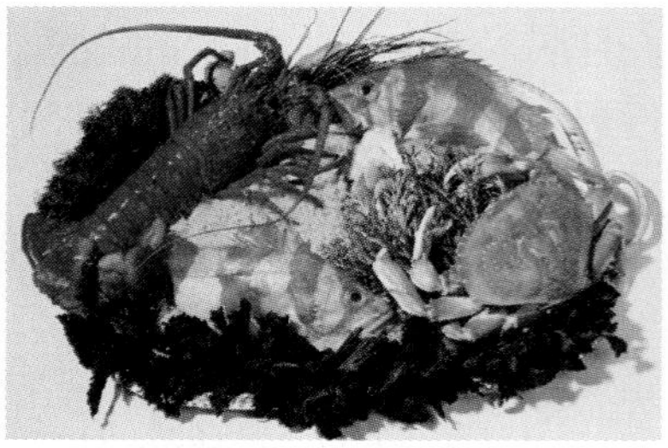

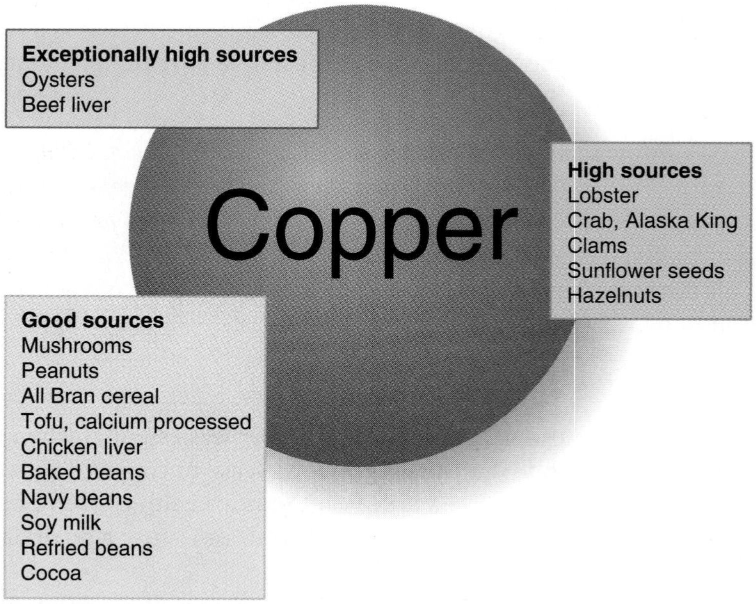

Figure 10.30 **Food sources of copper.** Copper is found in a limited variety of foods. The best sources are seafood, legumes, and nuts.

Copper Deficiency

Copper deficiency is rare and occurs most often in infants born prematurely, who have low copper stores at birth and a very rapid growth rate. Cow's milk has little copper, so infants who are inappropriately fed cow's milk rather than breast milk or formula could have low copper levels.

Copper deficiency reduces production of both red and white blood cells, causing anemia and poor immune function. Deficiency also causes bone abnormalities. Menkes' syndrome is an extremely rare (1 in 100,000 live births) genetic copper absorption disorder that usually is fatal in infancy or early childhood. Treatment within the first few days of life, however, may prevent irreversible damage.[68]

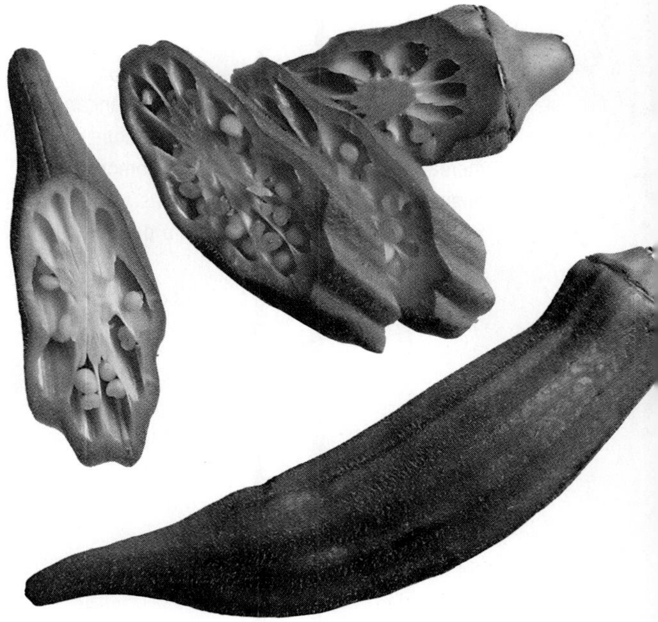

Copper Toxicity

Compared with other trace minerals, copper is relatively nontoxic. The UL for copper is 10 milligrams per day. However, in Wilson's disease, a rare (1 in 200,000) genetic disorder, excessive copper accumulates in the liver, brain, kidney, and eye. Like copper deficiency, copper excess causes anemia. People with Wilson's disease now avoid serious liver and neurologic problems with therapies that bind and remove copper and with zinc supplements, which inhibit copper absorption.

Key Concepts: *Copper is a component of ceruloplasmin, superoxide dismutase, and many other enzymes. Good food sources include organ meats, shellfish, nuts and seeds, legumes, peanut butter, and chocolate. Copper deficiency and toxicity are rare.*

Manganese

The body contains only 10 to 20 milligrams of manganese, yet manganese is a cofactor in reactions of key importance. It's involved in energy metabolism and in urea formation. (See Chapter 7, "Protein.") Manganese-containing enzymes are also required for building cartilage. Like zinc and copper, manganese is a component of the antioxidant enzyme superoxide dismutase.

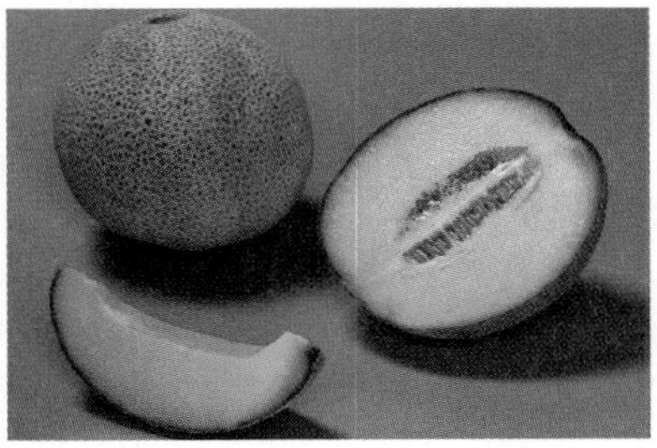

Absorption of manganese is very low, only 1 to 15 percent, probably a protection against toxicity. There is little storage, and any excess is excreted in bile and leaves via feces.

Dietary Recommendations and Sources of Manganese

Adequate Intake (AI) for manganese is 2.3 milligrams per day for men and 1.8 milligrams per day for women. Prior to 2001, manganese recommendations were higher: 2.0 to 5.0 milligrams per day. These recommendations were questioned because they were close to toxic levels determined by the Environmental Protection Agency. (The EPA defined maximum safe levels at no more than 10 milligrams manganese per day from food or no more than 4.2 milligrams per day from water.)[69]

Tea, coffee, nuts, cereals, and some fruits are the best food sources of manganese. (See **Figure 10.31**.) Meat, dairy products, poultry, fish, and refined foods are poor sources.

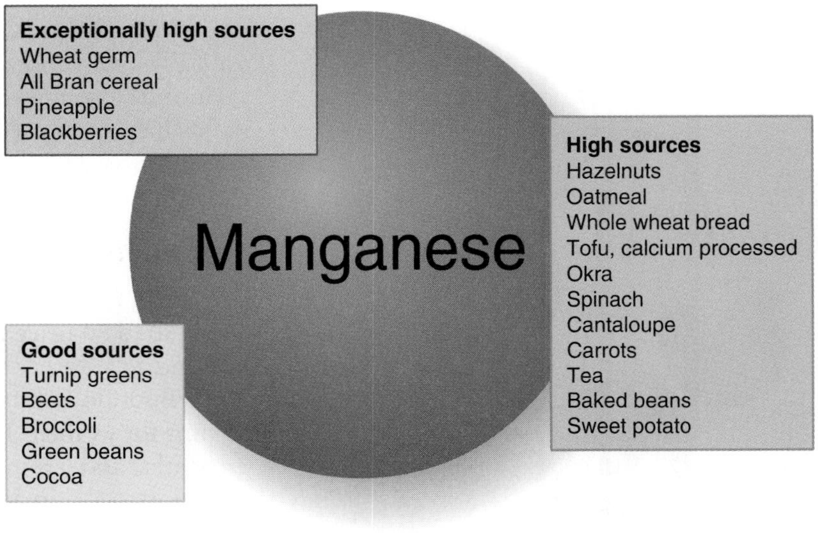

Figure 10.31 **Food sources of manganese.** Manganese is found mainly in plant foods such as grains, legumes, vegetables, and some fruits.

Quick Bites

Highway Harvest

Oil companies often add a type of manganese to modern gasoline as an antiknock compound to increase the octane rating for high-compression engines. It is now evident that plants along highways accumulate manganese from passing cars.

Manganese Deficiency and Toxicity

Most people are not at risk of manganese deficiency. However, some illnesses, such as **Lou Gehrig's disease** or **multiple sclerosis**, may cause suboptimal manganese status. In animal studies, manganese deficiency impairs growth, impairs energy metabolism, and produces bone abnormalities.

Manganese toxicity is a greater threat than manganese deficiency. However, incidents of toxicity have been due not to food, but to air pollutants. Foundry workers exposed to airborne manganese dust experience severe manganese toxicity. Their symptoms include irritability, hallucinations, and severe lack of coordination. Lower doses of airborne manganese can impair memory and motor coordination. The UL for manganese is 11 milligrams per day.

Key Concepts: *Manganese is a cofactor in several enzyme systems. Food sources for manganese are tea, coffee, cereals, and some fruits. Toxicity from airborne manganese is a greater threat than deficiency.*

Lou Gehrig's disease A syndrome marked by muscular weakness and atrophy due to a degeneration of motor neurons of the spinal cord. Technically known as amyotrophic lateral sclerosis (ALS).

multiple sclerosis A progressive disease that destroys the myelin sheath surrounding nerve fibers of the brain and spinal cord.

Fluoride

Fluoride is a form of the element fluorine. Large-scale studies undertaken during the 1940s convincingly demonstrated that fluoride has the ability to prevent dental caries. Since then, fluoride has been added to water supplies in many regions of the United States, and use of fluoridated toothpaste and mouthwash has become widespread.

Functions of Fluoride

Nearly 99 percent of the body's fluoride is in bones and teeth, where it promotes deposition of calcium and phosphate. Every day there is a battle in your teeth between normal mineral loss and mineral deposition. When your mouth contains food, bacteria multiply and produce acids that eat away tooth enamel, especially beneath plaque. Fluoride inhibits bacterial activity and shifts the balance toward depositing minerals. This action in teeth helps counter normal mineral loss, a loss that acid-forming bacteria accelerate. Fluoride therefore inhibits tooth decay and loss of tooth enamel.

During infancy and childhood, while new teeth are being formed, fluoride acts systemically. In other words, it arrives via the bloodstream to the site of new tooth formation. There it is incorporated into the tooth structure. Throughout life, the fluoride in toothpaste, mouth rinses, and other topically applied fluoride helps strengthen tooth surfaces.

Fluoride also may play a role in preventing bone loss.[70] Fluoride supplements have been used along with calcium and other medications to treat osteoporosis. Although the risk of fracture is reduced, optimal dosage is not clear, and fluoride is not an approved treatment for osteoporosis.

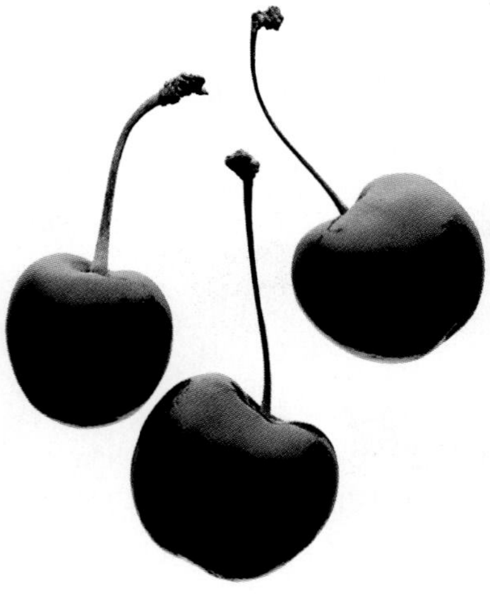

Dietary Recommendations and Sources of Fluoride

Your body absorbs almost all fluoride from water and other liquids, and about 50 to 80 percent of fluoride from food. Most excess fluoride is excreted in urine.

The fluoride AI for adults is 4 milligrams per day for men, and 3 milligrams for women. The AI is 0.01 milligram per day for infants up through 5 months, and 0.5 milligram for those aged 6 to 11 months. The American Dental Association and American Academy of Pediatrics recommend fluoride supplements for those over 1 year of age whose drinking water supplies less than 0.6 milligrams fluoride per liter.[71]

Water is the main source of fluoride. Water naturally may contain fluoride, or fluoride may be added to produce fluoridated water. Fluoride naturally present in drinking water varies from less than 0.1 milligram to more than 10 milligrams per liter. The Environmental Protection Agency requires public drinking water systems to remove excess fluoride so that it does not exceed 4.0 milligrams per liter.

Where naturally occurring fluoride levels are low, many water companies add fluoride, bringing levels up to 0.7 to 1.2 milligrams per liter. Communities must first vote their approval for fluoridation. Roughly 62 percent of the U.S. population now have fluoridated water.[72]

Other fluoride sources have emerged since we first began fluoridating water supplies. Today's fluoride sources include fluoride supplements, mouthwash, toothpaste, and some beverages.

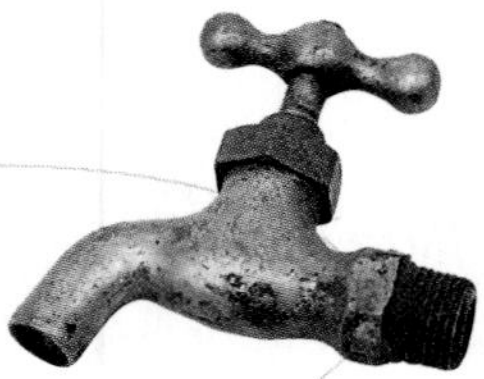

Quick Bites

Accidental Discovery

In the early 1900s people noticed that inhabitants of towns with naturally high levels of fluoride in their water had healthier teeth. To test the correlation between fluoride and tooth decay, in 1945 four cities in the United States and one in Canada took part in a controlled study of water fluoridation. The results were impressive, establishing that fluoride helps to prevent tooth decay.

When Fluoride Balance Goes Awry

Low fluoride intake is associated with tooth decay. Adequate fluoride intake during infancy and childhood cuts the incidence of tooth decay by up to 30 to 60 percent.

Prolonged excessive intake of fluoride causes **fluorosis**. (See **Figure 10.32**.) During tooth development, fluorosis damages teeth. In mild fluorosis, white specks form on the teeth. Severe fluorosis weakens teeth and produces permanent brownish stains. In adults fluorosis is associated with hip fracture; weak, stiff joints; and chronic stomach inflammation.

Fluorosis can occur in people living where water is naturally very high in fluoride, or in children who chronically swallow large amounts of fluoridated toothpaste. The UL for fluoride is 10 milligrams per day.

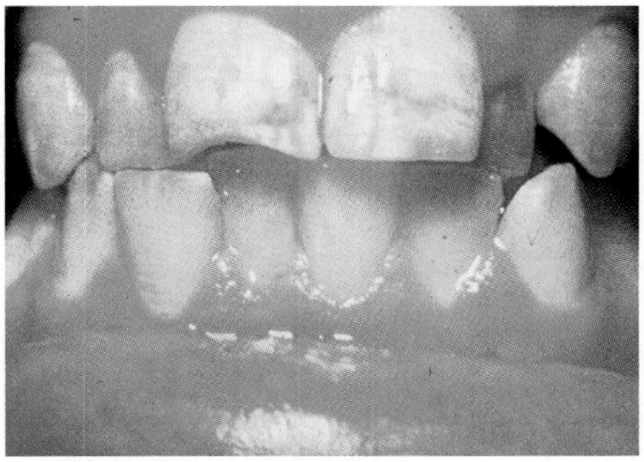

Figure 10.32 **Tooth mottling in fluorosis.** During tooth development, prolonged excessive fluoride intake can cause fluorosis, which discolors and damages teeth.

fluorosis Mottled discoloration and pitting of tooth enamel caused by prolonged ingestion of excessive fluoride.

The Fluoridation Debate

Think About It 4

In some communities, water fluoridation programs have been in place for over 50 years. It is indisputable that these programs have substantially reduced tooth decay, and more than 90 professional health organizations endorse fluoridation of the public water supplies as the most effective dental public health measure.[73] However, opponents argue that fluoridation is "mass, involuntary medication."[74] Among some opponents, the issue of fluoridation has taken on dark political tones.

Some argue that availability of fluoride supplements and fluoride-containing dental products makes fluoridation unnecessary. Others fear fluorosis or a connection with cancer and other illnesses, although well over 50 studies have proven there is no relationship.[75]

Proponents cite the substantial evidence of improved dental health and lack of evidence showing harm.[76] Bone health also may benefit. The presence of fluoride in water is not unnatural, and levels in fluoridated water are far less than the amount that occurs naturally in some sources. To retain benefits yet avoid overconsumption, the American Dental Association recommends the fluoridation of all water supplies and regulation of other fluoride sources.

The AI levels for infants and children have been reduced to account for increased fluoride in the food supply. Fluoride supplements are available only by prescription.

Quick Bites

Conspiracy Theory

Although the U.S. Public Health Service and the World Health Organization officially endorsed the fluoridation of water in the 1950s, some groups continue to oppose the practice. Objectors claim that water fluoridation violates civil rights, that fluoride is a "nerve poison," and that fluoride is unwanted compulsory medication that can have dangerous side effects. Some groups even claim that fluoridation is a component of a conspiracy for national destruction. So far, objectors have been unable to substantiate their claims, and the courts have upheld the constitutionality of fluoridation.

Key Concepts: *Bones and teeth contain 99 percent of body fluoride. Fluoride supports mineralization of bones and teeth, and adequate intake reduces tooth decay. The main dietary source is water. The majority of municipal water supplies con-*

Quick Bites

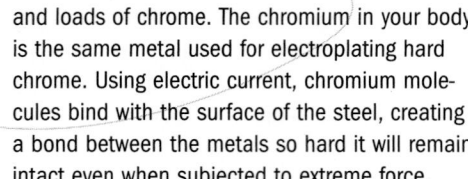

Chrome-Plated Cars

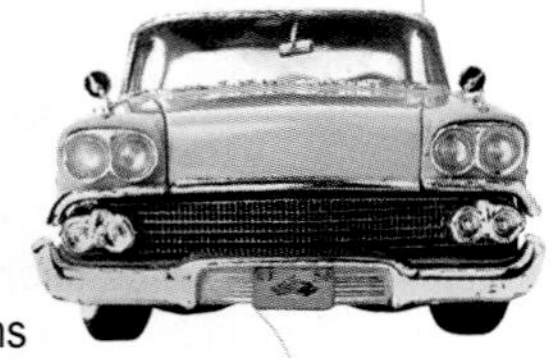

The cars of the 1950s sported fins and loads of chrome. The chromium in your body is the same metal used for electroplating hard chrome. Using electric current, chromium molecules bind with the surface of the steel, creating a bond between the metals so hard it will remain intact even when subjected to extreme force.

tain fluoride. Excess fluoride causes fluorosis with mottling of the teeth. Severe fluorosis causes weakened, brown-stained teeth.

Chromium

The best understood role of chromium is in glucose metabolism. Chromium appears to enhance the ability of insulin to move glucose into cells. Other functions of chromium involve nucleic acid metabolism, growth, and immune function. Athletes are especially interested in chromium because of claims that it has beneficial effects on body composition.

The amount of chromium in the body is exceedingly tiny—only about 4 to 6 milligrams total. And that amount appears to fall as people age. It's not clear whether the decline is normal or a negative effect that our diet has on chromium levels.[77] Some researchers speculate that chromium decline in aging may be partly responsible for type 2 diabetes.

Chromium absorption appears to increase with need and decrease as dietary intake rises. Absorption is probably better (10 to 25 percent) when chromium is combined with an organic acid, as it is in chromium picolinate. Excess is excreted in urine.

Dietary Recommendations and Sources of Chromium

The AI for adults 19 to 50 years of age is 35 micrograms per day for men and 25 micrograms per day for women, decreasing by 5 micrograms per day in older adults.

Rich sources of chromium are mushrooms, dark chocolate, prunes, nuts, asparagus, whole grains, wine, brewer's yeast, and some brands of beer. Animal products are poor sources. Cooking acidic foods in stainless steel containers leaches some chromium into the food.

Chromium Deficiency and Toxicity

It is difficult to detect chromium deficiency in the general population. In research settings, induced chromium deficiency inhibits glucose uptake by cells and raises blood glucose, insulin, and blood lipids. Patients who subsist on long-term intravenous feedings inadequate in chromium may suffer brain and nerve disorders.[78]

The only known cases of chromium toxicity are from airborne chromium compounds in industrial settings. To date, no UL has been set for chromium, but up to 200 micrograms of inorganic chromium appears to be a safe supplement dose.

Several years ago chromium picolinate supplements were hyped for weight loss. Popularity of the supplements faded because people did not lose weight and, in cell culture studies, large doses damaged DNA. Based on perceived but unfounded metabolic benefits, chromium supplements remain popular among athletes and bodybuilders.

Quick Bites

Molybdenum Takes a Stand Against the Elements

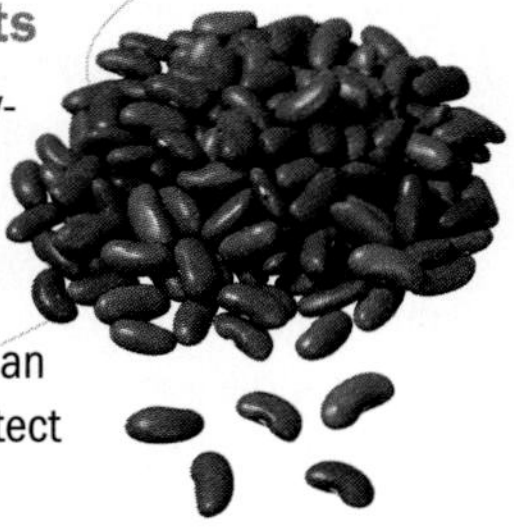

Molybdenum is a silvery-gray metal that is not found free in nature. It has properties similar to those of tungsten and is used as an alloy to strengthen and protect metal from corrosion.

Molybdenum

Molybdenum is essential to both plants and animals. In humans, molybdenum functions as a cofactor for several enzymes.

Molybdenum is efficiently absorbed, and it's excreted rapidly in urine and bile. Dietary copper can inhibit molybdenum absorption, and vice versa. Doctors exploit the competition between copper and molybdenum by using a form of molybdenum to treat patients with Wilson's disease.

The RDA for molybdenum is 45 micrograms per day for adults. Peas, beans, and some breakfast cereals are the richest food sources, and organ meats are also good sources.

Molybdenum deficiency does not occur in people who eat a normal diet. Deficiency symptoms of weakness, mental confusion, and night blindness have occurred in people on long-term intravenous feeding or people with a rare genetic disorder.

Although molybdenum is unlikely to cause toxicity in humans, a UL for molybdenum has been set at 2,000 micrograms per day.

Key Concepts: *Chromium is involved in glucose metabolism and probably has other important roles as well. Molybdenum is required in several important enzyme systems. Deficiency or toxicity of chromium and molybdenum are very unlikely.*

Other Trace Minerals and Ultratrace Minerals

Five of the minerals we have discussed—iodine, fluoride, manganese, molybdenum, and selenium—could be considered "ultratrace" minerals. They are found in the body in minuscule amounts; and for most of these, we need less than 1 milligram daily. While there is substantial research on these minerals, the functions of other trace and ultratrace minerals are less clear. Recent research and attention have focused on arsenic, boron, nickel, silicon, and vanadium. Although insufficient evidence exists to set an AI or RDA for these minerals, ULs have been established for boron, nickel, and vanadium.

Arsenic

Although arsenic (As) has been an infamous poison for centuries, inorganic arsenic may actually be an essential ultratrace element. As a colorless, tasteless toxin, arsenic trioxide can be fatal in a dose as low as 2 milligrams.[79] On the other hand, arsenic-deprived laboratory animals have poor growth and abnormal reproduction. The average man gets about 60 micrograms daily from foods. Some water supplies contain considerable arsenic, and standards for safe arsenic levels are hotly debated. A UL has not yet been established.

Boron

Boron appears to play a role in bone metabolism. In lab animals, boron deficiency impairs growth, and a vitamin D deficiency makes the problem worse. Conversely, boron supplementation reduces the bone abnormalities of vitamin D deficiency. We probably need about 1 milligram per day, an amount typically supplied by diet.[80]

Chronic boron toxicity symptoms include poor appetite, nausea, weight loss, decreased sex drive, and low sperm count. The UL for boron is 20 milligrams per day.

Nickel

A few nickel-containing enzymes have been identified, and nickel can activate or inhibit a number of other enzymes. Deficiency symptoms in humans have not been identified. Although dietary intake of nickel varies widely, an acceptable intake of 100 to 300 micrograms per day has been proposed.[81]

There is no known nickel deficiency in humans. Toxicity has occurred only in workers exposed to nickel dust or nickel carbonyl in industrial settings. The UL is 1 milligram per day.

Silicon

Experimental diets lacking silicon cause poor growth and skeletal abnormalities in baby chickens. Although there are no known deficiency symptoms in humans, silicon is believed to help strengthen collagen and elastin. An adequate amount in the diet may be 21 to 46 milligrams per day.[82]

Chronic inhalation of silicon causes serious illness, but there's no evidence of dietary silicon toxicity. No UL has been set for silicon.

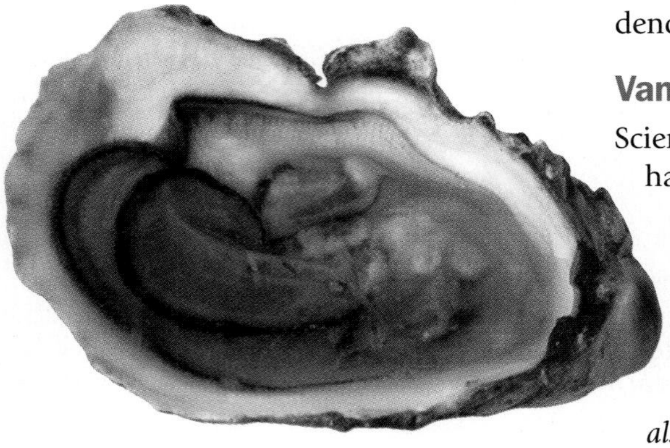

Vanadium

Scientists are not sure exactly what role vanadium plays in the body and have not observed deficiencies. Currently vanadium supplements are available in amounts many times greater than that found in the diet. They are promoted to athletes and people trying to gain muscle mass. The UL for vanadium is 1.8 milligrams per day.

Key Concepts: *Ultratrace minerals have very low estimated requirements. Although specific biochemical functions have not been defined for the minerals arsenic, boron, nickel, silicon, and vanadium, they are thought to be essential for humans.*

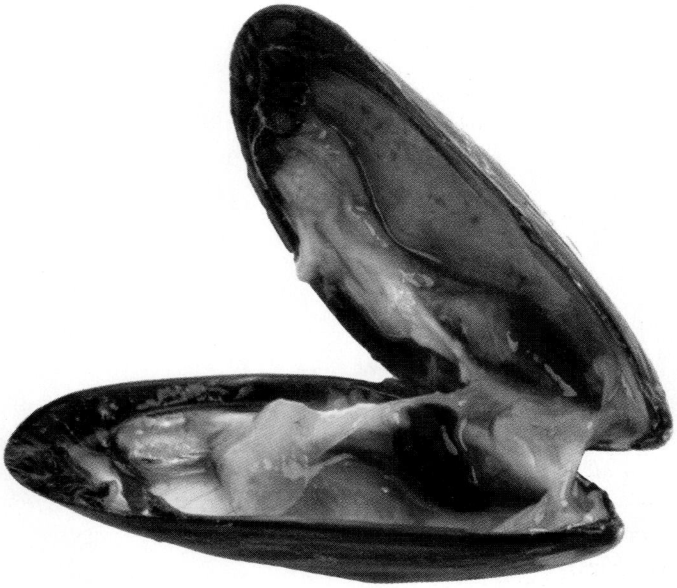

Label [to] Table

Have you ever noticed how many minerals are added to breakfast cereals these days? Take a look at the following Nutrition Facts label from a fortified breakfast cereal and see if you can find the major and trace minerals. You should be able to spot four major minerals (sodium, calcium, phosphorus, and magnesium) and three trace minerals (iron, zinc, and copper.) The bone minerals of calcium, phosphorus, and magnesium contribute 4 percent, 10 percent, and 8 percent, respectively, of the Daily Value. One serving of this cereal contributes 12 percent of the Daily Value for sodium, or 280 milligrams.

Looking at the Ingredients and Vitamins and Minerals lists, you can see that the iron and zinc were added (fortified), but the copper and major minerals appear to come naturally from the cereal. Why do you think these trace minerals are added to this cereal? Many people (especially children) eat marginal amounts of iron and zinc. The best sources of these minerals are meats, liver, shellfish, and eggs. Most children don't eat much shellfish or liver, so adding the minerals to cereals, which they do eat, is an easy way to make sure they get 45 percent and 25 percent of their iron and zinc Daily Values, respectively.

Nutrition Facts

Serving Size: 1 cup (30g)
Servings Per Container about 9

Amount Per Serving	Cereal	with ½ cup skim milk
Calories	110	150
Calories from Fat	15	20
		% Daily Value**
Total Fat 2g*	**3%**	**3%**
Saturated Fat 0g	**0%**	**3%**
Polyunsaturated Fat 0.5g		
Monounsaturated Fat 0.5g		
Cholesterol 0mg	**0%**	**1%**
Sodium 280mg	**12%**	**15%**
Total Carbohydrate 22g	**7%**	**9%**
Dietary Fiber 3g	**11%**	**11%**
Soluble Fiber 1g	**11%**	**11%**
Sugars 1g		
Other carbohydrates 1g		
Protein 3g		
Vitamin A	10%	15%
Vitamin C	10%	10%
Calcium	4%	20%
Iron	45%	45%
Vitamin D	10%	25%
Thiamin	25%	30%
Riboflavin	25%	35%
Niacin	25%	25%
Vitamin B_6	25%	25%
Folic Acid	50%	50%
Vitamin B_{12}	25%	35%
Phosphorus	10%	25%
Magnesium	8%	10%
Zinc	25%	30%
Copper	2%	2%

*Amount in Cereal. A serving of cereal plus skim milk provides 2g total fat (0.5g saturated fat, 1g monosaturated fat). less than 5mg cholesterol, 350mg sodium, 300mg potassium, 28g total carbohydrate (7g sugars) and 7g protein.

**Percent Daily Values are based on a 2,000 calorie diet. Your daily values may be higher or lower depending on your calorie needs:

Total Fat	Calories:	2,000	2,500
Sat Fat	Less Than	65g	80g
Cholesterol	Less Than	20g	25g
Sodium	Less Than	300mg	300mg
Potassium	Less Than	2,400mg	2,400mg
Total Carbohydrate		3,500mg	3,500mg
Dietary Fiber		300g	375g
	25g	30g	

INGREDIENTS: WHOLE GRAIN OATS (INCLUDES THE OAT BRAN), MODIFIED FOOD STARCH, SUGAR, SALT, OAT FIBER, TRISODIUM PHOSPHATE, CALCIUM CARBONATE, VITAMIN E (MIXED TOCOPHEROLS) ADDED TO PRESERVE FRESHNESS.

VITAMINS AND MINERALS: IRON AND ZINC (MINERAL NUTRIENTS), VITAMIN C (SODIUM ASCORBATE), A B VITAMIN (NIACINAMIDE), VITAMIN B_6 (PYRIDOXINE HYDROCHLORIDE), VITAMIN B_2 (RIBOFLAVIN), VITAMIN B_1 (THIAMIN MONONITRATE), VITAMIN A (PALMITATE), A B VITAMIN (FOLIC ACID), VITAMIN B_{12}, VITAMIN D.

LEARNING Portfolio chapter 10

Key Terms

	page
albumin	412
aldosterone [al-DOS-ter-own]	380
anions	378
antidiuretic hormone (ADH)	380
calmodulin	392
cations	378
ceruloplasmin	412
ciliary action	392
cretinism	411
diastolic	385
electrolytes [ih-LEK-tro-lites]	378
essential hypertension	385
ferritin	400
fibrin	391
fluorosis	415
galvanized	405
geophagia	405
goiter	411
goitrogens	410
heat capacity	379
heme	399
heme iron	400
hemochromatosis	404
hemosiderin	400
hydroxyapatite	391
hypertension	385
hypogonadism	405
hypothyroidism	408
insensible water loss	380
ions	378
iron overload	404
Keshan disease	408
Lou Gehrig's disease	414
major minerals	383
Menkes' syndrome	411
mineralization	391
multiple sclerosis	414
myoglobin	399
non-heme iron	400
osmosis	378
osteoblasts	391
osteoclasts	391
oxalate (oxalic acid)	385
phytate (phytic acid)	385
plasma	378
polyphenols	400
salts	378
systolic	385
thyroid-stimulating hormone (TSH)	411
trace minerals	383
transferrin	402
Wilson's disease	408

Study Points

- **Water is the most essential nutrient; we can live much longer without food than without water.**
- **Water is important for chemical reactions, temperature regulation, maintaining acid–base balance, and transporting nutrients and waste. Fluids in the body lubricate and cushion joints, cleanse the eyes, and moisten the food we eat.**
- **Water is lost through exhaled air, perspiration, feces, and urine. Insensible water loss is the continuous evaporation of water from the lungs and skin. Diuretics increase fluid excretion. When fluid loss exceeds intake, resulting dehydration can seriously impair physical and mental performance.**
- **Minerals are inorganic elements and are categorized as major or trace depending on the amount in the body and the amount needed in the diet.**
- **The bioavailability of minerals may be affected by excess intake of single-mineral supplements; phytate, oxalate, and fiber in plant foods; and mineral status in the body.**
- **Sodium helps regulate water distribution and blood pressure. Sodium needs (500 mg per day) are well below average intakes (3,000 to 6,000 mg per day).**
- **Potassium is necessary for nerve and muscle function. Unprocessed foods, including fruits and vegetables, provide most dietary potassium.**
- **Chloride is a component of stomach acid. Chloride deficiency is most often associated with prolonged vomiting.**
- **Calcium, the most abundant mineral in the body, is found mainly in bones and teeth. It's required for blood clotting, nerve and muscle function, and cellular metabolism. Major dietary sources of calcium are dairy products and calcium-fortified foods.**
- **Phosphorus is a key component of ATP, DNA, RNA, phospholipids, and lipoproteins. Because phosphorus is widespread in foods, inadequate phosphorus intake is rare.**

- **Plant foods like whole grains and vegetables are important sources of magnesium, which is a cofactor for hundreds of enzymes. Kidney disease, alcoholism, and overuse of diuretics may cause low magnesium levels.**
- **Sulfur does not function alone as a nutrient, but as a component of certain amino acids and the vitamins biotin and thiamin.**
- **Hypertension increases risk for heart disease, stroke, and kidney disease. Excessive sodium intake is linked to hypertension in people who are salt-sensitive. Other dietary factors linked to hypertension include low potassium, calcium, and magnesium intakes.**
- **Osteoporosis—weak, porous bones—results from excessive bone loss. Postmenopausal women are at highest risk for osteoporosis. Adequate dietary calcium, vitamin D, and physical activity throughout life reduce the risk for osteoporosis.**
- **Hemoglobin and myoglobin contain iron, which transports oxygen. Iron is also an enzyme cofactor, important for immune function and brain function.**
- **Due to menstruation, women of childbearing age need more iron than men do. Meats are the best source of iron, but enriched and whole grains are also significant sources in the American diet.**
- **Iron deficiency is the most common nutritional deficiency worldwide. Anemia is the most severe stage of deficiency, occurring after iron stores are depleted. Iron toxicity can be acute or chronic. Accidental iron overdose is a leading cause of poisoning deaths of young children in the United States. Hemochromatosis is a disease of chronic excessive iron absorption.**
- **Zinc is a cofactor for numerous enzymes and is crucial for normal growth, sexual development, and immune function. It is found in protein-rich foods, particularly meats. Deficiency results in poor growth, impaired taste, and impaired immune response.**
- **Selenium is considered an antioxidant nutrient. It is also needed for thyroid function. Good sources of selenium are Brazil nuts, organ meats, and seafood. Deficiency of selenium in the Keshan region of China is associated with Keshan heart disease.**
- **Iodine is required for thyroid function. Iodine deficiency causes enlarged thyroid or goiter. Severe deficiency during pregnancy can cause cretinism in the baby. Much of the iodine in the American diet comes from iodized salt.**
- **Copper functions in many enzyme systems involved with antioxidant protection, iron utilization, and immune function. The richest food sources of copper include organ meats, shellfish, nuts and seeds, peanut butter, and chocolate. Copper deficiency is rare.**
- **Manganese functions in many enzyme systems. The best food sources include tea, coffee, nuts, cereals, and some fruits. Manganese deficiency and toxicity are uncommon; toxicity is from manganese air pollutants.**
- **Fluoride promotes mineralization of bones and teeth and protects teeth from decay. Water, which contains fluoride naturally or is fluoridated, is our main fluoride source. Excessive fluoride causes fluorosis, which mottles teeth.**
- **Chromium is involved in glucose metabolism. Some good sources of chromium are mushrooms, dark chocolate, prunes, nuts, asparagus, and whole grains. Chromium toxicity is unlikely.**
- **Molybdenum functions as an enzyme cofactor. Good food sources are peas, beans, and some breakfast cereals. Molybdenum deficiency and toxicity are both rare.**
- **Ultratrace minerals are those required in extremely small amounts; the specific function of many of these nutrients is unknown. Some ultratrace minerals are arsenic, boron, nickel, silicon, and vanadium.**

Study Questions

Answers can be found at nutrition.jbpub.com/discovering.

1. **Name the main functions of water.**
2. **List two main factors that affect absorption of a mineral.**
3. **What three major minerals affect bone health?**
4. **What are the major functions of calcium, other than its relation to bone health?**
5. **How does the body compensate for low calcium intake?**
6. **Explain the differences between "heme" and "non-heme" iron. Which is absorbed better?**
7. **List the three stages of iron deficiency.**
8. **Describe the common causes of zinc deficiency.**
9. **What are the main functions of selenium?**
10. **Iodine is a component of which hormones? What are the functions of these hormones?**
11. **What are goitrogens and goiters?**
12. **How does fluoride prevent tooth decay? Other than water, what sources supply fluoride?**
13. **What are the food sources for chromium, and what is chromium's best understood role?**

Try This

Osmosis Experiment

Purchase some celery and let it sit for a week or two until it becomes limp. When the celery looks limp and lifeless, fill your sink with cold water and soak the celery. When it has soaked for several hours, take the celery out and examine its appearance. Notice anything different? Since the crispness of celery is due to osmotic pressure, when you soaked the limp celery, it absorbed water into its cells and became crisp again.

A Simple Check on Your Zinc

Reported in *Lancet* in the early 1980s, this simple test can provide a rough signal of your zinc status. Buy some zinc sulfate at a health food store. Dissolve it in distilled water to make a 0.1 percent zinc sulfate solution. Refrain from eating, drinking, and smoking for at least an hour before the test. Then swish a teaspoon of the solution around your mouth for 10 seconds. If it tastes unpleasant or metallic, your level of zinc is probably adequate. However, if the solution tastes like water, you may be consuming less zinc than you need.

What About Bobbie?

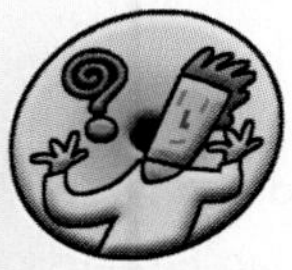

Let's take a look at Bobbie's intake of the minerals calcium, magnesium, sodium, iron, zinc, and selenium. Refer to Chapter 1 to refresh yourself regarding Bobbie's one-day intake. How do you think she did?

Calcium

Bobbie's calcium intake was quite low on the day she recorded her food intake. She consumed 745 milligrams, but the Adequate Intake (AI) for a 20-year-old woman is 1,000 milligrams per day. If this day reflects her usual intake, then she is at risk of poor bone mineralization and lower than average peak bone mass. This increases her risk of osteoporosis.

Magnesium

Bobbie's intake of magnesium was 330 milligrams, and the Recommended Dietary Allowance (RDA) for a woman her age is 320 milligrams per day. If this one-day record reflects her usual eating, she is consuming an adequate amount of magnesium and does not need to increase her intake of this mineral. Some of the best sources of magnesium in her diet were the banana, pizza, and spaghetti noodles.

Sodium

Bobbie's intake of 4,659 milligrams of sodium was much higher than the recommended amount (2,400 mg) and close to the average American's intake. This should not be a surprise since most of Bobbie's meals are either convenience items or prepared by someone else (e.g., the school's cafeteria), which makes it hard to control sodium content. The biggest contributors to her high intake of sodium were the sourdough bread, turkey lunchmeat, pickle (on sandwich), salsa, spaghetti sauce, and pizza. Bobbie would benefit from drinking extra water since her intake of sodium is so high.

Iron

Most of Bobbie's iron intake came from enriched grains and red meat: The spaghetti noodles, bagel, meatballs, and pizza were the four iron sources in her diet. Overall, she consumed 20 milligrams of iron, compared with the RDA of 18 milligrams per day for women her age.

Zinc

Bobbie's best source of zinc is red meat—the meatballs she had on her spaghetti. Other zinc sources were the pizza, spaghetti noodles, and bagel. Remember that zinc is much better absorbed from meats than from grains. Bobbie's intake of 14 milligrams of zinc was higher than the RDA of 8 milligrams per day.

Selenium

Bobbie's best sources of selenium are grain products and meats. Again, the spaghetti noodles, bagel, and meatballs were among the top sources in her day. Turkey also contributed a significant amount. Bobbie's overall selenium intake of 126 micrograms was well above the RDA of 55 micrograms per day for adults.

References

1 Institute of Medicine, Food and Nutrition Board, Commission on Life Sciences, National Research Council. *Recommended Dietary Allowances.* 10th ed. Washington, DC: National Academy Press; 1989.

2 Johnson R, Tulin B. *Travel Fitness.* Champaign, IL: Human Kinetics; 1995.

3 Kleiner SM. Water: an essential but overlooked nutrient. *J Am Diet Assoc.* 1999;2:200–206.

4 Guyton AC, Hall JE. *Textbook of Medical Physiology.* 10th ed. Philadelphia: W.B. Saunders; 2000.

5 Kleiner SM. Op. cit.

6 Institute of Medicine, Food and Nutrition Board. *Dietary Reference Intakes for Calcium, Phosphorus, Magnesium, Vitamin D, and Fluoride.* Washington, DC: National Academy Press; 1997.

7 Zemel MB. Dietary pattern and hypertension: the DASH study. *Nutr Rev.* 1997;55:303–308.

8 Ibid.

9 Sacks FM, Svetkey LP, Vollmer WM, et al. Effects on blood pressure of reduced dietary sodium and the Dietary Approaches to Stop Hypertension (DASH) diet. *N Engl J Med.* 2001;344:3–10.

10 Ibid.

11 Appel LJ, Moore TJ, Obarzanek E, et al. A clinical trial of the effects of dietary patterns on blood pressure. DASH Collaborative Research Group. *N Engl J Med.* 1997;336: 1117–1124.

12 National Institutes of Health (NIH). *Osteoporosis Prevention, Diagnosis, and Therapy.* NIH Consensus Statement Online, March 27–29, 2000;17(1):1–36. http://consensus.nih.gov/cons/111/111_statement.htm#introduction. Accessed 4/27/02.

13 Ibid.

14 McArdle WD, Katch FI, Katch VL. *Essentials of Exercise Physiology.* Baltimore: Lippincott Williams & Wilkins; 1999.

15 New SA, Bolton-Smith C, Grubb DA, Reid DM. Nutritional influences on bone mineral density: a cross-sectional study in premenopausal women. *Am J Clin Nutr.* 1997;65(6):1831–1839.

16 US Department of Agriculture, US Department of Health and Human Services. *Nutrition and Your Health: Dietary Guidelines for Americans.* 5th ed. Washington, DC: US Government Printing Office; 2000. Home and Garden Bulletin 232.

17 Institute of Medicine, Food and Nutrition Board. 1989. Op. cit.

18 Loria CM, Obarzanek E, Ernst ND. Choose and prepare foods with less salt: dietary advice for all Americans. *J Nutr.* 2001;131(suppl 2, pt 1):536S–551S.

19 Morris CD. Effect of dietary sodium restriction on overall nutrient intake. *Am J Clin Nutr.* 1997;65(suppl 2):687S–691S.

20 Guyton AC, Hall JE. Op. cit.

21 Ibid.

22 Fauci AS, Braunwald E, Isselbacher KJ, et al. *Harrison's Principles of Internal Medicine.* 14th ed. New York: McGraw-Hill; 1997.

23 Guyton AC, Hall JE. Op. cit.

24 Waltzer KB. Simple, sensible preventive measures for managed care settings. *Geriatrics.* 1998;53(10):65–68, 75–77, 81; quiz 82.

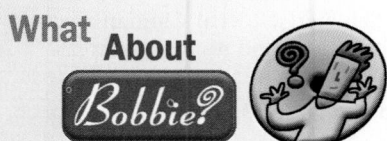

25 National Institutes of Health (NIH). *Optimal Calcium Intake.* NIH Consensus Statement, June 6–8, 1994; 12(4):1–31.

26 NIH. 2000. Op. cit.

27 Miller GD, Jarvis JK, McBean LD. The importance of meeting calcium needs with foods. *J Am Coll Nutr.* 2001;20(suppl 2): 168S–185S.

28 Institute of Medicine, Food and Nutrition Board. 1997. Op. cit.

29 NIH. 1994. Op. cit.

30 Institute of Medicine, Food and Nutrition Board. 1997. Op. cit.

31 NIH. 1994. Op. cit.

32 Institute of Medicine, Food and Nutrition Board. 1997. Op. cit.

33 Ibid.

34 Ibid.

35 Fauci AS, Braunwald E, Isselbacher KJ, et al. Op. cit.

36 Klevay LM, Milne DB. Low dietary magnesium increases supraventricular ectopy. *Am J Clin Nutr.* 2002;75(3):550–554.

37 Bothwell TH. Overview and mechanisms of iron regulation. *Nutr Rev.* 1995;53(9):237–245.

38 Oppenheimer SJ. Iron and its relation to immunity and infectious disease. *J Nutr.* 2001;131(suppl 2, pt 2):616S–633S; discussion 633S–635S.

39 Walter T, Olivares M, Pizarro F, Munoz C. Iron, anemia and infection. *Nutr Rev.* 1997;55(4):111–124.

40 Kretchmer N, Beard JL, Carlson S. The role of nutrition in the development of normal cognition. *Am J Clin Nutr.* 1996;63:997S–1001S.

41 De Andraca I, Castillo M, Walter T. Psychomotor development and behavior in iron-deficient anemic infants. *Nutr Rev.* 1997;55(4):125–132.

42 Recommendations to report and control iron deficiency in the United States. *MMWR.* 1998;7(RR-3).

43 Bothwell TH. Op cit.

44 Institute of Medicine, Food and Nutrition Board. *Dietary Reference Intakes for Vitamin A, Vitamin K, Arsenic, Boron, Chromium, Copper, Iodine, Iron, Manganese, Molybdenum, Nickel, Silicon, Vanadium, and Zinc.* Washington, DC: National Academy Press; 2001.

45 Minihane AM, Fairweather-Tait SJ. Effect of calcium supplementation on daily nonheme-iron absorption and long-term iron status. *Am J Clin Nutr.* 1998;68:96–102.

46 Institute of Medicine, Food and Nutrition Board. 2001. Op. cit.

47 Ibid.

48 Preventing iron poisoning in children. *FDA Backgrounder.* January 15, 1997.

49 Bulaj ZJ, Ajioka RS, Phillips JD, et al. Disease-related conditions in relatives of patients with hemochromatosis. *N Engl J Med.* 2000;343:1529–1535.

50 Prasad AS, Helstead JA, Nadami M. Syndrome of iron deficiency anaemia, hepatosplenomegaly, hypogonadism, dwarfism and geophagia. *Am J Med.* 1961;31:532–546.

51 Sandstead HH, Prasad AS, Schubert AR, et al. Human zinc deficiency endocrine manifestations and response to treatment. *Am J Clin Nutr.* 1967;20:422–442.

52 Institute of Medicine, Food and Nutrition Board. 2001. Op. cit.

53 Dibley MJ. Zinc. In: Bowman BA, Russell RM, eds. *Present Knowledge in Nutrition.* 8th ed. Washington, DC: ILSI Press; 2001.

54 Gibson RS. Content and bioavailability of trace elements in vegetarian diets. *Am J Clin Nutr.* 1994;59(suppl):1223–1232.

55 Krebs NF. Overview of zinc absorption and excretion in the human gastrointestinal tract. *J Nutr.* 2000;130:1374S–1377S.

56 Lonnerdal B. Dietary factors influencing zinc absorption. *J Nutr.* 2000;130:1378S–1383S.

57 Institute of Medicine, Food and Nutrition Board. 2001. Op. cit.

58 Tamura T, Goldenberg RL. Zinc nutriture and pregnancy outcome. *Nutr Res.* 1996;16:139–181.

59 Bogden JD, Oleske JM, Lavenhar MA, et al. Effects of one year of supplementation with zinc and other micronutrients on cellular immunity in the elderly. *J Am Coll Nutr.* 1990;9:214–225.

60 Hoogenraad T, Van den Hamer C, van Hattum J. Effective treatment of Wilson's disease with oral zinc sulphate: two case reports. *Br Med J.* 1984;289:273–276.

61 Institute of Medicine, Food and Nutrition Board. *Dietary Reference Intakes for Vitamin C, Vitamin E, Selenium, and Beta-Carotene, and other Carotenoids.* Washington, DC: National Academy Press; 2000.

62 Ibid.

63 Combs GF Jr. Selenium in global food systems. *B Jr Nutr.* 2001;85:517–547.

64 Hetzel BS. *The Story of Iodine Deficiency: An International Challenge in Nutrition.* Oxford: Oxford University Press; 1989.

65 World Health Organization sets out to eliminate iodine deficiency disorder. WHO press release; May 25, 1999.

66 Institute of Medicine, Food and Nutrition Board. 2001. Op. cit.

67 Bautista A. Effects of oral iodized salt on intelligence, thyroid status, and somatic growth in school-aged children from an area with endemic goiter. *Am J Clin Nutr.* 1982;35:127–134.

68 Kaler SG. Diagnosis and therapy of Menkes' syndrome, a genetic form of copper deficiency. *Am J Clin Nutr.* 1998;67(suppl):1029S–1034S.

69 Greger JL. Dietary standards for manganese: overlap between nutritional and toxicological studies. *J Nutr.* 1998;128: 368S–371S.

70 Fluoride for treating osteoporosis. *Cochrane Database Syst Rev.* 2000;(4):DC002825.

71 Institute of Medicine, Food and Nutrition Board. 1997. Op. cit.

72 Fluoridation of drinking water to prevent dental caries. *MMWR.* October 22, 1999.

73 Position of the American Dietetic Association: the impact of fluoride on health. *J Am Diet Assoc.* 2001;101:126–132.

74 Simko LC. Water fluoridation: time to reexamine the issue. *Pediatr Nurs.* 1997;23(2):155–159.

75 DePaola DP, Faine MP, Palmer CA. Nutrition in relation to dental medicine. In: Shils ME, Olson JA, Shike M, Ross AC, eds. *Modern Nutrition in Health and Disease.* 9th ed. Philadelphia: Lippincott Williams & Wilkins, 1999.

76 McDonagh MS, Whiting PF, Wilson PM, et al. Systematic review of water fluoridation. *BMJ.* 2000;321:855–859; and Padilla O, Davis MJ. Fluorides in the new millennium. *NY State Dent J.* 2001;67:34–38.

77 Davis S, McLaren HJ, Hunnisett A, Howard M. Age-related decreases in chromium levels in 51,665 hair, sweat, and serum samples from 40,872 patients: implications for the prevention of cardiovascular disease and type II diabetes mellitus. *Metabolism.* 1997;46:469–473.

78 Anderson RA. Effects of chromium on body composition and weight loss. *Nutr Rev.* 1998;56(9):266–270.

79 Nielsen FH. Ultratrace minerals. In: Shils ME, Olson JA, Shike M, Ross AC, eds. *Modern Nutrition in Health and Disease.* 9th ed. Philadelphia: Lippincott Williams & Wilkins; 1999.

80 Ibid.

81 Uthus EO, Seaborn CD. Deliberations and evaluations of the approaches, endpoints, and paradigms for dietary recommendations of the other trace elements. *J Nutr.* 1996;126:2452S–2459S.

82 Kelsay JL, Behall KM, Prather E. Effect of fiber from fruits and vegetables on metabolic responses in human subjects. II: Calcium, magnesium, iron, and silicon balances. *Am J Clin Nutr.* 1979;32:1876–1880.

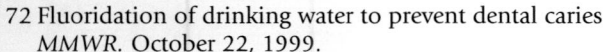

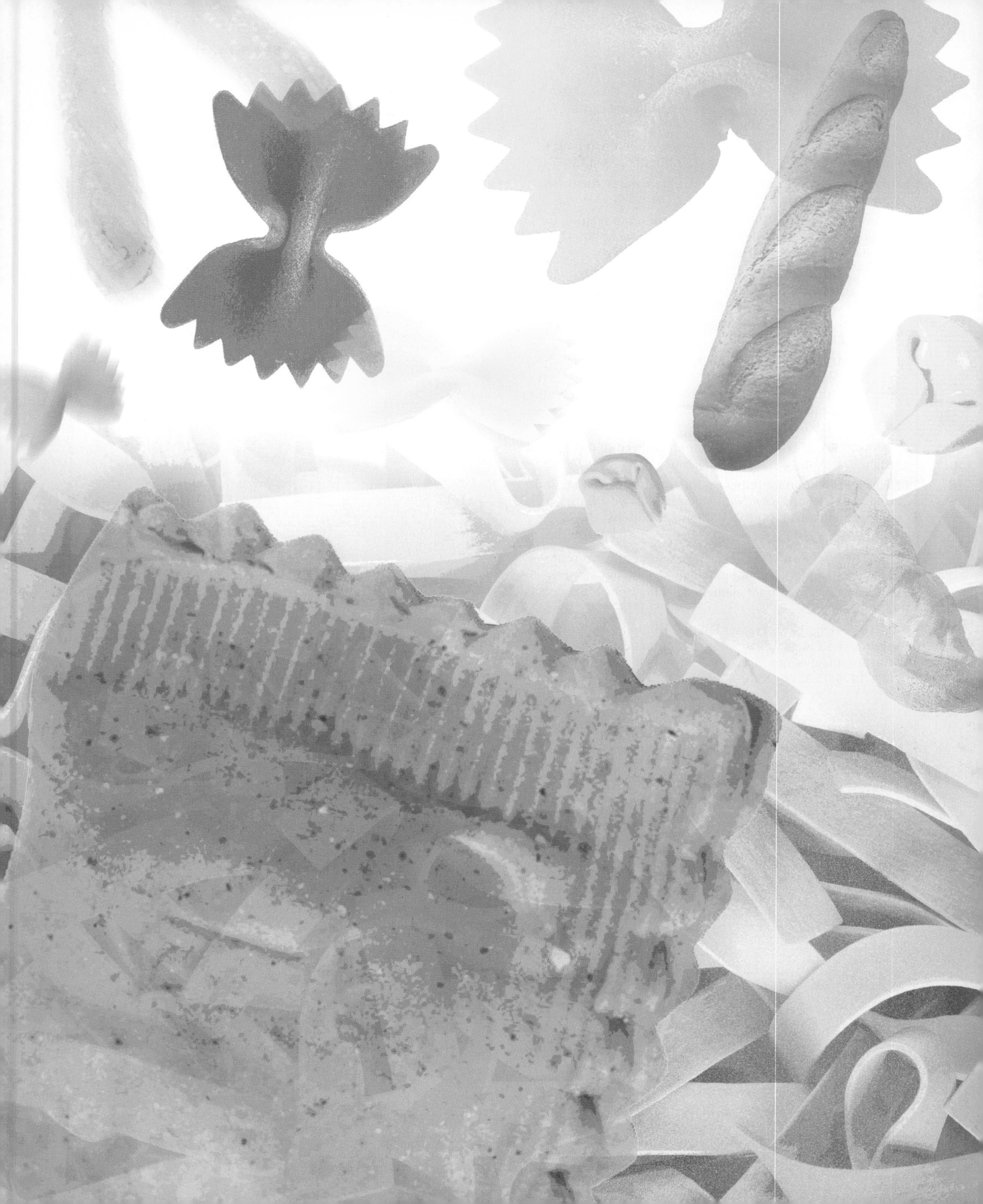

Chapter 11

Sports Nutrition: Eating for Peak Performance

Think About It

1. How much importance do you place on being physically active?
2. How often do you suffer from muscle fatigue? What do you think causes it?
3. How often do you think about food choices when you're planning a physical activity?
4. What kind of protein do you emphasize in your diet?

Fyi for your Information

This chapter's FYI boxes include practical information on the following topics:

- Lactate Is Not a Metabolic Dead End
- To Zone or Not to Zone? That Is the Question

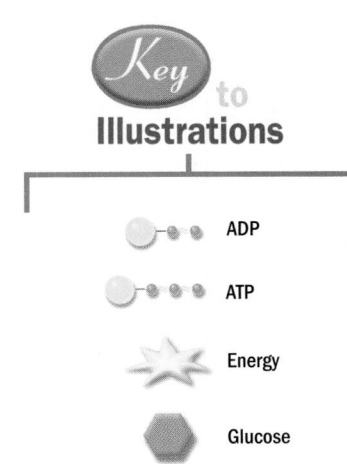

Key to Illustrations

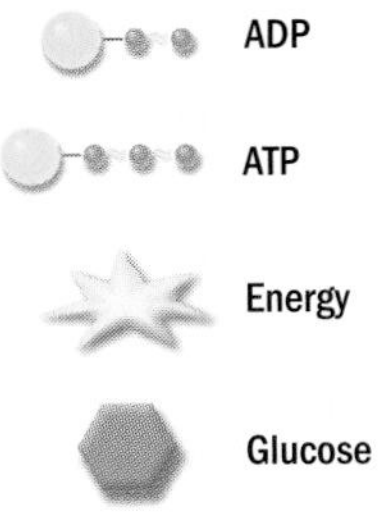

WWW

The Web site for this book offers many useful tools and is a great source for additional nutrition information for both students and instructors. For information on sports nutrition, visit the site at **nutrition.jbpub.com/discovering**. You'll find exercises that explore the following topics:

- Effective Training
- Sports Nutrition from a Sports Drink Company
- The EatRight Web Page of the ADA and CDA
- Scan SCAN

What About Bobbie?

Track the choices Bobbie is making with the EatRight Analysis software.

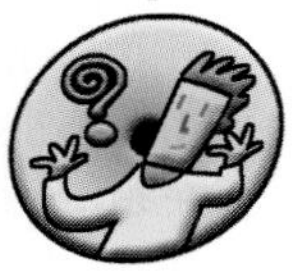

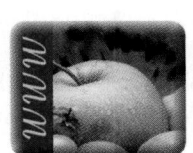

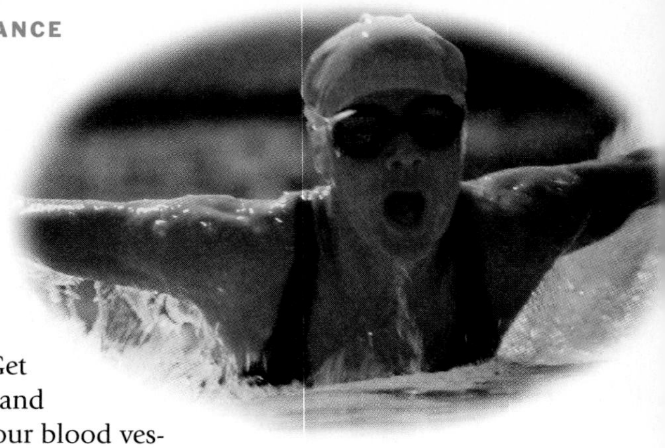

Today is the big 10,000-meter race. You've been training for months. The people in the crowd shade their eyes as they watch you and your competitors walk onto the track. "Ready," shouts the starter. "Get set." You toe the starting line and adrenaline courses through your blood vessels, increasing your heart rate, diverting blood to your muscles, and mobilizing energy stores in your liver, muscles, and fat. "Go!" Within a fraction of a second, a torrent of calcium flows into your muscle cells, causing your muscles to contract and launch you away from the starting line.

How do you expect to perform in this race? Will your breakfast help or hinder your performance? Will what you ate yesterday and the day before have any effect? Does it matter what you eat after you finish the race? Read on for the answers to these questions and learn about the links between nutrition and sports performance.

Nutrition and Physical Performance

Just how physically active do you need to be? (See **Figure 11.1**.) Both the National Institutes of Health (NIH) and Health Canada have found that just small to moderate amounts of physical activity can produce substantial health benefits. Physically active people have a lower risk of developing many chronic diseases, such as coronary heart disease, diabetes, hypertension, osteoporosis, and obesity. Active people also experience an increased sense of well-being and are much better equipped to cope with stress. Health Canada recommends choosing a variety of activities from three types of exercise: endurance, flexibility, and strength. (See **Figure 11.2**.) See Appendix C for *Canada's Physical Activity Guide to Healthy Active Living*.

Think About It 1

The American College of Sports Medicine (ACSM) notes an important distinction between physical activity as it relates to health and exercise for physical fitness.[1] According to the ACSM, the level of physical activity that may reduce the risk of various chronic diseases may not be enough—in quantity or quality—to improve physical fitness.

What is physical fitness? Measures of fitness may include such factors as strength, endurance, flexibility, and breathing capacity. The ACSM defines physical fitness as "the ability to perform moderate to vigorous levels of physical activity without undue fatigue and the capability of maintaining this level of activity throughout life."[2] **Table 11.1** shows guidelines for levels of physical activity to promote health and to achieve and maintain fitness.

Nutrition has taken its rightful place as a vital component of any program that seeks to enhance health, fitness, and athletic performance. In a joint position paper, the American Dietetic Association, Dietitians of Canada, and the American College of Sports Medicine state that "physical activity, athletic performance, and recovery from exercise are enhanced by optimal nutrition."[3] But just what is "optimal nutrition"? Is it the same for a child who plays recreational softball and for a senior citizen who takes daily walks to reduce the risk of type 2 diabetes? What about the competitive athlete who strives to maximize athletic performance and uses nutrition to gain a competitive edge? To understand the relationship between

Table 11.1 Guidelines for Physical Activity: Health and Fitness

Guidelines for Promoting Health

Frequency: daily activity
Intensity: any level of intensity
Duration: accumulation of a minimum of 30 minutes of total daily activity
Mode: any activity

Guidelines for Achieving and Maintaining Physical Fitness

Frequency: 3 to 5 days a week
Intensity: 50 to 90 percent of maximum heart rate
Duration: 20 to 60 minutes of continuous or intermittent aerobic activity (minimum of 10-minute bouts accumulated during the day)
Mode: activity using large muscle groups maintained continuously in a rhythmic and aerobic manner
Resistance training: minimum of 2 days a week to enhance strength and muscular endurance, and maintain fat-free mass
Flexibility training: minimum of 2 days a week, incorporated into overall fitness program to develop and maintain range of motion

Source: American College of Sports Medicine. Position stand: the recommended quantity and quality of exercise for developing and maintaining cardiorespiratory and muscular fitness and flexibility in healthy adults. *Med Sci Sports Exerc.* 1998;30:975–991.

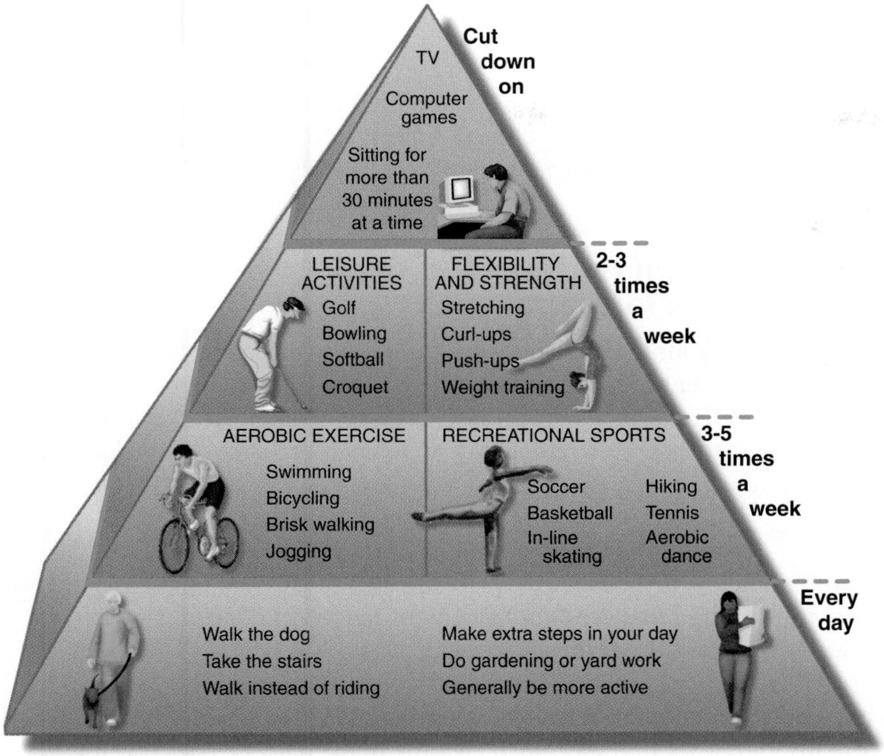

Figure 11.1 **The Physical Activity Pyramid.** Perhaps the most important aspect of increasing physical activity is to have fun.

Source: Adapted from Corbin CB, Pangrazi RD. Physical activity pyramid rebuffs peak experience. *ACSM's Health and Fitness Journal.* 1998;2(1):12–17.

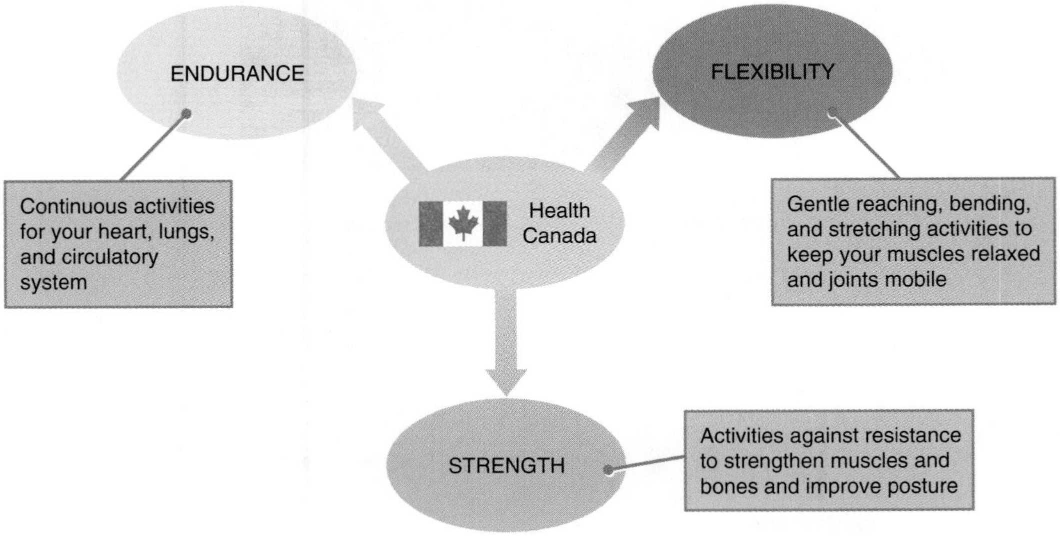

Figure 11.2 **Variety is the spice of life.** Health Canada recommends that you do a variety of activities from each group—endurance, flexibility, and strength—to receive the most health benefits.
Source: Adapted from *Canada's Physical Activity Guide to Healthy Active Living.*

physical activity and nutrition, you first need to appreciate how we use energy during exercise.

Key Concepts: *Exercise provides numerous health benefits, including reduced risk of chronic disease. Physical fitness includes strength, endurance, and flexibility. For optimal physical performance, nutrition is an essential part of all athletic training programs.*

Energy Systems, Muscles, and Physical Performance

Let's return to your race. As you leave the starting line, your body immediately ramps up energy production to meet the increased demand. Just as a rocket uses different fuel systems and stages to power its leap into space, your body uses three different energy systems to fuel launch, acceleration, and endurance.

ATP–CP Energy System

As you launch yourself from the starting line, it takes less than a second for your contracting muscles to burn their entire reserve of adenosine triphosphate (ATP), the immediate energy source for cells. Luckily, your body has a small reservoir of **creatine phosphate** (also called **phosphocreatine**) that your muscles can convert quickly to ATP. (See **Figure 11.3**.) Muscle cells contain four to six times as much creatine phosphate as ATP.[4] Together, your available ATP and creatine phosphate, the **ATP–CP energy system**, can power an all-out effort for only 3 to 15 seconds.[5] To continue the race, you must enlist carbohydrate stored as glycogen in your muscles and liver. Your cells rapidly disassemble glycogen to glucose, from which they can extract ATP.

Quick Bites

The First Sports Trainers

During the time of the ancient Olympic games, sports trainers demanded that their athletes follow strict training regimens: 10 months of regulated diet, bathing, exercise, rest, and massage. Until 480 B.C.E., Olympic athletes consumed a mostly vegetarian diet of cheese, porridge, figs, wine, and meal cakes. After twice winning the Olympic long race, however, Dromeus of Stymphalus revolutionized the ancient training diet by advocating mammoth amounts of meat and exercise.

creatine phosphate An energy-rich compound that supplies energy and a phosphate group for the formation of ATP. Also called phosphocreatine.

phosphocreatine See *creatine phosphate.*

ATP–CP energy system A simple and immediate anaerobic energy system that maintains ATP levels. Creatine phosphate is broken down, releasing energy and a phosphate group, which is used to form ATP.

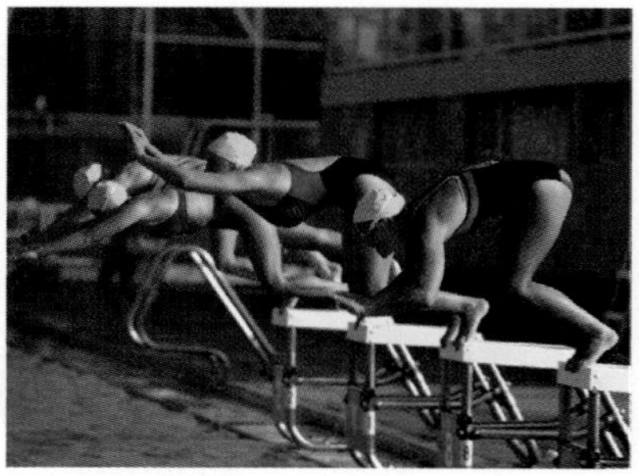

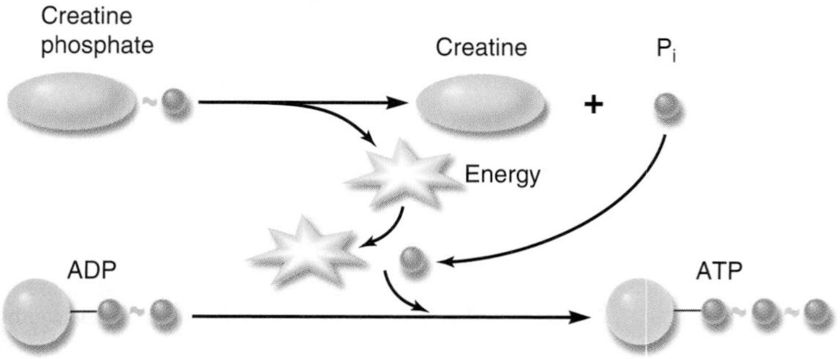

Figure 11.3 **ATP–CP energy system.** To maintain relatively constant ATP levels during an initial explosive burst of high-intensity activity, your body uses its ATP–CP energy system to generate ATP from creatine phosphate.

Lactic Acid Energy System

For the next minute or two, the acceleration stage, your body uses the simplest and speediest chemical pathways to produce ATP from glucose—the **lactic acid energy system**. (See **Figure 11.4**.) Like the ATP–CP energy system, these pathways are anaerobic—they do not require oxygen. The raw material, glucose, is much more plentiful than creatine phosphate, but its breakdown also produces a byproduct—lactate (lactic acid). Lactic acid pours into the bloodstream and begins to accumulate, making cells more acidic. A rise in acidity impairs the breakdown of glucose and inhibits calcium binding. Without calcium, muscles cannot contract. For years, coaches and athletes have blamed lactic acid for muscle fatigue. But it's the change in pH, rather than the lactic acid substance itself, that is the primary culprit.[6]

Think About It 2

To continue running beyond the first few minutes, your body employs a sophisticated, oxygen-based system to process lactic acid and squeeze out much more ATP from glucose.

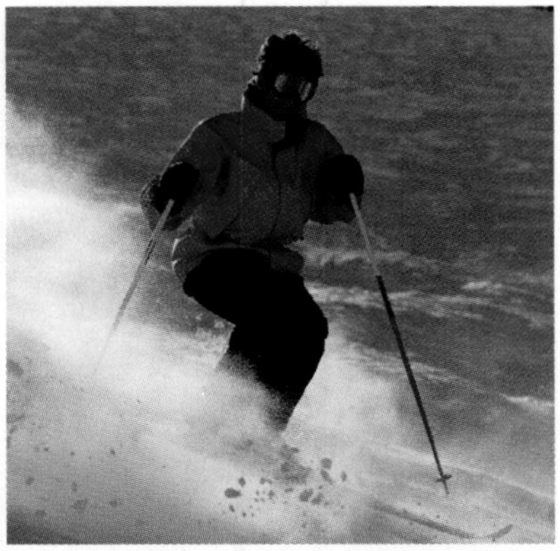

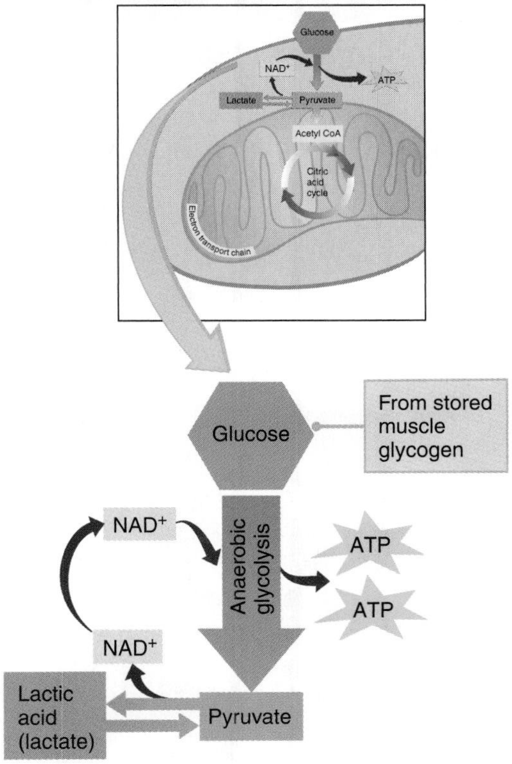

Figure 11.4 **Lactic acid energy system.** During short events requiring power and speed, the lactic acid energy system supplies much of the energy. Because the lactic acid system does not require oxygen, these events are anaerobic activities.

Oxygen Energy System

For the endurance stage, cells can use lengthy, complex chemical pathways in their mitochondria—small units within cells that function as power-generating plants—to convert food and oxygen to ATP. (See **Figure 11.5**.) These reactions are aerobic—they require abundant oxygen. In contracting muscle, blood vessels dilate and deliver a 20-fold increase in oxygen-rich blood to muscle cells,[7] a sufficient supply for mitochondria to produce ATP. In contrast to the two anaerobic systems (ATP–CP system and lactic acid system), the **oxygen energy system** can produce a tremendous amount of ATP. Another advantage is that the oxygen energy system can extract energy from fat as well as glucose. But since the required oxygen must travel a long distance—from lungs to blood to muscle cells to mitochondria—the oxygen energy system produces ATP at a much slower rate than the anaerobic systems do.

Teamwork in Energy Production

The anaerobic and aerobic energy systems work together to fuel athletic performance. (See **Figure 11.6**.) As the first two minutes of your race elapse, the oxygen energy system is supplying about half of your muscles' energy needs. (See **Figure 11.7**.) By the time you pass the 30-minute mark, this aerobic system is supplying 95 percent; and at two hours or more, the oxygen energy system is supplying 98 percent of your muscles' energy needs.[8] As long as ATP production by the mitochondria meets energy needs, you are exercising aerobically; highly trained athletes can sustain such exercise for hours. If the exercise rate exceeds your body's ability to supply oxygen to your muscles, you are exercising anaerobically, rapidly depleting your creatine phosphate and glycogen reserves. Once these are exhausted, if available oxygen cannot support the oxygen energy system, performance plummets.

Carbohydrate stores are limited. A 68-kilogram (150-pound) man with 10 to 20 percent body fat, for example, has carbohydrate stores of 1,800 to 2,000 kilocalories in muscle glycogen, liver glycogen, and blood glucose. Compare this with the energy he stores in fat. His fat tissue holds roughly 63,000 to 120,000 kilocalories.[9] While the body can burn protein for energy, in well-fed people protein probably provides no more than 5 percent of energy expended in exercise.[10]

lactic acid energy system Anaerobic energy system; using glycolysis, it rapidly produces energy (ATP) and lactate. Also called anaerobic glycolysis.

oxygen energy system A complex energy system that requires oxygen. To release ATP, it completes the breakdown of carbohydrate and fatty acids via the citric acid cycle and electron transport chain.

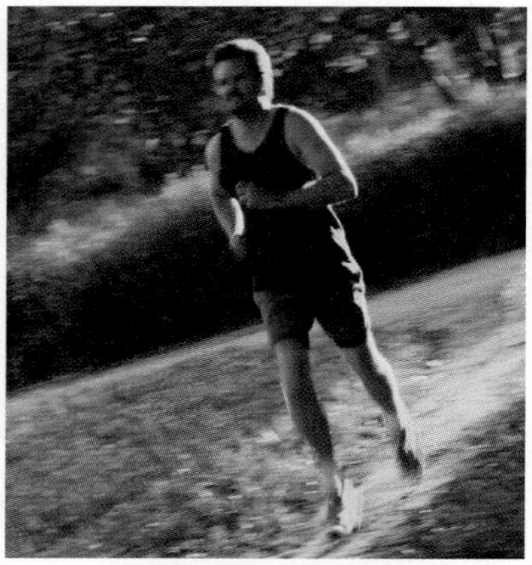

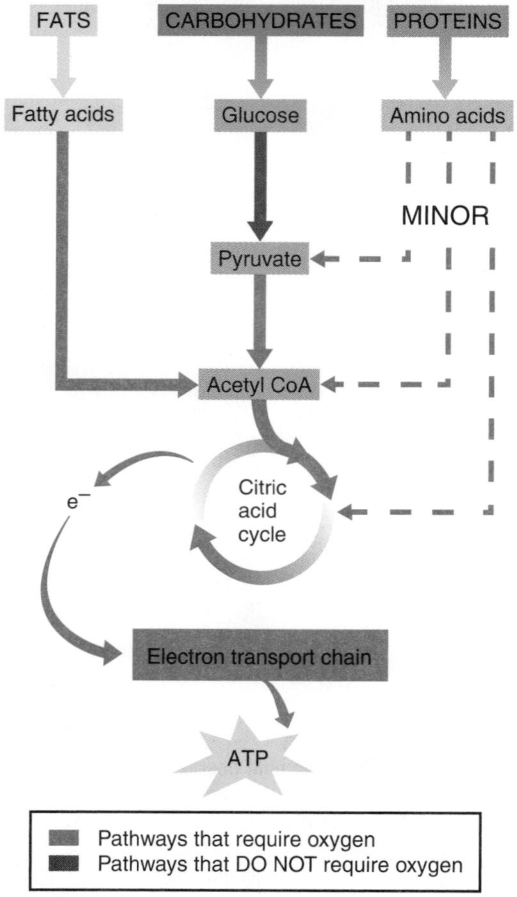

Figure 11.5 **Oxygen energy system.** During longer endurance events (aerobic events), the oxygen energy system supplies most of the energy. This energy system requires oxygen and primarily relies on carbohydrate and fat as fuels.

Glycogen Depletion

At the beginning of the race, your body rapidly uses muscle glycogen. But as the race grinds on, the rate of glycogen use markedly slows. During the first 1.5 hours, glycogen stores drop steadily to about one-third their starting levels. About 3 hours into the run, as glycogen stores are almost entirely depleted, you may "hit the wall." Your muscles become weak and heavy, your legs shake, and you become confused. Marathon runners commonly experience a sudden onset of exhaustive fatigue around the 18- to 20-mile mark. Drinking fluids that contain glucose can partially compensate for glycogen depletion and soften its effects. Dehydration can cause an even faster onset of fatigue, so drinking plenty of fluids is essential during endurance events.

As exercise intensity increases, glycogen depletion accelerates. Sprinting, for example, uses muscle glycogen 35 to 40 times faster than walking.[11] **Figure 11.8** illustrates how the sensation of fatigue relates to the depletion of muscle glycogen.

Training

Training builds endurance—as much as 500 percent in untrained people.[12] To increase endurance, training enhances aerobic capacity by increasing the number of mitochondria and improving the body's ability to deliver oxygen to them. This decreases the reliance on anaerobic energy systems, extending the availability of glycogen reserves and delaying fatigue.

Key Concepts: *Muscle cells use three different energy systems to produce ATP: the ATP–CP energy system, the lactic acid energy system, and the oxygen energy system. The ATP–CP and lactic acid energy systems rely on carbohydrate and do not require oxygen. The oxygen energy system requires oxygen and relies on carbohydrates and fats. During the early minutes of high-intensity exercise, the anaerobic*

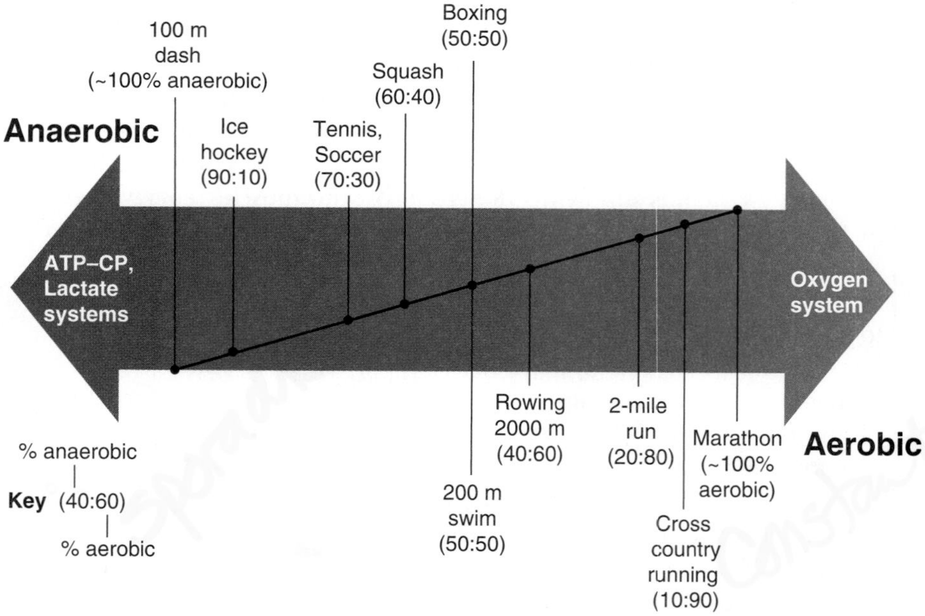

Figure 11.6 **The anaerobic–aerobic continuum.** Most activities use ATP from both anaerobic and aerobic energy systems. However, the 100-meter dash is considered completely anaerobic, and the marathon is considered completely aerobic.

creatine phosphate + ADP + H^+ $\leftrightarrow$ ATP + creatine

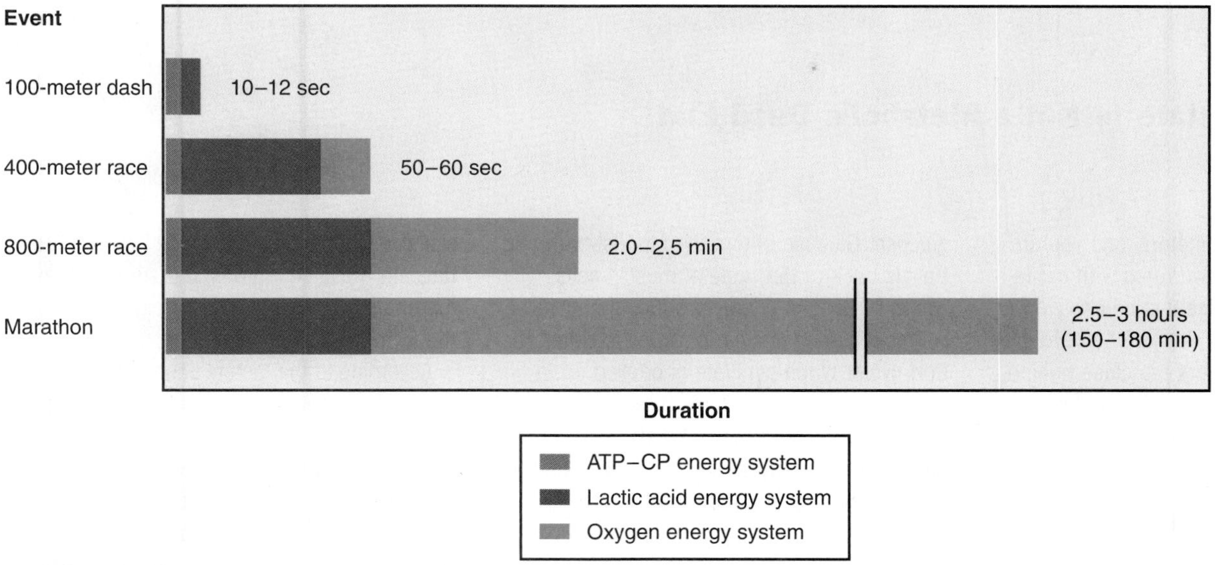

Figure 11.7 **Sports events and energy systems.** Short-term, explosive events rely upon the ATP–CP and lactic acid energy systems. For longer events, your body turns to the oxygen energy system. During endurance events, your body uses this system to burn fat as well as glucose.

systems are the predominant source of ATP. During lower-intensity endurance events, the third system supplies ATP, although at a much slower rate. Dehydration and depletion of glycogen stores are major factors in fatigue. Training increases the efficiency of oxygen delivery to muscle and increases the number of muscle mitochondria available for aerobic metabolism.

skeletal muscles Muscles composed of bundles of parallel, striated muscle fibers under voluntary control. Also called voluntary muscle or striated muscle.

Muscles and Muscle Fibers

Your body contains hundreds of muscles that help control a myriad of functions, from regulating blood pressure to climbing stairs. **Skeletal muscles** are bundles of parallel, striated fibers attached to your skeleton.

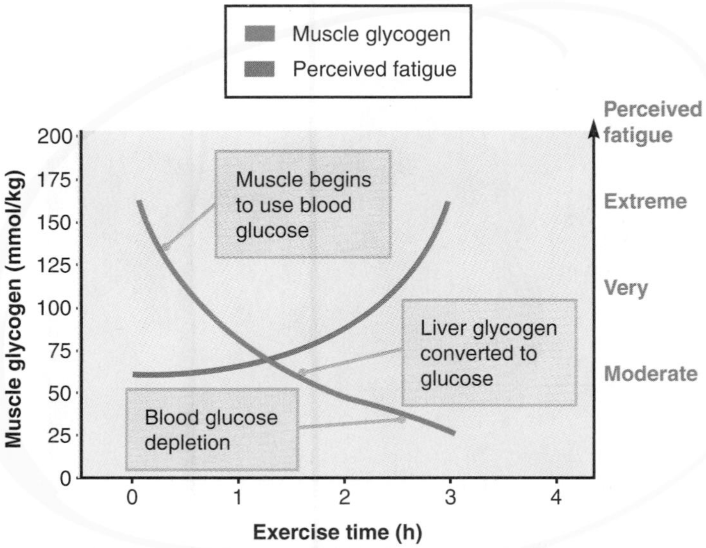

Figure 11.8 **Glycogen depletion and the sensation of fatigue.** As muscle glycogen levels decline, fatigue and eventually exhaustion set in.

Quick Bites

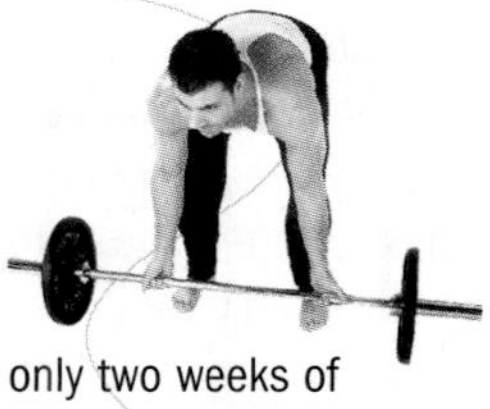

Use It or Lose It!

The benefits of training begin to disappear after only two weeks of inactivity. Muscular endurance (the ability of a muscle to avoid fatigue) declines, and activities of certain oxidative enzymes drop by as much as 40 percent. By the fourth week, muscle glycogen levels also may drop by 40 percent. Flexibility is quickly lost, and inactivity can substantially decondition the heart muscle and cardiovascular system.

Fyi Lactate Is Not a Metabolic Dead End

FOR YOUR INFORMATION

Today's race is 200 meters, and you are in the lead. The crowd roars with excitement and your coach screams hoarsely as your feet slam over and over on the hard gray cinder track. Other runners are close behind, and you can feel them breathing and pounding at your heels. Air whistles in and out of your wheezing lungs as you doggedly push to stay ahead. Your muscles are screaming, but they carry you across the finish line. A winner!

As you slump in exhaustion, you wonder how your limp muscles carried you through to the end. Each leg seemed to weigh a thousand pounds. As your muscles tire, lactate levels rise and the pH in your muscle cells drops. Scientists, coaches, and athletes have long believed that lactate was a useless, even toxic, dead-end substance. Recent research proves otherwise. It is the overall acidification of the muscle tissue, rather than a buildup of lactate, that primarily causes muscle fatigue. Also, lactate is now recognized as a fuel in its own right. In addition to acting as a metabolic shunt, lactate is a useful fuel produced and consumed under all conditions of oxygen availability, while exercising or at rest.

Without the energy supplied by the lactic acid energy system, you would never have crossed the finish line. While your body anaerobically burned muscle glycogen, it produced large amounts of lactate. Where does this lactate come from, and how does your body handle it?

Cori Cycle

During vigorous exercise, your contracting muscle cells quickly extract small amounts of ATP from glucose. This simple pathway, called glycolysis, splits glucose into pyruvate molecules faster than the oxygen energy system can accept them for further processing. Cells divert excess pyruvate to lactate to help alleviate the backup.

Lactate easily diffuses through muscle cell membranes into the bloodstream. The liver picks up the circulating lactate and converts it back to pyruvate. Using energy-demanding reactions, the liver transforms pyruvate to glucose. Glucose enters the bloodstream and travels back to the skeletal muscle cells, where it reenters energy-producing pathways.

This recurring circular pathway is called the *Cori cycle.* When pyruvate is backed up in muscle cells, the Cori cycle buys time with a detour through the liver. When oxygen becomes readily available, the oxygen energy system becomes the main pathway.

Lactate Shuttle

The pathways of the Cori cycle are an important, but incomplete, part of the lactate picture. The use of the Cori cycle as a holding pattern led to the mistaken belief that lactate was simply a metabolic dead end. Recent studies describe a more extensive role for this long-maligned substance.

Researchers now recognize lactate as an important means of distributing carbohydrate energy sources after a meal and during sustained physical exercise. Lactate's advantage is its ability to move rapidly between cells. It is a small molecule and, unlike glucose, does not need insulin to cross a cell membrane.

Under resting conditions of plentiful carbohydrate and oxygen, diverse tissues such as skeletal muscle, liver, and skin produce lactate.[1] In these conditions, the supply of raw materials, rather than limited oxygen, drives the formation of lactate.

According to the lactate shuttle hypothesis, lactate formed in muscle cells becomes an energy source at other sites, either adjacent or remote. Skeletal muscle, once thought simply to produce lactate, also directly uses lactate as a fuel. At times, skeletal muscle actually removes more lactate than it produces. The heart muscle is fully aerobic, but it both produces and consumes lactate. Studies suggest that during exercise lactate is the major fuel for the heart and the preferred fuel for certain muscle fibers.[2]

The next time you complain about sore, tired muscles, don't blame lactate. Instead, think about the daily usefulness of lactate and how this little-respected substance helped power you to the finish.

1 Brooks GA. Mammalian fuel utilization during sustained exercise. *Comp Biochem Physiol.* 1998;120:89–107.

2 Myers J, Ashley E. Dangerous curves: a perspective on exercise, lactate, and the anaerobic threshold. *Chest.* 1997;111:787–795.

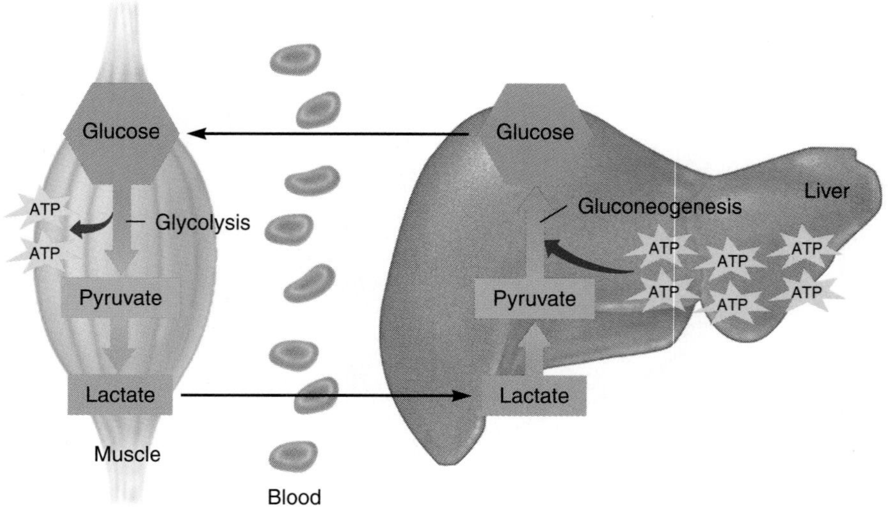

The Cori cycle. The Cori cycle shifts some of the metabolic burden of contracting muscle to the liver. Lactate formed in contracting muscle travels to the liver, which uses it to form glucose. This glucose returns to the muscle to fuel further contractions.

(See **Figure 11.9**.) These muscles are responsible for your physical movement and are under your conscious control. If you decide to bend your arm, for example, you consciously contract your biceps. Your body contains more than 600 skeletal muscles and uses 9 of them just to control your thumb!

Individual muscle cells are called **muscle fibers**; skeletal muscle has two primary types:

- **slow-twitch (ST) fibers**
- **fast-twitch (FT) fibers**

They derive their names from the difference in their speed of action. One type of fast-twitch fiber can contract 10 times faster than slow-twitch fibers.[13]

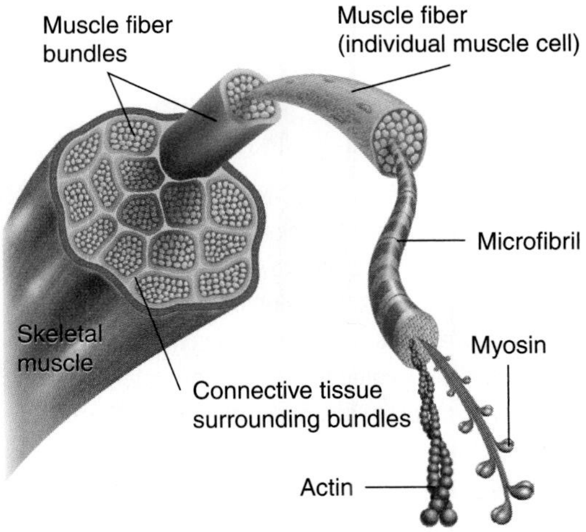

Figure 11.9 **Basic structure of skeletal muscle.** A muscle fiber is an individual muscle cell that usually extends the entire length of the muscle. Each muscle fiber contains hundreds to thousands of microfibrils. Each microfibril contains thousands of actin and myosin filaments, large protein molecules responsible for muscle contractions.

Slow-Twitch Fibers

To power their activity, slow-twitch fibers efficiently produce energy by breaking down carbohydrate and fat via aerobic pathways—metabolic reactions that require oxygen. As long as the aerobic pathways are active, ST fibers can produce energy to sustain their movement. With a sufficient supply of oxygen, ST fibers can maintain muscular activity for a prolonged time. This ability is known as **aerobic endurance**.

Because ST fibers have high aerobic endurance, your body predominantly relies on them during low-intensity endurance events, such as a marathon, and during everyday activities, such as walking.

Quick Bites

Pound for Pound?

Women's muscles have smaller muscle fiber cross-sections and less muscle mass than men. For a given amount of muscle, however, there is no difference in strength between men and women.

Fast-Twitch Fibers

Compared with ST fibers, fast-twitch fibers have poor aerobic endurance. They are optimized to perform anaerobically (when the oxygen supply is limited). FT fibers can efficiently produce energy for their use via metabolic pathways that do not require oxygen. Bundles of FT fibers exert considerably more force than bundles of ST fibers; but due to their limited endurance, FT fibers tire quickly.

The body recruits both ST and FT fibers during shorter, higher-intensity endurance events, such as the mile run or the 400-meter swim. During highly explosive events such as the 100-meter dash and the 50-meter sprint swim, the body relies mainly on FT fibers.

Fiber Type and the Athlete

Genes determine the relative proportion of muscle fiber types in athletes. Although distance runners who have a high percentage of ST fibers are well suited for endurance events, they will not succeed as elite sprinters. Conversely, sprinters who have predominantly FT fibers are better equipped for explosive events, but they will not become competitive marathon runners. (See **Figure 11.10**.)

Key Concepts: *A muscle cell is called a muscle fiber. The two main types of skeletal muscle fibers are slow-twitch and fast-twitch fibers. Slow-twitch fibers generate fuel through aerobic pathways, whereas fast-twitch fibers produce energy using anaerobic pathways. Fast-twitch fibers can exert more force, but have limited endurance.*

muscle fibers Individual muscle cells.

slow-twitch (ST) fibers Muscle fibers that develop tension more slowly and to a lesser extent than fast-twitch muscle fibers. ST fibers have high oxidative capacities and are slower to fatigue than fast-twitch fibers.

fast-twitch (FT) fibers Muscle fibers that can develop high tension rapidly. These fibers can fatigue quickly, but are well suited to explosive movements in sprinting, jumping, and weight lifting.

aerobic endurance The ability of skeletal muscle to obtain a sufficient supply of oxygen from the heart and lungs to maintain muscular activity for a prolonged time.

Quick Bites

Why Is Fish Meat White?

A large percentage (40 to 60 percent) of a fish's body weight is muscle tissue. Although it spends much of its life slowly cruising, a fish must be able to execute occasional quick bursts of high speed to escape predators or catch a meal. Thus, fish muscle is composed of approximately 75 to 90 percent fast-twitch fibers and fish flesh often is white. The slow-twitch fibers generally are concentrated just under the skin or near fins that are used during slow or high speeds. This arrangement is possible only because fish are buoyant. Land animals could not survive dragging around a large mass of muscle that they used only occasionally in extreme situations.

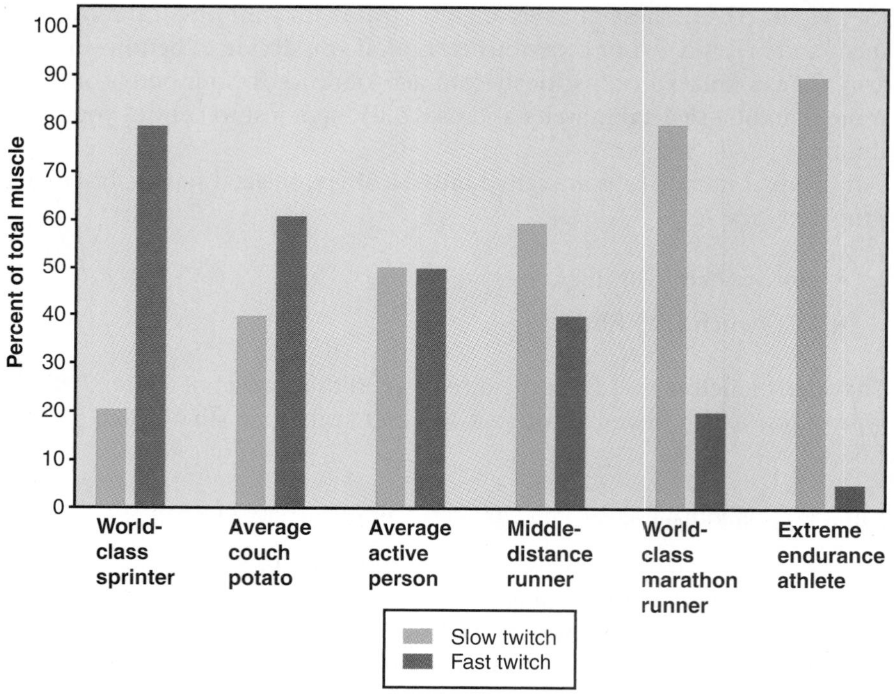

Figure 11.10 **What's your mix of muscle fibers?** If you are best at events requiring explosive movements, you may have a greater percentage of fast-twitch muscle fibers. If endurance events are your specialty, you may have more slow-twitch fibers.
Source: Adapted from Andersen JL, Scherling P, Saltin B. Muscle, genes and athletic performance. *Scientific American.* 2000;283(3):49.

Quick Bites

The Weaker Sex?

Prior to the 1960s, women were banned from running any race longer than 800 meters, and they could not officially participate in marathon competitions until 1970. The race authorities mistakenly believed that women could harm themselves and were unsuitable for distance running. Imagine their amazement during the 1984 Olympic Games when Joan Benoit won the gold medal for the women's marathon with a time of 02:24:52—a time that would have won 11 of the previous 20 men's Olympic marathons!

Optimal Nutrition for Athletic Performance

The optimal diet for most physically active people—from the college student who plays intramural basketball to the 50-year-old woman who enjoys walking during her lunch break—includes a variety of nutrient-dense foods from the Food Guide Pyramid. (See Chapter 2, "Nutrition Guidelines.") Food choices should be high in carbohydrate (more than 60 percent of calories), low in fat (less than 30 percent of calories), and moderate in protein. When energy needs are met by eating a variety of foods from each of the food groups, micronutrient (vitamins and minerals) needs are met as well.

Think About It 3

Optimal nutrition is an essential part of every athlete's training program and can make a difference when winning is measured in fractions of seconds or inches. General recommendations for competitive athletes include the following:[14]

- Consume adequate energy (calories) and nutrients to support health and performance.
- Maintain appropriate sports-specific ranges for percent body fat and fat-free body mass.
- Promote optimal recovery from training.
- Maintain hydration status.

The underlying foundations of a training diet are similar to the basic principles incorporated in the *Dietary Guidelines for Americans* and Canada's

Guidelines for Healthy Eating. The primary differences are increased fluid needs to cover an athlete's sweat losses, and increased energy needs to fuel physical activity. Studies indicate that athletes often are confused about nutrition and may not follow the dietary recommendations for peak sports performance.[15] Let's take a closer look at the nutritional needs of athletes.

carbohydrate loading Changes in dietary carbohydrate intake and exercise regimen before competition to maximize glycogen stores in the muscles. It is appropriate for endurance events lasting 60 to 90 consecutive minutes or longer. Also known as glycogen loading.

glycogen loading See *carbohydrate loading*.

Energy Intake and Exercise

Adequate energy intake is the first nutrition priority for athletes. Meeting energy needs is critical for athletic performance and for maintaining or increasing lean body mass. Sports nutritionists recommend eating small, frequent meals to maintain energy metabolism, improve nutrient intake, achieve desired body composition, support a training schedule, and reduce injuries.[16]

World-class athletes who train strenuously three to four hours each day can almost double their energy needs. The energy demand can be so high that some athletes have trouble consuming enough calories.[17] In contrast, athletes who compete in sports where they are judged by build and in sports with weight classifications often restrict energy intake to avoid weight gain. Energy intakes that are too low can lead to a loss of muscle mass, menstrual dysfunction, lower bone density, and increased risk of fatigue, injury, and illness.[18]

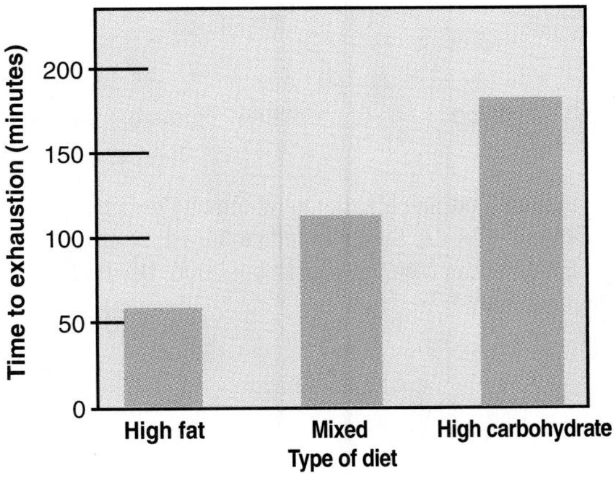

Figure 11.11 **Diet composition and endurance.** Athletes can exercise longer when eating a high-carbohydrate diet.

Carbohydrate and Exercise

Official dietary guidelines for athletes recommend high carbohydrate intakes during training.[19] A high-carbohydrate diet helps increase glycogen stores and extend endurance. (See **Figure 11.11**.) For endurance athletes, research studies suggest that carbohydrate should supply a minimum of 60 percent of total calories.[20] A high-carbohydrate diet also may prevent mental as well as physical fatigue and is important for stop-and-go sports such as basketball, football, and soccer.[21]

For all athletes, dietary carbohydrates should come mainly from complex carbohydrates, which provide many of the B vitamins necessary for energy metabolism, along with iron (if enriched) and fiber (if whole grain). Although added sugars should supply no more than 10 percent of the day's calories, some athletes may need to include more simple sugars to meet energy requirements.

Carbohydrate Loading

Just as you might top off the gas tank in a car before a long trip, athletes can fill their glycogen stores prior to training or competition. In a process called **carbohydrate loading**, or **glycogen loading**, athletes manipulate their carbohydrate intake and exercise regimen to maximize muscle glycogen stores. (See **Figure 11.12**.)

Current recommendations for carbohydrate loading include an intake of 60 to 70 percent of total calories from carbohydrate, along with a decrease in exercise intensity and duration prior to competition.[22] **Table 11.2** is a training plan for endurance athletes that includes carbohydrate

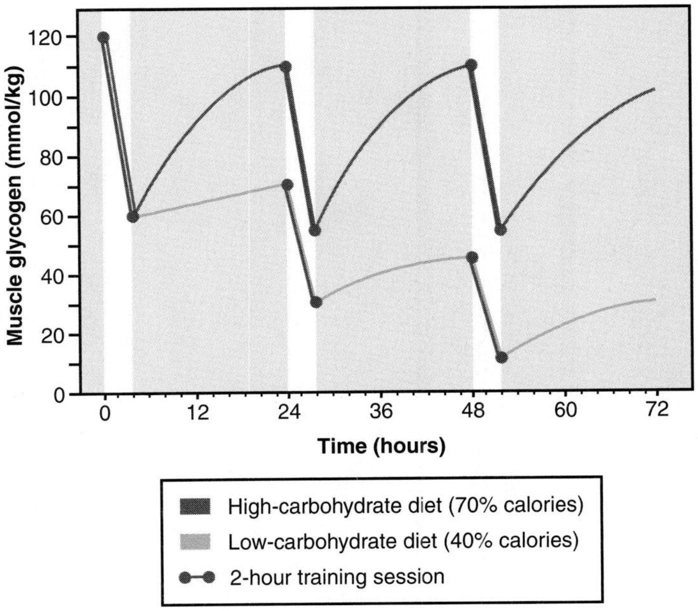

Figure 11.12 **Diet composition, training, and muscle glycogen.** A high-carbohydrate diet replenishes glycogen stores better than a low-carbohydrate diet.
Source: Adapted from Costill DL, Miller JM. Nutrition for endurance sport: carbohydrate and fluid balance. *Int J Sport Nutr.* 1980;1:2–14.

Table 11.2 Carbohydrate Loading for Endurance Athletes

Number of Days before Event	Exercise Duration (min)	Training Diet (g carbohydrate/ kg body weight)
6	90	5
5	40	5
4	40	5
3	20	10
2	20	10
1	Rest day	10
Race	Competition	Precompetition food and fluid

Source: Coleman MA. Carbohydrate and exercise. In: Rosenbloom CA. *Sports Nutrition.* 3rd ed. Chicago: The American Dietetic Association; 2000. Used with permission.

loading and exercise for the week before an event. The glycogen content of exercised muscles more than doubles in athletes who follow these recommendations, and this extends the duration of higher-intensity activity. For example, distance runners who carbohydrate-load may be able to keep a faster pace for a longer time and finish a race sooner.[23]

Even though "extra" glycogen prior to competition sounds like a perfect plan, there is a downside to carbohydrate loading. For each gram of glycogen stored in muscle tissue, the body also stores about 3 grams of water. Many athletes who carbohydrate-load complain about this weight gain and subsequent sluggishness. Some opt to train and compete without carbohydrate loading since, for them, the risk of physical discomfort outweighs the benefit of a greater carbohydrate store.

If you participate in an aerobic activity for fewer than 60 to 90 consecutive minutes, carbohydrate loading probably will provide no benefit. Instead, experts recommend that you taper your training program a few days before competition and eat a diet that provides 70 percent of its calories from carbohydrate for one or two days before the event.[24]

Carbohydrate Intake before Exercise

Eating carbohydrate two to four hours before morning exercise helps replenish glycogen stores and improve endurance. Since many athletes have problems with GI distress, the carbohydrate and caloric content of the meal should be smaller when eaten closer to a workout. While some athletes can tolerate solid foods, others prefer liquids to avoid GI distress. Since protein and fat take longer to digest and absorb, pre-exercise meals should contain no more than 10 to 15 percent of the total calories as protein and less than 20 percent of calories from fat. **Table 11.3** offers guidelines for timing of meals before an event.

Many athletes are confused about whether to eat less than an hour before exercise. To decrease hunger, delay fatigue, and improve performance, athletes who cannot fully refuel several hours prior to a workout must rely on "last-minute" carbohydrate intake. Although early research suggested that consuming carbohydrate within one hour before activity could cause low blood glucose levels and early fatigue, later studies report no effect or improved performance.[25]

Pre-Exercise Meals and the Glycemic Index

As you may recall from Chapter 5, individual foods have different effects on blood glucose levels independent of carbohydrate content. The glycemic index of foods is a measure of this effect and has attracted recent interest in relation to the diets of athletes. Current studies have produced mixed results, so it remains unclear whether the glycemic index of carbohydrate in pre-exercise meals affects performance.[26]

Carbohydrate Intake during Exercise

During exercise, athletes can maintain their carbohydrate supply to exercising muscle by consuming beverages with low to moderate amounts of simple carbohydrate.[27] When an event lasts at least one hour, drinking fluids with 4 to 8 percent carbohydrate, the amount in sports drinks, enables athletes to exercise longer and sprint harder at the finish. Current research now supports the benefits of this practice during events lasting less than one hour.[28] Consuming carbohydrate before and during an event improves performance more than either strategy alone.

Table 11.3 Timing Meals before Events

Time: 8 A.M. event, such as a road race or swim meet
Meals: The night before, eat a high-carbohydrate dinner and drink extra water. The morning of the event, about 6:00 or 6:30, have a light 200- to 400-calorie meal (depending on your tolerance), such as yogurt and a banana, or one or two sports bars, and extra water. Eat familiar foods. If you want a bigger meal, you might want to get up and eat by 5:00 or 6:00.

Time: 10 A.M. event, such as a bike race or soccer game
Meals: The night before, eat a high-carbohydrate meal and drink extra water. The morning of the event, eat a familiar breakfast by 7:00, to allow 3 hours for the food to digest. This meal will prevent the fatigue that results from low blood sugar. If your body cannot handle any breakfast, eat a late snack before going to bed the night before. This will boost liver glycogen stores and prevent low blood sugar the next morning.

Time: 2 P.M. event, such as a football or lacrosse game
Meals: An afternoon game allows time for you to have either a big, high-carbohydrate breakfast and a light lunch, or a substantial brunch by 10:00, allowing 4 hours for digestion. As always, eat a high-carbohydrate dinner the night before, and drink extra fluids the day before and up to noontime.

Time: 8 P.M. event, such as a basketball game
Meals: A hefty, high-carbohydrate breakfast and lunch will be thoroughly digested by evening. Plan for dinner, as tolerated, by 5:00 or have a lighter meal between 6:00 and 7:00. Drink extra fluids all day.

Time: All-day event, such as a 100-mile bike ride, triathlon training, or long, hard hike
Meals: Two days before, cut back on your exercise; the day before, take a rest day to allow your muscles the chance to replace depleted glycogen stores. Eat carbohydrate-rich meals at breakfast, lunch, and dinner. Drink extra fluids. The day of the event, eat breakfast according to your tolerance—whatever you usually have before exercising.

Throughout the day, plan to snack at least every 1.5 to 2 hours on wholesome carbohydrates to maintain a normal blood sugar. At lunchtime, eat a carbohydrate meal. Drink fluids before you get thirsty; you should need to urinate at least three times throughout the day.

Source: Reprinted by permission from Nancy Clark, 1997, *Nancy Clark's Sports Nutrition Guidebook*, 2nd ed. Champaign, IL: Human Kinetics, 169–170.

Carbohydrate Intake following Exercise

It can take 24 to 48 hours after an event to replenish glycogen stores, and the timing and type of carbohydrates are important factors in the refueling process. Athletes who delay the consumption of carbohydrates for more than four hours after exercising synthesize glycogen only half as fast as athletes who consume carbohydrates during the first two hours after exercising.[29] Some research shows that the first 15 minutes are critical.[30]

The best way to replenish glycogen stores after intense exercise is to consume 1 to 1.5 grams of carbohydrate per kilogram of body weight within 30 minutes after a workout, followed by an additional 1 to 1.5 grams per kilogram two hours later.[31] A 70-kilogram (154-pound) athlete who exercises vigorously for 90 minutes or more, for example, would consume 70 to 100 grams of carbohydrate immediately after exercise, followed by another 70 to 100 grams two hours later. Consuming high-glycemic-index foods enhances glycogen synthesis.[32] Among simple sugars, glucose and sucrose appear equally effective in replenishing glycogen, but fructose alone is not as effective.[33]

Carbohydrate intake after exercise also benefits protein metabolism. Several researchers have shown that these levels of carbohydrates taken immediately or one hour after resistance exercise decrease protein breakdown and enhance protein retention.[34]

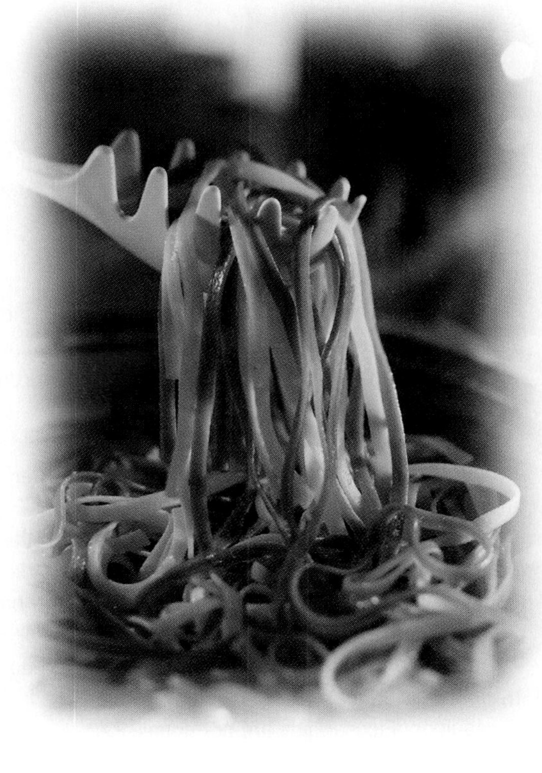

Key Concepts: *Energy intake is the most important element of the athlete's diet, and the major source of energy should be carbohydrates. Foods rich in complex carbohydrates, which also can provide fiber, iron, and B vitamins, are best. A high-carbohydrate diet prior to competition helps to maximize glycogen stores and*

endurance. Carbohydrate loading is a process of adjusting carbohydrate intake and training intensity to maximize glycogen stores just before an event. Consuming carbohydrates soon after exercise enhances the rebuilding of glycogen stores.

Dietary Fat and Exercise

During exercise, carbohydrates and fats are the two main fuel sources. Endurance (aerobic) training increases the capacity of your oxygen energy system, enhancing your body's ability to use fat as a fuel. Exercise intensity also affects fuel use. During low- to moderate-intensity exercise, fatty acids are the major fuel source. During high-intensity exercise, the predominant energy source is glucose.

This does not mean that endurance athletes should consume diets high in fat. High-fat diets usually are lower in carbohydrate, thus limiting muscles' ability to replenish glycogen stores. Insufficient carbohydrate also can impede processing of fat by the oxygen energy system. High-fat diets often are high in calories, saturated fat, and cholesterol; and your body digests fat more slowly than carbohydrate.

Fat Intake and the Athlete

Fat intake should not be overly restricted. There is no performance benefit in consuming a diet with less than 15 percent of energy from fat, compared with 20 to 25 percent of energy from fat.[35] Extreme fat restriction limits food choices, especially sources of protein, iron, zinc, and essential fatty acids. In addition, athletes with high caloric needs (greater than 5,000 kilocalories per day) may find it difficult to eat enough food without consuming more than 30 percent of their calories from fat, the upper limit recommended for the general population. Sports nutritionists recommend

[Fyi] To Zone or Not to Zone? That Is the Question

FOR YOUR INFORMATION

Barry Sears, creator of Eicotec bars and author of *Enter the Zone* and *Mastering the Zone*, puts forth the theory that insulin response to high-carbohydrate diets reduces performance by interfering with free fatty acid mobilization and lowering blood glucose. He further asserts that the insulin response facilitates the conversion of carbohydrate to fat and increases adipose tissue stores. The Zone diet books recommend a carbohydrate-restricted diet of exactly 40 percent carbohydrate, 30 percent protein, and 30 percent fat.

The Zone diet proponents assert that high insulin levels increase the production of "bad" eicosanoids. Eicosanoids are hormonelike compounds that help regulate inflammation, the tendency for blood to clot, and the immune system. The protein content of the Zone diet supposedly increases glucagon levels, which in turn support the production of "good" eicosanoids by counteracting the effects of insulin.

The scientific basis of the theory underlying the Zone diet has many faults. There is no evidence that insulin increases the amount of "bad" eicosanoids or that glucagon makes "good" eicosanoids.[1] A high-carbohydrate diet does elicit an insulin response because insulin is needed for the transport of glucose (energy) into the cells. With insulin-mediated glucose uptake, the synthesis of liver and muscle glycogen leads to a decrease in blood glucose. The body preferentially uses carbohydrates for energy and does not readily convert excess carbohydrate to fat. (See the FYI "Do Carbohydrates Turn into Fat?" in the "Spotlight on Metabolism.") During exercise, the release of catecholamines such as epinephrine and norepinephrine drives an increase in blood glucose and a decrease in insulin. Catecholamines also prompt the adipose tissue to release fatty acids into the bloodstream.

Consuming carbohydrate 30 to 60 minutes before exercise is associated with increased that any extra fat calories come from monounsaturated and polyunsaturated sources.

Protein and Exercise

Historically, many athletes believed they could become stronger by eating muscle from animals. Many bodybuilders and weightlifters still believe a meal of steak and eggs is their most important source of calories.[36] Current research suggests athletes require only slightly higher protein intakes than sedentary people.[37]

Enter the Zone, a popular book with an unscientific premise, recommends a diet of 40 percent carbohydrate, 30 percent fat, and 30 percent protein. With its success, athletes' interest in optimal protein intake surged. Athletes—from endurance runners to football players to weekend warriors—are asking the question, "Do I need to eat more protein and less carbohydrate for optimal performance?"[38] (See the FYI feature "To Zone or Not To Zone? That Is the Question.")

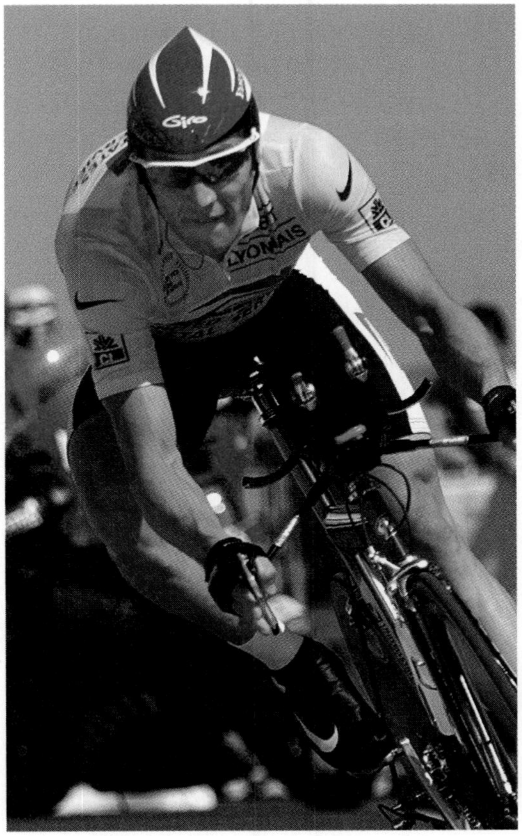

Optimal nutrition is an important part of Lance Armstrong's training.

Protein Recommendations for Athletes

The adult Recommended Dietary Allowance (RDA) for protein is 0.8 grams of protein per kilogram of body weight per day,[39] and people who regularly engage in low-intensity exercise do not need additional protein.[40]

Endurance athletes involved in heavy training require 1.2 to 1.4 grams of protein per kilogram of body weight per day.[41] Endurance athletes who are training for extreme events, such as the Tour de France, need up to 2 grams per kilogram.[42]

Strength athletes consuming 1.4 grams of protein per kilogram of body weight per day synthesize more body protein than athletes consuming 0.9

insulin and lowered blood glucose. However, those responses are temporary and do not adversely affect performance. In fact, a high-carbohydrate meal one hour before exercise can improve endurance by supplying the exercising muscles with glucose and sparing the loss of glycogen.

Carbohydrates—not fatty acids—are used preferentially for energy during exercise. Muscle glycogen is the body's predominant energy source for most sports. Because it takes longer for fat to become available to muscles as fuel in the form of free fatty acids, the duration of most athletes' workouts is not sufficient to burn significant amounts of fat. Rather, it is the calorie deficit resulting from the exercise session and negative energy balance during the day that promotes fat loss. When athletes restrict carbohydrate intake, they compromise the amount of carbohydrate stored in their muscles, which is needed to facilitate exercise performance. The Zone diet is a low-energy diet and does not increase the body's ability to burn fat.

It is not realistic to think that a diet composed of 30 percent protein would contain only 30 percent fat. If you use animal foods to meet these protein recommendations, it is not difficult to exceed the fat recommendations. And, with a restriction of carbohydrate foods, a vegetarian-based protein intake is largely ruled out.[2] There are some individuals for whom a high-carbohydrate diet is not recommended. But athletic individuals are not among them.

1 Coleman E. Carbohydrate and exercise. In: Rosenbloom CA. *Sports Nutrition* 3rd ed. Chicago: The American Dietetic Association; 2000.
2 Coleman E. Debunking the "Eicotec" myth. *Sports Med Dig.* 1993;15:6–7.

Table 11.4 Protein Requirements of Sedentary and Active People

Activity Level	Protein Requirements (g protein/kg body weight)
Sedentary	0.8
Strength athlete	1.6–1.7
Endurance athlete	1.2–1.4
Maximum usable amount for adults	2.0

Source: Adapted from Snyder AC, Naik J. Protein requirements of athletes. In: Berning JR, Steen SN, eds. *Nutrition for Sport and Exercise.* 2nd ed. Gaithersburg, MD: Aspen; 1998.

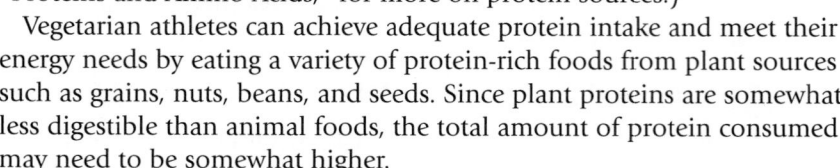

grams. Increased protein synthesis during training is an indicator of muscle growth. However, when protein intake was increased to 2.4 grams per kilogram, protein synthesis did not increase further.[43] After adjusting for safety, researchers recommend that strength athletes consume 1.6 to 1.7 grams of protein per kilogram per day.[44] A 91-kilogram (200-pound) strength athlete who wants to build muscle mass would consume about 150 grams of protein. **Table 11.4** shows the protein requirements of various levels of physical activity.

Protein Intake and the Athlete

Athletes don't need protein powders or amino acid supplements to meet the protein demands of athletic performance.[45] Their best protein sources are high-quality protein foods, including legumes, low-fat dairy products, egg whites, lean beef and pork, chicken, turkey, and fish. (See Chapter 7, "Proteins and Amino Acids," for more on protein sources.)

Think About It 4

Vegetarian athletes can achieve adequate protein intake and meet their energy needs by eating a variety of protein-rich foods from plant sources such as grains, nuts, beans, and seeds. Since plant proteins are somewhat less digestible than animal foods, the total amount of protein consumed may need to be somewhat higher.

Quick Bites

Lost in Space

Vigorous weight training can double or triple a muscle's size, whereas the lack of use during space travel can shrink it by 20 percent in two weeks.

Protein Intake after Exercise

Protein combined with carbohydrate in a postexercise meal increases glycogen synthesis more than carbohydrate alone.[46] Researchers suggest athletes consume 4 grams of protein for every 10 grams of carbohydrate (grams protein = 40% grams carbohydrate).[47] For example, using postexercise recommendations of 1.5 grams of carbohydrate per kilogram of body weight, a 55-kilogram female athlete would need 82.5 grams of carbohydrate ($55 \text{ g} \times 1.5 = 82.5 \text{ g}$) and 33 grams of protein ($82.5 \text{ g} \times 0.40 = 33 \text{ g}$). How does this translate to food? A bagel, 2 ounces of string cheese, and 8 ounces of low-fat yogurt would provide a portable snack to enjoy after a hard workout.

Dangers of High Protein Intake

diuresis The formation and secretion of urine.

Excessive protein intake from food or supplements enhances **diuresis** (loss of body water) as the body attempts to excrete excess nitrogen through the urine. This increases the risk for dehydration and may contribute to mineral losses. High-protein diets often are high in saturated and total fat and may contribute to obesity, osteoporosis, heart disease, and certain types of cancer. (See Chapter 7, "Proteins and Amino Acids.")

High intakes of single-amino-acid supplements may impair absorption of other amino acids. Further, the amount of amino acids contained in supplements is very small compared with the amount in food. For example, one pill may contain 500 milligrams of an amino acid, but 1 ounce of meat, poultry, or fish provides more than 7,000 milligrams of essential and nonessential amino acids! And, the cost of supplements is higher.

Key Concepts: *Although fat is an important fuel for exercise, a high-fat diet is not necessary. General recommendations that fat not exceed 30 percent of total energy intake are appropriate for athletes. Dietary protein is a source of energy and also a source of amino acids for body protein synthesis. The protein requirements of athletes are slightly higher than those of sedentary adults, but still within the normal range of protein consumption. High-protein diets are neither recommended nor* *necessary. Low-fat dairy products, egg whites, lean beef and pork, chicken, turkey, fish, and legumes are good sources of protein.*

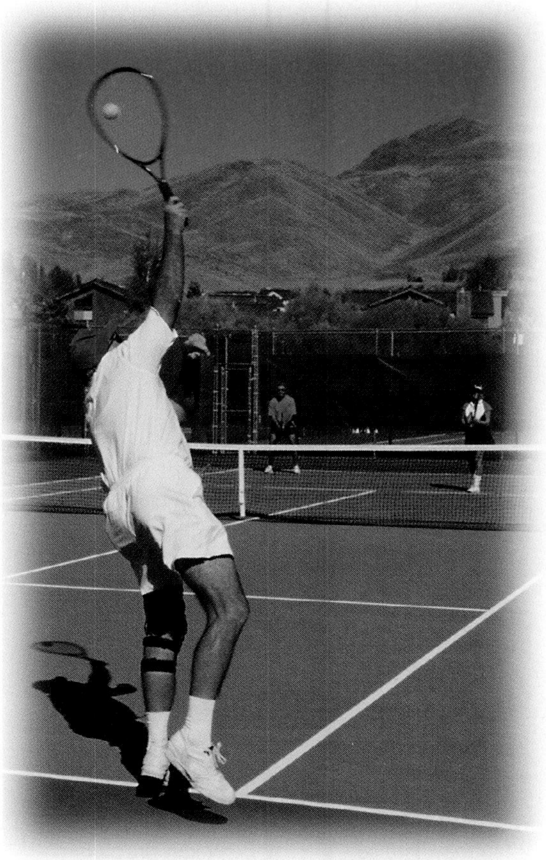

Vitamins, Minerals, and Athletic Performance

Many reactions that support exercise and physical activity require vitamins and minerals. They help extract energy from nutrients, transport oxygen, and repair tissues. Researchers have long debated whether physically active people have greater vitamin and mineral needs than sedentary people.

B Vitamins

Since B vitamins are essential for energy metabolism (see Chapter 9, "Vitamins"), wouldn't athletes, with their high energy needs, require more B vitamins? There is no need to run to the supplement counter. B vitamins are needed for chemical reactions that release energy. But if athletes consume adequate calories and ample complex carbohydrates, fruits, and vegetables, they eat plenty of B vitamins. However, if athletes consume too few calories or eat mostly refined sugars in lieu of complex carbohydrates, they can compromise their B vitamin intake.

Vegan athletes who do not include fortified foods, such as some soy products and ready-to-eat cereals, may have a problem with vitamin B_{12} intake. They should consult a medical advisor or registered dietitian to determine if they need B_{12} supplements.

Calcium

Calcium is essential for normal muscle function and strong bones. Adequate calcium intake coupled with regular exercise slows the deterioration of the skeleton with age and can reduce the risk of osteoporosis.

Inadequate calcium may increase the risk of stress fractures in athletes. This is of particular concern for the amenorrheic athlete (discussed in the "Female Athlete Triad" section later in this chapter). Athletes should strive to meet the Adequate Intake (AI) for calcium from a variety of low-fat dairy products and other calcium-rich foods. This is especially true for teens whose calcium needs (1,300 mg/day) are higher than those of adults (1,000 mg/day).

Iron

Iron is vital to oxygen delivery and energy production. As an essential part of hemoglobin and myoglobin, iron helps deliver oxygen to active muscle cells. It is also a key component of several enzymes vital to the production of ATP by the oxygen energy system. (For more details about iron's functional roles, see Chapter 10, "Water and Minerals.")

Because of menstrual losses and lower dietary iron intakes, female athletes have a greater risk of iron deficiency than male athletes. In endurance athletes, the impact of running can cause mechanical trauma to capillaries in the feet and increase the breakdown of red blood cells. The increased breakdown may contribute to low iron status.[48] Some studies suggest that athletes involved in heavy training may need 30 to 70 percent more iron than nonathletes.[49] Endurance training also increases the volume of plasma in the blood without initially changing the amount of hemoglobin. This dilutes the hemoglobin, even though training typically maintains or increases the amount of total hemoglobin. This condition, called **sports anemia,** is a false anemia for most athletes and can be remedied with a few days of rest.

sports anemia A lowered concentration of hemoglobin in the blood due to dilution. The increased plasma volume that dilutes the hemoglobin is a normal consequence of aerobic training.

Table 11.5 A Sample Training Diet

Athlete performs prolonged daily training
body weight = 70 kilograms
energy intake = 3,400 kilocalories

Macronutrients		
Carbohydrate	Protein	Fat
535 g	128 g	83 g
63% kcal	15% kcal	22% kcal
7.5 g/kg body weight*	1.8 g/kg body weight**	

Breakfast
8 oz orange juice
2 C Cheerios cereal
8 oz 1% milk
1 large bran muffin

Lunch
2 slices whole-wheat bread
2 oz turkey
2 slices tomato
Lettuce leaf
2 tsp mayonnaise
1 med apple
12 oz cranberry juice

Pre-exercise
8 oz Gatorade
1 cereal bar

Postexercise
1 bagel
2 oz string cheese
16 oz apple juice

Dinner
3 oz chicken breast
1 lg baked potato with 2 Tbsp low-fat sour cream
2 whole-wheat dinner rolls
1 tsp margarine
1 C cooked broccoli
1 C salad greens with 2 Tbsp Italian salad dressing
8 oz 1% milk
1 C low-fat frozen yogurt

* Recommended carbohydrate intake goals for prolonged daily training

** Recommended protein intake goals up to 2 g/kg body weight for extreme training loads

Although many elite athletes, especially endurance athletes, have mild iron deficiency, few are anemic.[50] Although anemia can seriously impair a person's capacity to perform activities, mild iron deficiency has little effect on performance.[51]

Other Trace Minerals

Strenuous exercise taxes the body's reserves of copper (essential for red blood cell synthesis) and zinc (vital to the work of many enzymes involved in energy production). During endurance events, increased fluid loss increases mineral losses—zinc in urine and relatively high amounts of both zinc and copper in sweat.

While these losses may cause marginal deficiencies, supplementation is not necessarily recommended. High-dose supplements of iron, copper, or zinc can interfere with the normal absorption of these and other minerals, so an excess of one can cause a deficiency of the others. **Table 11.5** is an example of a training diet that would meet an athlete's needs for vitamins and minerals through food, which is preferable to taking supplements.

Key Concepts: *Vitamins and minerals are important components of athletes' diets. B vitamins are necessary for normal energy metabolism. Adequate calcium intake can help protect against stress fractures and, coupled with exercise, delays the onset of osteoporosis. Iron is needed to carry oxygen. Strenuous exercise can tax the body's reserves of both copper and zinc.*

Fluid Needs during Exercise

Exercise generates heat, and heavy exercise can increase heat production 15- to 20-fold. (See **Figure 11.13**.) The increase in body heat triggers sweating, and sweat cools your body as it evaporates on your skin. The body of a well-trained athlete begins to cool itself soon after exercise begins. Even before core body temperature rises, the athlete's body starts to produce sweat. Sweating rates of elite athletes can range from 1 to 3 liters (4 to 12 cups) per hour.[52] Sweat rate is affected by environmental temperature (extreme heat or extreme cold), humidity (higher humidity increases the rate of sweat production but reduces efficiency of evaporation), type of clothing, fitness level, and initial fluid balance.

To keep the body from overheating, blood must flow to the skin, where evaporating sweat can dissipate heat. During exercise, the cooling demand for blood flow to the skin may compete with the cardiovascular demand for blood to deliver "fuel" to working muscles. Dehydration stresses both systems, making each less efficient. Without fluid replacement during heavy exercise, athletes can become dehydrated quickly. Signs of dehydration include

- elevated heart rate at a given exercise intensity
- increased rate of **perceived exertion** during activity
- decreased performance
- lethargy
- concentrated urine
- infrequent urination
- loss of appetite

Drinking enough fluid during exercise helps offset fluid loss, minimize cardiovascular changes, reduce perception of effort, and maintain a supply

Quick Bites

Sweating a World Record

When Alberto Salazar ran the Olympic marathon in 1984, he went down in the record books for sweat production. He lost 12 pounds during the 26.2-mile race, despite drinking about 2 liters. His sweat rate was approximately 3.7 liters per hour.

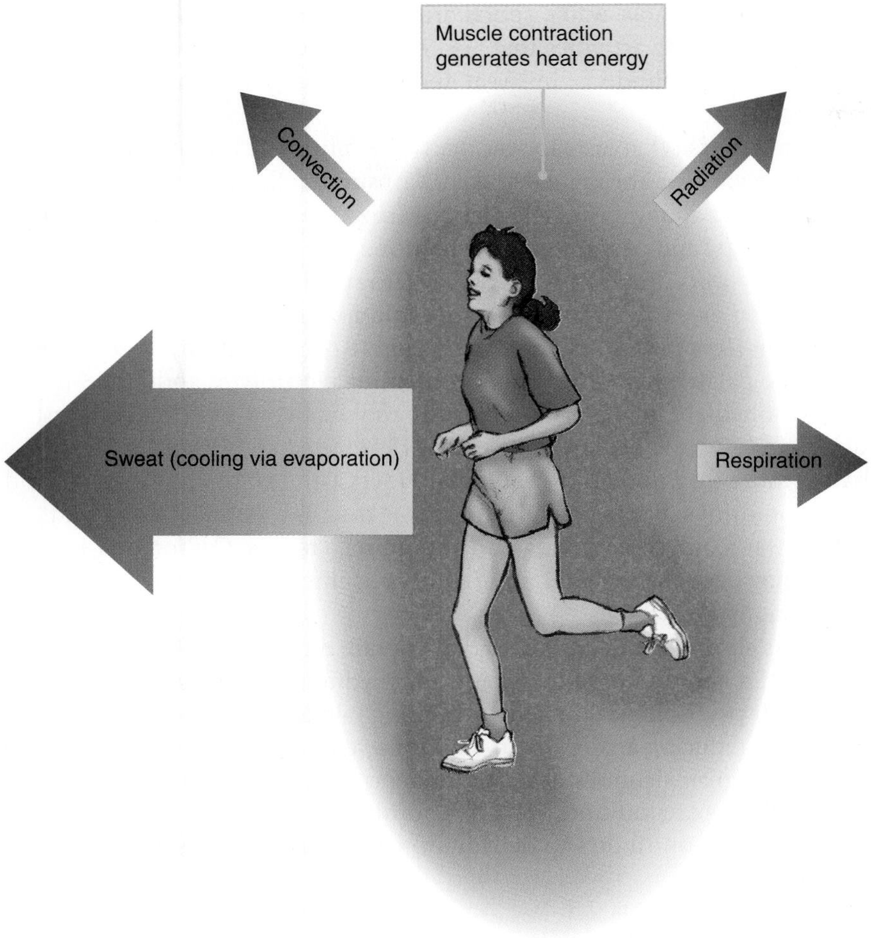

Figure 11.13 **Dissipation of heat during exercise.** During exercise, radiation, convection, and respiration are responsible for some heat loss, but evaporation of sweat dissipates more than 80 percent of the heat generated by increased physical activity.

perceived exertion The subjective experience of how difficult an effort is.

of fuel to working muscles. Because exercise inhibits the body's thirst signal, you probably won't take in enough fluid if you wait until you are thirsty to replenish your losses. Active people must train themselves to consume adequate amounts of fluid before, during, and after exercise. **Table 11.6** shows how much fluid a person should drink at various levels of physical activity.

Hydration: Drink More!

Athletes should be well hydrated before starting physical activity. The day before an event, the athlete should drink generous amounts of fluid. In the final two to three hours before exercise, the ACSM recommends drinking 400 to 600 milliliters (2 to 3 cups) of fluid.[53] Since even partial dehydration can compromise performance, athletes should maintain fluid balance during the event. After beginning exercise, drinking 150 to 350 milliliters (6 to 12 ounces) every 15 to 20 minutes helps facilitate optimal hydration. Most athletes are unable to replace all lost fluid, so they are somewhat dehydrated when the event ends. To make up for sweat losses and cover obligatory urine production, athletes may need to consume an amount of fluid equal to 1.5 times the body weight lost during the exercise session.

Table 11.6 **Typical Fluid Needs**

Activity Level	Environment	Fluid Requirements (liters per day)
Sedentary	Cool	2–3
Active	Cool	3–6
Sedentary	Warm	3–5
Active	Warm	5–10+

Note that fluid requirements include fluid from all sources—liquids, food, and metabolic water. See Chapter 10, "Water and Minerals," for more information.

Source: Murray R. Drink more! Advice from a world class expert. *ACSM's Health and Fitness Journal.* 1997;1:19–23, 50.

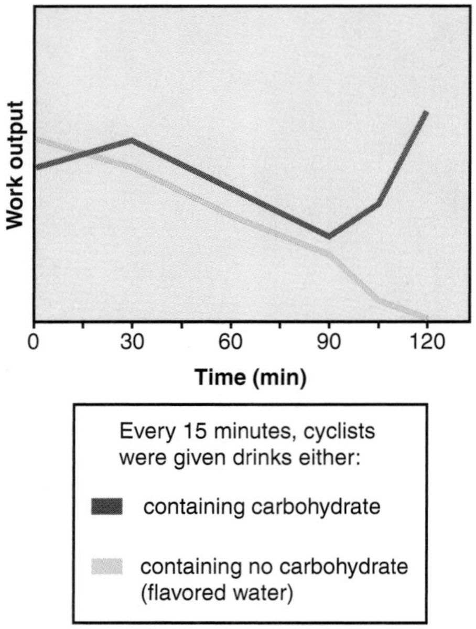

Figure 11.14 **Sports drinks and performance.** Consuming carbohydrate drinks dramatically increases power output after 90 minutes.

palatable Pleasant tasting.

Athletes may choose water, sports drinks, or other beverages to meet fluid needs. During activities that last fewer than 60 continuous minutes, water can replace fluid lost in sweat and help offset the rise in core temperature.

During exercise that lasts longer than 60 continuous minutes, muscle and liver glycogen stores become depleted. Consuming fluids that contain carbohydrate and sodium can delay fatigue (see **Figure 11.14**), enhance palatability of fluids, and promote fluid retention.[54]

Optimal sports drinks provide energy (from glucose, glucose polymers, or sucrose) and electrolytes in a **palatable** solution that promotes rapid absorption (less than 10 percent carbohydrate concentration). (See **Table 11.7.**) The palatability of beverages containing electrolytes and 4 to 8 percent carbohydrate may increase the voluntary intake of fluid.[55] Beverages such as fruit juices and soft drinks are concentrated sources of carbohydrates (more than 10 percent) and may slow gastric emptying. In juices and many soft drinks, the main carbohydrate is fructose, which is associated with slower stomach emptying and abdominal cramps. Carbonated soft drinks may decrease the volume of fluid consumed, although this effect varies among individuals.

Athletes should avoid beverages that contain alcohol or caffeine. These are diuretics and do not allow complete rehydration. Some athletes use alcohol for psychological benefits—calming nerves, improving self-confidence, and reducing anxiety, pain, and muscle tremor. This misguided effort fails to recognize alcohol's negative influence on physical performance. Alcohol slows reaction time, impairs coordination, and upsets balance. Its diuretic action contributes to dehydration and may impair regulation of body temperature.

For endurance events that last longer than four to five hours, athletes who do not replace electrolytes put themselves at risk for abnormally low levels of blood sodium. This life-threatening condition is associated with an excessive loss of electrolytes in sweat and with the excessive consumption of fluid, such as plain water, that does not replace electrolytes. See

Table 11.7 **Desirable Composition of Sports Beverages**

Characteristic	Comment
Fuel/Calories	Contains a source of carbohydrate: glucose, maltodextrin, sucrose, high-fructose corn syrup. Goal intake is 30–60 g/hr (2–4 cups of a 6 percent carbohydrate drink per hour).
Electrolytes	Enhances fluid uptake and palatability. Contains sodium, potassium, chloride, and phosphorus to replace sweat electrolyte loss in activity longer than four hours. Not an issue in exercise of shorter duration.
Rapid absorption	Carbohydrate concentration less than 10 percent. Carbohydrate concentration over 10 percent can slow gastric emptying. Fructose should not be main or sole form of carbohydrate.
Palatability	Flavor may be biggest key to amount consumed. Taste changes can occur during exercise. Carbonation may decrease amount of fluid consumed.

Source: Shi X, Gisolfi CV. Fluid and carbohydrate replacement during intermittent exercise. *Sports Med.* 1998;25:157–172.

Table 11.8 **American College of Sports Medicine Position on Fluid Replacement**

Before Activity or Competition

- Drink adequate fluids during the 24 hours before an event, especially during the meal before exercise, to promote proper hydration before exercise or competition.
- Drink about 500 milliliters (~17 ounces) of fluid about two hours before exercise to promote adequate hydration and allow time for excretion of excess ingested water.

During Activity or Competition

- Start drinking early and at regular intervals to consume fluids at a rate sufficient to replace all the water lost through sweating or consume the maximal amount that can be tolerated.
- Fluids should be cooler than ambient temperature and flavored to enhance palatability and promote fluid replacement.

During Competition That Lasts More Than One Hour

- To maintain blood glucose concentration and delay the onset of fatigue, the fluid replacement should contain 4 to 8 percent carbohydrate. Electrolytes (primarily salt) are added to make the solution taste better and reduce the risk of low blood levels of sodium. About 0.5 to 0.7 grams of sodium per liter of water replaces sodium lost by sweating.

Following Activity or Competition

- Complete restoration of the extracellular fluid compartment cannot be sustained without replacement of lost sodium.
- For each pound of body weight lost, consume at least 2 cups of fluid.
- Thirst sensation is *not* an adequate gauge of dehydration, and post exercise consumption stimulates obligatory urine losses. Research shows that drinking an amount of liquid that is 125 to 150 percent of fluid loss is usually enough to promote complete rehydration.

Source: Adapted from American College of Sports Medicine position stand. Exercise and fluid replacement. *Med Sci Sports Exerc.* 1996;28(1):i–vii. Reprinted by permission of Lippincott Williams & Wilkins.

Table 11.8 for a summary of the American College of Sports Medicine's position on the amount and type of fluid to consume before, during, and after activity.

Nutrition Needs of Youth in Sport

Young athletes (younger than 19 years) involved in competitive sports need to fuel both physical activity and continued growth. Studies indicate that diets in young athletes are often marginal or inadequate in energy intake.[56] The consequences of chronic low energy intake include[57]

- short stature and delayed puberty
- nutrient deficiencies and dehydration
- menstrual irregularities
- poor bone health
- increased incidence of injuries
- increased risk of developing eating disorders

Parents and youth need to understand the energy and nutrient demands of growth and training, and many need help in planning meals and snacks to meet those needs. Many sport activities for this age group take place after school, and some schools serve lunch as early as 10:45 A.M. To provide energy for the activity and nutrients for recovery, young people should have meals and snacks before and after exercise. Easily portable snacks include fruit, pretzels, dry cereal, cereal bars, yogurt, sports drinks, sandwiches, and milk. Young athletes must drink adequate fluids during the day as well as at practice and competition. This is especially important because youths have a high tolerance for exercising in heat, which puts them at increased risk for heat exhaustion and heat stroke.

Quick Bites

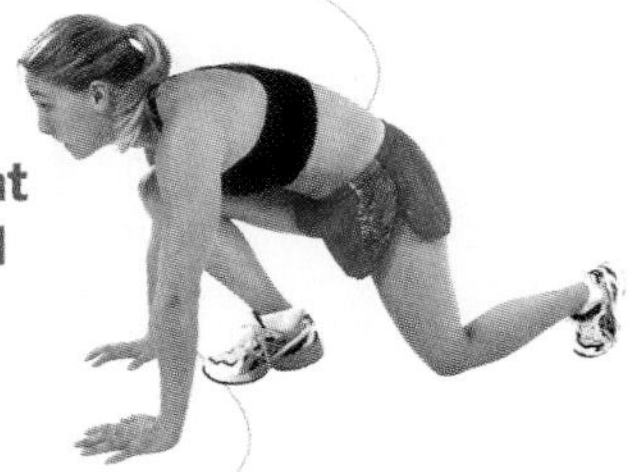

Training: Young at Heart or Skeletal Old Age?

With endurance training, younger athletes largely achieve improvements as a result of increased cardiac output. Older athletes show greater improvement in the activities of the oxidative enzymes in their skeletal muscles.

Quick Bites

Climbing with Age

Aging does not seem to impair a healthy person's ability to perform activities at a high altitude. On the other hand, aging reduces our ability to sweat; and so as we age, our ability to regulate body temperature declines, thus reducing our ability to exercise safely in hot environments.

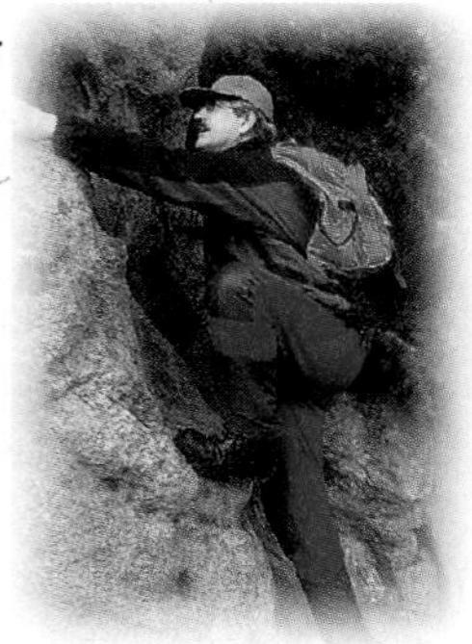

Key Concepts: *Exercise of any type increases fluid losses through sweat. Evaporation of sweat from the skin allows the body to cool itself. Fluid losses must be replaced in order to avoid dehydration. Athletes need to drink plenty of fluid before, during, and after exercise. Fluid choices depend on the duration of activity and the preferences of the athlete. Optimal sports drinks provide energy and electrolytes in a solution that promotes rapid absorption. Nutrient intakes by young athletes must support both competition and continued growth.*

Nutrition Supplements and Ergogenic Aids

The pressure to win contributes to athletes' search for a competitive edge. More than 75 percent of recreational and elite athletes use nutritional supplements and **ergogenic aids** with the expectation of improved performance.[58] Nutrition supplements and ergogenic aids include products that

- provide calories (e.g., liquid supplements and energy bars)
- provide vitamins and minerals (including multivitamin supplements)
- contribute to performance during exercise and enhance recovery after exercise (e.g., sports drinks and carbohydrate supplements)
- are believed to stimulate and maintain muscle growth (e.g., purified amino acids)[59]
- contain micronutrients, herbal, and/or cellular components that are promoted as ergogenic aids to enhance performance (e.g., caffeine, chromium picolinate, creatine, and pyruvate)[60]

ergogenic aids Substances that can enhance athletic performance.

Most nutrient supplements are unnecessary for athletes who select a variety of foods and meet their energy needs. However, iron and calcium supplements may be recommended for female athletes if their diets are low in these nutrients. Liquid supplements and sports bars that contain carbohydrates, proteins, and fats can provide an easy way to increase energy intake. Sports drinks, gels, and recovery drinks also can contribute to needed fluids and carbohydrates before, during, and after exercise. **Table 11.9** shows the nutrient content of some popular sports bars.

Dietary supplements marketed as performance enhancers are another matter. Herbals, glandulars, enzymes, hormones, and other compounds aimed at athletes carry many attractive claims. Although some products have been well researched, most lack vigorous clinical trials to evaluate efficacy, apply to only one gender (usually males), or are relevant to only one sport (e.g., weight lifting).

Table 11.9 Nutrient Content of Sports Bars

Bar	Calories	Carbohydrate (%)	Protein (%)	Fat (%)
Power Bar	225	75	17	8
X-Trainer	220	73	18	9
Tiger Sport	230	70	19	11
Ultra Fuel	490	82	12	6
GatorBar	220	87	5	8
PR Bar	190	40	30	30
Gatorade Energy Bar	260	72	11	17

Amino Acids

Researchers have studied the use of individual amino acids to enhance performance and have not found clear benefits. Some have proposed that branched-chain amino acids may provide energy and delay central nervous system fatigue, thus improving performance. Studies in humans, however, have shown inconsistent results. Because safety and effectiveness have not been established, they are not recommended.

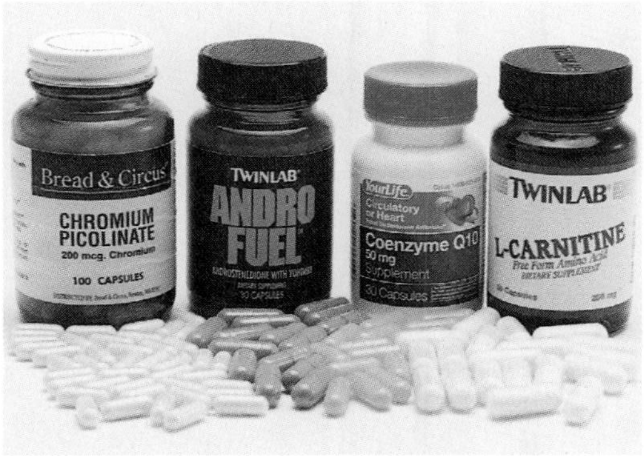

"Andro" and DHEA

The adrenal gland synthesizes the testosterone precursors **androstenedione** and **dehydroepiandrosterone (DHEA)**. Manufacturers claim that supplements of "andro" and DHEA increase testosterone levels and enhance muscle building—a kind of "natural" steroid. Studies of DHEA have found increases in androgen levels (including testosterone) in women, but not in men.[61] Two recent studies of androstenedione supplementation in men had mixed results. Low doses of andro (100 milligrams per day) did not raise serum testosterone levels, while 300 milligrams per day did.[62] In the one of these studies that looked at response to strength training, andro was not effective in improving strength or muscle gains.[63] In both studies, andro use caused estrogen levels to rise, a potentially serious side effect. No long-term studies have tested the safety of androstenedione or DHEA.[64] Despite the success reported anecdotally by a few high-profile athletes, hormone precursors are not recommended because they have many potentially negative effects. In fact, the International Olympic Committee, National Football League, **NCAA,** and U.S. Tennis Association ban the use of androstenedione.

Little is known about the side effects of these steroidal supplements, but if large quantities of these compounds substantially increase testosterone levels in the body, they also are likely to produce the same side effects as **anabolic steroids**. Anabolic steroid abuse has been associated with a wide variety of adverse side effects, ranging from some that are physically unattractive (e.g., acne and breast development in men) to others that are life-threatening (e.g., heart attacks and liver cancer). Most are reversible if the abuser stops taking the drugs, but some are permanent.

androstenedione (andro) A steroid precursor secreted by the testes, ovaries, and adrenal cortex.

dehydroepiandrosterone (DHEA) A steroid that is the precursor to androstenedione. DHEA is secreted primarily by the adrenal gland, but also by the testes.

NCAA National Collegiate Athletic Association.

anabolic steroids Several compounds derived from testosterone or prepared synthetically. They promote body growth and masculinization, and oppose the effects of estrogen.

Caffeine

Caffeine is a natural stimulant. Research suggests that caffeine may affect athletic performance by facilitating signals between the nervous system and the muscles as well as decreasing an athlete's perceived effort during exercise. Caffeine may also increase the body's ability to break down fat for energy. In one well-controlled study, subjects who ingested a high caffeine load one hour before exercise used less muscle glycogen and increased their endurance.[65]

How practical is this regimen? The dose used in the above study was 9 milligrams of caffeine per kilogram of body weight, which would be 630 milligrams of caffeine for a 70-kilogram person. Considering that one soda has about 30 milligrams of caffeine and one cup of regular coffee about 150 milligrams, that's quite a lot of caffeine! In fact, it's enough to be concerned about stomach discomfort and increasing the concentration of caffeine in the urine above amounts allowed by the International Olympic Committee—not to mention the fact that caffeine is a diuretic, and enhancing urine production is probably not the best course of action right before competition!

Quick Bites

Placebo Power!

Athletes involved in a heavy weight-lifting program volunteered to participate in a study where they would take what they thought were anabolic steroids. The results were dramatic—during four weeks of treatment these experienced weight lifters had a nearly 7.5-fold increase in the rate of their strength gain. However, they were taking a placebo—an inactive substance identical in appearance to the genuine drug. Because there was no pharmacological effect, gains were solely due to their belief in the treatment.

Carnitine

Carnitine, a natural compound in foods, is synthesized in the liver and kidneys from the amino acids lysine and methionine. Carnitine helps transport long-chain fatty acids into the mitochondria, where they are broken down. The appeal to athletes is the idea that supplemental carnitine could help move long-chain fatty acids into the mitochondria faster, so they will be metabolized more quickly, thus increasing the use of fat as an energy source. Short-term and long-term carnitine supplementation, however, has not been shown to augment muscle use of fatty acids.[66] Even though exercise increases carnitine excretion in the urine, its availability in foods and ready synthesis in the body make it unlikely that supplemental carnitine will benefit athletes.[67]

Chromium

The trace mineral chromium is vital to the movement of glucose into cells. Because of the link between chromium, glucose use, and insulin, chromium has become a popular supplement (typically in the form of chromium picolinate) for both weight loss and athletic performance. The theory is that by enhancing insulin action, chromium increases amino acid uptake, which then increases protein synthesis and promotes a gain in muscle mass.

Although the developers of the chromium picolinate supplements had promising results in several studies, subsequent controlled trials have not found chromium picolinate to be beneficial for body composition changes, strength gains, or performance.[68] Given these results and the potential risks from chromium picolinate supplementation (see Chapter 10, "Water and Minerals"), this supplement cannot be recommended.

Coenzyme Q_{10} (Ubiquinone)

In the mitochondria of muscle cells, **coenzyme Q_{10} (CoQ_{10})** actively helps transfer electrons in the electron transport chain. CoQ_{10} also may function as an antioxidant and spare vitamin E. In both athletes and sedentary people, supplementation with approximately 100 milligrams a day of CoQ_{10} has shown variable effects on aerobic performance. Early studies that showed positive results had poor study designs (no control group). Studies using control groups show no improvement in exercise performance or reduction in oxidative stress induced by exercise.[69]

coenzyme Q_{10} (CoQ_{10}) A compound abundant in cells and vital to the production of ATP in the electron transport chain. Also called ubiquinone.

creatine An important nitrogenous compound found in meats and fish, and synthesized in the body from amino acids (glycine, arginine, and methionine).

Creatine

Creatine, a nitrogenous compound in meats and fish, is synthesized by the liver, pancreas, and kidney. Muscles store creatine mainly as creatine phosphate, which functions as part of the ATP–CP energy system. Creatine has become a popular supplement based on the theory that increasing muscle creatine would prolong short-term energy availability and thus improve performance in short-term, high-intensity activities (such as weight lifting).[70] Several well-controlled studies have shown improvements in muscle strength when creatine supplementation was added to a strength training regimen.[71] Creatine supplements also may improve the explosive power needed for sprints.[72] But creatine supplements appear to have no benefit for aerobic training. The main side effect seems to be immediate weight gain attributable to water retention.

Although creatine appears to be effective in some sports situations, questions remain about its long-term use. Increases in muscle mass are probably a response to the increased stress that an athlete can put on muscle tissue by maximal exercise bursts—the supplement without weight training will have no effect. Also, the ability to store more CP may vary widely among people, so supplements may not be effective for everyone. Anecdotal reports of muscle cramps, muscle strains, kidney dysfunction, and GI distress have raised concerns. The American College of Sports Medicine has issued a cautionary statement regarding creatine supplementation and is awaiting the results of more studies that address risks of long-term use before giving the green light for use of creatine supplements.[73]

Ginseng

For thousands of years, the Chinese have used the root of the ginseng plant to treat and prevent numerous disorders. Modern-day use of **ginseng** continues because many people believe it combats a wide range of stressors.[74] Because some reports suggest it improves athletic performance by increasing stamina and aerobic capacity, ginseng also has become popular among athletes.[75]

ginseng A collective term that describes several species of plants of the genus *Panax*.

There is no known mechanism to explain how ginseng might work as an ergogenic aid, and controlled studies do not support ginseng use to improve exercise performance or reduce fatigue. Because the studies that showed an ergogenic benefit were poorly designed, many researchers question their results.[76] In a European study, for example, elite athletes experienced improved physical work capacity and physiological response after nine weeks of supplementation with 200 milligrams per day of *Panax ginseng*.[77] An American laboratory repeated this study using 200 or 400 milligrams per day of the same *Panax ginseng*, but found no effect on heart rate recovery, oxygen use, or aerobic ability.[78] While testimonials continue to drive ginseng supplementation, further research on this popular herb is needed to evaluate its effectiveness as an ergogenic aid.

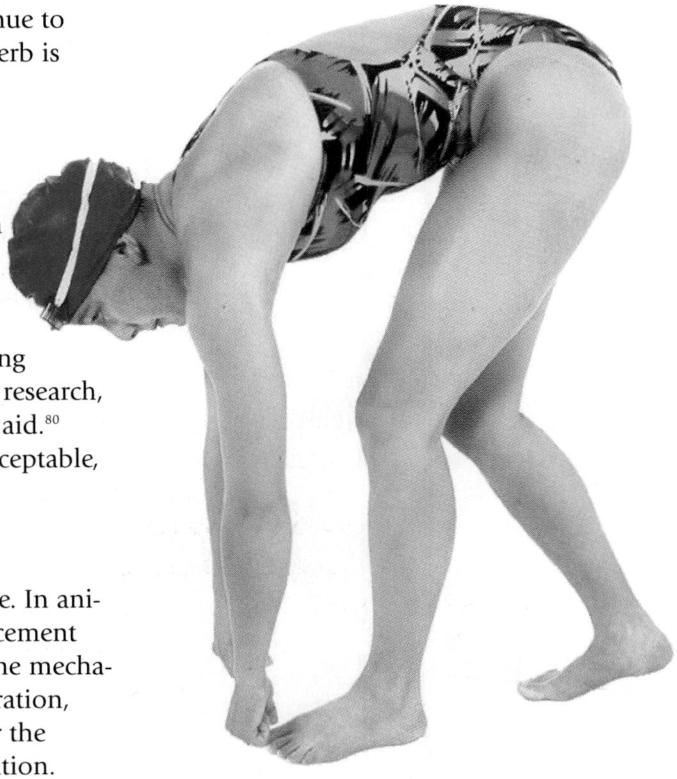

Medium-Chain Triglyceride Oil

Medium-chain triglycerides (MCT) are produced from plant oils, primarily coconut oil, and contain saturated fatty acids of medium length (6 to 10 carbons). As with carbohydrate, the body quickly absorbs MCT oil into the blood, where it can become an immediate energy source. One study shows that consumption of carbohydrate combined with MCT may improve cycling performance during endurance events that last more than two hours.[79] The majority of research, however, does not support MCT supplementation as an ergogenic aid.[80] A downside of MCT supplementation is that its taste may be unacceptable, and it may contribute to gastrointestinal distress.

Pyruvate

Carbohydrate breakdown produces pyruvate and dihydroxyacetone. In animal studies, pyruvate as a dietary supplement or as a partial replacement for dietary carbohydrate enhanced aerobic endurance capacity.[81] The mechanism of action is unclear, but an increased blood glucose concentration, which would spare muscle glycogen, appears to be responsible for the improvements seen after pyruvate–dihydroxyacetone supplementation. These studies looked only at the aerobic endurance of untrained subjects. A study of trained athletes found that pyruvate administered for five weeks had no beneficial effect on anaerobic exercise performance.[82] Pyruvate supplementation has been associated with GI distress. To support the claim that pyruvate enhances endurance, much more research is needed.[83]

soda loading Consumption of bicarbonate (baking soda) to raise blood pH. The intent is to increase the capacity to buffer acids, thus delaying fatigue. Also known as bicarbonate loading.

Sodium Bicarbonate

Some athletes consume sodium bicarbonate (baking soda) in the belief that it will help neutralize the buildup of lactic acid in muscles. Whether **soda loading** actually produces an ergogenic effect is controversial. No improvement in performance has been seen in short-term exercise of 30 to 100 seconds.[84] However, comparative studies that evaluate events lasting from 2 to 10 minutes, where lactic acid buildup is most likely, have shown some positive results related to interval training performance.[85]

Bicarbonate loading can also produce negative effects. Athletes who follow this regimen report side effects such as intestinal discomfort, stomach distress, nausea, cramping, diarrhea, and water retention. While bicarbonate loading is not banned, it does have serious health-related consequences. Bicarbonate loading increases blood alkalinity and influences blood pressure. Anyone with high blood pressure (hypertension) should not bicarbonate-load.

Quick Bites

The Burn to the Finish

The pain a runner feels when approaching the finish line and immediately after the event is called acute muscle soreness. The culprits include a buildup of metabolic byproducts, and tissue edema caused by fluid seeping from the bloodstream into surrounding tissues. The pain and soreness usually disappear within minutes or hours.

Key Concepts: *Numerous dietary supplements, such as caffeine, chromium, CoQ_{10}, and ginseng, are marketed for performance-enhancing effects. However, few have been subjected to rigorous clinical trials or long-term safety evaluation. Athletes should consult a physician before adding dietary supplements to their training regimen.*

Weight and Body Composition

Pete, a bodybuilder, wants to bulk up by gaining 15 pounds of muscle and not fat. Sarah, on the other hand, wants to compete as a lightweight rower and needs to lose 7 pounds. While some athletes struggle to lose weight, others find it nearly impossible to gain weight and muscle mass. Whether intentionally gaining or losing weight, weight change should be accomplished slowly—during the off-season or at the beginning of the season before competition starts.

Body composition and body weight are just two of many factors that affect exercise performance. Body composition can affect strength, agility, and appearance. Body weight can influence speed, endurance, and power. Because body fat adds weight without adding strength, many sports emphasize low body fat percentages. Yet, by themselves, body composition and body weight do not accurately predict athletic performance.[86]

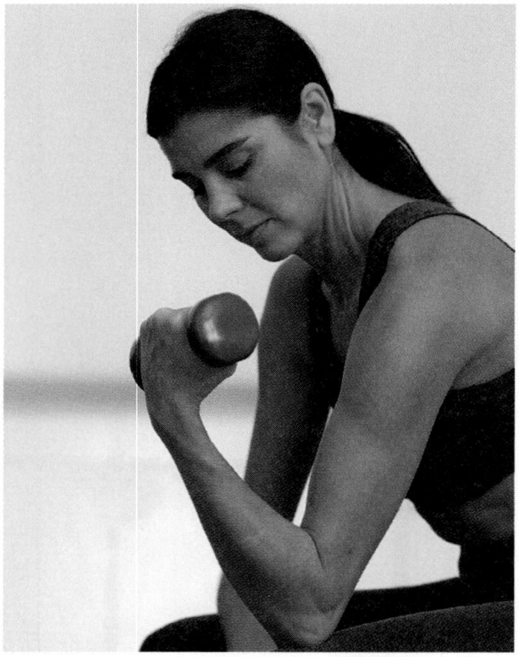

Weight Gain: Build Muscle, Lose Fat

Weight gain is influenced by genetics, stage of adolescent development, gender, body mass, diet, training program, prior resistance training, motivation, and use of supplements and anabolic steroids, among other factors. Complex interactions among these factors make it difficult to predict an athlete's ability to meet a weight goal. However, experience tells us the following:

- Untrained male athletes can gain approximately 3 pounds per month of lean body mass in the early stages of a rigorous resistance-training program. Because of their smaller muscle mass and lean tissue, young women can achieve only 50 to 75 percent of the gains seen in male counterparts.
- Approximately 20 percent of the increase in lean body mass occurs in the first year of resistance training, tapering to 1 to 3 percent in subsequent years. Scientists believe that the rate declines as muscle mass approaches the maximum potential amount determined by genetics.

- Some male athletes of high school age have difficulty gaining muscle mass. These athletes may be in the early stages of the adolescent growth spurt and may lack sufficient levels of the male hormones to stimulate muscle development.

Nutrition plays an important role in increasing lean body mass. Athletes must consume enough calories, along with adequate carbohydrate and protein, to gain the desired muscle mass.[87]

Key Concepts: *Athletes often seek to improve their power and strength by increasing muscle mass. Weight gain as muscle requires increased dietary calories, primarily as carbohydrate, combined with strength training.*

Weight Loss: The Panacea for Optimal Performance?

As the pressure to win increases, many coaches and athletes come to believe that weight loss and lower body fat composition will provide that competitive edge. Athletes strive for lower body weight and lower body fat for three reasons: (1) to improve appearance, especially in aesthetic sports (diving, figure skating, gymnastics), (2) to enhance performance where lower body weight may increase speed (race walking, running, pole vaulting, jumping, cross-country skiing), or (3) to qualify in a lower weight category (wrestling, boxing, and rowing).[88] **Figure 11.15** illustrates the key factors in a successful weight-loss program.

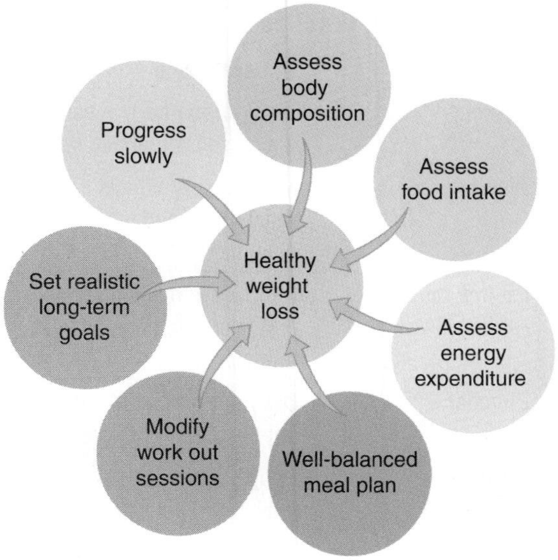

Figure 11.15 **Keys to successful weight loss.** Just as athletes focus on proper training techniques to avoid injury and improve performance, they should focus on proper weight-loss strategies to lose weight and maintain health.

As healthy young adults, men average 15 percent body fat and women average 25 percent.[89] While these averages provide starting points, recommendations for individual athletes must account for genetic background, age, gender, sport, health, and weight history. Male athletes should not go below 5 to 7 percent body fat. For female athletes, current research data suggest a minimum 13 to 17 percent body fat to maintain normal menstrual function, which in turn is important for maintaining bone health.[90]

Keeping accurate food and training records provides information on energy intake and expenditure. The best way for athletes to sustain a safe and sensible loss of body fat is to reduce calorie intake moderately and modify the training program. Experts recommend a modest decrease of about 500 kilocalories per day in total energy intake with an increase in aerobic activity to support a weight loss of 1 to 2 pounds per week.

Beware of "fad" weight-loss methods such as ketogenic diets, high-protein diets, and semistarvation diets. These practices can compromise energy reserves, body composition, and psychological well-being, thus leading to decreased performance and increased health risks. Athletes often are alert to the latest supplements to hit the market. Many claim to accelerate the burning of body fat and augment weight loss. In reality, studies show that most "fat burners" are ineffective or associated with only very modest weight loss in obese subjects.[91]

Quick Bites

What's the Best "Fat-Burning" Exercise?

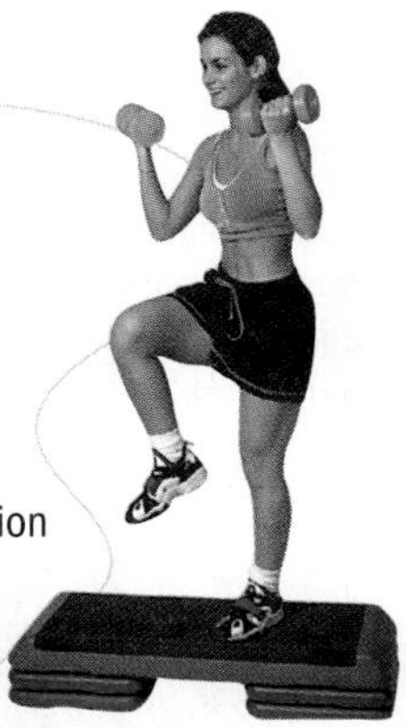

It's a common misconception that low-intensity exercise is superior for "fat burning." Aerobic activities do use a greater percentage of fat as fuel, but it is the total amount of calories expended during exercise that supports increased mobilization of fat in response to a caloric deficit. In terms of actual energy expenditure, higher-intensity exercise requires more calories for a given time period than exercise at a lower intensity. Thus, to lose body fat, the fuel (source of calories) is not as important as the amount of energy expended.

Key Concepts: *Before embarking on a weight-loss program, athletes should carefully evaluate their goals and set a realistic plan for weight loss and maintenance. Safe weight-loss practices include modest changes in food intake accompanied by gradual increases in aerobic activity.*

Weight Loss: Negative Consequences for the Competitive Athlete?

Changing body size and shape can have detrimental effects. An unrealistic perception of optimal body weight and a belief that weight loss is necessary

Table 11.10 Pathogenic Weight-Loss Practices

Behavior	Consequence
Fasting	Loss of lean body mass and decreased metabolic rate
Diet pills	Medical side effects and weight regained when discontinued
Fat-free diets	Deficient in macronutrients and micronutrients; difficult to maintain
Diuretics	Dehydration and electrolyte imbalance; no fat loss
Laxatives	Dehydration; no fat loss; may be addicting
Sweating	Dehydration; heat injury; no fat loss
Excessive exercise	Risk of injury and overtraining
Enemas	Dehydration and GI problems
Fluid restriction	Dehydration; heat injury
Self-induced vomiting	Dehydration; acid–base and electrolyte imbalances; esophageal tears and GI bleeding; erosion of dental enamel and swollen parotid glands

Source: Adapted from Otis CL. Too slim, amenorrheic, fracture-prone: the female athlete triad. *ACSM's Health and Fitness.* 1998;2:2–25.

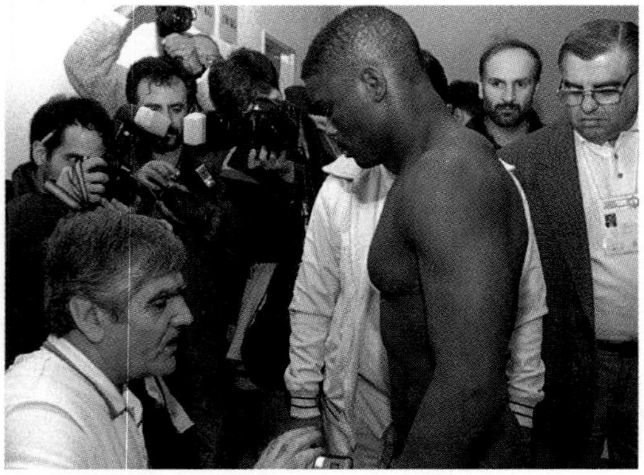

Figure 11.16 Weighing in. The NCAA discourages athletes from reducing their weight through intentional dehydration, a dangerous and potentially deadly practice.

for improved performance can contribute to unhealthy weight-loss practices.[92] Athletes risk medical problems when dieting goes awry.

Making Weight

Wrestlers, weight lifters, boxers, jockeys, rowers, and coxswains face competitive pressures to "make weight" in order to compete or to be certified in a lower weight classification. Such athletes often resort to the **pathogenic** weight-control behaviors summarized in **Table 11.10**. Repeated cycles of rapid weight loss and subsequent regain increase risk of disordered eating, fatigue, psychological distress (anger, anxiety, depression), dehydration, and sudden death.

Studies show that wrestlers, in attempts to gain a competitive advantage, will try to reduce weight a few days before or on the day of competition.[93] Athletes can achieve weight loss up to 22 pounds (10 kilograms) of body water in one day by fasting, restricting fluids, using diuretics, sitting in a sauna, and exercising in a hot environment using rubber suits. A fluid loss of only 2 percent of initial body weight (3 pounds for a 150-pound individual) can decrease athletic performance by elevating heart rate and lowering **cardiac output**. Moderate to severe dehydration (more than 3 to 5 percent of body weight) can be dangerous because of increased core body temperature, electrolyte imbalances, and cardiac and kidney changes. These conditions may result in heat illness, including heat cramps, heat exhaustion, or heatstroke.

Rapid weight loss can have serious health consequences. During one month in 1998, three previously healthy collegiate wrestlers died trying to make weight.[94] These athletes had not only dropped significant weight preseason—more than 20 pounds (9 kilograms)—but also lost between 3.5 to 9 pounds (1.6 to 4 kilograms) in the one to nine hours before their deaths. The wrestlers restricted food and fluid intake. To maximize sweat losses, they wore vapor-impermeable suits under cotton warm-up suits and exercised vigorously in hot environments. Dehydration and **hyperthermia** (elevated body temperature) led to their demise.

Since 1998, the NCAA has revised the guidelines for monitoring weight-loss practices and weigh-in procedures. (See **Figure 11.16**.) This includes educating coaches and athletic trainers about healthy weight-control strategies and limiting the amount of preseason and precompetition weight loss.[95]

Female Athlete Triad

While the majority of female athletes benefit from increased physical activity, there are those who go too far and risk developing a trio of medical problems. (See "Spotlight on Eating Disorders.") In 1991 the American College of Sports Medicine coined the term **female athlete triad** to describe the interaction of disordered eating, amenorrhea, and premature osteoporosis.[96] Female athletes who compete in endurance sports, sports judged by build, and sports with weight classifications are at the greatest risk.

Eating Disorders

Anorexia nervosa appears to be no more prevalent among female athletes than among nonathletes. On the other hand, the prevalence of bulimia nervosa or subclinical eating disorders is higher in athletes.[97]

Amenorrhea

In the general population, 2 to 5 percent of women have **amenorrhea**. However, the prevalence is much higher in athletes.[98] Research indicates that amenorrhea in athletic women is related to the combined effects of increased physical activity, weight loss, low body fat levels, and insufficient energy intake.

Premature Osteoporosis

Health consequences of amenorrhea include premature osteoporosis. Research shows that amenorrheic athletes experience rapid loss of bone mineral density in the spine, which can spread to other parts of the skeleton if amenorrhea continues for a long time.

Treatment involves replacing estrogen, which is low in amenorrheic females. Oral contraceptives are the most common method of estrogen replacement and can also serve as a reliable form of birth control. Calcium supplementation is also recommended. Although bone mineralization may never return to normal in amenorrheic athletes, studies indicate that reducing the intensity of training, improving dietary intake, and increasing body weight can help restore menstruation and increase bone density.[99]

Breaking the Triad

Female athletes at risk are perfectionists, driven to excel in a given sport, who believe that a specific athletic body image is required to excel as an athlete. Some reports estimate as many as 60 percent of female athletes in aesthetic sports (dance, skating, diving, gymnastics) and weight-dependent sports (rowing, martial arts, horse racing) may be at risk.[100]

Screening, referral, and education are keys to preventing the female athlete triad. Prevention and treatment are most successful when they are multidisciplinary efforts—carried out by a team of medical, athletic, nutrition, and mental health experts. Proactive sports education includes reducing the emphasis on body weight, eliminating group weigh-ins, treating each athlete individually, and facilitating healthy weight management. (See **Table 11.11**.)

Key Concepts: *Pathogenic weight-control practices increase risk of dehydration and compromise performance; they may have long-term serious consequences for athletes. The female athlete triad—disordered eating, amenorrhea, and premature osteoporosis—results from excessive weight loss. Often weight loss is driven by unrealistic ideas of appropriate body weight and shape for competition. Education of coaches and athletes is essential to prevent the female athlete triad.*

Quick Bites

Ouch! But I Felt Fine Yesterday. . .

After a bout of heavy exercise, a person may not feel muscle soreness for a day or two. We do not fully understand this painful phenomenon, which is called delayed-onset muscle soreness. Activities that lengthen muscles seem to be the primary cause. The muscles suffer damage with micro-tears in their structure. This leads to an inflammatory response, causing localized muscle pain, swelling, and tenderness.

pathogenic Capable of causing disease.

cardiac output The amount of blood expelled by the heart.

hyperthermia A much higher than normal body temperature.

female athlete triad A syndrome in young female athletes that involves disordered eating, amenorrhea, and lowered bone density.

amenorrhea [A-men-or-Ee-a] Absence or abnormal stoppage of menses in a female; commonly indicated by the absence of three to six consecutive menstrual cycles.

Table 11.11 Combating Eating Disorders in Athletes

De-emphasize body weight. Do not view the athlete's weight as the primary contributor to, or detractor from, athletic performance. Research indicates that athletes can achieve appropriate weight and fitness when the focus is on physical conditioning and strength development, as well as the cognitive and emotional aspects of performance.

Eliminate group weigh-ins. Often viewed as a way to motivate the team, the practice of group weigh-ins can be destructive to people who are struggling with their body image and disordered eating. If there is a legitimate reason for weighing an athlete, explain the reason and weigh the athlete privately.

Treat each athlete individually. Many athletes have an unrealistic perception of what an ideal body weight is, especially in sports for which leanness is considered important. Additionally, athletes may strive for weight and body composition that may be realistic in only a few genetically endowed people. It is important to understand that genetic and biological processes, rather than one's willpower to control food intake, affect a person's weight.

Facilitate healthy weight management. Be sensitive to issues related to weight control and dieting. Because many athletes have limited knowledge of sports nutrition, they resort to pathogenic weight-loss practices. Athletes can benefit from nutrition counseling by a sports nutritionist or a registered dietitian who has experience in working with athletes and disordered eating.

Source: Thompson RA, Sherman RT. Reducing the risk of eating disorders in athletics. *Eating Disorders: Journal of Treatment and Prevention.* 1993;1:65–78. Reproduced by permission of Taylor & Francis, Inc., http://www.routledge-ny.com.

Label [to] Table

Sports drinks are often recommended instead of plain water for those who engage in vigorous physical activity. Their proponents claim that they quickly replenish the body's supply of nutrients, particularly electrolytes. Let's take a look at the Nutrition Facts panel from a popular sports drink, Gatorade.

First, look closely at the serving size—it's not the whole container. This is worth noting because many people might drink the whole container and assume they were getting 50 calories. Not true! The whole container has 200 calories (50 × 4 servings). It's always a good idea to look at the serving size when you are studying a nutrition label.

So what makes this sports drink different from plain (and inexpensive) water? This one has added carbohydrate, sodium, and potassium. Replacing carbohydrate during long workouts prevents complete depletion of glycogen stores. Most sports drinks have between 5 and 8 percent simple sugar. Higher amounts would limit water absorption, and replacement of water is more critical than replacement of glucose.

Sodium and potassium are added to sports drinks to improve taste and help replace electrolytes that are lost during exercise. Gatorade contains 110 milligrams of sodium and 30 milligrams of potassium. For many athletes, and certainly for recreational exercisers, water really is the best fluid replacer. Although both sodium and potassium are lost in sweat, water is lost in greater quantities. Sports drinks have been shown to benefit only athletes who are strenuously exercising for longer than an hour. With prolonged exercise and sweat losses, large losses of electrolytes can make a person dizzy and weak, and may even lead to heat exhaustion or heatstroke.

The next time you head out for a bike ride, consider how long you'll be gone and how strenuous your ride will be, and then consider whether you'll need a sports drink. Also consider your personal taste—if a flavored sports drink will encourage you to replace fluids more than plain water will, that may be an important advantage. Just don't forget to read the label!

Nutrition Facts

Serving Size 8 fl oz (240mL)
Servings Per Container 4

Amount Per Serving	
Calories 50	
	% Daily Value*
Total Fat 0g	**0%**
Sodium 110mg	**5%**
Potassium 30mg	**1%**
Total Carbohydrate 14g	**5%**
Sugars 14g	
Protein 0g	

Not a significant source of Calories from Fat, Saturated Fat, Cholesterol, Dietary Fiber, Vitamin A, Vitamin C, Calcium, Iron.

* Percent Daily Values are based on a 2,000 calorie diet.

LEARNING Portfolio chapter 11

Key Terms

	page		page
aerobic endurance	435	ginseng	451
amenorrhea [A-men-or-Ee-a]	455	glycogen loading	437
anabolic steroids	449	hyperthermia	455
androstenedione (andro)	449	lactic acid energy system	431
ATP–CP energy system	430	muscle fibers	435
carbohydrate loading	437	NCAA	449
cardiac output	455	oxygen energy system	431
coenzyme Q_{10} (CoQ_{10})	450	palatable	446
creatine	450	pathogenic	455
creatine phosphate	430	perceived exertion	445
dehydroepiandrosterone (DHEA)	449	phosphocreatine	430
diuresis	442	skeletal muscles	433
ergogenic aids	448	slow-twitch (ST) fibers	435
fast-twitch (FT) fibers	435	soda loading	452
female athlete triad	455	sports anemia	443

Study Points

- Exercise promotes health and reduces risk of chronic diseases.
- The ACSM defines physical fitness as "the ability to perform moderate to vigorous levels of physical activity without undue fatigue and the capability of maintaining this level of activity throughout life."
- The muscular system contains three types of muscles: smooth, cardiac, and skeletal. There are two types of muscle fibers: slow-twitch (ST) and fast-twitch (FT). ST fibers have high aerobic endurance; FT fibers are optimized to perform anaerobically. Your body depends predominantly on ST fibers for low-intensity events and FT fibers for highly explosive events.
- The body uses three systems to produce energy for physical activity: (1) the ATP–CP energy system (anaerobic), (2) the lactic acid energy system (anaerobic), and (3) the oxygen energy system (aerobic).
- Anaerobic and aerobic metabolism work together to fuel all types of exercise. During the early minutes of high-intensity exercise, the ATP–CP energy system and the lactic acid energy system provide most of the energy. Endurance activities are fueled primarily by the metabolism of glucose and fatty acids in the oxygen energy system.
- Training improves use of fat as a fuel by enhancing oxygen delivery and increasing the number of mitochondria in muscle.
- Carbohydrates should be the major source of energy in the athlete's diet and should come from complex carbohydrates, which can provide fiber, iron, and B vitamins. Athletes need carbohydrates so that muscle glycogen stores and blood glucose concentrations will be adequate for training and competitive events. Likewise, carbohydrates are necessary to replenish glycogen stores after intense exercise.
- Carbohydrate loading is a process of reducing activity while increasing carbohydrate intake to maximize glycogen stores.
- Fat is a major fuel source for exercise, but high fat intake is not required or recommended.
- Protein needs of athletes are higher than for sedentary individuals, but generally athletes who consume adequate amounts of energy get enough protein. High-protein foods include low-fat dairy products, egg whites, lean beef and pork, chicken, turkey, fish, and legumes.
- Other nutrients important to the athlete's diet include B vitamins, iron, zinc, and calcium.
- Water is the most essential nutrient and is easily lost from the body with heavy sweating. Replacing fluid with water or sports drinks is important to prevent dehydration. Optimal sports drinks provide energy and electrolytes in a palatable solution that is rapidly absorbed.
- Athletes who are still growing have even higher energy and nutrient needs to support both physical activity and normal growth.

- **Many dietary supplements are promoted as ergogenic aids—substances that enhance performance. Few well-controlled studies on their efficacy and safety have been done, however.**
- **Many athletes strive to either gain or lose weight in order to improve performance. In both cases, realistic goals and gradual changes are necessary for long-term success. Gains in muscle mass require increased calorie intake and weight training. Successful weight loss requires modest reductions in energy intake and increases in aerobic activity.**
- **Weight-control efforts that involve fasting, excessive sweating, purging, diuretics, or laxatives are detrimental to health.**
- **Disordered eating accompanied by amenorrhea and premature osteoporosis is known as the female athlete triad.**

Study Questions

Answers can be found at nutrition.jbpub.com/discovering.

1. **What are muscle fibers and what are the two major types?**
2. **List the two anaerobic and one aerobic energy systems that your body uses to generate energy during exercise. When is each active during exercise?**
3. **What are the general recommendations for an athlete (compared with a nonathlete) in terms of the percentage of calories from carbohydrates, proteins, and fats?**
4. **What is carbohydrate loading?**
5. **How do protein recommendations for athletes vary from those for nonathletes?**
6. **Name three minerals that are of concern for athletes because they may not consume enough.**
7. **What is sports anemia and why does it happen? How does it compare with other anemias?**
8. **Define the term *ergogenic aid*. Is there a clear, research-based answer to whether ergogenic supplements work?**
9. **What is the nutritional strategy for athletes who want to gain muscle mass?**

[*Try*] This

The Popularity of Ergogenic Aids

Take a trip to a health food store to see just how popular (and expensive!) ergogenic aids are. Try to locate each of the supplements listed in this chapter. Are they all available? What are their prices? Ask a salesperson what he or she knows about each of them. Do their answers match what you read in the text?

Commit to Get Fit

Do you meet the American College of Sports Medicine's (ACSM) definition of fitness? Answer the questions below with a yes or no.

1. Do you exercise consistently three to five days per week?
2. When you exercise, does it include 20 to 60 minutes (20 minutes for intense activity and 60 minutes for less intense activity) of continuous aerobic activity?
3. Does your type of exercise use large muscle groups? Can you maintain it? Is it rhythmical and aerobic?
4. Does part of your activity include strength training of a moderate intensity (a minimum of one set of 8 to 12 repetitions of 8 to 10 exercises) at least two days per week?

If you answered no to any of these questions, you are not following the ACSM's suggestions to develop and maintain cardiorespiratory and muscular fitness. Choose a question to which you answered no and set a specific goal to include that factor in your exercise routine.

What About *Bobbie?*

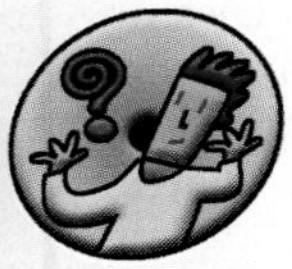

Imagine that Bobbie is training to do a marathon at the end of the semester. She has been exercising consistently and increasing her endurance and mileage times. She hasn't spent much time focusing on her diet, though, and wants to know what changes she could make to improve her nutrition and, therefore, performance. Assume that her current diet meets her calorie needs. How would you compare Bobbie's diet to the guidelines you read about in this chapter?

Macronutrient Contributions

Start with her overall contribution of carbohydrates, proteins, and fats. Compare Bobbie's macronutrient intake to the general sports nutrition recommendations.

	Bobbie's	Recommendations
Carbohydrates	*48%*	*60 to 70%*
Proteins	*16%*	*~ 15%*
Fats	*36%*	*~ 20%*

As you can see, Bobbie's diet is higher in fat and lower in carbohydrates than is recommended for an athlete. If she were to reduce her intake of cream cheese, mayonnaise, cookies, and salad dressing and increase her fruits, vegetables, and whole grains, her diet would come closer to the recommendations for sports nutrition.

Protein

Now let's calculate her protein need based on the athlete's guideline and see if she's consuming enough to maintain lean muscle mass and recover well from exercise.

The protein RDA for an athlete is approximately 1.2 to 1.4 grams per kilogram of body weight. Bobbie weighs 155 pounds, so her RDA is as follows:

$$155 \text{ lb} \div 2.2 \text{ kg per lb} = 70.45 \text{ kg}$$

$$70.45 \text{ kg} \times 1.3 \text{ g/kg} = 91.6 \text{ g protein}$$

Bobbie's protein intake was 97 grams, which makes her protein intake a near perfect match for her needs.

Minerals

Look at the two primary minerals that might be inadequate in diets of athletes, especially female athletes. Below is a comparison of Bobbie's calcium and iron intake and her daily recommendations.

	Bobbie's	Recommendations
Calcium	*745 mg*	*1,000 mg*
Iron	*20 mg*	*8 mg*

As you can see, Bobbie did a very good job of consuming iron, but she is short of her calcium need. If she were to replace the diet soda she had at lunch with 1 cup of nonfat or 1% milk, her intake of calcium would rise to just above 1,000 milligrams. Or she could change her afternoon snack of chips and salsa to a cup of yogurt to accomplish the same thing.

Hydration

Check out Bobbie's intake of fluids in Chapter 1. How many ounces of plain water did she consume? That's right, she had only 16 ounces! Bobbie is making the same mistake that many athletes do—she's not drinking enough water. Poor hydration status will probably affect her performance adversely. Bobbie's biggest change should be to increase her fluid intake. She'd be smart to drink at least 12 to 16 ounces of caffeine-free fluids at all of her meals and snacks. This way she'll stay hydrated and be able to perform at an optimal level!

References

1 American College of Sports Medicine. Position stand: the recommended quantity and quality of exercise for developing and maintaining cardiorespiratory and muscular fitness and flexibility in healthy adults. *Med Sci Sports Exerc.* 1998;30: 975–991.

2 Ibid.

3 Position of the American Dietetic Association, Dietitians of Canada, and the American College of Sports Medicine: nutrition and athletic performance. *J Am Diet Assoc.* 2000;100: 1543–1556.

4 Connolly-Schoonen J. Physiology of anaerobic and aerobic exercise. In: Rosenbloom CA, ed. *Sports Nutrition.* 3rd ed. Chicago: American Dietetic Association; 2000.

5 Wilmore JH, Costill DL. *Physiology of Sport and Exercise.* 2nd ed. Champaign, IL: Human Kinetics; 1999.

6 Brooks GA, Fahey TD, White T. *Exercise Physiology.* Mountain View, CA: Mayfield; 1996:705.

7 Brown GC. Speed limits. *The Sciences.* 2000;40(5):32–37.

8 McArdle WD, Katch FI, Katch VL. *Essentials of Exercise Physiology.* Baltimore, MD: Lippincott Williams & Wilkins; 1999.

9 Ibid.

10 Position of the American Dietetic Association, Dietitians of Canada, and the American College of Sports Medicine: nutrition and athletic performance. Op. cit.

11 Wilmore JH, Costill DL. Op. cit.

12 Brown GC. *The Energy of Life.* New York: Simon & Schuster; 1999.

13 Andersen JL, Scherling P, Saltin B. Muscle, genes and athletic performance. *Scientific American.* 2000;283(3):48–55.

14 Berning JR, Steen SN. *Nutrition for Sport and Exercise.* 2nd ed. Gaithersburg, MD: Aspen; 1998.

15 Hawley J, Dennis SC, Lindsay FH, Noakes TD. Nutritional practices of athletes: are they sub-optimal? *J Sports Sci.* 1995;13(suppl):S75–S87.

16 Benardot D, Thompson WR. Energy from food for physical activity: enough and on time. *ACSM's Health & Fitness.* 1999;3:14–18.

17 Vinci DM. Effective nutrition support programs for college athletes. *Int J Sports Nutr.* 1998;8:308–320.

18 Position of the American Dietetic Association, Dietitians of Canada, and the American College of Sports Medicine: nutrition and athletic performance. Op. cit.

19 Burke LM, Cox GR, Culmmings NK, Desbrow B. Guidelines for daily carbohydrate intake: do athletes achieve them? *Sports Med.* 2001;31:267–299.

20 Coleman EJ. Carbohydrate and exercise. In: Rosenbloom CA. Op. cit.

21 Shattuck D. Sports nutritionists fuel the competitive edge. *J Am Diet Assoc.* 2001;101:517–518.

22 Coleman EJ. Op. cit.

23 Ibid.

24 Walberg-Rankin J. Dietary carbohydrate as an ergogenic aid for prolonged and brief competitions in sport. *Int J Sport Nutr.* 1995;5:513–528.

25 Position of the American Dietetic Association, Dietitians of Canada, and the American College of Sports Medicine: nutrition and athletic performance. Op. cit.

26 Ibid.

27 Walton P, Rhodes EC. Glycemic index and optimal performance. *Sports Med.* 1997;23:164–172.

28 Position of the American Dietetic Association, Dietitians of Canada, and the American College of Sports Medicine: nutrition and athletic performance. Op. cit.

29 Ivy JL, Lee MC, Broznick JT, Reed MJ. Muscle glycogen storage after different amounts of carbohydrate ingestion. *J Appl Physiol.* 1988;65:2018–2023.

30 Storlie J. The art of refueling. *Training and Conditioning.* 1998;8:29–35.

31 Coleman EJ. Op. cit.

32 Hawley J, Burke L. *Peak Performance: Training and Nutritional Strategies for Sport.* Leonards, Australia: Allen & Unwin; 1998.

33 Position of the American Dietetic Association, Dietitians of Canada, and the American College of Sports Medicine: nutrition and athletic performance. Op. cit.

34 Roy B, Tarnopolosky M, MacDougall J, et al. Effect of glucose supplement timing on protein metabolism after resistance training. *J Appl Physiol.* 1997;82:1882–1888.

35 Ibid.

36 Kleiner SM, Bazarre TL, Ainsworth BE. Nutritional status of nationally ranked elite bodybuilders. *Int J Sport Nutr.* 1994;4:54–69.

37 Lemon PWR. Effects of exercise on dietary protein requirements. *Int J Sports Nutr.* 1998;8:426–447.

38 Clark N, Rosenbloom, C. To zone or not to zone: people respond to the Zone diet plan. *SCAN'S PULSE.* 1997;16:5–7.

39 Food and Nutrition Board. *Recommended Dietary Allowances.* 10th ed. Washington, DC: National Academy Press; 1989.

40 Carroll C. Protein and exercise. In: Rosenbloom CA. Op. cit.

41 Lemon PW. Dietary protein requirements in athletes. *J Nutr Biochem.* 1997;8:52.

42 Hawley J, Burke L. Op. cit.

43 Tarnopolosky MA, Atkinson SA, MacDougall JD, et al. Evaluation of protein requirements for trained strength athletes. *J Appl Physiol.* 1992;73:1986.

44 Lemon PW. Op. cit.

45 Hargreaves MH, Snow R. Amino acids and endurance exercise. *Int J Sport Nutr Exerc Metab.* 2001;11:133–145.

46 Storlie J. The art of refueling. *Training & Conditioning,* 1998;8:29–30, 32, 34–35; and Tipton KD, Wolfe RR. Exercise, protein metabolism, and muscle growth. *Int J Sport Nutr Exerc Metab.* 2001;11:109–132.

47 Storlie J. From fork to muscle. *Training & Conditioning.* 1998;8:26, 28–29, 32–33.

48 Clarkson PM, Haymes EM. Exercise and mineral status of athletes: calcium, magnesium, phosphorus, and iron. *Med Sci Sports Exerc.* 1995;27:831–843.

49 Institute of Medicine, Food and Nutrition Board. *Dietary Reference Intakes for Vitamin A, Vitamin K, Arsenic, Boron, Chromium, Copper, Iodine, Iron, Manganese, Molybdenum,*

Nickel, Silicon, Vanadium, and Zinc. Washington, DC: National Academy Press; 2001.

50 Fogelholm M. Indicators of vitamin and mineral status in athletes' blood: a review. *Int J Sport Nutr.* 1995;5:267–284.

51 Zhu YI, Haas JD. Iron depletion without anemia and physical performance in young women. *Am J Clin Nutr.* 1997;66: 334–341.

52 Guyton AC, Hall JE. *Textbook of Medical Physiology.* 10th ed. Philadelphia: W.B. Saunders; 2000.

53 Convertino VA, Armstrong LE, Coyle EF, et al. American College of Sports Medicine position stand: exercise and fluid replacement. *Med Sci Sports Exerc.* 1996;28:i–vii.

54 Ibid.

55 Burke LM. Nutritional needs for exercise in heat. *Comp Biochem Physiol A Mol Integr Physiol.* 2001;128:735–748.

56 Thompson JL. Energy balance in young athletes. *Int J Sports Nutr.* 1998;8:160–174.

57 Ibid.

58 Ahrendt DM. Ergogenic aids: counseling the athlete. *Am Fam Physician.* 2001;63:913–922.

59 Skinner R, Coleman E, Rosenbloom O. Ergogenic aids. In: Rosenbloom CA. Op. cit.

60 Ibid.

61 Clarkson PM, Rawson ES. Nutritional supplements to increase muscle mass. *Crit Rev Food Sci Nutr.* 1999;39: 317–328; and Kreider RB. Dietary supplements and the promotion of muscle growth with resistance exercise. *Sports Med.* 1999;27:97–110.

62 King DS, Sharp RL, Vukovich MD, et al. Effect of oral androstenedione on serum testosterone and adaptations to resistance training in young men. *JAMA.* 1999;281: 2020–2028; and Leder BZ, Longcope C, Catlin DH, et al. Oral androstenedione administration and serum testosterone concentrations in young men. *JAMA.* 2000;283: 779–782.

63 King DS, Sharp RL, Vukovich MD, et al. Op. cit.

64 Sarubin A. *The Health Professional's Guide to Popular Dietary Supplements.* Chicago: American Dietetic Association; 2000.

65 Spriet L. Caffeine and performance. *Int J Sport Nutr.* 1995;5(suppl):S84–S99.

66 Kanter M, Williams M. Antioxidants, carnitine and choline as putative ergogenic aids. *Int J Sport Nutr.* 1995;5(suppl): S120–S131.

67 Ibid.

68 Campbell WW, Joseph LJ, Davey SL, et al. Effects of resistance training and chromium picolinate on body composition and skeletal muscle in older men. *J Appl Physiol.* 1999;86:29–39.

69 Sarubin A. Op. cit.

70 Toler SM. Creatine is an ergogen for anaerobic exercise. *Nutr Rev.* 1997;55:21–25.

71 Engelhardt M, Neumann G, Berbalk A, Reuter I. Creatine supplementation in endurance sports. *Med Sci Sports Exerc.* 1998;30:1123.

72 Skare OC, Skalberg AR. Creatine supplementation improves sprint performance in male sprinters. *Scand J Med Sci Sports.* 2001;11:96–102.

73 American College of Sports Medicine. *Current comment: Creatine supplementation.* Indianapolis, IN: American College of Sports Medicine; 1998.

74 Williams MH. *The Ergogenics Edge: Pushing the Limits of Sports Performance.* Champaign, IL: Human Kinetics; 1998.

75 Engles HJ, Wirth JC. No ergogenic effects of ginseng (*Panax ginseng* C.A. Meyer) during graded maximal aerobic exercise. *J Am Diet Assoc.* 1997:97;1110–1115.

76 Sarubin A. Op. cit.

77 Engles HJ, Wirth JC. Op. cit.

78 Ibid.

79 Van Zyl CG, Lambert EV, Hawley JA, et al. Effects of medium-chain triglyceride ingestion on fuel metabolism and cycling performance. *J Appl Physiol.* 1996;80:2217–2225.

80 Skinner R, Coleman M, Rosenbloom C. Op. cit.

81 Ivy JL. Effect of pyruvate and dihydroxyacetone on metabolism and aerobic endurance capacity. *Med Sci Sports Exerc.* 1998;6:837.

82 Stone MH, Sanborn K, Smith LL, et al. Effects of in-season (5 weeks) creatine and pyruvate supplementation on anaerobic performance and body composition in American football players. *Int J Sport Nutr.* 1999;9:146–165.

83 Sarubin A. Op. cit.

84 Horswill CA. Effects of bicarbonate, citrate, and phosphate loading on performance. *Int J Sport Nutr.* 1995;5(suppl): S111–S119.

85 Ibid.

86 Houtkooper LB. Body composition. In: Manore MM, Thompson JL. *Sport Nutrition for Health and Performance.* Champaign, IL: Human Kinetics; 2000:199–219.

87 Storlie J. From fork to muscle. Op. cit.

88 McArdle WD, Katch FI, Katch VL. Op. cit.

89 Ibid.

90 Ibid.

91 Clarkson PM. The skinny on weight loss supplements and drugs. *ACSM's Health & Fitness.* 1998;2:18–26, 55.

92 Thompson JL. Op. cit.

93 Metz G. The NCAA weighs in. *Training & Conditioning.* 1998;8:16–17, 19, 21–23.

94 Rapid weight loss in wrestlers results in death. *MMWR.* 1998;47(6):105–108.

95 Metz G. Op. cit.

96 Otis CL, Drinkwater B, Johnson M, et al. American College of Sports Medicine. Position stand: the female athlete triad. *Med Sci Sports Exerc.* 1997;29:i–ix.

97 Sundgot-Borgen J. Risk and trigger factors for the developing of eating disorders in female elite athletes. *Med Sci Sports Exerc.* 1994;4:414–419.

98 Smith AD. The female athlete triad: causes, diagnosis, and treatment. *Physician Sportsmed.* 1996;24:67–70, 75–76, 86.

99 Dueck CA, Manore MM, Matt KS. Role of energy balance in athletic menstrual dysfunction. *Int J Sport Nutr.* 1996;6: 165–190.

100 Otis CL, Drinkwater B, Johnson M, et al. Op. cit.

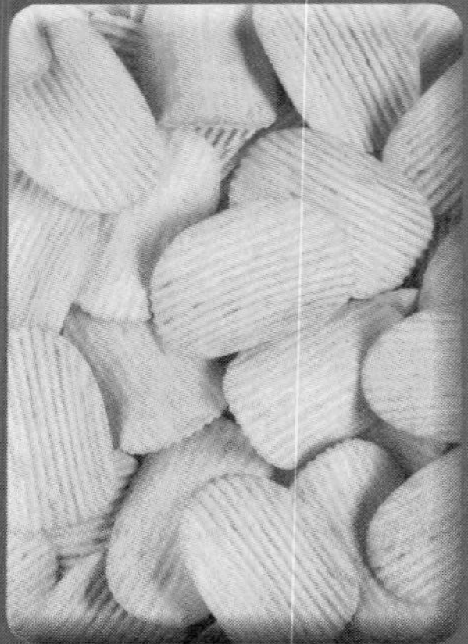
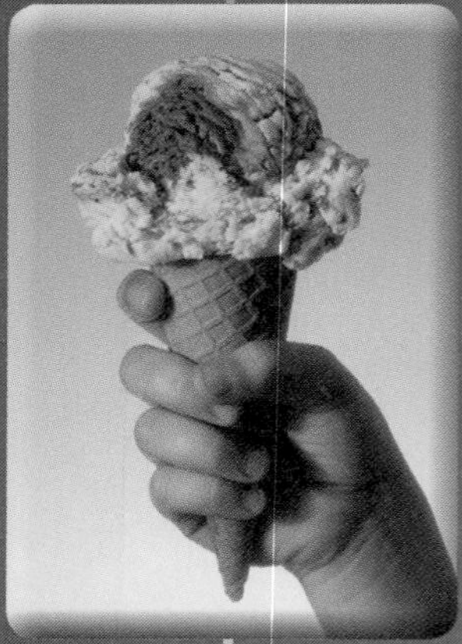
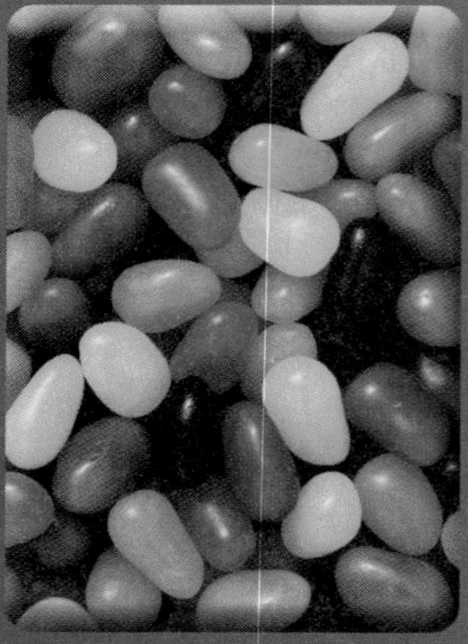
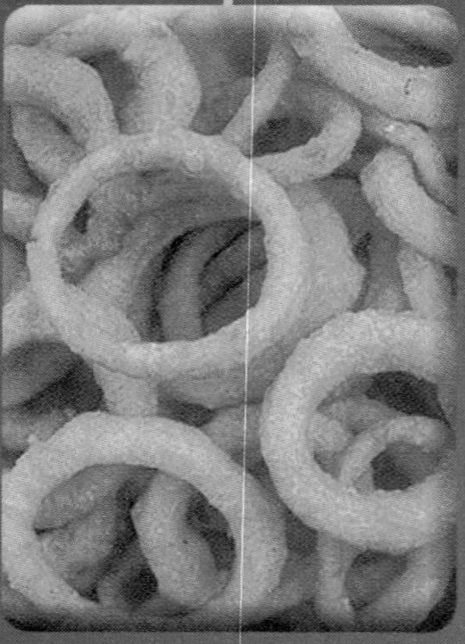
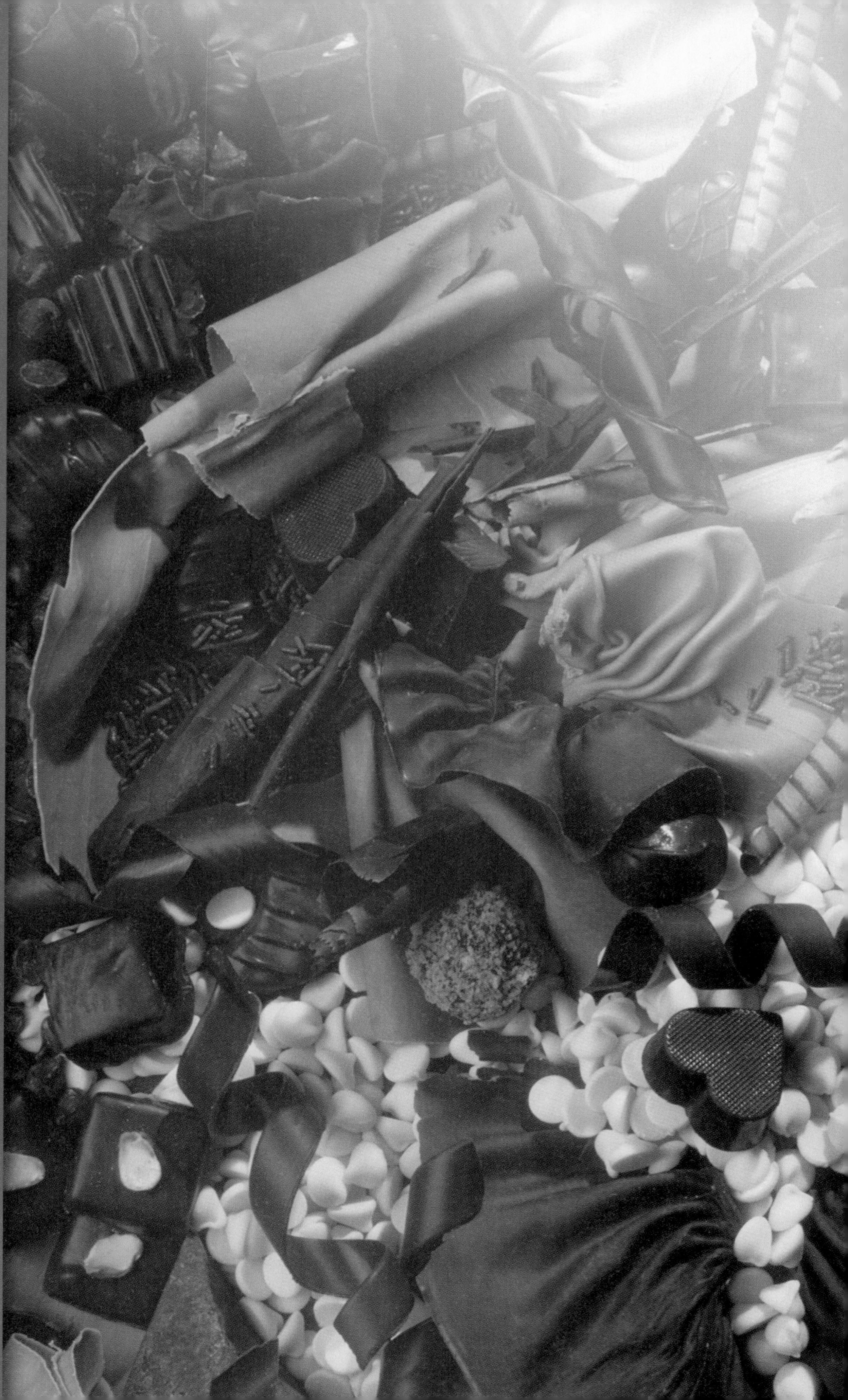

Spotlight on

Eating Disorders

Think About It

1. What's your view of the ideal female body?
2. When should you be concerned about obsessive dieting?
3. Given the right situation, what foods are you likely to binge on?
4. How many magazines do you read that promote dieting or encourage thinness?

Fyi for your Information

This chapter's FYI box includes practical information on the following topic:

- Diary of an Eating Disorder

www

The Web site for this book offers many useful tools and is a great source for additional nutrition information for both students and instructors. For information on eating disorders, visit the site at **nutrition.jbpub.com/discovering.** You'll find exercises that explore the following topics:

- Age and Eating Disorders
- Body Image
- The Genetics of Eating Disorders
- Cultural Roles

What About Bobbie?

Track the choices Bobbie is making with the EatRight Analysis software.

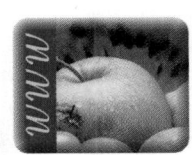

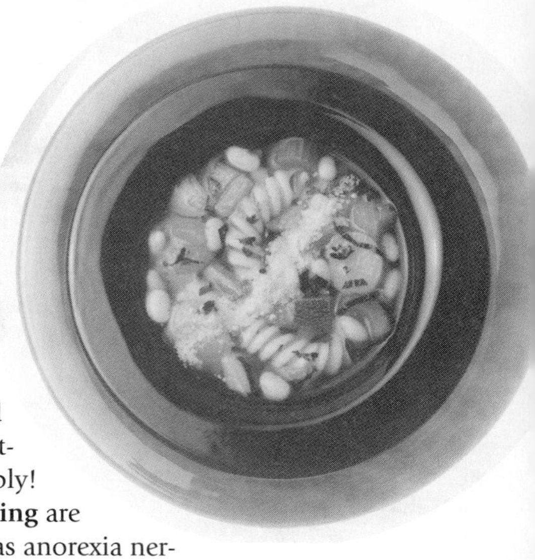

A gaunt, hollow-cheeked college freshman confides to her roommate that she feels chubby. After an enormous lunch, a secretary works her way through a bag of cookies, followed by a box of chocolates. A swimming champion who obsesses over every calorie becomes concerned that she hasn't had a period in two months. Disordered eating? Very likely! Eating disorder? Possibly!

Eating disorders and **disordered eating** are not the same. An eating disorder such as anorexia nervosa or bulimia nervosa is an illness that can seriously interfere with daily activities. Disordered eating is usually a temporary or mild change in eating patterns. Although it can occur after an illness or stressful event, it often is related to a dietary change intended to improve one's health or appearance. Unless disordered eating persists, it rarely requires professional intervention. Disordered eating, however, can lead to an eating disorder.

For most of us, eating is a pleasure. For people with an eating disorder, however, food is a source of continual stress and anxiety. (See **Figure SED.1**.) Eating disorders require professional intervention. They include a spectrum of emotional illnesses ranging from self-imposed starvation to chronic binge eating. These illnesses involve severe distortions of the eating process, with physical consequences that are often life-threatening.[1]

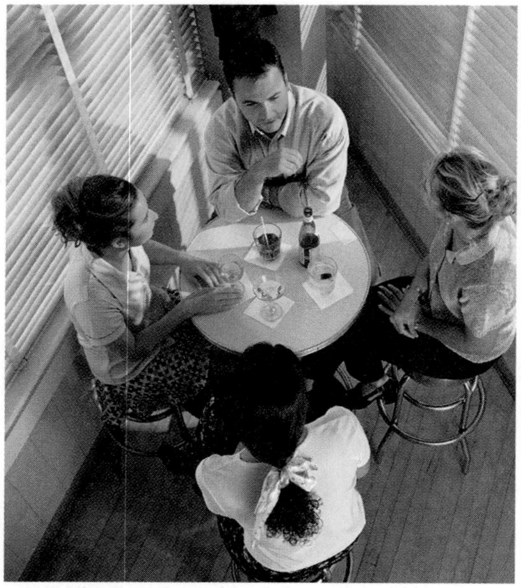

Figure SED.1 **Can you spot the person with the eating disorder?** Some people with eating disorders have normal body weights and are difficult to spot.

Most of us have eaten to the point of discomfort on particular occasions. (Thanksgiving dinner comes to mind.) And many of us have cut out desserts at one time or another, hoping to fit into a special outfit or to lose weight for an athletic event or job interview. But stuffing yourself at a holiday meal or going on an *occasional* diet does not constitute an eating disorder. According to the *Manual of Clinical Dietetics*, a defining characteristic of an eating disorder is a persistent inability to eat in moderation.[2]

eating disorders A spectrum of abnormal eating patterns that eventually may endanger a person's health or increase the risk for other diseases. Generally, psychological factors play a key role.

disordered eating An abnormal change in eating pattern related to an illness, a stressful event, or a desire to improve one's health or appearance. If it persists it may lead to an eating disorder.

anorexia nervosa [an-or-EX-ee-uh ner-VOH-sah] An eating disorder marked by prolonged decrease of appetite and refusal to eat, leading to self-starvation and excessive weight loss. It results in part from a distorted body image and intense fear of becoming fat, often linked to social pressures.

body image A person's mental concept of his or her physical appearance, constructed from many different influences.

The Eating Disorder Continuum

The 1994 edition of the American Psychiatric Association's *Diagnostic and Statistical Manual of Mental Disorders (DSM-IV)* divides eating disorders into three categories, with small but significant areas of overlap. These categories form a continuum, with self-starvation at one end and compulsive overeating at the other. (See **Figure SED.2**.) **Anorexia nervosa** is at the self-starvation end of the continuum. Anorexia is a self-imposed starvation syndrome that is triggered by a severely distorted **body image**. People with anorexia are at war with their bodies. Even when they are dangerously underweight, people with anorexia typically see themselves as fat. Severely restricted food

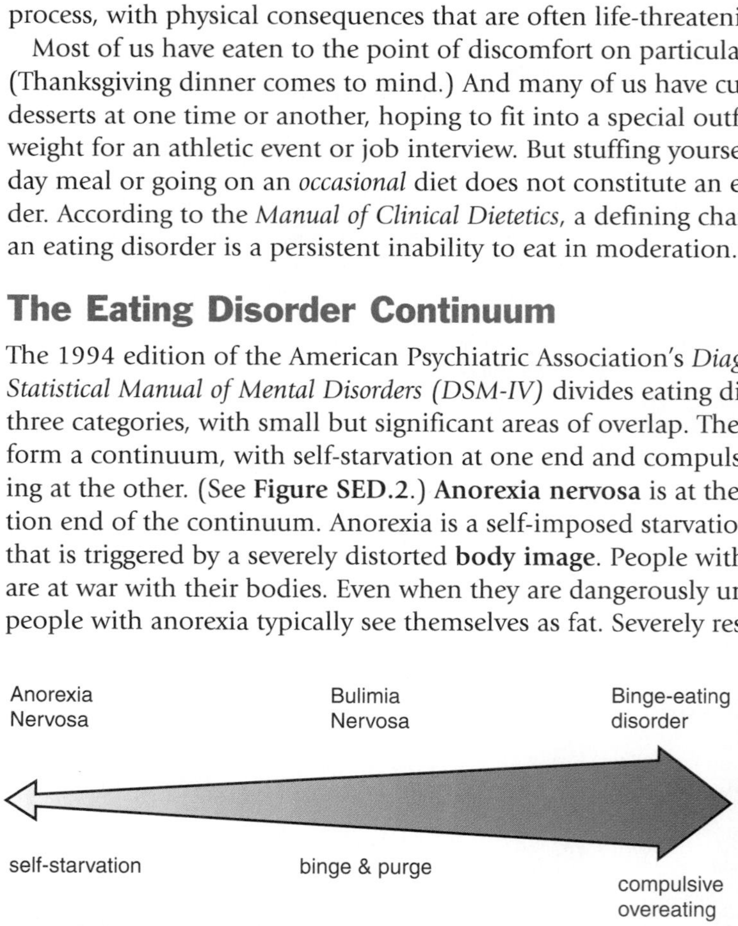

Figure SED.2 **The eating disorder continuum.**

intake is another symptom of anorexia nervosa. It may also involve purging (self-induced vomiting) and excessive exercise. Anorexia is most prevalent among adolescent females.

At the opposite end of the continuum is **binge-eating disorder**, formerly known as **compulsive overeating**. People with this disorder chronically consume massive quantities of food. Sufferers are typically obese; however, not all obese people binge eat. Diagnosis of binge-eating disorder is based on a person having an average of two binge-eating episodes per week for six months. Such episodes often are triggered by emotions such as frustration, anger, depression, and anxiety.[3]

In the middle of the continuum is **bulimia nervosa**. Like those with binge-eating disorder, people with bulimia nervosa compulsively gorge themselves. Like those with anorexia, people with bulimia desperately want to be thin and resort to purging to reach this goal. After gorging, people with bulimia often become disgusted with themselves and terrified of getting fat. To compensate, bulimic people make themselves vomit, use laxatives, exercise excessively, and take other action to avoid gaining weight. It is important to realize that few people who suffer from eating disorders are purely anorexic, bulimic, or binge eaters. Many swing from one disordered eating pattern to another, alternately starving and gorging themselves. People may suffer from binge-eating disorder at one point in their lives, and anorexia or bulimia at another.[4] **Table SED.1** shows the diagnostic criteria for these eating disorders.

binge-eating disorder An eating disorder marked by repeated episodes of binge eating and a feeling of loss of control. The diagnosis is based on a person's having an average of at least two binge-eating episodes per week for six months.

compulsive overeating See *binge-eating disorder.*

bulimia nervosa [bull-EEM-ee-uh] An eating disorder marked by consumption of large amounts of food at one time (binge eating) followed by a behavior such as self-induced vomiting, use of laxatives, excessive exercise, fasting, or other practices to avoid weight gain.

History of a Modern Malady

Contrary to public perception, eating disorders are not New Age diseases. In fact, the first formal report of anorexia nervosa appeared in the medical literature in the 1870s.[5] Informal reports of a "voluntary starvation syndrome" were published as early as 1694.[6] And some nutritional anthropologists argue that eating disorders can be traced to even more ancient times. During the Middle Ages, for instance, early Christian ascetics, who led lives of contemplation and rigorous self-denial, shunned worldly pleasures, including food, to show obedience and become closer to God. These people alternated periods of semistarvation with frequent fasts. Was this anorexia disguised as religious devotion? Some scholars think so.[7]

Early Greeks and Romans, in contrast, exhibited exaggerated bingeing and purging behavior at banquets that lasted for days. Guests gorged to the point of physical pain, then tickled the back of their throats with feathers to induce vomiting. Once their stomachs were empty, they returned to the table. Rather than finding this behavior repulsive or shameful, the ancient Romans glorified it. They even built areas known as vomitoriums into their banquet halls.[8] Interestingly, in ancient Rome only upper-class males attended banquets.[9]

Some scholars contend these ancient Romans had bulimia. Others disagree, arguing that the Roman men ate for pleasure in the company of others and purged only so they could rejoin the feast. In contrast, modern bulimia sufferers are usually females who gorge and purge in isolation—and in hopes of achieving an unrealistic cultural standard of beauty. Furthermore, today's bulimia sufferers invariably feel shame, low self-esteem, and even self-hate connected with their eating habits.

Although eating disorders are not an exclusively modern malady, it's clear that eating disorders have become increasingly common in the past four decades. A British model named Twiggy, nicknamed for her sticklike

Table SED.1 Diagnostic Criteria for Eating Disorders

Anorexia nervosa

- Body weight < 85% of expected weight (or BMI ≤ 17.5)
- Intense fear of weight gain
- Inaccurate perception of own body size, weight, or shape
- Amenorrhea (in females after menarche)

Bulimia nervosa

- Recurrent binge eating (at least two times per week for three months)
- Recurrent purging, excessive exercise, or fasting (at least two times per week for three months)
- Excessive concern about body weight or shape
- Absence of anorexia nervosa

Binge-eating disorder

- Recurrent binge eating (at least two times per week for six months)
- Marked distress with at least three of the following:
  - Eating very rapidly
  - Eating until uncomfortably full
  - Eating when not hungry
  - Eating alone
  - Feeling disgusted or guilty after a binge
- No recurrent purging, no excessive exercising, and no fasting
- Absence of anorexia nervosa

Source: Becker AE, Grinspoon SK, Klibanski A, Herzog DB. Eating disorders. *N Engl J Med.* 1999;340(14): 1092–1098. Adapted with permission.

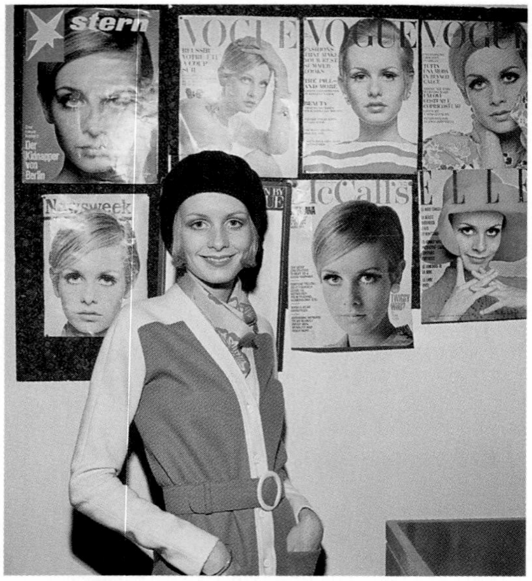

Figure SED.3 **Eye of the beholder.** In the 1960s, Twiggy became the new role model for young women who wanted to be thin and glamorous.

appearance, ushered in the epidemic in the early 1960s. Fashion magazine stories reported that she subsisted on water, lettuce, and a single daily serving of steak and that she had learned to suppress her hunger pangs. Rather than condemn these clearly dangerous eating habits, the magazines held Twiggy up as a model of self-control for girls and young women. (See **Figure SED.3**.)

Our national denial regarding the dangers of semistarvation ended abruptly and dramatically in 1983 with the highly publicized death of 32-year-old pop singer Karen Carpenter from complications of anorexia. Widespread media coverage of her death highlighted the lethal potential of eating disorders and made the terms anorexia and bulimia household words. Soon, other stars of film, TV, sports, and the fashion world revealed that they, too, suffered from eating disorders and described the physical, emotional, and social damage these diseases caused in their own lives. But, ironically, increased visibility and knowledge have not stemmed the tide of eating disorders. To the contrary, the prevalence of eating disorders and disordered eating continues to increase.[10]

Key Concepts: *Eating disorders are ancient conditions that have become alarmingly common in industrialized countries, particularly the United States. Eating disorders range from the self-starvation of anorexia nervosa to the compulsive overeating of binge-eating disorder.*

No Simple Causes

Certain people appear to have a predisposition to eating disorders. This vulnerability may be psychological. A person who suffers from depression or obsessive-compulsive disorder, for example, may have an increased risk of developing an eating disorder. The vulnerability also may be biological. Indeed, there is evidence that genetic factors may create an increased risk for eating disorders. Another important factor in the development of eating disorders is society's emphasis on extreme thinness. It is clear that eating disorders are complex problems, with multiple causes. Social, psychological, and biological factors all play roles.

Eating disorders can develop when people, especially women, feel social pressure to achieve an unrealistic standard of thinness. Modern Western culture would have women weigh less than what is considered healthy. This means that most women cannot attain what society considers the "ideal" female form without significant food deprivation. These pressures affect even very young girls, starting with their first Barbie doll and her unnatural shape (see **Figure SED.4**), if not before.[11]

Think About It 1

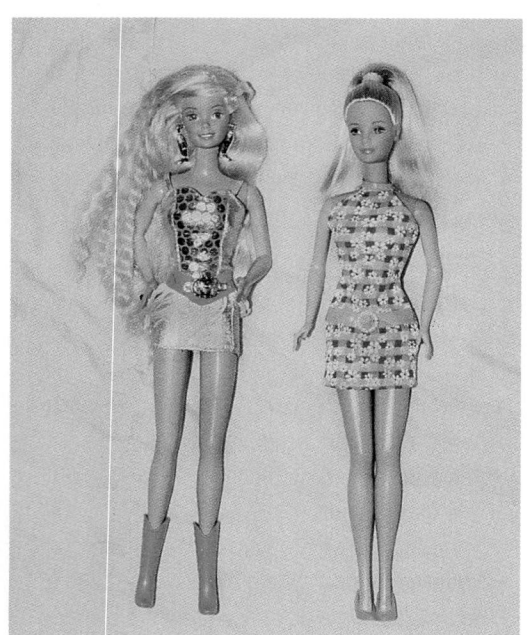

Figure SED.4 **Thin is in.** In 1998, Mattel overhauled Barbie's look for the millennium, giving her slimmer hips, a wider waist, and smaller breasts. Barbie's periodic overhauls are meant to fit the fashion of the times. Does the new Barbie (right) represent a realistic role model for today's young girls?

Psychological factors are important as well. These encompass everything from peer relationships to relationships with parents. In one recent study of peer relationships, L. Kris Gowen of the Stanford Center on Adolescence found that preadolescent girls who were teased or bullied by peers had a more negative image of their bodies and a greater concern about their weight than other girls.[12] This was true regardless of the girls' actual weight. Studies also have linked more severe forms of emotional trauma to disordered eating. For example, researchers at Texas A&M University detected symptoms of **post-traumatic stress disorder (PTSD)** in more than half of the anorexia and bulimia patients they studied.[13] PTSD occurs in people who have endured a significant trauma, such as child abuse or rape. Eating disorders also may be associated with dysfunctional family relationships. Some psychologists believe that people with anorexia and bulimia are trying to fulfill unrealistic parental expectations of perfection, in part by succumbing to societal pressure to be very thin.

In recent years, scientists have made major advances in understanding the biological foundation of eating disorders. Important studies link the neurotransmitters serotonin and norepinephrine to eating behavior. Researchers, for example, have shown that bulimia patients experience spontaneous improvement in eating habits when they take an antidepressant medication that increases brain levels of serotonin.[14] Interestingly, many anti-obesity drugs also affect serotonin levels.[15]

Quick Bites

Magazine Manipulations

When researchers studied fifth- through twelfth-grade girls in a working-class suburb in the Northeast, nearly 50 percent reported that they wanted to lose weight because of pictures in magazines. Frequent readers of fashion magazines were two to three times more likely to be influenced to diet or exercise to lose weight. Seventy percent of the girls reported that magazine pictures influenced their conception of the perfect body.

Neurotransmitters are just one focus of research into the biology of eating disorders. Another line of investigation focuses on genes. Recently, researchers have confirmed that eating disorders run in families. In addition, eating disorders occur most frequently in families with a history of obsessive-compulsive disorders, anxiety disorders, and depression.[16] Both depression and obsessive-compulsive behavior have been linked to atypical levels of serotonin and norepinephrine in the brain.[17]

It's likely that many genes are involved in the development of eating disorders. Two recently discovered genes are involved in the synthesis and release of the hormones leptin and **orexin**.[18] The leptin gene regulates the body's production of leptin, a hormone that causes rapid weight loss in genetically obese mice. (Unfortunately, leptin has not stimulated the same reaction in humans.) The orexin gene regulates production of two appetite-stimulating hormones, orexin A and orexin B (after the Greek word *orexis,* meaning "appetite"). In experiments, rodents injected with either hormone increased their food consumption 8- to 10-fold.[19]

post-traumatic stress disorder (PTSD) An anxiety disorder characterized by an emotional response to a traumatic event or situation involving severe external stress.

orexin A class of hormones in the brain that may affect food consumption.

The discoveries of leptin and orexin genes significantly advance our understanding of brain chemistry and eating disorders and may eventually lead to new classes of more effective drugs. Drugs that mimic orexins, for example, might help patients with anorexia or other wasting syndromes by increasing their appetites. Conversely, drugs that block orexins might help patients struggling with obesity and binge eating. Or a leptinlike drug may eventually be used to stimulate weight loss. At the very least, discovery of these genes supports the idea that biological factors probably contribute to the development of eating disorders in vulnerable people.

Key Concepts: *The precise causes of eating disorders remain obscure. Some researchers believe that eating disorders are primarily psychological in origin. Others have championed the theory that eating disorders have an important genetic basis. The current view is that eating disorders are a result of the complex interaction of social, biological, and psychological factors. In other words, eating disorders occur in biologically susceptible individuals exposed to particular types of environmental stimuli.*

Quick Bites

A Skinny Trend

In 1970 the average *Playboy* Playmate weighed 11 percent below the national average. Only 8 years later, in 1978, the average weight of *Playboy* Playmates was 17 percent below average. Today, the average model is 22 to 23 percent leaner than the average American woman.

Anorexia Nervosa

Until the 1960s, anorexia nervosa was a relatively obscure disease. Physicians learned about the condition in medical school, but few doctors ever saw a case in their own practices. By the mid-1970s, however, physicians were reporting many cases of anorexia, particularly among young women. Today an estimated 1 in 100 females between the ages of 13 and 19 suffer from anorexia. In comparison, fewer than 1 in 1,000 males younger than 20 have the problem.[20] Up to 10 percent of sufferers die from this disease.

The term *anorexia nervosa*, which translates to "nervous loss of appetite," is misleading. People diagnosed with anorexia don't lose their appetite except in the final stages of the disorder. Instead, they are obsessed with food. But their obsession with thinness is even greater. The German term for the disorder, *pubertätsmagersucht*, or "mania for leanness," more accurately reflects the nature of the disease.[21] The hallmark of anorexia nervosa is dramatic loss of weight, usually to less than 85 percent of the expected weight for height or a BMI of less than or equal to 17.5. (See **Figure SED.5**.)

Anorexia is more prevalent in industrialized societies that share an abundance of food and an attitude that equates beauty, particularly feminine beauty, with thinness. Nine of ten anorexia sufferers are female—probably because Western society emphasizes thinness more for women than for men.[22] Until recently, the typical anorexia sufferer was an upper-class Caucasian female adolescent. Unfortunately, during the past decade, anorexia has become more of an equal-opportunity disorder. Physicians have reported cases of the disorder in young women from all social and ethnic backgrounds; it is especially prevalent in women who participate in activities that emphasize leanness, including modeling, ballet, and gymnastics. In addition, anorexia has increased significantly among African American women.[23]

Quick Bites

Were Underweight Romans Dangerous?

Let me have men about me that are fat; ...
Yon Cassius has a lean and hungry look:
such men are dangerous...
I do not know the man I should avoid
So soon as that spare Cassius.

—Shakespeare, *Julius Caesar*, Act 1, Scene II

Perhaps Caesar should have listened to his instincts. He was stabbed to death by Cassius and other conspirators.

Causes of Anorexia Nervosa

On the surface, anorexia nervosa usually seems to result from a weight-loss program gone awry. A high school freshman may go on a diet after her boyfriend or gymnastics coach tells her she is too heavy. An eighth-grader may want to lose weight to be more popular at a new school. The diet may start out just fine, but it never stops.

Beneath the surface, psychological issues are typically at work. Because most cases of anorexia begin around the age of puberty, some psychologists theorize that anorexic behavior is an attempt to prevent or delay sexual maturation. By retaining a child's body, a young girl may hope to avoid the pressures of the teen years and the responsibilities of adulthood. In addi-

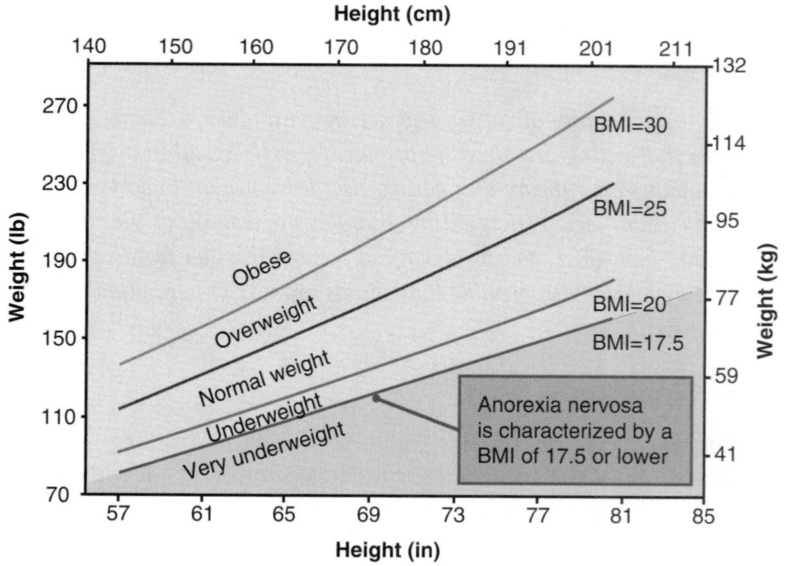

Figure SED.5 **BMI and underweight.** When managing eating disorders, BMI can help guide decisions about nutrition, medications, and psychotherapy.

Source: Reprinted with permission from the *Diagnostic and Statistical Manual of Mental Disorders*, Fourth Edition, Text Revision. Copyright © 2000 American Psychiatric Association.

tion, psychologists report that anorexia sufferers tend to be rigid, perfectionistic, all-or-nothing thinkers. Sufferers tend to lack a sense of independence and control over their own destiny. They may attempt to compensate for this through acts of intense self-discipline. Parents may facilitate this syndrome by being overly protective or rigid or by holding a child to excessively high standards of achievement.[24]

Some people probably are predisposed to anorexia. For example, obsessive-compulsive behaviors, depression, and anxiety frequently precede anorexia. In fact, half of anorexia sufferers also experience a major depression or **obsessive-compulsive disorder**.[25] All these disorders involve abnormalities in neurotransmitters, suggesting that brain chemistry contributes to anorexia. Although it is likely that biological factors predispose an individual to anorexia, psychological and social factors are critical in precipitating the disease. The current view is that complex biological, social, and psychological factors contribute to anorexia.[26]

obsessive-compulsive disorder A disorder in which a person attempts to relieve anxiety by ritualistic behavior and continuous repetition of certain acts.

emetics Agents that induce vomiting.

enema An infusion of fluid into the rectum usually for cleansing or other therapeutic purposes.

diuretics [dye-u-RET-iks] Drugs or other substances that promote the formation and release of urine. Diuretics are given to reduce body fluid volume in treating such disorders as high blood pressure, congestive heart disease, and edema. Both alcohol and caffeine act as diuretics.

laxatives Substances that promote evacuation of the bowel by increasing the bulk of the feces, lubricating the intestinal wall, or softening the stool.

Warning Signs

Parents and friends of people with anorexia often miss the early signs of the disease. It can be easy to mistake a loved one's obsession with dieting, avoidance of particular foods, or rigorous exercise schedule for a reasonable desire to lose weight.[27]

When asked about a child who has been diagnosed with anorexia, most parents will describe a "wonderful" daughter—one who has always been cooperative, obedient, an exceptional student, and unusually neat and organized. When she started to diet, she did so with the same zeal and dedication she exhibited in other areas of her life.[28]

Initially, someone with anorexia has a feeling of power. Sufferers enjoy a feeling of control as they learn to deny their hunger and limit their food intake. Early warning signs include obsessively counting calories; developing lists of "safe" foods and foods to avoid; cutting foods, even peas, into small pieces; and spending a great deal of time rearranging food on a plate. To suppress hunger, a person with anorexia may drink up to 30 cups of water or diet soda a day. Anorexia sufferers also may channel their obsessions with food into the preparation of elaborate meals for others without eating any of the food themselves.[29] **Table SED.2** shows the warning signs of anorexia.

Think About It 2

Table SED.2 Warning Signs of Anorexia

Anorexia nervosa is a disorder in which preoccupation with dieting and thinness leads to excessive weight loss. The person with anorexia may not acknowledge that weight loss or restricted eating are problems. Family and friends can help by recognizing that the following are warning signs:

- Loss of a significant amount of weight
- Continuing to diet (although thin)
- Feeling fat, even after losing weight
- Fear of weight gain
- Cessation of monthly menstrual periods
- Preoccupation with food, calories, nutrition, and/or cooking
- Preferring to eat in isolation
- Exercising compulsively
- Bingeing and purging

As the disease progresses, anorexia sufferers become increasingly disillusioned, withdrawn, and hostile. Success always seems beyond their grasp. No matter how thin they are, they see themselves as overweight. (See **Figure SED.6**.) When they eat more than they think they should, they may induce vomiting or use **emetics**, **enemas**, **diuretics**, or **laxatives**. Or they may exercise relentlessly. Eventually, their efforts to avoid obesity take over their lives. They start to avoid social situations that may expose their behaviors and so withdraw more and more from friends and family. Groggy and irritable from food deprivation and sleep disturbances, people with advanced anorexia spend so little time on their schoolwork or jobs that their performance deteriorates. Yet when confronted with their obsessive dieting or deteriorating behavior, they will deny that anything is unusual.[30]

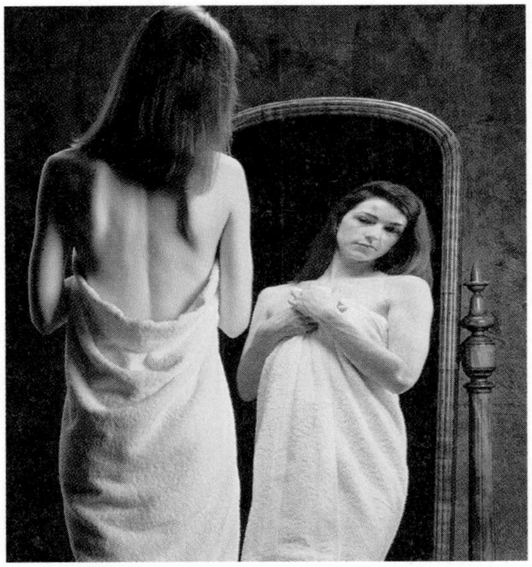

Figure SED.6 Distorted body image.

Treatment

Just as there is no one cause for anorexia nervosa, there is no single way to cure it. In fact, most experts doubt that patients with anorexia can ever be cured. Research suggests that with intensive therapy, most patients can achieve normal weight. However, they may struggle all their lives with a

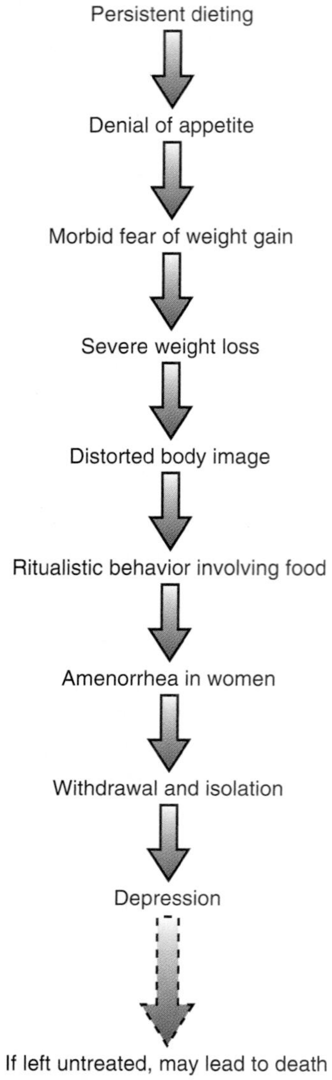

Figure SED.7 **The progression of anorexia.**

moderate to severe preoccupation with food and body weight, poor social relationships, and depression. The earlier a patient begins treatment, the better the prognosis.

The course of anorexia varies greatly. In rare instances, a sufferer recovers spontaneously without treatment. More typically, a patient recovers only after a variety of treatments or enters a cyclical pattern of weight gain and relapse. From 30 to 50 percent of anorexia patients also have symptoms of bulimia, which can complicate diagnosis and treatment.[31] Tragically, in 6 to 18 percent of cases, the disease proves fatal. (See **Figure SED.7**.) Patients who have other emotional disorders, such as major depression or substance abuse, are the most likely to die from complications of the disease. Potentially fatal complications of anorexia include starvation and suicide.[32]

As with many other behavioral disorders, people with anorexia usually deny the danger of their situation. And so family and friends must intervene to get sufferers to treatment—often by getting together and supportively confronting the person with evidence that something is seriously wrong. This common technique helps people accept the need for at least an initial medical screening. The complex and multifaceted nature of anorexia requires a team of experienced health care professionals, including physicians, clinical dietitians, and psychotherapists, so that both the physical and psychological aspects of the disorder can be addressed. One of the best places to find an experienced team of therapists is at an eating disorder clinic associated with a major medical facility.[33]

The first goal of treatment is to stabilize the patient's physical condition. The second is to convert the patient, who is typically reluctant, into a willing participant in the treatment plan. A combination of hospitalization, psychotherapy, and pharmacotherapy is often necessary.

Restoring the patient's nutritional status is of prime importance. Otherwise, dehydration, starvation, and electrolyte imbalances can lead to serious health problems and even death. (See **Table SED.3**.) If a patient has lost more than 30 percent of body weight over a three-month period or

Table SED.3 **Side Effects of Excessive Weight Loss in Anorexia Nervosa**

Emaciation

- Loss of fat stores and muscle mass
- Reduced thyroid metabolism
- Cold intolerance
- Difficulty maintaining core body temperature

Hematological

- Leukopenia (abnormal decrease of white blood cells)
- Iron-deficiency anemia

Other

- Growth of lanugo (fine, baby-like hairs) over the trunk
- Osteopenia (mineral depletion in bone)
- Premature osteoporosis

Neuropsychiatric

- Abnormal taste sensation
- Depression
- Impaired thought process

Cardiac

- Loss of cardiac muscle, resulting in a smaller heart
- Abnormal heart rhythm
- Increased risk of sudden death

Gastrointestinal

- Delayed gastric emptying
- Bloating
- Constipation
- Abdominal pain

weighs 70 percent or less of the standard weight considered healthy for height, hospitalization is essential. (See **Table SED.4.**) Once the patient's physical condition has stabilized and some of the physical symptoms of starvation have disappeared, psychotherapy can begin in earnest. Many therapists use a cognitive behavioral approach to help the patient challenge irrational beliefs and establish healthy attitudes and behaviors for gaining and maintaining weight.

The early phases of weight gain are fraught with challenges for both patient and clinician. Patients must gain a certain amount of weight to prevent death or permanent damage while the psychotherapeutic portion of their treatment is still in the very early phases. At first, the patient is encouraged to simply eat enough food to minimize or stop weight loss. Next, the patient is started on a very slow process of weight gain, all the while receiving intensive psychotherapy. The first sign of weight gain can precipitate a crisis. Phobia of obesity may return with renewed vengeance. Many patients refuse to eat. Others resist treatment in covert ways. If not restricted to bed and closely supervised, they may try to burn off calories through relentless exercise or by purging. To avoid detection, they adopt a series of behaviors to conceal their lack of weight gain. These include wearing concealing clothes or "bulking up" before weigh-ins by filling their pockets with coins or drinking large amounts of water or diet soda.[34]

Psychologists use a variety of psychotherapeutic techniques to help the patient deal with underlying emotional issues such as depression. Treatment programs generally use a combination of behavioral therapy, individual psychotherapy, patient education, family education, and family therapy. Frequently, therapists find family conflicts at the heart of the eating disorder. Ongoing therapy for the patient and family is key to successful recovery. As the patient's symptoms resolve, she or he must find new ways of relating to and communicating with family members. Family members must remain open and willing to change their behavior toward the person with the eating disorder.

Dietitians work closely with the psychotherapist to help patients develop a realistic view of food and to reshape their food selection and eating behaviors. Although no pharmaceutical agent has been developed specifically to treat anorexia, certain antidepressants have proved useful.

Most patients with anorexia nervosa require continued intervention after discharge from the hospital or treatment program. Support groups for people with eating disorders and their families can be an important link in the recovery process. Support groups also can be a useful technique for easing a resistant patient into treatment. With expert help and ongoing therapy, patients with anorexia can develop new mechanisms for coping with life's stresses, eventually replacing their disordered relationship with food with new, healthier interpersonal relationships.

Key Concepts: *The hallmark symptoms of anorexia nervosa are a mania for thinness and self-imposed starvation. Sufferers manifest a body weight as much as 15 percent below normal, a severely distorted body image, withdrawal from family and friends, and various physical and psychological changes related to starvation.*

Bulimia Nervosa

Although the behavior we now call bulimia was practiced in Greek and Roman times, it has been recognized as a psychiatric illness for only 20 years. Gerald Russell, a British psychiatrist, first coined the term *bulimia ner-*

Table SED.4 When Hospitalization Is Needed

Suggested criteria for hospitalization for individuals with anorexia nervosa include:

- Weight loss of greater than 30 percent over three months
- Severe metabolic disturbance
- Severe depression or suicide risk
- Severe bingeing and purging
- Failure to maintain outpatient weight contract
- Psychosis
- Family crisis

Source: American Psychiatric Association. *Diagnostic and Statistical Manual of Mental Disorders.* 4th ed. Washington, DC: American Psychiatric Association; 1994.

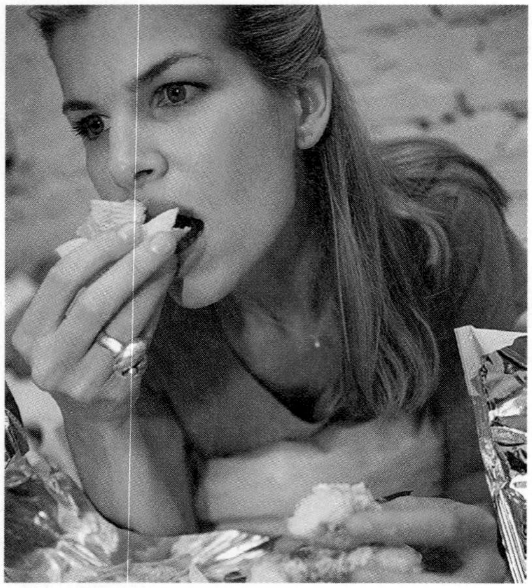

Figure SED.8 The typical person suffering from bulimia is an unmarried Caucasian woman in her twenties or thirties.

vosa in 1979 to describe a syndrome of bingeing and purging being reported in young Caucasian women.[35] The average patient with bulimia is an unmarried Caucasian woman in her twenties or thirties with a normal or near-normal body weight. (See **Figure SED.8**.) Patients with bulimia are more likely to be sexually active than are those with anorexia and often are involved in destructive relationships with members of the opposite sex. Almost anyone can be affected, however.

People with bulimia nervosa tend to feel very disorganized. They report suffering from depression and low self-esteem. Many were sexually abused as children. Food was often a source of comfort, and eating gradually evolved into a tool for dealing with every unpleasant event, from boredom to major life crises.

It is estimated that between 1 percent and 3 percent of American adolescent and young adult females have bulimia. But bulimia, particularly in its milder forms, often goes undetected. This is because people with bulimia are very secretive about their behavior, typically limiting their binge-and-purge episodes to the middle of the night or other times when they are assured of privacy. Also, unlike patients with anorexia or binge-eating disorder, whose body weights may hint at their underlying psychiatric disorder, the body weight of a patient with bulimia is usually average or only slightly above average. Several studies have found that as many as 40 percent of college-age women occasionally binge and purge—often enough to raise concern but too infrequently for an official diagnosis of bulimia.[36] **Table SED.5** lists the warning signs of bulimia.

Quick Bites

I'm So Hungry I Could Eat an Ox!

The term *bulimia* is derived from the Greek word *bous*, meaning "ox," and *limos*, meaning "hunger."

Causes of Bulimia

Bulimia seems to occur most often in people who have an intense desire to nurture themselves with food but are also strongly influenced by our societal obsession with thinness. One description of people with bulimia characterizes them as being obsessed with food but repulsed by fat. In contrast to people with anorexia, people with bulimia focus more on food than on thinness.

[Fyi] Diary of an Eating Disorder

FOR YOUR INFORMATION

Every time I leave one of my sessions I feel better. We talk about stuff; I feel, express, and even cry. Today was the third time since I left her office to come home and throw up. I think things are getting better despite the fact that my mind focuses 80 percent of the time on food during the 55 minutes. But it's like the kitchen is a refuge for my mind. I always know it will be there, waiting to embrace me when I get home.

Alone is how I hope to find it. I have been thinking of what I will sink my teeth into first. Usually I go for the fat-free chocolate cake, then to the frozen yogurt (which makes it all come up much smoother). I don't think this is normal, though I am not really concerned. I feel like a million-pound weight has been swept away by the effortless flush of the toilet. The hardest thing is to look in the mirror after I have thrown up. Sometimes I wipe my face before I look. Other times I leave the spit, bile, and food on my mouth and hands. I just stand there holding my hands up, with my shoulders slumped over. I produce this expression of absolute helplessness—then I laugh. I guess I am amazed by the act I've just committed. I can't explain why, I can't believe that it is really me doing this. Why would I do something like throw up? I really have no reason to torture myself. Bulimia was always *them*—I can't possibly be like that. I throw up, but I am not a bulimic. I sure as hell don't have an eating disorder.

I am totally for this whole counseling thing because I feel sad a lot and I want to feel better. But I can't leave there and not feel that I have to get this crap out. All this stuff that we talk about.

Table SED.5 Warning Signs of Bulimia

Bulimia nervosa involves frequent episodes of binge eating, almost always followed by purging and intense feelings of guilt or shame. The sufferer feels out of control and recognizes that the behavior is not normal. The signs that a person may have bulimia include:

- Bingeing, or eating uncontrollably
- Compensating for binges by strict dieting, fasting, vigorous exercise, vomiting, or abusing laxatives or diuretics in an attempt to lose weight
- Using the bathroom frequently after meals
- Preoccupation with body weight
- Depression or mood swings
- Irregular menstrual periods
- Dental problems, swollen cheeks or glands, heartburn, or bloating
- Personal or family problems with drugs or alcohol

Source: Adapted from the *National Eating Disorders Screening Program Body Weight Assessment Tool.*

Psychologists who have treated patients with bulimia have found that they typically did not receive sufficient nurturing during their formative years. Whereas families of anorexic patients tend to have a lot of rigidly defined roles and rules, families of bulimic patients tend to lack structure. Roles may be loosely defined. Parents are often described as distant and judgmental. Significant family conflict usually exists. Patients often feel that their families failed to provide an adequate sense of security and protection.

binge Consumption of a very large amount of food in a brief time (e.g., 2 hours) accompanied by a loss of control over how much and what is eaten.

purge Emptying of the GI tract by self-induced vomiting and/or misuse of laxatives, diuretics, or enemas.

Obsessed by Thoughts of Food

A person with bulimia chronically **binges** and **purges**. To meet the official definition of the disorder, bingeing and purging must occur at least twice a week for at least three months. Purging may be accompanied or replaced by

Today, Dr. Tant asked me when this all began. My first thought was, "Oh this throwing up thing? I can't remember." But I do recall one time when my ex-boyfriend Matt and I had gone to a really nice dinner. My recollection of the evening was that it was perfect. I remember thinking about how this food was really fattening, though, and how it would make me fat if I kept it down. I didn't know or have the willpower to just not eat it. Over and over I tortured and berated myself about the effects this dinner would have on my body. I couldn't bear it. This dinner was no longer one meal; it was going to ruin my body and make me fat. I couldn't stand that food being inside me another moment. Looking back I can't imagine how I could have thrown up right there on the side of the road. It was like I had no couth. I told Matt to pull over, and I just stuck my hand down my throat. Rationalizing the act while engaging in it, I then jumped back in the truck to carry on with the night. We never discussed my vile act other than Matt saying, "I can't believe you just did that."

"I know," I responded, "but it just was making me feel so sick. I mean, my stomach was really nauseous [*sic*]." Basically I don't know when I began this war with myself, but I know it caused me to fear myself. The rest is a blur–its beginning, its incentive. I heard Dr. Tant's question. I just didn't have the answer.

Chelsea Browning Smith

Source: Smith C. *Diary of an Eating Disorder.* Dallas, TX: Taylor Publishing Company; 1998. Reprinted by permission of Taylor Publishing, an imprint of Rowman & Littlefield Publishing Group.

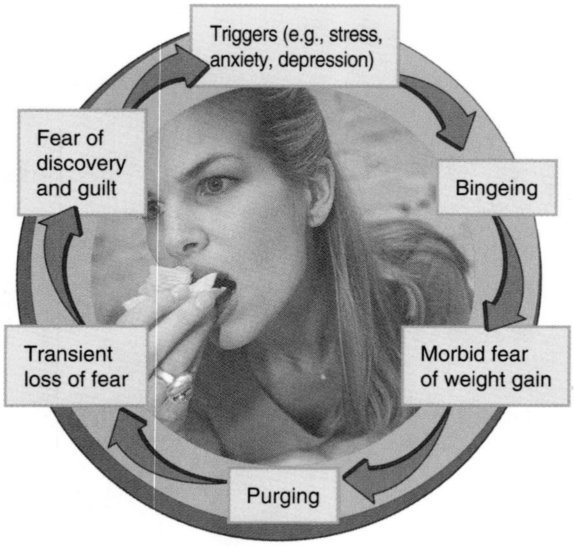

Figure SED.9 The binge-and-purge cycle of bulimia.

fasting, excessive exercise, or other behaviors that compensate for the binge episode. Between binges, people with bulimia typically restrict their dietary intake to a limited number of low-calorie foods they consider "safe." This dietary control is an illusion, however. The average bulimic sufferer is obsessed by thoughts of food and spends a great deal of time both planning the next binge and trying to resist the urge to binge.[37] **Figure SED.9** illustrates the binge-and-purge pattern of bulimia.

Just what triggers a binge is not clear. People with bulimia tend to be all-or-nothing thinkers. If they eat a single piece of food from their forbidden list, such as a cookie, they feel driven to consume the entire box. Some researchers believe that hunger caused by very restrictive dieting, combined with a buildup of everyday stresses, overwhelms the person's resolve and precipitates a binge.

During a binge, individuals with bulimia typically consume massive quantities of highly palatable "forbidden" foods like pastry, ice cream, and candy. This gorging takes place over a relatively short time span—say, an hour or two. Binges may contain up to 10,000 kilocalories. Afterward, feeling physically ill from overindulgence, sufferers use a variety of purging techniques, such as self-induced vomiting or excessive quantities of laxatives, to rid themselves of the food. Or they may follow a binge with a period of very strict fasting and heightened exercise.

Purging leads to a variety of physical symptoms. Over time, gastric acid in vomit burns the lining of the pharynx, esophagus, and mouth, erodes tooth enamel, and may even result in loss of teeth. Repeated vomiting also can enlarge the salivary glands and erode the lining of the stomach and esophagus.

Excessive self-induced vomiting and diarrhea can upset the body's delicate biochemical balance through loss of electrolytes and body water. Among other dangers, changes in electrolyte balance can trigger an irregular heartbeat and precipitate a life-threatening medical crisis. Excessive use of emetics (drugs to induce vomiting) and laxatives carries its own risks. Repeated use of emetics is toxic to the liver and kidneys, and abuse of laxatives can damage the lining of the large intestine. **Table SED.6** shows the side effects of bulimic purging.

Table SED.6 Side Effects of Purging in Bulimia Nervosa

Metabolic effects

- Electrolyte abnormalities
- Low blood magnesium

Gastrointestinal

- Inflammation of the salivary glands
- Pancreatic inflammation and enlargement
- Esophageal inflammation or ulcers
- Gastric erosion
- Dysfunctional bowel

Dental

- Erosion of dental enamel, particularly of front teeth, with corresponding decay

Neuropsychiatric

- Fatigue
- Weakness
- Impaired thought processes
- Seizures (related to large fluid shifts and electrolyte disturbances)
- Mild inflammation of peripheral nerves

Treatment

Little research has been done on the long-term course of bulimia. It appears, however, that bulimia is easier to treat than anorexia, perhaps because bulimic patients tend to recognize that their behavior is abnormal. Following treatment, more than half of patients report an improvement in their binge-eating and coping behaviors. About 30 percent of patients eventually become symptom-free. The rest, however, struggle with the disorder to some degree throughout their lives. To reduce the risk of relapse, therapists encourage patients to stay involved in support groups after completing formal therapy.

Cognitive behavior therapy is key to helping patients reshape their attitudes about food and identify situations that trigger bingeing. The therapist's goal is to help patients let go of their need to categorize foods as safe or dangerous, good or bad. Patients must learn techniques for dealing with stress and uncomfortable or painful memories and feelings. Depression, which typically accompanies this disorder, must be treated as well. Many patients with bulimia also require treatment for substance abuse. A patient is hospitalized only when severely depressed or when purging is so frequent that physical damage has occurred or is imminent.

Medication can be an effective adjunct to psychotherapy. Serotonin-enhancing antidepressants have been used successfully to treat bulimia. In 1997 the FDA approved the antidepressant Prozac for this purpose.

Key Concepts: *Key symptoms of bulimia nervosa are binge-eating episodes at least twice a week for three months, followed by behaviors that compensate for the binges, like severe dieting, purging, or a combination of dieting and purging. The body weight of people with bulimia is typically close to or slightly above that considered healthy for their heights.*

Binge-Eating Disorder

Overeating has been reported in the medical literature since scribes first put stylus to tablet. And over the generations, societies, including our own, have considered obesity a sign of good health, wealth, and even fertility.[38] But modern Western society is not among these. Binge eating is the most common eating disorder in industrialized nations. It occurs only in societies where people have access to an abundant supply of food. Its precise causes are unclear. However, the condition seems to be related to an intense desire to nurture oneself with food or to reduce stress by eating.[39] In 1994 the American Psychiatric Association recognized binge-eating disorder as an emotional illness.

Quick Bites

When Plumpness Was Valued

In centuries past, extra pounds displayed one's wealth and prosperity. The wealthy could afford abundant food and didn't perform physical labor.

Stress and Conflict Often Trigger Binge Eating

A person with binge-eating disorder consumes excessive quantities of food in a relatively short period of time at least twice a week. Unlike the bulimia sufferer, however, the person with binge-eating disorder does not attempt to compensate by purging or other means. In some instances, binge eaters adopt a grazing pattern. "Grazers" eat constantly for extended periods of time, eventually consuming an exceptionally large quantity of food. This pattern of overindulgence may be seen in people who restrict their food intake at work or school but seek solace in food at home.

Not all people who binge are obese. But bingeing is common among the severely obese and people with a history of weight cycling. In the United States, at least 30 percent of the people enrolled in weight-management

Table SED.7 Warning Signs of Binge-Eating Disorder

Binge eaters, like bulimia sufferers, experience periods of uncontrolled eating that they usually keep secret. Binge eaters often are depressed and sometimes have other psychological problems. Signs that a person may have a binge-eating disorder include:

- Episodes of binge eating
- Eating when not physically hungry
- Frequent dieting
- Feeling unable to stop eating voluntarily
- Awareness that eating patterns are abnormal
- Weight fluctuations
- Depressed mood
- Attribution of social and professional successes and failures to weight

programs report behaviors consistent with a diagnosis of binge-eating disorder, compared with only 3 to 5 percent of the general population.[40] (See **Table SED.7**, "Warning Signs of Binge-Eating Disorder.")

Many binge eaters begin dieting in grade school and start bingeing during adolescence or in their early twenties. Typically, they try numerous weight-loss programs without long-term success. Binge eaters exhibit many of the same characteristics as bulimic patients. More than 50 percent have clinical depression. Feelings of depression, loneliness, anxiety, or stress can precipitate a binge. Like other patients with eating disorders, those with binge-eating disorder are all-or-nothing thinkers. They tend to categorize foods as safe or dangerous. Eating even a small serving of a forbidden food can trigger a binge. Typical binge foods include sweets, pastries, ice cream, and high-fat snacks like nuts and chips. However, if junk foods aren't handy, binge eaters may eat large quantities of starchy foods, such as potatoes, bread, and pasta. **Figure SED.10** illustrates some factors that trigger binge eating.

Think About It 3

Most binge eaters are people who have not learned to express or even acknowledge their feelings. During therapy sessions, many binge eaters report feeling helpless to change the course of events or behaviors of others around them. Rather than acknowledge their feelings, they swallow them—aided by large quantities of food. They become addicted to the behavior itself because it is the only way they can get relief from stress. (See **Figure SED.11**.)

Binge eating often is a learned response to stress or conflict, passed down from one generation to the next. Parents may use food rather than affection and discussion to shape their children's behavior. Food is used for celebration and consolation, for reward and punishment. Children growing up in such environments learn to eat in response to emotions rather than hunger. As adults, they turn to food to satisfy all their emotional needs.

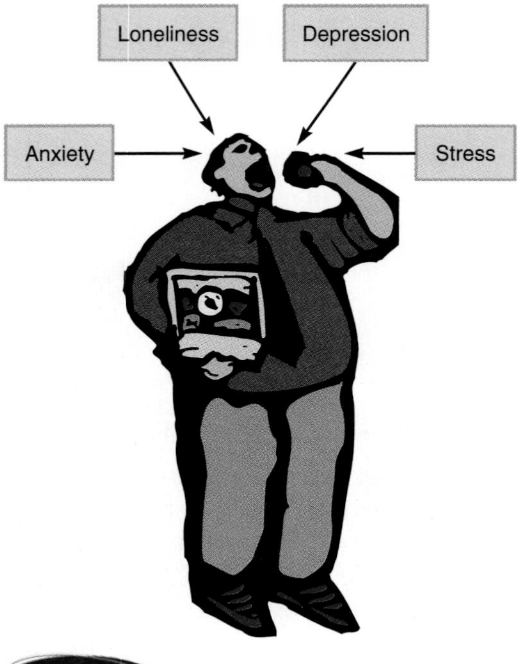

Figure SED.10 Feelings of loneliness, depression, anxiety, or stress can trigger a binge-eating episode.

Treatment

Little is known about the course and prognosis of binge-eating disorder. However, people who become obese as a result of this disorder are at risk of developing weight-related health problems, including type 2 diabetes, hypertension, degenerative joint disease, heart disease, and even certain cancers.

People who have binge-eating disorder are rarely able to control the condition themselves. They usually require therapy to help them identify their long-buried emotions and learn techniques for giving voice to their feelings. Therapists experienced in treating this disorder discourage patients from trying to lose weight initially. Any attempts to restrict food intake can backfire by creating anxiety and provoking a binge. The major focus of therapy is to help patients identify their emotions and separate true biological hunger from emotional hunger. Once significant progress is made in these areas, the patient is better equipped psychologically to address weight issues.

Long-term support is key to keeping binge eaters from relapsing. Self-help groups like Overeaters Anonymous are one source of support. These groups are organized according to the 12-step philosophy of Alcoholics Anonymous. In addition, many hospitals in large urban areas have support groups led by trained therapists. Hospitals and clinics that provide medically supervised fasting programs such as Optifast often supply this type of service as well. (See Chapter 8, "Energy Balance and Weight Management," for further information on this type of weight-control program.)

Many patients with binge-eating disorder benefit from antidepressant medications. These drugs reduce the urge to binge, most likely by altering the brain's serotonin level. Various weight-management medications are now in development. These also may curb the urge to binge.

Key Concepts: *Diagnostic criteria have recently been established for binge-eating disorder, the most common eating disorder. This disorder is seen in people of all ages and backgrounds. Like people with bulimia, those with binge-eating disorder consume significantly more food than is typically eaten in a given period of time. In contrast to individuals with bulimia, those with binge-eating disorder do not compensate by purging or fasting to limit weight gain. Not all binge eaters are obese, although many obese people binge. Some people with binge-eating disorder tend to graze; that is, they eat a large amount of food over a prolonged period of time, rather than all at once.*

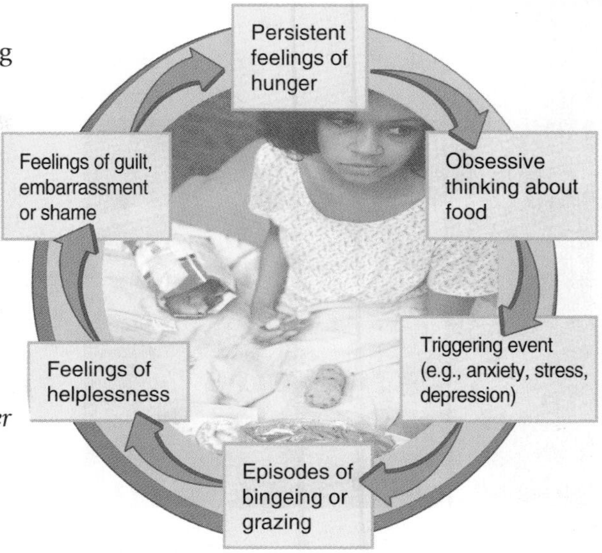

Figure SED.11 **The vicious cycle of binge eating.** Binge-eating disorder is the most common eating disorder.

Males: An Overlooked Population

As many as a million men struggle with eating disorders.[41] Yet males with eating disorders have been "ignored, neglected or dismissed because of statistical infrequency of the disease, combined with the pervasive myth that eating disorders are a female disease," according to Arnold E. Andersen, former director of the Eating and Weight Disorders Clinic at Johns Hopkins University and scientific editor of the book *Males with Eating Disorders*.[42]

Women who develop eating disorders may feel fat, but they typically are near average weight. In contrast, most men who develop these diseases are overweight. Many were seriously teased about their weight as children. While women are concerned primarily with weight, men are concerned with shape and muscle definition. Indeed, men often develop disordered eating habits while trying to improve their athletic performance. Finally, more men than women diet to prevent medical consequences associated with being overweight.

Why do fewer males than females develop full-blown eating disorders? Andersen contends there is a "dose-response" relationship between the amount of sociocultural pressure to be thin and the probability of developing an eating disorder. Consider that articles and advertisements that promote dieting usually are targeted at young women rather than young men. When men are exposed to activities that require leanness, such as wrestling, swimming, running, and horse racing, they exhibit a substantial increase in anorexic behavior. It seems clear that cultural conditioning, not gender, contributes to the incidence of eating disorders.[43]

Think About It 4

Furthermore, the degree of thinness held up as desirable for women is 15 percent below a healthy body weight, whereas the degree of thinness held up as desirable for men is well within the healthy limits of normal weight. Thus, women are more likely than men to alter their eating habits to achieve the desired appearance.

An Unrecognized Disorder

Like women, most men develop eating disorders during adolescence. But males can develop eating disorders during preadolescence and young adulthood as well. The diagnostic criteria for anorexia and bulimia in men and women are similar. But doctors are so conditioned to viewing eating disorders as a female phenomenon that they often miss eating disorders in males. Likewise, the patient, his family, and friends may not recognize disordered eating patterns. (See **Table SED.8**.) Because our culture accepts

Quick Bites

When Men Starve—A Starvation Study

During World War II, researchers at the University of Minnesota conducted a starvation study on 36 male volunteers, all conscientious objectors. Their typical food intake was cut in half and they lost about 25 percent of their body weight. Researchers noted significant psychological changes as well. The subjects began obsessing about food, collecting recipes and cookbooks, and hoarding food-related objects. They became apathetic, chronically exhausted, and lost all interest in sex. Most were afraid to leave the experimental conditions for fear of losing control in the outside world.

overeating among men more readily than in women, binge eating in particular may go unrecognized in men. In addition, anorexia may elude diagnosis in men more often than in women because malnourished men don't experience definitive symptoms, such as a woman's loss of menstrual periods, that can alert professionals and others to the problem. Men also tend to view an eating disorder as a "woman's disease," so they often are hesitant to seek medical attention.[44]

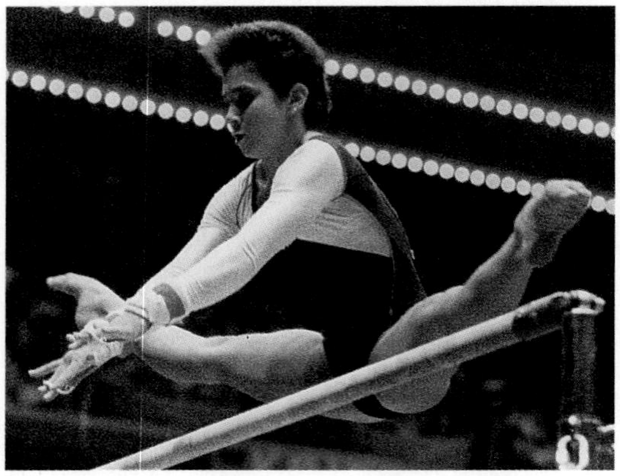

Christy Henrich, a top Olympic gymnast, weighed less than 60 pounds when she died in 1994 at age 22 of multiple organ failure, a complication resulting from anorexia and bulimia.

Key Concepts: *Men also suffer from eating disorders, although at rates much lower than those of women. Like women, men typically develop eating disorders during adolescence and young adulthood but are more often overweight and striving for a particular body shape and muscularity. Although the diagnostic criteria are the same, with the exception of amenorrhea, eating disorders in men are often undiagnosed due to societal conditioning that eating disorders are "female" diseases.*

Anorexia Athletica

Participation in competitive athletics seems to be a common link in the development of eating disorders among males and females, regardless of their social or ethnic backgrounds. Sports-related eating disorders are known as **anorexia athletica**. Some studies suggest that as many as 30 percent of competitive athletes exhibit some degree of disordered eating.[45] A study focusing on the incidence of eating disorders in female athletes found

anorexia athletica Eating disorder associated with competitive participation in athletic activity.

Table SED.8 Signs of an Undisclosed Eating Disorder

People with eating disorders usually exhibit several of the following signs.

Physical

- Arrested growth
- Marked change or frequent fluctuations in weight
- Inability to gain weight
- Fatigue
- Constipation or diarrhea
- Susceptibility to fractures
- Delayed menarche
- Calcium or phosphorus imbalances, abnormal blood pH, or high serum amylase levels

Behavioral

- Change in eating habits
- Difficulty in social settings
- Reluctance to be weighed
- Depression
- Social withdrawal
- Repeated absence from school or work
- Deceptive or secretive behavior
- Stealing (e.g., to obtain food)
- Substance abuse
- Excessive exercise

Source: Becker AE, Grinspoon SK, Klibanski A, Herzog DB. Eating disorders. *N Engl J Med.* 1999;340(14):1092–1098.

a higher incidence among gymnasts. Some 62 percent of college-age female gymnasts reported disordered eating patterns. Anorexia is also seen frequently in swimmers, dancers, wrestlers, and bodybuilders. Athletes who have anorexia athletica seek to achieve an unrealistic body size that they consider desirable for purposes of competition. In many cases, athletes with mild eating disorders are able to disguise their disease as attention to fitness. People who seem to be addicted to their exercise routine are at greater risk of developing eating disorders.[46]

According to the American College of Sports Medicine, coaches and trainers play a significant role in the development of eating disorders among athletes. The attitude that leanness equals performance, exemplified by sayings such as "get down to your fighting weight," still prevails.[47]

The Female Athlete Triad

Female athletes who fall prey to the "thin-at-any-cost" philosophy are at risk of developing a condition known as the female athlete triad. (See **Figure SED.12**.) This syndrome is characterized by disordered eating, amenorrhea (absence of menstruation), and abnormally low bone density. This triad occurs especially in young women involved in sports that involve appearance (e.g., gymnastics) and endurance (e.g., long-distance running).

Once body fat falls below 20 percent, a woman's estrogen levels often drop significantly. As a result, women's bodies enter a menopause-like state years ahead of time. Their periods become irregular or cease altogether. Bone loss accelerates, just as it would after natural menopause. Many female athletes who suffer from this triad have the bone density of women in their fifties and sixties. Weakened bones are more likely to fracture during exercise or daily activities. Stress fractures can be a red flag for female athlete triad. Because much of this bone loss is irreversible, women who suffer from the female athlete triad are at increased risk of developing osteoporosis.[48]

To help combat this alarming trend, the American College of Sports Medicine and the National Collegiate Athletic Association (NCAA) have established an eating disorders awareness campaign aimed at coaches and trainers. The NCAA also has a three-part video series, *Nutrition and Eating Disorders*, to acquaint coaches and trainers with the causes and effects of eating disorders as well as the steps to take when they suspect an athlete has an eating disorder.[49]

Key Concepts: *Athletics can be a gateway to eating disorders. Female athletes who develop restrictive eating habits are at risk for developing a more severe syndrome known as the female athlete triad. Disordered eating, amenorrhea, and abnormally low bone density characterize this syndrome. If not corrected, the female athlete triad can hinder athletic performance and set the stage for lifelong health problems.*

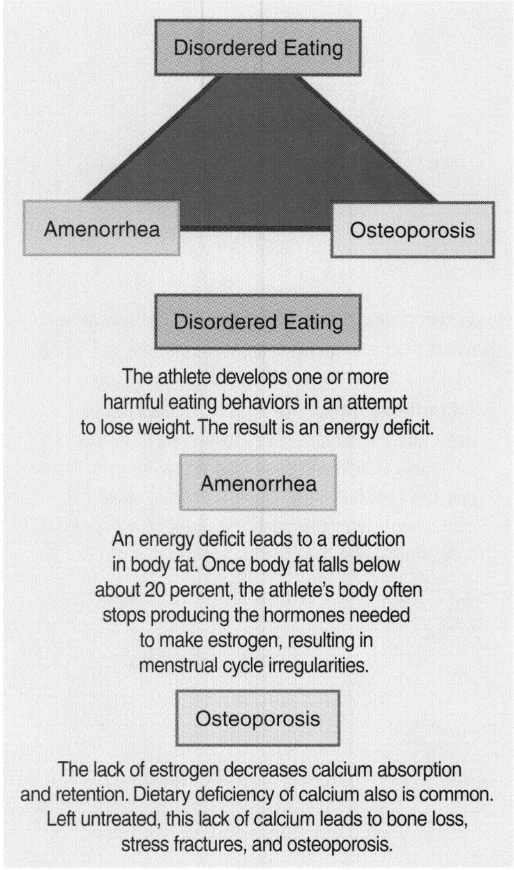

Figure SED.12 **Female athlete triad.** Disordered eating that results in excessive weight loss can lead to amenorrhea, which in turn leads to osteoporosis.

Vegetarianism and Eating Disorders

Some researchers have found a strong correlation between vegetarianism and eating disorders in teenagers. A recent study conducted in Minnesota schools found that 81 percent of the students who classified themselves as vegetarians were female. Compared with nonvegetarian peers, these self-described vegetarians were twice as likely to participate in frequent diets, four times as likely to report intentional vomiting, and eight times as likely to report laxative use.[50] Some people with eating disorders try to disguise a change in eating habits by adopting a strict vegetarian diet.

Smoking and Eating Disorders

British medical researcher Arthur Crisp recently described a new variation on eating disorders. His previous studies showed that smoking is more common among teens with eating disorders than in the general teenage population. His new research indicates that despite ample knowledge of the health risks of smoking, girls of average or slightly above average weight are taking up smoking in record numbers to cut their appetites. Though not frankly anorexic or bulimic, many of the young subjects report they periodically combine smoking with self-induced vomiting to enhance weight-control efforts.[51] This combined behavior is of particular interest and concern to researchers.

baryophobia [barry-oh-FO-bee-ah] An uncommon eating disorder that stunts growth in children and young adults as a result of underfeeding.

infantile anorexia Severe feeding difficulties that begin with the introduction of solid foods to infants. Symptoms include persistent food refusal for more than one month, malnutrition, parental concern about the child's poor food intake, and significant caregiver–infant conflict during feeding.

Baryophobia

Baryophobia, a disorder characterized by fear of fat, was virtually unheard of until the late 1970s, when pediatricians began reporting a surprising number of young patients from affluent backgrounds whose growth appeared to be stunted due to poor nutrition. In some instances, the stunting occurs when a child secretly starts to diet in order to fit in better with his or her trimmer classmates. More often, however, the child's parents are at the root of the problem.

Many well-intentioned parents underfeed their children in an attempt to "protect" them from inheriting their family's tendency toward obesity, heart disease, or diabetes. But the low-fat, high-carbohydrate diet beneficial to many adults may supply too few calories to meet the energy demands of active, growing children. In such instances, the entire family needs nutritional counseling to help them understand what constitutes a healthful diet and realistic body weight for a growing child.[52]

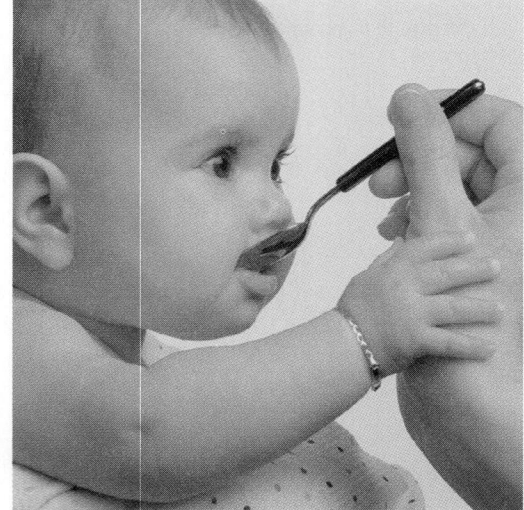

Infantile Anorexia

Unwitting parents can even create disordered eating in infants, perhaps setting the stage for eating disorders later in life.[53] Childhood nutrition specialist Ellyn Satter has analyzed videotapes of infant feedings. Satter examined whether parents responded to—or ignored—their babies' nonverbal eating readiness cues. She concluded that many parents fail to recognize their babies' body language: They feed their babies too rapidly or too slowly, they offer foods the baby doesn't care for, or they persist in trying to feed a clearly full baby who is turning away from food. These well-meaning parents may inadvertently teach their babies to ignore hunger and satiety (fullness) cues and, instead, to eat in response to outside influences.

Reports of a new disorder called **infantile anorexia** lend support to Satter's observations.[54] A team of child psychiatrists at the National Medical Center in Washington, D.C., described this disorder, in which severe feeding difficulties begin as an infant is introduced to solid foods. Symptoms include persistent food refusal for more than a month, malnutrition, parental concern about the child's poor food intake, and significant caregiver–infant conflict during feeding. The disorder typically starts or worsens during the transition from nursing to spoon-feeding and self-feeding, between ages 6 months and 3 years.

Babies with infantile anorexia should not be confused with picky eaters. Picky eaters may initially refuse all foods but allow themselves to be coaxed into eating. Picky eaters have strong food likes and dislikes but are not malnourished. And the relationship between the picky eaters and their parents or caregivers lacks the element of frustration and conflict seen in infantile anorexia.

Infantile anorexia has many serious consequences. Malnutrition can impair the developing brain and adds special stress to the parent–infant relationship. Furthermore, early conflict around meals may herald a lifelong unhealthy relationship with food.

Key Concepts: *Researchers are continuously recognizing associations between eating disorders and behaviors such as vegetarianism and smoking. Even babies and young children may suffer from disordered eating patterns.*

Combating Eating Disorders

Eating disorders are extremely difficult to treat, although advances in neurochemistry and scientific understanding of the mind–body connection may provide new avenues of treatment. Most experts agree that emphasis should be placed on preventing eating disorders.

The NIH believes that health care professionals should lead the eating disorder prevention effort by learning to promote self-esteem in their patients and teaching patients that people can be healthy at every size. Ideally, this approach would have a ripple effect: Patients would transmit these beliefs to others. A variety of public information campaigns aimed at parents and people who work with children and adolescents have evolved over the past decade to help promote eating disorder awareness. One of the most prominent examples is the Body Size Acceptance campaign coordinated through the University of California, Berkeley, under the direction of Joanne Ikeda.[55] (See **Table SED.9**.)

Quick Bites

Scary Statistics

About 5 million Americans have anorexia nervosa, bulimia, or binge-eating disorders. Researchers estimate that 15 percent of young women have disordered eating attitudes and behaviors. Every year an estimated 1,000 people die from anorexia nervosa.

Table SED.9 Preventing Eating Disorders

To join the effort to prevent eating disorders, follow these tips:

- Celebrate the diversity of human body shapes and sizes.
- Present accurate information about nutrition, weight management, and health.
- Discourage restrictive eating practices, including skipping meals.
- Encourage people to eat in response to hunger, not emotions.
- Reinforce messages about good eating and activity patterns at school and at home.
- Carefully phrase comments about a person's weight, body, or fitness level.
- Teach children and young people how to constructively express negative emotions.
- Encourage parents, teachers, coaches, and other professionals who work with children to do likewise.
- Encourage people of all ages to focus on personal qualities rather than physical appearance, of themselves and others.
- Find and promote images of fit people of all sizes and shapes.

LEARNING Portfolio

spotlight on
eating disorders

Key Terms

	page
anorexia athletica	478
anorexia nervosa [an-or-EX-ee-uh ner-VOH-sah]	464
baryophobia [bear-ee-oh-FO-bee-ah]	480
binge	473
binge-eating disorder	465
body image	464
bulimia nervosa [bull-EEM-ee-uh]	465
compulsive overeating	465
disordered eating	464
diuretics [dye-u-RET-iks]	469
eating disorders	464
emetics	469
enema	469
infantile anorexia	480
laxatives	469
obsessive-compulsive disorder	469
orexin	467
post-traumatic stress disorder (PTSD)	467
purge	473

Study Points

- An eating disorder is a complex emotional illness, the primary symptom of which is significantly altered eating habits. Eating disorders occur in biologically susceptible people exposed to particular types of environmental stimuli.
- Although eating disorders existed even in ancient times, they have become alarmingly common in industrialized countries.
- Eating disorders involve highly restrictive eating patterns (seen in anorexia nervosa), a combination of compulsive overeating and purging (seen in bulimia nervosa), or unrestricted binge eating.
- Eating disorders are common in people who participate in body-conscious activities such as dance, wrestling, gymnastics, and bodybuilding.
- From 1 to 5 percent of people with eating disorders are male.
- Anorexia nervosa is an obsession for thinness manifested in self-imposed starvation.
- The typical person with anorexia nervosa is a young Caucasian woman from an upper-class, achievement-oriented family.
- Victims of anorexia nervosa have a body weight at least 15 percent below normal, a distorted body image, and physical and psychological symptoms related to starvation.
- The body weight of people with bulimia nervosa is close to or even slightly above that considered healthy for their height.
- Key symptoms of bulimia nervosa are binge-eating episodes occurring at least twice a week for three months, followed by severe dieting, purging, or a combination of dieting and purging.
- Binge-eating disorder is the most common eating disorder.
- Like those with bulimia, people with binge-eating disorder consume more food than is typically eaten in a given period of time.
- Many competitive athletes, both male and female, have disordered eating behaviors.
- Disordered eating, amenorrhea, and abnormally low bone density characterize the female athlete triad.
- The best treatment for eating disorders is prevention. Once an eating disorder has become entrenched, intensive and prolonged treatment is typically required. Many people require lifelong support to maintain healthful eating and lifestyle habits.

Study Questions

Answers can be found at nutrition.jbpub.com/discovering.

1. **What three factors play a role in most, if not all, eating disorders?**
2. **What are the warning signs of anorexia nervosa?**
3. **What is the usual treatment for people with anorexia nervosa, and what do most experts say about their recovery?**
4. **What is the typical profile of a person with bulimia nervosa?**
5. **Describe an eating binge and all the behaviors that constitute purging.**
6. **List some common traits of people with binge-eating disorder.**
7. **What are the three components of the female athlete triad?**

[Try] This

Is There Any Help Out There?

How much help is available in your community for people with eating disorders? Scan the telephone directory (Yellow Pages) for eating disorder clinics, programs, and centers. Call them to inquire about their services. Do they have a psychologist, medical doctor, dietitian, nurse, and/or social worker on staff? Is it an inpatient or outpatient program? What is their philosophy of therapy? What is their success rate? What are their payment plans?

What About Bobbie?

Bobbie's friend Janet has been struggling with anorexia nervosa for some time. Bobbie recently expressed concern again and asked Janet about her eating habits. Janet told Bobbie she eats the following foods in a typical day:

"Breakfast"

1 head of iceberg lettuce, with salt and pepper but no dressing
(If she wakes up really hungry, she'll have another with vinegar on it.)

"Snack"

6 to 8 white mushrooms

"Lunch"

3 or 4 dill pickles

"Dinner"

1 12-ounce can artichoke hearts (rinsed)

Fluids include mineral water, diet cola, and/or caffeinated tea.

Let's compare this intake with Bobbie's (see Chapter 1 to review Bobbie's one-day diet). First, Janet's daily intake is just under 300 kilocalories compared with Bobbie's 2,440. Not only is Janet at risk due to her lack of calories, but her intake of protein is approximately 0 grams. Her body has already used any glycogen it had as reserve fuel. In addition, at 5 feet 3 inches and 98 pounds, she has very little reserve fat tissue for future energy needs. Without intake of dietary protein, her organ and muscle tissues have become prime targets for degradation. Even though Janet takes a multivitamin and a mineral supplement, if she doesn't seek help soon, she may suffer the typical symptoms and effects of starvation and malnutrition.

References

1 American Dietetic Association. Position of the American Dietetic Association: nutrition intervention in the treatment of anorexia nervosa, bulimia nervosa, and eating disorders not otherwise specified (EDNOS). *J Am Diet Assoc.* 2001;101: 810–819.

2 American Dietetic Association. *Manual of Clinical Dietetics.* 5th ed. Chicago: American Dietetic Association; 1996.

3 Crowther JH, Sanftner J, Bonifazi DZ, Sheperd KL. The role of daily hassles in binge eating. *Int J Eat Disord.* 2001;29: 449–454.

4 Westenhoefer J, Stunkard AJ, Pudel V. Validation of the flexible and rigid control dimensions of dietary restraint. *Int J Eat Disord.* 1999;26:53–64.

5 Leutwyler K. Treating eating disorders. The history of anorexia nervosa. http://www.sciam.com/explorations/1998/030298 eating/anorexia.html. Accessed 4/29/02.

6 Ibid.

7 Suraf M. Holy anorexia and anorexia nervosa: society and the concept of disease. *Pharo.* 1998;61(4):2–4.

8 Reid TR. The world according to Rome. *National Geographic.* 1997;8:54–83.

9 Casson L. *Everyday Life in Ancient Rome.* Baltimore: Johns Hopkins University Press; 1998.

10 National Institutes of Health, National Center for Health Statistics. http://www.nih.gov. Accessed 4/29/02.

11 Strauss R. Adolescents' perception of their body weight is dependent on social, cultural, and family pressures. *Arch Pediatr Adolesc Med.* 1998;153:741–747.

12 Gowan C. Teasing and body image: a predictor of eating disorders? Paper presented at: Annual Meeting of the American Psychiatric Association; August 1998; San Francisco.

13 Gleaves DH. Scope and significance of posttraumatic symptomatology among women hospitalized for an eating disorder. *Int J Eat Disord.* 1998;2:147–156.

14 Mayer LE, Walsh BT. The use of selective serotonin reuptake inhibitors in eating disorders [review]. *J Clin Psychiatry.* 1998;59(suppl 15):28–34.

15 Kaye W, Gendall K, Strober M. Serotonin neuronal function and selective serotonin reuptake inhibitor treatment in anorexia and bulimia nervosa [review]. *Biol Psychiatry.* 1998;44:825–838.

16 Lilenfeld LR, Kaye WH, Greeno CG, et al. A controlled family study of anorexia nervosa and bulimia nervosa: psychiatric disorders in first-degree relatives and effects of proband comorbidity. *Arch Gen Psychiatry.* 1998;55:603–610.

17 Aragona M, Vella G. Psychopathological considerations on the relationship between bulimia and obsessive-compulsive disorder. *Psychopathology.* 1998;31:197–205.

18 Leutwyler K. Treating eating disorders. http://www.sciam.com/explorations/1998/030298eating/index.html. Accessed 4/29/02.

19 Sakurai T, Amemiya A, Ishii M, et al. Orexins and orexin receptors: a family of hypothalamic neuropeptides and G protein-coupled receptors that regulate feeding behavior. *Cell.* 1998;92:573–585.

20 National Institutes of Health, National Center for Health Statistics. Op. cit.

21 Leutwyler K. Op.cit.

22 American Psychiatric Association. *Diagnostic and Statistical Manual of Mental Disorders.* 4th ed. Washington, DC: American Psychiatric Association; 1994.

23 le Grange D, Telch CF, Tibbs J. Eating attitudes and behaviors in 1,435 South African Caucasian and non-Caucasian college students. *Am J Psychiatry.* 1998;155:250–254.

24 Anderson AE. Recognizing eating disorders. *Nutrition & the MD.* 1998;24(7):5–7.

25 Logsdail S, Marks I, O'Sullivan G, et al. Eating disorders and obsessive-compulsive disorder. *Am J Psychiatry.* 1988;145:899.

26 Klump KL, Miller KB, Keel PK, et al. Genetic and environmental influences on anorexia nervosa syndromes in a population-based twin sample. *Psychol Med.* 2001;31:737–740.

27 Anderson AE. Op. cit.

28 Strauss R. Op. cit.

29 Anderson AE. Op. cit.

30 American Dietetic Association. 2001. Op. cit.

31 National Institutes of Health. Op. cit.

32 American Psychiatric Association. Op. cit.

33 Brownell K, Fairburn M. *Eating Disorders and Obesity: A Comprehensive Handbook.* New York: Guilford Press; 1995.

34 Anderson AE. Op. cit.

35 Leutwyler K. Op. cit.

36 Anderson AE. Op. cit.

37 French SA, Leffert N, Story M, et al. Adolescent binge/purge and weight loss behaviors: associations with developmental assets. *J Adolesc Health.* 2001;28:211–221.

38 Leutwyler K. Op. cit.

39 American Psychiatric Association. Op. cit.

40 Ibid.

41 Olivardia R, Pope HG Jr, Mangweth B, Hudson JI. Eating disorders in college men. *Am J Psychiatry.* 1995;152:1279–1284.

42 Andersen EA. *Males with Eating Disorders.* New York: Brunner Mazel; 1990.

43 Strober M, Freeman R, Lampert C, et al. Males with anorexia nervosa: a controlled study of eating disorders in first-degree relatives. *Int J Eat Disord.* 2001;29:263–269.

44 Olivardia R, et al. Op. cit.

45 Eating disorders and exercise: the connection. *Nutrition & the MD.* 1998;24(7):5–6.

46 Benyo R. *The Exercise Fix.* Berkeley, CA: Leisure Press; 1991.

47 Otis CI, Drinkwater B, Johnson M, et al. American College of Sports Medicine position stand. The female athlete triad. *Med Sci Sports Exerc.* 1997;29:i–ix.

48 Ruud JS, Woolsy MN, Dorfman L. Eating disorders in athletes. In: Rosenbloom CA, ed. *Sports Nutrition.* 3rd ed. Chicago: American Dietetic Association; 2000.

49 Mermel V. A review of contemporary sports nutrition. *Athletic Training.* 1995;1(3):228–244.

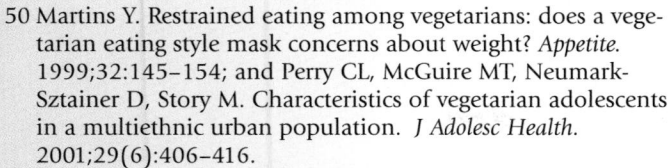

50 Martins Y. Restrained eating among vegetarians: does a vegetarian eating style mask concerns about weight? *Appetite.* 1999;32:145–154; and Perry CL, McGuire MT, Neumark-Sztainer D, Story M. Characteristics of vegetarian adolescents in a multiethnic urban population. *J Adolesc Health.* 2001;29(6):406–416.

51 Crisp AH, Halek C, Sedgewick P, et al. Smoking and pursuit of thinness in schoolgirls in London and Ottawa. *Postgrad Med J.* 1998;74:473–479.

52 Leifshiz F. Children on adult diets: is it harmful? Is it hurtful? *J Am Coll Nutr.* 1992;11:845–850.

53 Ibid.

54 Satter E. The feeding relationship: implications for dietitians. Paper presented at: Annual Meeting of the American Dietetic Association; October 1992; Washington, DC.

55 Parham ES. Promoting body size acceptance in weight management counseling. *J Am Diet Assoc.* 1999;99:920–925.

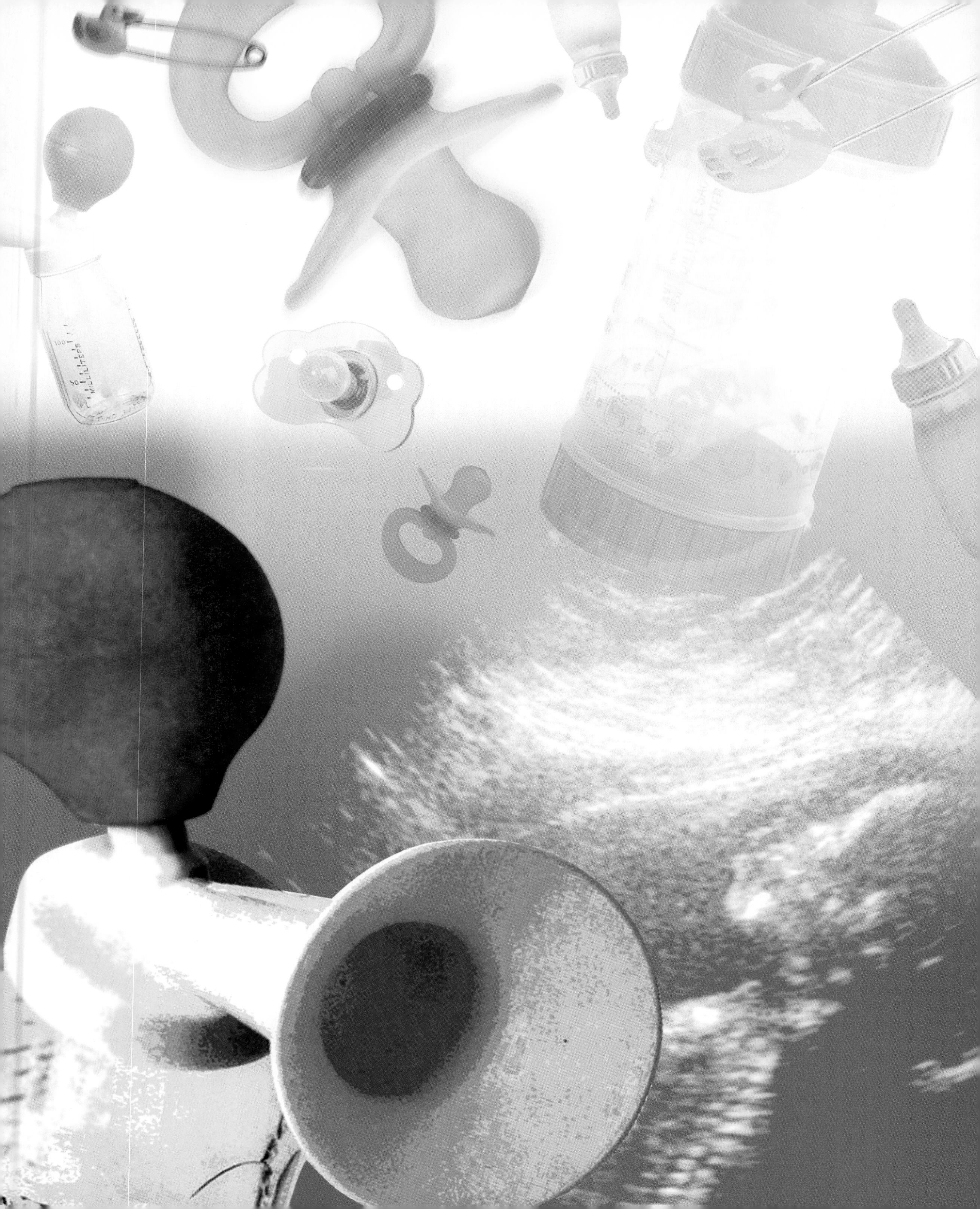

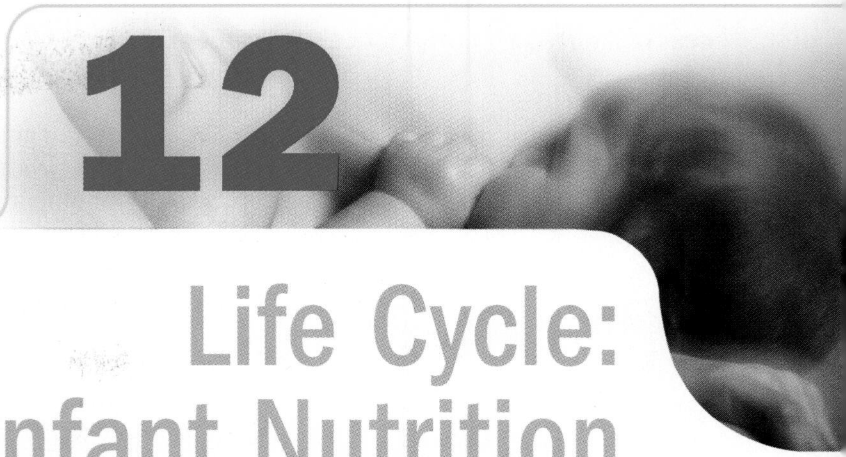

Chapter 12

Life Cycle: Maternal and Infant Nutrition

Think About It

1. Saying she is eating for two, your pregnant friend can't stop eating. What do you think about this?
2. Your best friend tells you she is pregnant. You know that she enjoys wine with dinner. What do you say to her?
3. Were you breastfed? Do you know of any benefits?
4. At a fast-food restaurant, you observe a man and woman giving a very young infant tiny pieces of french fries and a baby bottle filled with cola. Any thoughts?

Fyi for your Information

This chapter's FYI boxes include practical information on the following topics:

- Vegetarianism and Pregnancy
- Fruit Juices and Drinks

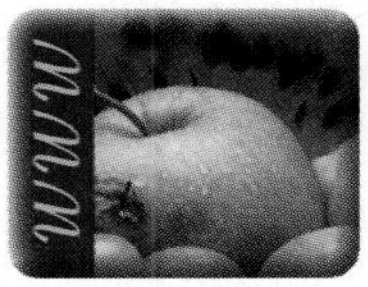

The Web site for this book offers many useful tools and is a great source for additional nutrition information for both students and instructors. For information on nutrition for pregnancy and lactation, visit the site at **nutrition.jbpub.com/discovering.** You'll find exercises that explore the following topics:

- Iron Supplementation in Canada
- Don't Even Mention Food: Eating during Morning Sickness
- Spicy Breast Milk?
- The Lactational Amenorrhea Method

Key to Illustrations

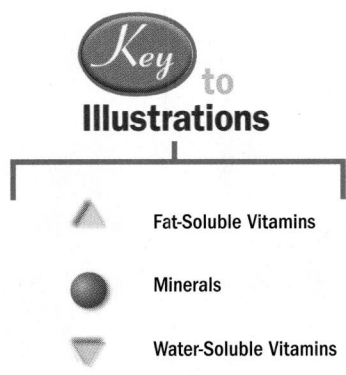

- ▲ Fat-Soluble Vitamins
- ● Minerals
- ▼ Water-Soluble Vitamins

What About Bobbie?

Track the choices Bobbie is making with the EatRight Analysis software.

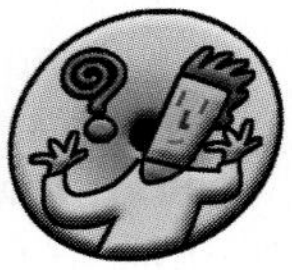

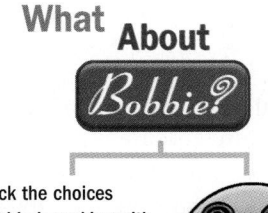

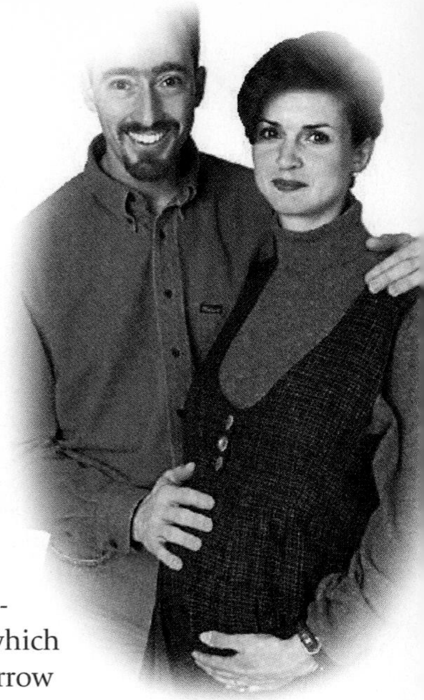

Imagine waking up tomorrow and finding a newborn baby in the house! Play along for a moment with the idea that it's *your* baby. Would your current eating habits have been sufficient to support the nutritional demands of pregnancy? If not, what changes should you have made and why? What about other aspects of your lifestyle that might need to be modified *before* pregnancy, such as smoking, alcohol use, exercise? How would you feed a new baby? Breastfeeding poses its own nutritional demands but has many benefits for the infant. If you've never shopped for infant formula or baby food before, you may be surprised at the variety of choices and confused as to which is best. So, while the likelihood of waking up tomorrow and finding a newborn in the house is remote, it's never too early to learn about the nutritional implications of pregnancy, breastfeeding, and infant feeding.

Pregnancy

Pregnancy is a time of tremendous physiological changes, and these changes demand healthful dietary and lifestyle choices. Energy and nutrient needs both increase, but the need for calories increases by a smaller percentage than the need for vitamins and minerals. As a result, food choices during pregnancy must be nutrient-dense.

What about tobacco and alcohol? Research clearly shows that both have damaging effects on a developing fetus, and it's essential to abstain from both during pregnancy. Although research about the effects of caffeine is less conclusive, most health care professionals also recommend limiting caffeine intake during pregnancy.

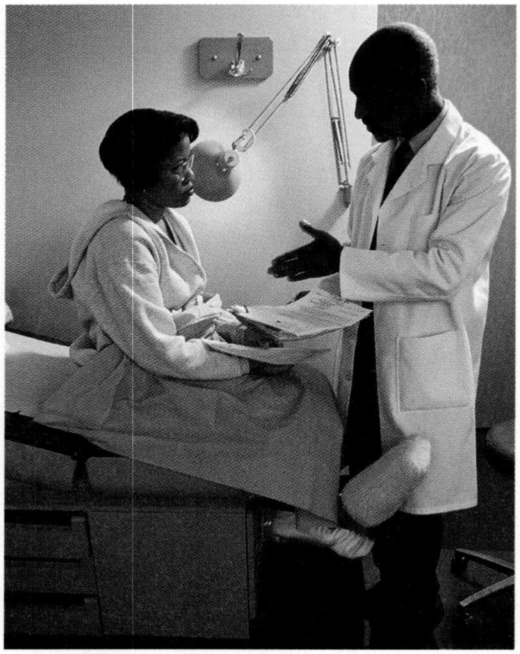

Figure 12.1 **Preconception care.** Planning and care before pregnancy are recommended for all prospective mothers.

Nutrition before Conception

Everyone knows a woman needs to eat well once she becomes pregnant. But her nutritional status at the moment of conception is also critical. Vitamin status at conception, for example, can mean the difference between a healthy baby and one with a devastating birth defect. In addition, a woman's weight at conception can influence her pregnancy and delivery and the baby's health.

For these reasons, it's important for a woman to get care before she gets pregnant; many experts recommend extending prenatal care—the routine health care that a woman receives during her pregnancy—to include the preconception period as well. (See **Figure 12.1**.) Preconception care has three main components: risk assessment, health promotion, and intervention. Nutrition is an important aspect of all three components. (See **Table 12.1**.)

Weight

Although everyone should be concerned about maintaining a healthful weight, a woman contemplating pregnancy needs to pay careful attention to weight. Maternal obesity can complicate pregnancy and delivery and may compromise a baby's health. Being too thin, meanwhile, carries its own risks.

Body mass index (BMI) is an indicator of a prospective mother's weight status. (See Chapter 8, "Energy Balance and Weight Management," to review

Table 12.1 Nutrition-Related Components of Preconception Care

Risk Assessment	
Age, diet, substance use (tobacco, alcohol, illicit drugs)	
Existing medical condition(s)	
Barriers to prenatal care and primary health care	
Health Promotion	
Healthful diet and refraining from substance use	
Compliance with prenatal care	
Interventions	
Referral to high-risk pregnancy programs if necessary	
Referral to treatment of adverse health behaviors	
Nutrition counseling, supplementation, or referral to improve diet as needed	

Source: Adapted in part from Jack B, et al. *Perspectives on Prenatal Care.* New York: Elsevier Science; 1990.

preterm delivery A delivery that occurs before the 37th week of gestation.

low-birth-weight infant A newborn who weighs less than 2,500 grams (5.5 lb) as a result of either premature birth or inadequate growth in utero.

morning sickness A persistent or recurring nausea that often occurs in the morning during early pregnancy.

how to calculate BMI.) Lean women with a BMI less than 20 kg/m^2 have increased risks of **preterm delivery** and delivering a **low-birth-weight infant**.[1] At the other end of the spectrum, overweight and obese women have increased risks of several problems, including preterm delivery and stillbirth.[2]

Of course, the time to lose or gain weight is well before a pregnancy begins. It is not a good idea for pregnant women, even obese pregnant women, to diet. And a thin woman who finds it hard to put on weight under normal circumstances is unlikely to find it any easier when she's pregnant, especially if she experiences **morning sickness**.

Women with eating disorders have special pregnancy-related risks. Ideally, anorexia nervosa or bulimia nervosa is diagnosed and treated well before conception, to give the prospective mother's body plenty of time to recover and prepare for the rigors of pregnancy, birth, and breastfeeding. A woman who begins her pregnancy with an active eating disorder may not gain enough weight—or may vomit too much—to sustain a growing fetus. Risks can include premature delivery, a low-birth-weight infant, and even fetal death.

Quick Bites

When D Gets a Failing Grade

New data provide irrefutable proof that vitamin D deficiency is a major unrecognized epidemic in adult women of childbearing age, according to Michael F. Holick of Boston University. In the July 2002 *American Journal of Clinical Nutrition*, a CDC study reports that 42 percent of 1,546 African American women and 4.2 percent of 1,426 white women lacked sufficient vitamin D. Infants born to these women could suffer major health problems. In the June 2002 *Canadian Medical Association Journal*, another study documents a high prevalence of vitamin D deficiency in healthy Canadians.

Vitamins

A good diet goes a long way toward meeting the demands of pregnancy, but even a diet that includes all the food groups may not contain enough of certain nutrients. This is especially true for folic acid, a nutrient needed to prevent neural tube defects, which are birth defects that involve the spinal column.[3] One of the most common neural tube defects is spina bifida, a birth defect in which part of the spinal cord protrudes through the spinal column, causing varying degrees of paralysis and lack of bowel and bladder control. (See **Figure 12.2**.) Spina bifida and other neural tube defects affect approximately 4,000 pregnancies each year in the United States.

The U.S. Public Health Service and the Institute of Medicine of the National Academy of Sciences both recommend that all women of childbearing age consume 400 micrograms of synthetic folic acid each day from fortified foods or supplements to reduce the risk of having a pregnancy affected with a neural tube defect. This recommendation covers all women

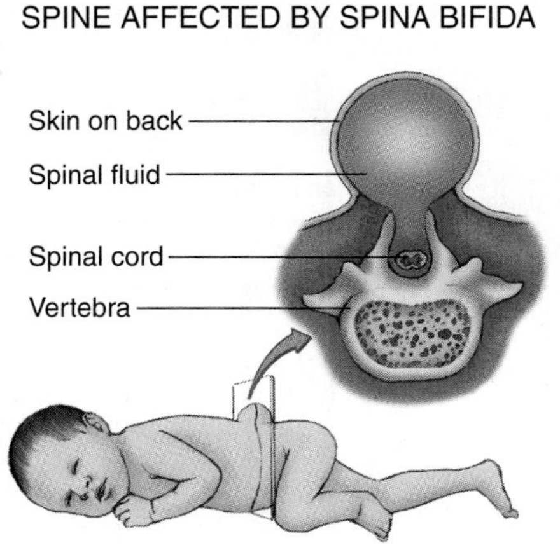

Figure 12.2 **Spina bifida: a neural tube defect.** Low folate status during the early stages of pregnancy can cause neural tube defects.

Table 12.2 **Folate in Grain Products**

Foods	Folate (μg DFE)
Ready-to-eat cereals (25% DV), 1 C	170
Pasta, enriched, cooked, 1 C	140–160
Rice, enriched, cooked, 1 C	170
Tortilla, flour, enriched, 1 (10" diameter)	140
Bagel, enriched, 2 oz (3" diameter)	70
Bread, white, enriched, 1 slice	25–40

Source: Data compiled from Suitor CW, Bailey LB. Dietary folate equivalents: interpretation and application. *J Am Diet Assoc.* 2000;100:88–94.

of childbearing age—not just pregnant women—because neural tube development occurs before the sixth week of fetal life. During this period, a woman may not know she is pregnant or may not have made appropriate dietary changes. This recommended intake of folic acid is in addition to folate (the natural form of the vitamin) consumed from other foods. **Table 12.2** presents the folate content of selected grain products.

While it's important to get enough folic acid, it is also crucial to avoid getting too much vitamin A (retinol) during pregnancy. Some vitamin A is good for you; too much may be teratogenic. A teratogen is a substance that causes birth defects—literally, the term means "monster-producing." The Institute of Medicine considered this link between excessive retinol intake and birth defects in setting the Tolerable Upper Intake Level (UL) of retinol for women of childbearing age. The UL is 3,000 micrograms (10,000 IU) of retinol from food and supplements for women over the age of 18. For teens, the UL is 2,800 micrograms (9,300 IU).

Any woman who might become pregnant must avoid using drugs that contain vitamin A or vitamin A analogs; examples are the acne medications isotretinoin (Accutane) and tretinoin (Retin-A). Because these medications are potent teratogens,[4] doctors typically prescribe such drugs to women of childbearing age only if tests show a woman is not pregnant, and she practices birth control.

Pregnant women can—and should—eat as much as they like of fruits and vegetables rich in beta-carotene and other carotenoids. These foods pose no risk of birth defects and offer many health benefits.

Substance Use

Many women plan to give up cigarettes, alcohol, or other drugs when they get pregnant. A better plan is to give up the substances well before becoming pregnant. (See **Figure 12.3**.) A woman who uses or abuses tobacco, alcohol, or illicit drugs prior to conception is likely to enter pregnancy with a low BMI and deficient nutritional stores.[5]

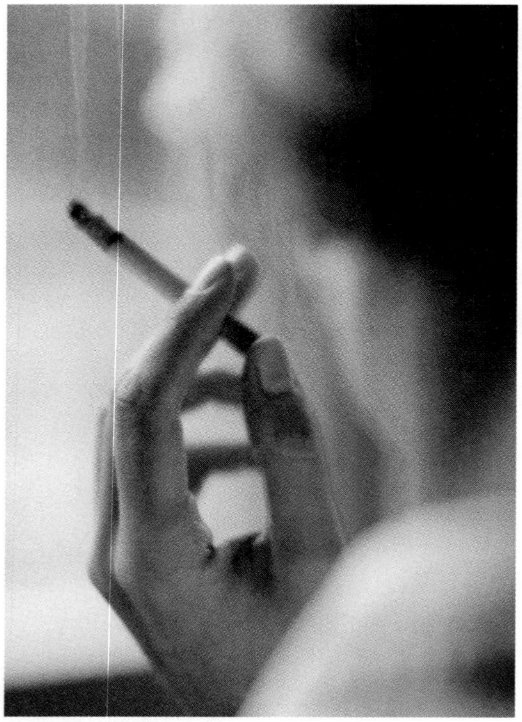

Figure 12.3 **Substance use.** Using tobacco, alcohol, or illicit drugs before and during pregnancy puts the baby at risk. If you use these substances, stop before becoming pregnant.

Key Concepts: *Ideally, the time to prepare nutritionally for pregnancy is well before conception. A woman who has adequate nutrient stores, particularly of folic acid, and is at a healthy weight can reduce the risk for maternal and fetal complications during pregnancy. In addition to healthful diet selections, avoiding cigarettes, alcohol, and other drugs is important when contemplating pregnancy.*

Physiology of Pregnancy

Pregnancy is an awe-inspiring process of growth and development that affects both mother and fetus. An understanding of the physiological changes that occur in the mother during pregnancy, and of the growth and development of the fetus, will help to explain the nutrient needs of a pregnant woman.

Stages of Human Fetal Growth

How long does pregnancy last? Nine months, right? Well, it depends on when you start counting. When a health care provider gives an expectant mother a due date, it is typically calculated as 40 weeks from the date of the start of her last menstrual period, roughly 10 to 14 days before the date of conception. This 40-week period is often divided into three **trimesters** of 13 or 14 weeks each; however, this division does not reflect specific stages

trimesters Three equal time periods of pregnancy, each lasting approximately 13 to 14 weeks.

in fetal development. **Figure 12.4** illustrates the early stages of pregnancy.

Following fertilization of the egg (ovum) comes the **blastogenic stage**—a period of rapid cell division. As these cells divide, they begin to differentiate. The inner cells in this growing mass will form the fetus; the outer layer of cells will become the **placenta**.

The next period of pregnancy, the **embryonic stage**, extends from the end of the second week through the eighth week after conception. The placenta, a vital organ that serves as a conduit between mother and child, forms on the uterine wall during this stage. Attached to the placenta by the umbilical cord, the embryo now receives its nourishment from its mother; and nearly everything the mother eats, drinks, or smokes reaches the embryo. This is the period of **organogenesis**. By the time the embryo is eight weeks old, all of the main internal organs have formed, along with the major external body structures. (See **Figure 12.5**.) Because nutrient deficiencies or excesses and intake of harmful substances can result in congenital abnormalities (birth defects) or spontaneous abortion (miscarriage), this stage is a **critical period of development.**

The longest period of pregnancy is the **fetal stage**, the period from the end of the embryonic period until the baby is born. During this time, the fetus is growing rapidly, with dramatic changes in body proportions. From the end of the third month of pregnancy until delivery at full term, fetal weight increases nearly 500-fold. The typical newborn is about 20 inches long and weighs approximately 7 pounds 7 ounces.

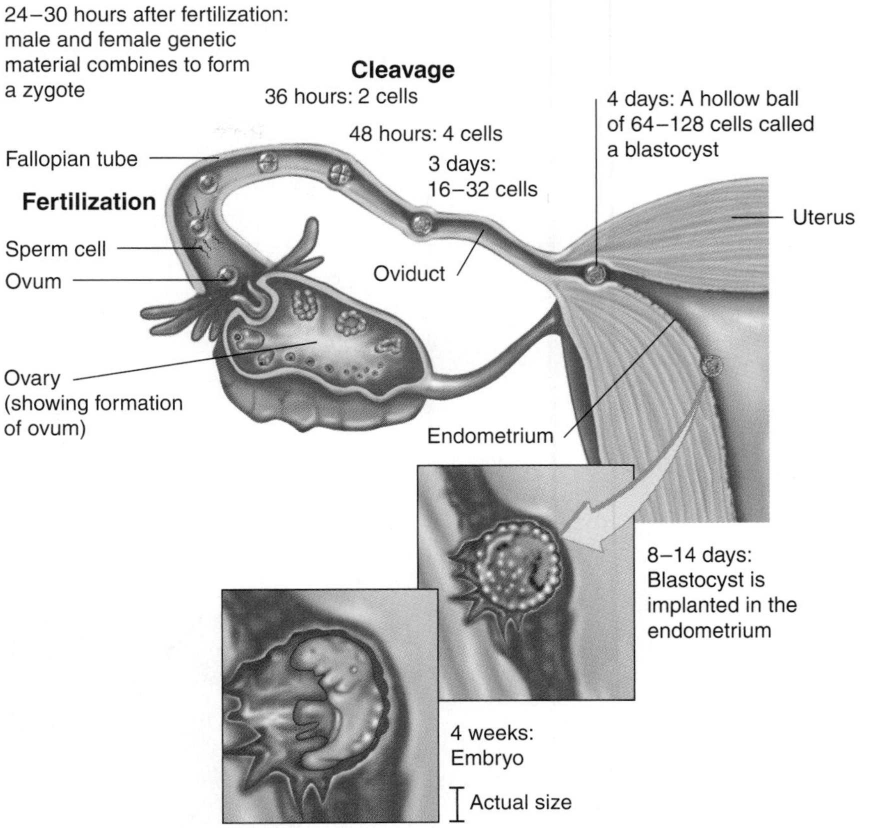

Figure 12.4 **Early stages of pregnancy.** The fertilized egg divides rapidly and begins to differentiate. The inner cells become the fetus, and the outer cells become the placenta.

Key Concepts: *From conception to full-term baby, the process of fetal development is typically divided into three stages. The blastogenic stage involves rapid cell division*

blastogenic stage The first stage of gestation, during which tissue proliferation by rapid cell division begins.

placenta The organ formed during pregnancy that produces hormones for the maintenance of pregnancy and across which oxygen and nutrients are transferred from mother to infant; it also allows waste materials to be transferred from infant to mother.

embryonic stage The developmental stage between the time of implantation (about two weeks after fertilization) through the seventh or eighth week; the stage of major organ system differentiation and development of main external features.

organogenesis The period of time when organ systems are developing in a growing fetus.

critical period of development Time during which the environment has the greatest impact on the developing embryo.

fetal stage The period of rapid growth from the end of the embryonic stage until birth.

Quick Bites

Would It Be Healthier to Menstruate *Less* Often?

Women in industrialized countries, who start menstruating at an average age of 12.5 years, will go through 350 to 400 menstrual cycles in their lifetimes. In populations where birth control is not used, however, women spend the majority of their fertile years either pregnant or lactating. Menarche in these populations occurs at an average age of 16. In addition, since menstrual cycles do not occur during pregnancy and may not occur during lactation, women in natural-fertility populations, like the Dogon of West Africa, experience only about 110 menstrual cycles in a lifetime. Women who go through fewer menstrual cycles are exposed to less estrogen and other steroid hormones. Researchers hypothesize that this may partly explain why nonindustrialized societies have lower cancer rates than industrialized societies.

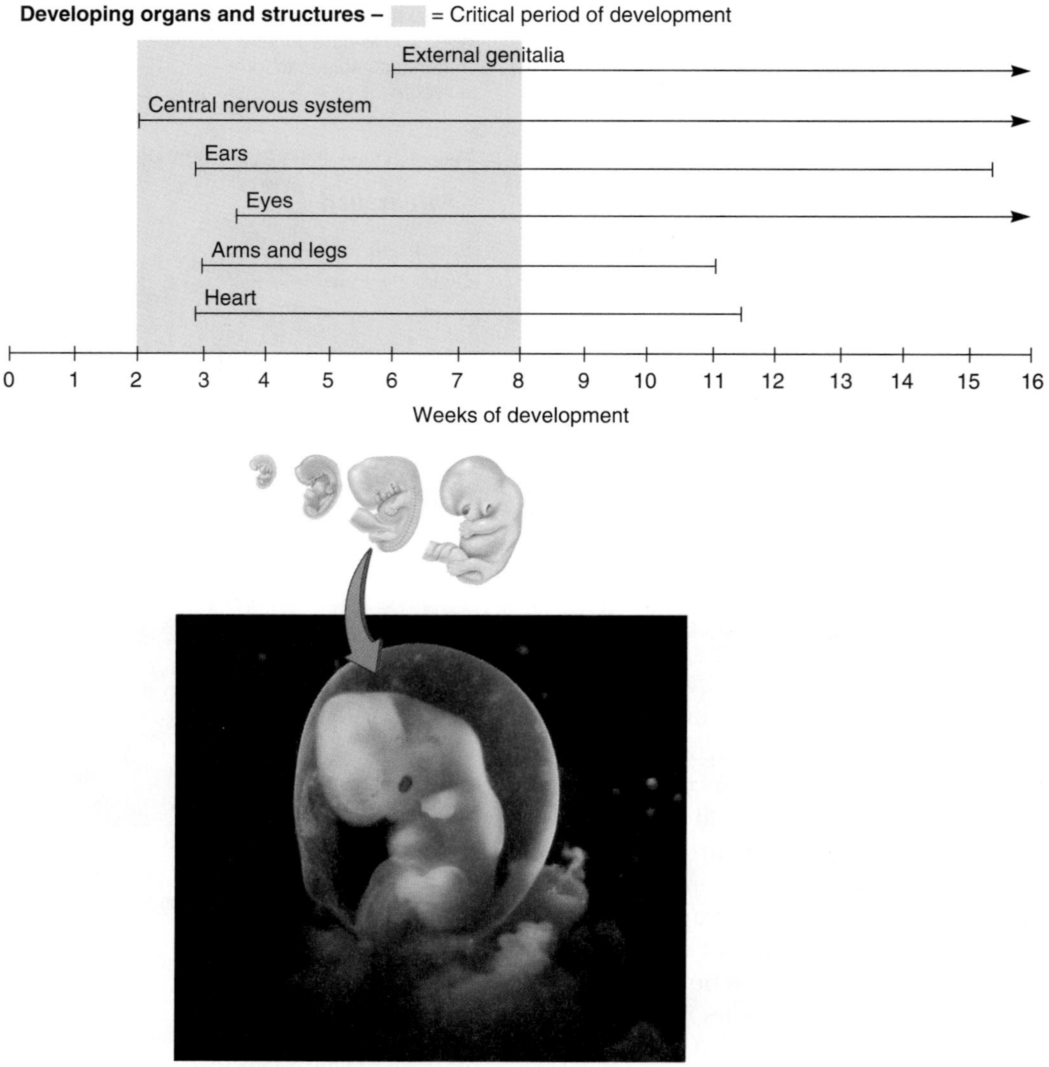

Figure 12.5 **Embryonic development.** During the embryonic stage—week 2 through week 8—all the major organ systems are forming. During this critical period of development, the embryo is highly vulnerable to nutrient deficiencies and toxicities as well as harmful substances like tobacco smoke.

Quick Bites

Who Am I?

Our entire collection of genes, the human genome, contains about 30,000 genes. These genes are made of building blocks called base pairs. The human genome contains about three billion base pairs. Your mother supplied half of your genes and your father supplied the other half to create your unique combination. Unless you are an identical twin, no other person has your exact combination of genes.

lactation The process of synthesizing and secreting breast milk.

of the fertilized ovum and its implantation in the uterine wall. Cells differentiate and organ systems and body structures are formed during the embryonic stage. The fetal stage, the longest stage of pregnancy, is marked by growth in size and change in body proportions.

Maternal Physiological Changes and Nutrition

While the fertilized ovum develops from blastocyst to embryo to fetus, changes are occurring in the mother's body as well. (See **Figure 12.6**.) These changes occur as the result of various hormones secreted mainly by the placenta.

Growth of Maternal Tissue

Maternal tissues, including the breasts, uterus, and adipose stores, increase in size during pregnancy. Hormones promote growth and changes in the breast tissue to prepare for **lactation**. Fat stores increase to provide energy for late pregnancy and for lactation and are a major component of maternal weight gain.

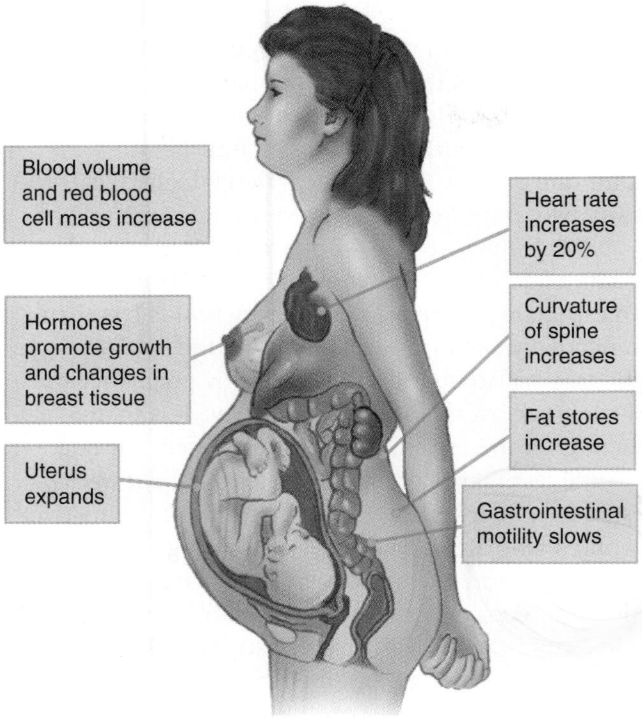
Blood volume and red blood cell mass increase
Heart rate increases by 20%
Hormones promote growth and changes in breast tissue
Curvature of spine increases
Fat stores increase
Uterus expands
Gastrointestinal motility slows

Figure 12.6 **Maternal changes during pregnancy.** Hormones released throughout pregnancy influence the growth of the baby and alter the way the mother's organs function.

Maternal Blood Volume

During the course of pregnancy, blood volume expands by nearly 50 percent. Production of red blood cells also increases. Iron, folate, and vitamin B_{12} are all key nutrients in red blood cell production.

Gastrointestinal Changes

During pregnancy, gastrointestinal motility slows, and food moves more slowly through the intestinal tract. On the plus side, nutrient absorption is increased because nutrients spend more time in the small intestine. On the other hand, slower motility can contribute to nausea, heartburn, constipation, and hemorrhoids.

Key Concepts: *The mother's body is undergoing various changes during pregnancy, guided by changing levels of hormones. Uterine, breast, and adipose tissues grow; blood volume expands; and gastrointestinal motility slows. All of these changes have nutritional and dietary implications for pregnant women.*

Maternal Weight Gain

How much weight should a woman gain during pregnancy? Doctors' recommendations have varied over the years from minimal weight gain to unlimited weight gain to more recent recommendations based on prepregnancy BMI, as shown in **Table 12.3**. For women of normal weight (BMI of 19.8–26 kg/m^2), the recommended weight gain is 25 to 35 pounds (12.5–18 kg).[6] For the

Table 12.3 Guidelines for Weight Gain during Pregnancy

Prepregnancy BMI	Weight Gain*	
(kg/m^2)	(lb)	(kg)
Low (< 19.8)	28–40	12.5–18
Normal (19.8–26)	25–35	11.5–16
High (> 26–29)	15–25	7.0–11.5
Obese (> 29)	≥ 15	≥ 6

*Young adolescents should strive for gains at the upper end of the recommended range. Short women (< 157 cm or 62 in.) should strive for gains at the lower end of the range.

Source: Adapted with permission from *Nutrition during Pregnancy.* Copyright 1990 by the National Academy of Sciences. Courtesy of the National Academy Press, Washington, DC.

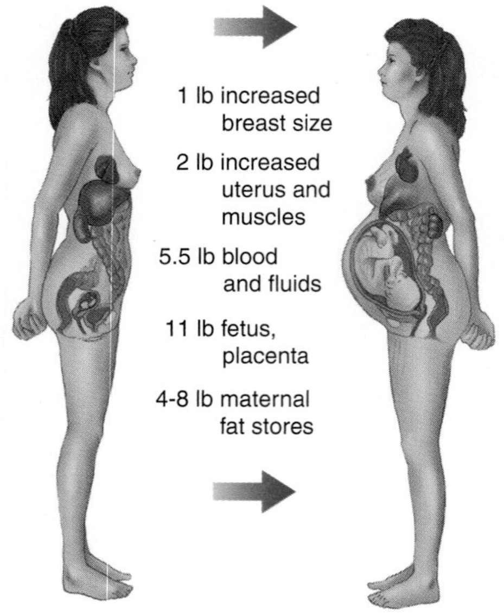

Figure 12.7 **Components of maternal weight gain.** During the first trimester, most women gain less than 5 pounds. Over the second and third trimesters, the suggested weight gain is a little less than 1 pound a week.

heaviest women—those with BMIs greater than 29 kg/m^2 at the start of pregnancy—a weight gain of at least 15 pounds (6 kg) is recommended. When maternal weight gain is within these limits, infants are more likely to be born normal weight and at term. However, weight gain varies widely among women who give birth to healthy, full-term infants.[7]

Twin births account for one of every 90 live births in the United States. Of course, women who carry two, or more, fetuses need to gain more weight, 35 to 45 pounds (16–20.5 kg), than women who carry just one. A higher weight gain is also recommended for women who were underweight prior to pregnancy. When an expectant mother's prepregnancy BMI is less than 19.8 kg/m^2, the recommended weight gain is 28 to 40 pounds (13–18 kg).

The pattern of weight gain is also important to a healthy pregnancy outcome. During the first trimester, average weight gain is low, less than 5 pounds for most women. Over the second and third trimesters, the suggested weight gain is a little less than 1 pound a week (0.4 kg per week), with more gain suggested for underweight women and those carrying twins and a lower gain for women who are overweight.[8] Monitoring the amount and rate of weight gain is an important component of prenatal care.

The weight gained during pregnancy can be divided into (1) the fetus and associated tissues and fluids and (2) maternal tissue growth. In a typical final weight gain of 27.5 pounds (12.5 kg), the fetus, placenta, and **amniotic fluid** account for nearly 40 percent of that weight. Maternal tissues (i.e., adipose stores, breast and uterine growth, and expanded blood and extracellular fluid volumes) account for the remaining 60 percent. (See **Figure 12.7**.)

Key Concepts: *Weight gained during pregnancy is a combination of fetal and maternal tissues and fluids. Weight gain recommendations are based on BMI prior to pregnancy. Women of normal weight (BMI = 19.8–26 kg/m^2) should gain 25 to 35 pounds over the course of pregnancy. Most of this weight gain occurs during the second and third trimesters.*

amniotic fluid The fluid that surrounds the fetus; contained in the amniotic sac inside the uterus.

Energy and Nutrition during Pregnancy

A pregnant woman requires added calories to grow and maintain not just her developing fetus, but also the placenta, increased breast tissue, and fat stores. Growth and development of the fetus also require protein, vitamins, and minerals.

Energy

The current RDA for energy suggests that during the second and third trimesters, pregnant women need 300 kilocalories per day more than they did prior to pregnancy. Recent evidence suggests that this recommendation is too simplistic and does not reflect the wide variation in energy expended by pregnant women.[9] Weight gain during pregnancy is probably the best indicator of adequate calorie intake. Think About It 1

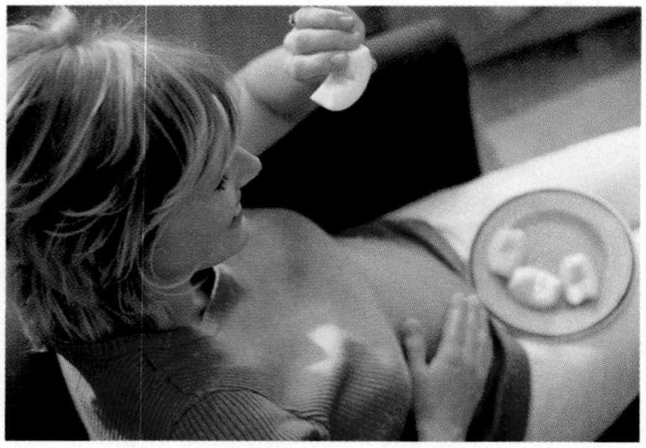

As mentioned in the discussion of preconception care, women should never diet to lose weight or sharply restrict weight gain during pregnancy. Inadequate energy intake during the first trimester is associated with higher rates of premature delivery, fetal death, and malformations of the infant's central nervous system. During the second and third trimesters, restricting intake results in slowed fetal growth so that the fetus is underdeveloped for his or her age.

Key Concepts: *The RDA for energy is increased by 300 kilocalories per day for pregnancy, although current evidence suggests that the actual increase in need varies substantially among women. The adequacy of energy intake can be measured by the amount of weight gained. Weight loss is not advised during pregnancy, even for obese women.*

Nutrients to Support Pregnancy

Most healthy women who eat a well-balanced diet have no trouble meeting the majority of their nutrient requirements in pregnancy without vitamin and mineral supplements. Essential nutrients can be divided into two broad categories: macronutrients (proteins, fats, and carbohydrates) and micronutrients (vitamins and minerals). **Table 12.4** shows the nutrient recommendations for pregnant women compared with nonpregnant women.

Macronutrients

Macronutrients supply energy and provide the building blocks for protein synthesis. The recommended balance of energy sources does not change during pregnancy. A low-fat, moderate-protein, high-carbohydrate diet is still appropriate.

Protein A pregnant woman's RDA for protein is 60 grams—about 10 to 15 grams a day higher than that recommended for women in the general population. This amount of protein is needed for the synthesis of new maternal, placental, and fetal tissues and is easily supplied in typical American diets consumed by nonpregnant women. Thus, many women need not increase their protein intake to reach the levels recommended for pregnancy. Pregnant women who are vegetarians, including vegans, also should be able to meet their protein needs from food sources alone—as long as they select a variety of protein sources and consume enough total calories. (See the FYI feature "Vegetarianism and Pregnancy.")

Fats Dietary fats provide vital fuel for the mother and for the development of placental tissues. The pregnant woman's body also stores fats to support breastfeeding after childbirth. Very-low-fat diets (in which fewer than 10 percent of daily calories come from dietary fats) are not recommended for pregnancy. Such diets are unlikely to supply sufficient amounts of essential fatty acids, fat-soluble vitamins, or calories.

Carbohydrates Carbohydrates provide the main source of extra calories during pregnancy. Food choices should emphasize complex carbohydrates such as whole-grain breads, fortified cereals, rice, and pasta. In addition to supplying vitamins and minerals, these foods can increase fiber intake substantially. A fiber-rich diet is recommended during pregnancy to help prevent constipation and hemorrhoids.

Key Concepts: *Most healthy women with well-balanced diets meet the majority of their nutrient requirements during pregnancy. Although protein needs increase during pregnancy, the basic balance of energy sources should still emphasize complex carbohydrates. As long as energy intake is adequate and a variety of foods are eaten, protein intake should be more than adequate to support prenatal growth and development.*

Micronutrients

A pregnant woman has an increased need for many vitamins and minerals that support growth and development. In addition, her increased energy needs mean she also requires higher amounts of nutrients such as the

Table 12.4 Nutritional Recommendations for Pregnancy

	Nonpregnant	Pregnant	% increase
Energy (kcal)	2,200	2,500	14
Protein (g)	46	60	30
Vitamin A (µg RAE)	700	770	10
Vitamin D (µg)	5	5	0
Vitamin E (mg)	15	15	0
Vitamin K (µg)	90	90	0
Thiamin (mg)	1.1	1.4	27
Riboflavin (mg)	1.1	1.4	27
Niacin (mg)	14	18	29
Vitamin B_6 (mg)	1.3	1.9	46
Folate (µg)	400	600	50
Vitamin B_{12} (µg)	2.4	2.6	8
Pantothenic acid (mg)	5	6	20
Biotin (µg)	30	30	0
Choline (mg)	425	450	6
Vitamin C (mg)	75	85	13
Calcium (mg)	1,000	1,000	0
Phosphorus (mg)	700	700	0
Magnesium (mg)	310	350	13
Iron (mg)	18	27	50
Zinc (mg)	8	11	38
Selenium (µg)	55	60	9
Iodine (µg)	150	220	47
Fluoride (mg)	3	3	0
Copper (µg)	900	1,000	11
Chromium (µg)	25	30	20
Manganese (mg)	1.8	2	11
Molybdenum (µg)	45	50	11

Needs for most nutrients increase during pregnancy. Generally, vitamin and mineral needs increase more than energy needs, which means that food choices should be nutrient-dense. Values shown are RDA or AI values for ages 19 to 24 (vitamins and minerals) or 19 to 30 (energy and protein).

B vitamins thiamin, riboflavin, niacin, and pantothenic acid that are essential for energy metabolism.

Needs for the other B vitamins (except biotin) also increase. Folate and vitamin B_{12} are used in synthesis of DNA and red blood cells, and vitamin B_6 is crucial for metabolism of amino acids. Of these vitamins, folate needs increase the most, from 400 micrograms per day to 600 micrograms per day during pregnancy. Vitamin C needs increase slightly during pregnancy, from 75 to 85 milligrams per day for women aged 19 to 50 years. For the fat-soluble vitamins, the RDA for vitamin A increases slightly during pregnancy, while the recommended intake levels for vitamins D, E, and K are unchanged.

For most minerals, recommended intakes are higher during pregnancy, most dramatically for iron. The RDA for iron increases from 18 milligrams per day to 27 milligrams per day. Iron is necessary to make red blood cells and is important for normal growth and energy metabolism. Iron deficiency

Fyi Vegetarianism and Pregnancy

FOR YOUR INFORMATION

Can pregnant women meet all of their nutritional needs on a vegetarian diet? A fair question. Common vegetarian practices include the avoidance of meat, poultry, and fish (lacto-ovo-vegetarian and lactovegetarian) and the avoidance of all animal foods (vegan). These foods are important sources of iron, zinc, calcium, vitamin B_{12}, and other nutrients. Although vegetarian diets can provide reasonable quantities of trace elements, animal-derived foods frequently contribute larger amounts that the body absorbs more easily. To meet the demands of pregnancy, supplementation may be in order.

Supplemental iron is generally recommended for all pregnant women. Supplemental vitamin B_{12} (2.0 micrograms per day) is also recommended for vegan mothers. If their sun exposure is limited, they also may need daily supplementation of 10 micrograms of vitamin D.[1] Vegetarians with low calcium intake (<600 milligrams per day) should consume a supplement that provides at least 500 milligrams per day. Some vegan foods, such as fortified soy milks, may contain these important nutrients. It is important to check the label to be sure.

The overall nutrient content of a vegetarian diet depends on both the energy content and the variety of the foods consumed. The suggested dietary patterns in Table A will meet the average energy levels recommended for pregnant women.

1 Institute of Medicine. *Dietary Reference Intakes for Calcium, Phosphorus, Magnesium, Vitamin D, and Fluoride.* Washington, DC: National Academy Press; 1997.

Table A Suggested Servings for Pregnant Vegans

Food Group	*2,200 kcal*	*2,800 kcal*
Bread, grains, cereals (50% whole-grain products)	10	12
Legumes, plant proteins	2	3
Vegetables	3	4
Dark-green leafy vegetables	2	2
Fruits	4	6
Nuts, seeds	1	1
Fortified soy drinks* and tofu	3	3
Added fats and oils	4	6
Approximate Composition		
Protein (g)	76	95
% kcal as fat	24	25
% kcal as carbohydrate	62	61

* Milk alternatives fortified with calcium, vitamin D, and vitamin B_{12}

Source: Adapted from Haddad EH. Development of a vegetarian food guide. *Am J Clin Nutr.* 1994;59(suppl):1248S–1254S.

and its associated anemia is the most common nutrient deficiency in pregnancy. **Table 12.5** lists the characteristics of women who are at particularly high risk for iron deficiency.

Key Concepts: *Needs for vitamins and minerals increase during pregnancy, some more than others. Extra vitamins and minerals are needed to support growth and development as well as increased energy use. Recommended intake levels increase most dramatically for folate and iron.*

Food Choices for Pregnant Women

You may be surprised to learn that the recommended diet for a pregnant woman is not much different from that for adults in the general population. The familiar Food Guide Pyramid recommendations apply to pregnant women:

Food Group	Food Pyramid Servings	2,200 kcal Servings	2,800 kcal Servings
Bread, cereal, rice, and pasta	6–11	9	11
Vegetables	3–5	4	5
Fruits	2–3	3	4
Milk, yogurt, and cheese	2–3	3	3
Meat, poultry, fish, dried beans, eggs, and nuts	2–3	6 oz	7 oz
Fats, oils, and sweets		——Use sparingly——	

Using the Food Guide Pyramid for 2,200 or 2,800 kilocalories, pregnant women can plan menus that meet all their nutrient needs, with the exception of folate and iron.[10] Variety is the key to a well-balanced diet. The extra calories needed for pregnancy are easy to obtain from an additional serving from each of the following food groups—grains, vegetables, fruits, and low-fat milk. Because the increased need for energy is proportionately less than the increased need for most nutrients, nutrient-dense foods are important. There is little room in the diet plan for high-calorie, high-fat, low-nutrient "extras."

Supplementation

Other than iron and folate, a pregnant woman can get all of the nutrients she needs by making healthful choices using the Food Guide Pyramid. In an ideal world, health care providers would evaluate the dietary intake of all prenatal patients and recommend dietary changes to improve nutrition where needed. In reality, this seldom happens, and pregnant women in the United States and Canada routinely receive prescriptions for prenatal vitamin/mineral supplements. The amount and balance of nutrients in prenatal formulations is appropriate for pregnancy. Because toxic levels can be reached quickly, especially for vitamins A and D, pregnant women should avoid high-dose and multiple supplements. In addition, because most herbal preparations have not been evaluated for safety during pregnancy, they are not recommended.

Foods to Avoid

With the exception of alcohol, no foods are completely off limits to pregnant women. If a mother-to-be is experiencing problems with nausea and vomiting, she may want to abstain for a while from foods that aggravate these symptoms. Cultural traditions may dictate changes in diet during

Table 12.5 Factors Associated with Increased Risk for Iron Deficiency during Pregnancy

Young age (e.g., 15 to 19 years)
Multiple pregnancies
Diets low in meat and ascorbic acid
Diets high in coffee and tea
Low socioeconomic status
Low level of education
Black or Hispanic ethnicity

Source: Adapted from Puolakka J, Janne O, Pakarinen A, Vihko R. Serum ferritin in the diagnosis of anemia during pregnancy. *Acta Obstet Gynecol Scand.* 1980;95(suppl):57–63.

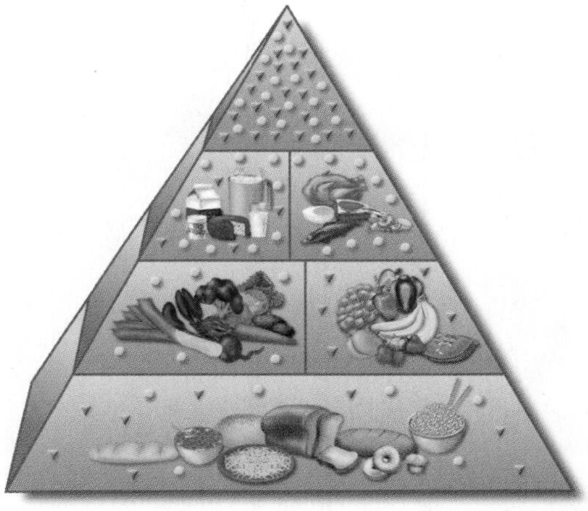

pregnancy, but these tend to reflect traditional beliefs and practices rather than health science.

The need to restrict or eliminate caffeine during pregnancy remains controversial. High caffeine intake has been shown to be teratogenic in animal studies and has been linked to low birth weight in humans. Recent studies suggest that low birth weight with high caffeine consumption occurs only in combination with smoking. Nonetheless, since caffeine sources tend to be low in nutrients, it is prudent to limit caffeine intake during pregnancy.

Key Concepts: *With the exception of iron and folate, a well-balanced, varied diet can easily meet all of a pregnant woman's nutrient needs. Pregnant women should choose nutrient-dense and high-carbohydrate foods in the proportions found in the Food Guide Pyramid. Although vitamin/mineral supplementation is common during pregnancy, it probably is not needed other than for iron and folate. When supplements are used, they should be designed for pregnant women. Pregnant women should avoid alcohol and moderate their intake of caffeine.*

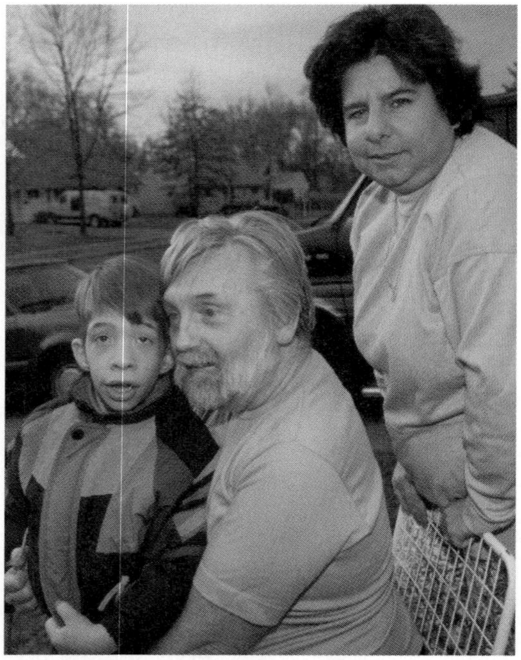

Figure 12.8 **Fetal alcohol syndrome.** The facial characteristics of a child with fetal alcohol syndrome include a short nose with a flattened bridge, eyelids with extra folds, and a thin upper lip with no groove below the nose.

Substance Use and Pregnancy Outcome

When a pregnant woman eats, she eats for two. When she smokes, drinks, or uses drugs, she does so for two as well. The consequences of these behaviors may be felt for generations.

Tobacco and Alcohol

Smoking during pregnancy increases the risks of miscarrying, delivering a stillborn infant, giving birth prematurely, and delivering a low-birth-weight baby.[11] Women in lower socioeconomic groups have the highest rates of cigarette use before, during, and after pregnancy. Women in the highest socioeconomic groups, meanwhile, are the most likely to quit smoking during pregnancy, but are just as likely as other women to take up the habit again after giving birth.

Fetal alcohol syndrome (FAS) describes a consistent pattern of physical, cognitive, and behavioral problems in infants born to women who use alcohol heavily during pregnancy. Children severely afflicted by the syndrome show marked growth deficiencies before and after birth; physical anomalies such as a small head, certain characteristic facial deformities (see **Figure 12.8**), heart defects, and joint and limb irregularities; mental retardation; and central nervous system disorders. The greater a mother's alcohol use during pregnancy, the more severe the symptoms of FAS tend to be in the child. There is no known safe threshold for alcohol use in pregnancy. The only way to avoid alcohol-related risks to a fetus is to avoid all alcohol during pregnancy.

Think About It 2

Drugs

A pregnant woman who smokes marijuana increases the risk for miscarriage, premature delivery, and low birth weight. In addition, maternal marijuana use may result in some of the same physical abnormalities seen in infants with FAS. Effects on the fetus vary, depending on the mother's diet and frequency of marijuana use and whether she uses other drugs.

Cocaine use has reached epidemic proportions among women of childbearing age in the United States, with the greatest use among African American and Hispanic women.[12] In addition to addicting the newborn, cocaine use increases risks of stroke, prematurity, fetal growth retardation, miscarriage, and certain birth defects.[13] Some of these problems may stem from nutritional deficiencies in the mother both before and during preg-

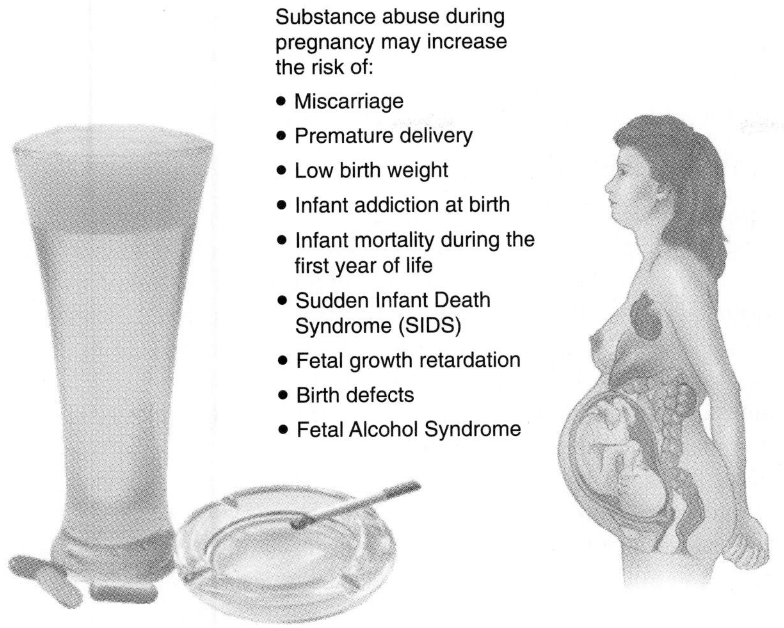
Substance abuse during pregnancy may increase the risk of:
• Miscarriage
• Premature delivery
• Low birth weight
• Infant addiction at birth
• Infant mortality during the first year of life
• Sudden Infant Death Syndrome (SIDS)
• Fetal growth retardation
• Birth defects
• Fetal Alcohol Syndrome

Figure 12.9 **Substance use can lead to birth defects.** When a pregnant woman smokes, drinks, or uses drugs, so does her growing baby. The consequences of these behaviors may be felt for generations.

nancy, as well as from concurrent tobacco and alcohol use, which is common among cocaine users. **Figure 12.9** illustrates the possible effects of a woman's use of drugs, alcohol, or tobacco while she is pregnant.

Key Concepts: *Smoking, alcohol, and illicit drug use during pregnancy can all have devastating effects on fetal development. Low birth weight, preterm delivery, and birth defects are some of the consequences. Fetal alcohol syndrome is a set of physical, mental, and behavioral consequences of alcohol consumption during pregnancy. A pregnant woman should avoid all these substances.*

Special Situations during Pregnancy

Most women progress through pregnancy with no more than a mild period of morning sickness or problems with constipation or heartburn. However, complications such as abnormal glucose tolerance or elevated blood pressure may affect dietary choices and nutritional status. In addition, some women have unique nutritional needs during pregnancy.

Gastrointestinal Distress

Morning sickness, or nausea associated with pregnancy, is most common early in pregnancy as the mother's body adjusts to changes in hormone levels. Many pregnant women find they experience less morning sickness if they eat dry cereal, toast, or crackers about half an hour before getting out of bed. (See **Figure 12.10**.) Keeping some food in the stomach throughout the day helps, too. This means eating smaller, more frequent meals, and drinking liquids between meals instead of with food. Avoiding food aromas that trigger nausea is another useful tactic.

Heartburn and constipation are the result of slowed GI movement. Remaining upright for at least an hour after eating and having smaller, more frequent meals may prevent heartburn. Getting plenty of fiber and fluids in the diet and getting

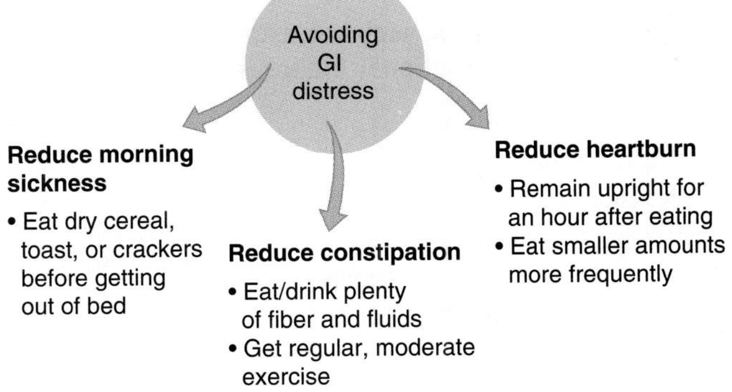
Avoiding GI distress
Reduce morning sickness
• Eat dry cereal, toast, or crackers before getting out of bed
Reduce constipation
• Eat/drink plenty of fiber and fluids
• Get regular, moderate exercise
Reduce heartburn
• Remain upright for an hour after eating
• Eat smaller amounts more frequently

Figure 12.10 **Strategies for avoiding GI distress.** During pregnancy, most women experience GI distress as morning sickness, constipation, or heartburn.

regular mild to moderate exercise can limit constipation. Of course, a pregnant woman should always consult her health care provider before using a prescription drug, over-the-counter medicine, herbal supplement, or home remedy for nausea, vomiting, heartburn, or constipation.

Food Cravings and Aversions

Many pregnant women experience specific food cravings and/or aversions, and we often laugh at stories about unusual combinations such as pickles and ice cream. These changes in food preferences may be linked to taste and metabolic changes, but they rarely are based on a nutrient deficiency or other physiological condition. Most cravings and aversions do not affect the quality of the diet unless food choices become very narrow.

Some pregnant women crave nonfood items such as starch or clay. The term *pica* describes routine consumption of nonfood items such as dirt, clay, laundry starch, ice, or burnt matches. Although this behavior may seem outlandish, in many cases it is a culturally accepted practice that affects significant numbers of pregnant women, especially in rural areas of the southeastern United States. Pica can be harmful if nonfood items crowd nutritious foods out of the diet. In addition, nonfood items may contain toxins, bacteria, and parasites; and in the case of laundry starch, a significant number of calories may be consumed without providing any vitamins and minerals.

Hypertension

Measurement of blood pressure is a routine part of prenatal care. When not accompanied by other symptoms, increased blood pressure during pregnancy is usually temporary and carries little risk. However, the combination of hypertension, edema, and proteinuria (protein in the urine) indicates the condition known as **preeclampsia**. If preeclampsia progresses to eclampsia, it can be life-threatening for both mother and baby.

preeclampsia A condition of late pregnancy characterized by hypertension, edema, and proteinuria.

gestational diabetes A condition that results in high blood glucose levels during pregnancy.

Diabetes

A woman with diabetes faces special challenges in pregnancy. She has an increased risk of developing preeclampsia and a greater-than-average chance of problems that affect the fetus, including fetal death. However, with early prenatal intervention and careful control of blood glucose levels, these risks can be reduced to the same level as in nondiabetic pregnancies.[14]

Gestational Diabetes

Gestational diabetes is a condition in which abnormal glucose tolerance exists only during pregnancy and resolves after delivery. The hormones of pregnancy tend to counteract insulin, and in about 4 percent of pregnancies, this results in a rise in blood glucose. Gestational diabetes often can be controlled through diet. **Table 12.6** lists factors associated with an increased risk of gestational diabetes.

Table 12.6 Factors Associated with Risk for Gestational Diabetes

Being older than 25 years
Obesity, at any age
Family history of diabetes mellitus
Previous poor pregnancy outcome
History of abnormal glucose tolerance
Ethnicity associated with high incidence of diabetes

AIDS

Women with AIDS are likely to have multiple nutrition problems, including protein-energy malnutrition, vitamin and mineral deficiencies, and inadequate weight gain. All of these can pose risks for the fetus. A pregnant woman with AIDS requires intensive nutrition management. Approximately 25 to 30 percent of pregnant women with HIV transmit the AIDS virus to their newborns, but medical intervention can reduce this number substantially.

Adolescence

Despite prevention efforts, adolescent pregnancy rates in the United States are among the highest in the developed world.[15] Pregnant adolescents are nutritionally at risk. Their own needs for growth and development are compromised by the extra demands posed by the growth and development of the fetus. Risks for preeclampsia, anemia, premature birth, low-birth-weight babies, infant mortality, and sexually transmitted diseases are all increased for pregnant adolescents under the age of 16.[16]

Even before becoming pregnant, many teenagers do not demonstrate healthful eating patterns. Their diets are likely to be inadequate in total calories, calcium, iron, zinc, riboflavin, folic acid, and vitamins A, D, and B_6. Poverty, smoking, and abuse of alcohol and other substances compound the negative effects of adolescent nutritional inadequacies.

Nutrition care for pregnant teens starts with determining daily energy needs. The Institute of Medicine recommends that pregnant adolescents be encouraged to strive for weight gains toward the upper end of the range recommended for adult mothers (Table 12.3).[17] Need for supplemental vitamins and minerals is also greater in this age group.

Key Concepts: *Numerous factors affect the dietary needs and choices of pregnant women. Routine prenatal care is important to identify unhealthful eating behaviors and potential complications such as preeclampsia and gestational diabetes. Pregnant women with diabetes or AIDS need special dietary intervention. Pregnant teens have especially high nutrient needs to fuel not only fetal growth, but also their own adolescent growth.*

Quick Bites

Breastfeeding and Birth Control

Does breastfeeding prevent pregnancy? No. But under certain conditions, breastfeeding can dramatically reduce the chances of becoming pregnant. During the first six months after giving birth, a woman who has not yet had a period and fully breastfeeds her baby (no other liquids or solids) has less than a 2 percent chance of pregnancy.

Lactation

During pregnancy, physiological changes in breast tissue and fat stores prepare the woman's body for the demands of lactation. Preparation for lactation also involves education. Although breastfeeding is one of the most natural functions of a woman's body, knowledge about lactation can make breastfeeding a success for both mother and infant. Parents should make decisions about feeding their infants based on accurate information; thus, providing information about the mechanics of breastfeeding as well as the benefits for both mother and baby should be an integral part of prenatal care.

Physiology of Lactation

Virtually every woman who wants to breastfeed her newborn can do so.[18] The size or shape of the breast has no impact on the lactation process. **Figure 12.11** shows the anatomy of a normal breast.

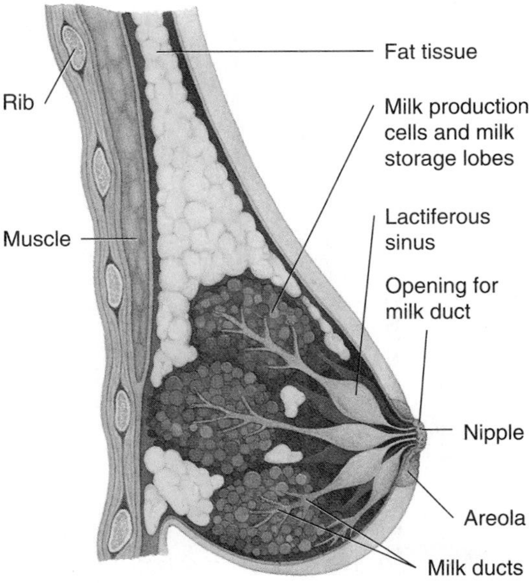

Figure 12.11 **Anatomy of the breast.** During pregnancy, breasts increase in size and undergo internal development. By the start of the third trimester, breasts are capable of producing milk.

Changes during Pregnancy

During pregnancy, the breast tissue changes so that milk production is possible. Not only does the breast change in size, but the structure of the glands and ducts also becomes more intricate, and secretory cells are formed. The mammary tissue is mature and capable of producing milk by the start of the third trimester.

After Delivery: Stages of Lactation

Although birth triggers a rapid increase in milk production and secretion, full lactation does not begin as soon as the baby is born. One of the best ways to establish lactation is to put the newborn to the breast as soon after delivery as possible. During the first two or three days after birth, a nursing infant receives **colostrum**, an immature milk that is quite high in protein and immunoglobulins (immunoprotective factors). If the newborn is fed regularly at the breast, lactation will be firmly established within two or three weeks after birth, and mature milk will be produced.

colostrum A thick yellow fluid secreted by the breast during pregnancy and the first days after delivery.

prolactin A pituitary hormone that stimulates the production of milk in the breast tissue.

oxytocin A pituitary hormone that stimulates the release of milk from the breast.

let-down reflex The release of milk from the breast tissue in response to the stimulus of the hormone oxytocin. The major stimulus for oxytocin release is the infant suckling at the breast.

Hormonal Controls

Maturation of breast tissue and the production and release of breast milk are controlled by several hormones. (See **Figure 12.12**.) During lactation, the pituitary gland produces two important hormones—**prolactin** and **oxytocin**. The infant suckling at the breast stimulates the release of prolactin from the pituitary gland. In turn, prolactin stimulates the production of milk in the breast tissue. Giving water or infant formula to the baby reduces the time spent nursing at the breast, and milk production declines.

The second hormone, oxytocin, allows milk to be released from the mammary glands to the nipple and therefore to the hungry infant. It would be inconvenient and messy if milk were released from the breast as soon as it was produced! So, the infant suckling at the breast signals the pituitary gland to release oxytocin, which in turn stimulates the release of milk. This process, often called the **let-down reflex**, may be accompanied by a tingling sensation in the breast that lets the mother know the infant is receiving milk. Let-down can be inhibited by anxiety, stress, and fatigue. It can also be stimulated by thoughts of the baby or hearing the baby cry.

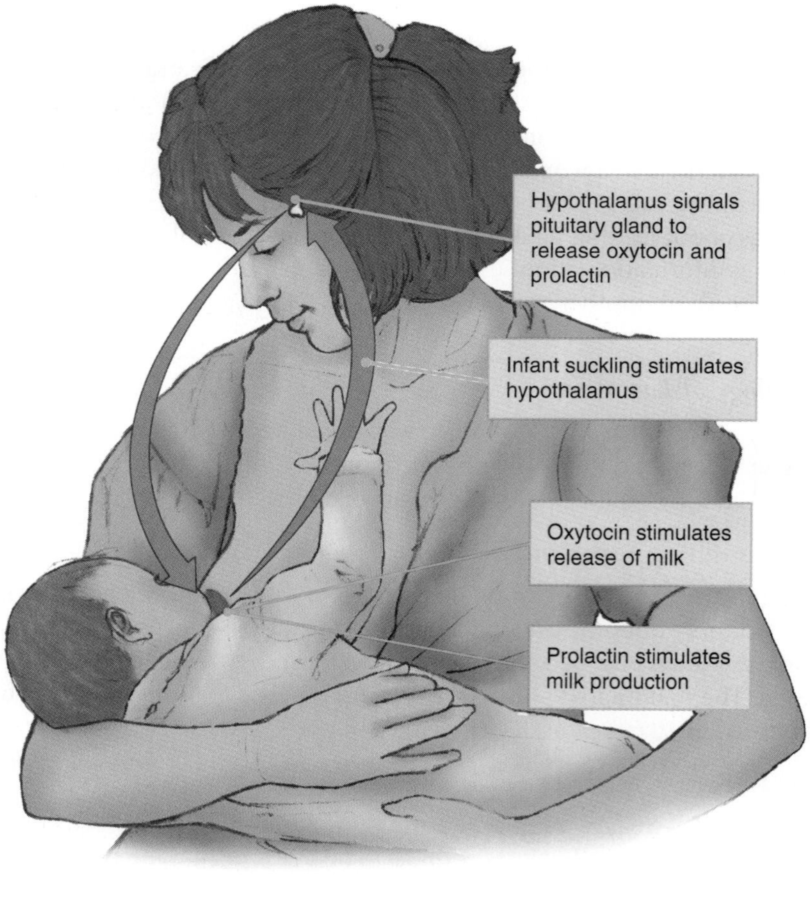
Hypothalamus signals pituitary gland to release oxytocin and prolactin
Infant suckling stimulates hypothalamus
Oxytocin stimulates release of milk
Prolactin stimulates milk production

Figure 12.12 Hormonal control of lactation. When an infant nurses, the infant's suckling stimulates the nipple, which sends nerve signals to the hypothalamus. In turn, the hypothalamus signals the pituitary gland to release hormones that stimulate milk production and release.

Key Concepts: *Changes in breast tissue that allow lactation culminate at delivery. Breast milk changes in the two or three weeks following the infant's birth. The first milk, colostrum, is high in protein and immune factors. Key hormones that regulate milk production and release are prolactin and oxytocin.*

Nutrition for Breastfeeding Women

To provide adequate nutrition for her baby while protecting her own nutritional status, a breastfeeding mother must choose a varied, healthful, nutrient-dense diet. Her needs for energy and most nutrients are higher or the same as for pregnancy.

Energy

The energy RDA for breastfeeding women is 500 kilocalories per day higher than the RDA for nonpregnant, nonlactating women, but this may be an overestimation of actual needs, especially for sedentary women. To ensure adequate milk production and avoid nutrient deficiencies, a nursing mother should consume at least 1,800 kilocalories a day.

Protein

Adequate protein intake is also important while nursing. The RDA for protein rises to 65 grams per day for the first six months of lactation and then is 62 grams per day for the second six months. This is only slightly higher than the 60 grams per day recommended during pregnancy. Unless calorie intake is very low, lack of dietary protein is uncommon among women in the United States and Canada.

Vitamins and Minerals

Vitamin needs for a woman who is breastfeeding are even greater than during pregnancy. Inadequate vitamin intake means that the vitamin content of breast milk can diminish, putting the infant at risk for deficiency.

The need for most minerals also increases during lactation (as compared with pregnancy). Iron needs decrease below nonpregnant values because iron losses from menstruation are not present during the early months of exclusive breastfeeding.

Water

Breastfeeding women require plenty of fluids. A nursing mother should drink about 2 liters (~8 cups) of water per day and at least 1 cup of water each time she breastfeeds her baby. Coffee and other caffeinated beverages are acceptable if limited to 1 or 2 cups a day—and if they do not replace other fluids. Because caffeine passes into the breast milk, caffeine can make some breastfed infants wakeful and jittery.

Key Concepts: *Energy and nutrient needs are usually even higher during lactation than during pregnancy. RDA values suggest an additional 500 kilocalories and 12 to 20 extra grams of protein each day above nonpregnant needs. Low vitamin intake affects the nutritional quality of breast milk. Recommended intake levels for minerals are generally higher during lactation than during pregnancy. Fluids are also important for adequate milk production.*

Food Choices

Choosing a variety of foods from the USDA Food Guide Pyramid is the best way to meet the nutritional demands of lactation. Following the Pyramid's

Quick Bites

Flavored Breast Milk

When lactating mothers exercise vigorously, the amount of lactic acid in breast milk can increase. Some babies dislike the taste and tend to nurse less. Alcohol can also cause a taste that babies dislike. What flavors do babies like? When mothers consume vanilla, mint, or garlic, some babies nurse more.

colic Periodic inconsolable crying in an otherwise healthy infant that appears to result from abdominal cramping and discomfort.

guidelines, diets of 2,200 to 2,800 kilocalories per day can easily meet most nutrient needs.

Nursing mothers should eat plenty of vegetables, the source of many essential micronutrients. Although vegetables in the cabbage family, including broccoli, cauliflower, kale, and Brussels sprouts, have long been considered causes of **colic** symptoms in breastfed infants, these cruciferous vegetables may have an unwarranted bad reputation. Scientific evidence that these vegetables cause distress for infants remains weak. Removal of numerous foods from the diet should be done only under the supervision of a registered dietitian.

Supplementation

In general, breastfeeding women do not need routine vitamin/mineral supplementation. The exceptions are those women who do not follow dietary guidelines and vegan women, who avoid all animal products. Vitamin B_{12} is likely to be too low in the milk of nursing vegans, and they should take a B_{12} supplement.[19] For breastfeeding women who do not get regular sun exposure and do not drink milk or other fortified products, a vitamin D supplement may be warranted.[20] For most nursing mothers, though, dietary counseling is the preferred way to address nutrient imbalances.

Practices to Avoid during Lactation

When a nursing mother smokes or uses alcohol or other drugs, these substances wind up in her breast milk. Cigarette smoking can decrease production of breast milk.[21] It is a myth that drinking alcohol enhances the let-down reflex, making it easier to nurse. Rather, alcohol inhibits the milk-ejection reflex so that the baby gets less milk with a higher concentration of alcohol.

Illicit drugs also show up in breast milk and can be transferred to the infant. If a new mother cannot abstain from using these drugs, she should not breastfeed. Legal drugs can be harmful to babies as well. A woman should discuss over-the-counter and prescription medicines and herbal products with her health care providers before taking them.

Key Concepts: *Food choices during lactation should follow the USDA Food Guide Pyramid and emphasize nutrient-dense foods. With good choices and adequate calories, a lactating woman may not need vitamin and mineral supplements. During pregnancy and lactation, a woman should avoid smoking, alcohol, and illicit drugs. She should consult a health care professional before taking medications or dietary supplements.*

Benefits of Breastfeeding

Breast milk is the optimal food for the health, growth, and development of infants.[22] Both mother and infant benefit from breastfeeding; in fact, the larger society benefits through reduced infant illness and health care costs. Think About It 3

Benefits for Infants

Human milk provides optimal nutrition for babies, as you will see in the section "Energy and Nutrient Needs of Infancy." Breast milk provides more than nutrients, however, and the health-promoting factors in breast milk are difficult, if not impossible, to replicate in infant formula.

Breast milk has been shown to reduce the incidence of respiratory, gastrointestinal, and ear infections; allergies; diarrhea; and bacterial meningitis. A recent well-designed study examined the relationship between the duration of breastfeeding and adult intelligence. It found that babies who are breastfed longer have higher intelligence scores as adults.[23] Breastfeeding promotes a close bond between mother and infant that may be important to normal psychological development.[24] It is important for mothers (and fathers) who bottle-feed to promote the same type of closeness while feeding.

As long as mother and baby are in reasonably close proximity, breast milk is always ready when the baby is ready to eat. There's nothing to prepare, mix, or heat; and for a hungry infant, that's an important advantage! Breast milk is always the perfect temperature and is sterile. In addition, links between breastfeeding and reduced risk of disorders such as type 1 diabetes and Crohn's disease have been suggested; these need further study. **Table 12.7** lists some of the possible protective benefits of human milk.

Table 12.7 Suggested Protective Benefits of Human Milk

Breastfeeding may reduce a baby's risk of these disorders during infancy or later in life:

- Sudden infant death syndrome (SIDS)
- Type 1 diabetes mellitus
- Crohn's disease
- Ulcerative colitis
- Chronic digestive diseases

Source: Adapted from Lawrence A. *A Review of the Medical Benefits and Contraindications to Breastfeeding in the United States.* Arlington, VA: National Center for Education in Maternal and Child Health; 1997. Maternal and Child Health Technical Information Bulletin.

Benefits for Mother

Breastfeeding stimulates uterine contractions, which help the uterus return to its normal size. If the baby is put to the breast immediately after delivery, these same contractions (an effect of oxytocin) also can help control blood loss. Although not an effective method of birth control, exclusive breastfeeding suppresses ovulation in many women.

Breastfeeding is as convenient for mother as it is for baby and is certainly less expensive than formula feeding. Although more comprehensive studies are needed, there is some evidence that breastfeeding will reduce a woman's risk of ovarian cancer, breast cancer, and osteoporosis.[25] If, as expected, a breastfed baby has fewer episodes of infectious illness, this saves health care costs and reduces employee absence and lost income for working mothers.

Quick Bites

Breastfeeding to Control Blood Pressure?

Oxytocin, the hormone produced while breastfeeding, can lower the blood pressure of nursing mothers. A recent study showed that breastfeeding mothers had lower blood pressures after nursing than did bottle-feeding mothers. When asked to discuss stressful events, nursing mothers also showed smaller increases in blood pressure than the bottle-feeders showed. Mothers often claim that they feel relaxed during breastfeeding, which may account for the difference in blood pressure.

Contraindications to Breastfeeding

Nearly all women who want to breastfeed can do so successfully, and breastfeeding is experiencing a resurgence in popularity.[26] There are times, however, when breastfeeding is inappropriate because of infant or maternal disease or drug use. Depending on the specifics of the operation, breast surgery may or may not preclude breastfeeding.[27]

Individual situations should be discussed with the health care provider. For example, because a woman with untreated tuberculosis may transmit the illness to her child, she should not breastfeed. In the United States and Canada, where safe feeding alternatives exist, women infected with the human immunodeficiency virus (HIV) are advised not to breastfeed because HIV can be transmitted to the baby through breast milk.

Some medications pass directly into human milk, and some prescribed medications may preclude breastfeeding. Illegal drugs pass into human milk as well. If the mother is using an illegal drug such as cocaine, she should not breastfeed. Women taking prescription or over-the-counter medicines or herbal supplements should discuss the effects of these products on breast milk with their health care providers.

Key Concepts: *Health benefits and convenience are key advantages of breastfeeding. For the infant, breastfeeding has been linked to reduced incidence of many infectious diseases, as well as other conditions. For a mother, breastfeeding speeds recovery of normal uterine size and may reduce her disease risk. Although breastfeeding is the preferred method of infant feeding, there are times when breastfeeding is contraindicated. These situations should be identified and discussed as part of prenatal care.*

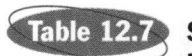

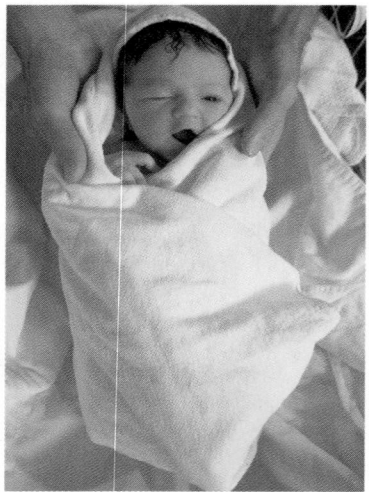

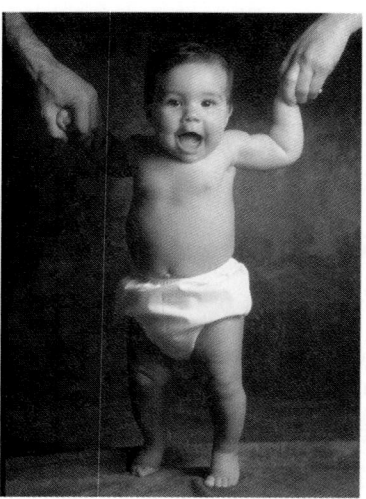

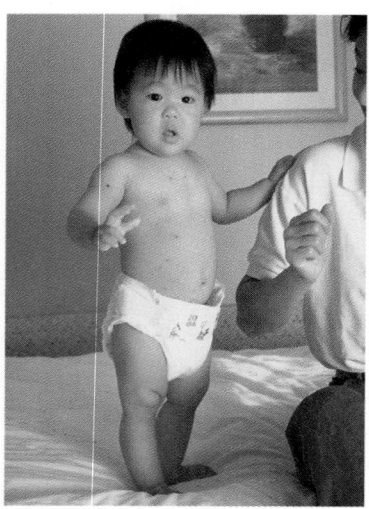

(a)

(b)

(c)

Figure 12.13 **Different stages of infancy.** (a) Newborn. (b) 4 to 6 months. (c) 12 months.

Resources for Pregnant and Lactating Women and Their Children

Many agencies support research and education programs that promote the health of pregnant and breastfeeding women and their children. You may be familiar with the March of Dimes and its efforts to reduce birth defects through optimal nutrition during pregnancy. La Leche League is a voluntary health and education organization that offers programs and educational materials to help breastfeeding mothers learn about the benefits and practice of breastfeeding.

The **Special Supplemental Nutrition Program for Women, Infants, and Children (WIC)** is a much-acclaimed program of the Food and Nutrition Service of the USDA. WIC provides food assistance, nutrition education, and referrals to health care services to low-income pregnant, postpartum, and breastfeeding women, as well as infants and children up to the age of 5. Compared with at-risk women and children who are eligible for WIC but do not participate in the program, WIC participants have significantly fewer problems such as low-birth-weight infants.[28]

WIC services include intensive breastfeeding education and support. Over the first six months of life, breastfed infants enrolled in WIC use about $500 less in WIC and Medicaid services than do formula-fed infants enrolled in WIC, according to a study conducted in Colorado.[29] Continued promotion of breastfeeding by WIC and other public health programs can have both health and economic benefits. Periodically, WIC participants are required to bring their infants into the local WIC office. These visits give WIC staff an opportunity to evaluate the infant's growth and provide the caregiver with additional nutrition education.

Infancy

Infancy is the period of a child's life between birth and 1 year. Because of the rapid growth that occurs during this time, nutritional needs are higher per unit of body weight than at any other time in the life cycle. Despite the critical importance of nutrition at this stage, feeding an infant is a fairly simple process. Human milk provides all of the nutrients an infant needs and is the model for infant formulas. By 4 to 6 months, the infant's physical development and physiological maturation signal readiness for the addition of "solid" foods to the diet.

Human infants need love as much as they need food. Without love and nurturing, a baby can fail to thrive even if she is offered all of the right nutrients. If an infant is not nourished emotionally, nutrition recommendations and requirements become meaningless.[30]

Infant Growth and Development

Birth weight is the best predictor of the child's health in the first year of life; however, it is important to correlate weight with **gestational age**. The risk profile of an infant who has a low birth weight because of **prematurity** is different from that of a **full-term baby** with a low birth weight.

Immediately after birth, an infant loses about 6 percent of his body weight. This is normal and expected. By 10 to 14 days, the infant should return to his birth weight. Over the next 12 months, his growth will be phenomenal. By the age of 4 to 6 months, a healthy infant will have doubled his birth weight. By his first birthday, the infant will have tripled his birth weight and increased his length by about 50 percent. The infant's body proportions change, too, so that by age 1 he is looking less like a baby and more like a **toddler**. (See **Figure 12.13**.)

Length (used instead of height because infants can't stand) and **head circumference** are more sensitive measures than weight for assessing a baby's growth and nutritional status. Weight alone reflects just recent nutritional intake. Head circumference measures brain growth and development. Chronic malnutrition can limit this growth and is reflected in inadequate gains in head size. Regular measurements of head circumference, therefore, can verify proper growth. Head circumference measurements are useful in infants and children up to age 2.

Growth Charts

During routine checkups throughout infancy (and during childhood and adolescence), health care practitioners measure weight, length or height, and head circumference and plot these values on **growth charts**. (See **Figure 12.14**.) Health care practitioners use growth charts to show the growth of an individual baby over time. These charts also allow comparison of one child's growth to that of children in the general population.

Key Concepts: *A typical infant doubles her birth weight by age 4 to 6 months and triples it by 12 months. Infant length increases about 50 percent during the first year. Health care practitioners use growth charts to follow and assess an infant's growth in weight, length, and head circumference.*

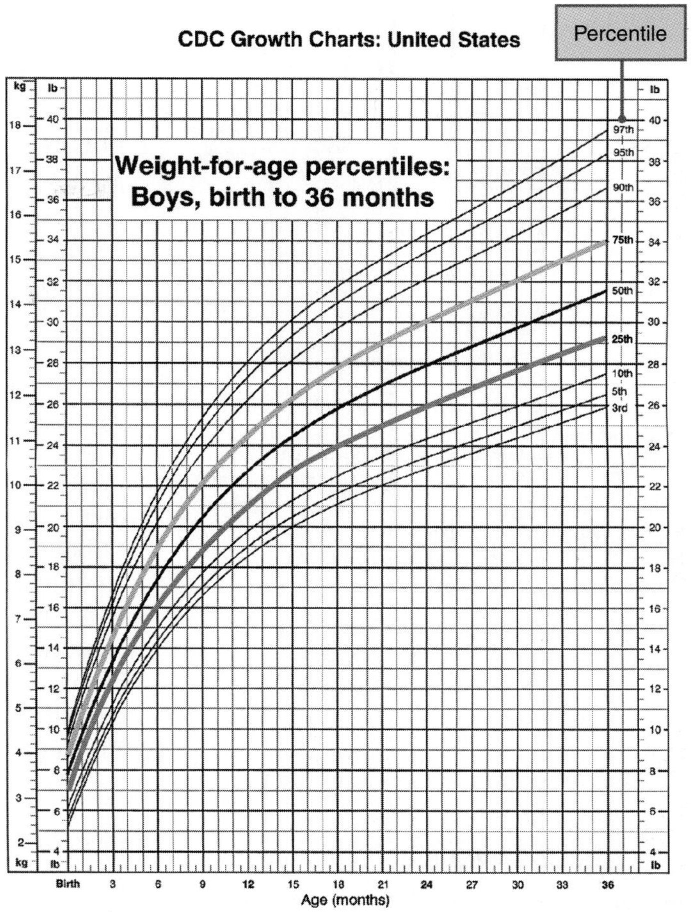

Figure 12.14 **Growth chart.** The CDC (Centers for Disease Control) has complete sets of growthcharts available on the Internet at www.cdc.gov/growthcharts. See Appendix H for full-scale samples of growth charts for boys and girls aged 2 to 20 years.
Source: Developed by the National Center for Health Statistics in collaboration with the National Center for Chronic Disease Prevention and Health Promotion (2000).

Energy and Nutrient Needs of Infancy

How do you suppose scientists determine the nutrient needs of newborns and young infants? Studies with babies as subjects are rare—the logistical and ethical questions are daunting! So how else can we know what babies need? It's simple; we just look at breast milk—the food that was designed especially for babies. The composition of human milk is the gold standard by which infant nutrient needs are determined. Babies who are not breastfed are given infant formula. In the United States, most infant formulas

Special Supplemental Nutrition Program for Women, Infants, and Children (WIC) A USDA program that provides federal grants to states for supplemental foods, health care referrals, and nutrition education for low-income pregnant, breastfeeding, and non-breastfeeding postpartum women, and to infants and children at nutritional risk.

infancy The period between birth and 12 months of age.

gestational age Age of the fetus measured from the first day of the mother's last menstrual period until birth.

prematurity Birth before 37 weeks of gestation.

full-term baby A baby delivered during the normal period of human gestation, between 38 and 41 weeks.

toddler A child between 12 and 36 months of age.

head circumference Measurement of the largest part of the infant's head (just above the eyebrow and ears); used to determine brain growth.

growth charts Charts that plot the weight, length, and head circumference of infants and children as they grow.

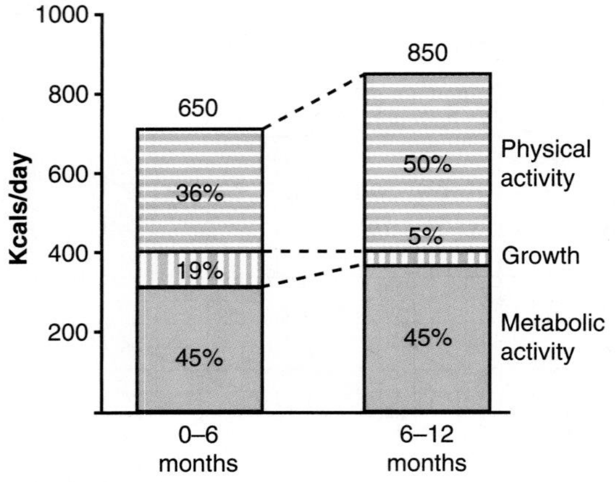

Figure 12.15 **Allocation of energy expenditure.** During the second six months, infants increase their energy expenditure for physical activity. **Source:** Adapted from Foman SJ, Bell EF. Energy. In: Foman SJ, ed. *Nutrition of Normal Infants.* St. Louis: Mosby; 1993.

have a base of modified cow's milk or soy protein. To assure that formula meets all of an infant's nutrient needs, federal regulations require that the formula's composition complies with nutritional standards.

Energy

An infant's energy need is the amount of energy she requires for basal functions such as respiration and metabolism, in addition to growth and activity. An infant's basal energy needs, relative to her size, are about twice that of an adult. The amount of energy an infant needs for activity varies throughout the first year of life, increasing as the child becomes more mobile. (See **Figure 12.15**.) In general, an infant requires about 100 kilocalories per kilogram of body weight.[31] **Table 12.8** lists the specific RDA values.

The appropriate balance of energy sources (carbohydrate, fat, and protein) is different for infants than for adults. (See **Figure 12.16**.) The best diet for infants (as modeled by human milk) is high in fat and moderate in carbohydrate. Infants have high calorie needs but can consume only a small amount at any one time. An infant's stomach is quite small; a newborn can consume only about 1 to 2 ounces of liquid at a feeding. Because fat is the most concentrated source of calories, a high-fat diet supplies adequate calories in a smaller volume. A high-fat diet also is necessary for normal brain growth, which continues until about 18 to 24 months of age. **Figure 12.17** shows the primary functions of energy-yielding nutrients in infants, which are discussed in the next sections.

Table 12.8 **Energy RDA for Infants**

Age (mo)	Median Weight lb	Median Weight kg	kcal/kg	kcal/d*
0–6	13	6	108	650
6–12	20	9	98	850

* The values for kilocalories per day are based on median weights of infants. Needs of individual infants vary.

Source: Food and Nutrition Board. *Recommended Dietary Allowances.* 10th ed. Washington, DC: National Academy Press; 1989.

Protein

Protein needs during infancy are higher than at any other time in the life cycle. In fact, protein needs (measured in grams per kilogram of body weight) throughout the first year of life are at least twice as high as an adult's needs. **Table 12.9** lists the protein RDA for infants. Both human milk and infant formula provide complete protein with all the essential amino acids. Because of the types of proteins found in human milk (as compared with cow's milk), human milk protein is more easily digested and absorbed.

Carbohydrate and Fat

Carbohydrates and triglycerides are the major energy sources for infants. This allows protein to be used primarily for growth and not as an energy source. Nearly all of the carbohydrate in human milk and in the infant formulas made from cow's milk is lactose. Infants digest lactose easily and tolerate it well.

Fat is the major energy source in the infant's diet and is important for central nervous system development and accumulation of body fat stores. Fats in milk also enhance a baby's sense of fullness between feedings. Although formula manufacturers try to mimic the composition of human milk, formula remains an imperfect copy. For example, *alpha*-linolenic acid, an essential *omega*-3 fatty acid, is missing from many formulas. In addition, formulas generally lack other related fats found in human milk: arachadonic acid (ARA), eicosapentaenoic acid (EPA), and docosahexaenoic acid (DHA).[32] However, two major infant formula makers began marketing formula with added ARA and DHA in 2002. Human milk also contains more cholesterol than infant formulas.

Table 12.9 **Protein RDA for Infants**

Age (mo)	g/kg	g/d*
0–6	2.2	13
6–12	1.6	14

* The values for grams per day are based on median weights of infants. Needs of individual infants vary.

Source: Food and Nutrition Board. *Recommended Dietary Allowances.* 10th ed. Washington, DC: National Academy Press; 1989.

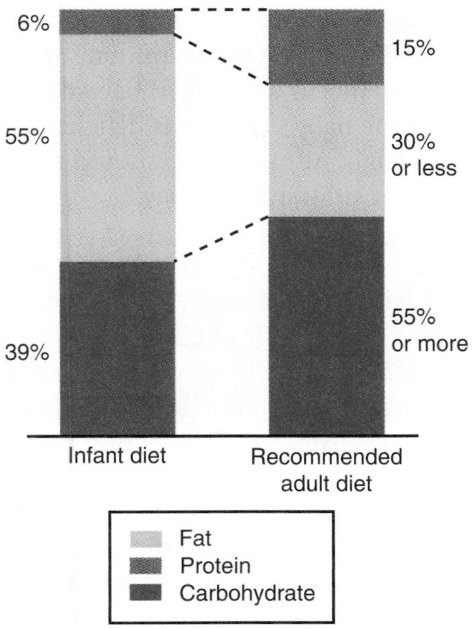

Figure 12.16 **Percentages of energy-yielding nutrients in infant and adult diets.** The best diets for infants are high in fat and moderate in carbohydrate. Infants need a high-fat diet for normal brain growth and to provide adequate calories in a smaller volume.

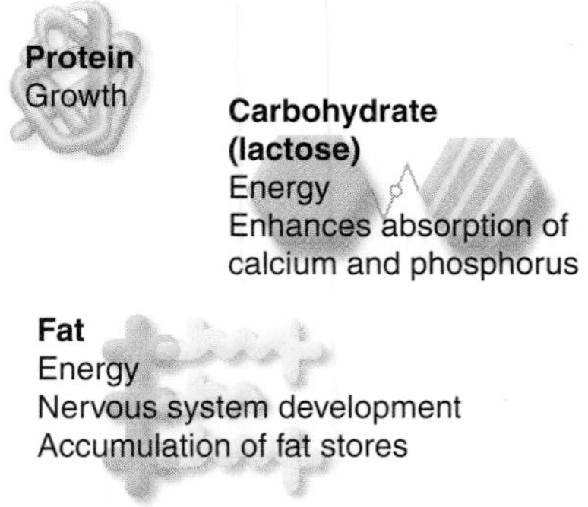

Figure 12.17 **Primary functions of energy-yielding nutrients for infants.** To support growth, protein needs (per kg body weight) are higher in infancy than in any other life stage.

neonate An infant from birth to 28 days.

Water

Because water as a percentage of body weight is higher in babies than adults, infants have higher fluid needs. Infants need 1.5 milliliters per kilocalorie consumed; the value for adults is 1.0 milliliters per kilocalorie. Human milk fulfills not only the nutrient needs of the **neonate**, but also the fluid requirements. Properly prepared formula accomplishes the same task. During the first 4 to 6 months, supplemental water is not necessary for healthy infants who are exclusively breastfed or who receive properly mixed formula. This is true even in hot, humid weather.[33] Once solid foods are introduced, a baby's water needs change, and additional water may be required.

Vitamins and Minerals

As long as an infant is receiving adequate calories from breast milk or infant formula, nearly all vitamin and mineral needs also are being met. Infant formula is fortified with all essential vitamins and minerals according to guidelines established by the American Academy of Pediatrics (AAP) and enforced by the Food and Drug Administration. Human milk is lower in a few nutrients (e.g., iron and vitamin D), but these nutrients are absorbed more efficiently from breast milk than from formula. This section focuses on a few vitamins and minerals that may be of concern for infants. (See **Figure 12.18**.)

Vitamin D Vitamin D is a key nutrient for calcium absorption and mineralization of bone. Human milk is low in vitamin D; however, inadequate vitamin D is rarely a problem because breastfed infants absorb it well and can make enough vitamin D from exposure to sunlight. It may be a concern, though, for infants who are not

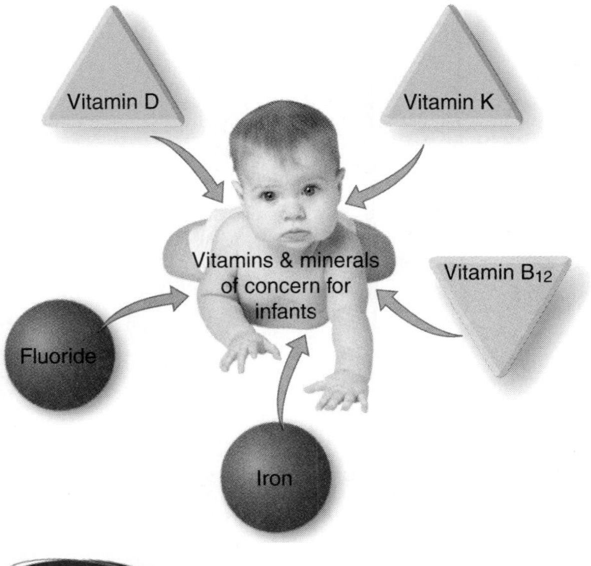

Figure 12.18 **Micronutrients of concern during infancy.** Infants who lack sun exposure can become deficient in vitamin D. A dose of vitamin K usually is given to babies at birth to ensure a sufficient supply. Because vegan mothers can have breast milk deficient in vitamin B_{12}, their babies may need a B_{12} supplement. By the age of 6 months, breastfed infants need additional iron. Formula-fed infants should consume iron-fortified formula. Human milk is low in fluoride.

exposed to sunlight, as well as those with darkly pigmented skin. These babies make less vitamin D from the same amount of sunlight exposure than do lighter-skinned infants. If a breastfed baby does not get adequate sunlight exposure and if the baby's mother is deficient in vitamin D, the infant's risk is especially high. At-risk babies should receive supplements of 10 micrograms (400 IU) of vitamin D per day.[34]

Vitamin K Vitamin K is necessary for the production of prothrombin, a substance needed in order for blood to clot. Although intestinal bacteria synthesize vitamin K, the gut is sterile at birth. Because babies are born with minimal stores of vitamin K, it is recommended that a single dose of vitamin K be given at birth. Both human milk and infant formula provide adequate vitamin K; and as feeding begins, helpful bacteria begin to flourish in the infant's intestinal tract.

Vitamin B_{12} Vitamin B_{12} is essential for cell division and normal folate metabolism. Mothers who include meat, fish, and dairy products in their diets produce milk that is adequate in vitamin B_{12}. This may not be true of strict vegetarians, whose diet—and milk—may be deficient in vitamin B_{12}. Breastfed infants of vegan mothers may need a vitamin B_{12} supplement.

Iron Iron is essential for growth and development, and iron-deficiency anemia is the most common nutritional deficiency in the United States. Human milk is not a rich source of iron, but it does not need to be. Approximately 50 percent of the iron in breast milk is absorbed, compared with only 4 percent of the iron in infant formula. If the mother has consumed an iron-rich diet during pregnancy, the fetus builds up large enough iron stores during gestation to meet most of its iron needs for the first few months of life. These stores begin to diminish during the fourth month of life. By the age of 6 months, a breastfed infant needs an additional iron source. Iron-fortified infant cereals can meet this need. For formula-fed babies, iron supplementation is needed from birth. The AAP therefore recommends iron-fortified formula for all formula-fed babies.[35]

Fluoride Human milk also is low in fluoride, a mineral important for dental health. Current research has led the American Dental Association and the AAP to recommend fluoride supplements for breastfed infants after the age of 6 months.[36] If the local water supply has adequate fluoride and the formula is mixed with tap water, formula-fed infants do not need fluoride supplements. If the water used to mix formula has inadequate fluoride, fluoride supplements are indicated. Fluoridation policies and the fluoride content of tap water vary among municipalities.

Key Concepts: *Energy and nutrient needs for infancy are estimated based on the composition of human milk. Because of their rapid growth and development, infants have high energy and nutrient needs per kilogram of body weight. Caregivers must give special attention to vitamin D, iron, and fluoride to ensure that the infant obtains enough. If breast milk or formula (properly mixed) is meeting energy needs, the fluid needs of the infant also are being met.*

Newborn Breastfeeding

The AAP has identified breastfeeding as the ideal method of feeding to achieve optimal growth and development[37] and recommends that breastfeeding begin as soon after birth as possible. Feedings should occur every two to three hours, for a total of 8 to 12 feedings a day. Duration of feedings is guided by the infant's behavior and may last from 10 to 15 minutes per breast. Hospitals should provide every opportunity for breastfeeding to begin before the baby goes home. Nurses or **lactation consultants** should be available to offer professional breastfeeding support to new mothers. The AAP recommends that no supplements of formula or water be given to breastfed neonates unless medically indicated.

Quick Bites

What's a Biberon?

Many people consider Dr. Nils Rosen von Rosenstein the father of pediatrics. In his 1764 textbook, he describes a "biberon," a leather nipple used for artificial infant feeding. He also describes 14 types of infant diarrhea.

Alternative Feeding: Infant Formula

Women may decide not to breastfeed or to breastfeed only briefly. Their infants need infant formulas designed to provide adequate nutrition.

Standard Infant Formulas

Standard infant formulas have cow's milk as a base. In making infant formula, manufacturers first remove the fat and replace it with vegetable oils. They add vitamins and minerals to approximate the nutritional content of human milk. Infant formulas are available with or without added iron, but because of the decreased bioavailability of iron in infant formulas and the infant's high needs, the AAP recommends using only iron-fortified formulas.

lactation consultants Health professionals trained to specialize in education about and promotion of breastfeeding; may be certified as an International Board Certified Lactation Consultant (IBCLC).

Soy-Based Formulas

Formula-fed infants who develop vomiting, diarrhea, constipation, abdominal pain, or colic are frequently switched to soy formulas. In these formulas, soy is the source of protein. To compensate for the inferior digestibility of soy protein, soy formulas contain more protein than formulas based on cow's milk. Soy formulas are lactose-free and iron-fortified. Corn syrup and sucrose are the carbohydrate sources.

Other Types of Formula

Special formulas are available for infants who are allergic to both cow's milk and soy protein, those who are premature, and those who have rare defects in metabolic pathways. These special formulas often have their protein content modified in either its digestibility or its amino acid composition. Many special formulas contain medium-chain triglycerides as the major fat source. This type of fat is very well digested and absorbed. These special formulas are expensive and often taste bad, but they are essential for many infants.

Formula Preparation

Formulas come in three forms: ready-to-feed, concentrate, and powdered. Although the ready-to-feed is the most convenient, it is also the most expensive. As the name implies, the formula can be poured directly from the can into a bottle and fed to the baby. Liquid concentrate formula is mixed with an equal amount of water before feeding. Powdered formula also is mixed with water and is the least expensive.

When using infant formulas, principles of food safety must be observed. Infants have an immature immune system and may develop infections from improperly prepared or stored formula. If not fed to the infant immediately, prepared formula should be refrigerated immediately and kept in the refrigerator until needed. If formula is not used within 48 hours, it should be discarded. For at least the first few months, the AAP recommends sterilizing all equipment used for feeding.

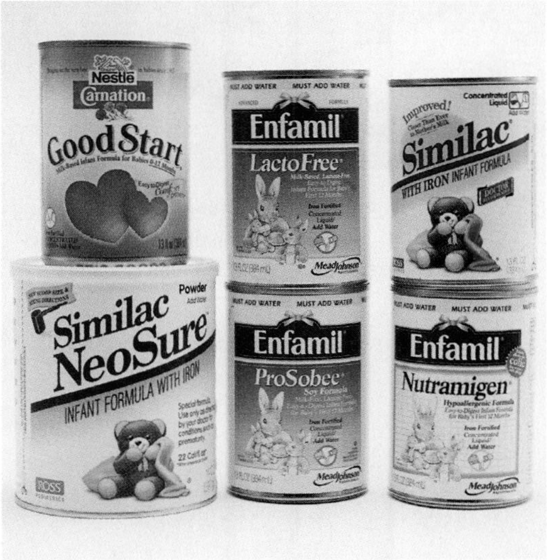

Improperly mixed formula is another danger, whether a result of ignorance in following instructions or of economics. Some caregivers on limited budgets might purposefully overdilute formula to make it last longer. This deprives the infant of necessary calories and protein and provides too much water. Other caregivers overconcentrate the formula in the misguided belief that this might encourage faster growth. Overconcentrated formula provides too much protein and too little water and may cause problems with an infant's kidney function and hydration.

Quick Bites

Ancient Baby Bottle

The earliest infant feeding vessel ever discovered is Egyptian and dates from 2000 B.C.E. A relief found in the ruins of the palace of King Sardanapalus of Nineveh, who died in 888 B.C.E., depicts a mother holding a modern-looking baby bottle.

Breast Milk or Formula: How Much Is Enough?

It's easy to keep track of how much formula an infant has consumed, but what about the breastfed baby? Although you can't see how much breast milk a nursing infant is consuming, there are other ways to tell that a baby is getting enough to eat. An adequately fed newborn will breastfeed 8 to 12 times, wet at least six diapers, and have at least three loose stools each day in the first week of life. The newborn will also regain its birth weight within the first two weeks. Normal growth, regular elimination patterns, and a satisfied demeanor are the best indicators that a baby is getting enough to eat.

Feeding Technique

Feeding should take place in a loving and warm environment. A breastfeeding mother holds her baby close, at a distance that encourages mother–baby eye contact. (See **Figure 12.19**.) During bottle-feeding, the caregiver needs to hold the baby close and make eye contact. Propping the bottle against a pillow or other object, so that the baby can feed alone, should be avoided.

Babies swallow air while feeding, whether at the breast or with a bottle, and they need to be burped. Babies generally need to be burped after 15 minutes or 2 to 3 ounces of formula. Just as the infant sends signals of readiness for feeding, she also signals fullness. Fullness cues include fussiness, playfulness, sleep, or just turning away. Parents need to learn these cues and respond to them.

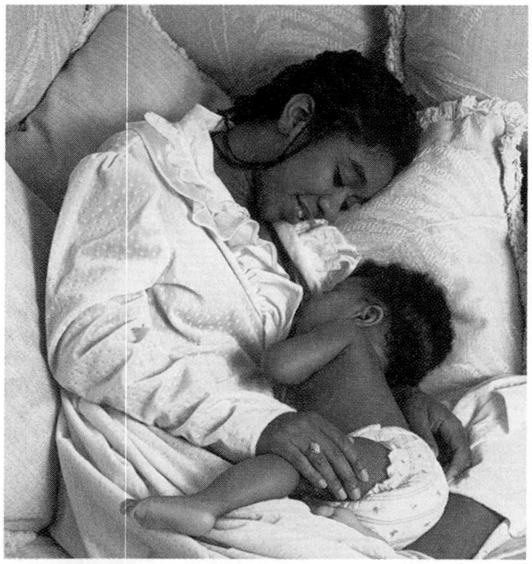

Figure 12.19 **Breastfeeding.** Breastfeeding nurtures an infant emotionally as well as physically. This intensely rewarding time helps to bond a mother and her child.

Key Concepts: *Human milk provides all necessary nutrients for growth and development and enhances the immune system of the maturing infant. Infants who are not breastfed receive infant formula, which should be fortified with iron. Careful preparation and storage of the formula ensures proper nutrient composition and food safety. Formula feedings should nourish the baby emotionally as well as nutritionally.*

Introduction of Solid Foods into the Infant's Diet

Solid foods are introduced based on an infant's physiological needs, such as depletion of iron stores, and physical development, such as the ability to sit up. To say that we are introducing solid foods is a bit of a misnomer; we are really referring to pureed and liquefied cereals, fruits, vegetables, and meats that are added to the infant's diet of breast milk or infant formula. Currently, the American Academy of Pediatrics recommends that solid foods be introduced between the age of 4 and 6 months.[38] This age range is purposefully broad to allow for differences in growth and development among babies.

Physiological Indicators of Infant Readiness for Solid Foods

Before a baby reaches 4 to 6 months of age, solid food is not necessary for nutrition; in fact, early introduction of supplemental foods can be detrimental. By the age of 4 to 6 months, however, an infant is physiologically

Think About It 4

ready to expand his diet. For example, at this age a baby has increased levels of digestive enzymes, so that foods other than human milk or formula can be digested with ease. However, solid food is a supplement to, not a replacement for, human milk or formula at this time.

It is wise to proceed slowly with the introduction of solid foods. Delaying—until age 1—the introduction of common food allergens, particularly cow's milk, egg whites, and wheat, can prevent food allergies for many infants. In addition to its allergic potential, whole cow's milk provides too much protein and too little iron, is low in essential fatty acids, may impair kidney function and lead to dehydration, and has been linked to development of insulin-dependent diabetes mellitus.[39] Although the existence of a link between early introduction of unmodified cow's milk and diabetes has not been clarified, the AAP recommended in 1994 that families with a strong history of type 1 diabetes mellitus breastfeed their infants and avoid introducing intact cow's milk protein during the first year of life.[40]

Developmental Readiness for Solid Foods

If you attempt to spoon-feed a very young infant, for example, at 3 weeks of age, the infant's tongue will push the spoon and food right back out. This **extrusion reflex** is a sign that the infant is not ready for solid foods. By 4 to 6 months of age, the infant will no longer push the food out and is capable of transferring food from the front of the mouth to the back, an ability necessary for swallowing solid foods. Also, the infant can purposefully bring her hand to her mouth, an ability necessary for self-feeding. In addition, if the baby is able to control her head and neck while sitting with minimal support, she is ready to be fed solids.

Feeding Schedule for Infants

The first food introduced is usually an iron-fortified, hypoallergenic infant cereal: baby rice cereal. The cereal should be mixed with human milk, formula, or water. Once the infant is taking rice cereal two or three times each day, caregivers can introduce other foods, such as vegetables and fruits. New foods are introduced one at a time, at intervals of about one week, to see how well the infant tolerates each food and to be on the lookout for allergic reactions. Throughout the first year, breast milk or infant formula still forms the major portion of the infant's diet. Ideally, however, the child has been introduced to a variety of foods by his first birthday.

By 6 to 7 months of age, the child will demonstrate advances toward self-feeding. Allowing the baby to hold an infant spoon and cup (preferably one with a cap and spout) during feeding helps to encourage eventual self-feeding. Babies of this age can hold and chew on large items such as infant teething biscuits, but picking up small pieces of food is still difficult.

At 8 months, the infant has more manual dexterity. He is able to participate in the feeding process and may be able to pick up small pieces of food. It is important that caregivers monitor the child's eating to make sure the youngster does not choke on food or on nonfood items.

By 9 to 12 months of age, a greater proportion of the child's nutrient needs are being met through solid foods, so consumption of human milk or formula decreases. Now the child is demonstrating a limited proficiency with both cup and spoon, and self-feeding is under way. If the texture is soft and the pieces are small, most table foods are appropriate for the child at this stage. The exceptions are cow's milk, egg whites, and wheat, which should be avoided.

Quick Bites

Pumping Iron

The use of cow's milk for children younger than 1 year is a common cause of iron deficiency. Cow's milk is low in iron, and drinking cow's milk can cause intestinal bleeding in infants. The amount of iron in breast milk is low, but this iron is highly bioavailable. Breast milk also contains proteins that bind iron, thereby inhibiting the growth of diarrhea-causing bacteria that feed on iron. If formula is used, the AAP recommends that it be iron-fortified.

extrusion reflex A young infant's response when a spoon is put in its mouth; the tongue is thrust forward, indicating that the baby is not ready for spoon feeding.

Quick Bites

But the Breast Milk Looks Weak...

Mature breast milk looks similar to nonfat milk—thin, pale, and bluish. Not to worry! This appearance is normal and breast milk always contains the right amount of nutrients for the baby. It is never too weak.

gastroesophageal reflux A backflow of stomach contents into the esophagus, accompanied by a burning pain because of the acidity of the gastric juices.

failure to thrive (FTT) Abnormally low gains in length (height) and weight during infancy and childhood; may result from physical problems or poor feeding, but many affected children have no apparent disease or defect.

Various caregivers may be involved in a child's nutrition. In today's society, it is inappropriate to assume that the caregiver is solely the mother, father, grandparent, or even a relative of the child. Many children spend the majority of their feeding time in a child-care setting. Nutrition education and training for child-care workers enhances the likelihood of proper feeding practices in these settings.[41]

Key Concepts: *Between the ages of 4 and 6 months an infant's physiological needs and developmental readiness usually indicate the appropriate time to introduce solid foods. Semisolid and solid foods are introduced slowly to check for food intolerances. The caregiver should choose foods that meet the child's nutritional needs and suit his or her developmental capabilities.*

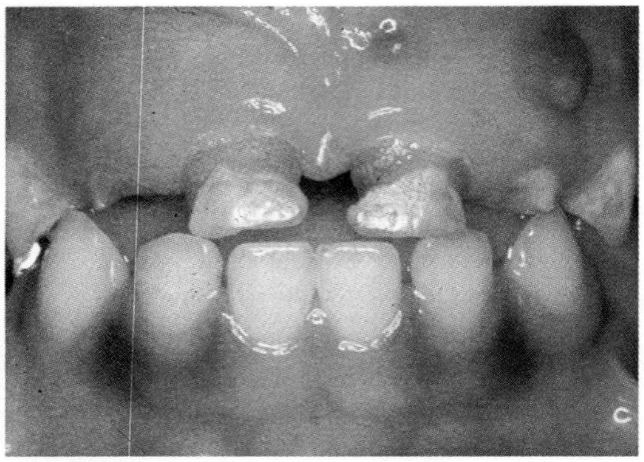

Figure 12.20 **Baby bottle tooth decay.** A baby routinely put to bed with a bottle can develop extensive tooth decay.

Feeding Problems during Infancy

Colic

The term *colic* refers to continuous crying and distress in a healthy infant—apparently due to abdominal cramping and discomfort. Infants with colic usually cry for hours, despite efforts to comfort them. In some cases, a change in formula or a change in the breastfeeding mother's diet provides some relief; however, diet is not considered a cause of colic. Most often, colic goes away on its own, usually by the age of 3 to 4 months.

Baby Bottle Tooth Decay

Extensive tooth decay (see **Figure 12.20**) can result if baby teeth are bathed too long in formula or juice, which nourish decay-producing bacteria. The problem usually occurs when a baby is routinely put to bed with a bottle, so that the baby's teeth are awash in formula or juice for much or all of the night.

Iron-Deficiency Anemia: Milk Anemia

Human milk and cow's milk both are low in iron. As discussed earlier, this is usually not a problem—the iron in breast milk is well absorbed, and regular cow's milk is not recommended for babies under the age of 1 year. Iron deficiency may develop in older infants who do not eat enough iron-rich foods.

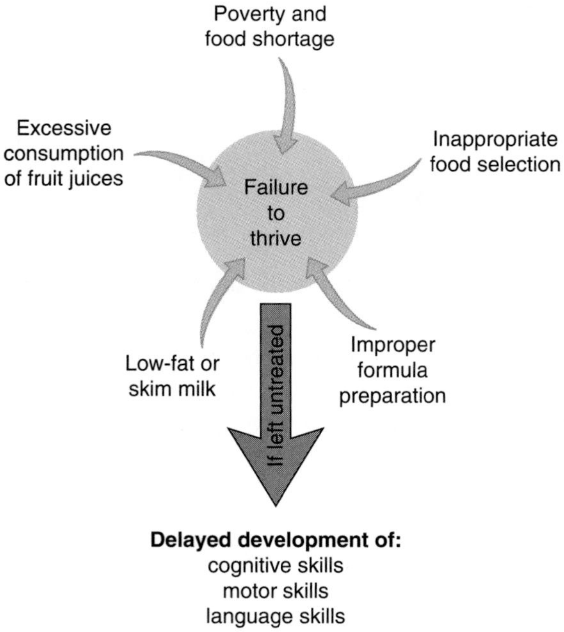

Figure 12.21 **Failure to thrive.** Failure to thrive can result from many different causes. If untreated, the effects are lifelong.

Gastroesophageal Reflux

Gastroesophageal reflux is the regurgitation of the stomach contents into the esophagus after a feeding. This type of spitting up occurs in 3 percent of newborns, usually males, and typically disappears within 12 to 18 months. Concern is warranted if reflux makes a child difficult to feed or results in coughing, choking, or frequent vomiting. Adding cereal to bottle feedings is *not* recommended for a baby who has reflux.

Diarrhea

Stool patterns vary from infant to infant, as well as in the same infant over time. Diarrhea, the frequent passage of loose, watery stools, can rapidly dehydrate an infant. Infants with diarrhea require increased fluids, and caregivers should consult the child's pediatrician for specific advice about how to meet this need.

Failure to Thrive

Full-term infants who experience poor growth in the absence of disease or physical defect suffer from **failure to thrive (FTT)**. (See **Figure 12.21**.)

Although this can occur at any age, in infancy it usually occurs in the second half of the first year. Common causes include poverty and a resulting shortage of food, inappropriate foods in an infant's diet, improper formula preparation, or excessive consumption of fruit juice or fruit drinks. (See the FYI feature "Fruit Juices and Drinks.") In addition, well-meaning parents may introduce low-fat or nonfat milk in an attempt to prevent obesity. Babies need a high-fat diet to support normal growth and brain development. As stated, regular cow's milk should not be introduced before age 1. Low-fat milks are inappropriate for children younger than 2 years.

[Fyi] Fruit Juices and Drinks

FOR YOUR INFORMATION

Fruit juices are popular beverages for children aged 6 months to 5 years. Juices do have benefits to the diet. They are refreshing and sweet, accessible and affordable, more healthful than soft drinks, and provide energy, water, and selected minerals and vitamins.[1] A glass of 100 percent fruit juice counts as one fruit serving. If juice is being used as a source of vitamin C, drinking just 3 to 6 fluid ounces per day meets vitamin C intake recommendations.

Fruit juices vary greatly in fiber, pectin, sorbitol, and carbohydrate composition. White grape juice is probably the easiest to digest (it contains similar amounts of glucose and fructose and no sorbitol). Apple and pear juice, while more popular, are less well absorbed due to higher amounts of sorbitol and fructose.[2]

Fruit juice consumption can be a factor in obesity, if excess juice is consumed on top of a well-rounded diet. Paradoxically, fruit juice consumption also can be a factor in failure to thrive. Failure to thrive may result if fruit juices replace other food sources (particularly milk), or if high amounts of sorbitol and fructose cause diarrhea and malabsorption.[3]

The vast array of juice drinks and fruit beverages available in the marketplace makes it difficult for parents to find nutritious choices. At best, these beverages contain added vitamin C and, in some cases, vitamin A and calcium. However, beverages that are less than 100 percent fruit juice are more like soft drinks than fruits and, as such, should be severely limited in the diets of young children.

To keep intake of fruit juices to a healthy level,

- Limit consumption of fruit juice to 12 fluid ounces per day and ideally no more than 3 to 6 fluid ounces per day
- Encourage caregivers to offer fruit rather than juice to children
- Dilute fruit juice with water
- Delay introduction of juices in the diet until the child can drink from a cup, thus avoiding using juice in bottles

1 Lifshitz F. Weaning foods...the role of fruit juice in the diets of infants and children. *J Am Coll Nutr.* 1996;15(suppl): 15–35.

2 Ibid.

3 Nobugrot T, Chasalow F, Lifshitz F. Carbohydrate absorption from one serving of fruit juice in young children: age and carbohydrate composition effects. *J Am Coll Nutr.* 1997;16: 152–158.

Untreated, FTT can delay cognitive, motor, and language development. Studies indicate, however, that intensive intervention can correct FTT. Such intervention includes nutrition education for caregivers, maintenance of food records by the caregiver, frequent weight checks of the infant, and perhaps social service intervention for the family.

While there is nothing complex about the nutrient needs and food choices appropriate for babies, it is important for caregivers to receive some education about proper feeding. Some of the practices we learn from friends, parents, and other family members, or remember from our own childhood, are inappropriate for babies. Studies show that even people who receive nutrition education in the WIC program introduce solid foods much too early and feed infants sweetened tea, soft drinks, and other inappropriate foods. Newborns don't come with instructions, but caregivers can always turn to a pediatrician or registered dietitian for answers to feeding questions.

Key Concepts: *Feeding-related problems of infancy include colic, baby bottle tooth decay, iron-deficiency anemia, gastroesophageal reflux, diarrhea, and failure to thrive. Usually minor adjustments in food choices or feeding techniques solve these problems; however, caregivers may need the guidance of a pediatrician or registered dietitian.*

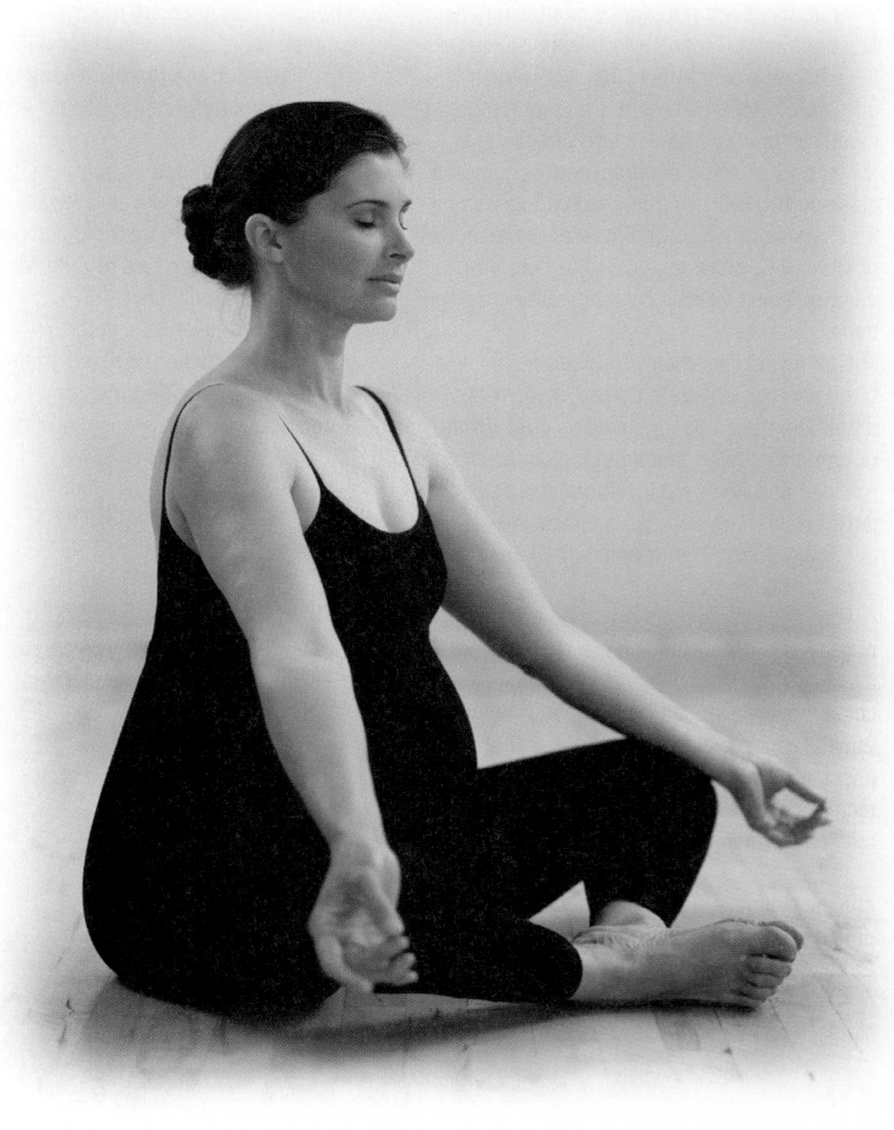

Label [to] Table

A pregnant woman requires more nutrients than usual. The RDA for both iron and folate increases by 50 percent during pregnancy. Iron, especially, is difficult to get in this quantity from the diet. Enriched grains and fortified foods, like cereals, make it easier to obtain these essential nutrients. Let's take a look at the Nutrition Facts label from a popular breakfast cereal.

Take a look at how much folic acid a 1-cup serving of this breakfast cereal contains—50% DV (DV = 400 micrograms). The DV for folate is the same as the RDA for nonpregnant women; for pregnancy, the RDA increases to 600 micrograms. If orange juice accompanies the cereal, another 15% DV (60 mg) is added for a 1-cup serving. So, these two foods provide a substantial amount of the folate that a pregnant woman would need.

Iron also is extremely important for pregnancy because of its role in growth and its importance as blood volume increases during pregnancy. One serving of this breakfast cereal provides almost half of the DV of 18 milligrams (45 percent of 18 milligrams equals 8 milligrams). However, during pregnancy, the RDA for iron is 27 milligrams. So, one serving of this cereal provides nearly one-third of the iron needed each day—a good start. Having orange juice with the cereal will enhance iron absorption.

Nutrition Facts

Serving Size: 1 cup (30g)
Servings Per Container about 9

Amount Per Serving	Cheerios	with ½ cup skim milk
Calories	110	150
Calories from Fat	15	20
		% Daily Value**
Total Fat 2g*	**3%**	**3%**
Saturated Fat 0g	**0%**	**3%**
Polyunsaturated Fat 0.5g		
Monounsaturated Fat 0.5g		
Cholesterol 0g	**0%**	**1%**
Sodium 280 mg	**12%**	**15%**
Total Carbohydrate 22g	**7%**	**9%**
Dietary Fiber 0g	**11%**	**11%**
Sugars 1g		
Protein 3g		
Vitamin A	10%	15%
Vitamin C	10%	10%
Calcium	4%	20%
Iron	45%	45%
Vitamin D	10%	25%
Thiamin	25%	30%
Riboflavin	25%	35%
Niacin	25%	25%
Vitamin B_6	25%	25%
Folic Acid	50%	50%
Vitamin B_{12}	25%	35%
Phosphorus	10%	25%

LEARNING Portfolio chapter 12

Key Terms

	page		page
amniotic fluid	494	lactation consultants	511
blastogenic stage	491	let-down reflex	502
colic	504	low-birth-weight infant	489
colostrum	502	morning sickness	489
critical period of development	491	neonate	509
embryonic stage	491	organogenesis	491
extrusion reflex	513	oxytocin	502
failure to thrive (FTT)	514	placenta	491
fetal stage	491	preeclampsia	500
full-term baby	507	prematurity	507
gastroesophageal reflux	514	preterm delivery	489
gestational age	507	prolactin	502
gestational diabetes	500	Special Supplemental Nutrition Program for Women, Infants, and Children (WIC)	507
growth charts	507		
head circumference	507		
infancy	507	toddler	507
lactation	492	trimesters	490

Study Points

- Nutritional status before pregnancy is an important part of having a healthy baby. Moreover, it is an integral part of all aspects of preconception care: risk assessment, health promotion, and intervention. Being either overweight or underweight prior to pregnancy increases risk of complications.
- Folic acid supplementation before pregnancy has been shown to reduce the risk of neural tube defects such as spina bifida.
- Excessive intake of some vitamins (vitamin A, in particular) and use of tobacco, alcohol, and drugs increase the risk of poor pregnancy outcomes; women should discontinue these practices before they become pregnant.
- Pregnancy can be divided into three stages: blastogenic, embryonic, and fetal. In the blastogenic stage, the fertilized ovum begins rapid cell division and implants itself in the uterine wall. During the embryonic stage, organ systems and other body structures form. During the fetal stage, the longest period of pregnancy, the fetus grows in size and changes in proportions.
- Women who enter pregnancy at a normal BMI should gain 25 to 35 pounds during pregnancy. Underweight women should gain more weight and overweight women less. The energy RDA during pregnancy increases by 300 kilocalories per day for the second and third trimesters.
- By using the Food Guide Pyramid to plan food intake, pregnant women who consume enough energy should be able to meet all their nutrient needs with the exception of iron and folate. They should get needed extra calories mainly from grains, fruits, and vegetables.
- Limiting caffeine intake during pregnancy is recommended. Smoking during pregnancy increases the risk of preterm delivery and low birth weight. Alcohol and drug use can interfere with normal fetal development and should be avoided during pregnancy.
- Gastrointestinal distress such as morning sickness, heartburn, and constipation are common during pregnancy and result from the action of various hormones on the GI tract. Although most food cravings or aversions present no problems, excessive consumption of nonfood items, known as pica, interferes with adequate nutrition.
- During pregnancy, hormones control the development of breast tissue in preparation for milk production. Colostrum, the first milk, which is rich in protein and antibodies, is produced soon after delivery. By two to three weeks after delivery, lactation is well established, and mature milk is being produced.
- The pituitary hormone prolactin stimulates milk production. Oxytocin, another pituitary hormone, stimulates milk release, which is known as the let-down reflex.
- Unless they reduce their physical activity, breastfeeding women need about 500 more kilocalories per day than they did when they were not pregnant. Obtaining adequate energy and using the Food Guide Pyramid to balance choices, most lactating women can obtain all the nutrients they need from their diet. Cigarettes, alcohol, and illicit drugs should not be used while breastfeeding.
- Mothers benefit from breastfeeding through enhanced physiologic recovery, convenience, and emotional bonding. Contraindications to breastfeeding include infec-

tion with HIV or active tuberculosis, and regular use of certain medications.

- Infants receive optimal nutrition from human milk. Breastfeeding can reduce the incidence of infectious diseases, allergies, and other problems during infancy.
- La Leche League, the March of Dimes, and the WIC program for low-income women are among the numerous resources for support and education of pregnant and breastfeeding women.
- Infancy is the fastest growth stage in the life cycle; infants double their birth weight in 4 to 6 months and triple it by 1 year of age. The nutritional status of infants is assessed primarily through measurements of growth.
- Infants' energy needs must be met through a high-fat diet, which provides the maximum calories in minimal volume. Infants' protein and fluid needs are also high.
- Human milk is low in vitamin D; breastfed babies need regular sun exposure or supplemental vitamin D. For breastfed infants, iron-fortified foods need to be introduced by 6 months of age. Formula-fed infants should be given iron-fortified formula.
- Infant formulas usually are based on either cow's milk or soy protein. Unmodified cow's milk is inappropriate for infants throughout the first year of life.
- The FDA regulates the vitamin and mineral composition of infant formulas to ensure adequate infant nutrition. Formula is available in ready-to-feed, liquid concentrate, and powdered forms.
- A nurturing environment is important to the feeding of infants, no matter what the milk source.
- Solid foods are introduced to the infant one at a time, usually beginning with iron-fortified infant cereal. Potential allergens, such as cow's milk, egg whites, and wheat, should be delayed until the baby is 12 months old. Developmental markers, such as head and body control and the absence of the extrusion reflex, show readiness for solid foods.
- Colic, although troublesome to infant and caregiver, is not caused by diet. Iron-deficiency anemia is common in infants who lack iron-rich foods. Infants are susceptible to dehydration, especially when diarrhea is prolonged. Failure to thrive describes an infant who is not growing well; intervention may be required to correct feeding practices of caregivers.

Study Questions

Answers can be found at nutrition.jbpub.com/discovering.

1. Describe the three stages of fetal growth.
2. What are some of the physiological changes that occur to a woman during pregnancy?
3. How do the RDA values for calories, protein, folate, and iron change for pregnancy?
4. What contributes to morning sickness, and how can a woman minimize its effects?
5. Is it okay for an infant to experience weight loss immediately after birth? If an infant does lose weight, does it mean he or she is at nutritional risk?
6. What are some of the nutritional benefits of breast milk?
7. How much water does a breastfed or formula-fed infant need each day?
8. Is it necessary to give breastfed infants supplements of vitamins and/or minerals? If so, which ones?
9. Describe the process for introducing solid foods into an infant's diet.
10. List the feeding problems that may occur during infancy.

Try This

For Just One Week, Can You Eat Like You're Expecting?

The purpose of this exercise is to see if you can follow the nutrition guidelines for pregnancy for just one week. Keep in mind that pregnant women attempt to do this for 38 to 40 weeks! Your goal is to reduce or eliminate caffeine, alcohol, and over-the-counter medications. If necessary, increase your Dairy Food Group servings to at least three per day. You should also take a basic multivitamin/mineral tablet (in place of a woman's prenatal supplement) daily. Make your choices from each food group wisely so that you select some of the most nutrient-dense foods. This will ensure that you consume the amounts of protein, vitamins, and minerals recommended for pregnancy.

Costs of Infant Formula

The purpose of this exercise is to find out how much it might cost to feed an infant. An average 3-month-old baby weighs about 13 pounds (6 kilograms) and would need about 650 kilocalories per day. Using standard infant formula, this baby would need about 32 ounces of formula each day. Now, go to a grocery store and find the infant formulas. If you were to purchase ready-to-feed formula, how much would it cost to feed this baby for one day? What if you were to use concentrated liquid formula? Powdered formula?

What About Bobbie?

Let's pretend that Bobbie is pregnant and in her second trimester. She wants to know whether she's meeting her basic nutrient needs by following her usual diet. Refer to Chapter 1 to review her one-day intake. How do you think she's doing? Let's compare Bobbie's intake of nutrients to the recommendations for pregnant women.

Calories

The recommended calorie intake for women in their second and third trimesters is an extra 300 kilocalories per day over the nonpregnant RDA. Using the RDA value for an average female, this is 2,500 kilocalories. Bobbie's intake for this one day was 2,440 kilocalories, which may already be enough for her growing baby. Bobbie's energy needs may be higher or lower than the RDA of 2,200 for her age group.

Protein

If you remember reviewing Bobbie's diet after reading Chapter 7, "Protein and Amino Acids," you may recall that it is quite high in protein. Her intake was 97 grams and her nonpregnancy RDA (based on her weight) was 51 grams. During pregnancy, however, Bobbie should have an extra 10 grams of protein to ensure her body can handle the demands of tissue growth. Even with the added protein needs of pregnancy (61 grams total protein per day), Bobbie's current intake is more than adequate and could be reduced.

Folate

Bobbie's intake of folate was 470 micrograms, which is short of her pregnancy RDA of 600 micrograms. Although she meets the nonpregnancy recommendations (400 micrograms per day), she would be advised to add folate-rich foods such as spinach, legumes, and orange juice. If Bobbie is adhering to proper prenatal/pregnancy care, then she is consuming a prenatal supplement with folic acid as well.

Iron

Bobbie's intake of iron for one day was 20 milligrams. This is substantially lower than her pregnancy RDA of 27 milligrams. This places Bobbie at greater risk for iron deficiency, a common condition in pregnancy. In addition to taking a prenatal supplement that contains iron, Bobbie is advised to continuing choosing iron-rich lean red meats like the beef meatballs for dinner. She would also benefit from adding more dark-green leafy vegetables to her diet, along with a squeeze of lemon (or other source of vitamin C) to increase the absorption of the non-heme iron. With these additions to her diet, Bobbie will lower her chances of having iron deficiency during her pregnancy.

References

1 Cnattingius S, Bergstrom R, Lipworth L, Kramer MS. Prepregnancy weight and the risk of adverse pregnancy outcomes. *N Engl J Med.* 1998;338:147–152.

2 Ibid.

3 Institute of Medicine, Food and Nutrition Board. *Dietary Reference Intakes for Thiamin, Riboflavin, Niacin, Vitamin B6, Folate, Vitamin B12, Pantothenic Acid, Biotin, and Choline.* Washington, DC: National Academy Press; 1998.

4 Worthington-Roberts B. The role of maternal nutrition in the prevention of birth defects. *J Am Diet Assoc.* 1997;97:S184.

5 Piyathilake CJ, Macaluso M, Hine RJ, et al. Local and systemic effects of cigarette smoking on folate and vitamin B_{12}. *Am J Clin Nutr.* 1994;60:559–566.

6 Institute of Medicine. *Nutrition during Pregnancy.* Washington, DC: National Academy Press; 1990.

7 Ibid.

8 Ibid.

9 Pitkin RM. Energy in pregnancy. *Am J Clin Nutr.* 1999;69(4): 583.

10 Shaw A, Fulton L, Davis C, Hogbin M. *Using the Food Guide Pyramid: A Resource for Nutrition Educators.* http://www.usda.gov/cnpp/using.htm. Accessed 5/11/02.

11 Lowe JB, Balanda KP, Clare G. Evaluation of antenatal smoking cessation programs for pregnant women. *Aust N Z J Public Health.* 1998;22:55.

12 Pamuk E, Makuc D, Heck K, et al. *Socioeconomic Status and Health Chartbook. Health, United States 1998.* Hyattsville, MD: National Center for Health Statistics; 1998. Updated October 1999.

13 Institute of Medicine. *Nutrition during Pregnancy.* Op. cit.

14 Story M, Alton I. Nutritional guidelines during pregnancy and lactation. In: Wolinsky I, Klimis-Tavantzis D, eds. *Nutritional Concerns of Women.* New York: CRC Press; 1996.

15 Assessing adolescent pregnancy. *MMWR.* 1998;47:433.

16 Story M, Alton I. Nutrition issues and adolescent pregnancy. *Nutr Today.* 1995;30:142.

17 Institute of Medicine. *Nutrition during Pregnancy.* Op. cit.

18 Neville MC. Anatomy and physiology of lactation. *Pediatr Clin North Am.* 2001;48:13–34.

19 Institute of Medicine. *Nutrition during Pregnancy.* Op. cit.

20 Greer FR. Do breastfed infants need supplemental vitamins? *Pediatr Clin North Am.* 2001;48:415–423.

21 Story M, Alton I. Nutritional guidelines during pregnancy and lactation. Op. cit.

22 American Dietetic Association. Position of the American Dietetic Association: breaking the barriers to breastfeeding. *J Am Diet Assoc.* 2001;101:1213–1220.

23 Mortensen EL, Michaelsen KF, Sanders SA, Reinisch JM. The association between duration of breastfeeding and adult intelligence. *JAMA.* 2002;287:2365–2371.

24 Worthington-Roberts BS, Williams SR. *Nutrition through the Life Cycle.* 4th ed. New York: McGraw-Hill; 1999.

25 Lawrence A. *A Review of the Medical Benefits and Contraindications to Breastfeeding in the United States.* Arlington, VA: National Center for Education in Maternal and Child Health; 1997. Maternal and Child Health Technical Information Bulletin.

26 Wright AL. The rise of breastfeeding in the United States. *Pediatr Clin North Am.* 2001;48:1–12.

27 Riordan J, Auerbach KG. *Breastfeeding and Human Lactation.* 2nd ed. Sudbury, MA: Jones and Bartlett; 1999.

28 Owen GM. Maternal nutrition. In: Owen AL, Splett PL, Owen GM, eds. *The Art and Science of Delivering Services.* 4th ed. Boston: WCB-McGraw-Hill; 1999:208.

29 Montgomery DL, Splett PL. Economic benefits of breastfeeding infants enrolled in WIC. *J Am Diet Assoc.* 1997;97: 379–386.

30 American Dietetic Association. Commentary. Why children must play while they eat: an interview with T. Berry Brazelton. *J Am Diet Assoc.* 1993;93:1385–1387.

31 Institute of Medicine, Food and Nutrition Board, Committee on Nutritional Status during Pregnancy and Lactation. *Nutrition during Lactation.* Washington, DC: National Academy Press; 1990.

32 Koletzko B, Agostoni C, Carlson SE, et al. Long chain polyunsaturated fatty acids (LC-PUFA) and perinatal development. *Acta Paediatr.* 2001;90:460–464.

33 Sachdev HP, Krishna J, Puri RK, et al. Water supplementation in exclusively breast-fed infants during summer in the tropics. *Lancet.* 1991;337:929–933.

34 American Academy of Pediatrics, Committee on Fetus and Newborn. *Guidelines for Perinatal Care.* 4th ed. Elk Grove Village, IL: American Academy of Pediatrics. 1997.

35 Ibid.

36 Ibid.

37 American Academy of Pediatrics. Breastfeeding and the use of human milk. *Pediatrics.* 1997;100:1035–1039.

38 Kleinman RE, ed. *Pediatric Nutrition Handbook.* 4th ed. Elk Grove, IL: American Academy of Pediatrics; 1998.

39 American Academy of Pediatrics. Infant feeding practices and their possible relationship to the etiology of diabetes mellitus. *Pediatrics.* 1994;94:752–754.

40 Ibid.

41 Nahikian-Nelms M. Influential factors of caregiver behavior at mealtime: a study of 24 child care programs. *J Am Diet Assoc.* 1997;97:505–509.

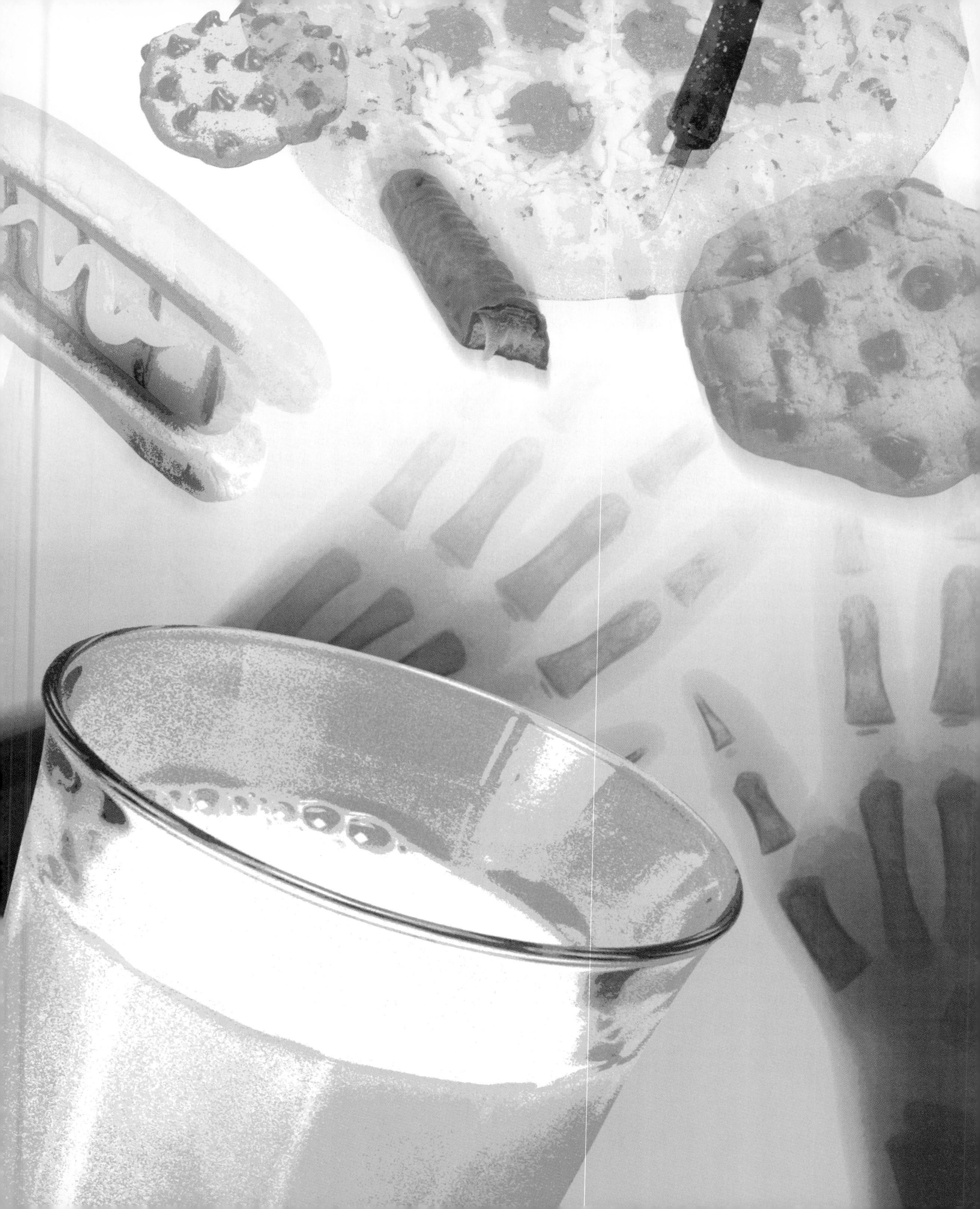

Chapter 13

Life Cycle: From Childhood through Adulthood

Think About It

1. Were you a "picky" eater as a child? What about now?
2. What's your experience with acne and eating particular foods?
3. What behavior changes would you consider making now that would help you live longer?
4. Your grandfather lives by himself and relies on frozen foods for his nutritional needs. How do you feel about this strategy?

Fyi for your Information

This chapter's FYI boxes include practical information on the following topics:
- Food Hypersensitivities and Allergies
- Are Dietary Recommendations to Lower Cholesterol Really Necessary for Elders?

Key to Illustrations

- Fat-Soluble Vitamins
- Minerals
- Water-Soluble Vitamins

www

The Web site for this book offers many useful tools and is a great source for additional nutrition information for both students and instructors. For information on nutrition during childhood, adolescence, and adulthood, visit the site at **nutrition.jbpub.com/discovering.** You'll find exercises that explore the following topics:
- Got Milk—Allergy?
- Lead
- Childhood Malnutrition
- The Elderly Nutrition Program
- Older Women and B_{12}
- Arthritis and Nutrition

What About Bobbie?

Track the choices Bobbie is making with the EatRight Analysis software.

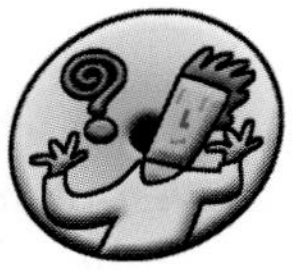

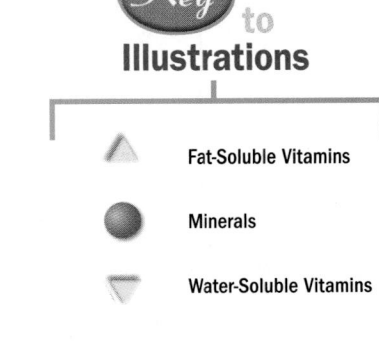

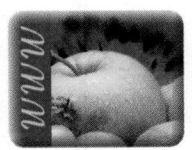

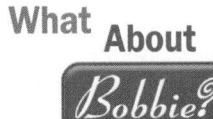

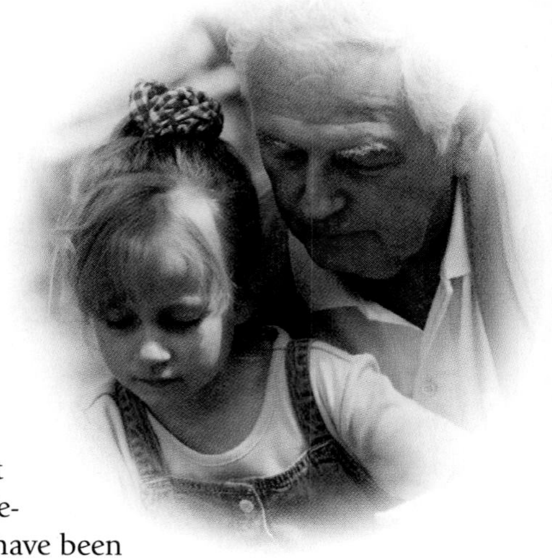

It's the year 2050. Who are you? Where do you live? What is your life like? How healthy are you? If projections made earlier in the century were accurate, you are part of the largest segment of the population—in 2050 between one-third and one-fourth of Americans are older than 65. Perhaps you have retired recently, or maybe you continue to work in your profession. Think about how technology has changed in your lifetime; new methods of communication have been developed that make e-mail and the Internet seem so old-fashioned, so late twentieth century!

Consider how much you have changed over the years. Throughout childhood and adolescence you were growing, sometimes quite rapidly! Whether you fueled that growth with burgers and fries, black beans and rice, chips and soft drinks, or yogurt and salads will have determined a lot about your health status in 2050. Did you continue the eating habits you had in college, and did these allow you to control your weight, blood cholesterol, and blood pressure? Or perhaps in the year 2050 these conditions are no longer of concern. Advances in genetics may have allowed gene therapy to replace diet therapy and medications for chronic diseases.

In the last chapter we explored the nutritional needs of pregnant and breastfeeding women and their babies. Now we will look at how continued growth in childhood and adolescence affects nutritional needs. In addition, we'll see how nutritional needs change as we age, and we'll consider feeding practices, meal planning, and obstacles to healthful eating for each age group.

Childhood

Childhood is the term that refers to the years from age 1 through the beginning of **adolescence**. Growth in childhood, while continuous, occurs at a significantly slower rate than in infancy. During the childhood years, a typical child will gain about 5 pounds and grow 2 to 3 inches annually. Children can be divided into three groups based on their age and development: toddlers (ages 1–3), preschoolers (ages 4–5), and school-aged children (ages 6–10).

childhood The period of life from age 1 to the onset of puberty.

adolescence The period between onset of puberty and adulthood.

Energy and Nutrient Needs during Childhood

Energy and Protein

An average 1-year-old requires about 1,000 to 1,300 kilocalories per day. This daily energy requirement gradually increases until it almost doubles by around age 10. (See **Table 13.1**.) While total energy requirements increase, the kilocalories needed per kilogram of body weight slowly decrease as children move through childhood. The same is true for protein requirements.

Vitamins and Minerals

As long as a healthy child cooperates by eating a variety of healthful foods, a well-planned diet should provide most of the nutrients a child needs. One exception is iron. Children aged 4 to 8 years require 10 milligrams of iron

Table 13.1 Energy and Protein RDAs for Children

Age (yr)	Kcal/kg	Kcal/d*	Protein g/kg	Protein g/d*
1–3	102	1,300	1.2	16
4–6	90	1,800	1.1	24
7–10	70	2,000	1.0	28

*The values per day are based on median weights of children. Individual needs vary.

Source: Food and Nutrition Board. *Recommended Dietary Allowances.* 10th ed. Washington, DC: National Academy Press; 1989. Reprinted with permission.

per day, but may not get that amount without careful meal planning. High consumption of milk, a low source of iron, can contribute to inadequate iron intake, and so milk intake during childhood should be limited to 3 to 4 cups per day. This allows room in the diet for high-iron food sources such as lean meats, legumes, fish, poultry, and iron-enriched breads and cereals. (See **Table 13.2.**) Iron deficiency not only affects growth, but also can impair the child's mood, attention span, focus, and ability to learn.

A child's diet also may be low in other micronutrients, especially zinc, vitamin D, and vitamin E. (See **Figure 13.1.**) Children often dislike vegetables or they may be following their parents' low-fat diets, which may be low in zinc and vitamin E.[1]

Vitamin and Mineral Supplements

Many caregivers would rather give a child a vitamin/mineral pill than plan and prepare the meals necessary to ensure an adequate diet. However, the balanced diet a child needs is not much different from the diet an adult needs. In fact, the USDA Food Guide Pyramid for children aged 2 to 6 years (**Figure 13.2**) shows approximately the same balance of food groups as is recommended for adults. Caregivers who understand this may be less tempted to rely on supplements to achieve a balanced diet.

Some children should receive supplements. Among them are children whose diets are restricted for medical reasons, those with chronic diseases, those who are malnourished, and those with food allergies that require them to avoid multiple foods or food groups.[2] (For more on food allergies, see the FYI feature "Food Hypersensitivities and Allergies.") Caregivers need to be reminded that vitamin and mineral supplements for children are dangerous in large doses. Vitamin and mineral preparations must be treated like all medicines and kept safely out of children's reach. Supplements containing iron in doses over 30 milligrams are especially dangerous to children. Accidental consumption of vitamin and mineral or iron supplements should be treated as a poisoning emergency.

Influences on Childhood Food Habits and Intake

Think About It 1

Children develop food preferences at an early age. But as their environment expands, more and more external factors influence their diet. It is estimated that children spend more time watching television than doing most other activities. Recognizing the influence that children have on household purchases, advertisers target commercials specifically at children during prime children's viewing hours. Saturday morning cartoons, for example, feature countless ads for sweetened cereals, fast foods, candy, and other foods high in sugar or fat, none of which are necessary or desirable.[3] When families make television watching a normal part of meal routines, children's diets

Table 13.2 Iron-Rich Foods and Snacks

Iron-Rich Foods

Ground beef
Poultry
Fish
Legumes
Dark-green vegetables
Enriched breads, cereals, rice, and pasta

Iron-Rich Snacks

Cream of Wheat
Cooked macaroni or pasta
Enriched cereals, either dry or with milk
Tortillas filled with refried beans
Dried apricots
Raisins (for older children)
Bean dip
Chili, mildly seasoned
Peanut butter on enriched bread or graham crackers
Sloppy Joe
Casseroles with meat (many children do not like plain meats)

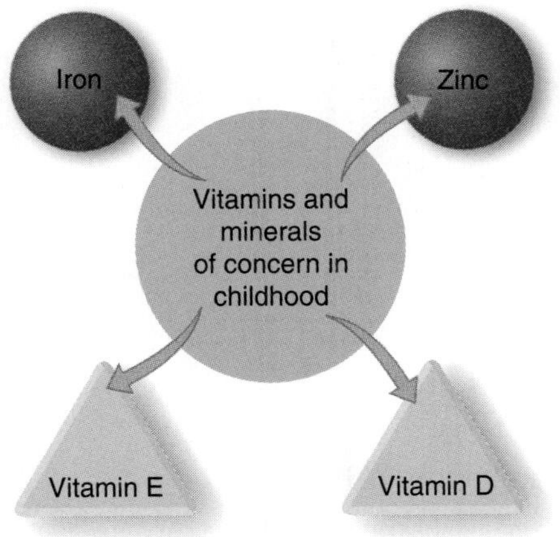

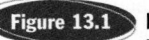

Figure 13.1 Micronutrients of concern in childhood. Milk is low in iron, and small children also may have low intakes of zinc, vitamin D, and vitamin E.

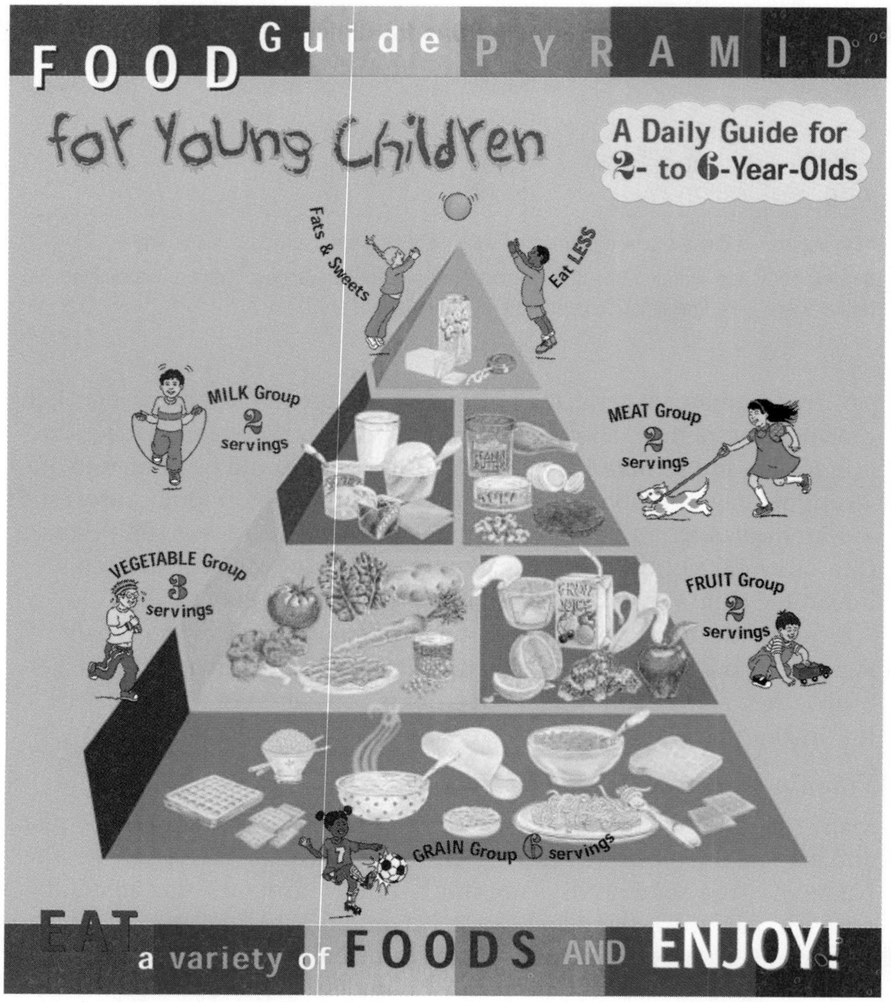

U.S. DEPARTMENT OF AGRICULTURE
CENTER FOR NUTRITION POLICY AND PROMOTION

WHAT COUNTS AS ONE SERVING?

GRAIN GROUP	FRUIT GROUP	MEAT GROUP
1 slice of bread ½ cup of cooked rice or pasta ½ cup of cooked cereal 1 ounce of ready-to-eat cereal	1 piece of fruit or melon wedge ¾ cup of juice ½ cup of canned fruit ¼ cup of dried fruit	2 to 3 ounces of cooked lean meat, poultry, or fish. ½ cup of cooked dry beans, or 1 egg counts as 1 ounce of lean meat. 2 tablespoons of peanut butter count as 1 ounce of meat.
VEGETABLE GROUP	**MILK GROUP**	**FATS AND SWEETS**
½ cup of chopped raw or cooked vegetables 1 cup of raw leafy vegetables	1 cup of milk or yogurt 2 ounces of cheese	Limit calories from these.

Four- to 6-year-olds can eat these serving sizes. Offer 2- to 3-year-olds less, except for milk. Two- to 6-year-old children need a total of 2 servings from the milk group each day.

Figure 13.2 **Food Guide Pyramid for Young Children.** Young children have unique food patterns and needs in comparison with older children and adults. Also, many young children are not eating healthful diets, and early food experiences are crucial to food preferences and patterns throughout life. To help improve the diets of young children 2 to 6 years old, the USDA has developed the Food Guide Pyramid for Young Children.

Quick Bites

Television Tubbies

The number of obese children in America doubled in the past 20 years, and one in five American children is now overweight. Today's kids spend more time watching TV and playing video games than engaging in physical activity. Advertisers know it. When programs for children are broadcast, 80 percent of commercials advertise food, most of it high in sugar or fat.

have fewer fruits and vegetables and more pizzas, snack foods, and sodas than the diets of children in families that separate television viewing and eating.[4]

Social events and parties often promote unhealthful eating habits. No matter what the occasion, the menu for children's parties rarely varies. The staples are pizza, ice cream, soft drinks, and candy. None of these foods alone is a problem, but the fact that these foods are offered at the majority

Fyi Food Hypersensitivities and Allergies

FOR YOUR INFORMATION

Food allergies, or food hypersensitivities, are allergic reactions to food proteins. Allergies are different from food intolerances (such as lactose intolerance) that may involve digestive problems rather than an immune response. Allergies are less likely than intolerances to be transient, and tend to have more serious consequences. Proteins that trigger allergies are known as allergens. The most common food allergens are found in milk, eggs, tree nuts, peanuts, soy, wheat, fish, and seafood.

Food allergies occur when the immune system mounts a specific reaction to a food protein. Surveys suggest that about 25 percent of people in the general population think they suffer from food allergies. But studies show that only 1 to 2 percent of adults and 6 to 8 percent of children under the age of 3 truly do.[1]

In a true allergic reaction, the immune system responds to an allergen with a cascade of chemical reactions that can cause wheezing, difficulty breathing, and hives, as well as a host of other symptoms. (See Table A, "Symptoms of Food Allergies.") Food allergy symptoms often affect more than one body system and may change in severity from one reaction to the next.

Anaphylaxis, the most severe allergic reaction, usually takes place within the first hour after eating the offending food. Shock and respiratory failure can rapidly ensue. Anaphylaxis can be fatal, so immediate emergency care is essential.

Allergy symptoms that occur immediately after a food is eaten make detective work easier. If symptoms are slow to evolve, a child may suffer chronic diarrhea and even experience failure to thrive before the problem is identified.

When identification of the food culprit isn't so obvious, an elimination diet can help. All suspected foods are eliminated from the diet and slowly reintroduced, one by one, on a specific schedule. Both intake and reactions are carefully recorded. Prolonged or improper use of such a diet can have severe nutritional consequences. A registered dietitian can help with diet planning to ensure nutritional adequacy.

The double-blind, placebo-controlled food challenge is the gold standard of food allergy testing. Although definitive, it can be dangerous for people prone to anaphylactic reactions. In this test, increasing amounts of a suspected food are given to the child under the supervision of a physician, who looks for allergy symptoms and signs. This test must be done by trained personnel with emergency equipment handy.

The treatment for food allergy is avoidance of the offending allergen. Each child with a food allergy needs a nutrition assessment that pays attention to the specific nutrients missing as a result of avoiding the offending foods. For example, if a toddler is avoiding milk and milk products due to a cow's milk allergy, the nutrients most at risk would be protein, vitamin D, and calcium. As a child's diet includes more and more foods, the key becomes careful label reading to identify allergen-containing foods. Organizations such as the Food Allergy & Anaphylaxis Network provide materials for deciphering food labels.[2] The Food Allergy & Anaphylaxis Network also offers tips for successful traveling and dining with a child who has food allergies.

Many children naturally outgrow food allergies by the time they are 3 years old. Once outgrown, the food allergy will not return.

1 Sampson HA. Food allergy. *JAMA.* 1997;278:1888–1894.
2 The Food Allergy & Anaphylaxis Network. http://www.foodallergy.org. Accessed 5/11/02.

Table A **Symptoms of Food Allergies**

Gastrointestinal Tract

Itching of the lips, mouth, and throat
Swelling of the throat
Abdominal cramping and distention
Diarrhea
Colic
Gastrointestinal bleeding
Protein-losing enteropathy

Skin

Hives
Swelling
Eczema, contact dermatitis

Respiratory Tract

Runny or stuffed-up nose, sneezing, postnasal discharge
Recurrent croup
Chronic pneumonia
Middle-ear infections

Systemic

Anaphylaxis
Heart rhythm irregularities
Low blood pressure

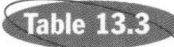

Table 13.3 Healthy Snacks

Cereal and milk
Yogurt shake: plain yogurt, fresh fruit
Peanut butter on celery
Popcorn sprinkled with Parmesan cheese
Fresh vegetables and a yogurt dip
Pretzels
Bananas with peanut butter
Graham crackers and peanut butter
Sliced apples with cheese
Bagel and melted cheese
Bran muffins
Pumpkin, banana, or zucchini bread
Mini pizza on English muffin
Homemade pita pocket sandwiches
Yogurt and mini bagel
Vegetable soup
Fresh fruit
Hot chocolate (made with milk)

of social gatherings is. Popular snacks and beverages also tend to be too high in sugar and fat. Serving more healthful, but still child-friendly, snacks, such as those in **Table 13.3**, breaks this tradition.

Key Concepts: *Children ages 1 through 10 grow at a slower rate than they did as infants, but still gain 2 to 3 inches and about 5 pounds per year. They should be able to obtain adequate energy and nutrients from their meals and snacks. Iron-deficiency anemia is the most common nutritional deficiency among American children. Cow's milk is not an adequate source of iron and should be limited to 3 or 4 cups per day to allow for other, high-iron foods. Outside influences, such as television viewing, affect children's preferences for foods with low nutrient density.*

Nutritional Concerns of Childhood

Malnutrition and Hunger in Childhood

Of all of the issues facing children with respect to growth and nutrition, none is so devastating as hunger and subsequent malnutrition. Throughout the world, hunger and malnutrition are responsible for nearly half of the deaths of preschool children. Deficiencies in vitamin A, zinc, iron, and protein also result in illness, stunted growth, limited development, and, in the case of vitamin A, possibly permanent blindness.

In the United States, an estimated 2.5 to 3 million people are homeless. Of this group, 43 percent are families with children.[5] About 25 percent of children younger than 3 years old live in poverty—a higher percentage than in any other age bracket of the population.[6] And children in families with low incomes have a higher prevalence of iron deficiency and poor health status than children in higher-income families.[7] Nearly 12 million children grow up in so-called **food-insecure households** (where calories are adequate, but diet quality has suffered), and more than 2.7 million children experience hunger.[8] Because their bodies need to grow, children are more vulnerable than adults to the effects of malnutrition.

Federal programs such as the WIC program, **National School Lunch Program, School Breakfast Program,** and **Summer Food Service Program** help to create a safety net for these children. (See **Figure 13.3**.) The WIC

food-insecure households Households whose members take in enough calories, but have diets of reduced quality that do not meet all daily nutritional requirements.

National School Lunch Program A USDA program that provides nutritious lunches and the opportunity to practice skills learned in classroom nutrition education; enacted in 1946 to provide U.S. children at least one healthful meal every school day.

School Breakfast Program A USDA program that assists schools in providing a nutritious morning meal to children nationwide.

Summer Food Service Program A USDA program that helps children in lower-income families to continue receiving nutritious meals during long school vacations when they do not have access to school lunch or breakfast.

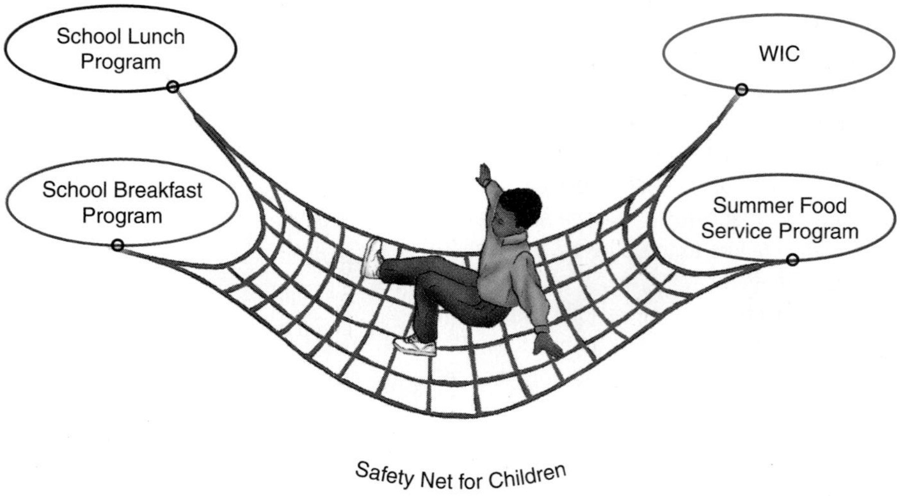

Figure 13.3 Federal safety net for children. Children are more vulnerable than adults to the effects of malnutrition. For many children, these federal programs provide the major and, in some cases, the only sources of calories and other nutrients.

program, designed to follow children through the fifth birthday, provides vouchers for milk, eggs, cereal, juice, cheese, and either peanut butter or dried beans. However, participation rates in WIC are less than they could be. Many caregivers do not understand that WIC is still available after a child is weaned off breast milk or formula or do not have transportation to the WIC site or grocery store.

The National School Lunch and School Breakfast programs offer free or reduced-cost breakfast and lunch at school. Lunches must provide at least one-third of a child's RDA for energy, protein, vitamins A and C, and the minerals iron and calcium; breakfasts must supply one-fourth of the RDA for these nutrients. In addition, school meals must now conform to the *Dietary Guidelines for Americans* and limit total fat calories to 30 percent and saturated fat calories to 10 percent. The Summer Feeding Program was created after many children who depend on the breakfast and lunch programs during the school year experienced hunger during the summer months. For many children, these meals are the major—and, in some cases, only—sources of calories and other nutrients. Those who plan and serve meals have the challenge of balancing popular foods that children will eat with foods that provide good nutrition.

Food and Behavior

Many parents and caregivers mistakenly believe that consuming sugar-laden foods causes **hyperactivity** in children. The myth persists even though a number of carefully controlled studies find no cause-and-effect relationship.[9] The term *hyperactivity* usually is defined as an abnormal increase in activity that is maladaptive and inconsistent with developmental level, but common usage has blurred its meaning. Parents often use this term to describe what they view as unruly behavior in children, particularly in social settings like parties. Many people also believe that certain food additives, including preservatives and colorings, can cause or exacerbate behavioral disorders. However, no studies conclusively link food to behavior. Children typically react to situations surrounding foods or parties (where high-sugar foods are often served) in excitable ways. This is not proof of a cause-and-effect relationship between those foods and those behaviors.

hyperactivity A maladaptive and abnormal increase in activity that is inconsistent with developmental levels. Includes frequent fidgeting, inappropriate running, excessive talking, and difficulty in engaging in quiet activities.

Caffeine products can make children jittery and interfere with their sleep. Because children have small body sizes, the effects of a caffeinated beverage are intensified. Many soft drinks are high in caffeine; examples include Mountain Dew (55 mg per 12-oz can), Surge (51 mg per 12-oz can), and Coca-Cola (47 mg per 12-oz can).

Nutrition and Chronic Disease in Childhood

When is it appropriate to adopt adult dietary guidelines for children? It is well documented that early signs of chronic disease appear in children. Evidence of early plaque development has been seen in the coronary arteries of adolescents and is associated with adult cardiovascular diseases. However, the low-fat, high-fiber diet advocated for adults may jeopardize a very young child's growth. Infants and toddlers younger than 2 years old need fat in their diets for growth, organ protection, and central nervous system development. Dietary restrictions at this age are not appropriate.

For children older than 3, however, efforts to lower fat, saturated fat, and cholesterol intake may reduce risks of chronic disease. The American Heart Association; National Heart, Lung and Blood Institute; and the American Academy of Pediatrics (AAP) all support such efforts.[10] But it's important that parents and caregivers do not misinterpret the recommendations and

Quick Bites

Are Minority Children at High Risk for Cardiovascular Disease?

Early risk factors for cardiovascular disease are increasing in America. African American and Mexican American children are more likely to exhibit high blood pressure and high body mass index and to consume a higher percentage of calories from fat than are Caucasian children. The three ethnic groups have similar blood cholesterol levels, however, and Caucasian children are more likely to smoke.

puberty The period of life during which the secondary sex characteristics develop and the ability to reproduce is attained.

restrict children's energy intake. During the preschool and school years, gradual changes can bring food choices in line with the *Dietary Guidelines for Americans.*

Many experts feel that before **puberty**, a low-fat diet has no demonstrated benefits for children. Health Canada, the Canadian government's health promotion department, recommends putting a priority on energy intake as well as the intake of nutrients required for proper growth. It recommends against restricting food choices during preschool and childhood. Health Canada recommends gradually adjusting fat intake so that it approaches adult recommendations at adolescence or puberty.[11] Caregivers should offer children healthful choices and, as they grow, educate them about proper adult nutrition.

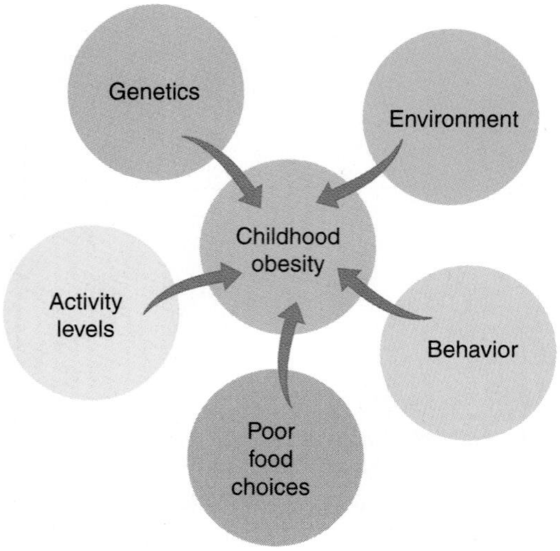

Figure 13.4 **Factors that contribute to childhood obesity.** Childhood obesity is on the rise and predisposes children to health problems when they become adults.

Childhood Obesity

In the United States, obesity in childhood is increasing at an alarming rate. Obese children run a high risk of becoming obese adults and suffering the ensuing health problems. An obese child is likely to reach maturity earlier than a child of normal weight, but perhaps at the expense of height. Some obese children already deal with cardiovascular consequences of obesity, such as lipid abnormalities and hypertension, and many obese children develop type 2 diabetes prior to the teen years. Finally, obese children experience the psychological trauma associated with obesity in our culture. Factors involved in the development of obesity in childhood include genetics, environment, behavior, and activity levels. (See **Figure 13.4**.)

Programs designed to treat childhood obesity generally provide behavior modification, exercise counseling, psychological support or therapy, family counseling, and family meal-planning advice. The goal is not weight loss, but allowing the child's height to catch up with his or her weight. Rather than restrict caloric intake or food choices, the usual strategy is to increase activity and improve food choices.

Lead Toxicity

Lead toxicity can result in slow growth and iron-deficiency anemia and can damage the brain and central nervous system, leading to a host of learning disabilities and behavior problems. Lead is present in the plumbing of old homes; old paint; house dust in homes with cracked or peeling lead-based paint; and, in some areas, the soil. Children can ingest lead by drinking contaminated water, eating paint chips, or sucking their fingers after playing in or around lead-contaminated house dust or soil. Lead toxicity occurs more frequently in areas of poverty, where lead contamination is more common and where iron-deficiency anemia is present.

Low intakes of iron, calcium, and zinc tend to result in increased lead absorption. Children with an adequate intake of these micronutrients show less incidence of lead toxicity. Therefore, many of the programs established to reduce the incidence of lead toxicity in children also promote good nutrition, with an emphasis on adequate iron, calcium, and zinc consumption.

Quick Bites

Tragedy in Lead

About 5 percent of American children demonstrate signs of lead toxicity, defined as a blood level of 10 micrograms of lead per deciliter. When children are exposed to lead on a continuous or regular basis, brain function is affected.

Vegetarianism in Childhood

A lacto- or lacto-ovo-vegetarian diet can supply adequate levels of protein, iron, calcium, vitamin B_{12}, and vitamin D. Without careful planning, however, a vegan diet, which contains no animal products, may not supply all of the nutrients needed to support a child's growth. For a vegan child, legumes and nuts should be substituted for meats, and calcium- and vitamin B_{12}-fortified soy milk should be substituted for cow's milk. At least

20 to 30 minutes of sunlight exposure three times a week should provide enough vitamin D.[12]

Key Concepts: *Hunger and malnutrition affect a significant number of our nation's children. To combat the growing number of hungry children, programs such as WIC, the National School Lunch Program, and the National School Breakfast Program are vital. Other concerns common to childhood include obesity, lead toxicity, and chronic disease prevention. Infants and toddlers should not be given low-fat, high-fiber diets; when children reach the age of 3, caregivers should begin to adjust children's diets to follow appropriate dietary guidelines. For children, strict vegetarian diets may be too limited in calcium, vitamin D, and vitamin* B_{12}.

Adolescence

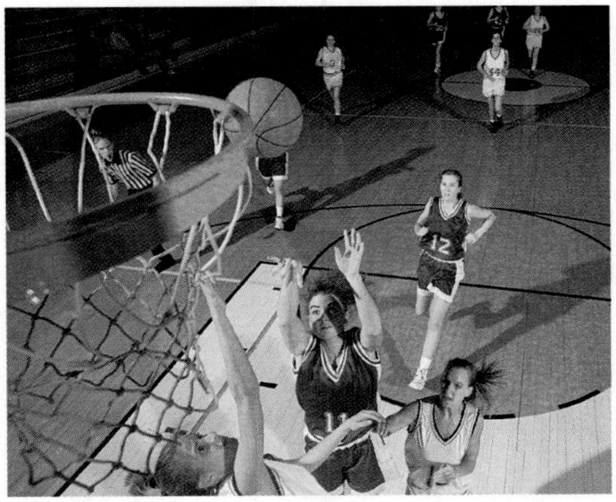

Adolescents seem to add inches overnight. Many caregivers complain that they cannot keep enough food in the house to satisfy an adolescent's appetite! Adolescence commonly is defined as the time between the onset of puberty and adulthood. This maturation process involves both physical growth and emotional maturation.

Physical Growth and Development

Hormones drive growth, which varies from child to child. In general, growth spurts begin between ages 10½ and 11 for girls, with a peak in the rate of growth at around age 12. For boys, growth spurts usually begin between ages 12½ and 13 and peak at around age 14. This spurt, or period of maximal growth, lasts about 2 years.

Height

The first phase of adolescent growth is linear. On average, boys grow 8 inches and girls grow 6 inches during puberty. This growth is uneven. The hands and feet enlarge first. The calves and forearms lengthen next, followed by expansion of the hips, chest, shoulders, and trunk. As a result, adolescents often appear awkward or clumsy. After the main growth spurt, growth continues for two to three years, but at a much slower rate.

For girls, peak growth occurs about one year before **menarche**, the onset of menstruation. A typical girl has achieved about 95 percent of her adult height by menarche and grows only 2 to 4 inches during the remainder of adolescence. Growth rates are closely related to sexual maturation, reflected in breast development (girls), change of voice (boys), development of sexual organs, and growth of pubic hair. When the growth plates at the ends of the long bones (**epiphyses**) close, skeletal growth is complete. This is a critical point in development. An adolescent who is malnourished and of small stature at the point of epiphysis closure may not achieve his or her full potential height.

menarche First menstrual period.

epiphyses The heads of the long bones that are separated from the shaft of the bone until the bone stops growing.

Weight

The second growth phase of adolescence involves lateral growth. Here, the adolescent "fills out," or gains weight. External factors such as diet and exercise affect weight gain more than linear growth, so weight gain can vary widely among adolescents. However, a typical healthy girl will gain 35 pounds during adolescence; a typical boy will gain 45 pounds. In our weight-sensitive society, adolescents should be prepared for this normal, expected weight gain. Although the bulk of an adolescent's lateral growth occurs after the linear growth spurt, a significant portion of the two growth stages overlap. For girls, for example, peak weight gain usually occurs around the time of menarche.

Body Composition

Before puberty, the body composition of boys and girls does not differ greatly. This changes dramatically during adolescence. Boys experience greater increases in lean body mass, resulting in more obvious muscle definition. Girls accumulate greater stores of body fat, specifically around the hips and buttocks, upper arms, breasts, and upper back. By adulthood, a typical woman's body composition is 23 percent fat; a typical man, in contrast, has 12 percent body fat.

Emotional Maturity: Developmental Tasks

Adolescence is a time not only of great physical growth, but also of tremendous emotional growth. This psychological development affects food choices, eating habits, and body image. Many teens become more interested in the healthful aspects of nutrition. Others experiment with unhealthful food choices, as an exercise in independence or in an attempt to achieve an idealized body.

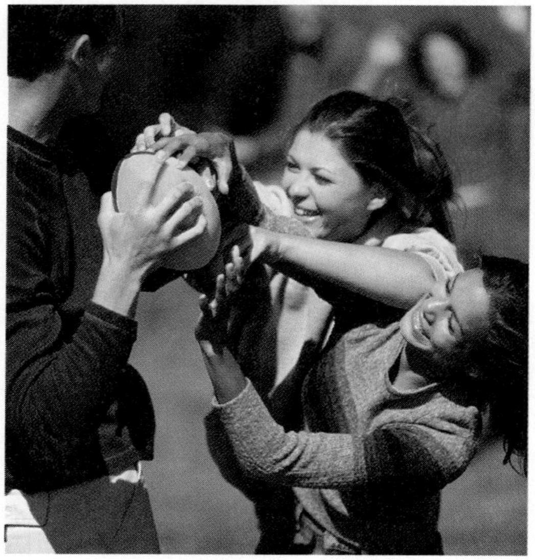

Nutrient Needs of Adolescents

Although growth, not age, should be the ultimate indicator of nutrient needs, RDAs are established based on age. Separate recommendations for males and females reflect their differences in growth rates and body composition seen during adolescence.

Energy and Protein

Energy needs, as total kilocalories per day, are greater during adolescence (**Table 13.4**) than at any other time of life, with the exception of pregnancy and lactation. Recommended energy intakes are guidelines only; adjustments often are needed to meet individual requirements. For example, the recommendations do not take activity levels into account. An active teen involved in regular exercise or sports will exceed the recommendations for energy. Conversely, a physically mature teen, with no regular exercise or fitness plan, will not need this much energy for weight maintenance.

To support growth, an adolescent's protein needs per unit body weight are higher than an adult's but less than a rapidly growing infant's. For teen girls aged 15 to 18, the protein RDA declines to adult levels (as g/kg body weight), reflecting the end of linear growth in most teen girls. American teens rarely have a problem with adequate protein intake, but teen girls risk a lack of protein if they cut calories too drastically in attempts to control weight.

Table 13.4 Energy and Protein RDAs for Adolescence

	Age (yr)	Kcal/kg	Kcal/d*	Protein g/kg	Protein g/d*
Males	11–14	55	2,500	1.0	45
	15–18	45	3,000	0.9	59
Females	11–14	47	2,200	1.0	46
	15–18	40	2,200	0.8	44

* The values per day are based on median weights of adolescents. Individual needs vary.

Source: Food and Nutrition Board. *Recommended Dietary Allowances.* 10th ed. Washington, DC: National Academy Press; 1989.

Vitamins and Minerals

Along with increased needs for energy and protein, adolescents have higher vitamin and mineral needs compared with people at most other life stages. Three nutrients of particular concern for adolescents are vitamin A, calcium, and iron, each of which plays an important role in growth. (See **Figure 13.5**.)

Teens can improve their vitamin A intake by including more fruits and vegetables in their diets. Adequate calcium, essential for bone formation and maximal bone density, can be harder to obtain. Many teens, especially girls, actually reduce their calcium intake by replacing calcium-rich milk in their diets with soft drinks.[13] During puberty, adolescents gain 15 percent of their full adult height and accumulate half of their ultimate adult bone mass. Adolescents who do not achieve sufficient bone density have a greater risk of developing osteoporosis later in life. The AI for calcium in adolescence is 1,300 milligrams of calcium every day. Dairy products are rich in calcium (about 300 milligrams per cup of milk or yogurt) and convenient to eat; without these or calcium-fortified products, meeting the AI is difficult indeed.

Adolescent boys need added iron to support growth of muscle and lean body mass. Teenage girls need added iron to replace blood lost during menstruation. The recommended intake for boys aged 14 to 18 is 11 milligrams per day throughout adolescence; for teen girls, it is 15 milligrams per day. As long as they take in enough calories, both groups should be able to obtain this iron from nutrient-dense foods. During adolescence, however, food selection often is less than optimal. Careful meal planning is required to maximize teenagers' iron consumption.

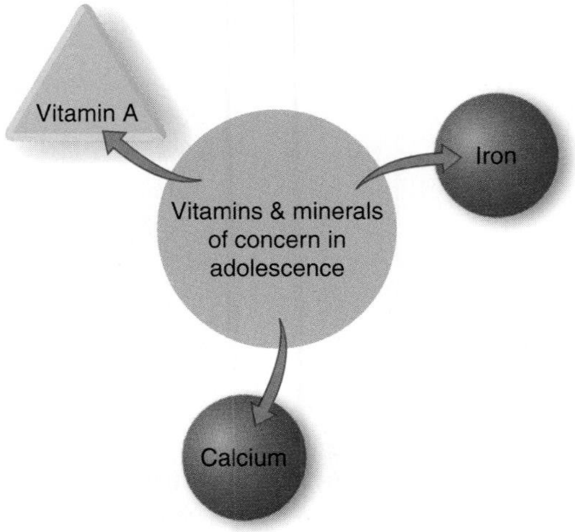

Figure 13.5 **Micronutrients of concern in adolescence.** Vitamin A is important for growth, and calcium is essential for building strong bones. Teen girls especially need adequate iron intake to replace iron lost due to menstruation.

Influences on Adolescent Food Intake

Teenagers want and need to make their own food choices and purchases and may want to take over preparation of their own food. While the parent can set a good example, parental influence is much weaker now. Factors that influence an adolescent's food selection and consumption include the desire to be healthy, fitness goals, amount of discretionary income, social practices, and peers. (See **Figure 13.6**.)

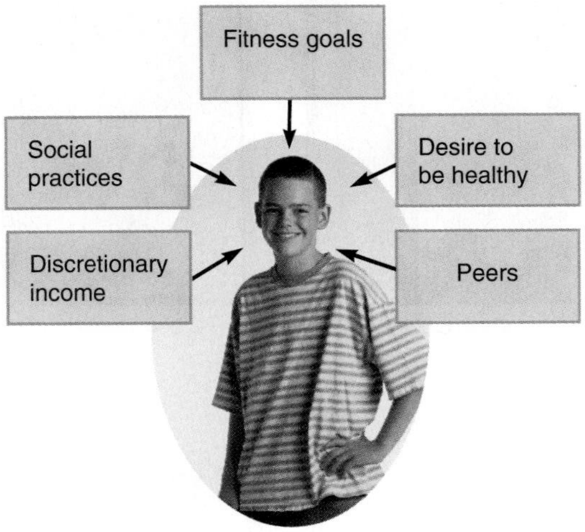

Figure 13.6 **Factors that influence adolescent food choices.** Social, cultural, and psychological factors, especially peer pressure, strongly influence adolescent food choices.

Key Concepts: *Humans need more calories and nutrients during adolescence than at any other stage of life, with the exception of pregnancy and lactation. Boys grow about 8 inches, gain about 45 pounds, and increase their lean body mass. Girls grow about 6 inches, gain about 35 pounds, and increase their body fat. As at earlier ages, calcium, iron, and vitamin A are often lacking in adolescent diets. Factors that determine food selection and consumption include the desire to be healthy, fitness goals, amount of discretionary income, social practices, and peers.*

Nutrition-Related Concerns for Adolescents

Fitness and Sports

For many adolescents, an interest in fitness becomes the catalyst for learning about nutrition and improving dietary habits. Some teens, unfortunately, become obsessed with their athletic performance, food intake, and body appearance and go to extremes that can jeopardize not only their current athletic performance but also their long-term health. For more information about nutritional needs of athletes, see Chapter 11, "Sports Nutrition."

acne An inflammatory skin eruption that usually occurs in or near the sebaceous glands of the face, neck, shoulders, and upper back.

Quick Bites

Early Abusers

These days, youngsters seem to start abusing substances earlier and earlier. Use of alcohol, cigarettes, and inhalants is increasing among fourth-, fifth-, and sixth-graders. By sixth grade, 15 percent of children have tried alcohol and cigarettes. Many children say that peer pressure is their reason for experimentation.

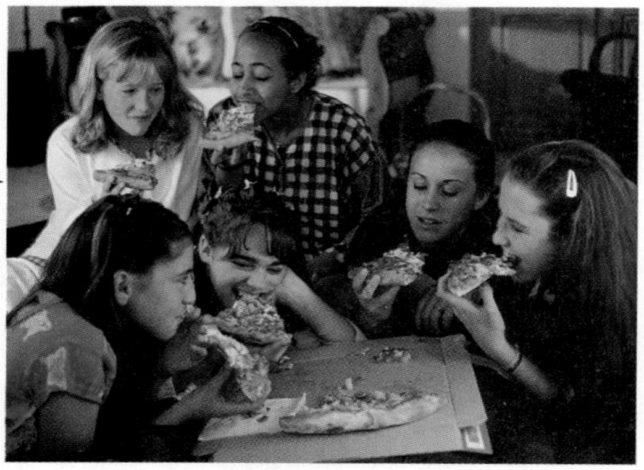

Acne

Many teens blame certain foods for their **acne**. Myths surrounding acne and diet abound, but research has not found any correlation between acne and chocolate, greasy foods, soft drinks, nuts, or milk. Unfortunately, acne cannot be cured or prevented through diet. People who suffer from acne, therefore, should not feel guilty about their food choices. Effective treatments for acne include topical benzoyl peroxide, low-dose oral antibiotics, and two medications derived from vitamin A—Retin-A and Accutane. Although both of these medications are derivatives of vitamin A, there is no correlation between dietary vitamin A and acne.

Think About It 2

Eating Disorders

Eating disorders, discussed more thoroughly in the "Spotlight on Eating Disorders," frequently begin during adolescence. Adolescents often become preoccupied with their weight, appearance, and eating habits. Although eating disorders still affect more girls than boys, the prevalence in males is increasing, so they shouldn't be ignored or dismissed as only a "girl's problem."

Obesity

As in childhood, obesity rates in adolescence are climbing. Obese adolescents have an increased risk of developing high blood pressure and abnormal glucose tolerance. They also suffer psychologically from teasing, being ostracized by peers, and from longing to be slimmer. In addition, adolescent obesity sets the stage for adult obesity, with all of its attendant health consequences. (See Chapter 8, "Energy Balance and Weight Management," for more on overweight and obesity.) Finally, adolescents who engage in unhealthful weight-loss methods are more likely to engage in other risky behaviors, such as tobacco, alcohol, or other drug use, unprotected sex, suicide attempts, and delinquency.[14] **Table 13.5** lists the factors that can put an adolescent at risk for obesity.

Table 13.5 Risk Factors for Obesity in Adolescents

Risk Factors	Explanations
Social Variables	
Socioeconomic status	Direct relationship for males; inverse relationship for females
Parental obesity	Strong correlation between obesity in parents and obesity in their children
Race	Higher in white children and African American female adolescents
Family size	Less obesity with larger family size
Television watching	Increased viewing correlates with increasing obesity
Physical Environment	
Region	Greater incidence of obesity in Northeast; urban areas
Seasonal	Higher in winter
Genetic and Metabolic Factors	
Reduced energy expenditure	

Source: Bandini L. Obesity in the adolescent. *Adolesc Med* 1992;3(3):459–472.

Tobacco, Alcohol, and Recreational Drugs

Developmentally, adolescence is a period of experimentation. Many adolescents experiment with illegal substances or drugs. Despite national efforts, tobacco use continues to grow, especially among young females who smoke to control appetite and weight. An adolescent who smokes tobacco often has a lower energy intake and subsequently decreased nutrient intake.

Marijuana has the opposite effect on hunger. Many teens who smoke marijuana will experience "the munchies," a desire to snack and munch—usually on snacks high in calories but with low nutrient density. Smoking marijuana carries the same risks as smoking tobacco. In addition, marijuana sometimes is laced with other drugs, including LSD and amphetamines.

Adolescents who drink alcohol are at greater risk of harming themselves or others through violence and accidental injury.[15] In addition, teens who drink are replacing needed nutrients with empty alcohol calories. Finally, alcohol can interfere with the absorption and metabolism of necessary nutrients. (For more information about nutrition and alcohol, see the "Spotlight on Alcohol," especially the section "Alcoholics and Malnutrition.") Growing adolescents cannot afford to have nutrients replaced or poorly absorbed during growth.

Other drugs, such as cocaine, pose further risks. In using illegal drugs, the adolescent becomes preoccupied with both the acquisition and use of the drug; these activities take priority over food intake or selection. Teens who use drugs are usually underweight and report poor appetites.

Key Concepts: *Adolescence can be an uncomfortable time for the teen who is concerned with body image, body changes, or athletic activities. Although many teens blame certain foods for their acne, research has not found a correlation between acne and diet. Many adolescents are preoccupied with their weight, appearance, and eating habits. Adolescent obesity is on the rise, and eating disorders frequently begin during adolescence. Use of tobacco, alcohol, or recreational drugs can influence nutrient intake and interfere with good nutrition.*

Quick Bites

The Dangers of Teenage Smoking

The Centers for Disease Control and Prevention estimate that one-third of high-school students smoke regularly. They predict that one-third of the 3 million teenage smokers in the United States will die of smoking-related diseases. New research shows that the earlier a person begins to smoke, the greater the damage.

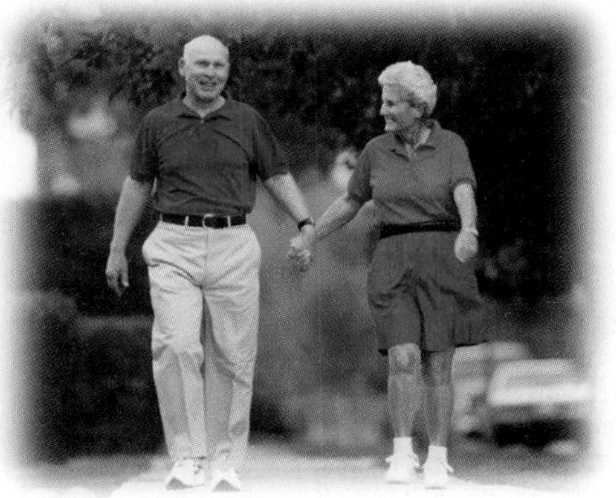

Staying Young while Growing Older

Just when does old age begin? The answer is increasingly elusive, as more people remain healthy and active well into their seventies, eighties, and even nineties. Today, older people represent the fastest-growing segment of the U.S. population, and the size of the older population (age 65 or older) is projected to double between 2000 and 2030. (See **Figure 13.7**.) It is estimated that by 2030, nearly one in four Americans will be older than 65. The population aged 85 and older is growing the fastest. In fact, the number of persons aged 100 or older is expected to increase nearly sixfold from 2000 to 2030.[16]

Age-related changes in body composition, sensory abilities, organ systems, and immune func-

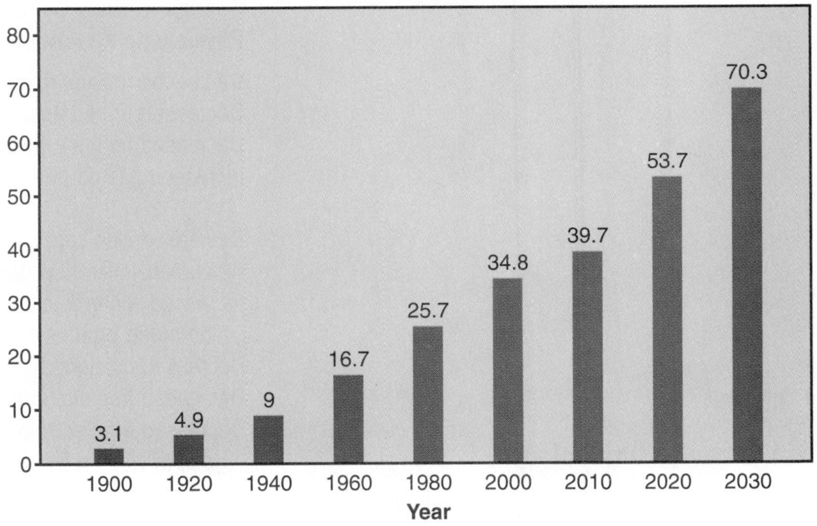

Figure 13.7 **The aging U.S. population.** The number of people over age 65 is growing rapidly.

Source: Department of Health and Human Services. A profile of older Americans 2000. http://www.aoa.gov/aoa/stats/profile/default.htm. Accessed 5/11/02.

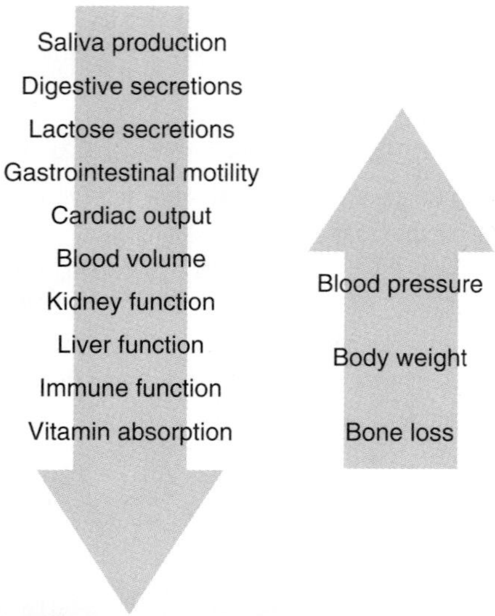

Figure 13.8 **Age-related physiological changes.** As we age, most physiological changes emerge gradually.

tion are normal. (See **Figure 13.8**.) We age at different rates, and many age-related declines will have little impact on our day-to-day lives. Other changes affect our nutrient needs and nutrient status (**Table 13.6**), so it becomes especially important to eat nutrient-dense food.

As we get older, many of us fear loss of mental function even more than loss of physical function. Yet, as the years advance, most people maintain cognitive function with only subtle changes. In most cases, slight changes involving sensory acuity, secondary memory, and information-processing speed do not affect quality of life or lead to progressive or rapid declines in mental function. On the other hand, when depression or dementia is suspected, professional evaluation becomes necessary. Overmedication or drug interactions, rather than disease, may be responsible for the changes in behavior.

Although it is not possible to stop the aging process, we can control aspects of our lifestyle that contribute to a healthier old age. Many of our choices—food, exercise, smoking, and alcohol—affect not only our risk for chronic disease (see **Figure 13.9**), but also the rate at which we age.

Weight and Body Composition

People who are overweight when they enter their later years or who gain weight after age 50 have a significantly increased risk of cardiovascular disease.[17] In addition, being overweight often is associated with diabetes, high blood pressure, and some types of cancer.

On the other hand, people who enter their mature years on the lean side—and who remain lean due to a healthy, active lifestyle—increase their chances of enjoying a healthy old age. But thinness alone is not always a health advantage. Obviously, older adults who lose weight due to illness enjoy no health benefits from losing these pounds. Weight loss puts them

Think About It 3

Quick Bites

Animal Lifetimes

In general, larger animals live longer than smaller animals, but there are many interesting exceptions. For instance, a mouse, a parakeet, and a bat are approximately the same size, but the mouse has a life span of 2 years, the parakeet 13 years, and the bat up to 50 years!

Quick Bites

Longevity Champions

In the United States, women live an average of seven years longer than men do.

Table 13.6 **Age-Related Changes and Nutrient Needs**

Change in Body Composition or Physiologic Function	Impact on Nutrient Requirement
Decreased muscle mass	Decreased need for energy
Decreased bone density	Increased need for calcium, vitamin D
Decreased immune function	Increased need for vitamin B_6, vitamin E, zinc
Increased gastric pH	Increased need for vitamin B_{12}, folic acid, calcium, iron, zinc
Decreased skin capacity for cholecalciferol synthesis	Increased need for vitamin D
Increased wintertime parathyroid hormone production	Increased need for vitamin D
Decreased calcium bioavailability	Increased need for calcium, vitamin D
Decreased hepatic uptake of retinol	Decreased need for vitamin A
Decreased efficiency in metabolic use of vitamin B_6	Increased need for vitamin B_6
Increased oxidative stress status	Increased need for beta-carotene, vitamin C, vitamin E
Increased levels of homocysteine	Increased need for folate, vitamin B_6, vitamin B_{12}

Source: Blumberg J. Nutritional needs of seniors. *J Am Coll Nutr.* 1997;16(6):517–523.

Chronic diseases	Dietary risk factors: High-fat diet	Excessive alcohol intake	Low complex carbohydrate/fiber	Low vitamin and/or mineral intake	High sugar intake	High intake of salty or pickled foods	Nondietary risk factors: Genetics	Age	Sedentary lifestyle	Smoking and tobacco use	Stress	Environmental contaminants
Cancers	?*	X	X	X		X	X	X	X	X		X
Hypertension	X	X		X		in salt sensitive people	X	X	X	X	X	
Diabetes (type 2)	X		X				X	X	X			
Osteoporosis		X		X			X	X	X	X		
Atherosclerosis	X		X	X			X	X	X	X	X	
Obesity	X	X	X		X		X		X			
Stroke	X		X				X	X	X	X	X	
Diverticulosis	X		X	X				X	X			
Dental and oral diseases				X	X		X			X		

* The Nurses' Health Study, a large prospective study, found no evidence linking higher total fat intake with increased risk of breast cancer. These results call into question theories that link dietary fat to other cancers.

Figure 13.9 **Risk factors for disease.** Diet, lifestyle choices, and genetics interact to shape a person's risk profile.

at increased risk for further illness, including cardiovascular disease and osteoporosis—especially if the original illness also limits activity. And, of course, leanness due to tobacco use or alcoholism increases a person's vulnerability to a decline in health.

Mobility

Muscle mass and strength decline naturally with age. Indeed, physiological functions that affect our mobility begin to decline at the rate of about 1 percent or more per year from about age 30.[18] Because of bad habits, bone loss, and a decrease in muscle tone, our posture begins to deteriorate in our fifties. This can affect lung and cardiovascular function, mobility, and balance. Diseases such as stroke, arthritis, and diabetes become more common and may cause severe physical disability. Medications and nutritional deficiencies may lead to impaired motor function.

Fortunately, exercise can offset much of this decline.[19] Canada, for example, addresses this issue in its *Physical Activity Guide for Older Adults*. (See **Figure 13.10** and Appendix C.) In fact, the benefits of physical activity and strength training may be most profound for those who are aging. Increased self-confidence, better balance and mobility, fewer falls and fractures,

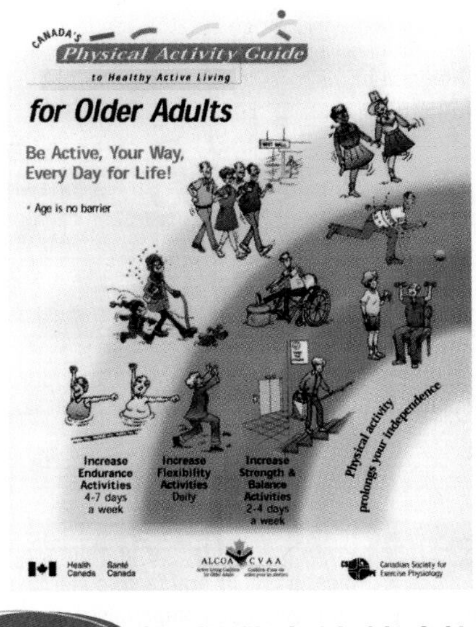

Figure 13.10 ***Canada's Physical Activity Guide for Older Adults.*** The guide explains why physical activity is important, offers tips for increasing physical activity, and recommends levels of activity necessary to good health and improved quality of living. See Appendix C for the complete guide.
Source: *Canada's Physical Activity Guide for Older Adults.* Reproduced with permission from Health Canada. ©Minister of Public Works and Government Services Canada, 2002.

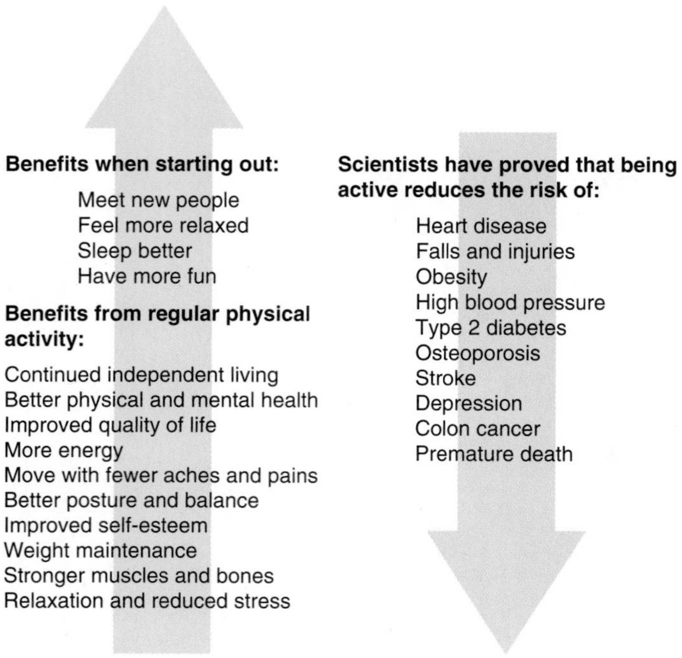

Figure 13.11 **Benefits from increased physical activity.** Physical activity helps adults maintain their health and independence as they age.
Source: *Canada's Physical Activity Guide for Older Adults.* Reproduced with permission from Health Canada. ©Minister of Public Works and Government Services Canada, 2002.

enhanced mental acuity, and improved appetite and nutrient intake are but a few of the physical and psychological benefits of exercise during our older years. (See **Figure 13.11.**)

Immunity

In the fifth decade of life, the body's defense mechanisms begin to weaken. The immune system loses some of its ability to fight viruses, bacteria, and other foreign bodies. Elders are more vulnerable to upper-respiratory infections such as influenza and pneumonia, urinary tract infections, pressure sores, and foodborne illnesses. Physical barriers to infectious agents, foreign bodies, and chemicals weaken as well. These barriers include the skin, the acid environment in the stomach, and swallowing and coughing reflexes.

Inadequate consumption of protein can compromise immunity and health in elders. Because of poor appetite, difficulty chewing, financial constraints, concerns about fat intake, or lactose intolerance, older people may reduce their intake of meat and dairy products, making it difficult for them to get all the calories, protein (see **Figure 13.12**), and other essential nutrients they need. Lack of protein and many of the vitamins and minerals commonly associated with animal foods (i.e., vitamins B_6, B_{12}, and D, calcium, iron, and zinc) can lead to suppressed immunity, decreased muscle mass, slowed wound healing, and osteoporosis.[20]

Key Concepts: *Lifestyle choices, such as diet and exercise, affect how we age. Control of body weight can reduce our risk for many chronic diseases associated with aging. Adequate protein, vitamins, and minerals can protect our immune status. Regular exercise not only enhances our mobility, but also reduces disease risk and improves mental health.*

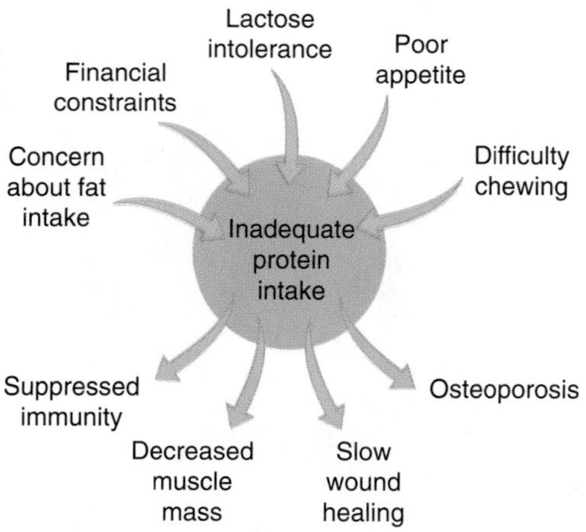

Figure 13.12 **Protein malnutrition in elders.** A combination of several factors can lead to inadequate protein intake that compromises immunity and health.

taste threshold The minimum amount of flavor that must be present for a taste to be detected.

Taste and Smell

In older adults, the **taste threshold**—the minimum amount of a flavor that must be present in order to detect the taste—is more than double that of college-aged adults. Sensitivity to sweet and salty tastes goes first, so older adults often increase their intake of foods high in sugar and sodium—increasing health problems that stem from overconsumption of these nutrients. Along with taste, our sense of smell also diminishes with age, especially in the seventh decade of life and beyond. Ideas that older people should be served bland foods are misguided. When food has stronger flavors and odors, both healthy and ill elders find it more palatable and eat more, thus increasing their nutrient intake.[21] (See **Figure 13.13.**)

Gastrointestinal Changes

Saliva production tends to decrease as we age, especially in people who take medications for conditions such as congestive heart failure. Lack of saliva affects the preparation of food for digestion and contributes to gum disease—a breach in one of the immune system's first lines of defense against infection.

With age, digestive secretions decline. Most significant are reductions in the stomach secretions of hydrochloric acid and pepsin. These reductions can allow the development of atrophic gastritis—a chronic inflammation of the stomach lining that is common among elders. Atrophic gastritis can affect protein digestion as well as interfere with normal absorption of iron, calcium, vitamin B_{12}, vitamin B_6, and folate.[22] Although reduced lactase production also is associated with aging, a complete intolerance to milk and dairy products is less common than older people often suspect. Most people with reduced lactase production can include some milk, cheese, and yogurt in their diets.

Constipation, gas, and bloating are common complaints of old age. These problems are due to a slowing of gastrointestinal motility with aging, along with decreased physical activity, a diet low in or lacking high-fiber fruits and vegetables, and low fluid intake. Feelings of fullness may cause older people to eat less. Reduced digestive secretions lower the amount of nutrients they absorb from the foods they do eat.

Myths and misinformation about GI effects of various foods, even among the medical community, may steer a person away from nutrient-dense foods such as dairy products, legumes, broccoli, cauliflower, tomatoes, and citrus products. While many elders mistakenly blame these foods for causing problems with gas, others may be sensitive to lactose in dairy products or may have had an adverse reaction to members of the cabbage family or "acid"-containing foods. GI distress also may be caused by factors totally unrelated to the food itself—inappropriate food preparation, lack of adequate fluid, and physical inactivity. Regardless of the cause, once people have an adverse reaction, they may associate it with a recently consumed food and become reluctant to try it again.

Key Concepts: *The perception of taste declines with age. To detect flavors, older people need food with stronger flavors and odors. This loss of taste may contribute to loss of appetite and poor food intake. Age-related changes in the GI tract reduce nutrient absorption. Decreased motility contributes to constipation.*

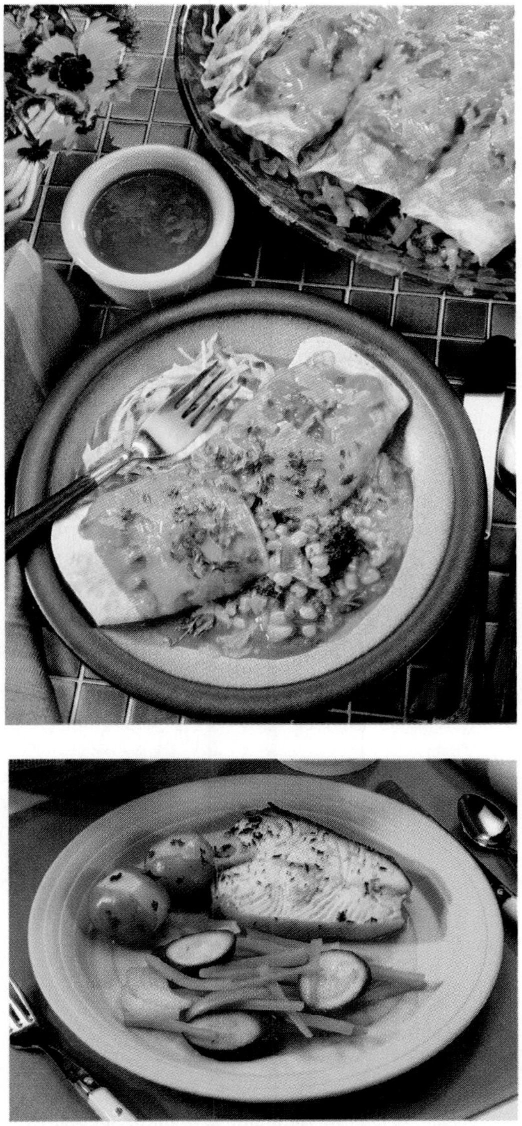

Figure 13.13 **Elders need stronger flavors.** More highly spiced meals rather than bland ones may encourage an elder to eat more.

Nutrient Needs of the Mature Adult

To live life to its fullest, you need good nutrition. A lifestyle that incorporates the *Dietary Guidelines for Americans*, together with regular physical activity, is essential to a long and productive life. **Figure 13.14** shows the Food Guide Pyramid modified for older adults.

Energy

Our energy requirements decline as we age, mainly because of reduced physical activity and loss of lean body mass. Physical activity can delay some of this loss, thus allowing us to eat more without gaining weight and increasing the likelihood that our diets will be adequate in essential nutrients.

The RDA for energy reflects the average requirement for people aged 51 and older. For men this value is 2,300 kilocalories per day, and for women the RDA is 1,900 kilocalories. Individual energy needs change based on activity, lean body mass, and the presence of disease; a person who is bed- or chair-ridden, for example, usually requires fewer calories than a mobile person.

Quick Bites

Losing Water

At birth, 75 percent of the body is composed of water. By the time a person reaches old age, that number has dwindled to 50 percent due to changes in body composition.

Protein

Protein needs (as grams per kilogram of body weight) do not change as we age, but may be somewhat harder for us to meet as our overall energy needs decrease and our tastes change. As our caloric needs decrease and our

Figure 13.14 Food Guide Pyramid for older adults. While not an official USDA pyramid, the Food Guide Pyramid for Older Adults reflects the nutrition needs of seniors. Its narrower profile reflects reduced energy needs, and the base recommends water to combat the chronic dehydration that is common in seniors.
Source: Adapted from Russell R, Rasmussen H, Lichtenstein A. Modified Food Guide Pyramid for people over 70 years of age. *J Nutr.* 1999;129:752.

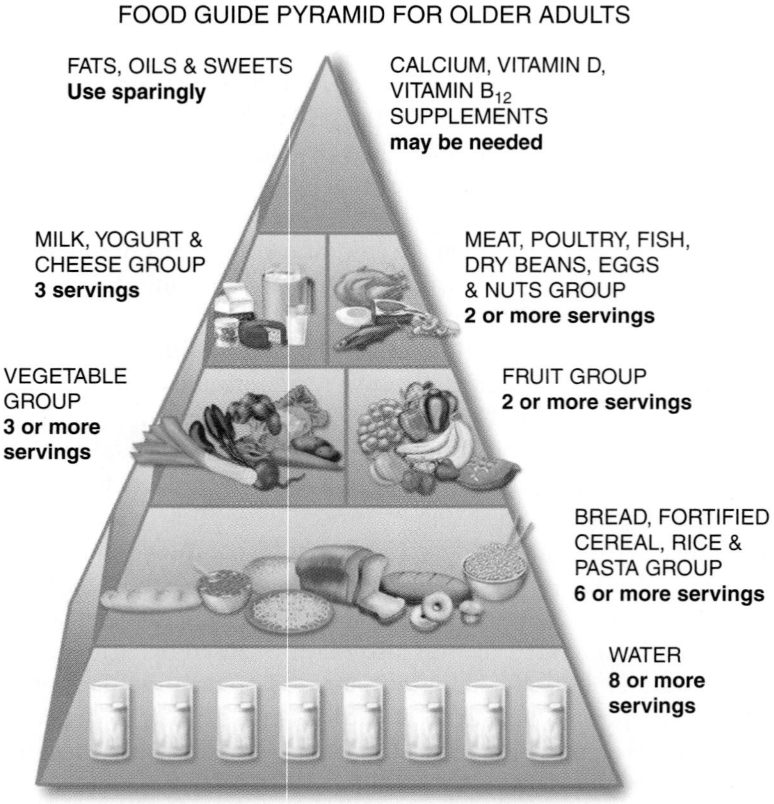

Quick Bites

Hardy Hearts

By the end of a normal life span, the human heart has pumped more than three billion times. Despite this heavy use, heart failures are usually caused by problems with blood vessels and valves; heart muscle itself rarely wears out.

protein needs remain constant, an adequate diet must contain relatively more protein. For healthy older people, the RDA for protein is 0.8 grams per kilogram of body weight, or on average 50 grams per day for women and 63 grams for men. Chronically ill individuals may need more protein to maintain nitrogen balance. Trauma, stress, and infection also may increase protein needs. However, there are risks associated with high protein intake, including dehydration, nitrogen overload, and adverse effects on the kidneys.

Carbohydrate

After infancy, carbohydrates should make up more than half of the calories in the diet. Because foods with primarily simple carbohydrates provide little nutrient value, the best choices are foods with complex carbohydrates.

Fiber, a complex carbohydrate, has many potential benefits, including preventing constipation and diverticulosis and possibly reducing the risk of colon cancer. (See Chapter 5, "Carbohydrates," for more information about fiber.) There are no specific fiber recommendations for elders; the typical recommendation for the general population is 20 to 35 grams per day. Fiber also can help to reduce blood cholesterol, making these recommendations especially important for those who are at risk for heart disease. Five or more servings of fruits and vegetables daily, accompanied by whole-grain breads or a serving of a cereal high in bran, will supply this amount easily. To avoid abdominal discomfort, increase dietary fiber intake gradually. When increasing dietary fiber intake, it is essential to consume adequate fluids—ideally water—to avoid dehydration and constipation.

Fat

Excess dietary fat can lead to obesity, which in turn increases the risk for diabetes, heart disease, and some types of cancer. Younger people should limit their dietary cholesterol and fat, but severe restrictions in elders may be counterproductive. (See the FYI feature "Are Dietary Recommendations to Lower Cholesterol Really Necessary for Elders?") Extreme fat phobia may contribute to nutritional deficiencies among older people who are afraid to drink milk, eat red meat, or even eat poultry or fish. Too few animal products in the diet may contribute to a lack of dietary protein; deficiency of minerals such as calcium, iron, and zinc; and poor vitamin B_{12} intake and absorption.

Healthy people who are at low risk for heart disease should obtain a maximum of 30 percent of their daily calories from fat, with no more than 8 to 10 percent of the calories from saturated fat. They should limit their cholesterol intake to 300 milligrams per day. People at increased risk for heart disease should limit saturated fat and cholesterol even more, according to their physicians' advice.

Water

Nutritionists often call water the forgotten nutrient. Water is essential to all body functions; and if intake is inadequate, cellular metabolism becomes difficult, if not impossible. In elders, a decreased thirst response and a

Quick Bites

Take Charge of Your Health

In June 2002, President George W. Bush announced *HealthierUS*, a new federal initiative to encourage healthier lifestyles. *HealthierUS* promotes four keys to a better and longer life:

- Be Physically Active Every Day
- Eat a Nutritious Diet
- Get Preventive Screening
- Make Healthy Choices

For more information on this new program, visit http://healthierus.gov.

Fyi FOR YOUR INFORMATION

Are Dietary Recommendations to Lower Cholesterol Really Necessary for Elders?

Coronary heart disease remains the number one cause of illness and death in the United States and Canada. While health care professionals continue to pay attention to cholesterol and fat intake in elders, some researchers speculate that overemphasizing restriction of these two dietary components may be unwarranted and, for some, unhealthful. People between the ages of 50 and 70 may benefit from blood lipid screening and intervention; however, those older than 70 may not.

Research has shown that there is little relationship between serum cholesterol values and coronary heart disease in those older than 70. Seniors who are overweight or who have coexisting chronic diseases such as diabetes may benefit more from controlling these conditions than from reducing cholesterol. Maintaining a healthful weight and controlling blood glucose may do more to bring cholesterol into line than a low-fat, low-cholesterol diet. Many older individuals are fat- and cholesterol-phobic, thanks to the media and popular press, and set themselves up for problems associated with osteoporosis and possibly protein-energy malnutrition.

Low blood cholesterol levels are associated with malnutrition, illness, and death, especially among frail elders. Adequate protein and calorie intake is necessary to prevent unintended weight loss. When older people restrict their intake of foods that are good sources of protein (e.g., meat, poultry, and dairy products) because they believe these foods are too high in fat, they risk depressing their immune system and causing irreversible, unintended weight loss.

For some, unintentional weight gain and associated health problems (e.g., increased triglycerides, blood glucose, and obesity) may arise from restricting fat in the diet. It is widely known that those who focus on fat-free and reduced-fat foods often increase their intake of carbohydrates, particularly sugar. These empty calories are of little use for those whose caloric needs are lower and nutrient needs higher.

Rather than focus on dietary restriction for those over the age of 70, it is more appropriate to focus on nutrients that are important for maintaining health and vitality; this, in turn, will reduce the risk of debilitation and disease. The proposed trend is away from diets that focus on reducing fat and cholesterol and toward those that include foods from all of the food groups in moderate amounts.

Sources: Heart disease in older adults: are dietary restrictions effective? Paper presented at: The American Dietetic Association 81st Annual Meeting and Exhibition; October 19, 1998; Kansas City, Missouri; and Position statement: liberalized diets for older adults in long-term care. *J Am Diet Assoc.* 1998;98:201.

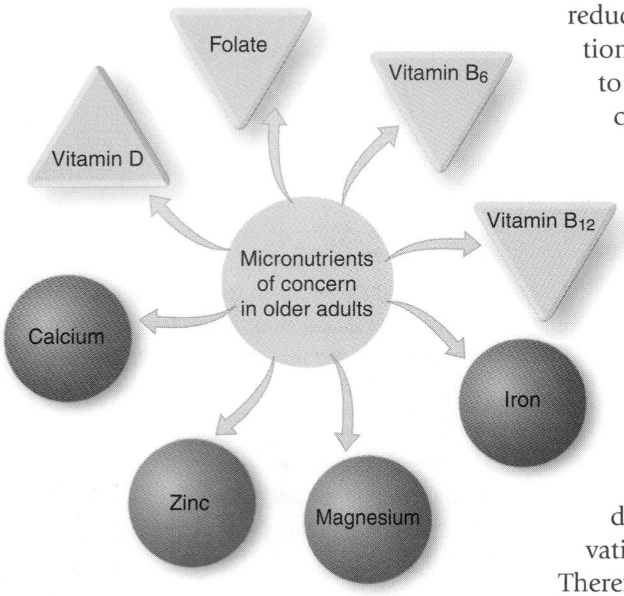

Figure 13.15 **Micronutrients of particular concern for older people.** As we age, our energy needs decline, but our vitamin and mineral needs remain stable. This makes nutrient-dense foods especially important for elders.

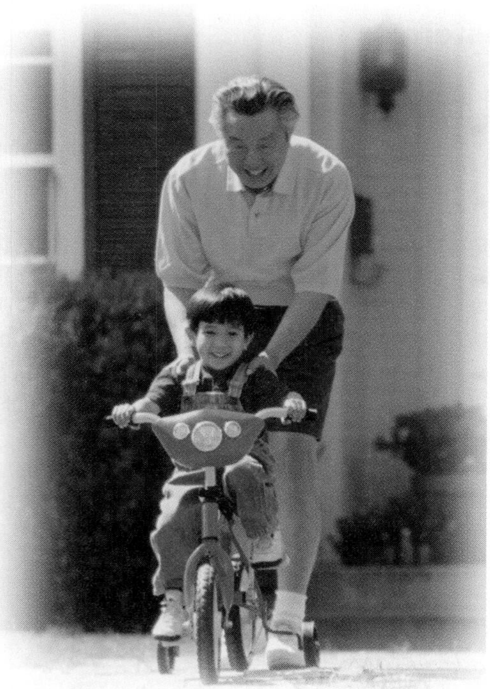

reduction in kidney function can lead to dehydration. Diuretic medications, alcohol, and caffeine all increase fluid excretion and can contribute to dehydration. Scientists estimate water needs at 1 milliliter per kilocalorie of food consumed.

Key Concepts: *Although caloric needs decline with loss of lean tissue and reduced physical activity, protein needs do not change for elders. A high-carbohydrate, moderate-fat diet is still recommended. Water is important, and because of their diminished thirst response, older people may not drink enough.*

Vitamins and Minerals

As we age, our micronutrient status changes, especially our needs for vitamin D, vitamin B_{12}, and calcium. (See **Figure 13.15**.) In many cases, our vitamin needs remain stable, while our energy needs decline. In other cases, age-related declines in absorption, use, or activation of nutrients lead to increased dietary vitamin and mineral needs. Therefore, it is especially important for elders to eat nutrient-dense foods. Adequate dietary calcium can reduce bone loss and risk of fractures. Although minerals such as zinc may be needed in larger amounts during late adulthood, conclusive evidence to support this view is lacking. The potential role of increased dietary magnesium in the reduction of high blood pressure, cardiovascular disease, and diabetes is a top research priority.

Vitamin D

Vitamin D promotes bone health; too little dietary vitamin D can lead to brittle and porous bones that are susceptible to fracture. Elders often have low vitamin D status. Not only are aging tissues less able to take up vitamin D from the blood, but aging skin also is less able to synthesize vitamin D when exposed to sunlight. In addition, many elders spend more time indoors and have reduced exposure to sunlight. When they go outside, many avoid the sun and use sunscreens—a good strategy for skin cancer prevention but one that reduces vitamin D synthesis. Elders with lactose intolerance often avoid dairy products, reducing their vitamin D intake and further compromising vitamin D status. The AI for vitamin D for adults aged 51 though 70 is 10 micrograms per day. For adults 70 and older, the AI is 15 micrograms per day. Younger adults only need 5 micrograms per day.

B Vitamins

The B vitamins deserve special consideration in adults and the aged. Extensive research links inadequate folate, vitamin B_6, and vitamin B_{12} to elevated levels of plasma homocysteine, which is associated with an increased risk for cardiovascular disease.[23] (See Chapter 9, "Vitamins.")

At least 15 percent of elders may have vitamin B_{12} deficiency.[24] Although most adults consume adequate amounts of dietary vitamin B_{12}, from 10 to 30 percent of elders lose their ability to absorb protein-bound vitamin B_{12} from foods. An intake of 2.4 micrograms per day of vitamin B_{12} is recommended for all adults older than 51 years. Because it is easier to absorb synthetic B_{12} than food-bound B_{12}, scientists suggest that adults older than 50 use fortified foods or B_{12}-containing supplements to meet their vitamin B_{12} requirements.

Key Concepts: *Vitamin D, folate, vitamin B_6, and vitamin B_{12} are key nutrients for elders. Vitamin D status can decline due to reduced intake, synthesis, and activa-*

tion. Poor folate, B_6, and B_{12} status may result in high homocysteine levels, a risk factor for heart disease. Vitamin B_{12} absorption declines with age; B_{12} is more easily absorbed from fortified foods and supplements, so these become important sources for elders.

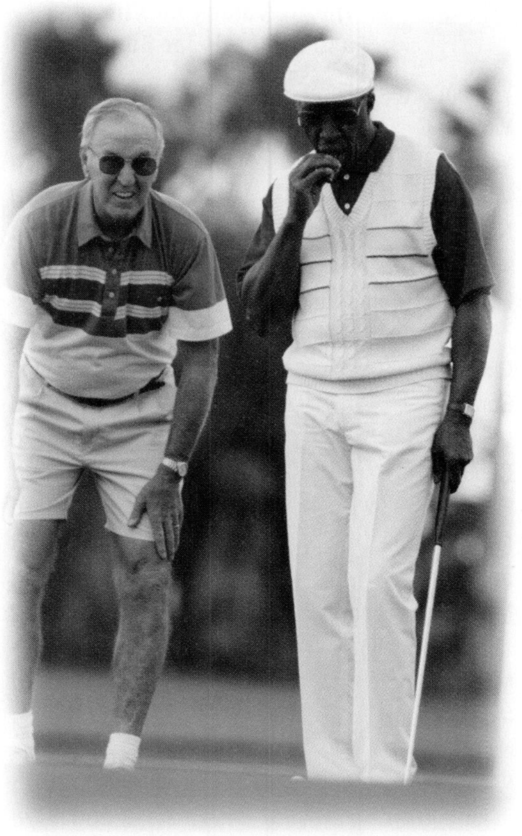

Calcium

Maintaining adequate calcium intake reduces the rate of age-related bone loss and the incidence of fractures, especially of the hip.[25] For all adults aged 51 and older, the AI for calcium is 1,200 milligrams per day, 200 milligrams per day higher than the AI for adults 31 to 50 years old.[26]

We are less able to absorb calcium as we age, partly because of a loss of vitamin D receptors in the gut. Stomach inflammation also reduces calcium absorption, as does an increase in the consumption of fiber—a practice that doctors recommend for its laxative effects. Because of real or perceived lactose intolerance, many older people have a low intake of dairy foods and therefore of calcium.

Zinc

Although clinical zinc deficiencies are uncommon, older adults frequently have marginal zinc intakes.[27] Stress, especially in hospitalized elders, appears to increase the risk of zinc deficiency and suppress immune function. Studies show that zinc supplementation hastens wound healing, but only in those who are zinc deficient. Because excess zinc may interfere with immune function and the absorption of other minerals and may work to lower HDL cholesterol, people of all ages should avoid excessive and continuous zinc supplementation.

Magnesium

Magnesium plays an essential role in many cellular reactions. Magnesium deficiency has been observed in people with malabsorption syndromes, those with malnutrition or alcoholism, and in elders. However, magnesium deficiency due to inadequate intake is rare.

Iron

Iron remains an important nutrient throughout the life cycle. Following menopause, the RDA for women drops to the same level as for men, 8 milligrams per day. Iron deficiency is a concern for elders who have limited intake of iron from the best sources—red meats, fish, and poultry. Reduced meat consumption may result from taste changes, economics, poor dentition, or a combination of factors.

To Supplement or Not to Supplement

Increased use of dietary supplements, including vitamins, minerals, and herbal and botanical products, is widespread. Although food is "the best medicine," some elders may feel they need a supplement in order to meet their nutrient needs. Food is more than the sum of its known nutrients, however, and replacing food with supplements may be a poor trade-off. In addition, some nutrients in large amounts can be toxic; they also can affect the absorption of other nutrients or interfere with the absorption and metabolism of prescription medications.

Excessive use of vitamin supplements by elders may result in **hypervitaminosis**. The need for vitamin A decreases with age, increasing the chances that supplementation may lead to liver dysfunction, bone and joint pain, headaches, and other problems. Also, taking large amounts of vitamin C

hypervitaminosis High levels of vitamins in the blood, usually a result of excess supplement intake.

Table 13.7 The UL Values for Vitamins and Minerals for Adults

Vitamin A (as retinol)	3,000 µg/d
Vitamin C	2,000 mg/d
Vitamin D	50 µg/d
Vitamin E	1,000 mg/d
Niacin	35 mg/d
Vitamin B_6	100 mg/d
Folic acid (from fortified foods and supplements only)	1,000 µg/d
Choline	3,500 mg/d
Boron	20 mg/d
Calcium	2,500 mg/d
Copper	10,000 µg/d
Fluoride	10 mg/d
Iodine	1,100 µg/d
Iron	45 mg/d
Magnesium (from nonfood sources only)	350 mg/d
Manganese	11 mg/d
Molybdenum	2,000 µg/d
Nickel	1 mg/d
Phosphorus	4,000 mg/d
for > 70 yr	3,000 mg/d
Selenium	400 µg/d
Vanadium	1.8 mg/d
Zinc	40 mg/d

can increase the likelihood of kidney stones and gastric bleeding. Because we know that many older people use vitamin supplements and that megadoses may have negative effects on health, it is important to inform elders of the ULs for micronutrients. The UL represents a level of intake from a combination of food and dietary supplements that should not be exceeded on a routine basis. (See **Table 13.7**.)

Key Concepts: *Important minerals for elders are calcium, zinc, magnesium, and iron. Calcium is important to reduce the risk for osteoporosis. Marginal zinc deficiency has been suspected in many elders and may be the result of reduced intake of red meats. Iron needs decline for women as they go through menopause. Excessive supplementation with certain vitamins or minerals can lead to health problems.*

Nutrition-Related Concerns of Mature Adults

Many factors can interfere with intake or use of nutrients by older adults. Therefore, caretakers, health-care practitioners, and seniors themselves must pay attention to nutritional status. To manage acute or chronic nutrition-related conditions, seniors may need to make specific dietary changes.

Drug–Drug and Drug–Nutrient Interactions

Drugs not only affect the way the body uses nutrients but also can alter the activities of other drugs. In turn, foods and nutrients can enhance or interfere with the effects of drugs. (See **Table 13.8**.) Some drugs interfere with appetite; others cause a dry mouth. Because many elders take several medications or are on long-term drug therapy, they may find themselves at increased nutritional risk.

People should view herbal supplements and vitamins or minerals in high doses as drugs, particularly when they take them in conjunction with prescription or over-the-counter medications. Although herbal products almost certainly interact with other medicines, such interactions are not well documented. In addition to the health and safety issues, many supplement therapies can be costly.

Depression

Many studies report high levels of well-being among elders, especially those who remain independent. Although depression is one of the most common psychological effects of aging, it is most common among institutionalized and low-income people. Researchers believe that depression is related to the loss of receptors for the neurotransmitter serotonin. Loss of these receptors also may cause cognitive difficulties.

In later life, life transitions and stressful events can become frequent companions that increase the likelihood and severity of depression. Among these stressors are the loss of loved ones, including spouse and friends; physical disability; perceived loss of physical attractiveness; inability to psychologically defend oneself from unpleasant events; inability to care for oneself, which forces one to depend upon caregivers and long-term care; social isolation; and, inevitably, the approach of death. In elders, depression often leads to malnutrition and may manifest itself as either anorexia (loss of appetite) or obesity. Anorectic elders lose weight and muscle mass, putting them at risk for chronic conditions such as osteoporosis.

Alcoholism is prevalent among socially isolated or depressed elders. People who consume excessive amounts of alcohol often have diets low in

Table 13.8 **Examples of Food–Drug Interactions**

Drug	Food That Interacts	Effect of the Food	What to Do
Analgesic			
Acetaminophen (Tylenol)	Alcohol	Increases risk for liver toxicity	Avoid alcohol.
Antibiotic			
Tetracyclines	Dairy products; iron supplements	Decreases drug absorption	Do not take with milk. Take 1 hr before or 2 hr after food or milk.
Amoxicillin, penicillin	Food	Decreases drug absorption	Take 1 hr before or 2 hr after meals.
Azithromycin (Zithromax), erythromycin	Food	Decreases drug absorption	Take 1 hr before or 2 hr after meals.
Nitrofurantoin (Macrobid)	Food	Decreases GI distress, slows drug absorption	Take with food or milk.
Anticoagulant			
Warfarin (Coumadin)	Foods rich in vitamin K	Decreases drug effectiveness	Limit foods high in vitamin K: liver, broccoli, spinach, kale, cauliflower, and Brussels sprouts.
Antifungal			
Griseofulvin (Fulvicin)	High-fat meal	Increases drug absorption	Take with high-fat meal.
Antihistamine			
Diphenhydramine (Benadryl), chlorphenira-mine (Chlor-Trimeton)	Alcohol	Increases drowsiness	Avoid alcohol.
Antihypertensive			
Felodipine (Plendil), nifedipine	Grapefruit juice	Increases drug absorption	Consult physician or pharmacist before changing diet.
Anti-inflammatory			
Naproxen (Aleve)	Food or milk	Decreases GI irritation	Take with food or milk.
Ibuprofen (Motrin)	Alcohol	Increases risk for liver damage or stomach bleeding	Avoid alcohol.
Diuretic			
Spironolactone (Aldactone)	Food	Decreases GI irritation	Take with food.
Psychotherapeutic (MAO inhibitors)			
Tranylcypromine (Parnate)	Foods high in tyramine: aged cheeses, Chianti wine, pickled herring, brewer's yeast, fava beans	Risk for hypertensive crisis	Avoid foods high in tyramine.

Note: Grapefruit juice contains a compound not found in other citrus juices. This compound increases the absorption of some drugs and can enhance their effects. Talk with your pharmacist or doctor to see if your medicine is affected by grapefruit juice before changing your routine.

Source: Bobroff LB, Lentz A, Turner RE. *Food/Drug and Drug/Nutrient Interactions: What You Should Know about Your Medications.* Gainesville, FL: University of Florida; March 1999. Publication FCS 8092 in a series of the Department of Family, Youth and Community Sciences, Florida Cooperative Extension Service, Institute of Food and Agricultural Sciences.

essential nutrients. Over time, excessive alcohol use can cause chronic liver disease, pancreatitis, secondary vitamin and mineral deficiencies, and protein-energy malnutrition.

Quick Bites

Who Discovered Atherosclerosis?

Leonardo Da Vinci offered the first detailed analysis of diseased blood vessels and was also the first to attribute this pathology to diet.

Anorexia of Aging

Poor food intake can lead to **anorexia of aging**. When older people become ill, anorexia puts them at high risk for developing protein-energy malnutrition.[28] Protein-energy malnutrition, in turn, can contribute to numerous problems, including immune deficiencies, anemia, falls, and cognitive deficits.[29]

anorexia of aging Loss of appetite and wasting associated with old age.

It can be difficult to pinpoint treatment strategies for anorexia in older people. However, treating even one aspect of the problem can provide at least temporary improvement. Unfortunately, lifelong inappropriate food habits, social factors, living conditions, and fear of injury may interfere with a person's ability and desire to stay or become healthy.

Key Concepts: *Among the problems elders face are lack of appetite and the side effects and interactions of medications they use. Medicines have the potential to interact with food and nutrients in the diet, and a lack of knowledge of these possibilities increases the risk for harmful effects. Although many elders have high levels of well-being, depression is common among institutionalized and low-income seniors.*

Arthritis

Arthritis is a general term that describes more than 100 diseases that cause pain and swelling of joints and connective tissue. (See **Figure 13.16**.) Arthritis is a chronic, lifelong affliction that, at its worst, can make movement difficult or even impossible. Unfortunately, there is no proven cure for arthritis. At best, appropriate treatment programs reduce symptoms. In terms of nutrition, arthritis pain may impair appetite or make it hard to prepare meals, and some arthritis medications may interfere with nutrient absorption. These factors underscore the importance of a nutrient-dense diet for arthritis sufferers.

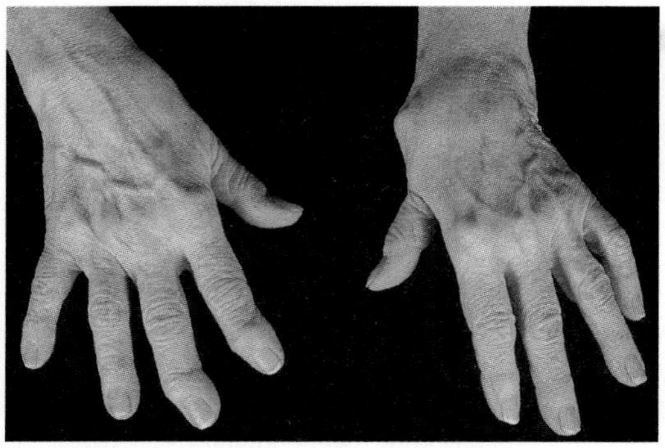

Figure 13.16 **Arthritis.** Degeneration of the finger joints can cause a debilitating lack of function.

Weight management is important in treating arthritis. Excess weight puts undue pressure on the hips and knees. Weight loss in overweight and obese individuals may reduce the risk of developing osteoarthritis, particularly of the knee.[30]

People who have rheumatoid arthritis may benefit from adding foods that are high in unsaturated fatty acids, particularly the *omega*-3 fatty acids in flaxseed and cold-water fish. There is some evidence that these fatty acids may have beneficial effects on the immune system of people with rheumatoid arthritis, thus helping reduce discomfort.[31]

Among the many kinds of arthritis, gout stands out because of the intensity of its pain. The classic attack occurs in someone who goes to bed feeling well and then awakens in the middle of the night with excruciating pain that has been likened to having someone walk on your eyeballs. This often leads to a visit to the emergency room.

Gout is directly linked to an excess of uric acid in the blood. Uric acid, a natural breakdown product of purines (organic compounds) found in all foods and body tissues, is normally dissolved in blood. But excess uric acid can accumulate as microscopic crystals in hand or foot joints, where it leads to painful inflammation, or gouty arthritis. Age-related degenerative osteoarthritis, particularly in the big toe, also enhances the risk of gout.

Certain medications, alcohol, overeating, and an unusual increase in exercise can trigger an attack of gout, but often it strikes without warning. After the attack passes, medications can help control uric acid levels. To reduce the risk of future attacks, overweight people should gradually lose weight, cut down on alcohol, and reduce their consumption of foods high in purines, such as organ meats, red meat, shellfish, and beans.

Bowel and Bladder Regulation

As a result of physiological and lifestyle changes, older people are susceptible to problems with their bowels and bladder. Hospitalized or institutionalized elderly patients who require catheters to urinate run an increased risk of **urinary tract infection (UTI)**, both during and after the procedure.

Inadequate hydration not only affects the bladder but also makes constipation more likely. Age-related decreases in intestinal motility and transit time, accompanied by poor food intake, may exacerbate the problem. In addition, lack of physical activity contributes to loss of muscle tone needed for elimination.

Chronic constipation is one of the most common health complaints among elders. If they do not have at least one bowel movement per day, many elders wrongly consider themselves constipated and quickly self-prescribe laxatives. However, excessive use of laxatives may cause nutritional deficiencies by decreasing transit time and preventing adequate absorption of nutrients. Decreased transit time also reduces water reabsorption by the GI tract and contributes to dehydration.

Increasing dietary fiber and fluid is one of the most effective treatments for bowel and bladder problems. Elders should gradually switch to—and then maintain—a high-fiber diet. They also should be careful to maintain adequate fluid intake.

urinary tract infection (UTI) An infection of one or more of the structures in the urinary tract; usually caused by bacteria.

macular degeneration Progressive deterioration of the macula, an area in the center of the retina, that eventually leads to loss of central vision.

Key Concepts: *Arthritis and changes in bowel and bladder habits are common problems in elders. Weight management is an important component of arthritis treatment. Because of an increased risk of dehydration and constipation, elders should be encouraged to follow a high-fiber diet and consume plenty of fluids.*

Dental Health

The mouth is the gateway to the rest of the gastrointestinal system. Poor oral health impairs the ability to eat and obtain adequate nutrition.[32] Missing teeth or poorly fitting dentures make some elders self-conscious about eating, which leaves them unable to eat comfortably in public. Mouth pain and difficulty swallowing interfere with the process of eating, and tooth loss can alter choices and quality of food. Oral infections affect the whole body and may increase the risk of other chronic diseases, including heart disease.

Quick Bites

Why Elephants Don't Need Dentures

Elephants are the only mammals with a built-in tooth replacement system. As they age, elephants go through six sets of teeth, changing about every 10 years. When elephants are around 70 years old, about the maximum life span, the last set of molars wears out.

Vision Problems

Poor vision and blindness interfere with the ability to buy and prepare food; visually impaired people cannot read food labels, cookbooks, or the settings on stoves or microwave ovens. **Macular degeneration** is a common disease of the eye that gradually leads to loss of vision. It affects about 6

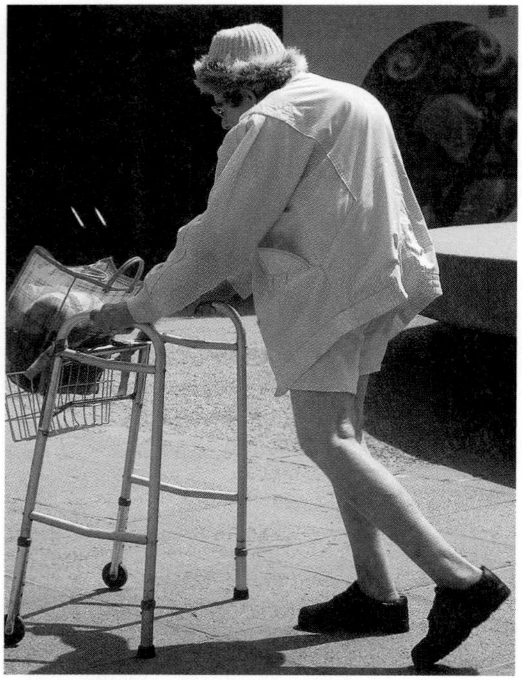

Figure 13.17 A hunched back due to collapsed vertebrae is a visible symptom of osteoporosis.

Alzheimer disease A presenile dementia characterized by accumulation of plaques in certain regions of the brain and degeneration of a certain class of neurons.

Quick Bites

Meno-What?

Most animal species do not go through menopause.

percent of people between the ages of 65 and 74, and about 20 percent of those aged 75 to 85. Research has found that people with a higher intake of green leafy vegetables are less likely to develop this sight-robbing disorder. Foods that contain antioxidants, including carotenoids but not vitamin E, are most strongly associated with a reduced risk. Greens, such as collards and spinach, show the most promise when consumed five or more times a week. By preventing free radical damage, antioxidants in these foods may protect the eye and the blood vessels that supply it. Retinol supplements do not appear to decrease risk of age-related macular degeneration, and vitamin C from foods had only a marginally beneficial effect on development of the disease.[33]

Osteoporosis

Although osteoporosis affects older adults of both genders, it is most common in postmenopausal women. Osteoporosis is the deterioration of bone structure (**Figure 13.17**) until, often without warning, the fragile bone breaks upon the slightest impact.

Nutritional factors, particularly early in life, are thought to play an important role in the development of osteoporosis. While regular weight-bearing exercise helps prevent osteoporosis, inactivity increases osteoporosis risk. Long periods of inactivity, such as may be imposed by complete bed rest or illnesses that limit mobility, can promote the disease. (See Chapter 10, "Water and Minerals," for more on osteoporosis, including risk factors.)

Although prevention is the best treatment for osteoporosis, many people enter later life with bad habits—poor nutrition and physical inactivity—that put them at risk. Adopting a diet that is rich in calcium and vitamin D and engaging in regular physical activity, particularly weight-bearing exercises, minimizes osteoporosis risks.

Alzheimer Disease

Among its other ravages, **Alzheimer disease (AD)** eventually destroys the ability to obtain, prepare, and consume an optimal diet. While genetic factors can affect the risk for Alzheimer disease, other risk factors include age, head trauma, and possibly exposure to environmental toxins. Although much more research is needed to determine their effects, estrogen and a combination of nonsteroidal anti-inflammatory drugs and antioxidants may offer some protection from the disease.[34]

Most cases of Alzheimer disease begin after age 70, but it can strike genetically predisposed people at a younger age. During the first stage of the disease, the afflicted person can have difficulty recalling names, frequently lose possessions, and easily become lost. Sensory sensitivity, such as loss of the sense of smell, begins to change gradually and so may not be readily noticed.

As the disease progresses, the person becomes unable to complete simple tasks that require learned motor movement, such as using a can opener. There is an increase in behavior problems, including wandering, aggression, and sleep disorders. These behaviors, if they occur frequently, can affect the person's ability to maintain weight and nutritional status.

The late stages of the disease are marked by inability to communicate, and about one-third of those with AD develop overactivity that drains the nutritional reserve and increases calorie needs. Eventually, people with AD become unable to walk and are restricted to a chair or bed. At this time, the caregiver must carefully plan the person's diet to meet psychological and physical needs, with particular attention to optimum nutrition without excess weight gain.

Key Concepts: *Oral health, vision, and bone health all decline with aging. Tooth loss and oral pain can reduce food intake and nutrient quality. Loss of vision can make food shopping and preparation difficult. Osteoporosis, most common in post-menopausal women, can cause debilitating fractures. Alzheimer disease eventually destroys the ability to obtain, prepare, and consume an optimal diet. Management of these conditions depends first on their identification by health care professionals.*

Meal Management for Mature Adults

Many elders are at nutritional risk because of economics, social isolation, physical restrictions, inability to shop for or prepare food, and medical conditions. Fortunately, there are a number of ways that older people can remain independent and have access to an adequate diet.

Meals on Wheels A voluntary, not-for-profit organization established to provide nutritious meals to homebound people (regardless of age) so they may maintain their independence and quality of life.

Elderly Nutrition Program (ENP) A federally funded program that provides older persons with nutritionally sound meals through meals-on-wheels programs or in senior citizen centers and similar congregate settings.

Food Stamp Program A USDA program that helps single people and families with little or no income to buy food.

Managing Independently

Independent and assisted-living programs allow people to live relatively carefree yet independent lives. Senior citizen apartment buildings and retirement villages offer a variety of services, including balanced meals. Programs like **Meals on Wheels** and the **Elderly Nutrition Program (ENP)** provide meals to homebound people, as well as those in congregate (group) settings. Most programs provide meals at least five times per week. The ENP is supported primarily with federal funds; volunteer time, in-kind donations, and participant contributions make up the remainder.

A recent evaluation of the ENP showed that program participants had higher nutrient intake levels than nonparticipants and had a higher level of regular social contacts—another important factor in eating well.[35] The **Food Stamp Program** is another option that provides low-income elderly households with the means to purchase food. Unfortunately, because Food Stamps carry a "welfare" stigma, some elders are reluctant to use them. In addition, many people who need some help buying food cannot meet the eligibility requirements.

Wise Eating for One or Two

Preparing meals that are healthful and tasty is a challenge for those living alone or in small households. As discussed earlier in this chapter, our nutrition needs—with the exception of calories—do not decrease as we age, but our ability to meet them does. Reliance on convenience foods, fast foods, and eating out can adversely affect the nutritional status of elders. Men who live alone are especially likely to eat out or skip meals rather than prepare foods for themselves. For both men and women, physical disability or illness can quash the desire to prepare and eat meals.

Think About It 4

Some simple changes in appliances and food-preparation techniques can help elders overcome common obstacles to food preparation. Those who can't or won't cook can use microwave or toaster ovens and small appliances to prepare simple meals. A meal based on a lower-sodium, low-fat convenience entree can meet nutritional needs if accompanied by vegetables, whole-grain bread, milk, and fruit.

Finding Community Resources

An older person's need for community support typically changes from decade to decade. Sometimes, identifying community resources can be challenging, and financial considerations may further limit access to resources that can assist older people in their own homes. Within local communities, area agencies on aging, social and rehabilitation services, cooperative extension services, churches, and extended-care facilities may have lists of resources and educational programs for elders. **Table 13.9** lists important resources for elders.

Key Concepts: *Older adults who obtain adequate food and nutrient intake while living independently may require assistance from time to time. This assistance may take the form of help with food shopping or preparation or identification of community resources that can stretch the food dollar. Because elders are at higher risk for foodborne illness due to weakened immune systems, food safety information is important. Numerous resources exist to assist elders in maintaining a productive, high-quality life.*

Table 13.9 Important Resources for Elders

Resource Directory for Older People

http://www.aoa.gov/directory/default.htm

The Resource Directory for Older People is a cooperative effort of the National Institute on Aging and the Administration on Aging. This directory provides resources for elders, their caregivers and family members, and those in the legal and health care professions. Available via the Internet, it provides telephone numbers (some toll-free), names, addresses, and fax numbers for organizations that work with older adults.

The Eldercare Locator

http://www.eldercare.gov
(800) 677-1116 (toll free)

The National Association of Area Agencies on Aging and the National Association of State Units on Aging administer the Eldercare Locator, a public service of the Administration on Aging, U.S. Department of Health and Human Services. The Eldercare Locator is a nationwide directory-assistance service that helps older persons and their families identify resources for aging Americans.

Label [to] Table

What is it about fruit snacks that attracts kids? The sweet flavors, bright colors, shapes, and logos of favorite movie or TV characters? Probably all of these. Parents may be attracted by claims for vitamins. So are these nutritious snacks or little more than candy? Let's have a look at the label.

On the positive side, this is a fat-free snack and contains little sodium. However, most of the calories, 56 of 80, come from sugar (14 g × 4 kcalories per gram), and the remainder from starch and protein. The ingredient list shows that the first three ingredients are sugars: corn syrup, sucrose, and fruit juice from concentrate.

The vitamins added to fruit snacks are the only redeeming feature of the product, providing 25% of the DV for vitamins A, C, and E. But is there a better way to get these nutrients? One-half cup of orange juice provides two-thirds of the DV for vitamin C and significant amounts of thiamin, folate, and potassium as well. Just a handful of baby carrots provides more than 100% DV for vitamin A, along with some fiber. Vitamin E is widespread in the food supply—a small amount of salad dressing as a dip for the carrots would add vitamin E.

So, the fruit snacks are not as devoid of nutrients as candy, but are not as nutrient-dense as fruits and vegetables. The fruit snacks may have some nutrient value, but they are high in sugar and, like all sugary snacks, should be used sparingly.

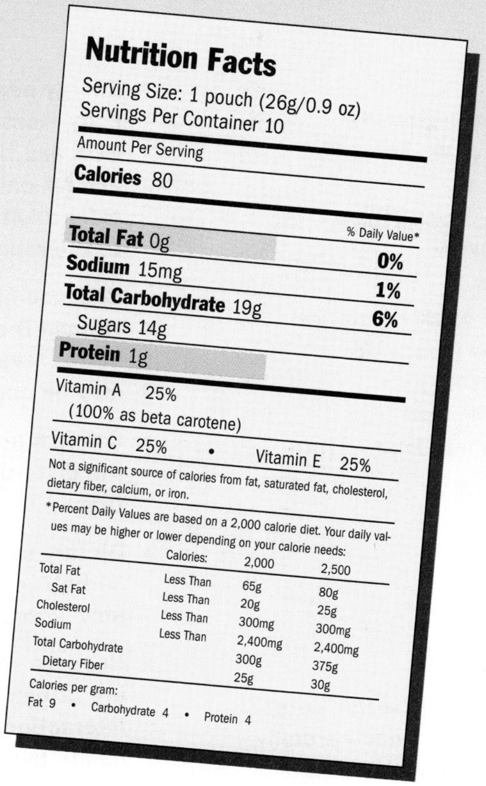

Nutrition Facts
Serving Size: 1 pouch (26g/0.9 oz)
Servings Per Container 10

Amount Per Serving
Calories 80

	% Daily Value*
Total Fat 0g	
Sodium 15mg	**0%**
Total Carbohydrate 19g	**1%**
Sugars 14g	**6%**
Protein 1g	

Vitamin A 25% (100% as beta carotene)
Vitamin C 25% • Vitamin E 25%

Not a significant source of calories from fat, saturated fat, cholesterol, dietary fiber, calcium, or iron.

*Percent Daily Values are based on a 2,000 calorie diet. Your daily values may be higher or lower depending on your calorie needs:

	Calories:	2,000	2,500
Total Fat	Less Than	65g	80g
Sat Fat	Less Than	20g	25g
Cholesterol	Less Than	300mg	300mg
Sodium	Less Than	2,400mg	2,400mg
Total Carbohydrate		300g	375g
Dietary Fiber		25g	30g

Calories per gram:
Fat 9 • Carbohydrate 4 • Protein 4

LEARNING Portfolio chapter 13

Key Terms

	page
acne	534
adolescence	524
Alzheimer disease	548
anorexia of aging	546
childhood	524
Elderly Nutrition Program (ENP)	549
epiphyses	531
food-insecure households	528
Food Stamp Program	549
hyperactivity	529
hypervitaminosis	543
macular degeneration	547
Meals on Wheels	549
menarche	531
National School Lunch Program	528
puberty	530
School Breakfast Program	528
Summer Food Service Program	528
taste threshold	538
urinary tract infection (UTI)	547

Study Points

- For children and adolescents, growth is the key determinant of nutrient needs. If diets are planned carefully, children do not need vitamin/mineral supplementation.
- Federally funded nutrition and feeding programs reduce malnutrition and hunger among American children.
- Adoption of adult-style diets to reduce risk of chronic disease should begin gradually after the age of 3.
- The prevalence of obesity and eating disorders is rising among American children and teens; treatment programs should address food choices and activity levels rather than impose strict calorie limits. Vegetarian diets for children need to be planned carefully to avoid nutrient deficiencies.
- Total energy and nutrient needs of adolescents are high in order to support growth and maturation. Girls need more iron than boys do to compensate for losses after the onset of menstruation. Active teens need more calories and nutrients than sedentary teens; fluid intake is also a priority.
- Nutrition and physical activity are two important, controllable components of a healthy life and healthful aging. Moreover, numerous physiological and psychological aspects of the aging process affect food intake and nutritional status.
- Energy needs decline with age, reflecting loss of lean body mass and reduced physical activity. The protein RDA and the recommended balance of carbohydrate and fat calories in the diet are similar for young and older adults. Fluid intake needs special attention due to the reduced thirst response that occurs with age.
- Because of reduced intake, synthesis, and activation, vitamin D status declines with age; recommended intake levels are therefore raised. Vitamin B_{12} status may be compromised due to inadequate absorption.
- Calcium and zinc intakes are likely to be marginal in the diets of elders. Magnesium and iron remain important.
- Dietary supplements, both vitamin/mineral and herbal/botanical, should be used with caution, preferably with professional advice.
- Because many elders take multiple medications, they are at risk for drug–nutrient, food–drug, and drug–drug interactions. Anorexia of aging is also a major public health problem.
- Arthritis is a prevalent chronic health problem in this age group. Weight management is a key element of arthritis treatment.
- Chronic constipation is a common complaint among older adults. Fluids, fiber, and regular exercise can reduce the likelihood of constipation.
- Both poor oral and visual health can compromise the ability of elders to consume a nutritionally adequate diet.
- Osteoporosis is a major health problem that can be addressed through adequate calcium, vitamin D, regular weight-bearing exercise, and medication if needed.
- Adults can maintain independence while aging but may require special assistance to obtain and prepare food. Community resources can help respond to the needs of elders and those of their caretakers and family.

Study Questions

Answers can be found at nutrition.jbpub.com/discovering.

1. **Which vitamins and minerals are most likely to be deficient in a child's diet?**
2. **Describe the hunger and malnutrition that occur in U.S. households. What federal programs help to address these problems?**
3. **Identify several chronic nutrition problems that can affect children. How can these problems be avoided?**
4. **What are typical nutritional concerns for adolescents?**
5. **What are some of the consequences of decreased immunity among elders?**
6. **How does the fact that most older people have less lean body mass affect their need for protein? Compared with a younger adult, does a person older than 65 need more, less, or about the same amount of protein?**
7. **Why are elders at risk of vitamin D deficiency?**
8. **Discuss minerals that may need special attention in assessment of an elder's nutrition status.**
9. **What problems might elders encounter with dietary supplements?**
10. **What is the role of physical activity in osteoporosis prevention? What nutritional factors are important?**
11. **List some of the meal/food programs that are available to assist older persons.**

[Try] This

Eat Like a Kid

Children, especially toddlers, tend to be exploratory, and take in the sensory nature of food—the textures, smells, and tastes. In fact, you were probably once this way. The purpose of this exercise is to eat a meal like a kid and gain an appreciation of food's textures and taste. Make some mashed potatoes, macaroni and cheese, buttered peas, or spaghetti (favorite "kid food") and eat it with your fingers. Explore your food and play with it. Try mixing foods. How does this experience make you feel?

Aging Simulation

The purpose of this exercise is to simulate what it can be like to age and experience age-related declines in health. Have you ever thought of how difficult it is to be an older person with health problems and do routine tasks? Invite a few friends over and do the following:

- Put gloves on to simulate the difficulty of losing sensitivity in your hands.
- Use cotton balls in your ears to decrease your hearing ability.
- Apply some petroleum jelly to a pair of glasses or sunglasses to give yourself poor vision.

Now try a simple activity. Make a salad or put a CD in your CD player and listen to it. After completing the activity, switch disabilities with your friends so that everyone has experienced each of the limitations. What is it like to do these everyday activities with your impairment?

What About *Bobbie?*

Let's pretend that Bobbie is in her sixties and just read a newspaper article about how older people may have low intakes of vitamins E and B_6, magnesium, calcium, and iron. How do you think her diet compares to the needs of a 65-year-old woman? You may want to review her one-day intake in Chapter 1. Although her calorie intake is probably much higher than that of most women in their sixties, let's look at her intake of these vitamins and minerals.

Bobbie met or exceeded her RDA or AI for each nutrient except vitamin E and calcium. Since Bobbie's fat intake was ample, this low value for vitamin E probably reflects a lack of complete data for the vitamin E content of foods. As is true of many women in their sixties who don't have an adequate intake of calcium, this increases Bobbie's risk of osteoporosis.

Vitamin E	
RDA	15 mg
Bobbie's intake	9 mg
Vitamin B_6	
RDA	1.5 mg
Bobbie's intake	1.9 mg
Magnesium	
RDA	320 mg
Bobbie's intake	330 mg
Calcium	
AI	1,200 mg
Bobbie's intake	745 mg
Zinc	
RDA	8 mg
Bobbie's intake	14 mg

References

1 Skinner JD, Carruth BR, Houck KS, et al. Longitudinal study of nutrient and food intakes of infants aged 2 to 24 months. *J Am Diet Assoc.* 1997;97:496–504.

2 Kleinman RE, ed. *Pediatric Nutrition Handbook.* 4th ed. Elk Grove, IL: American Academy of Pediatrics; 1998.

3 Kotz K, Story M. Food advertisements during children's Saturday morning television programming: are they consistent with dietary recommendations? *J Am Diet Assoc.* 1994;94: 1296–1300.

4 Coon KA, Goldberg J, Rogers BL, Tucker KL. Relationship between use of television during meals and children's food consumption patterns. *Pediatrics.* 2001;107:E7.

5 American Academy of Pediatrics, Committee on Community Health Services. Health needs of homeless children and families. *Pediatrics.* 1996;98:789–791.

6 Zuckerman B, Parker S. Preventive pediatrics: new models of providing needed health services [editorial]. *Pediatrics.* 1995;95:758–762.

7 Alaimo K, Olson CM, Frongillo EA Jr, Briefel RR. Food insufficiency, family income, and health in US preschool and school-aged children. *Am J Public Health.* 2001;91:781–786.

8 Andrews M, Nord M, Bickel G, Carlson S. *Household Food Security in the United States, 1999.* Washington, DC: US Department of Agriculture; 2000. Food Assistance and Nutrition Research Report No. 8 (FANRR-8).

9 Wolraich ML, Lindgren SD, Stumbo PJ, et al. Effects of diets high in sucrose or aspartame on the behavior and cognitive performance of children. *N Engl J Med.* 1994;330:301–307.

10 Gaull G, Giombetti T, Yeaton Woo R. Pediatric dietary lipid guidelines: a policy analysis. *J Am Coll Nutr.* 1995;14:411–418.

11 Zlotkin S, reviewer. Review of the Canadian nutritional recommendations update: dietary fat and children. *J Nutr.* 1996; 126(suppl):1022S–1027S.

12 Novak P. Nutrition counseling for the vegetarian child. *Pediatric Nutrition—A Building Block for Life.* 1991;14(4):5–9.

13 Lytle LA. Nutritional issues for adolescents. *J Am Diet Assoc.* 2002;102(3)(suppl):S8–S12.

14 Neumark-Sztainer D, Story M, French SA. Covariations of unhealthy weight loss behaviors and other high-risk behaviors among adolescents. *Arch Pediatr Adolesc Med.* 1996;150:304–308.

15 Wechsler H, Lee JE, Kuo M, Lee H. College binge drinking in the 1990s: a continuing problem. *J Am Coll Health.* 2000;48P: 199–210.

16 Federal Interagency Forum on Aging-Related Statistics. Older Americans 2000: key indicators of well-being. http://www.agingstats.gov/chartbook2000/population.html. Accessed 5/11/02.

17 Harris TB, Savage PJ, Grethe ST, et al. Carrying the burden of cardiovascular risk in old age: association of weight and weight change with prevalent cardiovascular disease, risk factors, and health statistics in the Cardiovascular Health Study. *Am J Clin Nutr.* 1997;66:837–844.

18 Worthington-Roberts BS, Williams SR. *Nutrition Throughout the Life Cycle.* 3rd ed. St. Louis: Mosby-Year Book; 1996.

19 Chin A, Paw MJ, DeJong N, et al. Physical exercise and/or enriched foods for functional improvement in frail, independently living elderly: a randomized controlled trial. *Arch Phys Med Rehabil.* 2001;82:811–817.

20 Lesourd BM. Nutrition and immunity in the elderly: modification of immune responses with nutritional treatments. *Am J Clin Nutr.* 1997;66(suppl):478S–484S.

21 Schiffman SS. Intensification of sensory properties of foods for the elderly. *J Nutr.* 2000;130(suppl):927S–930S; and Mathey MF, Siebelink E, de Graaf C, Van Staveren WA. Flavor enhancement of food improves dietary intake and nutritional status of elderly nursing home residents. *J Gerontol A Biol Sci Med Sci.* 2001;56:M200–M205.

22 Worthington-Roberts BS, Williams SR. Op. cit.

23 Blumberg J. Nutritional needs of seniors. *J Am Coll Nutr.* 1997;16:517–523; and Fairfield KM, Fletcher RH. Vitamins for chronic disease prevention in adults: scientific review. *JAMA.* 2002;287:3116–3126.

24 Stabler SP, Lindenbaum J, Allen RH. Vitamin B-12 deficiency in the elderly: current dilemmas. *Am J Clin Nutr.* 1997;66: 741–749.

25 Blumberg J. Op. cit.

26 Institute of Medicine, Food and Nutrition Board. *Dietary Reference Intakes for Calcium, Phosphorus, Magnesium, Vitamin D, and Fluoride.* Washington, DC: National Academy Press; 1997.

27 Blumberg J. Op. cit.

28 Morley JE. Anorexia, body composition, and ageing. *Curr Opin Clin Nutr Metab Care.* 2001;4:9–13.

29 Morley JE. Anorexia of aging: physiologic and pathologic. *Am J Clin Nutr.* 1997;66:760–773.

30 Arthritis Foundation. Osteoarthritis (OA). http://www.arthritis.org/conditions/DiseaseCenter/oa.asp. Accessed 5/11/02.

31 James MJ, Cleland LG. Dietary n-3 fatty acids and therapy for rheumatoid arthritis. *Semin Arthritis Rheum.* 1997;27:84–97.

32 Sheiham A, Steele JG, Marcenes W, et al. The relationship among dental status, nutrient intake, and nutritional status in older people. *J Dent Res.* 2001;80:408–413.

33 Pharmaceutical Information Associates Limited. Diets high in carotenoids may lower risk of macular degeneration. Reprinted from *Medical Science Bulletin*. February 1995. http://www.eyesight.org/Reports/Report-Carotenoids/report-carotenoids.html. Accessed 5/11/02.

34 Cyr M, Calon F, Morissette M, et al. Drugs with estrogen-like potency and brain activity: potential therapeutic application for the CNS. *Curr Pharm Des.* 2000;6:1287–1312; Prasad KN, Hovland AR, Cole WC, et al. Multiple antioxidants in the prevention and treatment of Alzheimer disease: analysis of biologic rationale. *Clin Neuropharmacol.* 2000;23:2–13; and Engelhart MJ, Geerlings MI, Ruitenberg A, et al. Dietary Intake of antioxidants and risk of Alzheimer disease. *JAMA.* 2002; 287:3223–3229.

35 Millen BE, Ohls JC, Ponza M, McCool AC. The Elderly Nutrition Program: an effective national framework for preventive nutrition interventions. *J Am Diet Assoc.* 2002;102: 234–240.

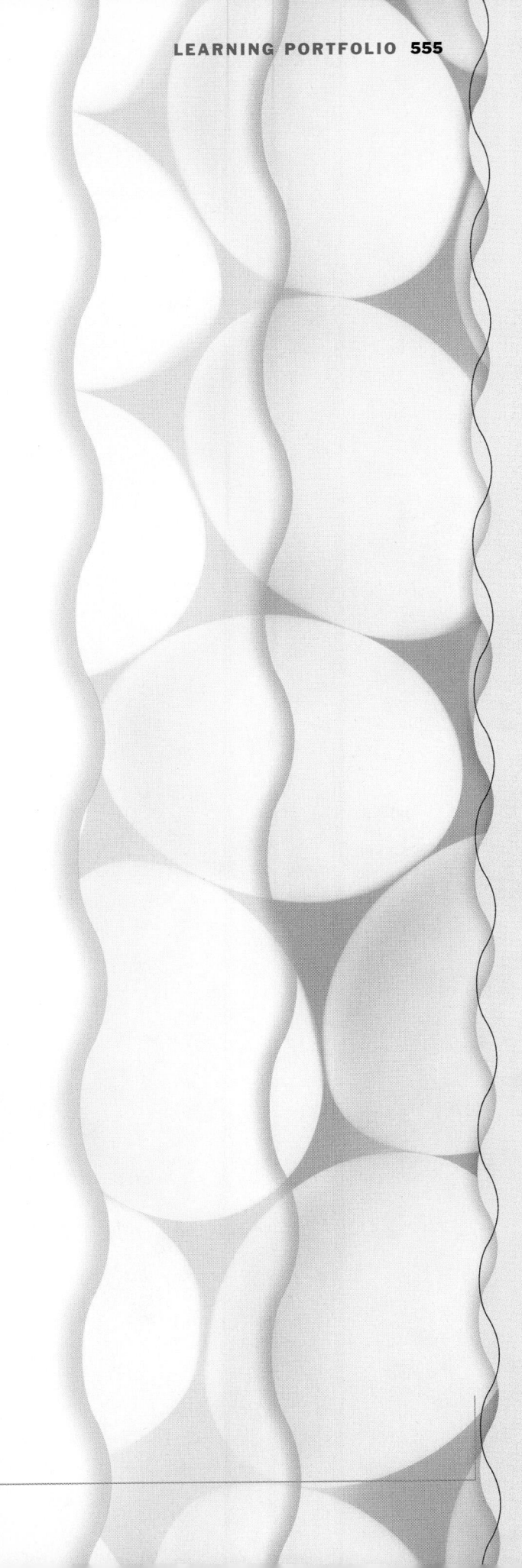

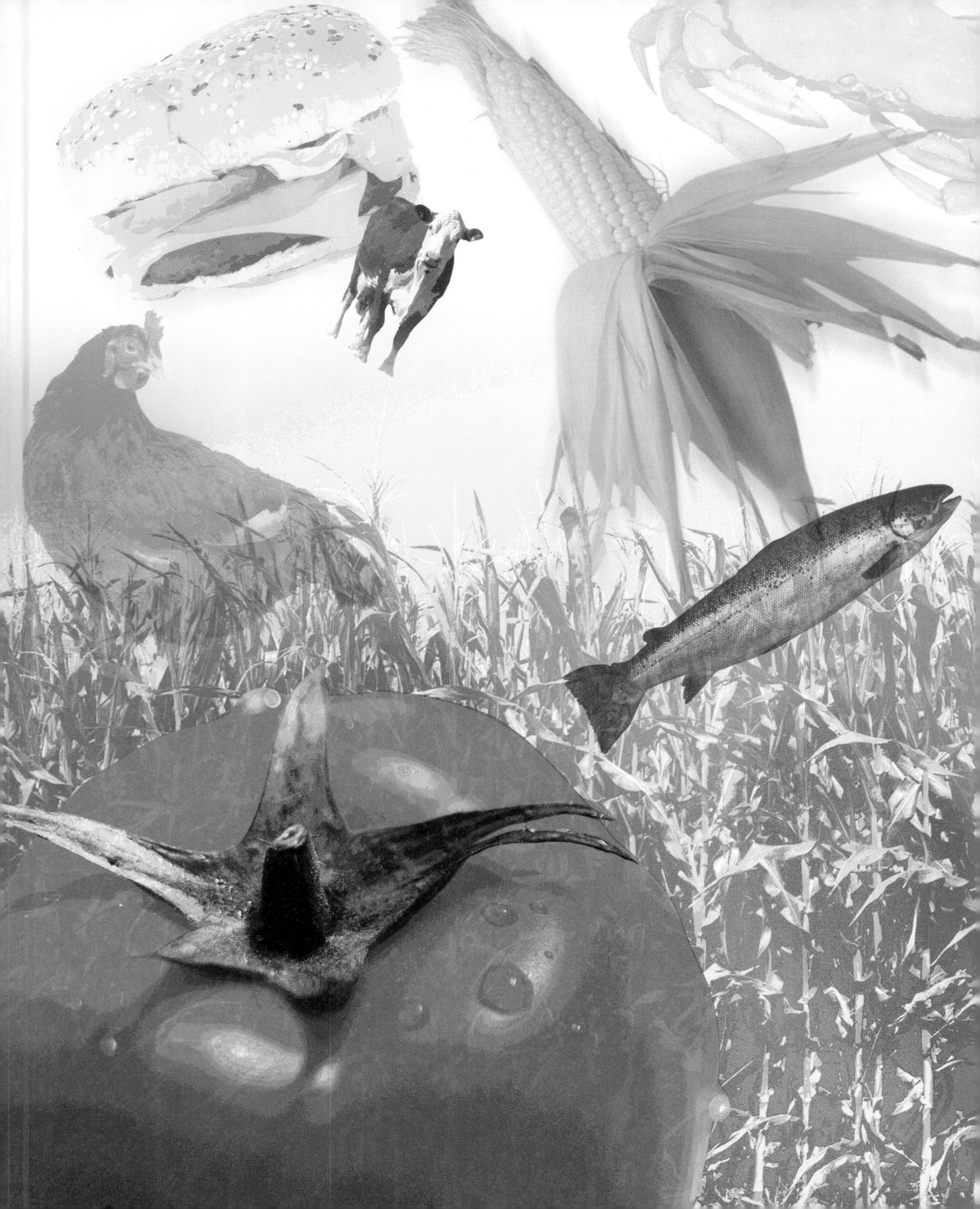

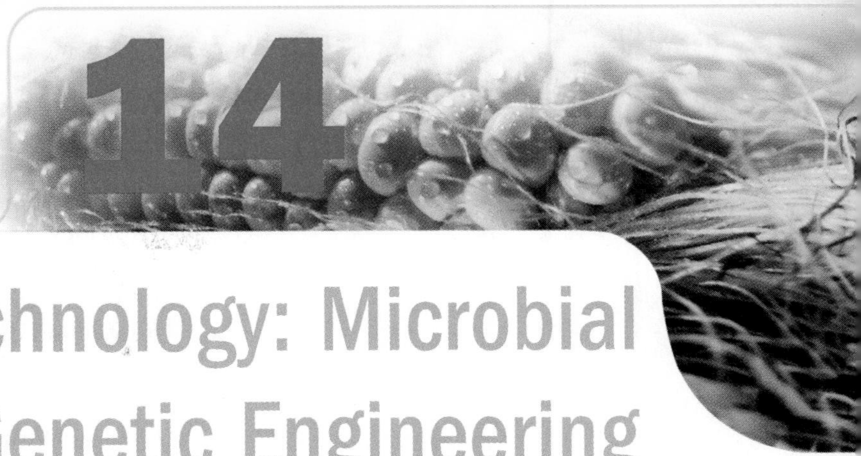

Chapter 14

Food Safety and Technology: Microbial Threats and Genetic Engineering

Think About It

1. Do you worry about getting sick from the food you eat?
2. To what extent do you rely on organically grown food to avoid pesticides?
3. What food safety measures, such as thawing meat in the refrigerator, do you practice at home?
4. Would genetically modified rice be welcome at your dinner table?

Fyi for your Information

This chapter's FYI boxes include practical information on the following topics:

- Safe Food Practices
- Seafood Safety
- At War with Bioterrorism

www

The Web site for this book offers many useful tools and is a great source for additional nutrition information for both students and instructors. For information on food safety and technology, visit the site at **nutrition.jbpub.com/discovering**. You'll find exercises that explore the following topics:

- The HACCP Approach to Food Safety
- Genetically Modified Food
- Irradiated Food
- What's Swimming with Your Seafood?

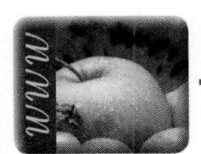

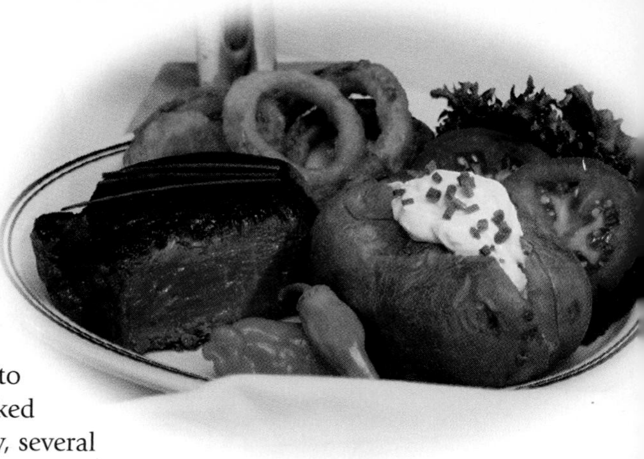

You pick up the newspaper and the headline screams, "POORLY COOKED HAMBURGER MEAT PROVES FATAL." You read further and discover that a child's death has been traced to thriving bacteria in undercooked hamburger meat. Additionally, several adults have become sick from the same source. This worries you. You hate well-done meat. You especially like your hamburgers blood red and your steaks rare. "Well," you ponder, "maybe I'll move my preferences up a notch to pink hamburgers and medium-rare steaks." Have you made the right choice? Or should you investigate this issue further?

Although it was once confined mainly to cookbooks and textbooks, today food safety advice shows up in many places—the popular press, the classroom, even the *Dietary Guidelines for Americans*. What has prompted such enthusiasm? Recent headlines tell part of the story. In the 1990s, microbial contamination of such foods as hamburger, apple juice, eggs, raw sprouts, and frozen berries seriously sickened thousands and killed many, especially those most susceptible: young children, people with compromised immune systems, and seniors.

Consumers are voicing their concerns about other food safety issues as well—including fears about excessive pesticide residues in plant foods, antibiotics and hormones in animals used for food, and hidden food allergens (e.g., nuts, milk, or eggs) in prepared foods. People often fail to recognize that a prepared food contains an ingredient they are allergic to (e.g., caseinates as milk protein); and sometimes an allergen may be an unintentional food additive (e.g., peanut material found in a milk chocolate candy might be residue left on machinery from earlier processing of peanut butter cups). Other less frequently discussed food hazards include physical contamination with glass fragments and other sharp objects, heavy metals, and naturally occurring toxins in seafood and some agricultural products. (See **Figure 14.1**.)

Quick Bites

A Morbid Margin Note

Every day 16,000 Americans get sick from something they ate. Twenty-five of them die.

Food Safety

This chapter reviews major food safety hazards and touches on controversial issues such as the merits of organic foods, the use of food irradiation, and the production of genetically modified foods.

Harmful Substances in Foods

Pathogens

In North America, most food safety experts agree that the chief cause of **foodborne illness** is pathogenic (disease-causing) microorganisms, including bacteria, viruses, and parasites. (See **Table 14.1** for a list of common foodborne microbes and the serious illnesses they cause.) Researchers at the Centers for Disease Control and Prevention (CDC) estimate that foodborne microbes cause 76 million illnesses, 325,000 hospitalizations, and 5,000 deaths in the United States each year.[1] These figures take into account the

Think About It 1

foodborne illness A sickness caused by food contaminated with microorganisms, chemicals, or other substances hazardous to human health.

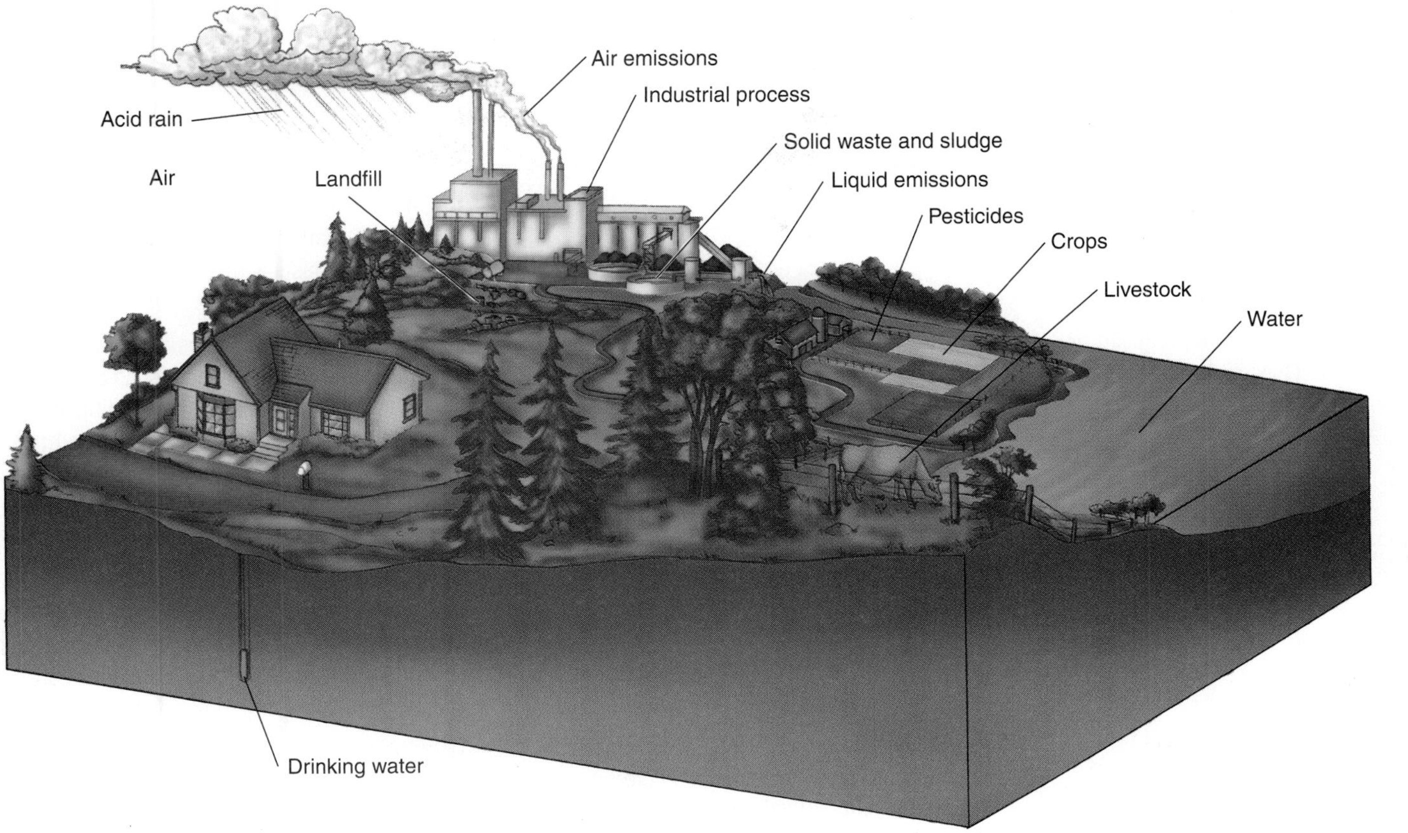

Figure 14.1 **Heavy metals and other contaminants can be found in foods.** Industrial plants and automobiles release heavy metals and other contaminants into the air. Rainfall carries these contaminants to the soil. Plants for food crops and animal feed absorb contaminants from the soil. Runoff can pick up contaminants from pesticides, fertilizers, and animal manure. This pollutes surface water (lakes and streams), groundwater, and coastal water. Polluted water contaminates seafood and other fish that people eat.

estimated number of unrecognized and unreported food-caused illnesses. The U.S. Department of Agriculture (USDA) estimates that the seven most common foodborne pathogens are responsible for $6.5 billion to $34.9 billion in medical costs and productivity losses each year.[2] Illnesses can range from relatively mild stomach upset to severe symptoms that can be fatal.

Development of foodborne illness results from the interaction of three factors: the pathogen, the host, and the environment in which they exist and interact.[3] Foodborne illnesses can result directly from infection with a pathogen or from toxins produced by a pathogenic microorganism. For example, the bacterium *Staphylococcus aureus* creates havoc with the gastrointestinal tract by producing a toxin. When food containing *S. aureus* stands unrefrigerated, the bacteria begin multiplying. After several hours the expanding bacterial population can produce enough of a nasty toxin to cause nausea, vomiting, and abdominal cramps. Staphylococcal food poisoning is extremely common, causing more than a million illnesses each year. Fortunately, the illness usually resolves after a day or so of vomiting and feeling miserable, with no further harmful effects. Another toxin-producing bacterium, *Clostridium botulinum*, causes the rare but deadly illness **botulism**. Improperly canned foods, as well as garlic in oil preparations, are sources of botulism. Honey can be contaminated with *botulinum*,

Quick Bites

Is It Stomach Flu or Food Poisoning?

Both can have similar symptoms—miserable vomiting, abdominal cramping, and diarrhea. Although we often do not know the exact cause, stomach flu tends to occur in the winter months and is preceded by other symptoms, such as sore throat. Food poisoning tends to occur in summer months, and symptoms usually appear suddenly without warning. Symptoms may not begin until 12 to 72 hours after eating tainted food. If many people who ate the same food get sick around the same time, it's probably food poisoning.

botulism An often fatal type of food poisoning caused by a toxin released from *Clostridium botulinum*, a bacterium that can grow in improperly canned low-acid foods.

Table 14.1 Common Foodborne Pathogens and Illnesses

Organism	Sources	Diseases and Symptoms
Bacteria		
Campylobacter jejuni	Raw poultry and meat and unpasteurized milk	Campylobacteriosis **Onset:** usually 2 to 5 days after eating **Symptoms:** diarrhea, stomach cramps, fever, bloody stools; lasts 7 to 10 days
Clostridium botulinum—illness is caused by a toxin produced by this organism	Improperly canned foods, such as corn, green beans, soups, beets, asparagus, mushrooms, tuna, and liver pate; also, luncheon meats, ham, sausage, garlic in oil, lobster, and smoked and salted fish	Botulism **Onset:** usually 4 to 36 hours after eating **Symptoms:** nerve dysfunction, such as double vision, inability to swallow, speech difficulty, and progressive paralysis of respiratory system; can lead to death
Escherichia coli O157:H7	Raw or undercooked meat, raw vegetables, unpasteurized milk, minimally processed ciders and juices, water	*E. coli* infection **Onset:** few days after eating **Symptoms:** watery and bloody diarrhea, severe stomach cramps, dehydration, colitis, neurological symptoms, stroke, and hemolytic uremic syndrome (HUS); a particularly serious disease in young children that can cause kidney failure and death
Listeria monocytogenes	Soft cheeses, unpasteurized milk, imported seafood products, frozen cooked crab meat, cooked shrimp, surimi (imitation shellfish) **Note:** resists salt, heat, nitrites, and acidity better than most microorganisms	Listeriosis **Onset:** from 7 to 30 days after eating, but symptoms have been reported 2 to 3 days after eating **Symptoms:** fever, headache, nausea, and vomiting; primarily affects pregnant women and their fetuses, newborns, older adults, people with cancer and compromised immune systems; can cause death in fetuses and babies
Salmonella	Meats, poultry; eggs; milk, ice cream, and other dairy products; seafood; fresh produce, including raw sprouts; coconut; pasta; chocolate; foods containing raw eggs	Salmonellosis **Onset:** usually 6 to 48 hours after eating **Symptoms:** nausea, abdominal cramps, diarrhea, fever, and headache
Shigella	Undercooked liquid or moist food that has been handled by an infectious person	Shigellosis (bacillary dysentery) **Onset:** 1 to 7 days after eating **Symptoms:** stomach cramps, diarrhea, fever, sometimes vomiting, and blood, pus, mucus in stools

Quick Bites

Saucy *Salmonella*

Hollandaise and Béarnaise sauces may pose health risks because of the infamous *Salmonella* bacteria. Cooks traditionally make these sauces with raw eggs, and even apparently pristine Grade A eggs may harbor the bacteria. Raw cookie dough and certain homemade salad dressings such as Caesar have the same problem.

but the acid in adult stomachs kills the bacteria. Infants produce insufficient amounts of stomach acid to kill *botulinum,* so even small amounts of contaminated honey can be fatal.

Salmonella bacteria cause an estimated 1.3 million cases of foodborne illness each year.[4] *Salmonella* bacteria are prevalent on poultry and in eggs as well as in a wide variety of other foods. Choosing eggs cooked "over easy" is potentially disastrous because inadequate cooking can leave you vulnerable to the misery of salmonellosis. (See the FYI feature "Safe Food

Table 14.1 Common Foodborne Pathogens and Illnesses—*continued*

Organism	Sources	Diseases and Symptoms
Bacteria		
Staphylococcus aureus—illness is caused by a toxin produced by this organism	Meat and poultry; egg products; tuna, potato, and macaroni salads; cream-filled pastries and other foods left unrefrigerated for long periods **Note:** *S. aureus* is frequently found in cuts on skin and in nasal passages	Staphylococcal food poisoning **Onset:** 30 minutes to 8 hours after eating **Symptoms:** diarrhea, vomiting, nausea, stomach pain, and cramps; lasts 1 to 2 days
Vibrio vulnificus	Raw seafood, especially raw oysters	*Vibrio* infection **Onset:** 6 hours to a few days **Symptoms:** chills, fever, nausea and vomiting, and possibly death, especially in people with underlying health problems
Viruses		
Hepatitis A	Raw shellfish from polluted water, food handled by an infected person	Hepatitis A **Onset:** average about 1 month after exposure **Symptoms:** at first, malaise, loss of appetite, nausea, vomiting, and fever; after 3 to 10 days, jaundice and darkened urine; severe cases can result in liver damage and death
Norwalk virus	Raw shellfish from polluted water; salads, sandwiches, and other ready-to-eat foods handled by an infected person	Gastroenteritis **Onset:** 1 to 3 days **Symptoms:** nausea, vomiting, diarrhea, stomach pain, headache, and low-grade fever
Protozoa		
Anisakis	Raw fish	Anisakiasis **Onset:** 12 to 24 hours **Symptoms:** abdominal pain, can be severe
Cryptosporidium	Food that comes in contact with sewage-contaminated water; foods handled by a person who did not wash hands after using the toilet	Cryptosporidiosis **Onset:** 1 to 12 days **Symptoms:** profuse watery stools, stomach pain, loss of appetite, vomiting, and low-grade fever
Giardia lamblia	Consumption of contaminated water, contamination of food by infected food worker	Giardiasis **Onset:** 1 to 3 days **Symptoms:** diarrhea, abdominal cramps, nausea
Toxoplasma gondii	Raw or undercooked meat and, under certain conditions, unwashed fruits and vegetables; also, cats shed cysts in their feces during acute infection—organism may be transmitted to humans, if feces are handled	Toxoplasmosis **Onset:** 10 to 13 days **Symptoms:** fever, headache, rash, sore muscles, diarrhea; can kill a fetus or cause severe defects, such as mental retardation

Practices" for more information on how to protect yourself from foodborne illness.)

Scientists long have known that pathogens like *Salmonella* and *Clostridium botulinum* cause foodborne illness, but other microbes, such as ***Escherichia coli (E. coli)***, did not emerge as foodborne pathogens until the past decade. Also, some foods that weren't previously recognized as harboring pathogenic microorganisms are now recognized as potential sources. Unpasteurized fruit and vegetable juices, for example, can contain harmful bacteria.

Salmonella Rod-shaped bacteria responsible for many foodborne illnesses.

Escherichia coli (E. coli) Bacteria that are the most common cause of urinary tract infections. Because they release toxins, *E. coli* can rapidly cause shock and death.

Contaminated water also has gained greater recognition as a source of foodborne pathogens.[5] Today we know that many foods, including eggs, dairy products, meat and poultry, seafood, fresh produce, juices, and cereal grains, can harbor disease-causing bacteria.

Because bacteria and other infectious organisms are pervasive in the environment, the contamination of food can occur anywhere from the farm to your plate. Many organisms capable of causing foodborne illness in humans are naturally present in food-producing animals and their environment. For example, *Salmonella enteritidis* bacteria enter eggs directly from the egg-laying hen,[6] and *E. coli* are normally present in the intestines of cattle. Microorganisms natural to the marine environment, but toxic to humans, can contaminate seafood. (See the FYI feature "Seafood Safety.")

Exposure to animal manure or sewage runoff can contaminate crops. Sewage runoff into rivers and streams also can contaminate fish that live there. In the food-processing stage, contamination can occur from dirty equipment, rodent droppings, improper food storage, and infectious employees who fail to wash their hands adequately or take proper precautions when handling food. Poor food safety practices in retail facilities and at home also can contaminate food.

Fyi Safe Food Practices

FOR YOUR INFORMATION

Because bacteria grow rapidly between 40°F and 140°F (4°C–60°C), most food should be kept out of this temperature range, known as the Danger Zone. Cold temperatures keep bacteria from multiplying; the fewer bacteria, the less the risk of illness. Proper cooking (or other heat treatment, such as pasteurization) kills the bacteria. These principles serve as the basis for many of the following recommended food-handling practices.

Buying Food

- Buy from reputable dealers and grocers who keep their selling areas and facilities clean and sanitary and maintain food at the appropriate temperature—for example, holding dairy foods, eggs, meats, seafood, and certain produce such as cut melons and raw sprouts at refrigerator temperatures.
- Don't buy canned goods with dents or bulges. Avoid torn, crushed, or open food packages. Also, avoid buying packages that are above the frost line in the store's freezer. If the package cover is transparent, look for frost or ice crystals, signs that the product has been stored for a long time or thawed and refrozen.

Storing Food

- Refrigerate perishable items as quickly as possible after purchase. The refrigerator temperature should be 40°F or colder. Check it periodically with a thermometer to make sure the correct temperature is being maintained.
- Keep eggs in their original carton and store them in the refrigerator itself, not the door, where the temperature is warmer.
- If raw meat, poultry products, or fresh seafood will be used within two days, store them in the coldest part of the refrigerator, usually under the freezer compartment or in a special "meat keeper." Store the packages loosely to allow air to circulate freely around each package, and be sure to wrap them tightly so that raw juices can't leak out and contaminate other foods.
- If raw meat, poultry, and seafood will not be used within two days, store them in the freezer, which should have a temperature of 0°F. Check this temperature periodically, too, and adjust as needed.
- Read label directions for storing other foods; for example, mayonnaise and ketchup need to be refrigerated after they have been opened.
- Store potatoes and onions in a cool dark place, but not under the sink because leakage from pipes can contaminate and damage them. Keep them away from household cleaning products and other chemicals as well.

Preparing Food

- Wash hands thoroughly with warm, soapy water for at least 20 seconds before beginning food preparation and every time you handle raw foods, including fresh produce.
- Defrost meat, poultry, and seafood products in the refrigerator, microwave oven, or in a water-tight plastic bag submerged

Patterns of foodborne illness have changed dramatically over the last several decades as our food production has become more centralized. When food animals and produce were grown, prepared, and eaten on the family farm, the consequences of errors in food handling were generally limited to a single family. Now, much of the food we eat is mass-produced at central locations and distributed widely to restaurant chains and supermarkets. Although most food poisoning cases arise from poor food handling in homes and restaurants, contamination at a processing plant can make hundreds or even thousands of people ill. This can have nationwide implications and, therefore, receives intense national media attention.

Quick Bites

How Many *Salmonella* Does It Take?

In 1994, 224,000 people in 41 states came down with *Salmonella* food poisoning from eating contaminated ice cream. The amazing part? The ice cream contained only about six *Salmonella* bacteria per serving.

Key Concepts: *Foodborne pathogens are a major cause of illness in the United States and Canada. Pathogenic (disease-causing) microorganisms include bacteria, viruses, and parasites. Contamination of food can occur at many points along the chain from farm to table.*

Chemical Contamination

Food safety experts view chemical contamination of food as a less significant public health hazard than contamination with pathogenic microorganisms.

in cold water (the water must be changed every 30 minutes). Never defrost at room temperature—an ideal temperature for bacteria to grow and multiply.

- Marinate foods in the refrigerator. Discard the marinade after use because it contains raw juices, which may harbor bacteria; make a separate batch for basting food while cooking.
- Always use a clean cutting board. Wash cutting boards with hot water, soap, and a scrub brush. Then sanitize them in an automatic dishwasher or by rinsing with a solution of 5 milliliters (1 teaspoon) chlorine bleach to about 1 liter (1 quart) of water. If possible, use one cutting board for fresh produce and a separate one for raw meat, poultry, and seafood. Once cutting boards become excessively worn or develop hard-to-clean grooves, you should replace them.
- Before opening canned foods, wash the top of the can to prevent dirt from coming in contact with the food.
- Wash fresh fruits and vegetables thoroughly with water only.
- Avoid eating dough or batter containing raw eggs because of the risk of *Salmonella enteritidis*, a bacterium that can live in shell eggs. Cooking the egg to at least 140°F (60°C) kills the bacteria.

Cooking Food

- Cook foods to the appropriate minimum internal temperature:
  Seafood
  145°F (63°C)
  Beef, lamb, and pork
  160°F (71°C)
  Ground chicken and turkey
  165°F (74°C)
  Poultry breasts
  170°F (77°C)
  Whole poultry and thighs
  180°F (82°C)
- Always use a thermometer to ensure that the product has reached the correct internal temperature. Color is not always a good guide.
- When microwaving foods, rotate the dish and stir its contents several times to ensure even cooking. Follow recommended standing times, then check meat, poultry, and seafood products with a thermometer to make sure they have reached the correct internal temperature.
- Cook eggs until the white is firm and the yolk begins to harden.

Serving Food

- Keep hot foods at 140°F (60°C) or higher and cold foods at 40°F (4°C) or lower.
- Do not keep leftovers at room temperature for more than two hours. Refrigerate as quickly as possible.
- Date leftovers so that they can be used within a safe time—generally, three to five days in the refrigerator.

Yet surveys and retail trends suggest that consumers think otherwise. To avoid foods exposed to chemicals, more and more people are turning to **organic foods**. (See the section "Organic Alternatives" in this chapter.) Chemical contaminants include pesticides, drugs, pollutants, and natural toxins.

organic foods Foods that originate from farms or handling operations that meet the standards set by the USDA National Organic Program.

pesticides Chemicals used to control insects, diseases, weeds, fungi, and other pests on plants, vegetables, fruits, and animals.

Pesticides

Pesticides play an important role in food production—controlling plant diseases, weeds, insects, and other pests. Pesticides protect crops and ensure a substantial yield, thus assuring consumers of a wide variety of foods at affordable prices. Without these chemicals, many argue that crop production would fall and prices for food would rise.

Every year, the U.S. Food and Drug Administration (FDA) collects about 10,000 samples of domestic and imported food and analyzes them for pesticide residues.[7] Since 1987, the FDA has found no illegal residues in more than 99 percent of domestic and more than 95 percent of imported samples. When a violation occurred, it usually involved the use of a pesticide on crops for which it was not approved, rather than an excessive level. In 1999, the FDA found no residues in over 60 percent of the samples.[8]

[Fyi] Seafood Safety

FOR YOUR INFORMATION

Seafood can be a delicious and heart-healthy part of our diets. However, as with all food, contamination can have serious consequences. Seafood is one of the most rapidly perishable foods, so proper refrigeration and rapid processing and transport to the consumer are essential. Although certain types of microbial contaminants and toxins are unique to seafood, properly handled and cooked seafood is as safe to eat as most other foods.

Eating raw seafood, on the other hand, is risky business. Despite the popularity of such dishes as sashimi, sushi, and raw oysters, uncooked fish, no matter how carefully prepared, poses a risk for infection. People with liver disease, diabetes, cancer, or other diseases that impair immune function should be especially careful to stay away from raw seafood. Pregnant women also should avoid uncooked seafood; some physicians recommend that pregnant women avoid seafood altogether. The rest of us should think twice before enjoying those raw oysters and sashimi and, at the very least, should make sure they are fresh and from a reliable source before letting those slippery delicacies pass our lips.

Seafood-related illness falls into several categories. Sources of infection include bacteria, viruses, and parasites. Toxins occur naturally in some fish, and human pollution may contaminate seafood. The following are several examples of seafood-caused illness:

- Raw or undercooked shellfish such as oysters, clams, and mussels may be contaminated with bacteria such as *Salmonella, Vibrio* species, and *Staphylococcus aureus.* Hepatitis A (caused by a virus) and gastroenteritis are other illnesses that can be contracted by eating uncooked shellfish from polluted waters.
- Fish such as mahi-mahi, tuna, and bluefish that have begun to spoil can cause scombroid poisoning. A toxin in these decomposing fish causes flushing, itching, and headache. Cooking does not destroy the toxin, so the best prevention is proper refrigeration and rapid use of fresh fish.
- Some tropical fish, such as red snapper and barracuda, may contain ciguatera toxin, which can cause gastrointestinal and neurological problems in humans. Larger warm-water fish are most often implicated in this illness. The toxin is actually produced by tiny plants that are eaten by small fish. When larger fish consume many small fish, the toxin can accumulate. The flesh of these large fish may contain enough of the toxin to make humans very ill. Heating or freezing does not destroy this toxin.
- *Anisakis* is a parasite found in raw fish. After a person eats an infected fish, the larvae of this roundworm can invade the human stomach, causing severe abdominal pain. Cooking or freezing the fish for at least 72 hours can kill this parasite.
- Red tide is a well-known phenomenon in which huge numbers of tiny toxic organisms called dinoflagellates infest seawater. Shellfish in the area become poisonous as a result. Respiratory paralysis and death are possible effects of eating shellfish from red tide areas.
- Human pollution is a serious problem, especially near population centers where industrial wastes and human sewage flow into the water. Heavy metals such as mercury can accumulate in

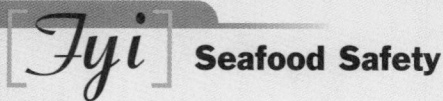

The FDA also samples and analyzes domestic and imported animal feeds for pesticide residues. This monitoring focuses on feeds for livestock and poultry—animals that become or produce foods for human consumption. In 1999 the FDA analyzed 463 domestic and 61 imported feed samples. Only two of these samples exceeded an established EPA tolerance or an FDA-requested maximum level.[9]

Despite these reassuring results, concerns about pesticides in food persist. Processing methods can either reduce or concentrate pesticide residues in foods. (See **Figure 14.2.**) Infants and young children are particularly susceptible to the hazards of pesticides. Their small size and rapid growth make them especially vulnerable to pesticide residues, which can accumulate in their bodies over their lifetimes. Enacted in 1996, the Food Quality Protection Act includes landmark protections for the young. For the first time, manufacturers must show that pesticide levels are safe for infants and children. In addition, when determining a safe level for a pesticide in a food, the Environmental Protection Agency (EPA) now must account for the cumulative effect of exposures to similar pesticides and toxic chemicals.[10]

larger fish (e.g., sharks and swordfish) that have been exposed to mercury in their environment for long periods. Since commercially caught fish generally contain minimal amounts of mercury, even large fish are safe to eat, although pregnant women are advised to avoid eating shark or swordfish more than once a month.

- Dioxin and polychlorinated biphenols (PCBs) also can accumulate in fish living in polluted water. Commercial seafood companies tend to avoid contaminated areas, but local fishers who frequently catch and eat fish from these waters may be at some risk.[1]

1 US Food and Drug Administration. *FDA and Seafood Safety.* Washington, DC: 1991.

Table A **Understanding Seafood Safety**

Condition	*Explanation*
Scombroid poisoning	Scombroid poisoning is a type of food intoxication caused by the consumption of scombroid and scombroid-like marine fish species that have begun to spoil with the growth of particular types of food bacteria. Fish most commonly involved are members of the *Scombridae* family (tunas and mackerels) and a few nonscombroid relatives (bluefish, mahi-mahi, and amberjacks). The suspect toxin is an elevated level of histamine generated by bacterial degradation of substances in the muscle protein.
Anisakis	*Anisakis simplex* (herring worm) and *Pseudoterranova (Phocanema, Terranova) decipiens* (cod or seal worm) are anisakid nematodes (roundworms) that have been implicated in human infections caused by the consumption of raw or undercooked seafood. *Anisakiasis* is the term generally used to refer to the acute disease in humans.
Red tide	When temperature, salinity, and nutrients reach certain levels, algae grow very fast or "bloom" and accumulate into dense, visible patches near the surface of the water. *Red tide* is a common name for such a phenomenon where certain species of phytoplankton contain reddish pigments and "bloom" such that the water appears to be colored red. The term is a misnomer because it is not associated with tides. A small number of species produce potent neurotoxins that can cause illness and even death.
Polychlorinated biphenols (PCBs)	A group of toxic, persistent chemicals used as insulation for electrical transformers and capacitors and as lubricants in gas pipeline systems. PCBs are a serious health problem because of their persistence in the environment, accumulation in the body, and potential for a long-term negative effect on health. In the United States, their manufacture was stopped in 1976.

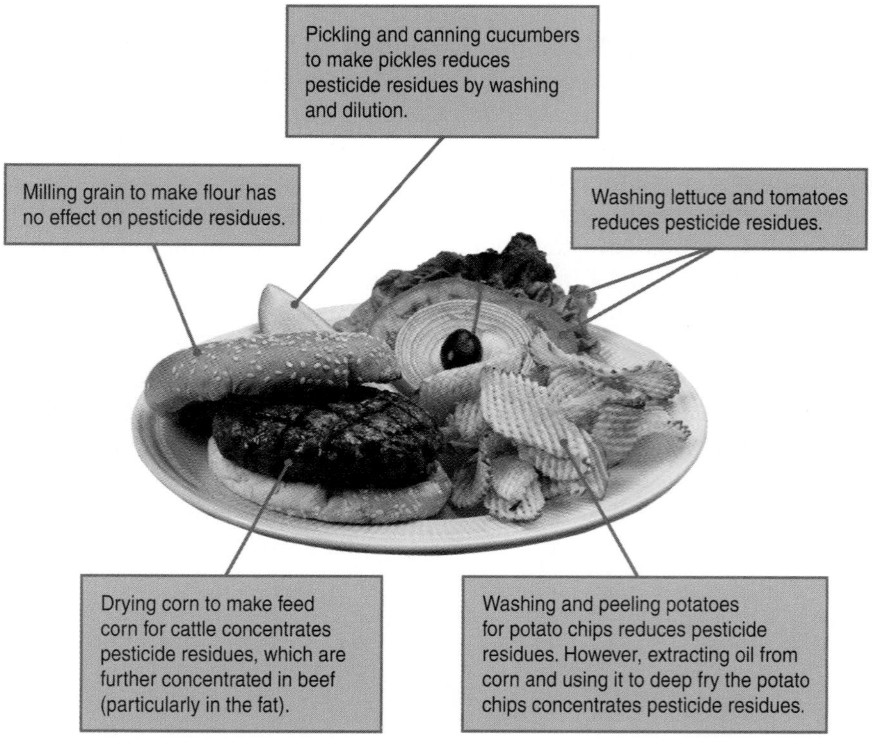

Pickling and canning cucumbers to make pickles reduces pesticide residues by washing and dilution.
Milling grain to make flour has no effect on pesticide residues.
Washing lettuce and tomatoes reduces pesticide residues.
Drying corn to make feed corn for cattle concentrates pesticide residues, which are further concentrated in beef (particularly in the fat).
Washing and peeling potatoes for potato chips reduces pesticide residues. However, extracting oil from corn and using it to deep fry the potato chips concentrates pesticide residues.

Figure 14.2 **Pesticide pathways to dinner.** Food processing and preparation methods can either reduce or concentrate pesticide residues in foods.

Consumers Union (the nonprofit publisher of *Consumer Reports*) has issued a report stating that legally permitted pesticide levels in some foods are much higher than the levels that scientific data show are safe for children.[11] Consumers Union analyzed data collected by the USDA's Pesticide Data Program and concluded that a relatively small number of highly toxic insecticides accounted for most of the toxicity in foods. Consumers Union suggests that focusing on reducing or eliminating these high-risk pesticides may be the best way to reduce toxicity from our foods.

To decrease pesticide intake, Consumers Union recommends washing and peeling (if possible) fruits and vegetables and eating a variety of produce.[12] Because the benefits of these foods far outweigh the risks from the pesticides they might contain, Consumers Union emphasizes that it *does not* recommend eating fewer fruits and vegetables.

Excessive use of synthetic pesticides, herbicides, and fertilizers contributes substantially to the pollution of soil and water. Overuse can be particularly hazardous to farm workers, whose exposure to these chemicals typically is much higher than consumers'. Overuse also threatens wildlife. Today, many farmers use **integrated pest management (IPM)** to reduce pesticide use. (See **Figure 14.3**.) IPM methods include crop rotation, use of natural rather than synthetic pesticides, and planting nonfood crops nearby that lure pests away from food crops. Releasing sterile fruit flies into orchards also allows reductions in pesticide use. Because fruit flies produce no offspring when they mate with sterile partners, the overall fruit fly population drops.

Organic Alternatives

Organic foods are grown or produced without synthetic pesticides and without synthetic fertilizer. Sales of organic foods totaled nearly $7 billion

integrated pest management (IPM) Economically sound pest control techniques that minimize pesticide use, enhance environmental stewardship, and promote sustainable systems.

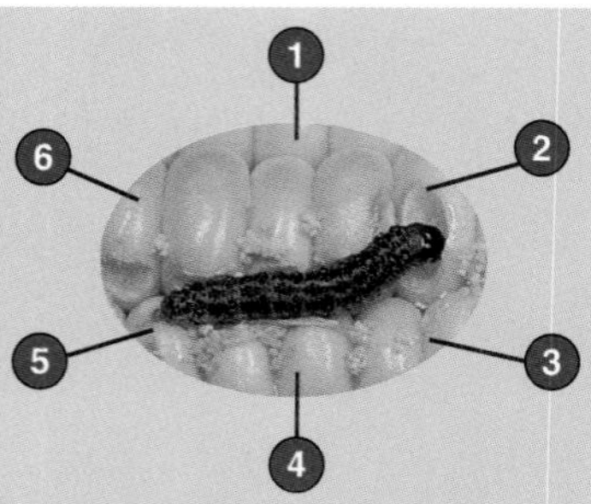

1. **Legal control**
   State and federal guidelines are designed to limit the spread of pests.
2. **Biological control**
   Beneficial organisms, such as predators, parasites, and viruses, are released into the environment to suppress pest organisms.
3. **Cultural control**
   Rotation, sanitation, and other good farming techniques are employed to help reduce pest populations.
4. **Physical control**
   Barriers, traps, and the location and timing of planting are all used to control pest infestations.
5. **Genetic control**
   Resistant plant strains are developed to reduce the impact of pests.
6. **Chemical control**
   Conventional pesticides, biopesticides, pheromones, and other chemicals are used to prevent or suppress pest outbreaks. The chemical controls are specific to a pest species and are ideally short-lived in the environment. In addition, the chemicals are used at their lowest effective rate and may be alternated to help prevent the development of pest resistance.

Figure 14.3 **Integrated pest management.** Integrated pest management is a sustainable approach that combines prevention, avoidance, monitoring, and suppression strategies in a way that minimizes economic, health, and environmental risks. It minimizes pesticide use and promotes economically sound practices.

in 2001, and the market is expected to surpass $20 billion by the year 2010.[13] Growth of the industry reflects, in part, America's distrust of technology and a desire to return to a simpler, more "natural" way of food production.

The Organic Foods Production Act and the National Organic Program (NOP) are intended to assure consumers that the organic foods they purchase are produced, processed, and certified to consistent national standards. The labeling requirements of the new program apply to raw, fresh produce and to processed foods that contain organic ingredients. Foods that are sold, labeled, or represented as organic must be produced and processed in accordance with the NOP standards.[14] **Table 14.2** outlines the requirements for labeling organic food.

Under the NOP, farm and processing operations that grow and process organic foods must be certified by the USDA. The certification process includes an on-site inspection that must verify that the applicant's operation complies with strict national organic standards. Certifying agents may collect and test soil, water, waste, plant and animal tissues, and processed products. A certified operation may label its products or ingredients as organic and may use the "USDA Organic" seal.

Even though there is no scientific evidence that genetic engineering and irradiation of foods present unacceptable risks, public opposition led the NOP to prohibit use of these technologies with organic foods. While irradiation and genetic engineering have been approved for use in agriculture

Table 14.2 Labeling Requirements for Organic Food

Labeling requirements are based on the percentage of a product's ingredients that are organic.

Foods labeled "100 percent organic" and "organic"

- Products labeled "100 percent organic" must contain only organically produced ingredients (excluding water and salt).
- Products labeled "organic" must consist of at least 95 percent organically produced ingredients (excluding water and salt). Any other ingredients must consist of nonagricultural substances approved on the National List maintained by the USDA National Organic Program or non–organically produced agricultural products that are not commercially available in organic form.
- Products that meet the requirements may display these terms and the percentage of organic content on their principal display panel.
- The USDA seal and the seal or mark of certifying agents may appear on product packages and in advertisements.
- Foods labeled "100 percent organic" and "organic" cannot be produced using excluded methods, sewage sludge, or ionizing radiation.

Processed products labeled "made with organic (specified ingredients)"

- Products that contain at least 70 percent organic ingredients can use the phrase "made with organic ingredients" and list up to three of the organic ingredients or food groups on the principal display panel. For example, soup made with at least 70 percent organic ingredients and only organic vegetables may be labeled either "soup made with organic peas, potatoes, and carrots" or "soup made with organic vegetables."
- Foods labeled "made with organic ingredients" cannot be produced using excluded methods, sewage sludge, or ionizing radiation.
- The percentage of organic content and the certifying agent's seal or mark may be used on the package. However, the USDA seal cannot be used anywhere on the package.

Processed products that contain less than 70 percent organic ingredients

- The packaging of these products can make no organic claim, except on the information panel, where they may identify the specific ingredients that are organically produced.

Other labeling provisions

- Any product labeled as organic must identify each organically produced ingredient in the ingredient statement on the information panel.
- The name and address of the certifying agent of the final product must be displayed on the information panel.
- There are no restrictions on the use of other truthful labeling claims, such as "no drugs or growth hormones used," "free range," or "sustainably harvested."

Source: USDA, National Organic Program. http://www.ams.usda.gov/nop/facts/index.htm. Accessed 5/11/02.

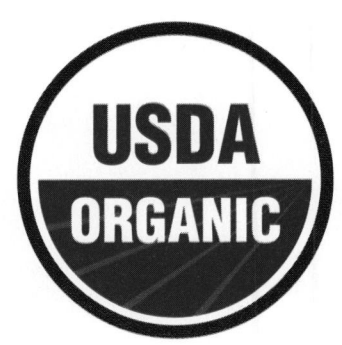

and may offer certain benefits for the environment and human health, consumers strongly oppose their use in organically grown foods. Because of consumer opposition, foods produced with these techniques are prohibited from carrying the organic label.[15]

Organic food advocates claim that using natural fertilizer, such as manure, produces a soil that is richer in a range of nutrients than a soil treated with chemical fertilizers, which typically contain only a few basic nutrients. They reason that organically fertilized soils produce foods that contain more nutrients. A recent review of 41 studies comparing organic and conventionally produced crops supports this idea, finding more iron, magnesium, phosphorus, and vitamin C in organic crops.[16] However, many of the studies reviewed are over 20 years old, and so more current evaluation of nutritional content is needed.

Organic farming has its drawbacks. The use of manure raises food safety concerns. The organic producer must manage animal and plant waste materials so they do not contribute to contamination of crops, soil, or water. Manure runoff can pollute nearby lakes and streams. Other critics charge that organic farming is "elitist," that synthetic fertilizers and pesticides are necessary to meet the food needs of an expanding world population. They also point out that complete freedom from pesticides cannot be guaranteed, no matter how carefully a food is produced, since pesticide residues may still exist in soil, water, and air.[17]

Organic foods are not pesticide-free foods. Organic farmers can use natural and approved synthetic pesticides to control weeds and insects.[18] Microbial contaminants that cause foodborne illness can be found in organic as well as conventional foods. Consumers must handle all food appropriately, whether organically or conventionally grown. Think About It 2

Animal Drugs

Current agricultural practice depends heavily on the use of drugs in food animals and food-producing animals raised specifically to provide meat, milk, and eggs. Producers use drugs to maintain animal health and well-being, as well as increase production. Keeping animals in good health reduces the chance that disease will spread from animals to humans, and healthy animals can use nutrients for growth and production rather than to fight infection. But there is a possibility that drugs used in animals could enter human food and possibly increase the risk of ill health in humans.

Many researchers fear that overuse of animal antibiotics will contribute to the emergence of antibiotic-resistant microorganisms that could threaten human health. Another potential problem, though with less widespread effects, is that humans with drug allergies could have reactions to drug residues in food-producing animals. Some people worry that the widespread use of hormones may impair animal health or the quality of the food obtained from treated animals.

There are five major classes of drugs used in animals raised for food:

1. topical antiseptics, bactericides, and fungicides used to treat skin or hoof infections, cuts, and abrasions
2. ionophores, which alter stomach microorganisms to more efficiently digest feeds and to help protect against some parasites
3. hormone and hormonelike production enhancers (anabolic hormones for meat production and bovine somatotropin for increased milk production in dairy cows)

4. antiparasitics
5. antibiotics used to prevent infections, treat disease, and promote growth[19]

The FDA is responsible for ensuring that drugs approved for use in animals are safe not only for the animals but also for humans who eat food produced from the animals. In addition, the FDA enforces regulations to ensure that drugs are used properly in cows, chickens, and seafood. However, FDA surveillance is not perfect; government investigations have revealed that a few U.S. veterinarians and farmers illegally use animal drugs that are known to be dangerous to humans.

Pollutants

Pollutants from animal manure and other wastes, factories, human sewage, and other runoff can contaminate food-production areas. For example, some scientists theorize that dioxin contamination of foods may cause human cancer. **Dioxins** are chemical compounds created in the manufacturing, combustion, and chlorine bleaching of pulp and paper and in other industrial processes.[20] Dioxins can accumulate in the food chain and are potent animal carcinogens. Fish from dioxin-polluted waters can contain significant amounts of dioxin.[21] The commercial fishing industry avoids areas of known dioxin pollution. Dioxins in tiny amounts are found in food packages, paper plates, and coffee filters made of bleached paper. Because the quantity of this toxic chemical is minimal, however, the FDA has concluded that use of these products poses no significant risk to human health.

Quick Bites

Well-Traveled Dioxin

In Nunavut, Canada's newest province, the breast milk of native Inuits has twice the average concentration of dioxin as does the milk of women in southern Quebec. Native Inuits primarily eat fatty animals high on the food chain. These animals accumulate dioxin, but where did the dioxin originate? Not Canada. Carried by the wind, most comes from industrial combustion in the eastern and midwestern United States and some originates as far away as Mexico.

Natural Toxins

Other chemical contamination of food can occur from **natural toxins**.[22] Examples include

- **aflatoxins**, found in contaminated food or animal feed. Aflatoxins are produced by certain strains of *Aspergillus* fungi under certain conditions of temperature and humidity. The most pronounced contamination has been found in tree nuts, peanuts, and other oilseeds, such as corn and cottonseed. Aflatoxins have been implicated as a factor in the development of liver cancer, particularly in parts of the world where food and water are frequently contaminated with this fungus.
- **ciguatera** and other marine toxins. These toxins can accumulate in seafood (mainly in large tropical fish) and, when ingested, cause serious problems, including paralysis, amnesia, and nerve toxicity. Commercial fishers avoid waters known to harbor ciguatera toxin. Ciguatera poisoning sometimes occurs when these fish are caught as part of recreational fishing. Cooking does not destroy these toxins.
- **methyl mercury**. Mercury occurs naturally in the environment and is produced by human activities. It is soluble in water, where bacteria can cause chemical changes that transform mercury to methyl mercury, a more toxic form. Fish absorb methyl mercury from water passing over their gills and by eating other contaminated aquatic species. Because larger predatory fish can consume many contaminated

pollutants Gaseous, chemical, or organic waste that contaminates air, soil, or water.

dioxins Chemical compounds created in the manufacturing, combustion, and chlorine bleaching of pulp and paper and in other industrial processes.

natural toxins Poisons that are produced by or naturally occur in plants or microorganisms.

aflatoxins Carcinogenic and toxic factors produced by food molds.

ciguatera A toxin found in more than 300 species of Caribbean and South Pacific fish. It is a nonbacterial source of food poisoning.

methyl mercury A toxic compound that results from the chemical transformation of mercury by bacteria. Mercury is water-soluble in trace amounts and contaminates many bodies of water.

poisonous mushrooms Mushrooms that contain toxins that can cause stomach upset, dizziness, hallucinations, and other neurological symptoms.

solanine A potentially toxic alkaloid that is present with chlorophyll in the green areas on potato skins.

Food Allergy & Anaphylaxis Network A nonprofit organization devoted to increasing public awareness of food allergy and anaphylaxis (a life-threatening allergic reaction), educating the public about food allergies, and advancing research on food allergies.

smaller fish, they accumulate higher levels of methyl mercury. (See **Figure 14.4**.)

- **poisonous mushrooms**. These plants produce toxic substances that can cause stomach upset, dizziness, hallucinations, and other neurological symptoms.[23] The more lethal mushroom species can cause liver and kidney failure, coma, and death.
- **solanine**, a toxic substance in raw potato skins.[24] Solanine develops in the greenish layer of improperly stored potatoes. It can be removed by thoroughly peeling the potato.

A variety of compounds in herbs and spices also can be toxic. However, foodborne illness caused by these and other natural toxins is relatively rare compared with illness from pathogenic microorganisms.

Other Food Contaminants

Because labeling will not identify a substance inadvertently added to a food, people who are allergic to it are at risk of severe illness. The most common food allergens, according to the **Food Allergy & Anaphylaxis Network**, are milk, eggs, peanuts, tree nuts (cashews, walnuts, etc.), fish, shellfish, soy, and wheat.[25] (See **Figure 14.5**.) In an allergic person, these

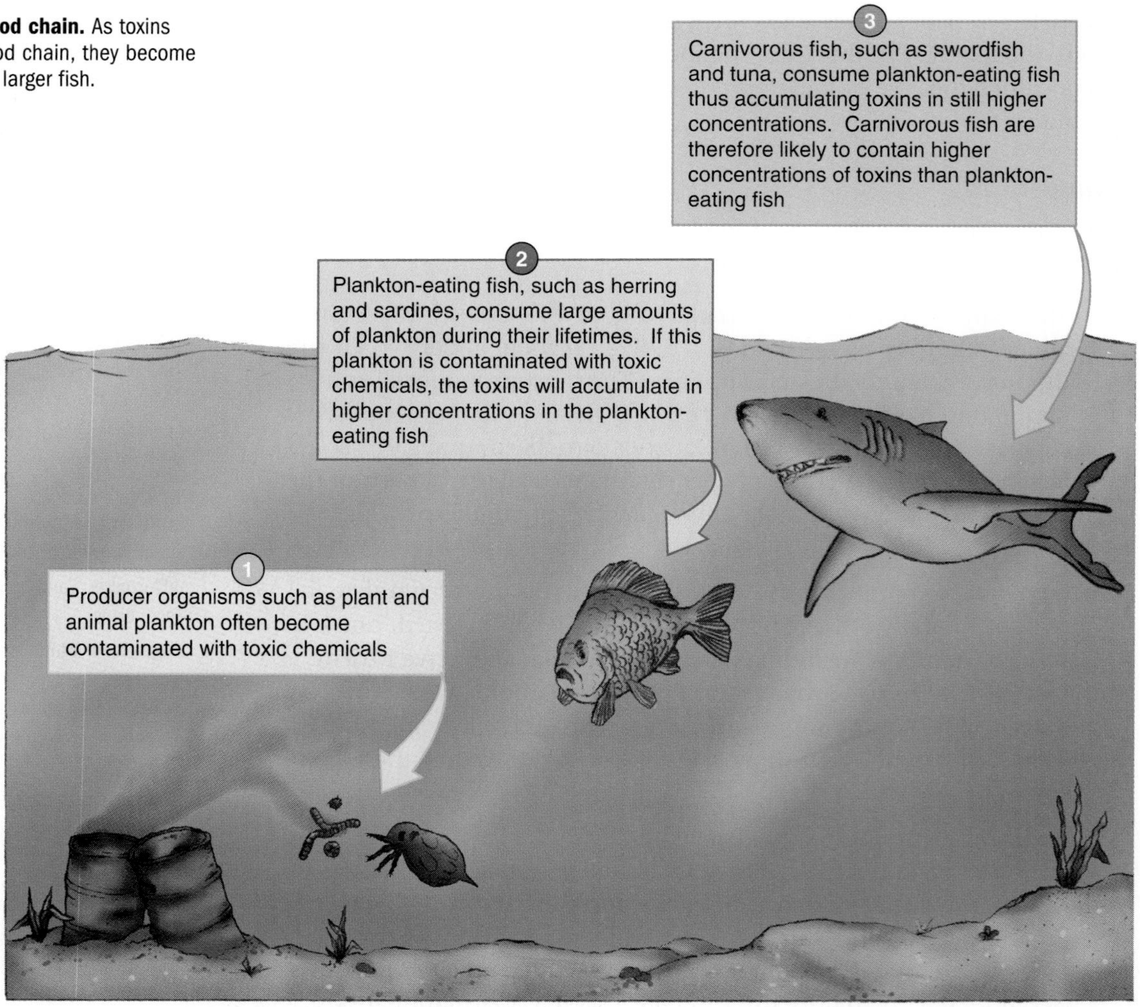
3
Carnivorous fish, such as swordfish and tuna, consume plankton-eating fish thus accumulating toxins in still higher concentrations. Carnivorous fish are therefore likely to contain higher concentrations of toxins than plankton-eating fish
2
Plankton-eating fish, such as herring and sardines, consume large amounts of plankton during their lifetimes. If this plankton is contaminated with toxic chemicals, the toxins will accumulate in higher concentrations in the plankton-eating fish
1
Producer organisms such as plant and animal plankton often become contaminated with toxic chemicals

Figure 14.4 **Toxins in the food chain.** As toxins travel up the food chain, they become concentrated in larger fish.

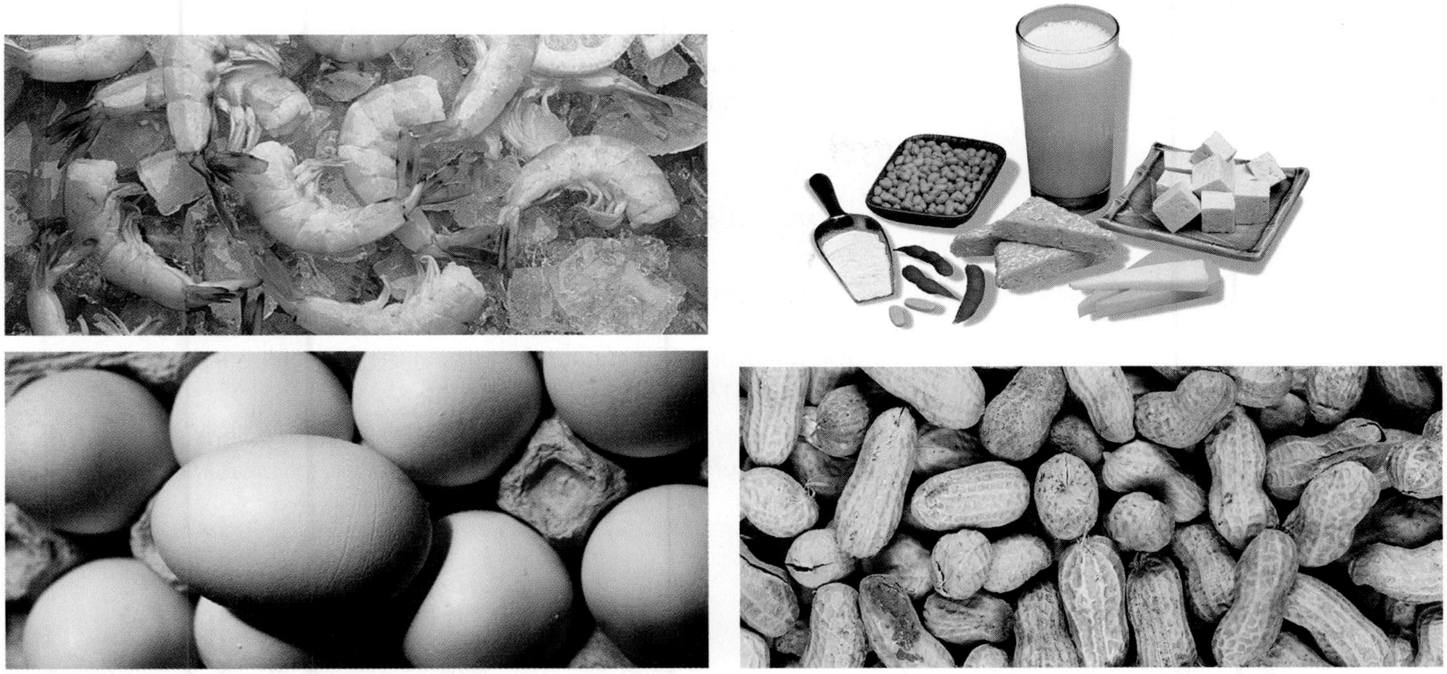

Figure 14.5 **Foods that commonly cause allergic reactions.** In sensitive people, an allergic reaction to food can be life threatening.

foods can cause a variety of reactions, including gastrointestinal problems, skin irritation, breathing difficulty, shock, and even death.

Whether intentionally added through tampering or unintentionally during food production, contaminants like glass, metal, and other objects can have serious health consequences. Misuse of cleaning agents in food-contact areas such as refrigerator trucks, food-production lines, and storage units can introduce undesirable chemicals into food. While generally not a health hazard, insects, dirt, and other undesirable items also can contaminate a food.

Key Concepts: *Chemical contaminants in foods include pesticides, natural toxins, and contamination related to pollution. Although organic foods are grown without synthetic pesticides or fertilizers, they still can contain chemical contaminants. Other potential food hazards are allergens and nonfood contaminants.*

Keeping Food Safe

The fifth edition of the *Dietary Guidelines for Americans,* released in 2000, contains a new guideline: "Keep food safe to eat." Having safe foods to eat requires the efforts of a great many people along the way from the farm to your plate. Imagine yourself enjoying a piece of broiled chicken. Consider that harmful contamination of that chicken could have occurred at the farm, in the processing plant, or during transportation to the supermarket. Once at the supermarket, the chicken might have been under-refrigerated or kept too long before being sold. After buying the chicken, you might have left it in a warm car or kept it in a refrigerator that was not cold enough. Your kitchen hygiene might not have been the best; and finally, you could have undercooked the chicken. Considering the many opportunities for

Quick Bites

Chill Out!

In 1939, Fred McKinley Jones, a prolific African-American inventor, and Joe Numero received a patent for a vehicle refrigeration device for large trucks. Their invention eliminated the problem of food spoilage during long shipping times and permitted year-round delivery of fresh produce across the country. Refrigerated shipping launched international markets for food, helped create new industries such as frozen foods, fast foods, and container shipping, and forever altered consumers' eating habits.

contamination, it is truly amazing that most of the time our food does not make us sick.

Keeping foods free from contamination is a job that falls to many parties. It is the responsibility not only of government officials at the national, state, and local levels, but also of everyone who comes in contact with food—the producer, the manufacturer, the retailer, and ultimately the consumer.

Government Agencies

The basis of modern food law is the Federal Food, Drug, and Cosmetic (FD&C) Act of 1938, which gives the Food and Drug Administration (FDA) authority over food and food ingredients and defines requirements for truthful labeling of ingredients. Today at the federal level, six agencies (**Figure 14.6**) share responsibility for food safety.

1. *The Food and Drug Administration (FDA)* enforces laws governing safety of domestic and imported food, except meat and poultry.

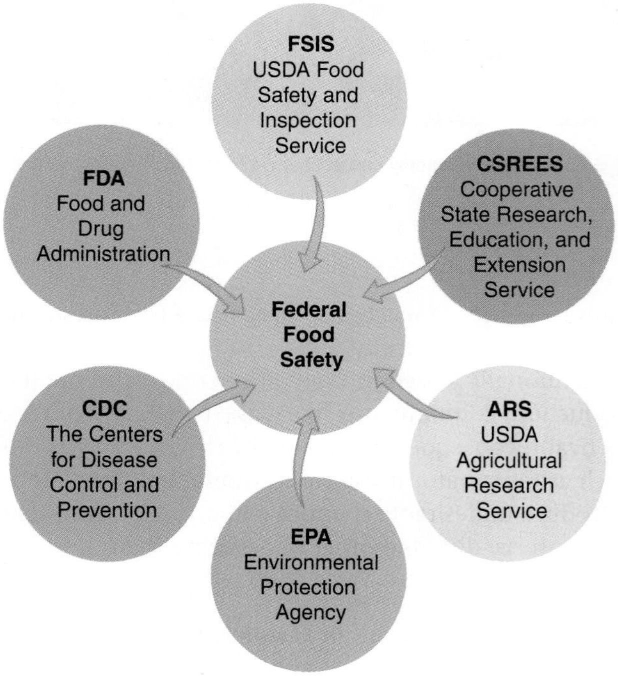

Figure 14.6 **Government agencies that help protect our food supply.** While the FDA has primary responsibility for the safety of much of our food supply, many government agencies provide oversight.

OTHER AGENCIES WITH FOOD SAFETY RESPONSIBILITIES

Federal Trade Commission (FTC)
- Regulates the advertising and marketing of food products.
- Has the authority to take legal action against unwarranted advertising claims.

Department of Justice
- Seizes products when federal food safety laws are violated.
- Prosecutes suspected violators of food safety laws.

Bureau of Alcohol, Tobacco and Firearms (BATF)
- Enforces laws that involve the production, distribution, and labeling of most alcoholic beverages.
- Sometimes shares responsibilities with FDA when alcoholic beverages are adulterated or contain food or color additives, pesticides, or contaminants.

National Marine Fisheries Service (NMFS)
- Responsible for seafood quality and identification, fisheries management and development, habitat conservation, and aquaculture production.

State and Local Governments
- Inspect restaurants, retail food outlet, dairies, grain mills, and other food establishments within their areas of jurisdiction.
- Embargo illegal food products in many situations.

2. *The Centers for Disease Control and Prevention (CDC)* monitor outbreaks of foodborne diseases, investigate their causes, and determine proper prevention.
3. *The USDA Food Safety and Inspection Service (FSIS)* enforces laws governing safety of domestic and imported meat and poultry products.
4. *The USDA Cooperative State Research, Education, and Extension Service (CSREES)* develops research and education programs on food safety for farmers and consumers.
5. *The USDA Agricultural Research Service (ARS)* conducts research to extend knowledge of various agricultural practices, including those involving animal and crop safety.
6. *The Environmental Protection Agency (EPA)* regulates public drinking water and approves pesticides and other chemicals used in the environment.

State and local health and agricultural departments oversee food safety in their jurisdictions, often in conjunction with federal agencies.

The public's heightened concern about food safety is evident in the creation of new consumer advocacy groups such as **S.T.O.P. (Safe Tables Our Priority)**, a national organization that works with government agencies and industry to prevent foodborne illnesses and deaths. In addition, the federal **Food Safety Initiative** calls on the federal government to take the lead in expanding research, training, and education about safety at all levels of food production.[26] The Food Safety Initiative has expanded the use of the food industry safety system called **Hazard Analysis Critical Control Point**, or **HACCP** (pronounced "hassip"). The Food Safety Initiative has also created a campaign to educate consumers, health professionals (such as doctors), and retail establishments about food safety. Other goals of the Food Safety Initiative include improved detection of foodborne pathogens and prevention of microbial growth during food production and distribution.[27]

Safe Tables Our Priority (S.T.O.P.) A national organization devoted to preventing illness and death from foodborne illness by working with government agencies and industry to encourage practices and policies that promote safe food.

Food Safety Initiative A 1996 presidential directive to three cabinet members to identify specific steps to improve the safety of the U.S. food supply.

Hazard Analysis Critical Control Point (HACCP) A modern food safety system that focuses on preventing contamination by identifying potential areas in food production and retail in which contamination could occur and taking steps to ensure contaminants are not introduced at these points.

critical control points (CCP) Operational steps or procedures in a process, production method, or recipe, at which control can be applied to prevent, reduce, or eliminate a food safety hazard.

Hazard Analysis Critical Control Point

Hazard Analysis Critical Control Point is a food industry program that focuses on preventing contamination by identifying areas in food production and retail where contamination could occur. HACCP also is an important line of defense against intentional contamination by bioterrorists. (See the FYI feature "At War with Bioterrorism.") HACCP is intended to replace the traditional system of spot checks at manufacturing sites and random sampling of final products. That system uncovered problems only after they had occurred, whereas HACCP works by preventing contamination.

Companies and retailers analyze their food-production processes and determine **critical control points (CCP)**—points at which hazards could occur. They then determine measures that they can institute at these points to prevent, control, or eliminate the hazards. (See **Table 14.3**.) Critical control points can occur anywhere in a food's production—from its raw state through processing and shipping to purchase by the consumer. Preventive measures can include proper cooking, chilling, and sanitizing, as well as preventing cross-contamination and improving employee hygiene.

The USDA requires HACCP for meat and poultry, the food products it regulates.[28] The FDA, which regulates all other foods, requires HACCP in the seafood and low-acid canned-food industries and recently added this requirement for the juice industry.[29] Also, the FDA has incorporated HACCP

Table 14.3 HACCP: Hazard Analysis and Critical Control Point

Step 1: Analyze hazards.	Identify the potential hazards associated with a food. The hazard could be biological (e.g., a microbe), chemical (e.g., mercury), or physical (e.g., ground glass or metal).
Step 2: Identify critical control points (CCPs).	Identify points in a food's production path—from its raw state through processing and shipping to consumption —where a potential hazard can be controlled or eliminated. Examples of CCPs are cooking, chilling, handling, cleaning, and storage.
Step 3: Establish preventive measures with critical limits for each control point.	An example is setting the minimum cooking temperature and time to ensure safety for a particular food (the temperature and time are critical limits).
Step 4: Establish procedures to monitor the control points.	Such procedures might include determining how and by whom cooking time and temperature should be monitored.
Step 5: Establish corrective actions to be taken when a critical limit has not been met.	For example, reprocessing or disposing of food if the minimum cooking temperature is not met.
Step 6: Establish effective record keeping to document the HACCP system.	For example, recording hazards and their control methods, the monitoring of safety requirements, and action taken to correct potential problems.
Step 7: Establish procedures to verify that the system is working consistently.	For example, testing time-recording and temperature-recording devised to verify that a cooking unit is working properly.

The HACCP method focuses on preventing hazards, relies heavily on scientific principles, permits efficient government oversight, and places greater responsibility on food operations to ensure food safety.

Source: HACCP: A state-of-the-art approach to food safety. *FDA Backgrounder.* October, 2001.http://www.cfsan.fda.gov/~lrd/bghaccp.html. Accessed 5/11/02.

Food Code A reference published periodically by the Food and Drug Administration for restaurants, grocery stores, institutional food services, vending operations, and other retailers on how to store, prepare, and serve food to prevent foodborne illness.

principles in its ***Food Code***, a reference for restaurants, grocery stores, institutional food services, vending operations, and other retailers on how to store, prepare, and serve food to prevent foodborne illness.[30] The FDA updates and publishes the *Food Code* periodically as a model for states to adopt and use to regulate retail food establishments in their jurisdictions.

Fyi At War with Bioterrorism

FOR YOUR INFORMATION

Late one afternoon, restaurant owner Dave Lutgens first felt nauseated, then experienced mild stomach cramps. By evening he was dizzy and disoriented. Suffering from diarrhea, he had to crawl to reach the toilet. Weak and dehydrated, he was wracked with chills, fever, and vomiting. Two days later his wife became ill with the same symptoms. By the end of the week, 13 employees were sick as well as dozens of customers. The culprit was *Salmonella typhimurium,* a rod-shaped bacteria responsible for many foodborne illnesses. But this was not a simple case of food poisoning. Occurring in 1984, this was a bioterrorist assault on the small Oregon town of Dalles. The Rajaneesh religious cult deliberately perpetrated this terrifying food experience by contaminating a number of self-service salad bars and coffee creamers with home-grown *Salmonella.* Ten restaurants were affected and more than 700 people fell ill from the biological attack.

Bioterrorists also have assaulted Canada. In 1970, four students in Montreal, Quebec, were admitted to the hospital after eating eggs inoculated with a parasitic nematode, *Ascaris suum.* They had signs of a parasitic infection and suffered from asthma and other lung problems. In 2000, 27 people suffered food poisoning after drinking coffee from a single vending machine at Lavalle University in Quebec City. The coffee had been laced with arsenic.

Bioterrorist attacks can range from making false statements or accusations to actively inflicting injury on people, animals, or crops. Threats can be as devastating as actual destruction. Just claiming that a product has been intentionally contaminated can be sufficient to trigger an expensive recall and harmful adverse publicity. Product tampering, whether a hoax or real, can provide notoriety to the perpetrator, who is attempting to terrorize people and businesses.

Our food supply is an obvious route for the delivery of certain chemical and biological agents. Food production and distribution is a complex system not protected easily from the deliberate introduction of toxic agents. The

Key Concepts: *Food safety is the responsibility of many agencies at the federal and state levels. The use of the Hazard Analysis Critical Control Point system allows government and industry to identify possible sites of food contamination and correct problems before they occur.*

The Consumer's Role in Food Safety

Food safety advice to consumers used to consist of a simple message: "Keep hot foods hot and cold foods cold." (See **Figure 14.7**.) Now food safety experts urge consumers to follow the following four rules (see **Figure 14.8**):

- *Clean.* Wash hands and surfaces often.
- *Separate.* Don't cross-contaminate.
- *Cook.* Cook to proper temperatures.
- *Chill.* Refrigerate promptly.[31]

Think About It 3

Once a consumer takes possession of a food, food safety becomes his or her responsibility. Unfortunately, studies show that many consumers fail to follow safe food practices in the home. Current public health efforts focus on teaching consumers—from young children to older Americans—safe food practices in the home. (See the FYI feature "Safe Food Practices.")

Some food-handling practices are so important that the federal government requires specific instructions or warnings on labels of certain foods. Following outbreaks of illness from *E. coli* O157:H7 in contaminated hamburger in 1993, the USDA mandated instructions on labels of raw meat and poultry to encourage consumers to follow recommendations for safe handling and cooking of these products.[32]

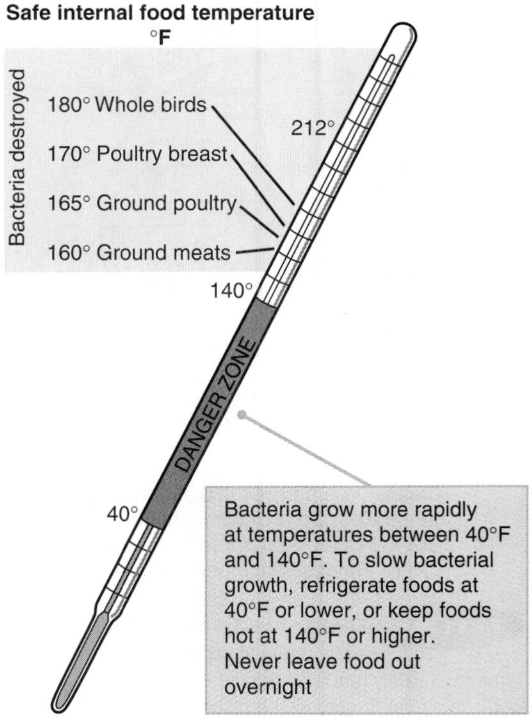
Safe internal food temperature
°F
Bacteria destroyed
180° Whole birds
170° Poultry breast
165° Ground poultry
160° Ground meats
212°
140°
DANGER ZONE
40°
Bacteria grow more rapidly at temperatures between 40°F and 140°F. To slow bacterial growth, refrigerate foods at 40°F or lower, or keep foods hot at 140°F or higher. Never leave food out overnight

Figure 14.7 **Temperature guide.** To prevent bacterial growth, keep hot food hot and cold food cold.

attacks on the World Trade Center and Pentagon and the anthrax assaults have increased the concern and vigilance of the United States and Canadian governments, who are acutely aware that public food and water supplies are among the most vulnerable avenues for terrorist attacks.

At ports of entry, food inspection facilities, and research labs and buildings, government personnel are at a heightened state of alert. To prevent the entry of animal or plant pests and diseases, they are carrying out intensified product and cargo inspections of travelers and baggage. Food safety inspectors have been given a mandate to be alert to any irregularities at food-processing facilities. Within processing facilities, specific plans for security should be developed. Such plans can be based on HACCP principles.[1]

What can consumers do to protect themselves from food contamination? We must be the final judges of the safety of the food we buy. At minimum we should:

1. Make sure the food package or can is intact before opening it. If it has been damaged or dented or opened prior to purchase, call it to the attention of the appropriate person.
2. Be alert to abnormal color, taste, and appearance of a food item. If you have any doubt, don't eat it.
3. If the food appears to be tampered with, report it immediately.
4. Follow safe food-handling practices. (See the FYI feature "Safe Food Practices.")

1 Bledsoe GE, Rasco BA. Addressing the risk of bioterrorism in food production. *Food Technol.* 2002;56(2):43–47.

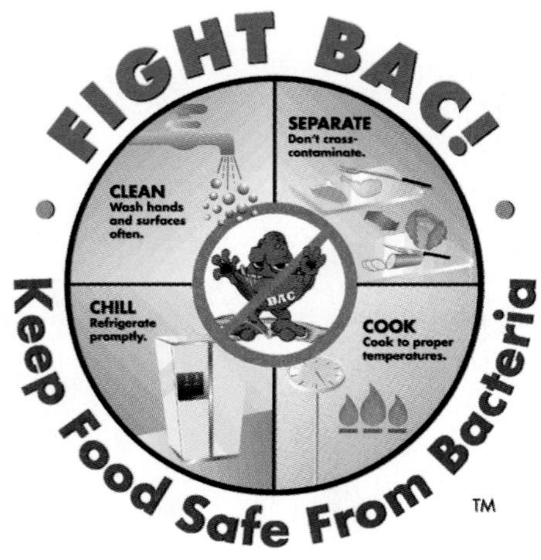

Clean: Wash hands and surfaces often
Separate: Don't cross-contaminate
Cook: Cook to proper temperatures
Chill: Refrigerate properly

Figure 14.8 Keeping harmful bacteria at bay. While our food supply generally is safe, home food safety practices are the weakest link in the food chain from farm to kitchen table. Be sure to follow the four basic practices: clean, separate, cook, and chill.

Because of a 1998 FDA rule, labels of unpasteurized or otherwise untreated packaged juice products carry a statement about the product's possible danger to children, older adults, and people with weakened immune systems.[33] The warning states that the product has not been pasteurized and therefore may contain harmful bacteria that can cause serious illness in these high-risk groups. This requirement was made after a number of people became seriously ill from drinking unpasteurized apple juice that was contaminated with *E. coli*.

In 2000 the FDA finalized rules requiring safe handling statements on egg cartons.[34] The proposed statement reads

> *SAFE HANDLING INSTRUCTIONS: To prevent illness from bacteria: keep eggs refrigerated, cook eggs until yolks are firm, and cook foods containing eggs thoroughly.*

Food manufacturers may voluntarily place other safe handling instructions on the label, such as proper cooking and storage of the item. Consumers should always follow these instructions.

Who's at Increased Risk for Foodborne Illness?

People with certain diseases and conditions need to be especially careful about following safe food practices. Their condition or the drugs they use may compromise their immune systems, making it more difficult for them to fight off infections. People who are at risk include those with these conditions:

- immune disorders, such as HIV infection
- cancer
- diabetes
- long-term steroid use, such as for asthma or arthritis
- liver disease
- hemochromatosis, an iron storage disorder that affects the liver
- stomach problems, including previous stomach surgery and low stomach acid (for example, from chronic antacid use)

Because these conditions are more common in older adults, seniors have an increased risk of foodborne illness. Young children do not have fully developed immune systems, so they are particularly vulnerable to serious illness from foodborne disease. Also, pregnant women and their fetuses are at special risk from the bacterium *Listeria monocytogenes* and the parasite *Toxoplasma gondii*. Both of these microorganisms can harm, even kill, fetuses and young babies.

Final Word on Food Safety

A totally risk-free system of food production is an unreasonable and unattainable goal. The United States and Canada enjoy a reputation as having food supplies that are among the safest in the world. We expect our food to be clean, fresh, and not contaminated with debris, chemicals, or organisms that cause sickness or discomfort. To make sure it stays that way, food safety experts are continually trying to ensure that every participant in the food production chain—from the farmer who produces the food to the manufacturer who processes it to the retailer who sells it and to the consumer who buys it—undertakes measures to help reduce and perhaps even elimi-

Quick Bites

How Good Are Your Food Safety Habits?

Do Americans practice food safety in their own kitchens? Apparently not. A study conducted by the FDA and the Centers for Disease Control and Prevention showed that one-half of people surveyed ate undercooked eggs in the past year. Twenty percent of people ate undercooked hamburger, and 25 percent of men and 14 percent of women failed to wash their hands with soap after handling raw meat.

nate foodborne disease. That's one reason food safety advice today is turning up in so many places—to ensure that everyone gets the word on food safety.

Key Concepts: *Consumers play a huge role in food safety. They can avoid foodborne illness by following a few simple food-handling and preparation rules: keep hands and food-preparation areas clean; avoid cross-contamination of foods; cook foods adequately; refrigerate foods promptly. People who have weak or less-developed immune systems are at higher risk for foodborne illnesses.*

Food Technology

At the start of the twenty-first century, technology is having a larger and larger impact on the food we eat. Our use of preservatives, other preservation techniques, and genetic engineering have implications for our food supply in the years to come and have triggered debates about their risks and benefits.

Food Preservation

In our modern society, few people grow their own vegetables, fruits, and grains, or keep livestock as a source of meat and milk. Rather, we shop for our food, typically at a large, full-service supermarket. Because we don't consume our food at the point of harvest or slaughter, we use food preservation methods to help maintain the quality of the foods we purchase. Among food preservation methods are the addition of chemical preservatives, canning or freezing, **pasteurization**, and more recent methods such as irradiation.

Preservatives

Preservatives are added to foods to prevent spoilage and increase shelf life. The most common antimicrobial agents are salt and sugar. Other preservatives, such as potassium sorbate and sodium propionate, extend the shelf life of baked goods and many other products. Antioxidants are a type of preservative that prevents the changes in color and flavor caused by exposure to air. Common antioxidants include vitamin C and vitamin E, sulfites, and BHA and BHT.

Preparation for Preservation

Some preservation techniques, such as salting and fermenting, date to ancient times and are still practiced along with their modern counterparts—freezing, canning, pasteurization, and the like. Salting, drying, or fermenting foods creates an environment in which bacteria cannot multiply and, therefore, cannot cause food spoilage. Canned foods are heated quickly to a temperature that kills microbes and then are sealed airtight to prevent both contamination and oxidative damage. Freezing temperatures not only keep bacteria from multiplying, but also prevent normal enzymatic changes in food that would cause spoilage. Pasteurization of milk or other beverages uses a very high temperature for a very short time to kill bacteria, but minimizes changes that would result from longer heating. The food industry and the North American public readily accept these food preservation methods. One of the most modern preservation techniques—irradiation—is also the most controversial, in part because of our fear of anything that has to do with radiation.

Quick Bites

Wood vs. Plastic: The Cutting Controversy

Which type of cutting board is safer to use while cutting meat: wood or plastic? They both have drawbacks. A wood cutting board tends to absorb bacteria, sucking them down into the wood fibers. This may be safer than a plastic board, which keeps bacteria on the surface, in an easy position to rub off onto food and other objects. But with use, wooden cutting boards tend to keep more on the surface than new wooden boards, acting more like plastic boards. What's the solution? Keep cutting boards clean by heating wooden boards in the microwave or putting plastic boards in the dishwasher.

pasteurization A process for destroying pathogenic bacteria by heating liquid foods to a prescribed temperature for a specified time.

preservatives Chemicals or other agents that slow the decomposition of a food.

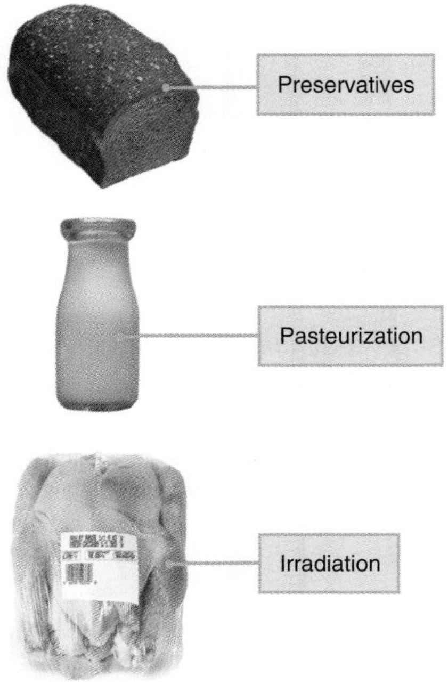

Preparing food for safe consumption.

irradiation A food preservation technique in which foods are exposed to measured doses of radiation to reduce or eliminate pathogens and kill insects, reduce spoilage, and, in certain fruits and vegetables, inhibit sprouting and delay ripening.

Quick Bites

Where Do *E. coli* Hang Out?

Ground beef is the most common source of *E. coli* bacteria, but *E. coli* also have been found on apples and lettuce.

Quick Bites

Bacteria at the Supermarket

Bacteria abound on the surface of supermarket meat. A piece of pork, on average, may harbor a few hundred bacteria per cubic centimeter, and a piece of chicken may have 10,000 in the same area.

Irradiation

Before it received official approval, food **irradiation** underwent over 40 years of scientific research and testing—more than any other food technology.[35] During irradiation, foods are exposed to a measured dose of radiation to reduce or eliminate pathogenic bacteria, including *E. coli* O157:H7, *Salmonella*, and *Campylobacter*, the chief causes of foodborne illness today.[36] Irradiation also can destroy insects and parasites, reduce spoilage, and inhibit sprouting and delay ripening of certain fruits and vegetables. Irradiation can reduce pathogens in raw poultry or meat by 99.9 percent.[37] Some people fear irradiation will make the food radioactive. This concern is unfounded. The energy used to irradiate foods passes through the food and leaves no residue—in the same way that microwaves pass through food. Despite its benefits, use of irradiation remains rare in North America.

Because food manufacturers fear consumer rejection, they have been reluctant to use irradiation on their products.[38] Some consumers and advocacy groups protest its use because they are concerned that irradiation may compromise a food's nutritional value and change its texture, taste, or appearance. According to the American Dietetic Association (ADA), the nutritive loss associated with irradiation is actually less than for most conventional methods of food preservation.[39] The ADA also states that at appropriate doses, irradiation of food does not significantly change its flavor, texture, or appearance. Many organizations, including the ADA, the American Medical Association, and the World Health Organization, endorse irradiation as a means of providing the public with a safer food supply.

The FDA has approved irradiation for

- spices and dry vegetable seasoning to decontaminate and control insects and microorganisms
- dry or dehydrated enzyme preparations to control insects and microorganisms
- fruits and vegetables to inhibit maturation
- poultry and red meat to control spoilage and pathogenic microorganisms
- all the foods above, to control insects, mites, and other arthropod pests

The FDA requires labels of irradiated foods to state that the product was "treated with irradiation" or "treated by irradiation" and display the international symbol for irradiation, the radura. (See **Figure 14.9**.) In May 2000, the USDA proposed the use of irradiation for fruits and vegetables imported into the United States in order to control fruit flies and mango seed weevil.

Some experts believe the time is right for food irradiation to become more widespread. News stories about deaths related to foodborne illness have made the public more aware of the need for protection against contamination of food. As more consumers become aware of the benefits of irradiation, the demand for irradiated foods is expected to increase. Studies have shown that education about irradiation significantly improves customers' attitudes.[40]

Key Concepts: *Various processing methods help protect us from contamination of food by pathogens. Drying, salting, canning, freezing, and pasteurizing are methods that consumers accept. Irradiation is a process in which foods are exposed to a*

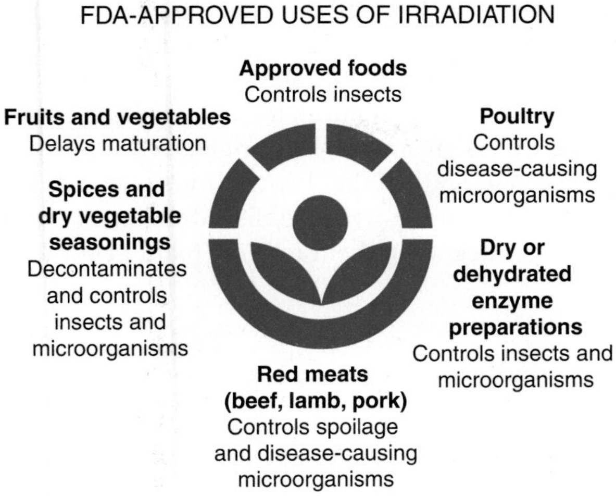

Figure 14.9 **Irradiation.** Irradiation can retard spoilage and reduce risk of foodborne illness.

measured dose of radiation to reduce or eliminate pathogenic bacteria. While government and professional organizations deem irradiation a safe procedure, consumers are still wary.

Genetically Modified Foods

Genetically modified (GM) foods have arrived, and most of us are already dining on them. When you prepare a dinner of broccoli and tofu, some of the soybeans used to make the tofu probably came from plants genetically modified to resist herbicide sprays or insect pests or both. And although your broccoli is currently "natural," you can be sure that in a lab somewhere genetically modified broccoli seeds are sprouting, perhaps with enhanced nutrient or other phytochemical levels. If you are eating tenderloin tonight, the steak probably came from a steer fed on genetically modified corn that had its DNA altered by the addition of foreign genes to allow the plant to resist insect pests and herbicides.

Should you be indignant that these new foods are showing up on your table without any indication on the label, or should you be grateful that these high-tech methods are keeping crop yields high and food costs low? An informed answer to this question requires some understanding of how genetic engineering works, how new crops and foods are regulated, and how gene modification of crops and animals differs from the classical methods of agricultural breeding that have been practiced for thousands of years.

Quick Bites

Biotechnology in the 1930s

One of the first examples of genetic theory successfully applied to food production was hybrid corn. When first introduced, it seemed miraculous and convinced skeptical farmers of the potential benefits of this emerging agricultural science. To this day, tougher and healthier new hybrids continue to outyield their predecessors.

A Short Course in Plant Genetics

How do GM food plants differ from those developed through traditional cross-pollination and hybridization? The answer, surprisingly, is that most crop modifications achieved by DNA manipulation and associated techniques of **biotechnology** could also be achieved with classical techniques, but the time scale and expense are very different.[41] (See **Figure 14.10**.)

The classical techniques for breeding a plant with new characteristics have been practiced for hundreds of years. They involve crossing two plants with different characteristics, then growing the resulting hybrid seeds and looking for plants with the desired combination of characteristics. Hybrid plants get half of their genes from one parent and half from the other. Though the hybrid may combine favorable qualities from both parents, a lot of undesir-

genetically modified (GM) foods Foods produced using plant or animal ingredients that have been modified using gene technology.

biotechnology The set of laboratory techniques and processes used to modify the genome of plants or animals and thus create desirable new characteristics. Genetic engineering in the broad sense.

genetic engineering Manipulation of the genome of an organism by artificial means for the purpose of modifying existing traits or adding new genetic traits.

genome The total genetic information of an organism, stored in the DNA of its chromosomes.

able genetic baggage must be sorted out after formation of such a hybrid. It usually takes dozens of additional crosses, and many years, to separate the desirable genes from the undesirable, and the process has a large element of chance. Due to human intervention, today virtually every domesticated crop plant species differs greatly from its original, wild form.[42]

Genetic engineering, on the other hand, allows scientists to transform a plant one gene at a time, using well-established methods for manipulating DNA sequences and integrating them into the plant **genome** (its set of

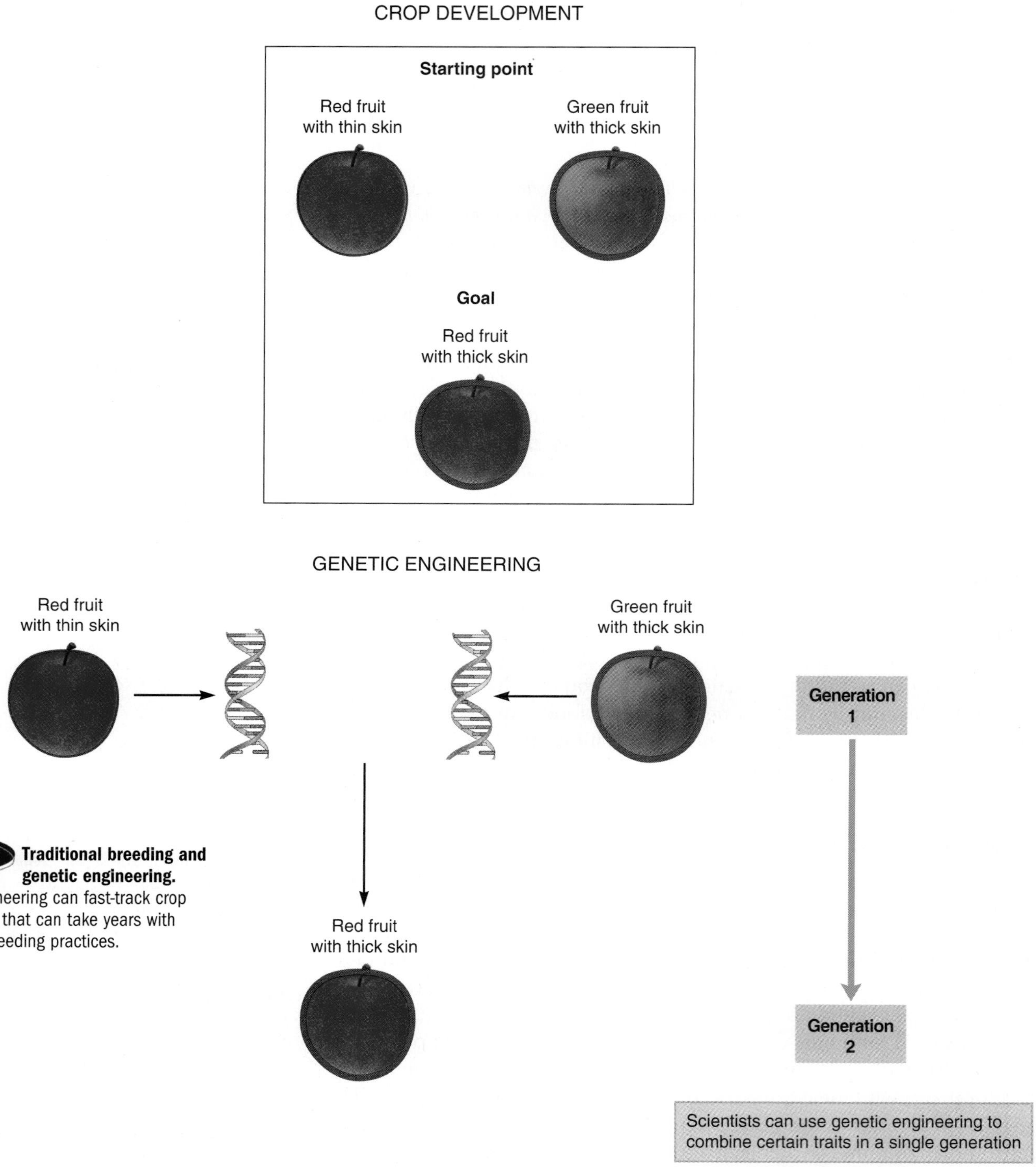

Figure 14.10 Traditional breeding and genetic engineering. Genetic engineering can fast-track crop development that can take years with traditional breeding practices.

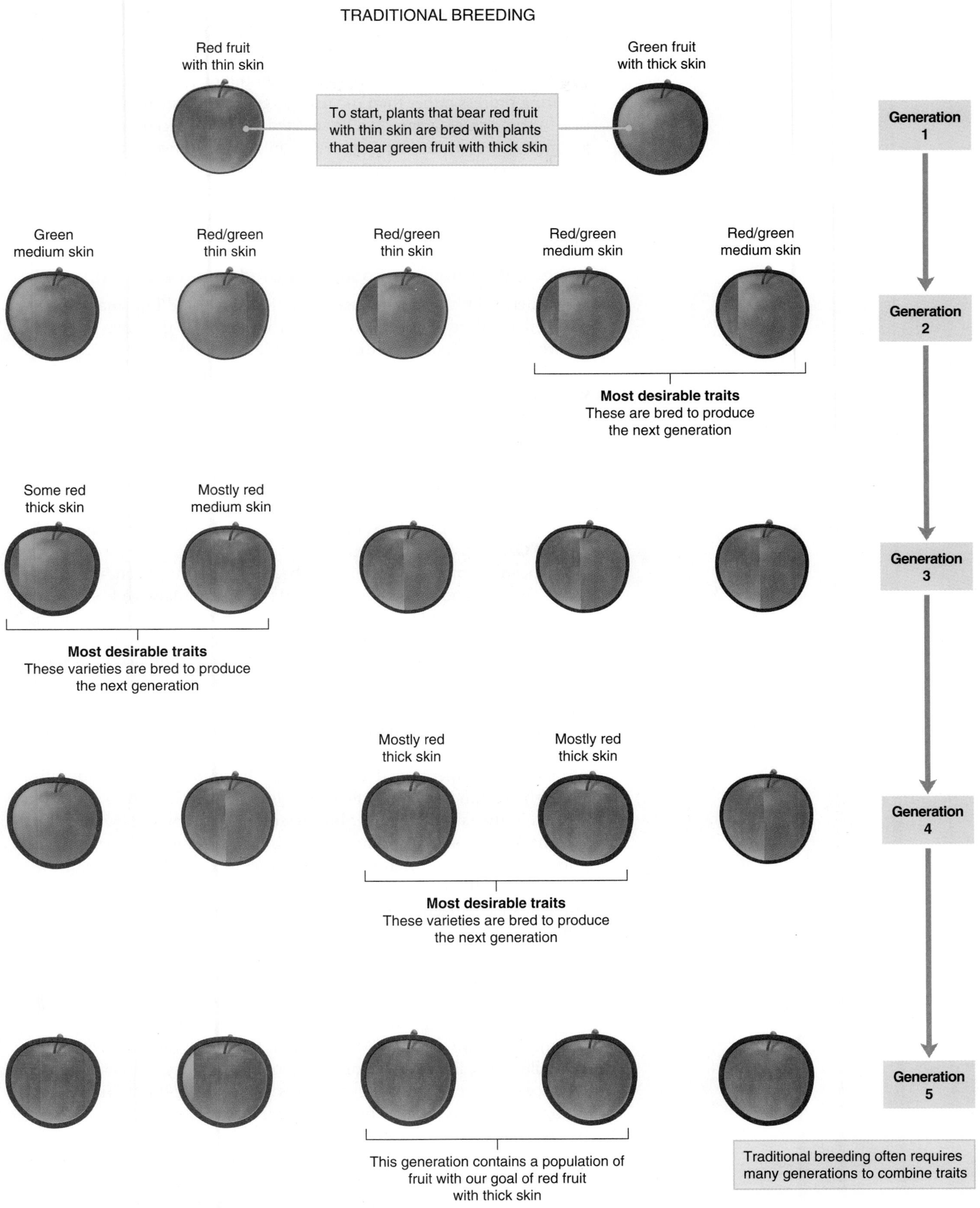
TRADITIONAL BREEDING
Red fruit with thin skin
To start, plants that bear red fruit with thin skin are bred with plants that bear green fruit with thick skin
Green fruit with thick skin
Generation 1
Green medium skin
Red/green thin skin
Red/green thin skin
Red/green medium skin
Red/green medium skin
Generation 2
Most desirable traits
These are bred to produce the next generation
Some red thick skin
Mostly red medium skin
Generation 3
Most desirable traits
These varieties are bred to produce the next generation
Mostly red thick skin
Mostly red thick skin
Generation 4
Most desirable traits
These varieties are bred to produce the next generation
Generation 5
This generation contains a population of fruit with our goal of red fruit with thick skin
Traditional breeding often requires many generations to combine traits

genes). Since many plant genes have already been identified, and complete DNA sequences of plant genomes will be available soon, we can anticipate that the genetic engineering of plants will become increasingly powerful and precise. Designing a new GM plant should come to resemble a manufacturing process rather than the tedious guessing game of classical genetics. In some cases, a gene can be selected and introduced into plant cells, and new GM seeds can be prepared within a year or two. When we consider that it took centuries of selection and breeding to transform the weedy wild maize plant of pre-Columbian Mexico into our modern varieties of corn, the scale and speed of the gene revolution in agriculture is both astounding and a little frightening.

Genetically Modified Foods: An Unstoppable Experiment?

How extensive is the shift to gene-modified crops, and how many different crops are involved? The United States produces more than two-thirds of the world's genetically modified crops, followed by Argentina (23 percent) and Canada (7 percent).[43] In the United States, about 50 percent of the soybean crop and over 33 percent of the cotton crop are genetically modified.[44] In addition to soybeans, the few types of genetically modified food crops in commercial production include corn, potatoes, and rapeseed (the source of canola oil). However, the amount of acreage involved is substantial, roughly equal to the land area of Oregon. The increased yields and lower costs associated with GM crops make them attractive to farmers. There is now strong, perhaps unstoppable, momentum to continue and expand GM crop plantings.

European countries, however, have been slow to accept gene-modified crops. They are concerned about possible ecological damage from such crops and fear potential unintended consequences of genetic "tampering" with the food supply. In 1999 the Gerber Products Company decided to stop using GM corn and soy in its baby foods. Heinz followed suit for its baby foods, and Frito-Lay has stopped using GM crops in its snack foods. While some consumer groups voice similar concerns, agribusiness and the U.S. federal government have been quite supportive of the trend toward GM foods.

The GM crops mentioned above are just the tip of the genetic modification iceberg; hundreds more are under development in university laboratories and in the labs of giant agribusinesses like Monsanto, Novartis, and DuPont. The goals of these modifications are higher yields, increased amounts of critical nutrients, and a healthier mix of plant oils. Many of these goals would be achievable with classical selection techniques; but with genetic engineering, they move from laboratory to table in decades, rather than centuries.

Genetic engineering also has affected the food-processing industry. The cheese-making industry uses genetically modified bacteria to produce the widely used enzyme chymosin. Chymosin has virtually replaced the natural milk-clotting enzyme rennet, which is extracted from the stomachs of calves.

In the future we will see GM plants that have been modified to yield better textile fibers, including colored cotton, or specialized proteins for use in human pharmaceuticals—or even plants that produce the starting materials for manufacture of plastics. In economic terms, these nonfood GM crops may become even more important than GM foods.

If only plant genes were involved in GM food production, there would be much less controversy. However, *any* gene, including genes from bacteria and animals, can be introduced into a plant genome. Some people find this frightening, and an imaginative term, *Frankenfoods*, has been coined to express the "unnatural" nature of some GM products. But how unnatural is the exchange of DNA between species? It may be reassuring to realize that organisms have been swapping DNA for eons, with no help from humans. Foreign DNA can be carried from one species to another by a variety of viruses, for example. Nature has already performed millions of "gene modifications" on its own, and exchange of DNA is an established part of the evolutionary process. Now that we can do our own experiments with DNA manipulation, we hope the benefits will be increased.

Benefits of Genetic Engineering

Whatever the risks, no one can argue with the success of these GM techniques. For instance, a bacterial gene was used to create Monsanto's new insect-resistant varieties of corn, potatoes, and soybeans. This gene, the **Bt gene**, was taken from the soil bacterium *Bacillus thuringiensis*. When inserted into a plant genome, the Bt gene directs the production of a protein in the plant that makes the plant toxic to insects. Such crops have been extremely successful and produce high yields without use of insecticides.

Bt-modified crops, which are now grown in the United States over an area larger than Rhode Island, are a boon to both the economy and the environment. Because chemical insecticides are not necessary, many benign insects are spared, and insect **biodiversity** is preserved. Similarly, other plants can be genetically modified to resist the effects of common herbicides. Chemical sprays that are lethal to most plant life have no effect on these GM plants. The crop plant grows larger in the absence of weeds, and the farmer gets a better yield with less effort and expense.

Bt gene *Bacillus thuringiensis* (Bt) is a bacterium that produces a protein called the Bt toxin. One of the bacterium's genes, the Bt gene, carries the information for the Bt toxin. Inserting a copy of the Bt gene into plants enables them to produce Bt toxin protein and resist some insect pests. The Bt protein is not toxic to humans.

biodiversity The countless species of plants, animals, and insects that exist on the earth. An undisturbed tropical forest is an example of the biodiversity of a healthy ecosystem.

The economic benefits of GM foods are clearly substantial. Increased yields of important food plants can help feed increasing populations without the need for putting more land under the plow or increasing the use of toxic insecticides. In the coming century, this may be the difference between starvation and adequate nutrition in many developing countries.

It is easy to imagine how manipulation of plant amino acids and plant oils could yield superior foods, which not only would be able to satisfy calorie requirements, but also would address protein and vitamin needs. A strain of rice, genetically modified to be rich in beta-carotene, could benefit the more than a million children in developing countries who die or are weakened by vitamin A deficiency.[45] In developed countries, where heart disease and cancer loom as greater risks than malnutrition, the ability to adjust the saturation level of plant lipids or to boost beneficial phytochemicals would be of great value to public health. But do these undoubted benefits outweigh the risks?

Think About It 4

Risks

What are the specific risks of GM foods? Many consumers are concerned about whether these new foods are safe to eat. The answer to this concern is a fairly unequivocal yes. When a new protein or other substance is introduced into a food, the FDA requires substantial testing to demonstrate its safety. With GM foods, the principal risk appears to be the possibility of introducing a new allergen into a GM food.[46] To be cautious, the FDA has focused on allergy issues. Under the law and the FDA's biotech food policy, companies must tell consumers on the food label when a product includes a gene from a food that commonly causes an allergic reaction. The only exception is when the company can show that the protein produced by the added gene does not make the genetically modified food cause allergies.[47]

Of greater concern, and more difficult to predict, are environmental effects, though no ecological disasters have occurred thus far. What if the Bt-containing plants lead to the development of insects resistant to Bt-modified plants and to other insecticides? Would the appearance of Bt-resistant insects spell the doom of a large portion of our crops of soybeans or maize? In a study of Bt cotton plants, scientists estimated that 1 in 350 pests carried resistance to the Bt gene,[48] but further research shows that genetic engineering can also be used to overcome or at least delay development of Bt resistance.[49] Scientists suggest that planting a certain percentage of normal plants alongside the Bt-modified plants should delay the appearance of such resistant mutants. If populations of such mutants became significant, farmers could fall back on conventional pest-control techniques. Meanwhile, we could have better crop yields with a reduction in pesticide use.

A related concern is the development of herbicide-resistant weeds, or "superweeds." When herbicide-resistant crops are planted in proximity to related wild plants, pollen may drift from food plant to weed, and the resistant genes might be passed to the weedy cousins of the GM plants. In the presence of herbicide, this might lead to the rapid selection of herbicide-resistant weeds. Although transfer of the herbicide-resistant gene to a related weed can occur, so far the effects have been minor, and the "superweeds" have rapidly lost the resistance gene once the herbicide was removed.

A final concern is that the herbicide-resistant food plants may become so successful that they are planted over a vast acreage in developing countries and sprayed with excessive amounts of herbicides. In the worst scenario, this could lead to a loss of many species of unmodified plants as well as the insect and animal communities that depend on them. Many scientists feel that the loss of biodiversity is one of the greatest threats to the planet today. Because of the complexity and interdependence of the biosphere, this is perhaps the greatest unknown and the greatest danger of unmonitored use of GM crops. **Table 14.4** summarizes current concerns and scientific research areas.

Table 14.4 GM Concerns and Current Research

1. GM crops will hurt innocent creatures.

Will crops engineered to contain insecticides harm nondestructive species important to biodiversity? While laboratory studies show that genetic modifications to plants can harm nontarget insects, such as monarch butterflies, field studies suggest the risk is small.

2. GM crops will lead to the emergence of superweeds.

Will genetic modifications that give crops the ability to kill insect pests or withstand certain herbicides migrate to weeds? Almost every crop has weedy relatives somewhere in the world. Despite anecdotal reports, studies have not found superweeds. Yet to avoid pollen spreading from modified genes to weeds, scientists warn that GM crops should not be grown near weedy relatives.

3. GM crops will have sudden failures.

Will target insect pests become tolerant to insecticides in GM plants and will weeds become immune to herbicides sprayed on herbicide-resistant GM crops? Could these threats become unstoppable? While there are no documented GM crop failures, scientists believe they are likely. Are current prevention measures adequate? Critics and proponents disagree.

Regulation

The FDA regulates foods and food safety, and it oversees genetically modified foods as well as conventional foods. For foods derived from new varieties of plants, the FDA takes the position that whether modified by traditional breeding or genetic engineering, testing for safe human consumption is the legal responsibility of the producer or manufacturer of the foods. Crops like Bt-modified soybeans do not require special testing, labeling, or FDA approval. Although the plant expresses the Bt protein, the beans do not contain it. Except for some foreign DNA sequences, the beans are identical to unmodified soybeans. However, when a new substance is added to a food, FDA review and approval are necessary. Thus, if a new substance is produced or introduced into a food by genetic means, it must be tested as though it were a food additive. (See Chapter 3, "Complementary Nutrition: Functional Foods and Dietary Supplements.")

Some consumer groups are pushing for mandatory labeling of GM foods. They believe consumers have the right to know if a food is bioengineered. Other groups desire labeling so they can adhere to cultural or religious beliefs that may ban certain animal foods. Because the FDA believes the way a food is developed or produced is irrelevant information, current FDA policy does not require labeling of GM foods. In its 1992 policy statement "Foods Derived from New Plant Varieties," the FDA describes four situations where changes in labels would be important to "reveal all material facts about the food":

- if a bioengineered food is significantly different from its traditional counterpart, such that the common or usual name no longer adequately describes the food, the name must be changed to describe the difference;
- if an issue exists for the food or a constituent of the food regarding how the food is used or consequences of its use, a statement must be made on the labeling to describe the issue;
- if a bioengineered food has a significantly different nutritional property, its labeling must reflect the difference;
- if a new food includes an allergen that consumers would not expect to be present based on the name of the food, the presence of that allergen must be disclosed in the labeling.[50]

In its 2001 draft guidance for industry regarding voluntary labeling, FDA asked for comments on how the terms "biotech free," "GM free," or "no genetically engineered materials" could be used without being false or misleading, and how these claims could be substantiated.[51] Considering that most, if not all, food crops have been genetically modified in some way, it would be very difficult to have a completely "GM" free food. Also, saying that a food or ingredient is not bioengineered may be misleading if there are no marketed bioengineered foods of that type. Before finalizing any further policy on labeling of foods that contain genetically engineered ingredients, additional work clearly needs to be done.

Similar to U.S regulations, Health Canada requires special labeling for genetically modified foods where there is a potential for allergic reactions, and a different name must be used for a GM food that is different in composition or nutritional value. Voluntary positive ("does contain") and voluntary negative ("does not contain") labeling is permitted provided the statements are factual and not misleading or deceptive.[52]

The generally conservative approach of the FDA is based on decades of experience with food plants, which contain thousands of different substances. The plants we eat every day produce a variety of compounds that, if eaten in sufficient quantity, are toxic to humans. Potatoes, for instance, produce variable amounts of solanine, a fairly toxic alkaloid. These naturally occurring toxins may be inadvertently increased by classical breeding, so monitoring levels of toxins in plants is neither new nor unusual.

If there are unexpected consequences of gene modification, the FDA is in an excellent position to evaluate them and alter food-testing procedures where necessary. Many groups, from government agencies like the FDA to professional organizations like the ADA to consumer advocacy groups, are monitoring developments in biotechnology. Web sites for these organizations can be a source of policy statements and breaking news in this area. Regardless of our views on genetic manipulation of food plants, research and development will continue. It remains to be seen how consumers will accept new GM foods in the coming years.

Key Concepts: *Genetic engineering allows scientists to transform a plant one gene at a time, using well-established methods for manipulating DNA sequences. The goals of genetic modification of foods are higher yields, lower costs, increased amounts of critical nutrients, and a healthier mix of plant oils. Because of the complexity and interdependence of the biosphere, loss of genetic biodiversity is perhaps the greatest unknown and the greatest danger of unmonitored GM crops.*

LEARNING Portfolio chapter 14

Key Terms

Term	page
aflatoxins	569
biodiversity	583
biotechnology	579
botulism	559
Bt gene	583
ciguatera	569
critical control points (CCP)	573
dioxins	569
Escherichia coli (E. coli)	561
Food Allergy & Anaphylaxis Network	570
Food Code	574
Food Safety Initiative	573
foodborne illness	558
genetic engineering	580
genetically modified (GM) foods	579
genome	580
Hazard Analysis Critical Control Point (HACCP)	573
integrated pest management (IPM)	566
irradiation	578
methyl mercury	569
natural toxins	569
organic foods	564
pasteurization	577
pesticides	564
poisonous mushrooms	570
pollutants	569
preservatives	577
Safe Tables Our Priority (S.T.O.P.)	573
Salmonella	561
solanine	570

Study Points

- Foodborne illness is extremely common; it affects millions of Americans each year. Estimates of the frequency of foodborne illness are difficult because the vast majority of foodborne illnesses go unreported.
- The incidence of foodborne illness may be on the rise in the United States and Canada. Many factors are responsible, including the increased centralization of food preparation, food imports, an increasing population of especially susceptible individuals (such as the elderly and those with weakened immune systems), and failure of consumers and retail establishments to follow appropriate food safety measures.
- Microorganisms cause most foodborne diseases in the United States and Canada. Most of these illnesses are preventable.
- *Staphylococcus aureus* is one of the most common causes of foodborne illness. Onset of illness is rapid, typically occurring between 30 minutes and a few hours after consuming the contaminated food.
- Common symptoms of foodborne illness are diarrhea, nausea, abdominal cramps, and sometimes fever. The severity of the illness depends on the type of organism and the amount of contaminant eaten.
- Ensuring a safe food supply is a farm-to-table continuum involving producers, manufacturers, retailers, and consumers.
- Pesticides, animal drugs, natural toxins, and pollutants are the major forms of chemical food contamination.
- The government monitors imported and domestic foods for pesticide residues by testing food samples for both amounts and types of pesticides. Efforts are under way to reduce the allowable amounts of certain pesticides to avoid harm to infants and children.
- The FDA evaluates drugs used in food-producing animals for safety in both animals and humans. Overuse of animal antibiotics could contribute to the emergence of antibiotic-resistant microorganisms that could threaten human health.
- The government and the food industry use the Hazard Analysis Critical Control Point system to prevent food contamination.
- Consumers must take responsibility for food safety in their homes. Cleaning hands and surfaces, avoiding cross-contamination, cooking adequately, and refrigerating foods promptly are important steps that prevent foodborne illness.
- Food preservation techniques inhibit growth of microorganisms. Canning, drying, freezing, fermentation, and pasteurization are common.

- Although the FDA has approved food irradiation for numerous uses, it is rarely used, mostly because of consumer fears. Food irradiation does not make foods radioactive. It can kill insects and most microorganisms. Appropriate doses of radiation extend the shelf life of many foods.
- Genetically modified (GM) foods are most likely already on your table. Soybeans, corn, and potatoes are some of the GM foods being commercially produced. Concerns about GM foods include worries about decreasing biodiversity and the development of herbicide-resistant weeds.

Study Questions

Answers can be found at nutrition.jbpub.com/discovering.

1. **What are the two main ways that pathogenic bacteria can cause foodborne illness?**
2. **Why shouldn't your 97-year-old great-grandmother drink homemade eggnog made from raw eggs?**
3. **How can you limit your intake of pesticides, according to the Consumers Union?**
4. **List four naturally occurring toxins.**
5. **List the most common food allergens. What are some symptoms of a food allergy?**
6. **What does "HACCP" stand for and what is its purpose?**
7. **The home kitchen can be a breeding ground for pathogenic bacteria; what are some ways to keep food safe at home?**
8. **List the most common food preservation techniques.**
9. **What are three major concerns about genetically engineered crops?**

[Try] This

Bacterial Detective

What sources of bacteria do you encounter in your everyday activities? Here's an experiment to find out.

First, you'll need ...

Cotton swabs

Six or more Petri dishes with agar

If you are unable to obtain a set of agar-filled Petri dishes from your school or local health department, you can make your own culture medium. Here's how:

- Add 2 teaspoons of unflavored gelatin (1 packet) and 2 teaspoons of sugar to $^2/_3$ cup of water.
- Bring the solution to a boil and stir for 1 minute until everything is dissolved. Pour $^1/_4$ inch of the solution into each Petri dish or other suitable container.

Then, using separate Petri dishes,

1. Pluck a hair and lay it in one Petri dish, labeled "Hair."
2. Sneeze or cough into another Petri dish, labeled "Cough."
3. Run a cotton swab around a nostril and carefully zigzag it across the agar in another Petri dish, labeled "Nose."
4. Run a cotton swab across a dampened kitchen sink sponge and carefully zigzag it across the agar in another Petri dish, labeled "Sponge."
5. Run a cotton swab around a clean kitchen countertop and carefully zigzag it across the agar in another Petri dish, labeled "Countertop."
6. Use the same procedure to collect additional samples from any other area in which bacteria may be present.
7. Finally, store the Petri dishes in a warm environment, at a constant temperature around 80°F. Check your specimens periodically. Within a week, you should see something growing!

Organic Foods

Organic foods are increasing in popularity. Are organic foods widely available in your neighborhood? What types of organic produce can you find? Go to either a natural food store or the local grocery store and look at the array of organic produce. Compare the prices of organic produce and nonorganic produce. Do you think the cost differences outweigh possible benefits? Compare the look of the organic and nonorganic produce. Do you see any differences? What other organic products can you find?

References

1 Mead PS, Slutsker L, Dietz V, et al. Food-related illness and death in the United States. *Emerg Infect Dis.* 1999;5:607–625; and Preliminary FoodNet data on the incidence of foodborne illnesses—selected sites, United States, 2000. *MMWR.* 2002;51(15):325–329.

2 US Environmental Protection Agency and US Departments of Health and Human Services and Agriculture. *Food Safety from Farm to Table: A National Food-Safety Initiative.* Washington, DC: FDA;1997.

3 Institute of Food Technologists. Emerging microbiological food safety issues: implications for control in the 21st century. http://www.ift.org/govtrelations/microfs. Accessed 5/11/02.

4 Ibid.

5 Position of the American Dietetic Association: food and water safety. *J Am Diet Assoc.* 1997;97:184–189.

6 Advance notice of proposed rulemaking. *Salmonella enteritidis* in eggs. *Federal Register.* 1998;63:27502–27511.

7 US Food and Drug Administration Pesticide Program. *Residue Monitoring 1999.* Washington, DC: April 2000. 13th annual report.

8 Ibid.

9 Ibid.

10 Food Quality Protection Act: Title III of Public Law 104–170; 1996.

11 Consumers Union. *Do You Know What You're Eating? Pesticide Residues in Food:* Yonkers, NY: Consumers Union of United States; 1999.

12 Ibid.

13 Sloan AE. The natural and organic foods marketplace. *Food Technol.* 2002;56(1):27–37.

14 US Department of Agriculture. Labeling and marketing information: National Organic Program fact sheet. Washington, DC; March 2000.

15 US Department of Agriculture. National Organic Program, Agricultural Marketing Service; June 2000.

16 Worthington V. Nutritional quality of organic versus conventional fruits, vegetables, and grains. *J Altern Complement Med.* 2001;7(2):161–173.

17 Greener greens? *Consumer Reports.* January 1998:12–18.

18 US Department of Agriculture. National Organic Program, Op. cit.; and US Department of Agriculture. Questions and answers about the National Organic Program proposed rule. Washington, DC: USDA; December 1997.

19 Institute of Medicine, Committee on Drug Use in Food Animals. *The Use of Drugs in Food Animals: Benefits and Risks.* Washington, DC: National Academy Press; 1999.

20 US Food and Drug Administration. FDA stops distribution of some eggs and catfish because of dioxin-contaminated animal feed. http://www.cfsan.fda.gov/~lrd/hhsdiox.html. Accessed 5/11/02.

21 Schecter A, Cramer P, Boggess K, et al. Intake of dioxins and related compounds from food in the U.S. population. *J Toxicol Environ Health A.* 2001;63:1–18.

22 US Food and Drug Administration. *Foodborne Pathogenic Microorganisms and Natural Toxins Handbook.* Washington, DC: FDA; 1992.

23 Segal M. Stalking the wild mushroom. *FDA Consumer.* October 1994;20–24.

24 US Food and Drug Administration. *Foodborne Pathogenic Microorganisms and Natural Toxins Handbook.* Op. cit.

25 The Food Allergy & Anaphylaxis Network. Common food allergens. http://www.foodallergy.org/allergens.html. Accessed 5/11/02.

26 US Environmental Protection Agency and US Departments of Health and Human Services and Agriculture. Op. cit.

27 Ibid.

28 Pathogen reduction: Hazard Analysis and Critical Control Point (HACCP) systems; final rule. *Federal Register.* 1996;61: 38805–38989.

29 Hazard Analysis and Critical Control Point (HAACP): procedures for the safe and sanitary processing and importing of juice; final rule. *Federal Register.* 2001;66:6137–6202.

30 US Department of Health and Human Services, Food and Drug Administration. *Food Code.* Washington, DC: FDA; 1997.

31 Partnership for Food Safety Education. Fight BAC! Four simple steps to food safety. http://www.fightbac.org. Accessed 5/11/02.

32 US Department of Agriculture. USDA issues final rule on safe handling labels for meat and poultry products. Press release 0860.93; October 8, 1993.

33 Food labeling: warning and notice statement: labeling of juice products; final rule. *Federal Register.* 1998;63:37029–37056.

34 Food labeling, safe handling statements, labeling of shell eggs; refrigeration of shell eggs held for retail distribution, final rule. *Federal Register.* 2000;65:76091–76114.

35 Wood OB, Bruhn CM. Position of the American Dietetic Association: food irradiation. *J Am Diet Assoc.* 2000;100: 246–253.

36 US Environmental Protection Agency and US Departments of Health and Human Services and Agriculture. Op. cit.

37 Wood OB, Bruhn CM. Op. cit.

38 Henkle J. Irradiation: a safe measure for safer food. *FDA Consumer,* May/June 1998.

39 Wood OB, Bruhn CM. Op. cit.

40 Pohlman A, Wood OB, Mason AC. Influence of audiovisuals and food samples on consumer acceptance of food irradiation. *Food Technol.* 1994;48(12):46–49.

41 Henkle J. Genetic engineering: fast forwarding to future foods. *FDA Consumer.* February 1998 update.

42 Formanek R Jr. Proposed rules issued for bioengineered foods. *FDA Consumer.* March–April 2001;35:9–11.

43 Brown K. Seeds of concern. *Scientific American.* April 2001;284: 52–61.

44 Overseeing biotech foods. *Genetic Engineering News.* 2000; 20(10):1,37.

45 Nash MJ. Grains of hope. *Time.* July 31, 2000;39–46; and Greger JL. Response: genetically engineered "golden" rice unlikely to overcome vitamin A deficiency. *J Am Diet Assoc.* 2001;101: 289–290.

46 Shewry PR, Tatham AS, Halford NG. Genetic modification and plant food allergies. *J Chromatogr B Biomed Sci Appl.* 2001;756:327–335; and Taylor SL, Hefle SL. Will genetically modified foods be allergenic? *J Allergy Clin Immunol.* 2001; 107:765–771.

47 Thompson. L. Are bioengineered foods safe? *FDA Consumer.* Jan/Feb 2000.

48 Gould F, Anderson A, Jones A, et al. Initial frequency of alleles for resistance to *Bacillus thuringiensis* toxins in field populations of *Heliothis virescens. Proc Natl Acad Sci.* 1997;94: 3519–3523.

49 Kota M, Daniell H, Varma S, et al. Overexpression of the *Bacillus thuringiensis* (Bt) Cry2Aa2 protein in chloroplasts confers resistance to plants against susceptible and Bt-resistant insects. *Proc Natl Acad Sci.* 1999;96:1840–1845.

50 Statement of policy: foods derived from new plant varieties. *Federal Register.* 1992;57:22984.

51 Draft guidance for industry: voluntary labeling indicating whether foods have or have not been developed using bioengineering: availability. *Federal Register.* 2001;66:4839–4842.

52 Health Canada. Novel foods (GMF). http://www.hc-sc.gc.ca/english/protection/novel_foods.html. Accessed 5/11/02.

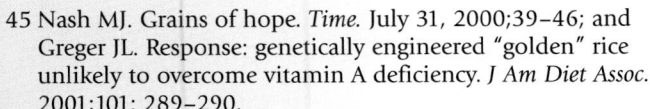

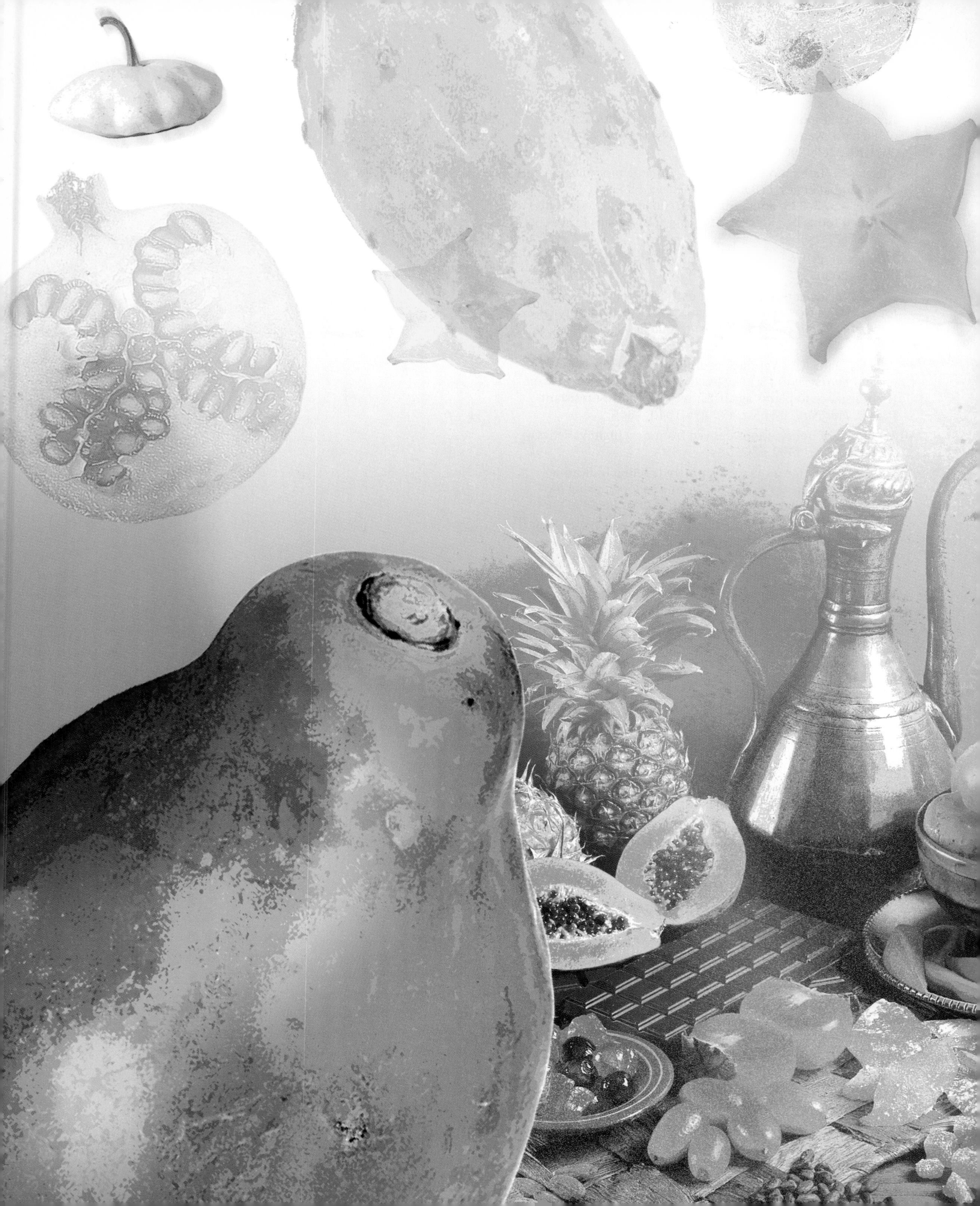

Chapter 15

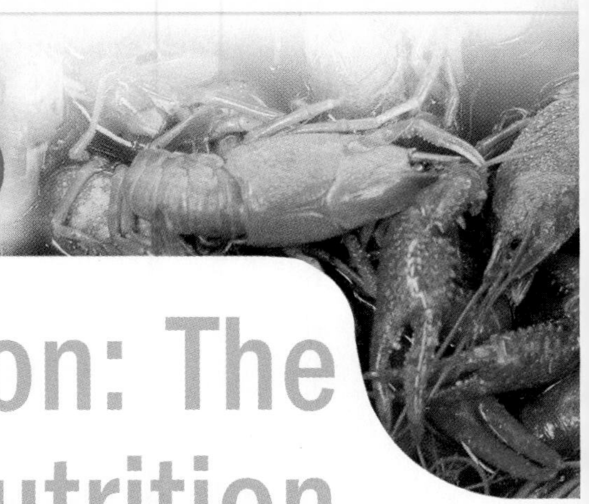

World View of Nutrition: The Faces of Global Malnutrition

Think About It

1. Have you ever experienced hunger without being able to satisfy it within a day?
2. Have you seen evidence of hunger or malnutrition in your community?
3. What can you do to help eliminate hunger in North America?
4. How do you feel about the United States sending food to impoverished nations?

Fyi for your Information

This chapter's FYI boxes include practical information on the following topics:

- Hungry and Homeless
- AIDS and Malnutrition
- Tough Choices

www

The Web site for this book offers many useful tools and is a great source for additional nutrition information for both students and instructors. For information on the world view of nutrition, visit the site at **nutrition.jbpub.com/discovering.** You'll find exercises that explore the following topics:

- The ADA and World Hunger
- U.S. Food Insecurity
- Individual Actions Count
- UNICEF

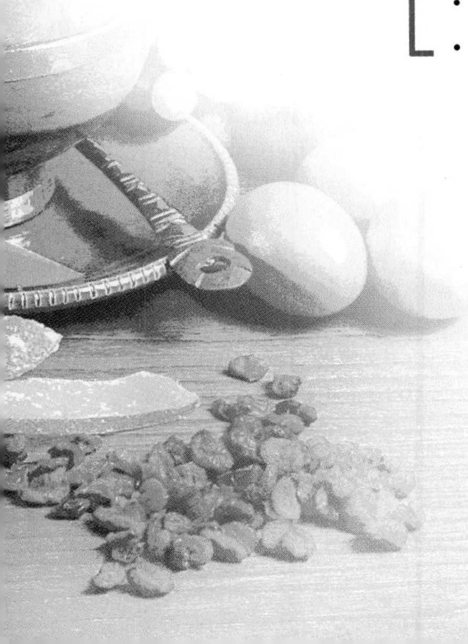

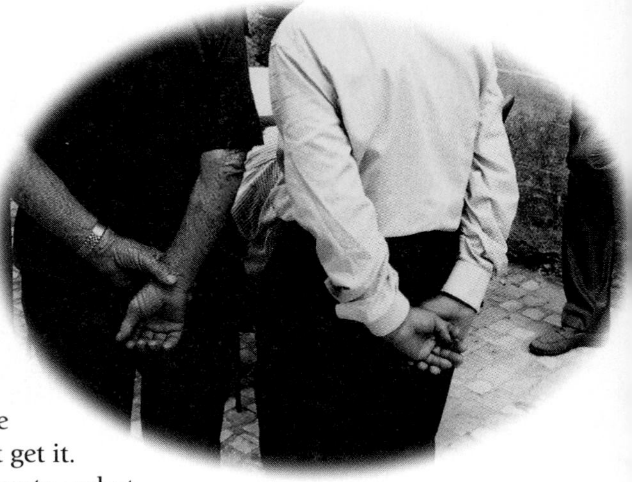

Each day on your way to class, you pass a soup kitchen. You look at the long line of men and women waiting to get their meals and wonder what brought them to this point. You wonder how many similar soup lines exist in your community and how many people need food assistance but can't get it. If **hunger** exists in our rich country, what about people living in poor countries?

hunger The uneasy or painful sensation caused by a lack of food; the recurrent and involuntary lack of access to food that may produce malnutrition over time.

malnutrition Failure to achieve nutrient requirements, which can impair physical and/or mental health. It may result from consuming too little food or a shortage or imbalance of key nutrients.

food insecurity (1) Limited or uncertain availability of nutritionally adequate and safe foods or (2) limited or uncertain ability to acquire acceptable foods in socially acceptable ways.

food security Access to enough food for an active, healthy life, including (1) the ready availability of nutritionally adequate and safe foods and (2) an assured ability to acquire acceptable foods in socially acceptable ways.

Almost 800 million people in the developing world do not have enough to eat. Another 34 million in industrialized countries worry regularly about having enough food.[1] And every day 35,000 people die, directly or indirectly, from **malnutrition**.[2]

In this chapter, we look at hunger and malnutrition. By *hunger* we don't mean that mildly empty feeling one gets before mealtime. We mean the inability, day after day, to satisfy basic nutrition needs, the gnawing emptiness that creates a constant focus on eating and how to obtain food. In contrast to the hunger dieters feel from cutting calories, this deprivation is involuntary and unwanted.

Technically speaking, *malnutrition* can be any kind of unhealthy nutritional status, including the result of imbalance and excess—obesity or toxicity from oversupplementation, for example. And although we touch on obesity as an emerging issue, even in developing countries, by and large in this chapter *malnutrition* means undernutrition resulting from hunger.

Along the spectrum of malnutrition and hunger is the less extreme condition of **food insecurity**, the ongoing worry about having enough to eat. At the opposite end of the spectrum is **food security**, access to nutritionally adequate and safe food. Most people in the industrialized world are food-secure. Overabundance and obesity are the primary problems in these populations, but malnutrition is a serious problem among certain groups such as the homeless and urban poor.

Malnutrition in the United States

The Face of American Malnutrition

In the food-rich United States, food insecurity remains a problem.[3] (See **Figure 15.1**.) It is characterized by anxiety about having enough to eat and about running out of food and having no money to purchase more. Some people actually go hungry in the United States: Almost 10 million people, over a third of them children, lived in a household in which at least one person experienced hunger during 1998.[4]

Households that are struggling to meet basic food needs tend to follow a typical pattern as their plight worsens. First, adults worry about having enough food. Then, they stretch resources and juggle other necessities, with more of the budget going for fixed expenses than for food. The quality and variety of the diet decline. Next, the adults eat less and less often. And finally, as food becomes more limited, the children also eat less. Think About It 1

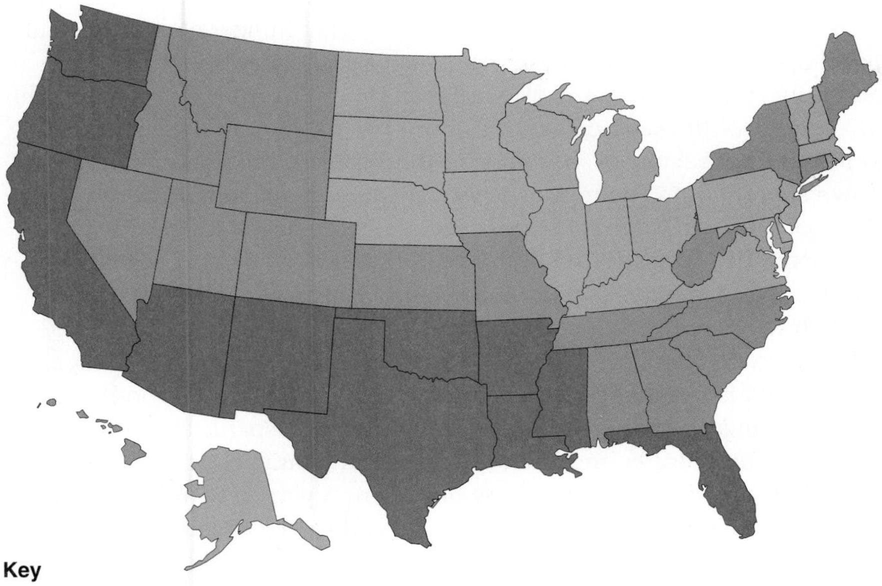

Figure 15.1 **Prevalence of food insecurity.** The National Health and Nutrition Examination Survey (NHANES III) found that food insecurity is as common among the working poor as the unemployed. Food insecurity is more common in southern and western states.
Source: Calculated by USDA Economic Research Service (ERS) based on Current Population Survey Food Security Supplement data, September 1996, April 1997, and August 1998.

Surprisingly, there is more obesity among low-income, food-insecure groups than among those with higher incomes. But the quality of those low-income diets is typically poor, and worsening food insecurity is accompanied by progressively more disordered eating patterns. Patterns such as binge eating can become habitual and contribute to obesity.[5]

Those who live in a state of food insecurity consume significantly fewer healthful foods and micronutrients. Although such suboptimal diets usually do not lead to overt deficiency diseases, more subtle effects are serious and costly, showing up years later as chronic illness or more immediately as reduced immune function. More illness, more medicines, more doctor visits and hospital stays, more missed days and poorer performance at school and work, poor pregnancy outcome, delayed growth and development—suboptimal nutrition contributes to them all.

Prevalence and Distribution

How much hunger and food insecurity exist in the United States? Until recently, it was difficult to measure. Estimates were based on the percentage of the population living in poverty, with the assumption that they were at risk of undernutrition. Such estimates are somewhat flawed because being *at risk* does not necessarily mean that people are poorly nourished. Many people with limited financial resources manage to eat well. On the other hand, under certain circumstances, such as loss of a

Food Recovery and Gleaning

Each year more than 96 billion pounds of food produced in this country go to waste. Programs throughout the country are rescuing much of this wholesome food and distributing it to people in need. "Gleaning" is harvesting excess food from farms, orchards, and packing houses. Perishable items are also salvaged from wholesale and retail markets; fresh foods that are wholesome but will spoil before they can be sold are given to local food pantries and meal providers. Canned goods and other staples are collected from groceries, distributors, food processors, and individual homes. Even surplus food from restaurants, caterers, and other food services is collected by some charities for local food programs.

job, people who live well above the poverty line (see **Table 15.1**) may be food-insecure.

In 1995 the U.S. Census Bureau began tracking hunger with an annual **Food Security Supplement Survey**, which asks about food availability and hunger in the household. (See **Table 15.2**.) From 1996 through 1998, 9.7 percent of households worried about having enough to eat, and 3.5 percent of households also experienced hunger.[6] These findings were down slightly from findings of 1995.[7] The figures are consistent with those of the large National Health and Nutrition Examination Survey (NHANES III), in which 3.5 percent of households reported not having enough to eat *sometimes*, and 0.6 percent said they *often* did not have enough to eat.[8]

Food Security Supplement Survey A federally funded survey that measures the prevalence and severity of food insecurity and hunger.

Personal Responsibility and Work Opportunity Reconciliation Act A 1996 federal welfare reform plan that dramatically changed the nation's welfare system into one that requires work in exchange for time-limited assistance. Also called the Welfare Reform Act.

Both surveys found that food insecurity is strongly associated with poverty and is interlinked with economic and social factors. Food insecurity and hunger were highest in the inner city, in Hispanic and African American households, and in households with young children, as well as those headed by women and those headed by a person with limited education. (See **Figure 15.2**.) Clearly then, to end food insecurity and hunger, nutrition programs must be accompanied by social and economic efforts.

Think About It 2

The Working Poor

Employment does not guarantee that families always have enough to eat. NHANES III found that food insecurity is as common among the working poor as the unemployed. Since the 1996 **Personal Responsibility and Work Opportunity Reconciliation Act**, commonly called welfare reform, thousands have left the welfare rolls for jobs. Often the pay is too little to lift households above poverty level,[9] and work-related expenses such as transportation or child care further deplete family budgets. Low-paid workers may be unaware that they still qualify for food-assistance programs. On the other hand, their work hours may preclude program participation.

Table 15.1 Poverty Guidelines: Income Levels Defined as Poverty for a Given Household Size

Size of Family Unit	48 Contiguous States and D.C.	Alaska	Hawaii
1	$8,860	$11,080	$10,200
2	11,940	14,930	13,740
3	15,020	18,780	17,280
4	18,100	22,630	20,820
5	21,180	26,430	24,360
6	24,260	30,330	27,900
7	27,340	34,180	31,440
8	30,420	38,030	34,980
For each additional person, add	3,080	3,850	3,540

Note: Despite the limits to the use of household income as a proxy for estimating food insecurity, poverty remains an intuitively reasonable indicator. Keep in mind that, in addition to food, income must cover housing, clothing, transportation, medical care, and other essentials.

Source: *Federal Register.* 2002;67(31):6931–6933.

Table 15.2 Sample Questions from the Food Security Questionnaire

Light Food Insecurity	
"We worried whether our food would run out before we got money to buy more." Was that often, sometimes, or never true for you in the last 12 months?	
"The food that we bought just didn't last and we didn't have money to get more." Was that often, sometimes, or never true for you in the last 12 months?	
Moderate Food Insecurity	
In the last 12 months did you or other adults in the household ever cut the size of your meals or skip meals because there wasn't enough money for food?	
In the last 12 months, were you ever hungry but didn't eat because you couldn't afford enough food?	
Severe Food Insecurity	
In the last 12 months did you or other adults in the household ever not eat for a whole day because there wasn't enough money for food?	
(For households with children) In the last 12 months did any of the children ever not eat for a whole day because there wasn't enough money for food?	

Source: Nord M, Jemison K, Bickel G. Prevalence of food insecurity and hunger, by state, 1996–1998. http://www.ers.usda.gov/epubs/pdf/fanrr2/fanrr2.pdf. Accessed 5/11/02.

The Isolated

People in remote rural areas may live far from food resources and lack access to transportation. Other people become isolated despite living in populated cities. Even though they live in a crowded neighborhood or apartment building, they are alone and are physically or mentally unable to obtain adequate food.

Elders

The infirmities of age, along with feelings of vulnerability, keep some elderly people homebound and lonely, conditions hardly conducive to a healthy appetite. Physical ailments may make cooking and eating difficult, while actually increasing nutrient needs. Elders often have small incomes, with little prospect for improvement. Like others with limited resources, they cut food purchases to pay for other necessities. Although food assistance may be available, pride or shame may keep an older person from participating in such programs.[10]

The Homeless or Inadequately Housed

The homeless rely on soup kitchens and other public programs for much of their food. Some resort to handouts and even forage through garbage. Many are mentally ill or substance abusers. The addict often has little interest in eating and may sell available food to buy more drugs. Many other people live in welfare hotels, single-room-occupancy facilities, or rooming houses without storage or cooking facilities. Budget-stretching strategies such as buying food in bulk and carefully using leftovers are out of the question for these people; as the monthly budget dwindles, they often rely on fast-food meals and then soup kitchens.

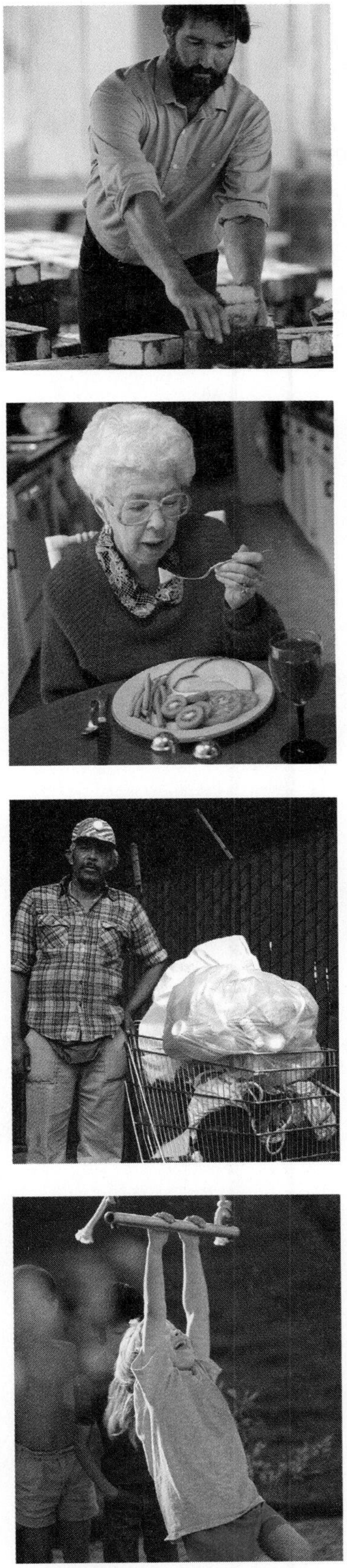

Figure 15.2 Americans at risk. Americans most at risk for hunger include working poor, elders, homeless people, and children.

Food Research and Action Center (FRAC)
Founded in 1970 as a public interest law firm, FRAC is a nonprofit child advocacy group that works to improve public policies to eradicate hunger and undernutrition in the United States.

Children

Perhaps no group is more vulnerable to hunger than the young. Growth and development are delayed in poorly nourished children. They get sick more often. It is harder for them to concentrate in school. Children are captives of their family circumstances; poverty and lack of nutritious food in the household are beyond a child's control. Approximately 4 million children under age 12 go hungry in the United States, and another 9.6 million are at risk of hunger.[11] These figures, based on the most comprehensive study of childhood hunger ever conducted in the United States, were estimated by the **Food Research and Action Center (FRAC)**, a nonprofit advocacy group that fights childhood hunger and undernutrition.

Attacking Hunger in America

Government efforts to fight hunger began during the Great Depression of the 1930s. From that modest beginning, federal efforts have grown to include at least 14 programs that address hunger. (See **Table 15.3**.) The School Lunch Program was created in 1946, after many young men had failed the physical requirements for military service in World War II because of poor nutrition. The Food Stamp Program, begun on a small scale years earlier, was greatly expanded in the early 1970s following an exposé of hunger in Appalachia and the Mississippi Delta and the television documentary "Hunger in America." The federal government initiated the Special Supplemental Nutrition Program for Women, Infants, and Children (WIC) in the 1970s as a response to concerns about maternal and child health. Other government programs have since been added to meet the special needs of the young, the elderly, the disadvantaged, and the disabled.

Table 15.3 U.S. Programs That Address Food Insecurity and Hunger

Food Stamp Program
Nutrition Assistance Program for Puerto Rico
National School Lunch Program
School Breakfast Program
Child and Adult Care Food Program
Summer Food Service Program
Special Milk Program
Special Supplemental Nutrition Program for Women, Infants, and Children (WIC)
Commodity Supplemental Food Program
Food Distribution Program on Indian Reservations
Elderly Nutrition Program
Disaster Feeding Program
The Emergency Food Assistance Program (TEFAP)
Food Distribution Program for Charitable Institutions and Summer Camps

Source: Position of American Dietetic Association: domestic food and nutrition security. *J Am Diet Assoc.* 1998;98:337–342.

Think About It 3

Nonprofit community agencies, charities, religious organizations, and similar groups were organized during hard economic times in the 1980s to create a large network of food pantries, soup kitchens, and services for home-delivered meals. Most of the federal government's programs for direct distribution of food or meals operate at the local level through these networks. Both laypeople and professionals, such as dietitians, work in these programs, either as volunteers or as staff, to fight hunger and malnutrition.

Food assistance programs have greatly reduced the prevalence of hunger, but not of food insecurity, which requires social and economic change. The following are among the federal government's most far-reaching programs against hunger.

The Food Stamp Program

The Food Stamp Program is our main food security program. Recipients can use food stamp benefits to purchase food, but not nonfood items

Fyi Hungry and Homeless

FOR YOUR INFORMATION

A shabbily dressed man slowly pushes a shopping cart along the sidewalk. It is laden with bottles and cans that he can redeem for cash. In front of a supermarket, a woman and child clutch a sign scrawled with the words "Hungry. Please help." On a street corner, a man confronts every passing car with a sign that says "Will work for food." When confronted by a homeless person, do you feel uncomfortable? Do you turn away? Or do you try to help?

Who are the homeless? Single men and families with children are the largest homeless groups. Roughly equal in size, they make up about 80 percent of the homeless population. Single women (13 percent) and unaccompanied minors (7 percent) account for the remainder. About 20 percent of the homeless are mentally ill—about the same number that are employed. Nearly one-third are substance abusers.[1]

Hunger in the homeless is caused by a number of interrelated factors, including low-paying jobs, unemployment and other employment-related problems, high housing costs, substance abuse, poverty or lack of income, and food stamp cuts. Family members—children and their parents—most frequently request emergency food assistance. Two-thirds of the adults requesting food assistance are employed.[2]

Complex challenges face the homeless, who may sleep in the streets or in emergency shelters. The homeless get food from many sources—shelters, drop-in centers, fast-food restaurants, and garbage bins. Soup kitchens are a primary source of meals, yet navigating this system to obtain adequate food can be a formidable and time-consuming task. Also, while homeless people often are eligible for food stamps, they are extremely limited in their ability to store and prepare food, and few restaurants are authorized to accept food stamps.

A major public health concern for homeless people is not only whether they are getting enough to eat but also the nutritional quality of their diet. This concern is complicated by the special needs of infants, children, and women, especially pregnant women. Diets of the homeless often are nutritionally inadequate. Studies of homeless women and children indicate that they consume less than half of the RDA for iron, zinc, magnesium, and folate daily.[3] Homeless adult males have diets low in calcium, zinc, vitamin B_6, and calories. Homeless adults consume less than 50 percent of the RDA for calcium. Poor diets put the homeless at an increased risk for illness and chronic conditions. Pregnant women, children, and people with compromised health status are particularly vulnerable.

Homeless families and individuals rely on emergency food assistance facilities not only during emergencies but also for extended periods. Unfortunately, these facilities are strained beyond their capacities—over 40 percent cannot provide an adequate quantity of food.[4] Some shelters have resorted to rationing to extend their food resources to a greater number of people. Because of a lack of resources, over half may be forced to turn people away. Addressing hunger is a top priority. Once access to food is secure, obtaining a nutritionally adequate diet and dealing with health issues become reasonable goals.

1 The United States Conference of Mayors. A status report on hunger and homelessness in America's cities, 1999. December 1999. http://www.usmayors.org/uscm/homeless/hunger99.pdf. Accessed 5/11/02.

2 Ibid.

3 Silliman K, Yamanoha M, Morrissey A. Evidence of nutritional risk in a population of homeless adults in rural Northern California. *J Am Diet Assoc.* 1998;98:908–910.

4 The United States Conference of Mayors. Op. cit.

Electronic Benefits Transfer (EBT) Electronic delivery of government benefits by a single plastic card that allows access to food benefits at point-of-sale locations.

Child and Adult Care Food Program A federally funded program that reimburses approved family child-care providers for USDA-approved foods served to preschool children; also provides funds for meals and snacks served at after-school programs for school-age children and to adult day care centers serving chronically impaired adults or people over age 60.

such as paper goods, pet food, and alcohol. The benefit amount varies according to household size and income level.

Actually, the term *food stamp* is becoming a misnomer. Almost half of the people who receive benefits use **Electronic Benefits Transfer (EBT)** cards. (See **Figure 15.3**.) The card resembles and functions like a debit card. Each month the household's benefit amount is credited to the card, which is then used at participating grocery stores.

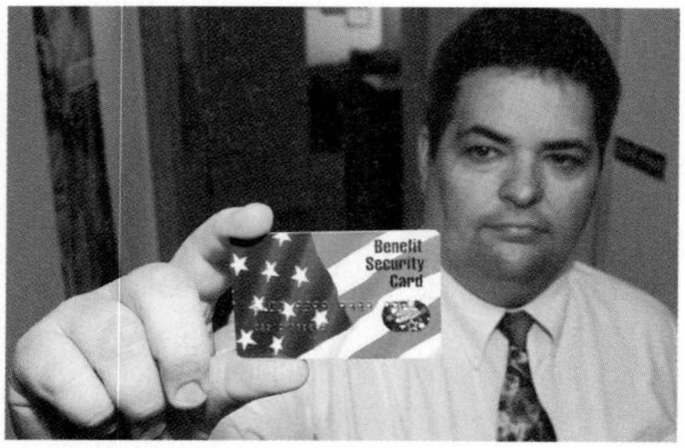

Figure 15.3 **Electronic Benefits Transfer card.** Electronic Benefits Transfer (EBT) is an electronic system that allows recipients to authorize transfer of their government benefits from a federal account to a retailer account to pay for products received.

Special Supplemental Nutrition Program for Women, Infants, and Children

The WIC program provides food to pregnant and breastfeeding women, infants, and preschoolers. In 1999 more than 7 million women and children received WIC benefits each month. To be eligible, the participant must be at nutritional risk, and household income must be less than 185 percent of the poverty level. For fiscal year 2002, the gross annual income for a family of four could not exceed $33,485.[12]

Nutrition assessment and nutrition education are important components of the WIC program. Participants receive coupons, or "checks," for specific categories of healthful foods, and they "cash" them at participating grocery stores. Unlike food stamps, the amount of the WIC benefit varies with nutritional need, not income.

National School Lunch Program

The National School Lunch Program ensures that children in primary and secondary schools receive at least one healthful meal every school day (supplemented in many areas by the School Breakfast Program). For a family of four in fiscal 2002, the child's meals are free if the household income is less than $23,530; the meals are reduced in price if household income is less than $33,485.[13] The lunch must provide one-third or more of dietary requirements for key nutrients. The program operates in more than 97,700 public and nonprofit private schools and residential child-care institutions. It provides nutritionally balanced, low-cost or free lunches to more than 27 million children each school day.[14] (See **Figure 15.4**.)

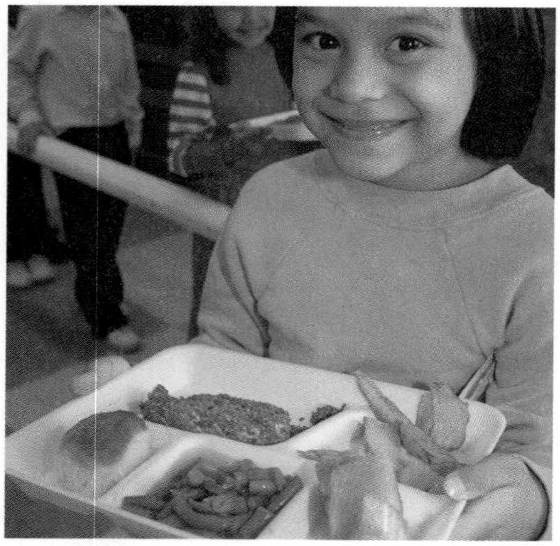

Figure 15.4 **National School Lunch Program.**

Child and Adult Care Food Program

The **Child and Adult Care Food Program** provides funds for children's meals and snacks at nonprofit licensed child-care centers, day care homes, after-school programs, and similar settings. Nutritious meals for elderly or disabled people are also funded at nonprofit facilities such as adult day care centers and recreation centers.

Key Concepts: *Overt malnutrition in the United States is uncommon. However, almost 10 percent of American households suffer food insecurity; and in more than 3 percent of American households, someone has gone hungry. Food insecurity and hunger are interlinked with poverty. Groups at risk include the working poor, the isolated, the homeless, children, and elders. A large network of individual volunteers, nonprofit agencies, and charities, together with major government programs such as Food Stamps, WIC, and School Lunch, have done much to reduce hunger. However, food insecurity, which continues among an unacceptably large number of people, must be overcome by social and economic improvements.*

Malnutrition in the Developing World

The numbers are staggering. In the developing world, 790 million people do not have enough to eat. Two out of five children are stunted by lack of food, one in three is underweight, and one in ten has significant wasting of muscle and fat tissue. The enormity of the problem can be overwhelming, until you learn that these statistics represent an improvement over former years. The proportion of undernourished people in developing countries has declined from 30 percent in 1979–1981 to 20 percent in 1990–1992 to 18 percent in 1995–1997—proof that progress is possible.[15]

But progress is much too slow and uneven. In the 98 countries monitored by the **World Health Organization (WHO)**, only 37 countries had declining numbers of hungry people during the 1990s. In 27 other countries, the proportion of undernourished people actually increased.[16] (See **Figure 15.5**.)

Think About It 4

Hunger in the developing world is chronic. "It is debilitating. Sometimes it is deadly. It blights the lives of all who are affected and undermines national economies and development processes where it is found on a large scale," says the **Food and Agriculture Organization (FAO)** of the United Nations.[17] Although food shortages severe enough to cause endemic starvation or famine have lessened significantly, natural disasters, epidemics, economic or political upheaval, or war can quickly precipitate famine.[18]

World Health Organization (WHO) A global organization that directs and coordinates international health work. Its goal is the attainment by all peoples of the highest possible level of health, defined as a state of complete physical, mental, and social well-being and not merely the absence of disease or infirmity.

Food and Agriculture Organization (FAO) The largest autonomous UN agency; the FAO works to alleviate poverty and hunger by promoting agricultural development, improved nutrition, and the pursuit of food security.

Figure 15.5 **Global hunger.** Although the proportion of the world's population that is chronically undernourished has been decreasing over the last few decades, undernutrition is still widespread, particularly in certain regions. Furthermore, projections to the year 2010 suggest that there is little change in the absolute number of chronically undernourished people.
Source: Food and Agriculture Organization of the United Nations, Luxembourg Income Study; First World Hunger, USDA; Second Harvest. http://www.fao.org/sd/eidirect/wfs/wfs1.htm.

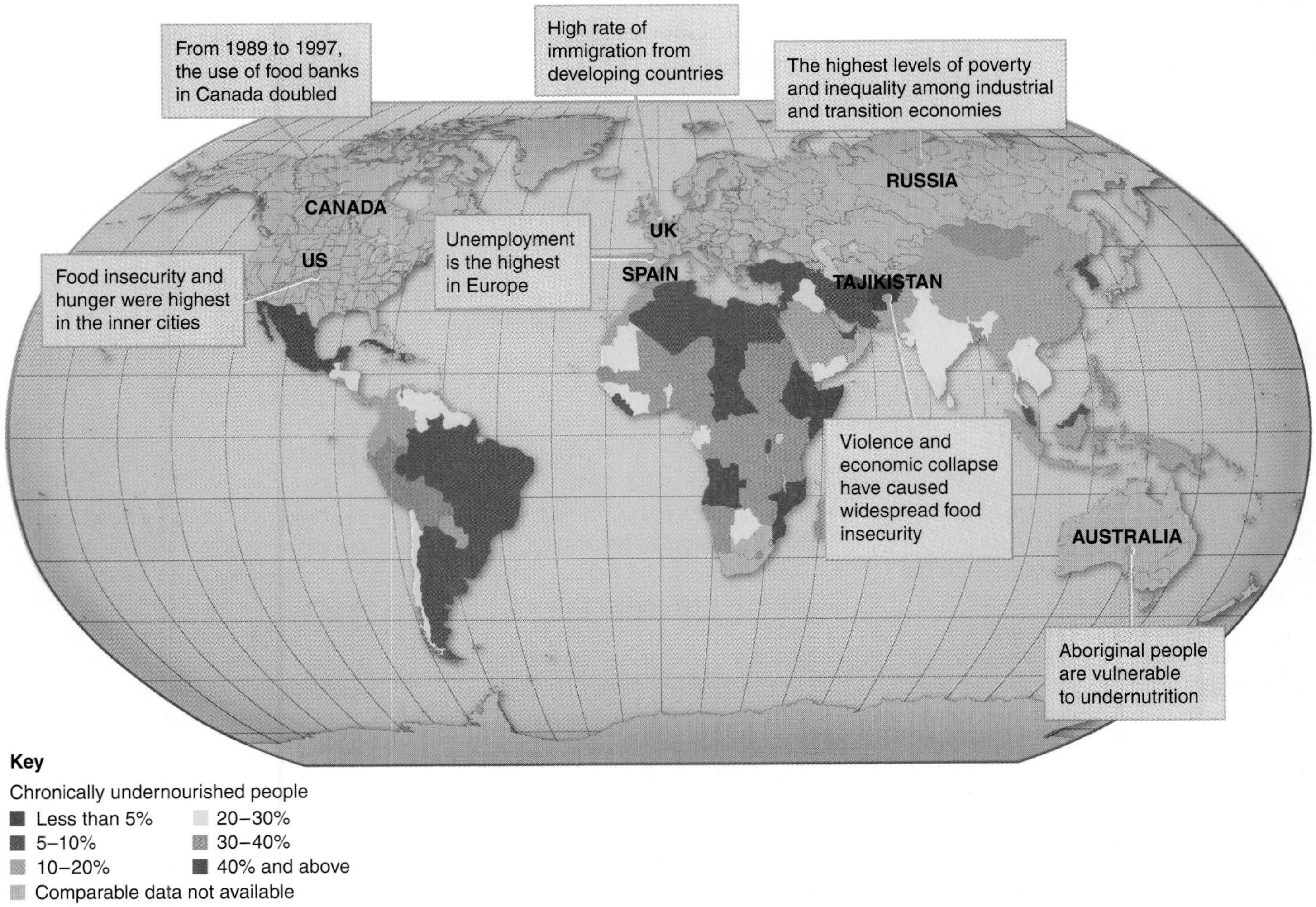
From 1989 to 1997, the use of food banks in Canada doubled
High rate of immigration from developing countries
The highest levels of poverty and inequality among industrial and transition economies
RUSSIA
CANADA
UK
US
Unemployment is the highest in Europe
SPAIN
TAJIKISTAN
Food insecurity and hunger were highest in the inner cities
Violence and economic collapse have caused widespread food insecurity
AUSTRALIA
Aboriginal people are vulnerable to undernutrition
Key
Chronically undernourished people
Less than 5%
5–10%
10–20%
20–30%
30–40%
40% and above
Comparable data not available

Why Hunger?

Why, in a world of plenty, does hunger still exist? The causes are simple, but the solutions are tremendously complex; they require economic, political, and social change, as well as improvements in nutrition, food production, and environmental safeguards. As you study the critical nutrient deficiencies in the developing world, you will see that poverty, infection, poor sanitation, and social upheaval interact with nutrient shortages to bring about the deficiencies.

Social and Economic Factors

Poverty, overpopulation, and the migration to overcrowded cities are closely interrelated causes of hunger. (See **Figure 15.6.**) Each situation worsens the effects of the others as they steadily drive a population toward malnutrition.

Poverty

Poverty is the most important underlying reason for chronic hunger. Obviously, it limits access to food. It limits purchase of farming supplies to grow food, boats and equipment to fish, and storage equipment to prevent spoilage. It limits access to medical care. It compromises efforts at sanitation. It discourages education and the chance for personal advancement.

For nations, poverty means paralyzed economic development and too few jobs; inadequate investments in infrastructure and basic housing; and too few resources to train doctors, nutritionists, nurses, and other health-care workers.

Population Growth

Population growth in many regions is outstripping gains in food production, education, employment, health care, and economic progress. The burgeoning numbers stress limited environmental resources, contributing

Quick Bites

Where Were You Born?

Your survival was greatly influenced by the location of your birth. Angola has the highest infant mortality rate (195 deaths per 1,000 live births), according to estimates for 2000. Other countries with high infant mortality rates include Sierra Leone (148 per 1,000), Afghanistan (149 per 1,000), and Liberia (134 per 1,000). At the other end of the spectrum is Finland (4 per 1,000). Canada (5 per 1,000) has a lower infant mortality rate than the United States (7 per 1,000).

Fyi AIDS and Malnutrition

FOR YOUR INFORMATION

Like other infections, HIV interacts with malnutrition in a vicious, devastating cycle. Left untreated, HIV infection progresses to acquired immunodeficiency syndrome (AIDS). The virus attacks by destroying its victim's immune system. When a person is unable to fight infections and malignancies, disease quickly depletes marginal nutrient stores, speeding the way to severe malnutrition and death. But malnutrition and HIV interact on several other levels, as well:

- Low vitamin A levels in pregnant women increase the rate of HIV transmission to their unborn babies.[1]
- HIV is transmitted to infants in breast milk; but in impoverished regions, substitutions for breast milk typically increase infantile diarrhea, malnutrition, and death.[2]
- AIDS leaves mothers too weak to feed and care for their children. Eventually AIDS turns children into orphans.
- AIDS disables parents so they cannot work to support and feed their families.
- Reduced levels of micronutrients in an HIV-infected person are associated with faster progression of HIV disease and AIDS.[3]
- Weight loss and muscle wasting in an infected person are associated with faster progression of HIV disease and AIDS.[4]
- Infections that accompany AIDS cause fever and diarrhea, making malnutrition worse. Nausea and loss of appetite also contribute to malnutrition.
- Severe protein-energy malnutrition (PEM) is characteristic of untreated AIDS and frequently the ultimate cause of death.

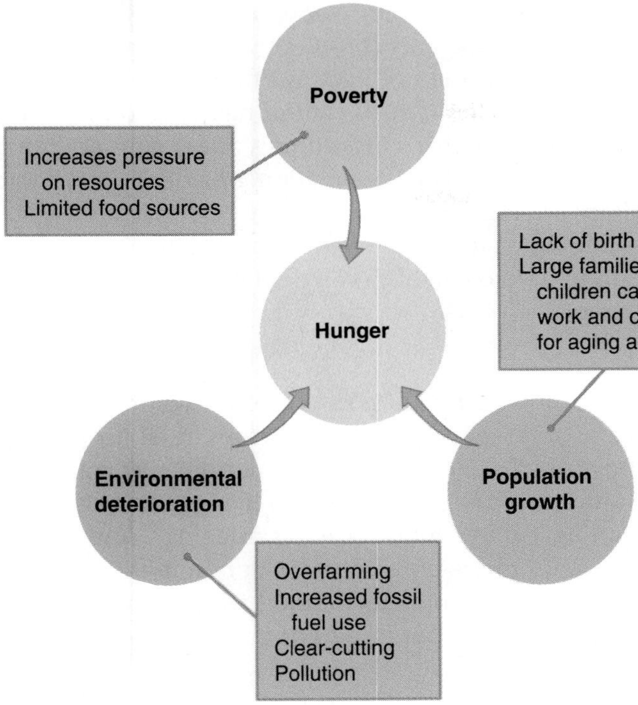

Figure 15.6 **Major problems causing hunger.** Poverty, population growth, and environmental degradation interact to make hunger worse.

to environmental degradation and pollution. In rural areas where farmland is limited, each small parcel of family land is subdivided with each generation, until there is too little land to support each family.

You might think that poverty would pressure parents to limit family size, but ironically, poverty and sickness do just the reverse. Where child mortality rates are high, having many babies is a guarantee some children

As of June 2000, sub-Saharan Africa had 24.5 million people infected with HIV. Southeast Asia had 5.6 million people infected with HIV, and Latin America had 1.3 million.[5] Without treatment or a cure, these people are doomed to death, usually within 10 years of the initial infection. The fate of severe PEM in millions of people appears unavoidable. If we do not arrest the continued transmission of HIV, the number of PEM victims will climb even higher.

1 Semba RD, Miotti PG, Chiphangwi JD. Maternal vitamin A deficiency and mother-to-child transmission of HIV-1. *Lancet.* 1994;343:1593–1597.

2 Desclaux A, Taverne B, Alfieri C, et al. Socio-cultural obstacles in the prevention of HIV transmission through breast-milk in West Africa. Program and abstracts of the 13th International AIDS Conference; July 9–14, 2000; Durban, South Africa. Abstract MoOrD205.

3 Tang AM, Graham NMH, Kirby AJ, et al. Dietary micronutrient intake and risk of progression to acquired immunodeficiency syndrome (AIDS) in human immunodeficiency virus type-1 (HIV-1)-infected homosexual men. *Am J Epidemiol.* 1993;138:937–951.

4 Coodley GO, Loveless MO, Merrill TM. The HIV wasting syndrome: a review. *J Acq Immune Def Syndr.* 1994;7:681–694.

5 Joint United Nations Programme on HIV/AIDS. *Report on the Global HIV/AIDS Epidemic.* Geneva, Switzerland: UNAIDS; 2000.

will survive. In countries that have no economic safeguards for disability, unemployment, or old age, parents consider their children a source of security and support in times of need. Many other factors contribute to large families, from ignorance of birth control methods to the attitude that big families reflect the father's masculinity. Some political groups also encourage high birth rates and fast population growth as a way to achieve political or military dominance.

To slow population growth, socioeconomic and cultural changes that make smaller family size acceptable, even desirable, must accompany access to birth control.

Urbanization

Urbanization is a worldwide trend. As rural lands become too crowded or exhausted farmland no longer supports good crops, rural people migrate to the city in hopes of jobs and a better life. Unfortunately, in fast-growing cities, social disorder, sanitary conditions, and living standards may be much worse. Hunting, fishing, foraging, and gardening—sources of accessible food in the rural setting—are seldom an option in the city. Breastfeeding becomes impractical for many mothers who could nurse their babies while doing farm work, but cannot do so with jobs in the city.

> **Quick Bites**
>
> **Food Supply versus Food Safety**
>
> Sometimes obtaining food is more important than safety. Food from street vendors is important in the diets of many urban populations, particularly the socially disadvantaged. Health authorities responsible for food safety should balance their risk management with issues of food availability and hunger. Rigorous application of codes and regulations suited to larger and permanent food-service establishments may cause the disappearance of the street vendors, with consequent aggravation of hunger and malnutrition. WHO encourages the development of regulations that empower vendors to take greater responsibility for the preparation of safe food.

Infection and Disease

Infection interacts with malnutrition, each making its victim more vulnerable to the other, each making the other worse, in a downward spiral. Nutrient deficiencies lower resistance to infections.[19] In turn, the fever of infection speeds depletion of calories and nutrients. Other symptoms (e.g., loss of appetite, weakness, nausea, and mouth lesions) limit ability to eat. Infectious diarrhea is especially dangerous, quickly wasting what few nutrients are consumed; infants and young children can die quickly from loss of electrolytes. Programs that prevent or control infection (e.g., immunizations, improvements in hygiene and sanitation, safe water supplies, and access to medicine and medical care) all indirectly improve nutrition status.

Today, infection with the human immunodeficiency virus (HIV) provides a dramatic demonstration of the interaction between malnutrition and infection. Transmission of the virus from mother to fetus is greater when the mother is deficient in vitamin A.[20] The infection progresses fastest in people who are poorly nourished.[21] And severe loss of weight and muscle are hallmarks of the advanced disease, acquired immune deficiency syndrome (AIDS). As of June 2000, 34.3 million people were infected with HIV—more than 90 percent of them in the developing world and more than 24 million of them in sub-Saharan Africa.[22] A nutrition disaster is on the horizon.

> **Quick Bites**
>
> **Rehydration Therapy for Diarrhea**
>
> Simple and inexpensive packets of carbohydrate and salts diluted with sterile water replace lost fluids and electrolytes. These packets are saving thousands of people each year.

Political Disruptions and Natural Disasters

Social upheavals and natural disasters such as floods and drought can leave famine in their wake. The resulting displacement of populations and inequitable food distribution usually lead to hunger and malnutrition.

War

Whereas poverty is the underlying cause of chronic mild to moderate malnutrition, war and its aftermath cause severe malnutrition and famine. War diverts limited financial resources from development efforts to expenditures for fighting and destruction. Men and women no longer farm, fish, or bring home a paycheck—they are in the army. Households become fatherless and sometimes motherless, often permanently. Crops and croplands are destroyed, along with irrigation systems, food-processing facilities, and transportation infrastructure, which may have taken decades to develop.

Refugees

Masses of refugees—many very young, old, infirm, and already weakened by chronic hunger—find themselves without the basic elements of sustenance. The resulting famine has become an all too common sight on the evening news. International relief agencies have learned to respond to these emergencies quickly and with great determination, but logistic difficulties (e.g., mobilizing manpower, obtaining foods, transporting supplies, setting up feeding stations) may slow relief until it is too late for the sickest or weakest. Some refugee groups are inaccessible, hidden, or intentionally kept hungry as part of a political plan; emergency food may never reach many of them.

Sanctions

International sanctions and embargoes create food shortages, both directly and indirectly, by limiting access to agricultural supplies, fuel, and food-processing supplies. Some people argue that shortages created by embargoes hurt powerless people rather than government officials; others say that such actions are preferable to war.

Floods, Droughts, Mudslides, and Hurricanes

Many countries are not equipped to deal with food shortages and hunger from natural disasters. International relief agencies and other governments step in to help when possible. Some U.S. agencies involved are the USDA, the U.S. State Department through its Agency for International Development, and the Centers for Disease Control and Prevention (CDC) through the Center for Communicable Diseases. These agencies offer both short-term, emergency efforts and long-term programs for repair and rebuilding.

Inequitable Food Distribution

Advances in agriculture have increased food production worldwide. Enough calories are now produced to supply the energy needs of every person on earth.[23] But distribution of these calories is uneven: among the continents, among nations, within nations, and even in families.

In some societies the father of the family may be wrongly perceived as having the greatest nutrition needs and will be given priority for the most nutritious, high-protein foods. In those societies, older boys will have second priority; pregnant and breastfeeding women, women in general, and small children will have the lowest priority. Nations may follow a similar pattern, ensuring that their soldiers or men of fighting age receive scarce foodstuffs.

Regional Trends

In sub-Saharan Africa, where the population is growing at an unprecedented rate of 3 percent per year, food production cannot keep pace; in fact, food availability per capita is declining.[24] Economic factors, violent regional conflicts, and the tremendous cost of the AIDS epidemic contribute to widespread, worsening hunger.

Quick Bites

Accidental Solution

Sometimes a solution to undernutrition is not planned. On October 9, 1998, the *Wall Street Journal* carried the headline, "In Guatemala, Organic Farms Sprout on Civil War Turf." During the country's 35-year civil war, local farmers abandoned their land. As the farmlands reverted to jungle and pesticide levels diminished, wild spices thrived. With the trend for "organic" spices, coffee, and natural dyes, the premium prices commanded by these new crops could be significant for the farmers' incomes.

Quick Bites

Emergency Management

Imagine a civil war in a developing country that displaces tens of thousands of people. What are the most important measures for preventing sickness and death among these refugees? Protection from violence heads the list, closely followed by adequate food rations, clean water and sanitation, diarrheal disease control, measles immunization, and maternal and child health care.

Quick Bites

Know Thine Enemy

Crops have a critical role in feeding the world's burgeoning population. "Responsible biotechnology is not the enemy; starvation is," says former President Jimmy Carter.

Among the former Communist countries of Eastern Europe and Eurasia, abrupt economic transition and political upheaval have led to severe food shortages, often made worse by violent conflicts. In Latin America, despite great progress, hunger remains in pockets of rural poverty and in inner-city slums.

There has been progress, however. Improved national economies have led to reduction in hunger in the Middle East. In the Asia-Pacific region, per capita food supplies have increased, partly because of austere birth control measures in China as well as improved food production. However, even in nations that have achieved food sufficiency, regions of impoverishment or isolation have food shortages.

Agriculture and Environment: A Tricky Balance

Advances in agriculture increase food supplies and reduce food costs. Because the economies of most developing countries are based on agriculture, improvements boost rural incomes and buying power, increase demand for agricultural labor, stimulate commerce among small vendors and food processors, and ultimately help a nation's economy.

Dramatic gains in agricultural productivity took place in the 1960s and 1970s with the development of new seed varieties, especially rice and corn. The seeds greatly increased crop yields. Expectations were so strong that these seeds would finally solve the world's food shortage that their development and use was dubbed the "Green Revolution." Despite its successes, the Green Revolution had limitations. The seeds required irrigation and heavy use of pesticides and fertilizers, which poor farmers could not afford. The farming techniques were sometimes hard on the environment. Gains from the Green Revolution have now about reached their limit and, if current trends continue, threaten to be lost to the population explosion.

Proponents of agricultural biotechnology see it as another step along the continuum of plant-breeding techniques and a promising tool to increase crop production. Some uses of biotechnology are well accepted—for example, diagnostic kits that identify plants and insects by DNA and

[Fyi] FOR YOUR INFORMATION

Tough Choices

Imagine you live in a poor village of a developing country. How would you make these choices?

- You've learned you must boil your drinking water to prevent diarrhea. But that means cutting young trees for firewood. You recently planted those trees to stop erosion. What do you do?
- You've recently given birth to your fourth child. Your husband was injured in an accident and is unable to work. But you can work at a nearby factory and use your pay to buy food and clothes for the older children. How would you feed the new baby?
- Your small herd of goats provides milk for your young children. You like the goats because they can survive in the rough, hilly countryside. But the goats are overgrazing the grasses on the hillside. What can you do?
- Insects have destroyed your crop. In the past, you burned fields after harvest to control insects, but you've learned that "slash and burn" is bad for the land. You've thought about using a chemical pesticide, but it is too expensive. You could clear the jungle for another growing field. Do you have other choices? What should you do?
- You can grow either vegetables to feed your family or a "cash crop" to sell for export. The cash crop would help pay for medicine and other necessities. Which should you grow?

tissue culture for plant reproduction, a technique already in widespread commercial use. More controversial is the modification of plant genetic material. The technology has the potential to improve plants' resistance to disease, tolerance to adverse conditions, yield, and nutritional quality. Chapter 14, "Food Safety and Technology," describes the techniques and controversies surrounding this application of biotechnology.

At the other end of the technology spectrum is a renewed appreciation and conservation of traditional seed varieties, those selected over the generations by local farmers because they do well in local conditions. In developing countries, farmers typically save some of these seeds at each harvest to use in the next planting season. The seeds grow well in the regions where they've evolved, whereas imported seeds, no matter how carefully bred, often fail.

In addition to seed selection, strategies to optimize agriculture include irrigation, soil preparation, improved planting and harvest methods, erosion prevention, fertilization, pest control, and flood control. The methods should be affordable, suitable for the level of local development, and protective of the environment. For example, where there is an abundant supply of willing farm laborers and gasoline is expensive, using heavy-duty farm machinery makes little sense. Other examples include mulching to conserve water and control weeds, and using manure (after composting to kill pathogens) to reduce the need for fertilizer.

Quick Bites

Vaccine Veggies

Genetic engineers are experimenting with inserting vaccine molecules into plants. William Landridge, a molecular biologist at the Loma Linda University School of Medicine in California, has successfully added anti–cholera toxin genes to the potato. Potatoes are a dietary staple in Peru, Bolivia, and India, where cholera causes dehydrating diarrhea and death. Every year, 2.2 million children die from dehydration due to diarrhea. Edible vaccines could overcome the problems of refrigeration and distribution that impede vaccination by injection. Next on the menu? Bananas and tomatoes may be even more effective vehicles than potatoes.

Environmental Degradation

Environmental degradation is a growing concern in both the developing and the industrialized world. In developing countries, there is pressure for more land to support rapidly expanding populations of the poor. In industrialized countries, there is pressure from the affluent for more land, more houses, larger properties, more recreation areas, and so on. Residents of the industrialized world consume vast amounts of resources (e.g., water, fuel, wood, paper, textiles, and food) without a thought and often without making the small effort to conserve or recycle. Residents of the developing world consume much less per person, but the impact of their numbers is greater.

Environmental degradation has nutritional consequences because it threatens food production. Urbanization and the expansion of cities reduce acreage available for farming. The pressure to supply food to growing populations leads to clear-cutting marginal land, eventually eroding hilly terrain or quickly exhausting fragile rain forest soils. Overdependence on irrigation can drain water, eventually creating deserts. The destruction of vast areas of natural ground cover can lead to global climate changes. Overuse of pesticides and fertilizers pollutes waterways, destroying fish and seafood.

Quick Bites

Who Produces the World's Soybeans?

Before 1900, the soybean was rarely grown in the United States. Today, it is the largest American crop. The United States produces 75 percent of the world's soybeans.

Key Concepts: *Despite gains in eradicating malnutrition, 18 percent of the people in the developing world continue to suffer from chronic hunger. Although world food supplies are adequate, factors that allow hunger to continue include poverty, poor sanitation, urbanization, and inefficient food distribution. Infection, especially AIDS, rapid population growth, wars, and environmental degradation threaten to reverse hard-won gains.*

Malnutrition: Its Nature, Its Victims, and Its Eradication

Previous chapters discussed the diseases of nutritional deficiency. Most of these diseases exist throughout the developing world, but seldom in isolation. Typically, the malnourished person has two or more coexisting deficiencies, each increasing the severity of the other. Keep the potential for this deadly synergy in mind as we discuss some of the major categories of malnutrition.

Protein-Energy Malnutrition

As you learned in Chapter 7, "Proteins and Amino Acids," lack of protein and also energy can have devastating consequences, especially on the young. In kwashiorkor, the body and face swell with excess fluid, the hair turns wispy and red, and a terrible rash develops; without treatment, the person dies. Marasmus paints an even more dramatic picture of sunken eyes, shriveled limbs, and a clearly visible outline of the skeleton; it is as deadly as kwashiorkor.

Protein-energy malnutrition (PEM) is most often a condition of infants and children. Their fast growth creates high nutrient demands, leaving them especially vulnerable to inappropriate food distribution in the family, inappropriate infant and child feeding practices, and interactions of infection with malnutrition.[25] PEM typically develops after a child is weaned from the breast. Men in the household may have priority for nutritious food. In big families, the young child must also compete for food with many siblings.

In the developing world, breastfeeding is almost always essential to an infant's survival. Inappropriate bottle-feeding puts a baby at grave risk. Relative to income, formula is usually very expensive and is often diluted to make it "stretch." Contaminated water and lack of other hygienic requirements for bottle preparation cause diarrhea. The combination of diarrhea and nutritional deficiency from watered-down formula is often fatal.

Quick Bites

Is Breastfeeding Always Best?

An HIV-positive mother can transmit the virus to her baby through breast milk. HIV-positive women whose infants were spared HIV transmission during pregnancy face the dilemma of how to feed those babies. In developing countries, the WHO is working to prevent HIV transmission through breastfeeding while continuing to protect, promote, and support breastfeeding as the best way to feed babies of women who are HIV-negative and women who do not know their status. Unfortunately, alternatives such as formula feeding are expensive, carry the risk of food poisoning from contaminated water, and often carry a social stigma.

A tremendous educational effort, including promotion of breastfeeding, has reduced the global prevalence and severity of infant and childhood PEM. Severe PEM typified by kwashiorkor or marasmus has become more sporadic, occurring mainly as a result of war or natural disaster. However, mild to moderate PEM continues to pose a grave problem in the developing world, putting children at risk of delayed growth, impaired psychological development, and the deadly interactions of disease and malnutrition. In fact, at least half of all deaths of children younger than 5 are still associated with PEM. Most of these deaths are from mild to moderate PEM interacting with other illness, rather than from severe malnutrition.[26] Moreover, with an epidemic of HIV infection raging in many developing countries, the return of widespread severe PEM threatens.

Iodine Deficiency Disorders

Iodine deficiency is the developing world's most common cause of preventable brain damage and impaired psychomotor development.[27] Its impairment of intellectual ability and work performance is potentially so widespread that **iodine deficiency disorders (IDD)** can actually slow a nation's social and economic development.

iodine deficiency disorders (IDD) A wide range of disorders that affect growth and development due to iodine deficiency.

Iodine deficiency is most devastating during pregnancy, causing spontaneous abortions, stillbirths, and birth defects, including cretinism, a disease of mental retardation that is often severe. Deafness and spastic paralysis are likely to accompany the retardation. In regions of Africa, dwarfism also occurs where diets rich in goitrogen-containing vegetables (e.g., cassava or cabbage) make the deficiency worse. Moreover, iodine deficiency is damaging at all ages, limiting mental development in infants and children and producing apathy and marginal mental function in adults. Localized iodine deficiency affects not only the human population, but also the fertility and survival of livestock, and thus can impede social and economic development.[28]

Iodine deficiency disorders are endemic throughout much of the developing world where the soil is low in iodine. These areas typically are mountainous or far from the oceans. They often are isolated and impoverished. Although imported food is a potential source of iodine, it often is not consumed. Iodine deficiency has been identified in 130 countries on all continents. Globally, about 740 million people have goiter and over 2 billion people are at risk of IDD.[29] (See **Figure 15.7**.)

Disturbing though these figures may be, great strides have been made in IDD prevention, mainly through iodizing salt. Countries with salt iodization programs have increased from 46 in 1990 to 93 in 1999; more than two-thirds of households in IDD-affected countries now use iodized salt.[30] The result is a dramatic improvement of iodine status in countries with salt iodization programs in place for 5 years or more. The cost is merely 5 cents per person per year.

Vitamin A Deficiency

Vitamin A deficiency is the leading cause of preventable childhood blindness. It is the leading cause of needless visual impairment in women and children. It also predisposes its victims to infection, and it worsens existing infections.

Vitamin A deficiency is most damaging to infants, children, and pregnant or lactating women. Among children in the developing world, 250,000 to 500,000 children each year become blind as a result of xerophthalmia (severe vitamin A deficiency); about half of them will die within a year of their blindness. Currently, some 3 million children under 5 years of age have signs of xerophthalmia.[31] **Table 15.4** gives WHO's estimates, by region, of the numbers of children younger than 5 who have clinical vitamin A deficiency.

Another 140 million to 250 million children have subclinical vitamin A deficiency, often coexisting with marginal PEM. The vitamin deficiency predisposes infants and children to diarrheal diseases, which in turn worsen the child's nutritional status, leading to severe PEM. Common childhood infections, most notably measles, are much more serious in vitamin A-deficient children, with a much greater risk of death or permanent damage from complications.

In communities where vitamin A deficiency exists, pregnant and breastfeeding women often experience night blindness, an early symptom of deficiency. Maternal death, poor pregnancy outcome, and failure to lactate are all increased with vitamin A deficiency. Vitamin A levels in the breast milk of these women are likely to be low as well, putting their infants at later risk of deficiency.

Many countries are taking a multipronged approach to vitamin A deficiency that includes promotion of breastfeeding, fortification of foods, supplementation, and nutrition education. Foods like eggs, dairy foods, and liver are promoted as important for women and children; educational programs also encourage growing and eating fruits and vegetables high in beta-carotene. However, dietary change can be difficult and slow. The best sources of vitamin A are often the most expensive or inaccessible. For absorption and conversion to vitamin A, beta-carotene requires dietary fat—another expensive item in many areas—and other factors not com-

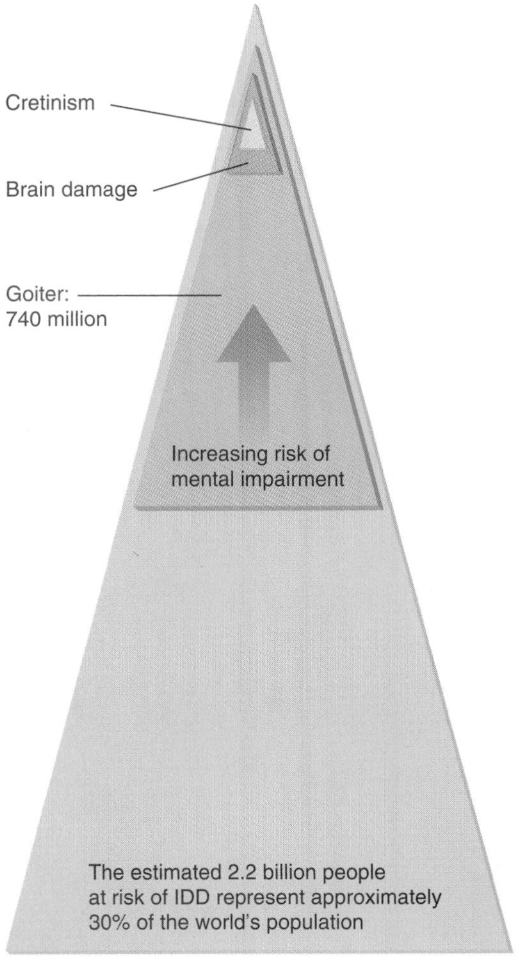

Figure 15.7 **The toll of iodine deficiency.** Iodine deficiency remains the single greatest cause of preventable brain damage and mental retardation worldwide.
Source: World Health Organization.

Table 15.4 **Estimated Number of Children under Age 5 with Clinical Vitamin A Deficiency**

Africa region	1,080,000
The Americas	60,000
Eastern Mediterranean region	60,000
Southeast Asia	1,300,000
Western Pacific region	100,000

Note: An estimated 140–250 million children under age 5 are at risk of sub-clinical vitamin A deficiency, mainly in Asia and Africa.

Source: World Health Organization. http://www.WHO. int/nut.

Quick Bites

The Importance of Rice

Rice is the principal food crop for one-half of the world's population.

pletely understood. Meanwhile, periodic single, large-dose vitamin A supplements, often given in tandem with maternal–child immunizations, are proving an effective short-term measure.

Biotechnology may have a significant impact on vitamin A deficiency. Through genetic engineering, scientists have developed a new strain of rice that is rich in beta-carotene. When these rice plants are crossed with locally grown strains of rice, they become suited to a particular region's climate and growing conditions. Such crops may play a critical role in feeding the world's burgeoning population and alleviating widespread vitamin A deficiency.[32]

Iron-Deficiency Anemia

WHO estimates that worldwide, 39 percent of preschool-aged children and 52 percent of pregnant women are anemic and that 90 percent of these people live in developing countries. Fast growth in young children and reproductive blood loss in women make them especially vulnerable to low-iron diets. However, iron deficiency occurs in all age groups. Like deficiencies discussed previously, anemia impairs psychomotor development, work capacity, learning capacity, and resistance to disease.[33] Anemia during pregnancy increases illness and death rates for mother and baby. For all groups of people, anemia can cause profound fatigue, and severe anemia causes death.

The anemias of the developing world demonstrate the interaction of multiple nutrient deficiencies, which in turn interact with infection, sanitation, and poverty. Supplying iron alone is seldom enough to correct the problem.

Iron-deficient diets are typically high in starch and cereal grains. During digestion, cereals may bind with the very limited iron the diet provides, preventing its absorption. Other blood-building nutrients, such as vitamins B_6 and B_{12} and folate, are in short supply as well.

Anemia-producing parasites are common in areas of iron deficiency, aggravating the effects of poor diet. Blood cells are destroyed by malarial infections. Intestinal malabsorption and intestinal bleeding are caused by hookworm, prevalent where human waste contaminates the fields where people walk barefoot, and by other parasites, acquired when human waste contaminates the water that people drink or in which people bathe.

People debilitated by anemia may be too weak to build outhouses, too poor to buy shoes or fuel to boil water, or too apathetic to clear standing water where malaria-carrying mosquitoes breed. Moreover, they often do not understand the connection between sanitation, infection, and malnutrition. Added to this mix are excessive blood loss from repeated pregnancies, inherited blood disorders such as sickle-cell disease, and chronic bacterial or viral infections such as HIV.

Efforts to increase intake of iron-rich foods have limited effectiveness because these foods are costly, and dietary improvements are likely to come too slowly. Supplementation targeted to women and children and food fortification are now the mainstays of anemia prevention and treatment, along with public health programs attacking anemia's other causes. Unfortunately, overcoming poverty and improving sanitation are not as easy as taking an iron pill, and so the prevalence of iron-deficiency anemia has remained essentially unchanged over the years.[34]

Deficiencies of Other Micronutrients

Deficiencies of zinc and calcium often coexist with other deficiencies, contributing to illness and death during periods of growth and threatening immune function and skeletal health in people who survive to old age.

Selenium deficiency, although limited to only a few countries, has serious consequences. It occurs where the soil is selenium-poor, in distinct regional patterns in China and Russia. In China, where the deficiency is most severe, it predisposes individuals to the fatal Keshan disease, in which heart muscle is destroyed. Keshan disease affects mainly women and children. The condition can be prevented by selenium supplementation or by fortification, as in programs undertaken in New Zealand, where soil is also low in selenium.

The classical deficiency diseases beriberi, pellagra, and scurvy still occur among the world's poorest and most underprivileged people. Most often, however, these diseases strike the victims of war and political strife—the refugees. Since 1990, at least 11 outbreaks of beriberi or pellagra have been reported among refugee populations, primarily in Africa.[35] Diets based on milled cereals and starchy roots, all poor thiamin sources, predispose populations to beriberi. People who rely on corn-based diets low in niacin and tryptophan are susceptible to pellagra. The disruption of refugee life can easily tip the balance from marginal deficiency to overt deficiency disease.

Overweight and Obesity

In some developing countries, obesity exists right alongside undernutrition. Obesity is more likely in areas of economic advancement and urban areas, less so in rural populations. Its prevalence is rising rapidly in Latin America and the Caribbean, but obesity still is relatively uncommon in Asia and Africa.

The factors leading to obesity in poor communities are different from those in affluent societies. Cultural attitudes toward overweight may be more accepting, even admiring. Calorie-dense foods that have few other nutrients are often cheap, satisfying, convenient, and heavily promoted; some are foreign brands that have become affordable status symbols. With urbanization and modernization, trends that typically reduce physical activity, comes a reduction in caloric expenditure that can be dramatic. Malnutrition itself may actually play a role; there is evidence that malnutrition during fetal development and early childhood predisposes people to obesity in adulthood.[36]

Key Concepts: *The most critical nutritional deficiencies in today's developing world are deficiencies of protein, calories, iodine, vitamin A, and iron. There have been gains in reducing the severity and prevalence of protein-energy malnutrition, through breastfeeding promotion, nutrition education, and improvements in food supplies. Fortification and supplementation programs are effectively attacking iodine and vitamin A deficiencies but have had less success overcoming iron deficiency. All of the underlying causes of malnutrition must be addressed to reduce and eliminate these and other deficiencies.*

Quick Bites

Undernutrition Cannot Be Blamed for Everything

In all populations in the developing world, low weight- and height-for-age affect 10 to 15 percent of preschool and school-aged children. Most experts attribute this shortfall to insufficiency of food. A study of African schoolchildren, however, found no significant difference between well-fed and underfed pupils on measures such as their class position, aptitude for games, and interest in education. Among children of school age, one must be careful not to overrate the effects of undernutrition nor the health disadvantages from mild to moderate malnutrition.

LEARNING Portfolio chapter 15

Key Terms

	page
Child and Adult Care Food Program	598
Electronic Benefits Transfer (EBT)	598
Food and Agriculture Organization (FAO)	599
food insecurity	592
Food Research and Action Center (FRAC)	596
food security	592
Food Security Supplement Survey	594
hunger	592
iodine deficiency disorders (IDD)	606
malnutrition	592
Personal Responsibility and Work Opportunity Reconciliation Act	594
World Health Organization (WHO)	599

Study Points

- Hunger and malnutrition continue to be problems in both industrialized and developing countries.
- Although most people in the United States are food-secure, malnutrition is a serious problem among the working poor, the rural poor, the homeless, elders, and children.
- According to the 1996–1998 Food Security Supplement Survey, almost 10 percent of American households worry about having enough to eat, and over 3 percent experience hunger.
- The Food Stamp Program; the Special Supplemental Nutrition Program for Women, Infants, and Children (WIC); the National School Lunch and Breakfast Programs; and the Child and Adult Care Food Program are among the many federal programs that address hunger in the United States.
- Although the rates of malnutrition and hunger in the developing world declined in the last three decades of the twentieth century, progress is still too slow and uneven. It is estimated that 790 million people in the developing world do not have enough to eat.
- Social and economic factors, infection, disease, political disruptions, natural disasters, and inequitable food distribution all contribute to hunger in the developing world.
- Advances in agricultural practices have increased food supplies and reduced food costs in the developing world; however, the increase in production has led to environmental degradation as a result of urbanization, clear-cutting, overirrigation, and soil erosion.
- Protein-energy malnutrition (PEM) refers to conditions, such as kwashiorkor and marasmus, that result from not having enough to eat.
- Infants and children are most likely to suffer from PEM. However, nutrition education efforts, including promotion of breastfeeding, have reduced the severity and prevalence of PEM.
- Iodine deficiency is the largest cause of preventable brain damage and impaired psychomotor development in the developing world. It can cause damage to people of all ages.
- Great strides have been made in preventing iodine deficiency disorders (IDD) through salt iodization programs. More than two-thirds of households in IDD-affected countries now use iodized salt.
- Vitamin A deficiency is the leading cause of preventable childhood blindness. It also makes its victims more vulnerable to infection, diarrheal diseases, and PEM.
- Pregnant and breastfeeding women with vitamin A deficiency are at increased risk of death, poor pregnancy outcomes, and lactation failure.
- Many countries are taking a multipronged approach to vitamin A deficiency that includes promotion of breastfeeding, fortification of foods, supplementation, and nutrition education.
- The best sources of vitamin A often are expensive and inaccessible to people in developing countries. Scientists have developed new bioengineered strains of rice that are rich in beta-carotene and that may play a critical role in alleviating widespread vitamin A deficiency.

- **The WHO estimates that, worldwide, 39 percent of preschool-aged children and 52 percent of pregnant women have iron-deficiency anemia, and that 90 percent of these people live in developing countries.**
- **The anemias of the developing world demonstrate the interaction of multiple nutrient deficiencies, which in turn interact with infection, poor sanitation, and poverty.**
- **Food fortification and iron supplementation for women and children are the mainstays of anemia prevention and treatment, along with efforts to overcome poverty and improve sanitation.**
- **The classical deficiency diseases beriberi, pellagra, and scurvy still occur among the world's poorest and most underprivileged people.**
- **In some developing countries, obesity exists right alongside undernutrition.**

Study Questions

Answers can be found at nutrition.jbpub.com/discovering.

1. **What's the difference between food insecurity and hunger?**
2. **What is food security?**
3. **List four common nutritional deficiencies worldwide.**
4. **List four causes of malnutrition worldwide.**
5. **List some of the organizations and programs fighting hunger and food insecurity in the United States.**
6. **What populations are at increased risk of nutritional deficiencies, and why?**

[Try] This

Try Giving Up Your Stove and Refrigerator

A homeless person has no kitchen facilities to store or prepare food. For one day, eat a balanced diet without resorting to cooking or using your refrigerator. Some of the foods you could eat include the following:

breads, bagels, tortillas, rolls

cereals

crackers

milk—canned, evaporated, or aseptic packaging

cheese—hard cheeses keep well

pudding cups (single-serve, nonrefrigerated type)

tuna/chicken—canned

sardines, salmon—canned

nuts, peanut butter

beans—canned

fruits and vegetables—fresh, canned, dried fruits

How satisfying did you find this eating pattern? What did you miss most? What would it be like to eat this way for an extended time?

Community Food Programs

The purpose of this exercise is to see how you can contribute to decreasing or eliminating food insecurity in your community. Look in the phone book (under "Food Programs" and "Human Services") to see what programs are available. Consider volunteering at your local food bank or another community program to help feed people who do not have the means to feed themselves.

References

1 Food and Agriculture Organization of the United Nations. The state of food insecurity in the world 1999. http://www.fao.org/NEWS/1999/img/SOFI99-E.PDF. Accessed 5/11/02.

2 Position of the American Dietetic Association: world hunger. *J Am Diet Assoc.* 1995;95:1160–1162.

3 Kendall A, Kennedy E. Position of the American Dietetic Association: domestic food and nutrition security. *J Am Diet Assoc.* 1998;98:337–342.

4 US Department of Agriculture. Office of Analysis, Nutrition and Evaluation, Food and Nutrition Service. *Household Food Security in the United States 1995–1998.* Alexandria, VA: USDA; 2000. Advance Report.

5 Kendall A, Olson CM, Frongillo EA. Relationship of hunger and food insecurity to food availability and consumption. *J Am Diet Assoc.* 1996;96:1019–1024.

6 Nord M, Jemison K, Bickel G. *Prevalence of Food Insecurity and Hunger, by State, 1996–98.* Alexandria, VA: USDA, Economic Research Service, Food and Nutrition Service; 1999. Food Assistance and Nutrition Research report 2 (FANRR-2).

7 Hamilton WL, Cook JT, Thompson WW, et al. *Household Food Security in the United States in 1995.* Alexandria, VA: USDA, Office of Analysis and Evaluation, Food and Consumer Service; 1997.

8 Alaimo K, Briefel RR, Frongillo EA, Olson C. Food insufficiency exists in the United States: results for the third National Health and Nutrition Examination Survey (NHANES III). *Am J Public Health.* 1998;88:419–426.

9 Schlesinger JM. Working full time is no longer enough. *Wall Street Journal.* June 29, 2000:A2, 12.

10 Wellman NS, Weddle DO, Kranz S, Brain CT. Elder insecurities: poverty, hunger, and malnutrition. *J Am Diet Assoc.* 1997;97(suppl):S120–S122.

11 Food Research and Action Center. Hunger in the U.S. http://www.frac.org/html/hunger_in_the_us/hunger_index.html. Accessed 5/11/02.

12 USDA Food and Nutrition Service Online. WIC frequently asked questions. http://www.fns.usda.gov/wic/MENU/FAQ/FAQ.HTM#1. Accessed 5/11/02.

13 USDA Food and Nutrition Service Online. School programs: income eligibility guidelines. http://www.fns.usda.gov/cnd/Lunch/Governance/Notices/02-03iegs.htm. Accessed 5/11/02.

14 USDA Food and Nutrition Service Online. School Lunch Program. http://www.fns.usda.gov/cnd/Lunch/. Accessed 5/11/02.

15 Food and Agriculture Organization of the United Nations. Op. cit.

16 Ibid.

17 Food and Agriculture Organization of the United Nations. Undernourishment around the world. http://www.FAO.org/focus/e/sofi/under-e.htm. Accessed 5/11/02.

18 Uvin P. The state of world hunger. In: Uvin P, ed. *The Hunger Report 1993.* Newark, NJ: Gordon and Breach; 1994:1–42.

19 Mata LJ, Urrutia JJ, Albertazzi C. Influence of recurrent infections on nutrition and growth of children in Guatemala. *Am J Clin Nutr.* 1972;25:1267–1275.

20 Semba RD, Miotti PG, Chipangwi JD, et al. Maternal vitamin A deficiency and mother-to-child transmission of HIV-1. *Lancet.* 1994;343:1593–1597.

21 Tang AM, Graham NMH, Kirby AJ, et al. Dietary micronutrient intake and risk of progression to acquired immunodeficiency syndrome (AIDS) in human immunodeficiency virus type 1 (HIV-1)-infected homosexual men. *Am J Epidemiol.* 1993;138: 937–951.

22 Joint United Nations Programme on HIV/AIDS. Report on the *Global HIV/AIDS Epidemic.* Geneva, Switzerland: UNAIDS; 2000.

23 Position of the American Dietetic Association: world hunger. Op. cit.

24 Ibid.

25 Keusch GT, Scrimshaw NS. Selective primary health care: strategies for control of disease in the developing world. XXIII. Control of infection to reduce the percentile of infantile and childhood malnutrition. *Rev Infect Dis.* 1986;8:349–353.

26 World Health Organization. Nutrition for health and development activities and outputs. http://www.who.int/nut/pem.htm. Accessed 5/11/02.

27 Ibid.

28 Stanbury JB, Dunn JT. Iodine and the iodine deficiency disorders. In: Bowman BA, Russell RM, eds. *Present Knowledge in Nutrition.* 8th ed. Washington, DC: International Life Sciences Institute; 2001:344–351.

29 International Council for Control of Iodine Deficiency Disorders. Global IDD status. *IDD Newsletter.* 1999;15(2). http://www.people.virginia.edu/~jtd/iccidd/newsletter/may1999.htm. Accessed 5/11/02.

30 World Health Organization. Micronutrient deficiencies. http://www.who.int/nut/idd.htm. Accessed 5/11/02.

31 Ibid.

32 Nash M. Grains of hope. *Time.* 2001:156(5):38–46; and Greger JL. Response: genetically engineered "golden" rice unlikely to overcome vitamin A deficiency. *J Am Diet Assoc.* 2001;101: 289–290.

33 Stoltzfus RJ. Iron-deficiency anemia: reexamining the nature and magnitude of the public health problem. *J Nutr.* 2001; 131(suppl 2, pt 2):697S–701S.

34 World Health Organization. Nutrition for health and development activities and outputs. Op. cit.

35 Ibid.

36 Pena M, Bacallao J. *Obesity and Poverty: A New Public Health Challenge.* Geneva, Switzerland: World Health Organization; 2000. PAHO scientific publication 576.

Appendices

APPENDIX A Food Composition Tables

ERA CODE	FOOD DESCRIPTION	AMT	UNIT	WT (g)	WTR (g)	CAL (kcal)	PROT (g)	CARB (g)	FIBR (g)	FAT (g)	SATF (g)	MONO (g)	POLY (g)
Beverage and Beverage Mixes													
Alcoholic Beverages													
22500	Beer	1.5	cup	356.4	329	146	1	9	1	0	0	0	0
22512	Beer, light	1.5	cup	29.5	28	8	<1	<1	0	0	0	0	0
20276	Beer, nonalcoholic	1.5	cup	355.5		58	<1	12		0	0	0	0
22519	Coffee liqueur, 53 proof	1.5	fl oz	52.2	16	175	<1	24	0	<1	<0.1	0.1	0.1
22521	De menthe liqueur, 72 proof	1.5	fl oz	50.4	14	187	0	21	0	<1	<0.1	<0.1	0.1
22543	Gin, rum, vodka, whiskey, 100 prf	1.5	fl oz	41.7	24	123	0	0	0	0	0	0	0
22514	Gin, rum, vodka, whiskey, 80 prf	1.5	fl oz	41.7	28	96	0	0	0	0	0	0	0
22516	Gin, rum, vodka, whiskey, 86 prf	1.5	fl oz	41.7	27	104	0	<1	0	0	0	0	0
22542	Gin, rum, vodka, whiskey, 94 prf	1.5	fl oz	41.7	25	115	0	0	0	0	0	0	0
22601	Sangria wine drink	0.5	cup	118	102	79	<1	11	<1	<1	0	0	<0.1
22509	Sherry, dry	0.5	cup	117	104	82	<1	2	0	0	0	0	0
22518	Wine, dessert, dry	0.5	cup	118	94	149	<1	5	0	0	0	0	0
22507	Wine, dessert, sweet	0.5	cup	118	86	181	<1	14	0	0	0	0	0
20077	Wine, light, nonalcoholic	0.5	cup	116	114	7	1	1	0	0	0	0	0
20076	Wine, nonalcoholic	0.5	cup	116	114	7	1	1	0	0	0	0	0
22501	Wine, red	0.5	cup	118	104	85	<1	2	0	0	0	0	0
22502	Wine, rosé	0.5	cup	118	105	84	<1	2	0	0	0	0	0
22504	Wine, white, medium	0.5	cup	118	106	80	<1	1	0	0	0	0	0
Carbonated Drinks													
20006	Club soda	1.5	cup	355	355	0	0	0	0	0	0	0	0
20054	Cola, caffeine free	1.5	cup	360		160	0	41	0	0	0	0	0
20030	Cola, diet	1.5	cup	355	354	4	<1	<1	0	0	0	0	0
20056	Cola, diet, caffeine free	1.5	cup	360		0	0	0	0	0	0	0	0
20005	Cola, regular	1.5	cup	372	333	153	0	39	0	0	0	0	0
20028	Cream soda	1.5	cup	371	321	185	0	49	0	0	0	0	0
20189	Cream soda, diet	1.5	cup	360		0	0	0	0	0	0	0	0
20007	Diet soda, assorted flavors	1.5	cup	355	354	0	0	<1	0	0	0	0	0
20027	Dr. Pepper-type soda	1.5	cup	368	329	151	0	38	0	<1	0.3	0	0
20008	Ginger ale	1.5	cup	366	334	124	0	32	0	0	0	0	0
20031	Grape soda	1.5	cup	372	330	160	0	42	0	0	0	0	0
20032	Lemon-lime soda	1.5	cup	368	330	147	0	38	0	0	0	0	0
20029	Orange soda	1.5	cup	372	326	178	0	46	0	0	0	0	0
20009	Root beer	1.5	cup	370	330	151	0	39	0	0	0	0	0
Coffee and Substitutes													
20012	Coffee, brewed	1	cup	237	235	5	<1	1	0	<1	<0.1	0	<0.1
20065	Coffee, decaf, brewed	1	cup	240	238	5	<1	1	0	0	<0.1	0	<0.1

< = Trace amount present   Blank = Not available

ERA, EatRight Analysis CD-ROM; **AMT,** amount; **WT,** weight; **WTR,** water; **CAL,** calories; **PROT,** protein; **CARB**, carbohydrate; **FIBR,** fiber; **FAT,** fat; **SATF,** saturated fat; **MONO,** monounsaturated fat; **POLY,** polyunsaturated fat; **CHOL,** cholesterol; **V,** vitamin; **THI,** thiamin; **RIB,** riboflavin; **NIA,** niacin; **FOL,** folate; **CALC,** calcium; **PHOS,** phosphate; **SOD,** sodium; **POT,** potassium; **MAG,** magnesium

CHOL (mg)	V-A (RE)	THI (mg)	RIB (mg)	NIA (mg)	V-B6 (mg)	FOL (μg)	V-B12 (μg)	V-C (mg)	V-E (mg)	CALC (mg)	PHOS (mg)	SOD (mg)	POT (mg)	MAG (mg)	IRON (mg)	ZINC (mg)
0	0	<0.1	0.1	1.6	0.2	12	0.1	0	0	18	43	18	89	21	0.1	0.1
0	0	<0.1	<0.1	0.1	<0.1	1	<0.1	0	0	1	4	1	5	1	<0.1	<0.1
0							0					3				
0	0	<0.1	<0.1	0.1	0	0	0	0	0	1	3	4	16	2	<0.1	<0.1
0	0	0	0	<0.1	0	0	0	0	0	0	0	3	0	0	<0.1	<0.1
0	0	<0.1	<0.1	<0.1	0	0	0	0	0	0	2	<1	1	0	<0.1	<0.1
0	0	<0.1	<0.1	<0.1	0	0	0	0	0	0	2	<1	1	0	<0.1	<0.1
0	0	<0.1	<0.1	<0.1	0	0	0	0	0	0	2	<1	1	0	<0.1	<0.1
0	0	<0.1	<0.1	<0.1	0	0	0	0	0	0	2	<1	1	0	<0.1	<0.1
0	2	<0.1	<0.1	0.1	<0.1	3	0	5	<0.1	5	5	8	42	4	0.1	0.1
0	0	<0.1	<0.1	0.1	<0.1	1	<0.1	0	0	9	16	9	104	12	0.5	0.1
0	0	<0.1	<0.1	0.2	0	<1	0	0	0	9	11	11	109	11	0.3	0.1
0	0	<0.1	<0.1	0.2	0	<1	0	0	0	9	11	11	109	11	0.3	0.1
0	0	0	<0.1	0.1	<0.1	1	0	0	0	10	17	8	102	12	0.5	0.1
0	0	0	<0.1	0.1	<0.1	1	0	0	0	10	17	8	102	12	0.5	0.1
0	0	<0.1	<0.1	0.1	<0.1	2	<0.1	0	0	9	17	6	132	15	0.5	0.1
0	0	<0.1	<0.1	0.1	<0.1	1	<0.1	0	0	9	18	6	117	12	0.4	0.1
0	0	<0.1	<0.1	0.1	<0.1	<1	0	0	0	11	17	6	94	12	0.4	0.1
0	0	0	0	0	0	0	0	0	0	18	0	75	7	4	<0.1	0.3
0							0				49	45	0			
0	0	<0.1	0.1	0	0	0	0	0	0	14	32	21	0	4	0.1	0.3
0							0				49	55	54			
0	0	0	0	0	0	0	0	0	0	11	45	15	4	4	0.1	<0.1
0	0	0	0	0	0	0	0	0	0	19	0	44	4	4	0.2	0.3
0							0				0	55	0			
0	0	0	0	0	0	0	0	0	0	14	39	57	7	4	0.1	0.2
0	0	0	0	0	0	0	0	0	0	11	41	37	4	0	0.1	0.1
0	0	0	0	0	0	0	0	0	0	11	0	26	4	4	0.6	0.2
0	0	0	0	0	0	0	0	0	0	11	0	56	4	4	0.3	0.3
0	0	0	0	<0.1	0	0	0	0	0	7	0	41	4	4	0.3	0.2
0	0	0	0	0	0	0	0	0	0	19	45	45	7	4	0.2	0.4
0	0	0	0	0	0	0	0	0	0	18	0	48	4	4	0.2	0.3
0	0	0	0	0.5	0	<1	0	0	0	5	2	5	128	12	0.1	<0.1
0	0	0	0	0.5	0	<1	0	0	0	5	2	5	130	12	0.1	<0.1

ERA, EatRight Analysis CD-ROM; **AMT,** amount; **WT,** weight; **WTR,** water; **CAL,** calories; **PROT,** protein; **CARB**, carbohydrate; **FIBR,** fiber; **FAT,** fat; **SATF,** saturated fat; **MONO,** monounsaturated fat; **POLY,** polyunsaturated fat

ERA CODE	FOOD DESCRIPTION	AMT	UNIT	WT (g)	WTR (g)	CAL (kcal)	PROT (g)	CARB (g)	FIBR (g)	FAT (g)	SATF (g)	MONO (g)	POLY (g)
Beverage and Beverage Mixes (continued)													
Coffee and Substitutes (continued)													
20044	Cappucino, prep from mix	0.75	cup	192	178	61	<1	11	0	2	1.8	0.1	<0.1
20048	Postum coffee substitute	1	cup	240	237	12	<1	2	0	<1	<0.1	<0.1	0.1
20093	Coffee+chicory, instant, prep	1	cup	179	177	7	<1	1	0	<1	<0.1	0	<0.1
20023	Coffee, prep from instant	1	cup	238.4	236	5	<1	1	0	0	0	0	0
20091	Coffee, decaf, instant, prep	1	cup	179	177	4	<1	1	0	<1	<0.1	0	<0.1
20063	Espresso coffee	1	cup	240	235	22	<1	4	0	<1	0.2	0	0.2
20064	Espresso coffee, decaf	1	cup	240	235	22	<1	4	0	<1	0.2	0	0.2
20108	French coffee-mix+water	0.75	cup	189	178	57	1	7	0	3	2.9	0.2	0.1
22517	French van coffee, prep from mix	1	ea	14	<1	65	<1	10	<1	3	0.6		
20109	Mocha coffee, prep from mix	0.75	cup	188	177	51	1	8	<1	2	1.6	0.1	<0.1
Dairy Mixes and Drinks													
73	Cocoa, prep from mix	0.75	cup	209	178	119	2	24	1	3	1.8	1	0.1
21	Cocoa, prep w/ whole milk	1	cup	250	202	192	10	29	2	6	3.6	1.7	0.2
46	Cocoa, sugar free, prep from mix	0.75	cup	192	177	48	4	8	<1	<1	0.2	0.1	<0.1
27	Instant Breakfast+skim milk	1	cup	282		216	16	36	<1	1	0.7	0.3	<0.1
101	Instant Breakfast+1% milk	1	cup	281		233	15	36	<1	3	2	0.9	0.1
26	Instant Breakfast+2% milk	1	cup	281		252	15	36	<1	5	3.3	1.5	0.2
25	Instant Breakfast+whole milk	1	cup	281		280	15	36	<1	9	5.4	2.5	0.3
41	Nestle's Quik, strawberry+milk	1	cup	266	215	234	8	33	0	8	5.1	2.4	0.3
38	Ovaltine drink-choc flavor	1	cup	265	215	225	9	29	<1	9	5.5	2.6	0.4
62006	SlimFast straw pwdr scoop	1	ea	28	1	100	5	20	2	1			
62652	UltraSlimFast choc pwdr scoop	1	ea	33	2	120	5	22	5	1	0		
Fruit Flavored Drinks													
20421	All Sport drink, fruit punch	1	cup	240		53	0	15	0	0	0	0	0
20314	Crystal Light drink, citrus	1	cup	238.4		5	0	0	0	0	0	0	0
20052	Five Alive citrus drink	1	cup	248	218	114	1	29	0	<1	0	0	<0.1
20024	Fruit punch drink, canned	1	cup	248	218	116	0	30	<1	<1	<0.1	<0.1	<0.1
20035	Fruit punch drink, prep from frozen	1	cup	247	218	114	0	29	<1	<1	<0.1	<0.1	<0.1
20648	Gatorade	1	cup	240.9	225	60	0	15	0	0	0	0	0
20101	Grape drink, canned	1	cup	250	221	112	<1	29	0	<1	<0.1	0	<0.1
20158	Hi-C fruit punch	1	cup	250.1		130	0	34	0	0	0	0	0
20016	Koolade, dry+sugar+water	1	cup	262	237	97	0	25	0	<1	<0.1	<0.1	<0.1
20017	Koolade, sugar free, dry+water	1	cup	240	228	43	0	11	0	0	0	0	0
20000	Lemonade, prep from frozen	1	cup	248	221	99	<1	26	<1	<1	<0.1	<0.1	<0.1
20045	Lemonade, prep from mix	1	cup	266	237	112	0	29	0	<1	<0.1	<0.1	<0.1
20047	Lemonade, lo cal, prep from mix	1	cup	237	235	5	0	1	0	0	0	0	0
20002	Limeade, prep from frozen	1	cup	247	220	101	0	27	<1	<1	<0.1	<0.1	<0.1
20004	Orange drink, prep from mix	1	cup	248	218	114	0	29	0	0	<0.1	<0.1	<0.1
20025	Pineapple orange drink, canned	1	cup	250	217	125	3	30	<1	0	0	0	0
20117	Pink lemonade, prep from frozen	1	cup	247	220	99	<1	26	0	<1	<0.1	<0.1	<0.1
20070	Sunny Delight orange ade	1	cup	248	216	126	0	32	<1	<1	<0.1	<0.1	<0.1
62020	UltraSlimFast fruit pwdr w/OJ	1	cup	279		200	11	44	6	<1			

< = Trace amount present   Blank = Not available

CHOL, cholesterol; **V,** vitamin; **THI,** thiamin; **RIB,** riboflavin; **NIA,** niacin; **FOL,** folate;
CALC, calcium; **PHOS,** phosphate; **SOD,** sodium; **POT,** potassium; **MAG,** magnesium

CHOL (mg)	V-A (RE)	THI (mg)	RIB (mg)	NIA (mg)	V-B6 (mg)	FOL (μg)	V-B12 (μg)	V-C (mg)	V-E (mg)	CALC (mg)	PHOS (mg)	SOD (mg)	POT (mg)	MAG (mg)	IRON (mg)	ZINC (mg)
0	0	<0.1	<0.1	0.3	0	0	0	0	0.1	8	27	104	119	10	0.2	0.1
0	0	<0.1	<0.1	0.5	<0.1	1	0	0	0	7	17	10	58	10	0.1	0.1
0	0	0	<0.1	0.4	0	0	0	0	0	5	5	11	61	5	0.1	0.1
0	0	0	0	0.7	0	0	0	0	0	7	7	7	86	10	0.1	0.1
0	0	0	<0.1	0.5	0	0	0	0	0	5	5	5	63	7	0.1	0.1
0	0	<0.1	0.4	12.5	<0.1	2	0	<1	0	5	17	34	276	192	0.3	0.1
0	0	<0.1	0.4	12.5	<0.1	2	0	<1	0	5	17	34	276	192	0.3	0.1
0	0	0	<0.1	0.7	0	0	0	0	0	8	42	30	136	2	<0.1	<0.1
0	0							0		2	28	56	76		<0.1	
0	0	<0.1	<0.1	0.3	0	0	0	0	<0.1	8	28	36	118	9	0.2	0.2
0	150	0.2	0.2	2	<0.1	0	0.4	6	0.1	104	111	207	405	23	1.8	0.3
20	138	0.1	0.4	0.4	0.1	15	0.9	2	0.3	315	292	128	500	70	1.1	1.5
2	<1	<0.1	0.2	0.2	<0.1	2	0.3	0	0.1	90	134	173	405	33	0.7	0.6
9	703	0.4	0.4	5.5	0.5	118	1.6	31	7.5	407	406	268	755	112	4.8	4.1
14	698	0.4	0.5	5.5	0.5	118	1.5	31	7.6	406	393	266	731	118	4.9	4.1
23	693	0.4	0.5	5.5	0.5	118	1.5	31	7.5	401	390	264	726	118	4.9	4.1
38	630	0.4	0.5	5.5	0.5	118	1.5	31	7.5	396	385	262	719	117	4.9	4.1
32	74	0.1	0.4	0.2	0.1	12	0.9	2	0.3	293	229	128	370	32	0.2	0.9
34	901	0.7	1.3	10.9	1	32	0.9	34	0.3	384	313	244	620	53	3.8	1.2
5	75	0.4	0.2	7	0.6	100	1.2	18	10.1	150	100	130	210	100	6.3	4.5
5	225	0.4	0.2	10	0.6	100	2.1	27	20.1	150	100	140	200	100	6.3	4.5
0	0						0	0		0	7	37	37		0	
0	0						0	6		0		0	45		0	
0	10	<0.1	<0.1	0.4	<0.1	5	0	67	0	22	25	7	278	15	2.8	0.1
0	3	0.1	0.1	0.1	0	3	0	73	0	20	2	55	62	5	0.5	0.3
0	2	<0.1	<0.1	0.1	<0.1	2	0	108	0	10	2	10	32	5	0.2	0.1
0	0	<0.1	0	0	0	0	0	0	0	0	22	96	26	2	0.1	<0.1
0	<1	<0.1	<0.1	0.1	<0.1	1	0	85	0	8	2	15	12	5	0.4	0.3
	0						0	100				30				
0	0	0	<0.1	<0.1	0	<1	0	31	0	42	52	37	3	3	0.1	0.1
0	2	<0.1	<0.1	<0.1	0	5	0	78	0	17	5	50	50	5	0.6	0.3
0	5	<0.1	0.1	<0.1	<0.1	5	0	10	0	7	5	7	37	5	0.4	0.1
0	0	0	<0.1	0	0	0	0	34	0	29	3	19	3	3	0.1	0.1
0	0	0	0	0	0	<1	0	6	0	50	24	7	0	2	0.1	0.1
0	0	<0.1	<0.1	0.1	0	2	0	7	0	7	2	5	32	2	0.1	<0.1
0	550	<0.1	<0.1	0	0	143	0	121	0	62	37	12	50	2	0.2	0.1
0	132	0.1	<0.1	0.5	0.1	27	0	56	0	12	10	8	115	15	0.7	0.2
0	<1	<0.1	0.1	<0.1	<0.1	5	0	10	0	7	5	7	37	5	0.4	0.1
0	5	<0.1	<0.1	0.1	<0.1	5	0	85	0	15	2	40	45	5	0.7	0.2
	250	0.5	0.6	7	0.7	140	2.1	60		400	400	30	590	140	6.3	5.2

ERA, EatRight Analysis CD-ROM; **AMT,** amount; **WT,** weight; **WTR,** water; **CAL,** calories; **PROT,** protein; **CARB**, carbohydrate; **FIBR,** fiber; **FAT,** fat; **SATF,** saturated fat; **MONO,** monounsaturated fat; **POLY,** polyunsaturated fat

ERA CODE	FOOD DESCRIPTION	AMT	UNIT	WT (g)	WTR (g)	CAL (kcal)	PROT (g)	CARB (g)	FIBR (g)	FAT (g)	SATF (g)	MONO (g)	POLY (g)
Beverage and Beverage Mixes (continued)													
Teas													
20118	Chamomile tea, brewed	1	cup	237	236	2	0	<1	0	<1	<0.1	<0.1	<0.1
20036	Herbal tea, brewed	0.75	cup	178	177	2	0	<1	0	<1	<0.1	<0.1	<0.1
20014	Tea, brewed	1	cup	237	236	2	0	1	0	<1	<0.1	<0.1	<0.1
20020	Tea, prep from instant	1	cup	237	236	2	<1	<1	0	0	0	0	0
20079	Tea, decaf, lo cal, prep from instant	1	cup	245	243	6	<1	2	0	<1	<0.1	<0.1	<0.1
20038	Tea, lemon, prep from instant	1	cup	238	236	5	<1	1	0	<1	0	0	<0.1
20040	Tea, lemon, lo cal, prep from inst	1	cup	237	235	5	<1	1	0	<1	0	0	<0.1
20022	Tea, sweet, prep from instant	1	cup	259	236	88	<1	22	0	<1	<0.1	<0.1	<0.1
Water													
20050	Bottled water, Perrier	1	cup	237	237	0	0	0	0	0	0	0	0
20051	Bottled water, Poland Springs	1	cup	237	237	0	0	0	0	0	0	0	0
20010	Tonic/Quinine water	1	cup	244	222	83	0	21	0	0	0	0	0
20121	Tonic water, sugar free	1	ea	355	354	0	0	<1	0	0	0	0	0
20041	Water	1	cup	237	237	0	0	0	0	0	0	0	0
Breakfast Cereals													
Cereals, Hot, Cooked													
40094	Corn grits, white, cooked	1	cup	242	206	145	3	31	<1	<1	0.1	0.1	0.2
40093	Corn grits, white, enriched, cooked	1	cup	242	206	145	3	31	<1	<1	0.1	0.1	0.2
40078	Cream of Rice cereal, cooked	1	cup	244	214	127	2	28	<1	<1	0.1	0.1	0.1
40014	Malt O Meal, pl/choc, cooked	1	cup	240	210	122	4	26	1	<1	0.1	0.1	<0.1
40015	Maypo cereal, cooked	0.75	cup	180	149	128	4	24	4	2	0.3	0.5	0.7
40138	Multigrain cereal, cooked	1	cup	246	194	202	7	40	4	2	0.3	0.5	1.1
40000	Oatmeal, cooked, no salt	1	cup	234	200	145	6	25	4	2	0.4	0.7	0.9
40072	Oatmeal, instant, pkt, prepared	1	ea	177	151	104	4	18	3	2	0.3	0.6	0.7
40075	Oatmeal, inst, flavored, pkt, prep	1	ea	155	116	153	4	31	3	2	0.4	0.6	0.7
40088	Ralston cereal, cooked	1	cup	253	218	134	6	28	6	1	0.1	0.1	0.4
40002	Rolled Wheat, cooked	1	cup	240	201	149	5	33	4	1	0.1	0.1	0.5
40016	Roman Meal cereal, cooked	0.75	cup	181	150	110	5	25	6	1	0.1	0.1	0.3
40080	Wheatena cereal, cooked	1	cup	243	208	136	5	29	7	1	0.2	0.2	0.6
Cereals, Ready to Eat													
40063	100% Natural cereal	1	cup	104	3	462	11	71	8	17	7.4	7.4	2.2
40003	All-Bran cereal	0.75	cup	32		119	4	24	3	2	0.3	0.5	0.6
40246	AlphaBits cereal, frosted	1	cup	32	<1	130	3	27	1	1	0.3		
40123	Amaranth Flakes cereal	1	cup	38	1	134	4	27	4	4	0.8	1.2	1.6
40029	Bran Buds cereal	0.33	cup	30	1	83	3	24	12	1	0.1	0.2	0.4
40031	C.W. Post cereal+raisins	1	cup	103	4	446	9	74	14	15	11	1.7	1.4
40030	C.W. Post cereal, plain	1	cup	97	2	421	9	73	7	13	1.7	6	4.7
40032	Cap'n Crunch cereal	1	cup	37	1	147	2	32	1	2	0.5	0.4	0.3
40037	Cocoa Pebbles cereal	1	cup	33	1	129	1	29	1	1	0.4	0.6	0.2
40036	Corn Bran cereal	1	cup	36	1	120	2	30	6	1	0.3	0.3	0.4
40039	Corn Flakes, Honey Crisp cereal	0.75	cup	30		112	2	27	1	<1	<0.1	0.1	0.1
40040	Crispy Wheat 'n Raisins cereal	1	cup	43	3	150	3	35	3	1	0.1	0.1	0.1
40043	Frosted Mini-Wheats cereal	1	cup	55	3	186	5	45	6	1	0.2	0.1	0.6
40025	Frosted Flakes cereal	0.75	cup	31	1	116	1	28	1	<1	<0.1	0.1	0.1

< = Trace amount present

Blank = Not available

CHOL, cholesterol; **V,** vitamin; **THI,** thiamin; **RIB,** riboflavin; **NIA,** niacin; **FOL,** folate;
CALC, calcium; **PHOS,** phosphate; **SOD,** sodium; **POT,** potassium; **MAG,** magnesium

CHOL (mg)	V-A (RE)	THI (mg)	RIB (mg)	NIA (mg)	V-B6 (mg)	FOL (µg)	V-B12 (µg)	V-C (mg)	V-E (mg)	CALC (mg)	PHOS (mg)	SOD (mg)	POT (mg)	MAG (mg)	IRON (mg)	ZINC (mg)
0	5	<0.1	<0.1	0	0	1	0	0	0.2	5	0	2	21	2	0.2	0.1
0	0	<0.1	<0.1	0	0	1	0	0	0	4	0	2	16	2	0.1	0.1
0	0	0	<0.1	0	0	12	0	0	0	0	2	7	88	7	<0.1	<0.1
0	0	0	<0.1	0.1	<0.1	1	0	0	0	5	2	7	47	5	<0.1	0.1
0	0	0	<0.1	0	0	13	0	0	0	<1	2	7	90	7	<0.1	<0.1
0	0	0	<0.1	0.1	<0.1	1	0	0	0	5	2	14	50	5	<0.1	0.1
0	0	0	<0.1	0.1	<0.1	5	0	0	0	5	2	24	40	5	0.1	0.1
0	0	0	<0.1	0.1	<0.1	10	0	0	0	5	3	8	49	5	0.1	0.1
0	0	0	0	0	0	0	0	0	0	33	0	2	0	0	0	0
0	0	0	0	0	0	0	0	0	0	2	0	2	0	2	<0.1	0
0	0	0	0	0	0	0	0	0	0	2	0	10	0	0	<0.1	0.2
0	0	0	0	0	0	0	0	0	0	14	39	57	7	4	0.1	0.2
0	0	0	0	0	0	0	0	0	0	5	0	7	0	2	<0.1	0.1
0	0	<0.1	<0.1	0.5	0.1	2	0	0	0.1	0	29	0	53	10	0.5	0.2
0	0	0.2	0.1	2	0.1	75	0	0	0.1	0	29	0	53	10	1.5	0.2
0	0	0	0	1	0.1	7	0	0	<0.1	7	41	2	49	7	0.5	0.4
0	0	0.5	0.2	5.8	<0.1	5	0	0	0.3	5	24	2	31	5	9.6	0.2
0	527	0.5	0.5	7	0.7	7	2.2	22	1.3	94	185	7	158	38	6.3	1.1
0	116	0.4	0.5	4.4	0.5	17	0	0	3.4	69	184	2	138	66	5.4	0.9
0	5	0.3	<0.1	0.3	<0.1	9	0	0	0.2	19	178	2	131	56	1.6	1.1
0	453	0.5	0.3	5.5	0.7	97	0	0	0.7	163	133	285	99	42	6.3	0.9
0	302	0.3	0.3	4	0.4	81	0	0	0.2	105	132	234	112	39	3.9	0.9
0	0	0.2	0.2	2	0.1	18	0.1	0	0.3	13	147	5	154	58	1.6	1.4
0	0	0.2	0.1	2.1	0.2	26	0	0	2.2	17	166	0	170	53	1.5	1.2
0	0	0.2	0.1	2.3	0.1	18	0	0	0.7	22	161	2	226	81	1.6	1.3
0	0	<0.1	<0.1	1.3	<0.1	17	0	0	0.9	10	146	5	187	49	1.4	1.7
1	1	0.4	0.2	1.8	0.2	26	0.1	<1	2.2	100	322	28	456	109	3.1	2.5
0	5	0.1	0.1	0.6	<0.1	13	0	0	0.7	21	147	202	157	46	1.3	1
0	225	0.4	0.4	5	0.5	100	1.5	0		10	67	212	62	25	2.7	1.5
0	3	<0.1	<0.1	1	<0.1	4	0	1	3.2	6	126	13	134	10	0.7	0.1
0	225	0.4	0.4	5	0.5	90	0	15	0.5	20	166	200	270	83	4.5	6.4
<1	1363	1.3	1.5	18.1	1.9	364	5.5	0	0.7	50	232	161	260	74	16.4	1.6
<1	1284	1.3	1.5	17.1	1.7	342	5.1	0	0.7	47	224	167	198	67	15.4	1.6
0	5	0.5	0.6	6.9	0.7	137	0	0	0.2	7	39	286	47	13	6.2	5.1
0	330	0.4	0.5	5.5	0.5	110	0	13	0.3	9	55	133	71	18	4.9	4.1
0	5	0.1	0.6	6.7	0.7	134	0	0	0.2	27	48	338	75	19	10.1	5
0	75	0.4	0.4	5	0.5	100	0	15	<0.1	<1	14	261	27	5	4.5	0.1
0	293	0.3	0.3	3.9	0.4	78	0	0	0.4	54	110	223	180	33	3.5	0.8
0	0	0.4	0.4	5.4	0.5	110	1.6	0	0.5	20	160	2	183	56	15.4	1.6
0	225	0.4	0.4	5	0.5	100	0	15	<0.1	1	17	281	34	8	4.7	0.1

ERA, EatRight Analysis CD-ROM; **AMT,** amount; **WT,** weight; **WTR,** water; **CAL,** calories; **PROT,** protein; **CARB,** carbohydrate; **FIBR,** fiber; **FAT,** fat; **SATF,** saturated fat; **MONO,** monounsaturated fat; **POLY,** polyunsaturated fat

ERA CODE	FOOD DESCRIPTION	AMT	UNIT	WT (g)	WTR (g)	CAL (kcal)	PROT (g)	CARB (g)	FIBR (g)	FAT (g)	SATF (g)	MONO (g)	POLY (g)
Breakfast Cereals (continued)													
Cereals, Ready to Eat (continued)													
40038	Fruitangy Ohs cereal	1	cup	31	1	122	2	27	1	1	0.3	0.5	0.3
40245	Golden Crisp cereal	0.75	cup	27	1	107	1	25	0	<1	0.1		
13343	Granola, low fat	0.5	cup	53		210	5	40	3	3	1		
40045	Granola, low fat w/raisins	0.66	cup	55		213	5	44	3	3	0.8	1.3	0.6
40009	Granola, oats, honey, raisin	0.5	cup	51		225	5	34	3	9	3.6	3.8	1.1
40265	GrapeNut Flakes cereal	0.75	cup	29	1	106	3	24	3	1	0.2	0.2	0.5
40129	Heartwise Cereal	1	cup	39	1	113	4	31	9	1	0.2	0.2	0.4
40052	Honey Bran cereal	1	cup	35	1	119	3	29	4	1	0.3	0.1	0.3
40051	Honey Nut Cheerios cereal	1	cup	33	1	126	3	27	2	1	0.2	0.5	0.2
40134	Just Right cereal	1	cup	43	1	160	3	36	2	1	0.1	0.2	0.8
40053	Kashi GoodFriends cereal	0.75	cup	30		90	3	24	8	1			
5014	Kashi Medley cereal	0.5	cup	30		100	4	20	2	1			
40054	King Vitamin cereal	1	cup	21	<1	81	2	18	1	1	0.2	0.3	0.2
40010	Kix cereal	1.5	cup	28.35	1	108	2	24	1	1	0.2	0.1	<0.1
40011	Life cereal	1	cup	44	2	167	4	35	3	2	0.3	0.6	0.8
40124	Mueslix Five Grain cereal	1	cup	82	7	289	6	63	6	5	0.7	2	1.8
40275	Post Bran'ola Raisin cereal	0.5	cup	55		200	4	44	5	3	0.5		
40018	Puffed Rice cereal	1	cup	14	1	54	1	12	<1	<1	<0.1	<0.1	<0.1
40023	Puffed Wheat cereal	1	cup	12	<1	44	2	9	1	<1	<0.1	<0.1	0.1
40066	Quisp cereal	1	cup	30	1	121	1	26	1	2	0.5	0.4	0.2
40393	Raisin Nut Bran cereal	1	cup	55	2	209	5	41	5	4	0.7	1.9	0.5
40017	Rice Krispies cereal	1	cup	28	1	111	2	25	<1	<1	<0.1	<0.1	<0.1
40062	Shredded Wheat, lg biscuit	1	ea	23.6	1	85	3	19	2	<1	0.1	0.1	0.2
40022	Shredded Wheat, sm biscuit	0.75	cup	32	2	114	4	26	3	1	0.1	0.1	0.3
40068	Sugar Smacks cereal	0.75	cup	27	1	103	2	24	1	1	0.3	0.1	0.2
40070	Tasteeos cereal	1	cup	24	1	94	3	19	3	1	0.2	0.2	0.2
40024	Toasted Oat cereal	1	cup	30		114	3	23	2	2	0.3	0.5	0.4
40021	Total Wheat cereal	0.75	cup	30	1	105	3	24	3	1	0.2	0.1	0.1
Condiments, Sauces, and Gravies													
Condiments													
27000	Catsup/ketchup	1	cup	245	163	255	4	67	3	1	0.1	0.1	0.4
27001	Catsup/ketchup, packet	1	ea	6	4	6	<1	2	<1	<1	<0.1	<0.1	<0.1
27012	Dill pickle	1	ea	65	60	12	<1	3	1	<1	<0.1	<0.1	0.1
27013	Dill pickle, slices	10	pce	60	55	11	<1	2	1	<1	<0.1	<0.1	<0.1
27004	Horseradish, prepared	1	tsp	5	4	2	<1	1	<1	<1	<0.1	<0.1	<0.1
27009	Olives, large, ripe, pitted	10	ea	44	35	51	<1	3	1	5	0.6	3.5	0.4
27042	Olives, green, stuffed	10	ea	40	32	41	1	1	<1	4	0.6	3.2	0.4
27016	Pickle, sweet, medium	1	ea	35	23	41	<1	11	<1	<1	<0.1	<0.1	<0.1
435	Mustard, yellow, prepared	1	cup	250	204	165	10	19	8	8	0.4	5.4	1.5
Gravies													
53023	Beef gravy, canned	1	cup	233	204	123	9	11	1	5	2.7	2.2	0.2
53006	Beef gravy, homemade	1	cup	270	231	213	5	15	1	15	3.8	6.9	4.1
53027	Brown gravy, dry mix+water	1	cup	258	237	75	2	13	<1	2	0.8	0.7	0.1

< = Trace amount present   Blank = Not available

CHOL, cholesterol; **V,** vitamin; **THI,** thiamin; **RIB,** riboflavin; **NIA,** niacin; **FOL,** folate;
CALC, calcium; **PHOS,** phosphate; **SOD,** sodium; **POT,** potassium; **MAG,** magnesium

CHOL (mg)	V-A (RE)	THI (mg)	RIB (mg)	NIA (mg)	V-B6 (mg)	FOL (μg)	V-B12 (μg)	V-C (mg)	V-E (mg)	CALC (mg)	PHOS (mg)	SOD (mg)	POT (mg)	MAG (mg)	IRON (mg)	ZINC (mg)
0	311	0.4	0.4	5.2	0.5	104	0	12	0.3	3	55	152	59	18	4.7	3.9
0	225	0.4	0.4	5	0.5	100	1.5	0		4	37	40	34	16	1.8	1.5
0	200							0		20		50			1.8	
1	2	0.2	0.1	1	0.1	13	0	<1	0.3	33	130	145	189	44	1.4	1
1	1	0.1	0.1	0.8	0.1	14	0.1	<1	0.5	59	152	19	250	49	1.2	1
0	225	0.4	0.4	5	0.5	100	1.5	0	0.1	11	88	140	99	30	8.1	1.2
0	310	0.5	0.6	7	0.7	136	2	0	<0.1	30	154	168	265	55	6.2	2.1
0	463	0.5	0.5	6.2	0.6	23	1.9	19	0.8	16	132	202	150	46	5.6	0.9
0	248	0.4	0.5	5.5	0.6	110	0	16	0.3	22	113	285	94	32	4.9	4.1
0	294	0.3	0.3	3.9	0.4	80	1.2	0	1.8	11	83	264	95	27	12.7	0.7
0	0	<0.1	<0.1	1.2	0.1	7		0		0	102	70	119		0.4	
0	0	0.1	0.1	1.1	0.1	7		0		0	84	50	108		0.4	
0	212	0.3	0.3	3.5	0.4	71	1.1	8	6.7	3	54	176	58	18	5.9	2.7
0	355	0.4	0.4	4.7	0.5	94	0	14	0.1	41	40	249	39	9	7.7	3.5
0	2	0.6	0.6	7.3	0.7	147	0	0	0.2	134	186	240	109	43	12.3	5.5
0	747	0.7	0.8	9.8	1	197	3.3	1	8.9	67	215	107	369	82	8.9	7.5
0	375	0.4	0.4	5	0.5	100	1.5	0		0	100	220	220	40	4.5	1.5
0	0	0.1	<0.1	0.9	0	1	0	0	<0.1	1	17	1	16	4	0.4	0.2
0	<1	<0.1	<0.1	1.4	<0.1	4	0.1	0	0.1	3	40	1	44	16	0.6	0.4
0	4	0.4	0.5	5.7	0.6	113	0	0	0.2	6	47	216	40	15	5.1	4.2
0	0	0.4	0.4	5	0.5	100	0	0	2	74	163	246	218	54	4.5	1.1
0	371	0.5	0.6	6.9	0.7	138	0.1	15	0.1	5	31	206	27	12	0.7	0.5
0	0	0.1	0.1	1.1	0.1	12	0	0	0.1	10	86	<1	77	40	0.7	0.6
0	0	0.1	0.1	1.7	0.1	16	0	0	0.5	12	113	3	116	42	1.4	1.1
0	225	0.4	0.4	5	0.5	100	0	15	0.1	3	40	51	42	16	1.8	0.4
0	318	0.3	0.4	4.2	0.4	85	1.3	13	0.2	11	96	183	71	26	6.9	0.7
0	102	0.4	0.4	5.1	0.5	103	0	12	0.8	12	116	284	87	29	8.5	4.4
0	375	1.5	1.7	20.1	2	400	7.7	60	23.5	258	211	199	97	32	18	15
0	250	0.2	0.2	3.3	0.4	37	0	37	3.6	47	96	2905	1178	54	1.7	0.6
0	6	<0.1	<0.1	0.1	<0.1	1	0	1	0.1	1	2	71	29	1	<0.1	<0.1
0	21	<0.1	<0.1	<0.1	<0.1	1	0	1	0.1	6	14	833	75	7	0.3	0.1
0	20	<0.1	<0.1	<0.1	<0.1	1	0	1	0.1	5	13	769	70	7	0.3	0.1
0	0	0	<0.1	<0.1	<0.1	3	0	1	0	3	2	16	12	1	<0.1	<0.1
0	18	<0.1	0	<0.1	<0.1	0	0	<1	1.3	39	1	384	4	2	1.5	0.1
0	25	0	<0.1	<0.1	<0.1	1	0	5	1.1	21	7	826	28	8	0.6	0.1
0	5	<0.1	<0.1	0.1	<0.1	<1	0	<1	0.1	1	4	329	11	1	0.2	<0.1
7	0	0.1	0.1	1.5	<0.1	5	0.2	0	0.6	14	70	1304	189	5	1.6	2.3
5	300	<0.1	0.1	1.2	<0.1	5	0.3	0	0.4	54	78	1558	294	5	1.3	2.2
3	0	<0.1	0.1	0.8	0	0	0	0	0.3	67	44	1075	57	10	0.2	0.3

ERA, EatRight Analysis CD-ROM; **AMT,** amount; **WT,** weight; **WTR,** water; **CAL,** calories; **PROT,** protein; **CARB**, carbohydrate; **FIBR,** fiber; **FAT,** fat; **SATF,** saturated fat; **MONO,** monounsaturated fat; **POLY,** polyunsaturated fat

ERA CODE	FOOD DESCRIPTION	AMT	UNIT	WT (g)	WTR (g)	CAL (kcal)	PROT (g)	CARB (g)	FIBR (g)	FAT (g)	SATF (g)	MONO (g)	POLY (g)
Condiments, Sauces, and Gravies (continued)													
Gravies (continued)													
53022	Chicken gravy, canned	1	cup	238	203	188	5	13	1	14	3.4	6.1	3.6
53028	Chicken gravy, dry+water	1	cup	260	238	83	3	14	<1	2	0.5	0.9	0.4
53005	Chicken gravy, homemade	1	cup	260	221	194	12	13	1	10	2.8	4.3	2.6
53026	Mushroom gravy, canned	1	cup	238	212	119	3	13	1	6	1	2.8	2.4
53039	Mushroom gravy, dry+water	1	cup	258	237	70	2	14	1	1	0.5	0.3	<0.1
53033	Turkey gravy, canned	1	cup	238	211	121	6	12	1	5	1.5	2.1	1.2
53045	Turkey gravy, dry+water	1	cup	261	237	86	3	15	1	2	0.5	0.8	0.4
Sauces													
53388	Alfredo sauce, DiGiorno	0.25	cup	62		230	4	2	0	22	10		
53396	Alfredo sauce, low fat, DiGiorno	0.25	cup	69		170	5	16	0	10	6		
53000	Barbecue sauce	1	cup	250	202	188	4	32	3	4	0.7	1.9	1.7
53015	Cheese sauce	0.5	cup	101	64	221	10	9	<1	16	9.3	4.9	2.2
53016	Curry sauce	0.5	cup	115	102	74	3	3	<1	6	1	2.6	1.7
53103	Enchilada sauce, green	1	cup	250	217	187	4	13	4	14	8.1	3.9	1.2
53102	Enchilada sauce, red	1	cup	250	205	321	3	10	2	31	16.7	10.1	2.8
53351	Hoisin sauce	2	Tbs	34		70	1	14	0	2	0		
53110	Hollandaise sauce, mix+water	1	cup	259.2	217	238	5	14	1	20	11.6	5.9	0.9
53098	Horseradish sauce	1	Tbs	14	10	30	<1	1	<1	3	1.8	0.8	0.1
7563	Miso sauce	1	cup	248	141	389	13	73	6	7	1	1.5	3.8
53106	Pesto sauce	1	cup	232	48	1240	45	16	7	114	30.5	69.6	8
53466	Salsa, ready-to-serve	1	cup	259	234	73	3	16	4	1	0.1	0.1	0.3
53002	Soy sauce	1	Tbs	16	11	9	1	1	<1	<1	0	<0.1	<0.1
53267	Soy sauce, lite	1	Tbs	18	13	15	1	2	0	<1	0		
53011	Spaghetti sauce w/meat, canned	1	cup	250	212	178	7	19	4	8	1.8	3.3	1.8
53010	Spaghetti sauce w/meat, recipe	1	cup	248	189	287	16	21	4	17	4.5	6.2	4.3
53014	Spaghetti sauce+mushroom, can	0.75	cup	185	155	162	2	19	2	4	0.6	2.3	1.2
53008	Spaghetti/marinara sauce	1	cup	250	217	142	4	21	4	5	0.7	2.2	1.8
53001	Szechuan sauce	1	cup	250	202	188	4	32	3	4	0.7	1.9	1.7
53085	Tabasco sauce/pepper sauce	1	Tbs	15.6	15	2	<1	<1	<1	<1	<0.1	<0.1	<0.1
53415	Tartar sauce, nonfat, Kraft	2	Tbs	32		25	0	5	<1	0	0	0	0
53004	Teriyaki sauce	1	Tbs	18	12	15	1	3	<1	0	0	0	0
53025	White sauce, dry mix+milk	1	cup	264	215	240	10	21	<1	13	6.4	4.7	1.7
53007	White sauce, recipe	1	cup	250	192	355	9	20	<1	27	7.8	9.1	8.8
53099	Worcestershire sauce	1	cup	272	190	182	0	45	0	0	0	0	0
Dairy Products and Substitutes													
Creams and Substitutes													
501	Cream, coffee/table	1	cup	240	177	469	6	9	0	46	28.8	13.4	1.7
500	Cream, Half & Half	1	cup	242	195	315	7	10	0	28	17.3	8	1
502	Cream, heavy whipping, liq	1	cup	238	137	820	5	7	0	88	54.8	25.4	3.3
503	Cream, hvy whipping, whipped	2	cup	239	138	824	5	7	0	88	55	25.5	3.3
511	Cream, light whipping, liq	1	cup	239	152	699	5	7	0	74	46.2	21.7	2.1
527	Cream, medium fat, 25%	1	cup	239	164	583	6	8	0	60	37.3	17.2	2.2
540	Cremora NonDairy Creamer	1	tsp	2	<1	12	<1	1	0	1	0.7	<0.1	0

< = Trace amount present   Blank = Not available

CHOL, cholesterol; **V,** vitamin; **THI,** thiamin; **RIB,** riboflavin; **NIA,** niacin; **FOL,** folate;
CALC, calcium; **PHOS,** phosphate; **SOD,** sodium; **POT,** potassium; **MAG,** magnesium

CHOL (mg)	V-A (RE)	THI (mg)	RIB (mg)	NIA (mg)	V-B6 (mg)	FOL (μg)	V-B12 (μg)	V-C (mg)	V-E (mg)	CALC (mg)	PHOS (mg)	SOD (mg)	POT (mg)	MAG (mg)	IRON (mg)	ZINC (mg)
5	264	<0.1	0.1	1.1	<0.1	5	0.2	0	0.4	48	69	1373	259	5	1.1	1.9
3	0	0.1	0.1	0.8	<0.1	3	0.2	3	0.1	39	47	1133	62	10	0.3	0.3
110	653	0.1	0.4	3.2	0.1	98	4.7	1	0.6	31	124	1365	302	9	3.1	2.9
0	0	0.1	0.1	1.6	<0.1	29	0	0	0.2	17	36	1356	252	5	1.6	1.7
0	0	0.1	0.1	0.8	<0.1	3	0.2	2	<0.1	49	44	1400	57	8	0.3	0.3
5	0	<0.1	0.2	3.1	<0.1	5	0.2	0	0.1	10	69	1373	259	5	1.7	1.9
3	0	0.1	0.1	1	<0.1	3	0.3	2	0.1	50	50	1495	65	10	0.3	0.3
45	80	0	0.1	0				0		100	100	550	75	0	0	
30	80	0	0.1	0				0		150	100	600	80	8	0	
0	218	0.1	0.1	2.2	0.2	10	0	18	2.8	48	50	2037	435	45	2.2	0.5
36	167	0.1	0.2	0.5	<0.1	10	0.4	1	1.2	267	202	515	126	17	0.6	1.1
0	61	<0.1	0.1	1.6	<0.1	3	0.1	<1	1	9	38	392	104	3	0.5	0.1
43	156	0.1	0.2	2.9	0.2	13	0.1	23	0.9	77	118	30	540	41	1.2	0.6
91	349	0.1	0.1	0.7	0.1	17	0.1	20	1.6	55	76	36	336	20	0.6	0.3
0	0							0		0		500			0	
52	220	0.1	0.2	0.1	0.5	21	0.8	<1	0.6	124	127	1565	124	8	0.9	0.8
6	27	<0.1	<0.1	<0.1	<0.1	2	<0.1	<1	0.1	16	12	10	20	2	<0.1	<0.1
0	10	0.1	0.3	1	0.2	37	0	0	<0.1	77	173	4061	208	53	3.2	3.7
80	336	0.1	0.4	1.6	0.3	58	1.4	18	11.3	1762	908	1904	726	126	8.5	4.3
0	155	0.1	0.1	2.1	0.3	41	0	36	1.6	78	67	1124	552	34	2.5	0.6
0	0	<0.1	<0.1	0.4	<0.1	3	0	0	0	3	20	871	64	7	0.3	0.1
0	0							0		3		505			0.1	
15	176	0.1	0.1	3.5	0.3	25	0.5	19	3	54	104	982	742	43	2.1	1.3
46	487	0.2	0.3	6	0.5	30	1.4	37	5.3	59	173	868	1098	62	3.5	3.4
0	362	0.1	0.1	1.4	0.2	19	0	14	2.9	22	45	744	500	22	1.5	0.5
0	95	0.1	0.1	2.7	0.3	25	0	20	3.1	55	80	1030	738	42	1.8	0.4
0	218	0.1	0.1	2.2	0.2	10	0	18	2.8	48	50	2037	435	45	2.2	0.5
<1	65	<0.1	<0.1	0.1	<0.1	<1	9.4	<1	0.1	4	3	92	20	1	0.4	<0.1
0	0							0		0		210	15		0	
0	0	<0.1	<0.1	0.2	<0.1	4	0	0	0	4	28	690	40	11	0.3	<0.1
34	92	0.1	0.4	0.5	0.1	16	1.1	3	10	425	256	797	444	264	0.3	0.5
29	310	0.2	0.4	1	0.1	14	0.8	2	3.4	260	216	368	343	32	0.7	0.9
0	30	0.2	0.4	1.9	0	0	0	35	0	291	163	2665	2176	35	14.4	0.5
159	437	0.1	0.4	0.1	0.1	6	0.5	2	0.4	231	192	95	292	21	0.1	0.6
89	259	0.1	0.4	0.2	0.1	6	0.8	2	0.3	254	230	98	314	25	0.2	1.2
326	1001	0.1	0.3	0.1	0.1	9	0.4	1	1.5	154	148	89	179	17	0.1	0.5
328	1006	0.1	0.3	0.1	0.1	9	0.4	1	1.5	154	149	90	180	17	0.1	0.5
265	705	0.1	0.3	0.1	0.1	9	0.5	1	1.4	166	146	82	231	17	0.1	0.6
209	554	0.1	0.3	0.1	0.1	5	0.5	2	1.4	216	169	88	275	20	0.1	0.6
0	<1		0									6				

ERA, EatRight Analysis CD-ROM; **AMT,** amount; **WT,** weight; **WTR,** water; **CAL,** calories; **PROT,** protein; **CARB**, carbohydrate; **FIBR,** fiber; **FAT,** fat; **SATF,** saturated fat; **MONO,** monounsaturated fat; **POLY,** polyunsaturated fat

ERA CODE	FOOD DESCRIPTION	AMT	UNIT	WT (g)	WTR (g)	CAL (kcal)	PROT (g)	CARB (g)	FIBR (g)	FAT (g)	SATF (g)	MONO (g)	POLY (g)
Dairy Products and Substitutes (continued)													
Creams and Substitutes (continued)													
517	Mocha mix creamer	1	Tbs	14.2		19	<1	1	0	2	0.3	0	0.7
504	Sour cream, cultured	1	cup	230	163	493	7	10	0	48	30	13.9	1.8
505	Sour cream, imitation	1	cup	230	164	479	6	15	0	45	40.9	1.4	0.1
515	Sour cream, low cal	1	Tbs	15	12	20	<1	1	0	2	1.1	0.5	0.1
526	Whip topping, low cal, from mix	1	cup	80	66	42	1	8	0	5	2.5	1.1	0.9
Milks and Nondairy Milks													
7	Buttermilk, cultured, skim	1	cup	245	221	99	8	12	0	2	1.3	0.6	0.1
19	Chocolate milk, 1% fat	1	cup	250	211	158	8	26	1	2	1.5	0.8	0.1
18	Chocolate milk, 2% fat	1	cup	250	209	179	8	26	1	5	3.1	1.5	0.2
59	Chocolate milk, nonfat	1	cup	250	211	144	9	27	1	1	0.7	0.3	<0.1
20	Chocolate milk, whole	1	cup	250	206	208	8	26	2	8	5.3	2.5	0.3
98	Eggnog, 2% fat	1	cup	254	215	191	12	17	0	8	3.7	2.7	0.7
17	Eggnog, whole milk	1	cup	254	189	342	10	34	0	19	11.3	5.7	0.9
80	Evaporated milk, 2% fat	1	cup	252	196	232	19	28	0	5	3.1	1.4	0.2
10	Evaporated milk, skim	1	cup	256	203	199	19	29	0	1	0.3	0.2	<0.1
23	Goat milk	1	cup	244	212	168	9	11	0	10	6.5	2.7	0.4
54	Lactose reduced milk, 1% fat	1	cup	246	222	103	8	12	0	3	1.6	0.8	0.1
56	Lactose reduced milk, nonfat	1	cup	245	222	86	8	12	0	<1	0.3	0.1	<0.1
4	Milk, 1% fat	1	cup	244	220	102	8	12	0	3	1.6	0.7	0.1
2	Milk, 2% fat	1	cup	244	218	121	8	12	0	5	2.9	1.4	0.2
6	Milk, nonfat	1	cup	245	222	86	8	12	0	<1	0.3	0.1	<0.1
1	Milk, whole, 3.3% fat	1	cup	244	215	150	8	11	0	8	5.1	2.4	0.3
57	Nonfat dry milk powder+water	1	cup	245	223	82	8	12	0	<1	0.1	<0.1	<0.1
20033	Soy milk	1	cup	245	228	81	7	4	3	5	0.5	0.8	2
7801	Soy milk bev, carob (Eden)	1	cup	244		150	6	23	0	4	0.5		
7775	Soy milk bev, vanilla (VitaSoy)	1	cup	228.3		190	7	27		6	1	1	3
11	Sweetened condensed milk	1	cup	306	83	982	24	166	0	27	16.8	7.4	1
82	Vitamite imitation milk	1	cup	244	220	112	4	13	0	5	0.6	1.2	2.9
Natural Cheeses													
1029	Asiago cheese, shredded	1	cup	108	40	406	31	4	0	30	19.2	7.9	1
1003	Blue cheese	1	cup	135	57	477	29	3	0	39	25.2	10.5	1.1
1037	Brick cheese, shredded	1	cup	113	46	419	26	3	0	34	21.2	9.7	0.9
1004	Brie cheese, sliced	1	cup	144	70	480	30	1	0	40	25.1	11.5	1.2
1006	Camembert cheese	1	cup	246	127	737	49	1	0	60	37.5	17.3	1.8
1227	Cheddar cheese, fat free (Lifetime)	0.25	cup	31	18	44	9	1	0	0	0	0	0
1423	Cheddar cheese, low fat	0.25	cup	31	15	89	10	1	0	5	3.3		
1091	Cheddar cheese, low fat, low sod	1	cup	113	73	195	27	2	0	8	5	2.3	0.2
1105	Cheddar cheese, low sod	1	cup	113	44	450	28	2	0	37	23.5	10.4	1.1
1008	Cheddar cheese, shredded	1	cup	113	42	455	28	1	0	37	23.8	10.6	1.1
1010	Colby cheese, shredded	1	cup	113	43	445	27	3	0	36	22.8	10.5	1.1
1047	Cottage cheese, 1% Lowfat	1	cup	226	186	164	28	6	0	2	1.5	0.7	0.1
1014	Cottage cheese, 2% lowfat	1	cup	226	179	203	31	8	0	4	2.8	1.2	0.1
1013	Cottage cheese, crm, lg curd	1	cup	225	178	232	28	6	0	10	6.4	2.9	0.3
1012	Cottage cheese, crm, sm curd	1	cup	210	166	217	26	6	0	9	6	2.7	0.3

< = Trace amount present   Blank = Not available

CHOL, cholesterol; **V,** vitamin; **THI,** thiamin; **RIB,** riboflavin; **NIA,** niacin; **FOL,** folate;
CALC, calcium; **PHOS,** phosphate; **SOD,** sodium; **POT,** potassium; **MAG,** magnesium

CHOL (mg)	V-A (RE)	THI (mg)	RIB (mg)	NIA (mg)	V-B6 (mg)	FOL (μg)	V-B12 (μg)	V-C (mg)	V-E (mg)	CALC (mg)	PHOS (mg)	SOD (mg)	POT (mg)	MAG (mg)	IRON (mg)	ZINC (mg)
0										1	8	7	20	0		
102	448	0.1	0.3	0.2	<0.1	25	0.7	2	1.5	268	195	122	331	26	0.1	0.6
0	0	0	0	0	0	0	0	0	0.3	6	102	235	369	15	0.9	2.7
6	17	<0.1	<0.1	<0.1	<0.1	2	<0.1	<1	0.1	16	14	6	19	2	<0.1	0.1
0	0	0	0	0	0	0	0	0	<0.1	2	24	85	21	1	<0.1	<0.1
9	20	0.1	0.4	0.1	0.1	12	0.5	2	0.2	285	218	257	371	27	0.1	1
7	148	0.1	0.4	0.3	0.1	12	0.9	2	0.1	287	256	152	426	33	0.6	1
17	142	0.1	0.4	0.3	0.1	12	0.8	2	1.5	284	254	150	422	33	0.6	1
4	142	0.1	0.3	0.3	0.1	14	0.9	2	0.1	292	265	121	486	45	0.7	1.2
30	72	0.1	0.4	0.3	0.1	12	0.8	2	0.2	280	251	149	417	33	0.6	1
194	197	0.1	0.6	0.2	0.1	30	1.2	2	0.6	270	270	155	368	32	0.7	1.3
149	203	0.1	0.5	0.3	0.1	2	1.1	4	0.6	330	278	138	420	47	0.5	1.2
20	331	0.1	0.8	0.4	0.1	21	0.6	3	0.1	717	482	285	821	67	0.7	2.2
9	300	0.1	0.8	0.4	0.1	22	0.6	3	0.2	741	499	294	849	69	0.7	2.3
28	137	0.1	0.3	0.7	0.1	1	0.2	3	0.2	326	270	122	499	34	0.1	0.7
10	145	0.1	0.4	0.2	0.1	13	0.9	2	0.1	302	237	124	384	34	0.1	1
4	149	0.1	0.3	0.2	0.1	13	0.9	2	0.1	302	247	126	406	28	0.1	1
10	144	0.1	0.4	0.2	0.1	12	0.9	2	0.1	300	235	123	381	34	0.1	1
18	139	0.1	0.4	0.2	0.1	12	0.9	2	0.2	297	232	122	377	33	0.1	1
4	149	0.1	0.3	0.2	0.1	13	0.9	2	0.1	302	247	126	406	28	0.1	1
33	76	0.1	0.4	0.2	0.1	12	0.9	2	0.2	291	228	120	370	33	0.1	0.9
4	162	0.1	0.4	0.2	0.1	11	0.9	1	<0.1	284	224	132	388	29	0.1	1.1
0	7	0.4	0.2	0.4	0.1	4	0	0	<0.1	10	120	29	345	47	1.4	0.6
0	0	0.9	0.1	1.2	0.1	40		0		60	100	105	330	40	1.8	0.6
0		0.2	0.2							80		130	210		0.7	
104	248	0.3	1.3	0.6	0.2	34	1.4	8	0.7	868	775	389	1136	78	0.6	2.9
0	149	0	0	0.2	0	0	0	0	0	200	244	134	366	2	0.2	0.2
99	273	<0.1	0.4	0.1	0.1	7	1.8	0	0.5	1037	653	281	120	39	0.2	4.2
102	308	<0.1	0.5	1.4	0.2	49	1.6	0	0.9	712	523	1883	346	31	0.4	3.6
107	341	<0.1	0.4	0.1	0.1	23	1.4	0	0.6	761	510	632	153	27	0.5	2.9
144	262	0.1	0.7	0.5	0.3	94	2.4	0	0.9	265	271	906	219	29	0.7	3.4
177	620	0.1	1.2	1.5	0.6	153	3.2	0	1.6	953	853	2070	459	49	0.8	5.9
3	95									443		244				
17	95							1		277		105			0.4	
24	70	<0.1	<0.1	0.1	0.1	20	0.9	0	0.2	794	547	24	126	31	0.8	3.5
113	325	<0.1	0.4	0.1	0.1	20	0.9	0	0.4	794	547	24	126	31	0.8	3.5
118	314	<0.1	0.4	0.1	0.1	21	0.9	0	0.4	815	579	701	111	31	0.8	3.5
107	311	<0.1	0.4	0.1	0.1	21	0.9	0	0.4	774	516	683	143	29	0.9	3.5
10	25	<0.1	0.4	0.3	0.2	28	1.4	0	1.5	138	302	918	193	12	0.3	0.9
19	45	0.1	0.4	0.3	0.2	30	1.6	0	0.1	155	340	918	217	14	0.4	0.9
34	108	<0.1	0.4	0.3	0.2	27	1.4	0	1.4	135	296	911	190	12	0.3	0.8
31	101	<0.1	0.3	0.3	0.1	26	1.3	0	1.3	126	277	850	177	11	0.3	0.8

ERA, EatRight Analysis CD-ROM; **AMT,** amount; **WT,** weight; **WTR,** water; **CAL,** calories; **PROT,** protein; **CARB**, carbohydrate; **FIBR,** fiber; **FAT,** fat; **SATF,** saturated fat; **MONO,** monounsaturated fat; **POLY,** polyunsaturated fat

ERA CODE	FOOD DESCRIPTION	AMT	UNIT	WT (g)	WTR (g)	CAL (kcal)	PROT (g)	CARB (g)	FIBR (g)	FAT (g)	SATF (g)	MONO (g)	POLY (g)
Dairy Products and Substitutes (continued)													
Natural Cheeses (continued)													
1015	Cream cheese	1	cup	232	125	810	18	6	0	81	51	22.8	2.9
1115	Cream cheese, fat free	2	Tbs	33		30	5	2	0	0	0	0	0
1098	Cream cheese, low fat	1	Tbs	15	10	35	2	1	0	3	1.7	0.7	0.1
1083	Cream cheese, soft	2	Tbs	30		100	2	1	0	10	7		
1050	Edam cheese	1	cup	132	55	471	33	2	0	37	23.2	10.7	0.9
1016	Feta cheese, shredded	1	cup	150	83	395	21	6	0	32	22.4	6.9	0.9
1052	Fontina cheese, shredded	1	cup	108	41	420	28	2	0	34	20.7	9.4	1.8
1078	Goat cheese, hard	1	oz	28.35	8	128	9	1	0	10	7	2.3	0.2
1080	Goat cheese, soft type	1	cup	246	149	659	46	2	0	52	35.8	11.8	1.2
1054	Gouda cheese	1	cup	132	55	470	33	3	0	36	23.2	10.2	0.9
1074	Gruyere cheese, shredded	1	cup	108	36	446	32	<1	0	35	20.4	10.8	1.9
1038	Havarti cheese, diced	1	cup	132	54	490	31	4	0	39	24.8	11.3	1
1223	Jack cheese, fat free (Lifetime)	1	cup	124	72	177	35	4	0	0	0	0	0
1017	Monterey Jack cheese, shredded	1	cup	113	46	422	28	1	0	34	21.5	9.9	1
1056	Mozzarella cheese, whole, shred	1	cup	113	61	318	22	3	0	24	14.9	7.4	0.9
1058	Mozzarella, part skim, shredded	1	cup	113	61	287	27	3	0	18	11.4	5.1	0.5
1021	Muenster cheese, shredded	1	cup	113	47	416	26	1	0	34	21.6	9.8	0.7
1060	Neufchatel cheese	1	cup	232	144	603	23	7	0	54	34.3	15.7	1.5
1075	Parmesan cheese, grated	1	cup	100		456	42	4	0	30	19.1	8.7	0.7
1112	Parmesan cheese, shredded	1	Tbs	5	1	21	2	<1	0	1	0.9	0.4	<0.1
1062	Port du Salut cheese, shredded	1	cup	113	51	397	27	1	0	32	18.9	10.6	0.8
1023	Provolone cheese, diced	1	cup	132	54	464	34	3	0	35	22.5	9.8	1
1024	Ricotta cheese, part skim	1	cup	246	183	340	28	13	0	19	12.1	5.7	0.6
1064	Ricotta cheese, whole milk	1	cup	246	176	428	28	7	0	32	20.4	8.9	0.9
1066	Romano cheese, grated	1	cup	100		387	32	4	0	27	17.1	7.8	0.6
1026	Roquefort cheese, crumbled	1	cup	135	53	498	29	3	0	41	26	11.4	1.8
1059	String cheese, stick	1	ea	28.35	15	72	7	1	0	5	2.9	1.3	0.1
1428	Swiss cheese, low fat	0.25	cup	31	13	100	9	1	0	7	4.4		
1027	Swiss cheese, shredded	1	cup	108	40	406	31	4	0	30	19.2	7.9	1
Processed Cheese and Cheese Substitutes													
1001	American cheese food	1	oz	28.35	12	94	6	2	0	7	4.4	2	0.2
1000	American processed cheese	1	pce	21	8	79	5	<1	0	7	4.1	1.9	0.2
1002	Cheez Whiz/cheese spread	1	cup	244	116	709	40	21	0	52	32.5	15.2	1.5
1081	Kraft Free Singles cheese	1	pce	19		30	4	3	0	0	0	0	0
1069	Pimento proc cheese, shred	1	cup	113	44	424	25	2	0	35	22.2	10.1	1.1
1071	Swiss cheese food, slice	1	pce	21	9	68	5	1	0	5	3.3	1.4	0.1
1272	Velveeta cheese spread	1	oz	28	13	85	5	3	0	6	4		
1094	Velveeta, low fat, low sod	1	pce	34	21	61	8	1	0	2	1.5	0.7	0.1
1420	White American cheese, fat free	0.25	cup	31	19	27	5	1	0	0	0	0	0
Yogurt													
7546	Tofu yogurt	1	cup	262	203	254	9	43	1	5	0.7	1	2.7
2428	Yogurt, custard type, berry	6	oz	170		180	7	30		4			
2014	Yogurt, low fat, coffee/vanilla	1	cup	245	194	209	12	34	0	3	2	0.8	0.1

< = Trace amount present

Blank = Not available

CHOL, cholesterol; **V,** vitamin; **THI,** thiamin; **RIB,** riboflavin; **NIA,** niacin; **FOL,** folate;
CALC, calcium; **PHOS,** phosphate; **SOD,** sodium; **POT,** potassium; **MAG,** magnesium

CHOL (mg)	V-A (RE)	THI (mg)	RIB (mg)	NIA (mg)	V-B6 (mg)	FOL (μg)	V-B12 (μg)	V-C (mg)	V-E (mg)	CALC (mg)	PHOS (mg)	SOD (mg)	POT (mg)	MAG (mg)	IRON (mg)	ZINC (mg)
254	886	<0.1	0.5	0.2	0.1	31	1	0	2.2	185	242	686	277	15	2.8	1.3
2	143		0.3				0.1	0		100	150	160	65	0	0	0.3
8	33	<0.1	<0.1	<0.1	<0.1	3	0.1	0	0.1	17	22	44	25	1	0.3	0.1
30	86		<0.1				0	0		20	20	100	40	0	0	0
118	334	<0.1	0.5	0.1	0.1	21	2	0	1	965	707	1273	248	39	0.6	4.9
134	192	0.2	1.3	1.5	0.6	48	2.5	0	<0.1	739	506	1674	93	29	1	4.3
125	313	<0.1	0.2	0.2	0.1	6	1.8	0	0.4	594	374	864	69	15	0.2	3.8
30	135	<0.1	0.3	0.7	<0.1	1	<0.1	0	0.2	254	207	98	14	15	0.5	0.4
113	696	0.2	0.9	1.1	0.6	30	0.5	0	1.1	344	630	905	64	39	4.7	2.3
150	230	<0.1	0.4	0.1	0.1	28	2	0	0.5	924	721	1081	159	38	0.3	5.1
119	325	0.1	0.3	0.1	0.1	11	1.7	0	0.4	1091	654	363	87	39	0.2	4.2
125	399	<0.1	0.5	0.2	0.1	27	1.7	0	0.7	889	595	739	179	32	0.6	3.4
13	380									1771		974				
100	286	<0.1	0.4	0.1	0.1	21	0.9	0	0.4	843	502	606	91	31	0.8	3.4
89	272	<0.1	0.3	0.1	0.1	8	0.7	0	0.7	584	419	422	76	21	0.2	2.5
65	200	<0.1	0.3	0.1	0.1	10	0.9	0	0.7	730	523	526	95	26	0.2	3.1
108	357	<0.1	0.4	0.1	0.1	14	1.7	0	0.5	810	528	709	152	31	0.5	3.2
176	696	<0.1	0.5	0.3	0.1	26	0.6	0	2.2	175	316	927	265	18	0.6	1.2
79	173	<0.1	0.4	0.3	0.1	8	1.4	0	0.8	1375	807	1861	107	51	0.9	3.2
4	9	<0.1	<0.1	<0.1	<0.1	<1	0.1	0	<0.1	63	37	85	5	3	<0.1	0.2
139	420	<0.1	0.3	0.1	0.1	21	1.7	0	0.6	734	407	603	153	27	0.5	2.9
91	348	<0.1	0.4	0.2	0.1	14	1.9	0	0.5	998	655	1155	182	36	0.7	4.3
76	278	0.1	0.5	0.2	<0.1	32	0.7	0	1.6	669	449	307	308	36	1.1	3.3
124	330	<0.1	0.5	0.3	0.1	30	0.8	0	1.6	509	389	207	257	28	0.9	2.9
104	141	<0.1	0.4	0.1	0.1	7	1.1	0	0.7	1063	760	1200	86	41	0.8	2.6
122	404	0.1	0.8	1	0.2	66	0.9	0	2.7	893	529	2442	122	40	0.8	2.8
16	50	<0.1	0.1	<0.1	<0.1	2	0.2	0	0.2	183	131	132	24	7	0.1	0.8
22	95							1		277		39			0.4	
99	273	<0.1	0.4	0.1	0.1	7	1.8	0	0.5	1037	653	281	120	39	0.2	4.2
18	57	<0.1	0.1	<0.1	<0.1	2	0.4	0	0.2	141	113	274	103	8	0.2	0.9
20	61	<0.1	0.1	<0.1	<0.1	2	0.1	0	0.1	129	156	300	34	5	0.1	0.6
135	461	0.1	1.1	0.3	0.3	17	1	0	1.7	1371	1737	3282	590	70	0.8	6.3
2	86		0.1					0	0	150	714	290	55		0	
106	364	<0.1	0.4	0.1	0.1	9	0.8	3	0.5	694	840	1613	183	25	0.5	3.4
17	51	<0.1	0.1	<0.1	<0.1	1	0.5	0	0.1	152	110	326	60	6	0.1	0.7
22	89		0.1					<1		130	242	420	94		0.1	0.5
12	22	<0.1	0.1	<0.1	<0.1	3	0.3	0	0.2	232	281	2	61	8	0.1	1.1
5	62							1		164		459			0.4	
0	8	0.2	0.1	0.6	0.1	16	0	7	0.8	309	100	92	123	105	2.8	0.8
15	21	0.1	0.3				0.4			200	150	95	310			
12	32	0.1	0.5	0.3	0.1	26	1.3	2	0.1	420	330	161	537	40	0.2	2

ERA, EatRight Analysis CD-ROM; **AMT,** amount; **WT,** weight; **WTR,** water; **CAL,** calories; **PROT,** protein; **CARB**, carbohydrate; **FIBR,** fiber; **FAT,** fat; **SATF,** saturated fat; **MONO,** monounsaturated fat; **POLY,** polyunsaturated fat

ERA CODE	FOOD DESCRIPTION	AMT	UNIT	WT (g)	WTR (g)	CAL (kcal)	PROT (g)	CARB (g)	FIBR (g)	FAT (g)	SATF (g)	MONO (g)	POLY (g)
Dairy Products and Substitutes (continued)													
Yogurt (continued)													
2001	Yogurt, low fat, fruit	1	cup	245	182	250	11	47	0	3	1.7	0.7	0.1
2000	Yogurt, low fat, plain	1	cup	245	208	155	13	17	0	4	2.5	1	0.1
2034	Yogurt, nonfat, low cal sweetener	1	cup	241	208	122	11	19	1	<1	0.2	0.1	<0.1
2012	Yogurt, nonfat, plain	1	cup	245	209	137	14	19	0	<1	0.3	0.1	<0.1
2099	Yogurt, nonfat, vanilla/coffee	1	cup	245	187	223	13	43	0	<1	0.3	0.1	<0.1
2013	Yogurt, whole milk, plain	1	cup	245	215	150	9	11	0	8	5.1	2.2	0.2
Desserts													
Cakes													
46004	Angel food cake	1	pce	28.35	9	73	2	16	<1	<1	<0.1	<0.1	0.1
46098	Applesauce cake, no icing	1	pce	87	20	313	3	52	2	12	2.4	5	3.5
46103	Banana cake, no icing	1	pce	87	29	262	3	46	1	8	1.6	3.6	2.1
46010	Carrot cake, cream chz icing	1	pce	111	23	484	5	52	1	29	5.4	7.2	15.1
49001	Cheesecake, mix, prepared	1	pce	99	44	271	5	35	2	13	6.6	4.5	0.8
49004	Cheesecake (pce=1/12)	1	pce	80	36	257	4	20	<1	18	7.9	6.9	1.3
49017	Cheesecake, chocolate	1	pce	128	37	505	8	49	2	32	15.5	11.3	3.6
46115	Choc sponge cake, no icing	1	pce	66	20	197	5	36	1	4	1.4	1.5	0.5
46013	Chocolate cake+choc icing	1	pce	64	15	235	3	35	2	10	3.1	5.6	1.2
46118	Chocolate cake+ van icing	1	pce	103		358	4	58	1	14	3.6	6.4	3.2
46093	Coffee cake, cinn+crumb top	1	pce	63	14	263	4	29	1	15	3.7	8.2	2
46097	Coffee cake, fruit	1	pce	50	16	156	3	26	1	5	1.2	2.8	0.7
46106	Date pudding cake	1	pce	42	14	131	2	19	1	6	3	1.9	0.3
45562	Funnel cake, 6 inch diam	1	pce	90	38	278	7	29	1	14	2.7	4.4	6.3
46066	German choc cake mix, prep+icing	1	pce	111	30	404	4	55	2	21	5.3	8.7	5.5
46000	Gingerbread cake, homemade	1	pce	74	21	263	3	36	1	12	3	5.3	3.1
42209	Hoecake, 1/8th pone	1	pce	61	31	129	2	24	2	3	0.6	1.2	1.1
46109	Ice cream cake roll (pce=1/10)	1	pce	34	13	101	1	14	<1	5	2.1	1.8	0.8
46111	Lemon cake+icing-2 layer	1	pce	109	24	385	3	71	1	11	1.9	4.8	3.4
46070	Pineapple upside down cake	1	pce	115	37	367	4	58	1	14	3.4	6	3.8
46107	Plum pudding cake	1	pce	42	14	131	2	19	1	6	3	1.9	0.3
46016	Pound cake w/butter	1	pce	28.35	7	110	2	14	<1	6	3.3	1.7	0.3
46077	Shortcake biscuit, recipe	1	ea	65	18	225	4	32	1	9	2.5	3.9	2.4
46011	Snack cake/choc+filling	1	ea	50	10	188	2	30	<1	7	1.4	2.8	2.6
46116	Spice cake w/icing	1	pce	109	29	368	5	62	1	12	3.2	5.9	1.9
46078	Sponge cake, recipe	1	pce	63	19	187	5	36	<1	3	0.8	1	0.4
46008	Twinkie snack cake	1	ea	42.5	9	155	1	27	<1	5	1.1	1.7	1.4
46017	White cake w/white icing	1	pce	71	14	266	2	45	1	10	4.3	3.8	1
46007	White cake w/choc icing	1	pce	100		364	3	64	1	12	5.2	3.6	1.8
46012	Yellow cake w/choc icing	1	pce	64	14	242	2	35	1	11	3	6.1	1.4
Cookies, Brownies, and Bars													
47073	Almond cookie	2	ea	20	1	103	2	10	1	6	1	3.4	1.6
47000	Brownie+nuts+icing, commerc	1	ea	61	8	247	3	39	1	10	2.6	5.5	1.4
47019	Brownie, fudge nut, recipe	1	ea	24	3	112	1	12	1	7	1.8	2.6	2.3
47005	Butter cookie, thin	5	ea	25	1	117	2	17	<1	5	2.8	1.4	0.2

< = Trace amount present

Blank = Not available

CHOL, cholesterol; **V,** vitamin; **THI,** thiamin; **RIB,** riboflavin; **NIA,** niacin; **FOL,** folate;
CALC, calcium; **PHOS,** phosphate; **SOD,** sodium; **POT,** potassium; **MAG,** magnesium

CHOL (mg)	V-A (RE)	THI (mg)	RIB (mg)	NIA (mg)	V-B6 (mg)	FOL (μg)	V-B12 (μg)	V-C (mg)	V-E (mg)	CALC (mg)	PHOS (mg)	SOD (mg)	POT (mg)	MAG (mg)	IRON (mg)	ZINC (mg)
10	27	0.1	0.4	0.2	0.1	23	1.1	2	0.1	372	292	143	476	36	0.2	1.8
15	39	0.1	0.5	0.3	0.1	27	1.4	2	0.1	447	352	172	573	43	0.2	2.2
3	6	0.1	0.4	0.5	0.1	32	1.1	26	0.2	370	291	139	550	41	0.6	1.8
4	5	0.1	0.6	0.3	0.1	30	1.5	2	<0.1	488	383	187	624	47	0.2	2.4
4	4	0.1	0.5	0.3	0.1	27	1.3	2	<0.1	436	343	168	559	42	0.2	2.1
31	74	0.1	0.3	0.2	0.1	18	0.9	1	0.2	296	232	114	379	28	0.1	1.4
0	0	<0.1	0.1	0.2	<0.1	10	<0.1	0	<0.1	40	9	212	26	3	0.1	<0.1
22	10	0.1	0.1	1.1	0.1	6	<0.1	1	1.6	17	45	141	144	11	1.4	0.2
32	83	0.1	0.2	1.2	0.2	11	0.1	3	1.2	26	50	181	168	15	1.1	0.3
60	426	0.2	0.2	1.1	0.1	13	0.1	1	11.3	28	79	273	124	20	1.4	0.5
29	98	0.1	0.3	0.5	0.1	30	0.3	<1	1.1	170	232	376	209	19	0.5	0.5
44	117	<0.1	0.2	0.2	<0.1	14	0.1	<1	2.2	41	74	166	72	9	0.5	0.4
118	296	0.2	0.3	1.3	0.1	14	0.2	<1	2	71	144	239	189	37	2.2	0.9
138	62	0.1	0.2	0.7	0.1	14	0.3	1	0.4	21	89	42	98	20	1.7	0.6
27	16	<0.1	0.1	0.4	<0.1	11	0.1	<1	4.7	28	78	214	128	22	1.4	0.4
35	102	0.1	0.1	0.6	<0.1	7	0.1	0		71	147	404	168	22	2.1	0.4
20	21	0.1	0.1	1.1	<0.1	38	0.1	<1	2.2	34	68	221	77	14	1.2	0.5
4	10	<0.1	0.1	1.3	<0.1	24	<0.1	<1	0.4	22	59	192	45	8	1.2	0.3
15	10	0.1	0.1	0.5	0.1	3	0.1	<1	0.2	46	36	66	199	23	1	0.2
63	58	0.2	0.3	1.9	0.1	14	0.2	<1	2.4	128	137	116	155	18	1.9	0.6
53	23	0.1	0.1	1.1	<0.1	4	0.1	0	1.2	53	173	368	151	19	1.2	0.5
24	10	0.1	0.1	1.3	0.1	24	<0.1	<1	6.9	53	40	242	325	52	2.1	0.3
0	0	0.1	0.1	1	0.1	5	0	0	0.4	70	98	132	87	39	1.2	0.6
15	22	<0.1	0.1	0.3	<0.1	2	0.1	<1	0.3	42	40	45	57	9	0.5	0.2
34	62	0.1	0.1	0.7	<0.1	6	0.1	1	1.6	67	154	359	53	6	0.8	0.2
25	75	0.2	0.2	1.4	<0.1	30	0.1	1	2.1	138	94	367	129	15	1.7	0.4
15	10	0.1	0.1	0.5	0.1	3	0.1	<1	0.2	46	36	66	199	23	1	0.2
63	44	<0.1	0.1	0.4	<0.1	12	0.1	0	0.2	10	39	113	34	3	0.4	0.1
2	12	0.2	0.2	1.7	<0.1	34	<0.1	<1	1.3	133	93	329	69	10	1.7	0.3
8	2	0.1	0.1	1.2	<0.1	14	<0.1	0	1.7	36	46	212	61	20	1.7	0.3
50	39	0.1	0.2	1.1	<0.1	9	0.1	<1	2.2	76	209	281	136	13	1.5	0.4
107	49	0.1	0.2	0.8	<0.1	25	0.2	0	0.3	26	63	144	89	6	1	0.4
7	2	0.1	0.1	0.5	<0.1	12	<0.1	<1	0.9	19	79	155	37	3	0.5	0.1
6	23	0.1	0.1	0.6	<0.1	4	<0.1	<1	1.3	34	46	166	41	4	0.6	0.1
18	58	0.1	0.1	0.4	<0.1	3	0.1	<1	1	78	132	308	72	5	0.7	0.2
35	21	0.1	0.1	0.8	<0.1	14	0.1	0	1.9	24	103	216	114	19	1.3	0.4
9	41	0.1	0.1	0.5	<0.1	4	<0.1	<1	1.6	15	35	47	44	15	0.5	0.2
10	4	0.2	0.1	1	<0.1	13	<0.1	0	1.3	18	62	190	91	19	1.4	0.4
18	48	<0.1	<0.1	0.2	<0.1	7	<0.1	<1	0.7	14	32	82	42	13	0.4	0.2
29	42	0.1	0.1	0.8	<0.1	10	0.1	0	0.1	7	26	88	28	3	0.6	0.1

ERA, EatRight Analysis CD-ROM; **AMT,** amount; **WT,** weight; **WTR,** water; **CAL,** calories; **PROT,** protein; **CARB**, carbohydrate; **FIBR,** fiber; **FAT,** fat; **SATF,** saturated fat; **MONO,** monounsaturated fat; **POLY,** polyunsaturated fat

ERA CODE	FOOD DESCRIPTION	AMT	UNIT	WT (g)	WTR (g)	CAL (kcal)	PROT (g)	CARB (g)	FIBR (g)	FAT (g)	SATF (g)	MONO (g)	POLY (g)
Desserts (continued)													
Cookies, Brownies, and Bars (continued)													
47075	Butterscotch brownie	1	ea	34	4	152	2	20	<1	8	1.4	3.3	2.5
47032	Choc chip cookie, commerc	1	ea	10	<1	45	1	7	<1	2	0.4	0.6	0.5
47035	Choc chip cookie, mix, prep	1	ea	16	1	79	1	10	<1	4	1.3	2.1	0.4
47002	Choc chip cookie, recipe, marg	1	ea	16	1	78	1	9	<1	5	1.3	1.7	1.3
47041	Chocolate wafer cookie	2	ea	12	1	52	1	9	<1	2	0.5	0.6	0.5
47042	Coconut macaroons, recipe	1	ea	24	3	97	1	17	<1	3	2.7	0.1	<0.1
47012	Fig bar cookie	1	ea	16	3	56	1	11	1	1	0.2	0.5	0.4
47043	Fortune cookie	1	ea	8	1	30	<1	7	<1	<1	0.1	0.1	<0.1
47376	Fruit cookie, no fat (Archway)	1	ea	28		90	2	21	0	0	0	0	0
47045	Gingersnap cookie	1	ea	7	<1	29	<1	5	<1	1	0.2	0.4	0.1
47009	Lady finger cookie	4	ea	44	9	161	5	26	<1	4	1.5	1.8	0.7
47078	Lemon bar cookie	1	ea	16	2	69	1	10	<1	3	0.6	1.4	0.8
47046	Marshmallow cookie, choc dip	1	ea	13	1	55	1	9	<1	2	0.6	1.2	0.3
47109	Molasses cookie	1	ea	15	1	64	1	11	<1	2	0.5	1.1	0.3
47171	Nilla Wafer cookie (Nabisco)	8	ea	32		140	1	24	<1	5	1	1.5	0
47054	Oatmeal cookie, homemade	1	ea	15	1	67	1	10	<1	3	0.5	1.1	0.8
47051	Oatmeal cookie, mix, prep	1	ea	16	1	74	1	10	1	3	0.8	1.7	0.4
47496	Oatmeal raisin cookie (Archway)	1	ea	26	3	107	1	17	1	4	0.8	1.3	0.3
47010	Peanut butter cookie, homemade	1	ea	20	1	95	2	12	<1	5	0.9	2.2	1.4
47062	Pecan shortbread cookie	1	ea	14	<1	76	1	8	<1	5	1.1	2.6	0.6
23171	Rice Krispies bar	1	ea	28	4	107	1	20	<1	3	0.6	1.3	0.8
47038	Sandw cookie, choc, choc dip	1	ea	17	<1	82	1	11	1	4	1.3	2.5	0.5
47006	Sandwich cookie, all types	4	ea	40	1	189	2	28	1	8	1.5	3.4	2.9
47180	Sandwich cookie, Oreo	3	ea	33		160	2	23	1	7	1.5	3	0.5
47059	Sandwich cookie, peanut butter	1	ea	14	<1	67	1	9	<1	3	0.7	1.6	0.5
47071	Sandwich cookie, vanilla	1	ea	10	<1	48	<1	7	<1	2	0.3	0.8	0.8
47007	Shortbread cookie	4	ea	32	1	161	2	21	1	8	2	4.3	1
47153	Snackwell dev fd cookie, svg	1	ea	16	3	49	1	12	<1	<1	0.1	<0.1	<0.1
47160	Snackwell van san cookie, svg	2	ea	26	1	109	1	21	1	2	0.5	0.8	0.2
47164	Snackwell choc san cookie, svg	3	ea	33	1	135	2	26	1	3	0.8	1	0.2
47011	Snickerdoodle cookie	1	ea	20	4	81	1	12	<1	3	2.1	1	0.2
47064	Sugar cookie	1	ea	15	1	72	1	10	<1	3	0.8	1.8	0.4
47068	Sugar cookie, made w/marg	1	ea	14	1	66	1	8	<1	3	0.7	1.4	1
47069	Sugar wafers, creme filled	1	ea	9	<1	46	<1	6	<1	2	0.3	0.9	0.8
Dessert Toppings													
23069	Butterscotch topping	2	Tbs	41	13	103	1	27	<1	<1	<0.1	<0.1	0
23070	Caramel topping	2	Tbs	41	13	103	1	27	<1	<1	<0.1	<0.1	0
23013	Chocolate syrup, thin	1	cup	300	93	837	6	195	5	3	1.6	0.9	0.1
509	Dessert topping/Dream Whip	1	cup	80	53	151	3	13	0	10	8.5	0.7	0.2
508	Frzn dessert topping/Cool Whip	1	cup	75	38	239	1	17	0	19	16.3	1.2	0.4
23014	Hot fudge chocolate topping	1	cup	340	74	1190	16	214	10	30	13.5	13.1	0.9
23071	Marshmallow creme topping	2	Tbs	38	8	122	<1	30	<1	<1	<0.1	<0.1	<0.1
23162	Nuts in syrup topping	2	Tbs	41	8	167	2	22	1	9	0.8	2	5.6
510	Whipped cream, pressurized	1	cup	60	37	154	2	7	0	13	8.3	3.8	0.5

< = Trace amount present　　　Blank = Not available

CHOL, cholesterol; **V,** vitamin; **THI,** thiamin; **RIB,** riboflavin; **NIA,** niacin; **FOL,** folate;
CALC, calcium; **PHOS,** phosphate; **SOD,** sodium; **POT,** potassium; **MAG,** magnesium

CHOL (mg)	V-A (RE)	THI (mg)	RIB (mg)	NIA (mg)	V-B6 (mg)	FOL (μg)	V-B12 (μg)	V-C (mg)	V-E (mg)	CALC (mg)	PHOS (mg)	SOD (mg)	POT (mg)	MAG (mg)	IRON (mg)	ZINC (mg)
21	67	0.1	0.1	0.5	<0.1	5	<0.1	<1	1	24	31	90	72	10	0.8	0.2
0	<1	<0.1	<0.1	0.3	<0.1	7	0	0	0.2	2	8	38	12	3	0.3	0.1
7	3	<0.1	<0.1	0.3	<0.1	1	<0.1	0	0.4	8	15	47	34	6	0.3	0.1
5	26	<0.1	<0.1	0.2	<0.1	5	<0.1	<1	0.5	6	16	58	36	9	0.4	0.1
<1	<1	<0.1	<0.1	0.3	<0.1	6	<0.1	0	0.2	4	16	70	25	6	0.5	0.1
0	0	<0.1	<0.1	<0.1	<0.1	1	<0.1	0	0.1	2	10	59	37	5	0.2	0.2
0	1	<0.1	<0.1	0.3	<0.1	4	<0.1	<1	0.2	10	10	56	33	4	0.5	0.1
<1	<1	<0.1	<0.1	0.1	<0.1	4	0	0	<0.1	1	3	22	3	1	0.1	<0.1
0	0							0	<0.1	0		95			0.4	
0	<1	<0.1	<0.1	0.2	<0.1	5	0	0	0.1	5	6	46	24	3	0.4	<0.1
161	73	0.1	0.2	0.9	0.1	34	0.3	2	0.6	21	76	65	50	5	1.6	0.5
12	32	<0.1	<0.1	0.2	<0.1	2	<0.1	1	0.4	7	12	42	11	1	0.2	0.1
0	<1	<0.1	<0.1	0.1	<0.1	2	<0.1	<1	0.3	6	13	22	24	5	0.3	0.1
0	0	0.1	<0.1	0.5	<0.1	11	0	0	0.3	11	14	69	52	8	1	0.1
2										20		100	30		1.1	
5	27	<0.1	<0.1	0.2	<0.1	5	<0.1	<1	0.4	16	25	90	27	6	0.4	0.1
7	3	<0.1	<0.1	0.2	<0.1	2	<0.1	<1	0.4	5	28	75	30	8	0.4	0.1
3	1	0.1	<0.1	0.4				0		8		98	60		0.6	
6	31	<0.1	<0.1	0.7	<0.1	11	<0.1	<1	2.5	8	23	104	46	8	0.4	0.2
5	<1	<0.1	<0.1	0.3	<0.1	9	<0.1	0	0.5	4	12	39	10	3	0.3	0.1
0	85	0.1	0.1	1.3	0.1	28	<0.1	4	0.4	2	12	123	12	4	0.5	0.1
0	<1	<0.1	<0.1	0.2	<0.1	3	<0.1	0	0.6	6	15	55	41	7	0.5	0.1
0	<1	<0.1	0.1	0.8	<0.1	17	<0.1	0	1.7	10	39	242	70	18	1.6	0.3
0												220	60		0.7	
0	<1	<0.1	<0.1	0.5	<0.1	6	<0.1	<1	0.5	7	26	52	27	7	0.4	0.1
0	0	<0.1	<0.1	0.3	<0.1	6	0	0	0.4	3	8	35	9	1	0.2	<0.1
6	4	0.1	0.1	1.1	<0.1	19	<0.1	0	1	11	35	146	32	5	0.9	0.2
0	<1	<0.1	<0.1	0.2	<0.1	3	<0.1	<1	0	5	11	28	18	4	0.4	0.1
<1	<1	<0.1	0.1	0.7	<0.1		<0.1	0		17	36	95	28	5	0.6	0.2
<1	<1	<0.1	0.1	0.7	<0.1		<0.1	0		18	67	253	53	16	0.9	0.2
9	32	0.1	<0.1	0.4	<0.1	2	<0.1	<1	0.2	8	10	74	24	2	0.5	0.1
8	4	<0.1	<0.1	0.4	<0.1	7	<0.1	<1	0.4	3	12	54	9	2	0.3	0.1
4	35	<0.1	<0.1	0.3	<0.1	7	<0.1	<1	0.5	10	13	69	11	2	0.3	0.1
0	0	<0.1	<0.1	0.2	<0.1	4	0	0	0.4	2	5	13	5	1	0.2	<0.1
<1	11	<0.1	<0.1	<0.1	<0.1	1	<0.1	<1	0	22	19	143	34	3	0.1	0.1
<1	11	<0.1	<0.1	<0.1	<0.1	1	<0.1	<1	0	22	19	143	34	3	0.1	0.1
0	9	<0.1	0.2	1	<0.1	12	0	1	3	42	387	216	672	195	6.3	2.2
8	39	<0.1	0.1	<0.1	<0.1	3	0.2	1	0.1	72	69	53	120	8	<0.1	0.2
0	64	0	0	0	0	0	0	0	0.1	5	6	19	14	1	0.1	<0.1
7	14	0.2	0.8	1	0.2	14	0.7	1	9.9	275	459	1176	1230	173	4.4	2.3
0	<1	0	0	<0.1	0	<1	0	0	0	1	3	19	2	1	0.1	<0.1
0	2	0.1	<0.1	0.2	0.1	9	0	<1	0.4	16	46	17	86	26	0.4	0.4
46	124	<0.1	<0.1	<0.1	<0.1	2	0.2	0	0.4	61	54	78	88	6	<0.1	0.2

ERA, EatRight Analysis CD-ROM; **AMT,** amount; **WT,** weight; **WTR,** water; **CAL,** calories; **PROT,** protein; **CARB**, carbohydrate; **FIBR,** fiber; **FAT,** fat; **SATF,** saturated fat; **MONO,** monounsaturated fat; **POLY,** polyunsaturated fat

ERA CODE	FOOD DESCRIPTION	AMT	UNIT	WT (g)	WTR (g)	CAL (kcal)	PROT (g)	CARB (g)	FIBR (g)	FAT (g)	SATF (g)	MONO (g)	POLY (g)
Desserts (continued)													
Doughnuts													
45505	Cake doughnut	1	ea	47	10	198	2	23	1	11	1.7	4.4	3.7
45524	Cake doughnut, choc icing	1	ea	43	6	204	2	21	1	13	3.5	7.5	1.6
45508	Chocolate eclair+custard	1	ea	100		262	6	24	1	16	4.1	6.5	3.9
45509	Cream puff+custard	1	ea	130	70	335	9	30	1	20	4.8	8.5	5.4
45563	Cream-filled yeast doughnut	1	ea	85	32	307	5	26	1	21	4.6	10.3	2.6
45527	French cruller doughnut	1	ea	41	7	169	1	24	<1	8	1.9	4.3	0.9
45507	Jelly-filled doughnut	1	ea	85	30	289	5	33	1	16	4.1	8.7	2
45559	Mexican crueller	1	ea	26	6	116	1	12	<1	7	2	4.1	0.9
45560	Oriental doughnut/Okinawan	1	ea	18	3	76	1	10	<1	4	0.9	2	0.4
45506	Yeast doughnut, plain	1	ea	60	15	242	4	27	1	14	3.5	7.7	1.7
Frozen Desserts													
2070	Banana split w/whip cream	1	ea	425	217	1088	15	124	1	65	37.5	18.7	5.3
23174	Frozen fruit juice bar	1	ea	77	60	63	1	16	0	<1	<0.1	0	<0.1
2043	Frozen yogurt bar, choc coat	1	ea	41	21	109	1	12	<1	7	5.3	0.8	0.2
2035	Frozen yogurt, choc, soft	0.5	cup	72	46	115	3	18	2	4	2.6	1.3	0.2
2071	Frozen yogurt, low fat, choc	1	cup	193	134	219	10	42	3	4	2.4	1.1	0.1
2075	Frozen yogurt, low fat, van, fruit	1	cup	193	143	203	9	37	0	3	1.7	0.7	0.1
2039	Frozen yogurt, nonfat, choc	1	cup	193	135	207	11	43	3	2	1	0.5	0.1
2079	Frozen yogurt, nonfat, van, fruit	1	cup	193	143	191	10	38	0	<1	0.2	0.1	<0.1
2064	Frozen yogurt, vanilla	0.5	cup	72	47	114	3	17	0	4	2.5	1.1	0.2
23094	Frozen juice bar w/cream	1	ea	65	43	86	1	19	<1	1	0.8	0.4	0.1
2032	Hot fudge sundae	1	ea	158	94	284	6	48	0	9	5	2.3	0.8
2055	Ice cream bar, choc, Dove	1	ea	101	38	339	3	36	2	23	13.8	7.2	0.7
2028	Ice cream bar, Creamsicle	1	ea	66	44	91	2	18	<1	2	1.2	0.6	0.1
2029	Ice cream bar, Drumstick	1	ea	60	29	159	3	18	1	9	4.4	3.1	1
2030	Ice cream bar, Fudgesicle	1	ea	73	48	104	3	18	1	3	2.1	1	0.1
2084	Ice cream bar, Heath	1	ea	68	33	206	2	17	<1	15	11.6	2.3	0.4
2089	Ice cream sandwich, Chipwich	1	ea	59	28	144	3	22	1	6	3.2	1.7	0.4
2087	Ice cream sandwich	1	ea	59	28	144	3	22	1	6	3.2	1.7	0.4
2050	Ice cream, hard, choc	0.5	cup	66	37	142	3	19	1	7	4.5	2.1	0.3
2008	Ice cream, soft, French vanilla	0.5	cup	86	51	185	4	19	0	11	6.4	3	0.4
2063	Ice cream, strawberry	0.5	cup	66	40	127	2	18	<1	6	3.4	1.6	0.2
2004	Ice cream, vanilla	0.5	cup	66	40	133	2	16	0	7	4.5	2.1	0.3
2006	Ice cream, vanilla, rich	0.5	cup	74	42	178	3	17	0	12	7.4	3.4	0.4
2057	Ice milk, chocolate	1	cup	131	86	189	6	34	1	4	2.6	1.2	0.2
2009	Ice milk, hard, vanilla	0.5	cup	66	45	92	3	15	0	3	1.7	0.8	0.1
23051	Ice slushy	1	cup	193	129	247	1	63	0	0	0	0	0
2216	Ice cream, ch chip cook do, rich	0.5	cup	106		270	4	30	0	17	9		
2105	Ice cream, cookies & crm, low fat	0.5	cup	71		120	3	21	1	2	1	1	0
49013	Ice cream cone, cake/wafer	1	ea	4	<1	17	<1	3	<1	<1	<0.1	0.1	0.1
49014	Ice cream cone, sugar/rolled	1	ea	10	<1	40	1	8	<1	<1	0.1	0.1	0.1
2020	Milkshake, chocolate	1	cup	166	119	211	6	34	1	6	3.8	1.8	0.2
2011	Orange sherbet	0.5	cup	99	65	137	1	30	0	2	1.1	0.5	0.1
70308	Orange sorbet+van ice crm, rich	0.5	cup	106		190	2	24	0	9	5		

< = Trace amount present

Blank = Not available

CHOL, cholesterol; **V,** vitamin; **THI,** thiamin; **RIB,** riboflavin; **NIA,** niacin; **FOL,** folate; **CALC,** calcium; **PHOS,** phosphate; **SOD,** sodium; **POT,** potassium; **MAG,** magnesium

CHOL (mg)	V-A (RE)	THI (mg)	RIB (mg)	NIA (mg)	V-B6 (mg)	FOL (μg)	V-B12 (μg)	V-C (mg)	V-E (mg)	CALC (mg)	PHOS (mg)	SOD (mg)	POT (mg)	MAG (mg)	IRON (mg)	ZINC (mg)
17	8	0.1	0.1	0.9	<0.1	22	0.1	<1	1.9	21	126	257	60	9	0.9	0.3
26	5	0.1	<0.1	0.6	<0.1	12	0.1	<1	1.9	15	87	184	84	17	1.1	0.3
127	191	0.1	0.3	0.8	0.1	28	0.3	<1	2.1	63	107	337	117	15	1.2	0.6
174	259	0.2	0.4	1.1	0.1	36	0.5	<1	2.9	86	142	443	150	16	1.5	0.8
20	16	0.3	0.1	1.9	0.1	54	0.1	0	2.3	21	65	263	68	17	1.6	0.7
5	1	0.1	0.1	0.9	<0.1	14	<0.1	0	1	11	50	141	32	5	1	0.1
22	14	0.3	0.1	1.8	0.1	53	0.2	0	2.1	21	72	249	67	17	1.5	0.6
2	6	<0.1	<0.1	0.4	<0.1	1	<0.1	0	1	2	8	7	8	2	0.3	0.1
13	7	<0.1	0.1	0.4	<0.1	2	<0.1	<1	0.5	24	22	38	15	2	0.4	0.1
4	2	0.2	0.1	1.7	<0.1	26	0.1	<1	2.4	26	56	205	65	13	1.2	0.5
204	531	0.1	0.9	0.5	0.2	19	1.4	2	0.5	466	484	360	783	92	1.6	2.7
0	2	<0.1	<0.1	0.1	<0.1	5	0	7	0	4	5	3	41	3	0.1	<0.1
1	18	<0.1	0.1	0.1	<0.1	2	0.1	<1	<0.1	46	43	28	74	6	0.1	0.2
4	31	<0.1	0.2	0.2	0.1	8	0.2	<1	0.1	106	100	71	188	19	0.9	0.4
10	25	0.1	0.4	0.4	0.1	21	0.9	1	0.1	300	300	113	621	75	1.7	2.1
10	27	0.1	0.4	0.2	0.1	19	0.9	1	0.1	307	241	118	393	29	0.1	1.5
3	3	0.1	0.4	0.4	0.1	22	1	1	<0.1	326	321	123	655	78	1.7	2.2
3	3	0.1	0.4	0.2	0.1	20	1	1	<0.1	334	263	129	428	32	0.2	1.6
1	41	<0.1	0.2	0.2	0.1	4	0.2	1	<0.1	103	93	63	152	10	0.2	0.3
5	8	<0.1	0.1	0.1	<0.1	3	0.1	8	<0.1	29	5	20	64	2	0.1	<0.1
21	57	0.1	0.3	1.1	0.1	9	0.6	2	0.7	207	228	182	395	33	0.6	0.9
38	95	<0.1	0.2	0.3	<0.1	2	0.2	<1	0.7	74	139	56	260	63	1.1	1.1
6	20	<0.1	0.1	0.1	<0.1	3	0.3	2	<0.1	62	48	43	99	7	0.1	0.3
21	55	<0.1	0.1	0.9	<0.1	8	0.2	<1	0.4	66	82	44	145	21	0.4	0.7
10	33	<0.1	0.2	0.1	<0.1	5	0.5	1	<0.1	101	98	60	221	24	0.5	0.5
24	63	<0.1	0.1	0.1	<0.1	3	0.2	<1	<0.1	70	62	43	126	11	0.2	0.4
20	53	<0.1	0.1	0.2	<0.1	5	0.2	<1	0.1	60	64	36	122	13	0.3	0.4
20	53	<0.1	0.1	0.2	<0.1	5	0.2	<1	0.1	60	64	36	122	13	0.3	0.4
22	79	<0.1	0.1	0.1	<0.1	11	0.2	<1	1.1	72	71	50	164	19	0.6	0.4
78	132	<0.1	0.2	0.1	<0.1	8	0.4	1	0.3	113	100	52	152	10	0.2	0.4
19	51	<0.1	0.2	0.1	<0.1	8	0.2	5	0.2	79	66	40	124	9	0.1	0.2
29	77	<0.1	0.2	0.1	<0.1	3	0.3	<1	0	84	69	53	131	9	0.1	0.5
45	136	<0.1	0.1	0.1	<0.1	4	0.3	1	0	87	70	41	118	8	<0.1	0.3
12	35	0.1	0.2	0.2	0.1	8	0.6	1	0.1	189	156	82	310	26	0.3	0.8
9	31	<0.1	0.2	0.1	<0.1	4	0.4	1	0	92	72	56	139	10	0.1	0.3
0	0	<0.1	0	<0.1	<0.1	0	0	2	0	4	2	42	6	2	0.3	<0.1
80	150							1		100		95			1.1	
5	40	<0.1	0.2					0		100	141	90	254			
0	0	<0.1	<0.1	0.2	<0.1	4	0	0	0.1	1	4	6	4	1	0.1	<0.1
0	0	0.1	<0.1	0.5	<0.1	8	0	0	0.1	4	10	32	14	3	0.4	0.1
22	38	0.1	0.4	0.3	0.1	6	0.6	1	0.4	188	169	161	332	28	0.5	0.7
6	14	<0.1	0.1	0.1	<0.1	5	0.2	3	0.1	53	40	46	95	8	0.1	0.5
60	60	<0.1	0.1	0.9				9		80	64	45	114		0	

ERA, EatRight Analysis CD-ROM; **AMT,** amount; **WT,** weight; **WTR,** water; **CAL,** calories; **PROT,** protein; **CARB,** carbohydrate; **FIBR,** fiber; **FAT,** fat; **SATF,** saturated fat; **MONO,** monounsaturated fat; **POLY,** polyunsaturated fat

ERA CODE	FOOD DESCRIPTION	AMT	UNIT	WT (g)	WTR (g)	CAL (kcal)	PROT (g)	CARB (g)	FIBR (g)	FAT (g)	SATF (g)	MONO (g)	POLY (g)
Desserts (continued)													
Frozen Desserts (continued)													
23050	Popsicle/ice pops, double	1	ea	128	102	92	0	24	0	0	0	0	0
2026	Pudding pop, chocolate	1	ea	47	30	72	2	12	<1	2	2.1	0	0
2027	Pudding pop, vanilla	1	ea	47	30	75	2	13	0	2	2.1	0	0
2066	Sorbet, citrus	1	cup	200	152	184	1	46	<1	0	0	0	0
2065	Sorbet, fruit	1	cup	200	157	164	2	40	0	<1	0	0	0.1
Fruit Desserts													
49031	Apple crisp	0.5	cup	141	87	230	3	46	2	5	1	2.2	1.6
49006	Apple dumpling	1	ea	151	78	357	2	53	2	16	3.6	8.2	3.4
49015	Apple strudel	1	pce	71	31	194	2	29	2	8	1.5	2.3	3.8
49002	Cherry cobbler, 3x3 in piece	1	pce	129	85	198	2	34	1	6	1.2	2.8	1.9
49018	Fruit-filled blintz	1	ea	70	44	124	4	17	<1	4	1.3	1.8	0.9
49008	Peach cobbler, 3x3 in piece	1	pce	130	84	204	2	36	2	6	1.2	2.8	1.9
Gelatin Desserts													
23052	Gelatin/Jello, prepared	0.5	cup	135	114	80	2	19	0	0	0	0	0
23156	Gelatin/Jello dessert w/fruit	0.5	cup	106	86	73	1	18	1	<1	0.1	<0.1	0.1
23093	Gelatin/Jello, sug free, prepared	0.5	cup	117	115	8	1	1	0	0	0	0	0
Pastries and Sweet Rolls													
45515	Apple fritter	1	ea	24	9	87	1	8	<1	6	1.2	2.4	1.6
45550	Apple turnover	1	ea	82	27	290	3	37	1	15	3	6.5	4.6
45516	Baklava, 2x2x2.5 in piece	1	pce	78	19	336	5	29	2	23	9.3	8.1	4.2
45523	Cheese croissant	1	ea	57	12	236	5	27	1	12	6.1	3.7	1.4
45552	Cherry turnover	1	ea	78	32	240	3	31	1	12	2.4	5.2	3.7
45557	Chinese pastry	1	oz	28	13	67	1	13	<1	2	0.2	0.5	0.8
42166	Cinnamon roll, bkd, frosted	1	ea	30	7	109	2	17	1	4	1	2.2	0.5
45555	Guava turnover	1	ea	78	34	234	2	28	3	13	2.5	5.5	3.9
42188	Jelly-filled sweet roll	1	ea	55	13	202	3	29	1	8	2.2	4.7	1.1
48057	Lemon meringue tart	1	ea	117	58	301	4	41	1	14	2.9	5.9	3.9
42094	Pan dulce w/topping	1	ea	79	17	291	5	48	1	9	1.8	4	2.5
45540	Popover, mix, prepared	1	ea	33	18	67	3	10	<1	1	0.4	0.6	0.2
45504	Pop tart, fruit filled	1	ea	52	6	204	2	37	1	5	0.8	2.2	2
45604	Pop tart, fruit filled, frosted	1	ea	52	6	205	2	37	1	6	1	3.2	1.3
Pies													
48151	Apple pie	1	pce	126		350	2	41	2	21	4	6	0.5
70557	Boston cream pie	1	pce	106		240	3	48	1	4	1.5	1.7	0.8
48153	Cherry pie	1	pce	120		340	3	45	1	22	4	7	0.5
48154	Chocolate crème pie	1	pce	124		280	4	36	1	14	4	4	0
48155	Lemon meringue pie	1	pce	119		250	2	41	<1	9	2	3	0
48058	Pecan pie, single, bama pie	1	ea	85	14	363	4	46	2	20	2.8	10.4	5.3
48156	Pumpkin pie	1	pce	121		260	3	34	1	13	3	4	0
Puddings and Custards													
2617	Bread pudding+raisins	0.5	cup	126	79	212	7	31	1	7	2.9	2.7	1.2

< = Trace amount present

Blank = Not available

CHOL, cholesterol; **V,** vitamin; **THI,** thiamin; **RIB,** riboflavin; **NIA,** niacin; **FOL,** folate;
CALC, calcium; **PHOS,** phosphate; **SOD,** sodium; **POT,** potassium; **MAG,** magnesium

CHOL (mg)	V-A (RE)	THI (mg)	RIB (mg)	NIA (mg)	V-B6 (mg)	FOL (μg)	V-B12 (μg)	V-C (mg)	V-E (mg)	CALC (mg)	PHOS (mg)	SOD (mg)	POT (mg)	MAG (mg)	IRON (mg)	ZINC (mg)
0	0	0	0	0	0	0	0	0	0	0	0	15	5	1	0	<0.1
1	16	<0.1	0.1	0.1	<0.1	1	0.3	<1	<0.1	66	53	78	105	10	0.2	0.2
1	24	<0.1	0.1	<0.1	<0.1	2	0.2	<1	<0.1	61	47	50	65	5	<0.1	0.2
0	54	<0.1	0.1	0.3	<0.1	44	0	51	0.1	18	26	16	200	16	0.9	<0.1
0	6	<0.1	<0.1	0.3	0.1	12	0	19	0	10	12	8	106	8	0.4	0.1
0	44	0.1	0.1	1.1	0.1	7	0	3		39	35	257	137	10	1.1	0.2
0	93	0.1	0.1	0.8	0.1	6	<0.1	5	5.9	50	38	302	212	17	1.3	0.2
4	6	<0.1	<0.1	0.2	<0.1	10	0.2	1	2.2	11	23	191	106	6	0.3	0.1
1	135	0.1	0.1	0.8	0.1	9	<0.1	2	1.3	28	34	294	133	9	1.8	0.2
53	73	0.1	0.1	0.4	<0.1	8	0.2	1	0.5	35	59	93	78	7	0.8	0.3
1	105	0.1	0.1	1.2	<0.1	6	<0.1	3	1.5	24	40	291	159	10	0.9	0.2
0	0	0	<0.1	<0.1	<0.1	0	0	0	0	3	30	57	1	1	<0.1	<0.1
0	3	<0.1	<0.1	0.2	0.1	4	0	4	0.1	5	22	30	110	7	0.1	0.1
0	0	0	<0.1	<0.1	<0.1	0	0	0	0	2	32	56	0	1	<0.1	<0.1
20	13	<0.1	0.1	0.3	<0.1	3	0.1	<1	0.7	13	22	10	34	3	0.3	0.1
0	3	0.2	0.1	1.5	<0.1	5	0	1	1.9	6	33	4	56	7	1.3	0.2
36	124	0.2	0.2	1.4	<0.1	11	<0.1	1	2	33	93	292	144	35	1.7	0.5
32	112	0.3	0.2	1.2	<0.1	42	0.2	<1	0.6	30	74	316	75	14	1.2	0.5
0	26	0.1	0.1	1.2	<0.1	6	0	1	1.6	8	28	8	59	7	1.6	0.2
0	<1	<0.1	<0.1	0.3	<0.1	1	0	0	0.3	6	15	3	25	7	0.2	0.2
0	<1	0.1	0.1	1.1	<0.1	16	<0.1	<1	0.5	10	104	250	19	4	0.8	0.1
<1	32	0.1	0.1	1.5	0.1	6	<0.1	48	2	13	33	13	120	9	1.1	0.2
34	33	0.2	0.1	1.2	0.1	12	0.1	1	1.5	39	43	196	86	10	0.9	0.3
69	31	0.1	0.2	1.1	<0.1	10	0.1	3	1.7	13	52	23	50	7	1.2	0.3
26	67	0.2	0.2	2	<0.1	19	0.1	<1	1.2	13	56	75	57	9	1.8	0.3
37	16	0.1	0.1	0.4	<0.1	6	0.1	<1	0.4	9	30	143	25	5	0.6	0.2
0	150	0.2	0.2	2	0.2	34	<0.1	<1	10.1	14	58	218	58	9	1.8	0.3
0	100	0.2	0.2	2	0.2	52	0	0	0	11	46	211	44	8	1.8	0.6
0								1				220	75		1.1	
4	7	<0.1	0.1	0.3	0.1			1		43		240	105		0.5	
0								1				220	90		1.4	
45	20									80		300	130		1.1	
35												180	25		0.7	
38	19	0.2	0.2	1.2	<0.1	11	0.1	<1	1.7	14	80	54	90	25	1.4	1
55	200							2		60		210	180		1.4	
83	82	0.1	0.3	0.8	0.1	16	0.3	1	5.1	144	137	291	282	24	1.4	0.7

ERA, EatRight Analysis CD-ROM; **AMT,** amount; **WT,** weight; **WTR,** water; **CAL,** calories; **PROT,** protein; **CARB**, carbohydrate; **FIBR,** fiber; **FAT,** fat; **SATF,** saturated fat; **MONO,** monounsaturated fat; **POLY,** polyunsaturated fat

ERA CODE	FOOD DESCRIPTION	AMT	UNIT	WT (g)	WTR (g)	CAL (kcal)	PROT (g)	CARB (g)	FIBR (g)	FAT (g)	SATF (g)	MONO (g)	POLY (g)
Desserts (continued)													
Puddings and Custards (continued)													
2613	Egg custard, mix+whl milk	0.5	cup	133	97	162	5	23	0	5	3	1.7	0.3
2625	Flan carm custard, mix+whl mlk	0.5	cup	133	99	150	4	25	<1	4	2.5	1.2	0.2
2628	Pudding, instant+2% milk	0.5	cup	147	110	153	4	29	0	2	1.5	0.7	0.2
2605	Pudding, instant+whole milk	0.5	cup	147	108	163	5	28	1	5	2.7	1.4	0.3
2614	Pudding, low cal (D-Zerta)	0.5	cup	130	110	81	4	12	0	2	1	0.5	0.1
2636	Pudding, reg mix+2% milk	0.5	cup	142	105	150	5	28	<1	3	1.8	0.8	0.1
2604	Pudding, reg mix+whole milk	0.5	cup	142	106	158	5	26	1	5	3	1.4	0.2
48044	Pumpkin pie mix, canned	1	cup	270	193	281	3	71	22	<1	0.2	<0.1	<0.1
2653	Tapioca pudding+2% milk	0.5	cup	141	105	147	4	28	0	2	1.5	0.7	0.1
Eggs, Substitutes, and Egg Dishes													
19539	Deviled egg, 1/2+filling	1	ea	31	22	63	4	<1	0	5	1.2	1.7	1.5
19581	Egg Beaters, egg substitute	0.25	cup	61		30	6	1	0	0	0	0	0
19522	Egg white, cooked	1	ea	33.4	29	17	4	<1	0	0	0	0	0
19507	Egg white, raw, fresh	1	cup	243	213	122	26	3	0	0	0	0	0
19506	Egg white, raw, fresh, large	1	ea	33.4	29	17	4	<1	0	0	0	0	0
19523	Egg yolk, cooked	1	ea	16.6	8	59	3	<1	0	5	1.6	1.9	0.7
19508	Egg yolk, raw, fresh, large	1	ea	16.6	8	59	3	<1	0	5	1.6	1.9	0.7
19511	Egg, hard boiled, chopped	1	cup	136	101	211	17	2	0	14	4.4	5.5	1.9
19510	Egg, hard cooked/boiled	1	ea	50	37	78	6	1	0	5	1.6	2	0.7
19509	Egg, large, fried in marg	1	ea	46	32	92	6	1	0	7	1.9	2.7	1.3
19517	Egg, poached, large	1	ea	50	38	74	6	1	0	5	1.5	1.9	0.7
19516	Egg, scrambled+milk+marg	1	ea	61	45	101	7	1	0	7	2.2	2.9	1.3
19500	Egg, whole, raw, fresh, large	1	cup	243	183	362	30	3	0	24	7.5	9.3	3.3
19535	Omelet, 1 egg+cheese & ham	1	ea	78	52	156	11	2	0	11	4.5	4.4	1.4
19543	Omelet, 1 egg+mushroom	1	ea	69	54	88	6	2	<1	6	1.8	2.4	1
19537	Omelet, 3 eggs+on+pep+tom+ms	1	ea	145	116	178	8	6	1	14	3.4	5.9	3
19534	Omelet, plain (1 lrg egg)	1	ea	61	46	93	6	1	0	7	1.9	2.8	1.3
Fast Foods/Restaurants													
Arby's													
6432	Arby's curly fries	3.5	oz	99		337	4	43		18	7.4	7.6	1.5
69045	Arby's Q sandwich	1	ea	190		389	18	48		15	5.4	6.3	3.5
53256	Arby's sauce	0.5	oz	14		15	<1	3		<1	0	0.1	0.1
69056	Beef'nCheddar sandwich	1	ea	194		508	25	43		26	7.7	12	6.8
57015	Cheddar fries, serving	5	oz	142		399	6	46		22	9	10	1.7
69046	Grilled chicken deluxe sandwich	1	ea	230		430	24	42		20	3.5	5.1	4.4
69048	Italian sub sandwich	1	ea	297		671	34	47		39	12.8	15.7	8.5
69051	Roast beef sandwich, lt, deluxe	1	ea	182		294	18	33		10	3.4	4.6	2
69052	Roast chick sandwich, lt, deluxe	1	ea	195		276	24	33		7	1.7	2.9	2.5
69055	Philly Beef'nSwiss sandwich	1	ea	197		467	24	38		25	9.6	10.6	5.1
56336	Roast beef sandwich, reg	1	ea	155		383	22	35	1	18	6.9	7.9	3.4
56337	Roast beef sandwich, Jr	1	ea	89		233	12	23	<1	11	3.8	4.8	2.3
69049	Roast beef sub sandwich	1	ea	305		623	38	47		32	11.5	13	6.8
69042	Roast chicken club sandwich	1	ea	238		503	30	37		27	6.9	9.8	10.4

< = Trace amount present   Blank = Not available

CHOL, cholesterol; **V,** vitamin; **THI,** thiamin; **RIB,** riboflavin; **NIA,** niacin; **FOL,** folate;
CALC, calcium; **PHOS,** phosphate; **SOD,** sodium; **POT,** potassium; **MAG,** magnesium

CHOL (mg)	V-A (RE)	THI (mg)	RIB (mg)	NIA (mg)	V-B6 (mg)	FOL (μg)	V-B12 (μg)	V-C (mg)	V-E (mg)	CALC (mg)	PHOS (mg)	SOD (mg)	POT (mg)	MAG (mg)	IRON (mg)	ZINC (mg)
81	44	0.1	0.3	0.2	0.1	11	0.6	1	0.1	194	174	198	283	25	0.3	0.7
16	35	<0.1	0.2	0.1	<0.1	5	0.3	1	0.1	150	114	65	192	16	0.1	0.5
9	66	<0.1	0.2	0.1	0.1	6	0.4	1	0.1	150	318	435	192	18	0.1	0.5
16	31	<0.1	0.2	0.1	0.1	6	0.4	1	0.1	150	351	417	244	26	0.4	0.6
7	71	<0.1	0.2	0.1	<0.1	5	0.4	1	0.1	152	212	302	195	17	0.1	0.5
10	68	<0.1	0.2	0.2	0.1	6	0.4	1	0.1	160	138	149	240	30	0.5	0.7
17	37	<0.1	0.2	0.1	0.1	6	0.4	1	0.1	158	132	146	231	21	0.5	0.6
0	2241	<0.1	0.3	1	0.4	94	0	9	2.2	100	122	562	373	43	2.9	0.7
8	69	<0.1	0.2	0.1	0.1	6	0.4	1	0.1	149	117	172	189	17	0.1	0.5
122	50	<0.1	0.1	<0.1	<0.1	13	0.3	0	0.6	15	50	50	37	3	0.3	0.3
0	60		0.9		0.1	32	0.6	0	0.8	20		125	85		1.1	0.6
0	0	<0.1	0.1	<0.1	<0.1	1	0.1	0	0	2	4	55	48	4	<0.1	<0.1
0	0	<0.1	1.1	0.2	<0.1	7	0.5	0	0	15	32	398	347	27	0.1	<0.1
0	0	<0.1	0.2	<0.1	<0.1	1	0.1	0	0	2	4	55	48	4	<0.1	<0.1
213	97	<0.1	0.1	<0.1	0.1	18	0.4	0	0.5	23	81	7	16	1	0.6	0.5
213	97	<0.1	0.1	<0.1	0.1	24	0.5	0	0.5	23	81	7	16	1	0.6	0.5
577	228	0.1	0.7	0.1	0.2	60	1.5	0	1.4	68	234	169	171	14	1.6	1.4
212	84	<0.1	0.3	<0.1	0.1	22	0.6	0	0.5	25	86	62	63	5	0.6	0.5
211	114	<0.1	0.2	<0.1	0.1	17	0.4	0	0.8	25	89	162	61	5	0.7	0.5
212	95	<0.1	0.2	<0.1	0.1	18	0.4	0	0.5	24	88	140	60	5	0.7	0.6
215	119	<0.1	0.3	<0.1	0.1	18	0.5	<1	0.8	43	104	171	84	7	0.7	0.6
1032	464	0.2	1.2	0.2	0.3	114	2.4	0	2.6	119	432	306	294	24	3.5	2.7
198	133	0.1	0.3	0.6	0.1	17	0.6	<1	0.8	113	179	372	145	12	0.8	1.2
177	102	<0.1	0.2	0.3	0.1	17	0.4	<1	0.7	42	100	147	97	9	0.7	0.6
220	211	0.1	0.4	0.8	0.2	30	0.5	19	2	60	142	170	269	16	1.2	0.8
214	114	<0.1	0.2	<0.1	0.1	18	0.4	0	0.8	26	90	165	62	5	0.7	0.6
0	0	0.1	0.1	2			0			20		167	724		1.4	0.6
29		0.3	0.4	9.2						70		1268	456		9.2	
0												113	28		0.4	
52		0.4	0.6	9.8				1		150		1166	321		6.1	3
9		0.1	0.1	2			0			80		443	742		1.4	0.9
44	80	0.3	0.3	13.6				8		70		901	659		2.5	
69	100	0.9	0.5	8.2				11		410		2062	565		4.3	
42	40	0.3	0.5	8.4				8		130		826	392		4.5	
33	40	0.4	0.7	9.4				7		130		326	392		2.9	
53		0.3	0.5	8.8				19		290		1144	409		4.1	3.8
43	0	0.3	0.5	11	0.2	14		1		60	120	936	422	16	4.9	3.8
22		0.2	0.3	6.6	0.1	7				40	60	519	201	8	2.7	1.5
73	100	0.6	0.7	10.1				9		410		1847	708		7.7	
46		0.5	0.7	10.6				8		180		1143	534		2.9	2.2

ERA, EatRight Analysis CD-ROM; **AMT,** amount; **WT,** weight; **WTR,** water; **CAL,** calories; **PROT,** protein; **CARB**, carbohydrate; **FIBR,** fiber; **FAT,** fat; **SATF,** saturated fat; **MONO,** monounsaturated fat; **POLY,** polyunsaturated fat

ERA CODE	FOOD DESCRIPTION	AMT	UNIT	WT (g)	WTR (g)	CAL (kcal)	PROT (g)	CARB (g)	FIBR (g)	FAT (g)	SATF (g)	MONO (g)	POLY (g)
Fast Foods/Restaurants (continued)													
Arby's (continued)													
69050	Tuna sub sandwich	1	ea	284		663	74	50		37	8.2	11.8	17
69044	Turkey sub sandwich	1	ea	277		486	33	46		19	5.3	6	7
Burger King													
57002	BK broiler chicken sandwich	1	ea	248		550	30	41	2	29	6		
56360	Chicken sandwich	1	ea	229		710	26	54	2	43	9		
57001	Double cheeseburger	1	ea	210		600	41	28	1	36	17		
56362	Ocean Catch fish filet	1	ea	255		700	26	56	3	41	6		
56363	Onion rings, serving	1	ea	124		310	4	41	6	14	2	8	4
57000	Whopper Jr sandwich+cheese	1	ea	177		460	23	29	2	28	10		
56999	Whopper Jr sandwich	1	ea	164		420	21	29	2	24	8		
56354	Whopper sandwich	1	ea	270		640	27	45	3	39	11		
56355	Whopper sandwich+cheese	1	ea	294		730	33	46	3	46	16		
Dairy Queen													
2131	Banana split	1	ea	369		510	8	96	3	12	8		
2132	Blizzard, Heath bar flavor	1	ea	404		820	14	119	1	33	20		
2227	Blizzard, strawberry, regular	1	ea	383		570	12	95	1	16	11		
2239	Breeze, Heath bar, regular	1	ea	404		710	15	123	1	18	11		
2237	Breeze, strawberry, regular	1	ea	383		460	13	99	1	1	1	0	0
2133	Buster bar	1	ea	149		450	10	41	2	28	12		
2222	Cone, chocolate, regular	1	ea	213		360	9	56	0	11	8		
2135	Dilly bar	1	ea	85		210	3	21	0	13	7	3	3
2136	Dipped cone, regular	1	ea	234		510	9	63	1	25	13		
69027	Double bacon cheeseburger	1	ea	269		670	40	29	2	43	19		
13236	Hot dog, super, 1/4 lb	1	ea	198		590	20	41		38	16	16	4
56374	Hot dog	1	ea	99		240	9	19	1	14	5		
56375	Hot dog+cheese	1	ea	113		290	12	20	1	18	8	8	2
2141	Hot fudge brownie delight	1	ea	305		710	11	102	1	29	14	12	2
2051	Ice cream, chocolate, soft	1	cup	173	100	355	6	48	1	17	10.3	4.8	0.6
2145	Malt, regular, vanilla	1	ea	418		610	13	106	<1	14	8	2	2
2147	Mr. Misty, regular	1	ea	330		250	0	63	0	0	0	0	0
2151	Peanut buster parfait	1	ea	305		730	16	99	2	31	17		
2224	Shake, chocolate, regular	1	ea	539		770	17	130	0	20	13		
56371	Single cheeseburger	1	ea	152		340	20	29	2	17	8		
56368	Single hamburger	1	ea	138		290	17	29	2	12	5	6	1
2154	Sundae, chocolate, regular	1	ea	241		410	8	73	0	10	6		
Dominos Pizza													
57025	Pepperoni pizza, deep dish	2	pce	218	94	622	26	63	3	29	11.3		
57016	Pepperoni pizza, hand tossed	2	pce	159.4	72	406	18	50	3	15	6.5		
57019	Pepperoni pizza, thin crust	2	pce	156.7	69	447	20	40	2	23	9.2		
57028	Saus mushrm pizza, deep dish	2	pce	235.7	110	618	26	66	4	28	10.8		
57029	Veggie pizza, deep dish	2	pce	235.7	117	576	24	65	4	25	9.2		
57017	Veggie pizza, hand tossed	2	pce	176	95	360	15	52	3	10	4.6		
57023	Veggie pizza, thin crust	2	pce	178.7	99	386	17	43	3	17	6.4		

< = Trace amount present   Blank = Not available

CHOL, cholesterol; **V,** vitamin; **THI,** thiamin; **RIB,** riboflavin; **NIA,** niacin; **FOL,** folate;
CALC, calcium; **PHOS,** phosphate; **SOD,** sodium; **POT,** potassium; **MAG,** magnesium

CHOL (mg)	V-A (RE)	THI (mg)	RIB (mg)	NIA (mg)	V-B6 (mg)	FOL (μg)	V-B12 (μg)	V-C (mg)	V-E (mg)	CALC (mg)	PHOS (mg)	SOD (mg)	POT (mg)	MAG (mg)	IRON (mg)	ZINC (mg)
43	100	0.6	0.7	14.2				9		410		1847	708		7.7	
51	20	13.2	0.5	18.8						400		2033	500		4.7	
80	60							6		60		480			5.4	
60	0							0		100		1400			3.6	
135	80							0		200		1060			4.5	
90	20							1		60		980			2.7	
0	0						0	0		100		810			1.4	
75	80							5		150		770			3.6	
60	40							5		60		530			3.6	
90	100	0.3	0.4	7	0.3			9		80		870			4.5	
115	150	0.3	0.5	7	0.3			9		250		1350			4.5	
30	200	0.2	0.3	0.4	0.2			15		250	40	180	860		1.8	
60	300	0.2	0.8					1		450	450	580	730		1.8	
50	300	0.2	0.7					9		450	350	260	700		1.8	
20	20	0.1	0.8					2		450	479	580	575		2.7	
10	0	0.1	0.7					9		450	378	270	530		2.7	
15	80	0.1	0.2	3	0.1			0		150	250	280	400		1.1	
30	200	0.1	0.4					1		250	300	180	525		1.8	
10	60	<0.1	0.1		0.1			0		100	80	75	170		0.4	
30	150	0.1	0.4	0.2	0.1			2		300	225	200	435		1.8	
135	40	0.4	0.5	7.7				4		600	389	1210	467		2.7	
60		0.4	0.3	5						100	150	1360	340		2.7	
25	20	0.2	0.1	2				4		60	60	730	170		1.8	
40	60	0.2	0.2	2				4		150	150	950	180		1.8	
35	80	0.2	0.7	0.3	0.2			1		300	600	340	510		5.4	
43	147	0.1	0.3	0.2	0.1	9	0.6	1	0.5	206	184	89	384	37	0.7	1
45	80	0.1	0.6	0.8	0.2			<1		400	350	230	570		1.4	
0	0	0	0		0			2		0		10			0	
35	150	0.2	0.5	3	0.2			1		300	450	400	660		1.8	
70	400	0.2	0.8	1.1				2		600	543	420	814		2.7	
55	60	0.3	0.3	3.9				4		150	243	850	263		3.6	
45	40	0.3	0.2	3.9				4		60	145	630	252		2.7	
30	150	0.1	0.3	0.4	0.2			0		250	204	210	394		1.4	
44	155							3		456		1382			5	
32	94							3		282		1179			4.3	
43	116							4		428		1276			1.9	
43	158							4		460		1355			5.2	
32	160							13		460		1232			5.2	
19	99							13		286		1028			4.4	
26	123							17		433		1076			2	

ERA, EatRight Analysis CD-ROM; **AMT,** amount; **WT,** weight; **WTR,** water; **CAL,** calories; **PROT,** protein; **CARB**, carbohydrate; **FIBR,** fiber; **FAT,** fat; **SATF,** saturated fat; **MONO,** monounsaturated fat; **POLY,** polyunsaturated fat

Fast Foods/Restaurants (continued)

Generic Fast Food

ERA CODE	FOOD DESCRIPTION	AMT	UNIT	WT (g)	WTR (g)	CAL (kcal)	PROT (g)	CARB (g)	FIBR (g)	FAT (g)	SATF (g)	MONO (g)	POLY (g)
56606	Croissant+egg & cheese	1	ea	127	58	368	13	24		25	14.1	7.5	1.4
5463	Hashbrown potatoes, svg	0.5	cup	72	43	151	2	16		9	4.3	3.9	0.5
56667	Hot dog+chili	1	ea	114	54	296	14	31		13	4.9	6.6	1.2
66004	Hot dog/frankfurter & bun	1	ea	98	53	242	10	18		15	5.1	6.9	1.7
56639	Nachos, chips+cheese	7	pce	113	46	346	9	36		19	7.8	8	2.2
6176	Onion rings, serving	8.5	pce	83	31	276	4	31		16	7	6.7	0.7

Hardees

ERA CODE	FOOD DESCRIPTION	AMT	UNIT	WT (g)	WTR (g)	CAL (kcal)	PROT (g)	CARB (g)	FIBR (g)	FAT (g)	SATF (g)	MONO (g)	POLY (g)
56407	Big country breakfast+bacon	1	ea	217		740	25	81		43	13	22	8
56411	Biscuit 'n gravy	1	ea	221		510	10	55		28	9	14	5
2247	Cool twist cone, van/choc	1	ea	118		180	4	34		2	0.7	1.3	0
2158	Cool twist sundae, hot fudge	1	ea	156		290	7	51		6	3	1.6	0.2
69061	Frisco hamburger	1	ea	242		760	36	43		50	18		
56420	Hot ham 'n cheese sandwich	1	ea	201		530	18	49		30	9		
56417	Mushroom & swiss burger	1	ea	203		520	30	37		27	13	12	2
56418	Roast beef sandwich, regular	1	ea	124		270	15	28		11	5	4	2
2250	Shake, peach	1	ea	345		390	10	77		4	3		

Jack in the Box

ERA CODE	FOOD DESCRIPTION	AMT	UNIT	WT (g)	WTR (g)	CAL (kcal)	PROT (g)	CARB (g)	FIBR (g)	FAT (g)	SATF (g)	MONO (g)	POLY (g)
69032	Bacon cheeseburger	1	ea	242		710	35	41	0	45	15	15.7	8.7
1215	Beef teriyaki bowl	1	ea	440		640	28	124	7	3	1		
56430	Breakfast Jack sandwich	1	ea	121		300	18	30	0	12	4.8	4.8	2.4
56441	Chicken fajita pita	1	ea	189		290	24	29	3	8	3	3.6	1.4
69035	Chicken sandwich	1	ea	160		400	20	38	0	18	4		
69063	Chicken Caesar pita sandwich	1	ea	237		520	27	44	4	26	6		
90094	Cinnamon churritos, svg	1	ea	75		330	3	34	3	21	5		
69036	Country fried steak sandwich	1	ea	153		450	14	42	0	25	7		
69033	Grilled sourdough burger	1	ea	223		670	32	39	0	43	16	17.8	7.9
56436	Jumbo Jack burger	1	ea	229		560	26	41	0	32	10	13	8
56437	Jumbo Jack burger+cheese	1	ea	242		610	29	41	0	36	12	15	9
69064	Monterey roast beef sandwich	1	ea	238		540	30	40	3	30	9		
69040	Sourdough breakfast sandwich	1	ea	147		380	21	31	0	20	7		

KFC

ERA CODE	FOOD DESCRIPTION	AMT	UNIT	WT (g)	WTR (g)	CAL (kcal)	PROT (g)	CARB (g)	FIBR (g)	FAT (g)	SATF (g)	MONO (g)	POLY (g)
15169	Chicken breast, extra crispy	1	ea	168		470	39	17	1	28	8	16.7	3.3
15163	Chicken breast, original	1	ea	153		400	29	16	1	24	6	14.4	3.6
15170	Chicken leg, extra crispy	1	ea	67		195	15	7	1	12	3	7.4	1.6
15165	Chicken leg, original	1	ea	61		140	13	4	0	9	2	5.3	1.7
15177	Hot wings, pieces	6	pce	135		471	27	18	2	33	8		
15184	Hot & spicy chicken drumstick	1	ea	64		175	13	9	1	10	3		
15187	Hot & spicy chicken wing	1	ea	55		210	10	9	1	15	4		

Long John Silvers

ERA CODE	FOOD DESCRIPTION	AMT	UNIT	WT (g)	WTR (g)	CAL (kcal)	PROT (g)	CARB (g)	FIBR (g)	FAT (g)	SATF (g)	MONO (g)	POLY (g)
15199	Chicken plank, 2 pce	1	ea	112		240	16	22		12	3.2	8.4	0.2
56459	Clam dinner	1	ea	361		990	24	114		52	10.9	31.3	9.9

< = Trace amount present   Blank = Not available

CHOL, cholesterol; **V,** vitamin; **THI,** thiamin; **RIB,** riboflavin; **NIA,** niacin; **FOL,** folate;
CALC, calcium; **PHOS,** phosphate; **SOD,** sodium; **POT,** potassium; **MAG,** magnesium

CHOL (mg)	V-A (RE)	THI (mg)	RIB (mg)	NIA (mg)	V-B6 (mg)	FOL (μg)	V-B12 (μg)	V-C (mg)	V-E (mg)	CALC (mg)	PHOS (mg)	SOD (mg)	POT (mg)	MAG (mg)	IRON (mg)	ZINC (mg)
216	255	0.2	0.4	1.5	0.1	47	0.8	<1		244	348	551	174	22	2.2	1.8
9	2	0.1	<0.1	1.1	0.2	8	<0.1	5	0.1	7	69	290	267	16	0.5	0.2
51	6	0.2	0.4	3.7	<0.1	73	0.3	3		19	192	480	166	10	3.3	0.8
44	0	0.2	0.3	3.6	<0.1	48	0.5	<1	0.3	24	97	670	143	13	2.3	2
18	92	0.2	0.4	1.5	0.2	10	0.8	1		272	276	816	172	55	1.3	1.8
14	1	0.1	0.1	0.9	0.1	55	0.1	1	0.3	73	86	430	129	16	0.8	0.3
305										166		1800	530		5	
15										150		1500	210		2	
10										123		120	180		2	
20										152		310	173		0.4	
70												1280				
65										288		1710	300		3	
45										294		890	370		5	
25										105		780	260		4	
25												290				
110	80	0.2	0.5	8.8	0.4			9		250		1240	540		5.4	
25	1000							6		150		930	430		4.5	
185	80	0.5	0.4	3				9		200		890	220		2.7	
35	100	0.8	0.2	6				6		250		700	430		2.7	
45	40							0		150		1290	180		1.8	
55	80							2		250		1050	490		2.7	
20	0							0		20		200	170		5.4	
35	20							5		60		890	270		2.7	
110	150	0.6	0.5	8	0.3			6		200		1140	510		4.5	
65	40	0.4	0.3	1.8				6		100		700	450		4.5	
80	60	0.4	0.4	1.6				6		200		780	460		5.4	
75	80							5		300		1270	500		3.6	
235	150							9		250		1120	260		3.6	
	160	20							1		20		874			1.1
135	20							1		40		1116			1.1	
77	20							1		20		375			0.7	
75	20							1		20		422			0.7	
150	20							1		40		1230			1.4	
77	20							1		20		360			0.7	
55	20							1		20		350			0.7	
30		0.2	0.3	7								790	320		1.1	0.6
75	40	0.8	0.4	12				12		200		1830	910		4.5	3

ERA, EatRight Analysis CD-ROM; **AMT,** amount; **WT,** weight; **WTR,** water; **CAL,** calories; **PROT,** protein; **CARB**, carbohydrate; **FIBR,** fiber; **FAT,** fat; **SATF,** saturated fat; **MONO,** monounsaturated fat; **POLY,** polyunsaturated fat

ERA CODE	FOOD DESCRIPTION	AMT	UNIT	WT (g)	WTR (g)	CAL (kcal)	PROT (g)	CARB (g)	FIBR (g)	FAT (g)	SATF (g)	MONO (g)	POLY (g)
Fast Foods/Restaurants (continued)													
Long John Silvers (continued)													
56462	Fish & More	1	ea	407		890	31	92		48	10.1	28.5	9.5
69030	Fish sandwich batter dip	1	ea	159		340	18	40		13	3.1	8.9	1
57009	Fish, shrimp, chicken dinner	1	ea	513		1160	45	113		65	14.2	40.3	9.6
57010	Fish, shrimp, clams dinner	1	ea	512		1240	44	123		70	15.2	44.2	9.9
56467	Fish+fries, 2 pce, batter dip	1	ea	261		610	27	52		37	7.9	23.5	5.3
57004	Fish+lem crumb dinner, 2 pce	1	ea	334		330	24	46		5	0.9	1.6	1.2
57003	Fish+lem crumb dinner, 3 pce	1	ea	493		610	39	86		13	2.2	3.9	5.3
56461	Fish, batter fried, serving	1	ea	88		180	12	12		11	2.7	8.1	0.2
15198	Lt herb chicken, a la Carte	1	ea	100		120	22			4	1.2	1.7	1.1
27110	Malt vinegar, serving	1	ea	8		1	0	0	0				
19118	Seafood gumbo w/cod	1	ea	198		120	9	4		8	2.1	3.2	2.6
McDonalds													
69010	Big Mac sandwich	1	ea	216		560	26	45	3	31	10		
42332	Biscuit+biscuit spread	1	ea	84		290	5	34	1	15	3		
56675	Breakfast burrito	1	ea	117		320	13	23	2	20	7		
69009	Cheeseburger	1	ea	121		320	15	35	2	13	6		
15174	Chicken McNuggets	1	ea	71		190	12	10	0	11	2.5		
42335	Danish, apple	1	ea	105		360	5	51	1	16	5		
69005	Egg McMuffin	1	ea	136		290	17	27	1	12	4.5		
42064	English muffin+butter	1	ea	63	21	189	5	30	2	6	2.4	1.5	1.3
69013	Filet-O-Fish sandwich	1	ea	156		450	16	42	2	25	4.5		
2166	Frozen yogurt cone, vanilla	1	ea	90		150	4	23	0	4	3		
4732	Grill chick dlxe sand w/o mayo	1	ea	205		300	27	38	4	5	1		
69008	Hamburger	1	ea	107		260	13	34	2	9	3.5		
4730	Hamburger, deluxe, w/bacon	1	ea	247		590	32	39	4	34	12		
6155	Hashbrown potatoes	1	ea	53		130	1	14	1	8	1.5		
45069	Hotcakes+marg+syrup	1	ea	228		610	9	104	2	18	3.5		
47147	McDonaldland cookies	1	ea	42		180	3	32	1	5	1		
69011	Quarter Pounder	1	ea	172		420	23	37	2	21	8		
69012	Quarter Pounder+cheese	1	ea	200		530	28	38	2	30	13		
69006	Sausage McMuffin	1	ea	112		360	13	26	1	23	8		
19579	Scrambled eggs, 1 svg	1	ea	102		160	13	1	0	11	3.5		
2167	Shake, low fat, choc	1	ea	294.6		360	11	60	1	9	6		
2168	Shake, low fat, strawberrry	1	ea	294		360	11	60	0	9	6		
2169	Shake, low fat, vanilla	1	ea	293.4		360	11	59	0	9	6		
Pizza Hut													
56481	Cheese pizza, pan style	1	pce	108		261	12	28	2	11	5	3.4	1.7
56490	Pepperoni pizza, hand tossed	1	pce	103.8		238	12	29	2	8	4		
56482	Pepperoni pizza, pan style	1	pce	103.8		265	11	28	2	12	4	5	1.9
56493	Pepperoni pizza, pers pan	1	ea	255.2		637	27	69	5	28	10	11.8	4.5
56483	Supreme pizza, pan style	1	pce	136.4		311	15	28	3	15	6	6	2.1
56494	Supreme pizza, pers pan	1	ea	327.4		722	33	70	6	34	12	14.8	5.6
56487	Supreme pizza, thin/crispy	1	pce	115.9		257	14	21	2	13	5		

< = Trace amount present   Blank = Not available

CHOL, cholesterol; **V,** vitamin; **THI,** thiamin; **RIB,** riboflavin; **NIA,** niacin; **FOL,** folate;
CALC, calcium; **PHOS,** phosphate; **SOD,** sodium; **POT,** potassium; **MAG,** magnesium

CHOL (mg)	V-A (RE)	THI (mg)	RIB (mg)	NIA (mg)	V-B6 (mg)	FOL (μg)	V-B12 (μg)	V-C (mg)	V-E (mg)	CALC (mg)	PHOS (mg)	SOD (mg)	POT (mg)	MAG (mg)	IRON (mg)	ZINC (mg)
75	40	0.5	0.5	12				9		200		1790	1230		3.6	2.2
30		0.4	0.3	6				1		80		890	370		3.6	1.5
135	40	0.8	0.7	16				9		200		2590	1450		4.5	3.8
140	40	0.9	0.7	16				9		200		2630	1390		5.4	3.8
60		0.4	0.3	8				9		40		1480	900		1.8	1.2
75	1000	0.3	0.3	14				18		80		640	440		1.8	0.9
125	700	0.8	0.6	24				6		200		1420	990		5.4	2.2
30		0.2	0.2	3								490	260		0.4	0.3
60		0.1	0.3									570	270		0.7	0.6
												15	10			
25	200	0.2	0.2	3						100		740	310		1.8	1.5
85	60	0.5	0.4	6.1	0.3	49	2.3	4	1	250	267	1070	455	46	4.5	4.8
0	2	0.3	0.3	2.5	<0.1	5		0	0.9	60	390	780	116	10	1.8	0.3
195	100							9		150		600			1.8	
40	60	0.3	0.3	3.8	0.1	24	1.2	2	0.5	200	176	820	279	27	2.7	2.6
40	0	0.1	0.1	5	0.2		0.2	0	0.9	9	194	340	204	17	0.7	0.7
40	100	0.3	0.2	2				1		80	0	290	113		1.1	
235	100	0.5	0.4	3.3	0.1	33	0.7	1	0.8	200	268	790	197	23	2.7	1.5
13	33	0.3	0.3	2.6	<0.1	57	<0.1	1	0.1	103	85	386	69	13	1.6	0.4
50	40	0.3	0.2	2.8	0.1	32	0.6	0	1.6	150	197	870	286	34	1.8	0.8
20	60							1		100		75			0.4	
50	40							5		60		930			2.7	
30	22	0.3	0.3	3.8	0.1	21	1	2	0.2	150	111	580	258	24	2.7	2.2
100	100							6		150		1150			4.5	
0	0	0.1	<0.1	0.9	0.1	8	0	2	0.6	7	51	330	212	11	0.4	0.2
25	80	0.2	0.3	1.9	0.1	<1	0.3	<1	1.2	150	516	680	292	28	1.1	0.5
0	0	0.2	0.1	1.5	<0.1			0	0.7	20	52	190	46	8	1.8	0.3
70	20	0.4	0.3	6.8	0.2	28	2.6	2	0.4	150	208	820	408	34	4.5	4.7
95	100	0.4	0.4	6.8	0.3	33	2.9	2	0.8	300		1290			4.5	
45	40	0.6	0.3	3.8	0.1	16	0.5	0	0.7	200	156	740	191	22	1.8	1.5
425	135	0.1	0.5	0.1	0.1	44	1.1	0	0.9	40	172	170	126	10	1.1	1.1
40	73	0.1	0.5	0.4	0.1			1		350	354	250	542		0.7	
40	73	0.1	0.5	0.4	0.1			6		350	329	180	542		0.7	
40	73	0.1	0.5	0.3				1		350	327	250	534		0.4	
25	105	0.3	0.3	2.7	0.1			4		144		501	168	32	1.5	2.2
24	93	0.4	0.3	3.8				6		101		689	305	42	1.6	3
24	95	0.3	0.2	2.7	0.1	0		4		103		569	199	28	1.6	2.1
55	233	0.6	0.7	8.2	0.2			10		250		1340	407	60	4	3.8
30	98	0.4	0.4	3.2	0.2			5		117		764	310	41	2.3	3
66	240	0.7	0.8	9.9	0.4			14		276		1760	604	74	5.2	4.7
31	99	0.3	0.3	3.1				6		119		795	315	39	1.8	2.7

ERA, EatRight Analysis CD-ROM; **AMT,** amount; **WT,** weight; **WTR,** water; **CAL,** calories; **PROT,** protein; **CARB**, carbohydrate; **FIBR,** fiber; **FAT,** fat; **SATF,** saturated fat; **MONO,** monounsaturated fat; **POLY,** polyunsaturated fat

ERA CODE	FOOD DESCRIPTION	AMT	UNIT	WT (g)	WTR (g)	CAL (kcal)	PROT (g)	CARB (g)	FIBR (g)	FAT (g)	SATF (g)	MONO (g)	POLY (g)
Fast Foods/Restaurants (continued)													
Subway													
52127	Chicken taco salad	1	ea	370		250	18	15	2	14	5		
69117	Club sandwich (6-inch)	1	ea	246		297	21	40	3	5	1		
52120	Cold cut salad	1	ea	330		191	13	11	1	11	3		
69123	Italian sandwich (6-inch)	1	ea	232		467	20	38	3	24	9		
69129	Meatball sandwich (6-inch)	1	ea	260		404	18	44	3	16	6		
52121	Pizza salad	1	ea	335		277	12	13	2	20	8		
52116	Seafood/crab salad	1	ea	331		161	13	11	2	8	1		
52118	Tuna salad	1	ea	331		205	12	11	1	13	2		
69107	Tuna sandwich (6-inch)	1	ea	178		279	11	38	2	9	2		
69109	Veggie sandwich (6-inch)	1	ea	175		222	9	38	3	3	0		
Taco Bell													
56691	7-layer burrito	1	ea	283		530	16	66	13	23	7		
56690	Big Beef Burrito Supreme	1	ea	298		520	24	54	11	23	10		
56688	Chicken burrito	1	ea	171		345	17	41		13	5		
56689	Chicken soft taco	1	ea	121		200	14	21	2	7	2.5		
45585	Cinnamon twists, 1 svg	1	ea	28		140	1	19	0	6	0		
56531	Mexican pizza	1	ea	220		570	21	42	8	35	10		
56534	Nachos Bellgrande, 1 svg	1	ea	312		770	21	84	17	39	11		
56684	Nachos Supreme, 1 svg	1	ea	198		450	14	45	9	24	8		
56536	Pintos+cheese+red sauce	1	ea	120		190	9	18	10	9	4		
56526	Soft Taco Supreme	1	ea	142		260	12	23	3	14	7		
56693	Steak soft taco	1	ea	128		230	15	20	2	10	2.5		
56524	Taco	1	ea	78		180	9	12	3	10	4		
56692	Taco Supreme	1	ea	113		220	10	14	3	14	7		
Taco Time													
56540	Crispy bean burrito	1	ea	164.2	77	427	15	53	9	18	5		
56541	Crispy meat burrito	1	ea	162.8	58	552	34	39	7	30	10		
56553	Mexican fries, serving	1	ea	114.2	67	266	3	27		17			
56546	Natural super taco	1	ea	312.4	186	609	40	58	14	26	12.6		
56544	Soft combo burrito	1	ea	272		617	39	66	18	23	10		
Wendy's													
56571	Bacon cheeseburger	1	ea	166		380	20	34	2	19	7	10.2	1.4
56574	Big classic burger+cheese	1	ea	282		580	34	46	3	30	12		
2177	Frosty dairy dessert, med	1	ea	298		440	11	73	0	11	7		
69059	Grilled chicken sandwich	1	ea	189		310	27	35	2	8	1.5		
69058	Junior cheeseburger deluxe	1	ea	180		360	18	36	3	17	6		
69057	Junior hamburger	1	ea	118		270	15	34	2	10	3.5		
56566	Single burger, deluxe	1	ea	219		420	25	37	3	20	7		
Fats, Oils, Margarines, Shortenings, and Substitutes													
Fat Substitutes													
8133	Butter Buds	1	Tbs	5	<1	19	<1	4	0	<1	<0.1	<0.1	<0.1
8002	Pam cking spray, btr flav, 1/3 sec	1	ea	0.266		2	<1	<1		<1	<0.1		

< = Trace amount present　　Blank = Not available

CHOL, cholesterol; **V,** vitamin; **THI,** thiamin; **RIB,** riboflavin; **NIA,** niacin; **FOL,** folate;
CALC, calcium; **PHOS,** phosphate; **SOD,** sodium; **POT,** potassium; **MAG,** magnesium

CHOL (mg)	V-A (RE)	THI (mg)	RIB (mg)	NIA (mg)	V-B6 (mg)	FOL (μg)	V-B12 (μg)	V-C (mg)	V-E (mg)	CALC (mg)	PHOS (mg)	SOD (mg)	POT (mg)	MAG (mg)	IRON (mg)	ZINC (mg)
52	361							35		115		990			3	
26	120							15		29		1341			4	
64	282							33		46		1127			2	
57	169							15		40		1592			4	
33	142							16		32		1035			4	
50	390							33		100		1336			2	
32	284							32		25		599			2	
32	298							32		29		654			2	
16	126							14		26		583			3	
0	120							15		25		582			3	
25	300							6		200		1280			3.6	
55	600							5		150		1520			2.7	
57	440							1		140		854			2.5	
35	60							1		80		540			0.7	
0	40	0.1	<0.1	0.6	<0.1			0		0		190	22		0.4	
45	400	0.3	0.3	2.9	1.1	59		5		250		1040	403	79	3.6	5.3
35	150	0.1	0.4	2.4				4		200		1310	733		3.6	
30	100							4		150		810			2.7	
15	250	0.1	0.1	0.4	0.2	64	0	0		150		650	360	103	1.8	2
35	150							4		100		590			1.8	
25	40							0		80		1020			1.4	
25	100	0.1	0.1	1.2	0.1			0		80		330	159		1.1	
35	150							0		100		350			1.1	
12	24	0.4	0.2	2.2	0.4	14				158	238	453	382		4.4	2.2
58	60	0.3	0.4	5.5	0.4	74		2		197	276	1000	506		4.4	4.4
0	0	0.1	<0.1	0.9			0	3		11	40	798	277		0.9	
80	118	0.5	0.5	5.5	0.6	82		6		331	457	889	827		7.7	5.5
63	96	0.5	0.5	5.3	0.6	75		5		292	418	1343	760		7.5	5.3
60	80	0.3	0.3	6.4	0.3	28	2	6		170	334	850	375	38	3.4	5.9
100	150	0.4	1.5	6				15		250		1460	578		5.4	
50	200	0.1	0.6	0.4	0.2	23	1.1	0		410	328	239	714	60	1.4	1.3
65	40							6		100		790			2.7	
50	100							6		180		890			3.4	
30	20							1		110		610			3.1	
70	60	0.4	0.3	5.8				6		130		920	468		4.7	
<1	0	0	0	0	0	0	0	0	0	1	<1	60	<1	0	0.1	0
	0												0			

ERA, EatRight Analysis CD-ROM; **AMT,** amount; **WT,** weight; **WTR,** water; **CAL,** calories; **PROT,** protein; **CARB**, carbohydrate; **FIBR,** fiber; **FAT,** fat; **SATF,** saturated fat; **MONO,** monounsaturated fat; **POLY,** polyunsaturated fat

ERA CODE	FOOD DESCRIPTION	AMT	UNIT	WT (g)	WTR (g)	CAL (kcal)	PROT (g)	CARB (g)	FIBR (g)	FAT (g)	SATF (g)	MONO (g)	POLY (g)
Fats, Oils, Margarines, Shortenings, and Substitutes (continued)													
Fats, Oils, Spreads													
8004	Beef fat/tallow, drippings	1	cup	205	0	1849	0	0	0	205	102	85.7	8.2
8826	Benecol spread, serving	1	ea	8		27	0	0		3	0.4	0.9	1.7
8825	Benecol spread, tablespoon	1	Tbs	14		48	0	0		5	0.7	1.6	3
8031	Butter oil/ghee	1	cup	205	<1	1795	1	0	0	204	126.9	58.9	7.6
8001	Butter, pat	1	ea	5	1	36	<1	<1	0	4	2.5	1.2	0.2
8000	Butter, regular, salted, cup	1	cup	227	36	1627	2	<1	0	184	114.8	54.5	6.8
8000	Butter, regular, salted, tbsp	1	Tbs	14.19	2	102	<1	<1	0	12	7.2	3.4	0.4
8025	Butter, unsalted, cup	1	cup	227	41	1627	2	<1	0	184	114.6	53.2	6.8
8025	Butter, unsalted, tablespoon	1	Tbs	14.19	3	102	<1	<1	0	12	7.2	3.3	0.4
8142	Butter, whipped	1	cup	151	24	1082	1	<1	0	122	76.2	35.4	4.5
8084	Canola oil, cup	1	cup	218	0	1927	0	0	0	218	15.5	128.4	64.5
8084	Canola oil, tablespoon	1	Tbs	13.6	0	120	0	0	0	14	1	8	4
8005	Chicken fat	1	cup	205	<1	1845	0	0	0	204	61.1	91.6	42.8
8037	Coconut oil, cup	1	cup	218	0	1879	0	0	0	218	188.5	12.6	3.9
8037	Coconut oil, tablespoon	1	Tbs	13.6	0	117	0	0	0	14	11.8	0.8	0.2
8067	Cod liver oil (fish oil)	1	Tbs	13.6		123	0	0	0	14	3.1	6.4	3.1
8009	Corn oil, cup	1	cup	218	0	1927	0	0	0	218	27.7	52.8	127.9
8009	Corn oil, tablespoon	1	Tbs	13.6	0	120	0	0	0	14	1.7	3.3	8
8081	Cottonseed oil, cup	1	cup	218	0	1927	0	0	0	218	56.5	38.8	113.1
8081	Cottonseed oil, tablespoon	1	Tbs	13.6	0	120	0	0	0	14	3.5	2.4	7.1
8012	Crisco/Wesson oil, cup	1	cup	218	0	1923	0	0	0	218	31.3	50.7	126
8012	Crisco/Wesson oil, tablespoon	1	Tbs	13.6	0	120	0	0	0	14	2	3.2	7.9
8179	Margarine, hard, stick, cup	1	cup	225.6	35	1621	2	2	0	182	29.5	84.8	59.1
8179	Margarine, hard, stick, tbsp	1	Tbs	14.1	2	101	<1	<1	0	11	1.8	5.3	3.7
8165	Margarine, liquid	1	Tbs	14.2	2	102	<1	0	0	11	1.9	4	5.1
8168	Margarine, soft, tub	1	Tbs	14.1	2	101	<1	<1	0	11	1.9	5.1	3.8
8134	Margarine, unsalted, cup	1	cup	225.6	42	1610	1	1	0	181	33.8	82.8	56.4
8134	Margarine, unsalted, tablespoon	1	Tbs	14.1	3	101	<1	<1	0	11	2.1	5.2	3.5
8008	Olive oil, cup	1	cup	216	0	1909	0	0	0	216	29.2	159.1	18.1
8008	Olive oil, tablespoon	1	Tbs	13.6	0	119	0	0	0	14	1.8	9.9	1.1
8083	Palm kernel oil, cup	1	cup	218	0	1879	0	0	0	218	177.6	24.9	3.5
8083	Palm kernel oil, tablespoon	1	Tbs	13.6	0	117	0	0	0	14	11.1	1.5	0.2
8082	Palm oil, cup	1	cup	218	0	1927	0	0	0	218	107.4	80.7	20.3
8082	Palm oil, tablespoon	1	Tbs	13.6	0	120	0	0	0	14	6.7	5	1.3
8026	Peanut oil, cup	1	cup	216	0	1909	0	0	0	216	36.5	99.8	69.1
8026	Peanut oil, tablespoon	1	Tbs	13.6	0	119	0	0	0	14	2.3	6.2	4.3
8010	Safflower oil, cup	1	cup	218	0	1927	0	0	0	218	13.5	31.3	162.6
8010	Safflower oil, tablespoon	1	Tbs	13.6	0	120	0	0	0	14	0.9	2	10.2
8027	Sesame oil, cup	1	cup	218	0	1927	0	0	0	218	31	86.5	90.9
8027	Sesame oil, tablespoon	1	Tbs	13.6	0	120	0	0	0	14	1.9	5.4	5.7
8176	Shedd's spread, tub	1	Tbs	14.5	8	60	<1	<1	0	6	0.8	2.4	2.4
8007	Shortening (Crisco)	1	cup	205	0	1812	0	0	0	205	51.2	91.2	53.5
8028	Soybean+cottonseed oil, cup	1	cup	218	0	1927	0	0	0	218	39.2	64.3	104.8
8028	Soybean+cottonseed oil, tbsp	1	Tbs	13.6	0	120	0	0	0	14	2.5	4	6.6

< = Trace amount present   Blank = Not available

CHOL, cholesterol; **V,** vitamin; **THI,** thiamin; **RIB,** riboflavin; **NIA,** niacin; **FOL,** folate; **CALC,** calcium; **PHOS,** phosphate; **SOD,** sodium; **POT,** potassium; **MAG,** magnesium

CHOL (mg)	V-A (RE)	THI (mg)	RIB (mg)	NIA (mg)	V-B6 (mg)	FOL (μg)	V-B12 (μg)	V-C (mg)	V-E (mg)	CALC (mg)	PHOS (mg)	SOD (mg)	POT (mg)	MAG (mg)	IRON (mg)	ZINC (mg)
223	0	0	0	0	0	0	0	0	6.2	0	0	<1	<1	0	0	0
0	50								0.8							
0	88								1.4							
525	1896	<0.1	<0.1	<0.1	<0.1	<1	<0.1	0	6.2	8	6	3	10	1	<0.1	<0.1
11	38	0	<0.1	<0.1	0	<1	<0.1	0	0.1	1	1	41	1	<1	<0.1	<0.1
497	1711	<0.1	0.1	0.1	<0.1	7	0.3	0	3.6	54	52	1875	59	5	0.4	0.1
31	107	<0.1	<0.1	<0.1	<0.1	<1	<0.1	0	0.2	3	3	117	4	<1	<0.1	<0.1
497	1711	<0.1	0.1	0.1	<0.1	6	0.3	0	3.6	53	52	25	59	5	0.4	0.1
31	107	<0.1	<0.1	<0.1	<0.1	<1	<0.1	0	0.2	3	3	2	4	<1	<0.1	<0.1
330	1138	<0.1	0.1	0.1	<0.1	4	0.2	0	2.4	35	34	1248	39	3	0.2	0.1
0	0	0	0	0	0	0	0	0	45.8	0	0	0	0	0	0	0
0	0	0	0	0	0	0	0	0	2.9	0	0	0	0	0	0	0
174	0	0	0	0	0	0	0	0	6.2	0	0	0	0	0	0	0
0	0	0	0	0	0	0	0	0	0.6	0	0	0	0	0	0.1	0
0	0	0	0	0	0	0	0	0	<0.1	0	0	0	0	0		0
78	4080	0	0	0	0	0	0	0	3	0	0	0	0	0	0	0
0	0	0	0	0	0	0	0	0	181.3	0	0	0	0	0	0	0
0	0	0	0	0	0	0	0	0	11.3	0	0	0	0	0	0	0
0	0	0	0	0	0	0	0	0	142.1	0	0	0	0	0	0	0
0	0	0	0	0	0	0	0	0	8.9	0	0	0	0	0	0	0
0	0	0	0	0	0	0	0	0	203.8	<1	1	0	0	<1	<0.1	0
0	0	0	0	0	0	0	0	0	12.7			0	0			0
0	1802	0	<0.1	<0.1	0	3	0.2	<1	34.9	67	52	2128	96	6	0	
0	113	0	<0.1	<0.1	0	<1	<0.1	<1	2.2	4	3	133	6	<1	0	
0	113	<0.1	<0.1	<0.1	<0.1	<1	<0.1	<1	10.6	9	7	111	13	1	0	0
0	113	0	<0.1	0	0	<1	<0.1	<1	5.8	4	3	152	5	<1	0	0
0	1802	0	<0.1	0	0	2	0.1	<1	106	39	30	5	56	3	0	0
0	113	0	<0.1	0	0	<1	<0.1	<1	6.6	2	2	<1	3	<1	0	0
0	0	0	0	0	0	0	0	0	27.2	<1	3	<1	0	<1	0.8	0.1
0	0	0	0	0	0	0	0	0	1.7							
0	0	0	0	0	0	0	0	0	13.5	0	0	0	0	0	0	0
0	0	0	0	0	0	0	0	0	0.8	0	0	0	0	0	0	0
0	0	0	0	0	0	0	0	0	83.7	0	<1	0	0	0	<0.1	0
0	0	0	0	0	0	0	0	0	5.2	0	<1	0	0	0	<0.1	0
0	0	0	0	0	0	0	0	0	54	<1	0	<1	<1	<1	0.1	<0.1
0	0	0	0	0	0	0	0	0	3.4	<1	0	<1	<1	<1	<0.1	<0.1
0	0	0	0	0	0	0	0	0	93.9	0	0	0	0	0	0	0
0	0	0	0	0	0	0	0	0	5.9	0	0	0	0	0	0	0
0	0	0	0	0	0	0	0	0	63.4	0	0	0	0	0	0	0
0	0	0	0	0	0	0	0	0	4	0	0	0	0	0	0	0
0	144	0	<0.1	<0.1	0	<1	<0.1	<1	1.4	3	2	110	4	<1	0	0
0	0	0	0	0	0	0	0	0	201.5	0	0	0	0	0	0	0
0	0	0	0	0	0	0	0	0	216.2	0	0	0	0	0	0	0
0	0	0	0	0	0	0	0	0	13.5	0	0	0	0	0	0	0

ERA, EatRight Analysis CD-ROM; **AMT,** amount; **WT,** weight; **WTR,** water; **CAL,** calories; **PROT,** protein; **CARB**, carbohydrate; **FIBR,** fiber; **FAT,** fat; **SATF,** saturated fat; **MONO,** monounsaturated fat; **POLY,** polyunsaturated fat

ERA CODE	FOOD DESCRIPTION	AMT	UNIT	WT (g)	WTR (g)	CAL (kcal)	PROT (g)	CARB (g)	FIBR (g)	FAT (g)	SATF (g)	MONO (g)	POLY (g)
Fats, Oils, Margarines, Shortenings, and Substitutes (continued)													
Fats, Oils, Spreads (continued)													
8132	Touch of Butter spread, tub	1	Tbs	14.2	5	77	<1	0	0	9	2	4.4	1.9
8085	Walnut oil, cup	1	cup	218	0	1927	0	0	0	218	19.8	49.7	137.9
8085	Walnut oil, tablespoon	1	Tbs	13.6	0	120	0	0	0	14	1.2	3.1	8.6
8011	Wesson Sunlite/sunflr oil, cup	1	cup	218	0	1927	0	0	0	218	22.5	42.5	143.2
8011	Wesson Sunlite/sunflr oil, tbsp	1	Tbs	13.6	0	120	0	0	0	14	0.2	2.7	8.9
8038	Wheat germ oil, cup	1	cup		0	1923	0	0	0	218	40.9	32.8	134.3
8038	Wheat germ oil, tablespoon	1	Tbs	13.6	0	120	0	0	0	14	2.6	2.1	8.4
Fish, Seafood, and Shellfish													
19086	Abalone, cooked	2	oz	56.7	28	119	19	7	0	1	0.2	0.1	0.1
17124	Anchovies+oil, canned	5	ea	20	10	42	6	0	0	2	0.4	0.8	0.5
17128	Catfish, steamed/poached	1	cup	132	91	223	26	0	0	13	2.9	5.9	2.6
17034	Caviar, granular, black/red	1	Tbs	16	8	40	4	1	0	3	0.6	0.7	1.2
19049	Clams, baked/broiled, small	15	ea	150	109	210	23	5	0	11	1.9	4.4	2.9
19002	Clams, canned, drained	1	cup	160	102	237	41	8	0	3	0.3	0.3	0.9
17000	Cod, batter fried	4	pce	64	43	111	11	4	<1	5	1	2	1.7
17001	Cod, steamed/poached	1	cup	132	101	135	30	0	0	1	0.1	0.1	0.4
19420	Crab cakes, blue crab	1	ea	60	43	93	12	<1	0	5	0.9	1.7	1.4
19036	Crab leg, Alaska, king, boiled	1	ea	134	104	130	26	0	0	2	0.2	0.2	0.7
19052	Crab, baked/broiled	1	cup	118	87	163	22	<1	0	8	1.3	3	2.3
19038	Crayfish/crawdads, steam/boiled	3	oz	85	67	70	14	0	0	1	0.2	0.2	0.3
17003	Fish patty, frozen sq, heated	1	ea	57	26	155	9	14	0	7	1.8	2.9	1.8
17002	Fish sticks, frozen, heated	1	ea	28	13	76	4	7	0	3	0.9	1.4	0.9
17040	Fried fish cakes, frzn, heated	1	ea	85	45	230	8	15	1	15	5.9	3.4	3.4
17103	Gefilte fish, sweet, commercial	1	pce	42	34	35	4	3	0	1	0.2	0.3	0.1
17071	Grouper fillet, baked/broiled	1	ea	202	148	238	50	0	0	3	0.6	0.5	0.8
17090	Haddock fillet, bkd/brld	1	ea	150	111	168	36	0	0	1	0.2	0.2	0.5
17047	Herring fillet, baked/broiled	1	ea	143	92	290	33	0	0	17	3.7	6.8	3.9
17012	Herring, pickled	1	pce	20	11	52	3	2	0	4	0.5	2.4	0.3
19057	Lobster, baked/broiled, pieces	1	cup	145	108	169	29	2	0	4	2.4	1.3	0.3
19044	Mussels, steamed/boiled	3	oz	85	52	146	20	6	0	4	0.7	0.9	1
19048	Octopus, cooked, moist	3	oz	85	51	139	25	4	0	2	0.4	0.3	0.4
19025	Octopus, raw	3	oz	85	68	70	13	2	0	1	0.2	0.1	0.2
17121	Orange roughy, baked/broiled	3	oz	85	59	76	16	0	0	1	<0.1	0.5	<0.1
19027	Oysters, Eastern, boiled/steamed	6	ea	42	30	58	6	3	0	2	0.6	0.3	0.8
19009	Oysters, Eastern, breaded, fried	6	ea	88	57	173	8	10	<1	11	2.8	4.1	2.9
19026	Oysters, Eastern, raw	1	cup	248	211	169	17	10	0	6	1.9	0.8	2.4
19012	Prawns/lrg shrimp, steamed	4	ea	22	17	22	5	0	0	<1	0.1	<0.1	0.1
18807	Salmon croquette	1	ea	63	38	137	9	7	1	8	1.9	3.4	2.4
17123	Salmon fillet, baked/broiled	1	ea	308	184	560	78	0	0	25	3.9	8.3	10
17059	Salmon, canned, drained, cup	1	cup	150	103	230	31	0	0	11	2.5	4.7	2.8
17060	Sardines+oil, can, drained	1	ea	12	7	25	3	0	0	1	0.2	0.5	0.6
19061	Scallops, baked/broiled	4	ea	100		134	20	3	0	4	0.7	1.5	1.2
19070	Scallops, battered, fried	10	ea	80	45	185	14	11	<1	9	1.9	3.8	2.7
17086	Sea bass fillet, baked/broiled	1	ea	101	73	125	24	0	0	3	0.7	0.5	1

< = Trace amount present   Blank = Not available

CHOL, cholesterol; **V,** vitamin; **THI,** thiamin; **RIB,** riboflavin; **NIA,** niacin; **FOL,** folate;
CALC, calcium; **PHOS,** phosphate; **SOD,** sodium; **POT,** potassium; **MAG,** magnesium

CHOL (mg)	V-A (RE)	THI (mg)	RIB (mg)	NIA (mg)	V-B6 (mg)	FOL (µg)	V-B12 (µg)	V-C (mg)	V-E (mg)	CALC (mg)	PHOS (mg)	SOD (mg)	POT (mg)	MAG (mg)	IRON (mg)	ZINC (mg)
1	113	<0.1	<0.1	<0.1	0	<1	<0.1	<1	1.2	3	2	140	4	<1	0	0
0	0	0	0	0	0	0	0	0	70	0	0	0	0	0	0	0
0	0	0	0	0	0	0	0	0	4.4	0	0	0	0	0	0	0
0	0	0	0	0	0	0	0	0	138.6	0	0	0	0	0	0	0
0	0	0	0	0	0	0	0	0	8.7	0	0	0	0	0	0	0
0	0	0	0	0	0	0	0	0	418.7	0	0	0	0	0	0	0
0	0	0	0	0	0	0	0	0	26.2	0	0	0	0	0	0	0
96	2	0.2	0.1	1.3	0.1	4	0.5	2	4.5	33	151	290	198	46	3.3	0.9
17	4	<0.1	0.1	4	<0.1	2	0.2	0	1	46	50	734	109	14	0.9	0.5
78	21	0.5	0.1	3.2	0.2	13	3.5	1	2	15	300	79	419	34	0.8	1.2
94	90	<0.1	0.1	<0.1	0.1	8	3.2	0	1.1	44	57	240	29	48	1.9	0.2
60	223	0.1	0.3	3	0.1	27	82.9	22	3.1	84	301	202	559	16	24.7	2.4
107	274	0.2	0.7	5.4	0.2	46	158.2	35	3	147	541	179	1004	29	44.7	4.4
32	6	<0.1	0.1	1.5	0.2	6	0.5	1	0.8	19	116	58	245	16	0.5	0.3
61	11	<0.1	0.1	2.9	0.5	9	1.3	4	0.4	12	258	105	565	36	0.4	0.7
90	49	0.1	<0.1	1.7	0.1	32	3.6	2	0.9	63	128	198	194	20	0.6	2.5
71	12	0.1	0.1	1.8	0.2	68	15.4	10	1.2	79	375	1436	351	84	1	10.2
111	57	0.1	0.1	3.7	0.2	56	8.1	4	1.9	118	230	375	363	37	1	4.7
113	13	<0.1	0.1	1.9	0.1	37	1.8	1	1.3	51	230	80	252	28	0.7	1.5
64	18	0.1	0.1	1.2	<0.1	10	1	0	0.8	11	103	332	149	14	0.4	0.4
31	9	<0.1	<0.1	0.6	<0.1	5	0.5	0	0.4	6	51	163	73	7	0.2	0.2
22	17	<0.1	0.1	1.4	<0.1	10	0.9	0	0.9	9	142	150	296	15	0.3	0.3
13	11	<0.1	<0.1	0.4	<0.1	1	0.4	<1	0.1	10	31	220	38	4	1	0.3
95	101	0.2	<0.1	0.8	0.7	21	1.4	0	1.3	42	289	107	960	75	2.3	1
111	28	0.1	0.1	6.9	0.5	20	2.1	0	1.8	63	362	130	598	75	2	0.7
110	44	0.2	0.4	5.9	0.5	16	18.8	1	1.9	106	433	164	599	59	2	1.8
3	52	<0.1	<0.1	0.7	<0.1	<1	0.9	0	0.3	15	18	174	14	2	0.2	0.1
111	70	<0.1	0.1	1.5	0.1	16	4.4	0	1.5	87	261	570	496	49	0.6	4.1
48	77	0.3	0.4	2.5	0.1	64	20.4	12	1.2	28	242	314	228	31	5.7	2.3
82	69	<0.1	0.1	3.2	0.6	20	30.6	7	2	90	237	391	536	51	8.1	2.9
41	38	<0.1	<0.1	1.8	0.3	14	17	4	1	45	158	196	298	26	4.5	1.4
22	20	0.1	0.2	3.1	0.3	7	2	0	0.5	32	218	69	327	32	0.2	0.8
44	23	0.1	0.1	1	<0.1	6	14.7	3	0.7	38	85	177	118	40	5	76.3
71	79	0.1	0.2	1.5	0.1	27	13.8	3	2	55	140	367	215	51	6.1	76.7
131	74	0.2	0.2	3.4	0.2	25	48.3	9	2.1	112	335	523	387	116	16.5	225.2
43	15	<0.1	<0.1	0.6	<0.1	1	0.3	<1	0.2	9	30	49	40	7	0.7	0.3
30	14	<0.1	0.1	2.9	0.2	10	1.2	2	1.3	95	145	266	203	17	0.5	0.5
219	40	0.8	1.5	31	2.9	89	9.4	0	3.9	46	788	172	1934	114	3.2	2.5
66	80	<0.1	0.3	8.2	0.4	15	0.4	0	2.4	358	489	807	566	44	1.6	1.5
17	8	<0.1	<0.1	0.6	<0.1	1	1.1	0	<0.1	46	59	61	48	5	0.3	0.2
40	46	<0.1	0.1	1.3	0.2	18	1.8	3	1.7	30	266	231	392	68	0.4	1.2
66	29	0.1	0.1	1.4	0.1	14	1	2	1.8	35	184	171	253	44	1	0.9
54	65	0.1	0.2	1.9	0.5	6	0.3	0	0.6	13	250	88	331	54	0.4	0.5

ERA, EatRight Analysis CD-ROM; **AMT,** amount; **WT,** weight; **WTR,** water; **CAL,** calories; **PROT,** protein; **CARB**, carbohydrate; **FIBR,** fiber; **FAT,** fat; **SATF,** saturated fat; **MONO,** monounsaturated fat; **POLY,** polyunsaturated fat

ERA CODE	FOOD DESCRIPTION	AMT	UNIT	WT (g)	WTR (g)	CAL (kcal)	PROT (g)	CARB (g)	FIBR (g)	FAT (g)	SATF (g)	MONO (g)	POLY (g)
Fish, Seafood, and Shellfish (continued)													
19013	Shrimp, small, boiled/steamed	10	ea	40	31	40	8	0	0	<1	0.1	0.1	0.2
19000	Small clams, steamed/boiled	20	ea	190	121	281	49	10	0	4	0.4	0.3	1
17022	Snapper fillet, baked/broiled	1	ea	170	120	218	45	0	0	3	0.6	0.5	1
17004	Sole/flounder, fillet, breaded/fried	1	ea	81	48	179	16	7	<1	9	2	3.8	2.7
17068	Sole/flounder, fillet, broiled	1	ea	127	93	148	31	0	0	2	0.5	0.3	0.8
19068	Squid/calamari, baked	1	cup	140	99	194	26	5	0	7	1.4	2.2	2.1
17080	Surimi	3	oz	85	65	84	13	6	0	1	0.2	0.1	0.4
17066	Swordfish, broiled/baked	1	pce	106	73	164	27	0	0	5	1.5	2.1	1.3
17101	Tuna, bluefin, baked/broiled	3	oz	85	50	156	25	0	0	5	1.4	1.7	1.6
17025	Tuna, lt, oil, can, drnd, cup	1	cup	146	87	289	43	0	0	12	2.2	4.3	4.2
17027	Tuna, lt, wat, cnd, drnd, cup	1	cup	154	115	179	39	0	0	1	0.4	0.2	0.5
19040	Whelk, steamed/boiled	3	oz	85	27	234	41	13	0	1	0.1	<0.1	<0.1
17145	Whiting, baked/broiled	1	cup	132	99	153	31	0	0	2	0.5	0.6	0.8
Fruits													
3005	Apple rings, dried	10	ea	64	20	156	1	42	6	<1	<0.1	<0.1	0.1
3000	Apple+peel, medium	1	ea	138	116	81	<1	21	4	<1	0.1	<0.1	0.1
3308	Apple, baked, unsweetened	1	ea	161	133	102	<1	26	5	1	0.1	<0.1	0.2
3003	Apple, peeled, medium	1	ea	128	108	73	<1	19	2	<1	0.1	<0.1	0.1
3147	Applesauce, canned, sweet	1	cup	255	203	194	<1	51	3	<1	0.1	<0.1	0.1
3006	Applesauce, canned, unsweet	1	cup	244	216	105	<1	28	3	<1	<0.1	<0.1	<0.1
3013	Apricot halves, dried, each	1	ea	3.5	1	8	<1	2	<1	<1	<0.1	<0.1	<0.1
3151	Apricots+juice, can	1	cup	244	211	117	2	30	4	<1	<0.1	<0.1	<0.1
3157	Apricots, fresh, pitted	1	ea	35	30	17	<1	4	1	<1	<0.1	0.1	<0.1
3016	Avocado, fresh	1	ea	201	149	324	4	15	10	31	4.9	19.3	3.9
3307	Banana chips	1	cup	92	4	477	2	54	7	31	26.6	1.8	0.6
3020	Banana, fresh	1	ea	118	88	108	1	28	3	1	0.2	<0.1	0.1
3024	Blackberries, fresh	1	cup	144	123	75	1	18	8	1	<0.1	0.1	0.3
3028	Blackberries, frozen	1	cup	151	124	97	2	24	8	1	<0.1	0.1	0.4
3029	Blueberries, fresh	1	cup	145	123	81	1	20	4	1	<0.1	0.1	0.2
3031	Blueberries, frozen	1	cup	155	134	79	1	19	4	1	0.1	0.1	0.4
3231	Blueberries, fz, sweet, thaw	1	cup	230	178	186	1	50	5	<1	<0.1	<0.1	0.1
3239	Breadfruit	1	cup	220	155	227	2	60	11	1	0.1	0.1	0.1
3076	Cantaloupe melon	1	ea	552	496	193	5	46	4	2	0.4	<0.1	0.6
3075	Cantaloupe melon, cubes	1	cup	160	144	56	1	13	1	<1	0.1	<0.1	0.2
3240	Carambola/starfruit, fresh	1	ea	127	115	42	1	10	3	<1	<0.1	<0.1	0.2
3079	Casaba/crenshaw melon	1	ea	1640	1508	426	15	102	13	2	0.4	<0.1	0.6
3078	Casaba/crenshaw melon, cubes	1	cup	170	156	44	2	11	1	<1	<0.1	<0.1	0.1
3039	Cranberries, fresh	1	cup	95	82	47	<1	12	4	<1	<0.1	<0.1	0.1
3040	Cranberry sauce, strained	1	cup	277	168	418	1	108	3	<1	<0.1	0.1	0.2
3043	Dates, chopped	1	cup	178	40	490	4	131	13	1	0.3	0.3	0.1
3044	Dates, whole, each	10	ea	83	19	228	2	61	6	<1	0.2	0.1	<0.1
3162	Dried figs	1	ea	19	5	48	1	12	2	<1	<0.1	<0.1	0.1
3271	Feijoa fruit, raw	1	ea	50	43	24	1	5	2	<1	0.1	<0.1	0.2
3160	Figs, medium, fresh	1	ea	50	40	37	<1	10	2	<1	<0.1	<0.1	0.1
3045	Fruit cocktail+heavy syrup	1	cup	248	199	181	1	47	2	<1	<0.1	<0.1	0.1

< = Trace amount present   Blank = Not available

CHOL, cholesterol; **V,** vitamin; **THI,** thiamin; **RIB,** riboflavin; **NIA,** niacin; **FOL,** folate;
CALC, calcium; **PHOS,** phosphate; **SOD,** sodium; **POT,** potassium; **MAG,** magnesium

CHOL (mg)	V-A (RE)	THI (mg)	RIB (mg)	NIA (mg)	V-B6 (mg)	FOL (μg)	V-B12 (μg)	V-C (mg)	V-E (mg)	CALC (mg)	PHOS (mg)	SOD (mg)	POT (mg)	MAG (mg)	IRON (mg)	ZINC (mg)
78	26	<0.1	<0.1	1	0.1	1	0.6	1	0.3	16	55	90	73	14	1.2	0.6
127	325	0.3	0.8	6.4	0.2	55	187.8	42	3.7	175	642	213	1193	34	53.1	5.2
80	60	0.1	<0.1	0.6	0.8	10	5.9	3	1.4	68	342	97	887	63	0.4	0.7
55	15	0.1	0.1	2.8	0.2	9	1.1	1	2.2	38	164	148	306	29	0.9	0.5
86	14	0.1	0.1	2.8	0.3	12	3.2	0	2.9	23	367	133	437	74	0.4	0.8
395	57	<0.1	0.6	3.5	0.1	8	2.1	8	2.7	56	376	124	420	56	1.2	2.6
26	17	<0.1	<0.1	0.2	<0.1	1	1.4	0	0.2	8	240	122	95	37	0.2	0.3
53	43	<0.1	0.1	12.5	0.4	2	2.1	1	0.7	6	357	122	391	36	1.1	1.6
42	643	0.2	0.3	9	0.4	2	9.2	0	1.1	8	277	42	274	54	1.1	0.7
26	34	0.1	0.2	18.1	0.2	8	3.2	0	1.8	19	454	517	302	45	2	1.3
46	26	<0.1	0.1	20.5	0.5	6	4.6	0	0.8	17	251	520	365	42	2.4	1.2
110	42	<0.1	0.2	1.7	0.6	10	15.4	6	0.2	96	240	350	590	146	8.6	2.8
111	45	0.1	0.1	2.2	0.2	20	3.4	0	0.5	82	376	174	573	36	0.6	0.7
0	0	0	0.1	0.6	0.1	0	0	2	0.7	9	24	56	288	10	0.9	0.1
0	7	<0.1	<0.1	0.1	0.1	4	0	8	0.9	10	10	0	159	7	0.2	0.1
0	7	<0.1	<0.1	0.1	0.1	3	0	8	0.6	12	12	0	179	9	0.3	0.1
0	5	<0.1	<0.1	0.1	0.1	1	0	5	0.1	5	9	0	145	4	0.1	0.1
0	3	<0.1	0.1	0.5	0.1	2	0	4	2.3	10	18	8	156	8	0.9	0.1
0	7	<0.1	0.1	0.5	0.1	1	0	3	0.6	7	17	5	183	7	0.3	0.1
0	25	0	<0.1	0.1	<0.1	<1	0	<1	0.1	2	4	<1	48	2	0.2	<0.1
0	412	<0.1	<0.1	0.8	0.1	4	0	12	2.2	29	49	10	403	24	0.7	0.3
0	91	<0.1	<0.1	0.2	<0.1	3	0	4	0.3	5	7	<1	104	3	0.2	0.1
0	123	0.2	0.2	3.9	0.6	124	0	16	4.6	22	82	20	1203	78	2	0.8
0	7	0.1	<0.1	0.7	0.2	13	0	6	5	17	52	6	493	70	1.1	0.7
0	9	0.1	0.1	0.6	0.7	23	0	11	0.4	7	24	1	467	34	0.4	0.2
0	23	<0.1	0.1	0.6	0.1	49	0	30	1	46	30	0	282	29	0.8	0.4
0	17	<0.1	0.1	1.8	0.1	51	0	5	1.1	44	45	2	211	33	1.2	0.4
0	14	0.1	0.1	0.5	0.1	9	0	19	2.7	9	14	9	129	7	0.2	0.2
0	12	<0.1	0.1	0.8	0.1	10	0	4	3.1	12	17	2	84	8	0.3	0.1
0	9	<0.1	0.1	0.6	0.1	15	0	2	4.6	14	16	2	138	5	0.9	0.1
0	9	0.2	0.1	2	0.2	31	0	64	2.5	37	66	4	1078	55	1.2	0.3
0	1777	0.2	0.1	3.2	0.6	94	0	233	1.7	61	94	50	1705	61	1.2	0.9
0	515	0.1	<0.1	0.9	0.2	27	0	68	0.5	18	27	14	494	18	0.3	0.3
0	62	<0.1	<0.1	0.5	0.1	18	0	27	0.5	5	20	3	207	11	0.3	0.1
0	49	1	0.3	6.6	2	279	0	262	2.5	82	115	197	3444	131	6.6	2.6
0	5	0.1	<0.1	0.7	0.2	29	0	27	0.3	8	12	20	357	14	0.7	0.3
0	5	<0.1	<0.1	0.1	0.1	2	0	13	0.9	7	9	1	67	5	0.2	0.1
0	6	<0.1	0.1	0.3	<0.1	3	0	6	0.4	11	17	80	72	8	0.6	0.1
0	9	0.2	0.2	3.9	0.3	22	0	0	0.2	57	71	5	1160	62	2	0.5
0	4	0.1	0.1	1.8	0.2	10	0	0	0.1	27	33	2	541	29	1	0.2
0	2	<0.1	<0.1	0.1	<0.1	1	0	<1	0	27	13	2	135	11	0.4	0.1
0	0	<0.1	<0.1	0.1	<0.1	19	0	10		8	10	2	78	4	<0.1	<0.1
0	7	<0.1	<0.1	0.2	0.1	3	0	1	0.4	18	7	<1	116	8	0.2	0.1
0	50	<0.1	<0.1	0.9	0.1	6	0	5	2.1	15	27	15	218	12	0.7	0.2

ERA, EatRight Analysis CD-ROM; **AMT,** amount; **WT,** weight; **WTR,** water; **CAL,** calories; **PROT,** protein; **CARB**, carbohydrate; **FIBR,** fiber; **FAT,** fat; **SATF,** saturated fat; **MONO,** monounsaturated fat; **POLY,** polyunsaturated fat

ERA CODE	FOOD DESCRIPTION	AMT	UNIT	WT (g)	WTR (g)	CAL (kcal)	PROT (g)	CARB (g)	FIBR (g)	FAT (g)	SATF (g)	MONO (g)	POLY (g)
Fruits (continued)													
3163	Fruit cocktail+lite syrup	1	cup	242	204	138	1	36	2	<1	<0.1	<0.1	0.1
3164	Fruit cocktail, juice pack	1	cup	237	207	109	1	28	2	<1	<0.1	<0.1	<0.1
3313	Fruit cocktail, water pack	1	cup	237	215	76	1	20	2	<1	<0.1	<0.1	<0.1
3048	Grapefruit, fresh, pieces	1	cup	230	209	74	1	19	3	<1	<0.1	<0.1	0.1
3047	Grapefruit, fresh, white	0.5	ea	118	107	39	1	10	1	<1	<0.1	<0.1	<0.1
3060	Grapes, Concord	1	cup	92	75	62	1	16	1	<1	0.1	<0.1	0.1
3057	Grapes, red, cup	1	cup	160	129	114	1	28	2	1	0.3	<0.1	0.3
3054	Grapes, white, seedless, cup	1	cup	160	129	114	1	28	2	1	0.3	<0.1	0.3
3207	Guava, fresh	1	ea	90	77	46	1	11	5	1	0.2	<0.1	0.2
3081	Honeydew melon (1/10th)	1	pce	160	143	56	1	15	1	<1	<0.1	<0.1	0.1
3080	Honeydew melon, cubes	1	cup	170	152	60	1	16	1	<1	<0.1	<0.1	0.1
3065	Kiwifruit	1	ea	76	63	46	1	11	3	<1	<0.1	<0.1	0.2
3066	Lemon, fresh, peeled	1	ea	58	52	17	1	5	2	<1	<0.1	<0.1	0.1
3071	Lime, fresh, peeled	1	ea	67	59	20	<1	7	2	<1	<0.1	<0.1	<0.1
3257	Lychees	1	ea	9.6	8	6	<1	2	<1	<1	<0.1	<0.1	<0.1
3221	Mango, fresh, whole	1	ea	207	169	134	1	35	4	1	0.1	0.2	0.1
3215	Nectarine, fresh	1	ea	136	117	67	1	16	2	1	0.1	0.2	0.3
3082	Orange, fresh, medium	1	ea	131	114	62	1	15	3	<1	<0.1	<0.1	<0.1
3083	Orange, fresh, sections, cup	1	cup	180	156	85	2	21	4	<1	<0.1	<0.1	<0.1
3089	Oranges, mandarin, canned	1	cup	249	223	92	2	24	2	<1	<0.1	<0.1	<0.1
3171	Papaya, fresh	1	ea	304	270	118	2	30	5	<1	0.1	0.1	0.1
3098	Peaches, canned+heavy syrup	1	cup	262	208	194	1	52	3	<1	<0.1	0.1	0.1
3173	Peaches, canned+light syrup	1	cup	251	213	136	1	37	3	<1	<0.1	<0.1	<0.1
3096	Peach, fresh, medium	1	ea	98	86	42	1	11	2	<1	<0.1	<0.1	<0.1
3103	Pears, Bartlett, fresh, med	1	ea	166	139	98	1	25	4	1	<0.1	0.1	0.2
3107	Pears, canned+heavy syrup	1	cup	266	214	197	1	51	4	<1	<0.1	0.1	0.1
3179	Pears, canned+juice	1	cup	248	214	124	1	32	4	<1	<0.1	<0.1	<0.1
3177	Pears, canned+light syrup	1	cup	251	212	143	<1	38	4	<1	<0.1	<0.1	<0.1
3115	Pineapple, canned+heavy syrup	1	ea	49	39	38	<1	10	<1	<1	<0.1	<0.1	<0.1
3183	Pineapple, canned+juice	1	cup	250	209	150	1	39	2	<1	<0.1	<0.1	0.1
3181	Pineapple, canned+light syrup	1	cup	252	216	131	1	34	2	<1	<0.1	<0.1	0.1
3113	Pineapple, fresh, slices	1	pce	84	73	41	<1	10	1	<1	<0.1	<0.1	0.1
5632	Plantain, fried, ripe	1	cup	169	81	425	2	61	4	22	3	6.8	11.5
3121	Plum, medium, fresh	1	ea	66	56	36	1	9	1	<1	<0.1	0.3	0.1
3126	Prunes, dried	10	ea	84	27	201	2	53	6	<1	<0.1	0.3	0.1
3129	Raisins, seedless, packed	1	cup	165	25	495	5	130	7	1	0.2	<0.1	0.2
3130	Raisins, seedless, unpacked	1	cup	145	22	435	5	115	6	1	0.2	<0.1	0.2
3131	Raspberries, fresh	1	cup	123	106	60	1	14	8	1	<0.1	0.1	0.4
3235	Raspberries, frozen, sweet	1	cup	250	182	258	2	65	11	<1	<0.1	<0.1	0.2
3133	Rhubarb, fzn, cooked+sugar	1	cup	240	163	278	1	75	5	<1	<0.1	<0.1	0.1
3209	Rhubarb, raw, diced	1	cup	122	114	26	1	6	2	<1	0.1	<0.1	0.1
3664	Starfruit, raw, cube, cup	1	cup	137	124	45	1	11	4	<1	<0.1	<0.1	0.3
3236	Strawberries, frzn/sweet/thaw	1	cup	255	187	245	1	66	5	<1	<0.1	<0.1	0.2
3136	Strawberries, medium size	1	ea	12	11	4	<1	1	<1	<1	<0.1	<0.1	<0.1
3135	Strawberries, sliced, cup	1	cup	166	152	50	1	12	4	1	<0.1	0.1	0.3
3037	Sweet cherries, fresh, cup	1	cup	145	117	104	2	24	3	1	0.3	0.4	0.4

< = Trace amount present   Blank = Not available

CHOL, cholesterol; **V,** vitamin; **THI,** thiamin; **RIB,** riboflavin; **NIA,** niacin; **FOL,** folate;
CALC, calcium; **PHOS,** phosphate; **SOD,** sodium; **POT,** potassium; **MAG,** magnesium

CHOL (mg)	V-A (RE)	THI (mg)	RIB (mg)	NIA (mg)	V-B6 (mg)	FOL (μg)	V-B12 (μg)	V-C (mg)	V-E (mg)	CALC (mg)	PHOS (mg)	SOD (mg)	POT (mg)	MAG (mg)	IRON (mg)	ZINC (mg)
0	51	<0.1	<0.1	0.9	0.1	7	0	5	2.1	15	27	15	215	12	0.7	0.2
0	73	<0.1	<0.1	1	0.1	6	0	6	2.1	19	33	9	225	17	0.5	0.2
0	59	<0.1	<0.1	0.9	0.1	6	0	5	0.7	12	26	9	223	17	0.6	0.2
0	28	0.1	<0.1	0.6	0.1	23	0	79	0.6	28	18	0	320	18	0.2	0.2
0	1	<0.1	<0.1	0.3	0.1	12	0	39	0.3	14	9	0	175	11	0.1	0.1
0	9	0.1	0.1	0.3	0.1	4	0	4	0.3	13	9	2	176	5	0.3	<0.1
0	11	0.1	0.1	0.5	0.2	6	0	17	1.1	18	21	3	296	10	0.4	0.1
0	11	0.1	0.1	0.5	0.2	6	0	17	1.1	18	21	3	296	10	0.4	0.1
0	71	<0.1	<0.1	1.1	0.1	13	0	165	1	18	22	3	256	9	0.3	0.2
0	6	0.1	<0.1	1	0.1	10	0	40	0.2	10	16	16	434	11	0.1	0.1
0	7	0.1	<0.1	1	0.1	10	0	42	0.3	10	17	17	461	12	0.1	0.1
0	14	<0.1	<0.1	0.4	0.1	29	0	74	0.9	20	30	4	252	23	0.3	0.1
0	2	<0.1	<0.1	0.1	<0.1	6	0	31	0.5	15	9	1	80	5	0.3	<0.1
0	1	<0.1	<0.1	0.1	<0.1	5	0	19	0.2	22	12	1	68	4	0.4	0.1
0	0	<0.1	<0.1	0.1	<0.1	1	0	7	0.1	<1	3	<1	16	1	<0.1	<0.1
0	805	0.1	0.1	1.2	0.3	29	0	57	2.3	21	23	4	323	19	0.3	0.1
0	101	<0.1	0.1	1.3	<0.1	5	0	7	1.2	7	22	0	288	11	0.2	0.1
0	28	0.1	0.1	0.4	0.1	40	0	70	0.3	52	18	0	237	13	0.1	0.1
0	38	0.2	0.1	0.5	0.1	55	0	96	0.4	72	25	0	326	18	0.2	0.1
0	212	0.2	0.1	1.1	0.1	11	0	85	1.2	27	25	12	331	27	0.7	1.3
0	85	0.1	0.1	1	0.1	116	0	188	3.4	73	15	9	781	30	0.3	0.2
0	86	<0.1	0.1	1.6	<0.1	8	0	7	2.6	8	29	16	241	13	0.7	0.2
0	88	<0.1	0.1	1.5	<0.1	8	0	6	2.2	8	28	13	243	13	0.9	0.2
0	53	<0.1	<0.1	1	<0.1	3	0	6	1	5	12	0	193	7	0.1	0.1
0	3	<0.1	0.1	0.2	<0.1	12	0	7	0.8	18	18	0	208	10	0.4	0.2
0	0	<0.1	0.1	0.6	<0.1	3	0	3	1.3	13	19	13	173	11	0.6	0.2
0	2	<0.1	<0.1	0.5	<0.1	3	0	4	1.2	22	30	10	238	17	0.7	0.2
0	0	<0.1	<0.1	0.4	<0.1	3	0	2	1.3	13	18	13	166	10	0.7	0.2
0	<1	<0.1	<0.1	0.1	<0.1	2	0	4	<0.1	7	3	<1	51	8	0.2	0.1
0	10	0.2	<0.1	0.7	0.2	12	0	24	0.2	35	15	2	305	35	0.7	0.2
0	3	0.2	0.1	0.7	0.2	12	0	19	0.3	35	18	3	265	40	1	0.3
0	2	0.1	<0.1	0.4	0.1	9	0	13	0.1	6	6	1	95	12	0.3	0.1
0	162	0.1	0.1	1.2	0.5	21	0	25	4.7	5	65	8	858	71	1.1	0.3
0	21	<0.1	0.1	0.3	0.1	1	0	6	0.6	3	7	0	114	5	0.1	0.1
0	167	0.1	0.1	1.6	0.2	3	0	3	2.1	43	66	3	626	38	2.1	0.4
0	2	0.3	0.1	1.3	0.4	5	0	5	1.2	81	160	20	1239	54	3.4	0.4
0	1	0.2	0.1	1.2	0.4	5	0	5	1	71	141	17	1088	48	3	0.4
0	16	<0.1	0.1	1.1	0.1	32	0	31	0.6	27	15	0	187	22	0.7	0.6
0	15	<0.1	0.1	0.6	0.1	65	0	41	1.1	38	42	2	285	32	1.6	0.4
0	17	<0.1	0.1	0.5	<0.1	13	0	8	0.5	348	19	2	230	29	0.5	0.2
0	12	<0.1	<0.1	0.4	<0.1	9	0	10	0.2	105	17	5	351	15	0.3	0.1
0	67	<0.1	<0.1	0.6	0.1	19	0	29	0.5	5	22	3	223	12	0.4	0.2
0	5	<0.1	0.1	1	0.1	38	0	106	0.4	28	33	8	250	18	1.5	0.2
0	<1	<0.1	<0.1	<0.1	<0.1	2	0	7	<0.1	2	2	<1	20	1	<0.1	<0.1
0	5	<0.1	0.1	0.4	0.1	29	0	94	0.4	23	32	2	276	17	0.6	0.2
0	30	0.1	0.1	0.6	0.1	6	0	10	1.3	22	28	0	325	16	0.6	0.1

ERA, EatRight Analysis CD-ROM; **AMT,** amount; **WT,** weight; **WTR,** water; **CAL,** calories; **PROT,** protein; **CARB**, carbohydrate; **FIBR,** fiber; **FAT,** fat; **SATF,** saturated fat; **MONO,** monounsaturated fat; **POLY,** polyunsaturated fat

ERA CODE	FOOD DESCRIPTION	AMT	UNIT	WT (g)	WTR (g)	CAL (kcal)	PROT (g)	CARB (g)	FIBR (g)	FAT (g)	SATF (g)	MONO (g)	POLY (g)
Fruits (continued)													
3158	Sweet cherries, frozen	1	cup	259	196	230	3	58	5	<1	0.1	0.1	0.1
3087	Tangelo, medium	1	ea	95	82	45	1	11	2	<1	<0.1	<0.1	<0.1
3138	Tangerine, fresh	1	ea	84	74	37	1	9	2	<1	<0.1	<0.1	<0.1
3142	Watermelon, fresh pieces	1	cup	152	139	49	1	11	1	1	0.1	0.2	0.2
Grains and Grain Products													
Bagels													
42100	Bagel, cinnamon raisin	1	ea	71	23	194	7	39	2	1	0.2	0.1	0.5
42041	Bagel, egg, 3.5 inch diam	1	ea	71	23	197	8	38	2	1	0.3	0.3	0.5
42103	Bagel, oat bran	1	ea	71	23	181	8	38	3	1	0.1	0.2	0.3
42000	Bagel, plain, 3.5 in diam	1	ea	71	23	195	7	38	2	1	0.2	0.1	0.5
42092	Bagel, whole wheat	1	ea	55	16	145	6	31	5	1	0.1	0.1	0.3
Biscuits													
42206	Biscuit, cheese, 2 in diam	1	ea	30	8	113	3	13	<1	6	1.7	2.3	1.4
42110	Biscuit, low-fat dough, baked	1	ea	21	6	63	2	12	<1	1	0.3	0.6	0.2
42002	Biscuit, mix, enr+milk, baked	1	ea	57	16	191	4	28	1	7	1.6	2.4	2.5
42001	Biscuit, recipe	1	ea	60	17	212	4	27	1	10	2.6	4.2	2.5
42205	Biscuit, whole wheat, 3 inch	1	ea	63	18	198	6	30	5	7	1.7	3	2.2
42203	Crumpet, 3.75 inch	1	ea	45	24	80	3	17	1	<1	0.1	<0.1	0.2
42071	Scone	1	ea	42	12	150	4	19	1	6	2	2.6	1.3
42072	Scone, whole wheat	1	ea	42	11	144	5	18	3	7	2.1	2.6	1.4
Breads and Rolls													
42171	Armenian bread	1	pce	20	7	54	2	10	1	1	0.2	0.2	0.3
42039	Banana bread, recipe w/marg	1	pce	60	18	196	3	33	1	6	1.3	2.7	1.9
42052	Boston brown bread, canned	1	pce	45	21	88	2	19	2	1	0.1	0.1	0.3
42090	Challah/egg bread	1	pce	40	14	115	4	19	1	2	0.6	0.9	0.4
42115	Cornbread, dry mix, prep	1	ea	60	19	188	4	29	1	6	1.6	3.1	0.7
42116	Cornbread, recipe w/2% milk	1	pce	65	25	173	4	28	2	5	1	1.2	2.1
42042	Cracked wheat bread, slice	1	pce	25	9	65	2	12	1	1	0.2	0.5	0.2
42015	Croissant, 4.5x4x2 inch	1	ea	57	13	231	5	26	1	12	6.6	3.1	0.6
42173	Cuban/Spanish/Portug bread	1	pce	20	7	55	2	10	1	1	0.1	0.2	0.1
42157	Dinner roll/bun	1	ea	28	9	84	2	14	1	2	0.5	1	0.3
42160	Dinner roll/bun, wheat	1	ea	36	13	98	3	17	1	2	0.5	1.1	0.4
42169	Dinner roll, bran	1	ea	28	10	76	3	14	1	2	0.2	0.6	0.6
42091	Egg bread/challah, toasted	1	pce	37	10	116	4	19	1	2	0.6	1.1	0.4
42043	French/Vienna bread	1	pce	25	9	68	2	13	1	1	0.2	0.3	0.2
42368	Garlic bread, frozen	1	pce	47		160	5	14	1	10	3	4	1.5
42184	Garlic roll	1	ea	35	11	105	3	18	1	3	0.6	1.3	0.4
42020	Hamburger bun	1	ea	43	15	123	4	22	1	2	0.5	0.4	1.1
42022	Hard roll, white	1	ea	57	18	167	6	30	1	2	0.3	0.6	1
42021	Hot dog/frankfurter bun	1	ea	40	14	114	3	20	1	2	0.5	0.3	1
49012	Hush puppies, recipe	1	ea	22	6	74	2	10	1	3	0.5	0.7	1.6
42118	Indian fry bread	1	pce	90	24	296	6	48	2	9	2.1	3.6	2.3
42046	Italian bread	1	pce	30	11	81	3	15	1	1	0.3	0.2	0.4
42185	Mexican bolillo roll	1	ea	117	43	307	10	61	2	2	0.4	0.2	0.6

< = Trace amount present Blank = Not available

CHOL, cholesterol; **V,** vitamin; **THI,** thiamin; **RIB,** riboflavin; **NIA,** niacin; **FOL,** folate;
CALC, calcium; **PHOS,** phosphate; **SOD,** sodium; **POT,** potassium; **MAG,** magnesium

CHOL (mg)	V-A (RE)	THI (mg)	RIB (mg)	NIA (mg)	V-B6 (mg)	FOL (μg)	V-B12 (μg)	V-C (mg)	V-E (mg)	CALC (mg)	PHOS (mg)	SOD (mg)	POT (mg)	MAG (mg)	IRON (mg)	ZINC (mg)
0	49	0.1	0.1	0.5	0.1	11	0	3	0.3	31	41	3	515	26	0.9	0.1
0	20	0.1	<0.1	0.3	0.1	29	0	51	0.2	38	13	0	172	10	0.1	0.1
0	77	0.1	<0.1	0.1	0.1	17	0	26	0.3	12	8	1	132	10	0.1	0.2
0	56	0.1	<0.1	0.3	0.2	3	0	15	0.2	12	14	3	176	17	0.3	0.1
0	0	0.3	0.2	2.2	<0.1	64	0	<1	0.1	13	71	229	105	20	2.7	0.8
17	23	0.4	0.2	2.4	0.1	62	0.1	<1	1.9	9	60	358	48	18	2.8	0.5
0	<1	0.2	0.2	2.1	<0.1	58	0	<1	0.2	9	78	360	82	22	2.2	0.6
0	0	0.4	0.2	3.2	<0.1	62	0	0	1.9	53	68	379	72	21	2.5	0.6
0	0	0.2	0.1	2.9	0.2	33	0	<1	0.5	16	159	296	190	58	1.8	1.3
4	16	0.1	0.1	0.8	<0.1	3	0.1	<1	0.6	91	68	150	46	6	0.8	0.3
0	0	0.1	<0.1	0.7	<0.1	14	0	0	0.2	4	98	305	39	4	0.6	0.1
2	15	0.2	0.2	1.7	<0.1	30	0.1	<1	1.6	105	268	544	107	14	1.2	0.3
2	14	0.2	0.2	1.8	<0.1	37	<0.1	<1	2.7	141	98	348	73	11	1.7	0.3
2	14	0.1	0.1	2.2	0.1	13	0.1	<1	1.3	155	199	210	200	57	1.7	1.2
0	0	0.1	<0.1	0.4	<0.1	4	0	0	<0.1	50	72	324	37	7	0.4	0.2
49	69	0.1	0.2	1.2	<0.1	8	0.1	<1	0.7	80	74	171	49	7	1.3	0.3
0	71	0.1	0.1	1.3	0.1	11	0.1	<1	0.9	86	126	174	114	33	1.1	0.8
0	0	0.1	0.1	0.9	<0.1	6	0	0	0.1	16	21	117	22	5	0.6	0.2
26	72	0.1	0.1	0.9	0.1	20	0.1	1	1.1	13	35	181	80	8	0.8	0.2
<1	5	<0.1	0.1	0.5	<0.1	5	<0.1	0	0.3	32	50	284	143	28	0.9	0.2
20	9	0.2	0.2	1.9	<0.1	42	<0.1	0	0.3	37	42	197	46	8	1.2	0.3
37	26	0.1	0.2	1.2	0.1	33	0.1	<1	0.7	44	226	467	77	12	1.1	0.4
26	35	0.2	0.2	1.5	0.1	42	0.1	<1	0.6	162	110	428	96	16	1.6	0.4
0	0	0.1	0.1	0.9	0.1	15	<0.1	0	0.2	11	38	134	44	13	0.7	0.3
38	106	0.2	0.1	1.2	<0.1	35	0.1	<1	0.5	21	60	424	67	9	1.2	0.4
0	0	0.1	0.1	0.9	<0.1	6	0	0	<0.1	9	21	122	23	5	0.5	0.2
<1	0	0.1	0.1	1.1	<0.1	27	<0.1	<1	0.2	33	32	146	37	6	0.9	0.2
0	0	0.2	0.1	1.5	<0.1	18	0	0	0.4	63	37	122	41	13	1.3	0.3
0	<1	0.1	0.1	1.1	<0.1	18	0	<1	0.2	6	55	1	53	14	0.9	0.3
21	9	0.1	0.2	1.8	<0.1	33	<0.1	0	0.3	38	43	200	47	8	1.2	0.3
0	0	0.1	0.1	1.2	<0.1	24	0	0	0.1	19	26	152	28	7	0.6	0.2
30	0	0.2	0.1	1.6				0		0		250			3.6	
<1	0	0.2	0.1	1.4	<0.1	10	<0.1	<1	0.3	42	41	181	47	8	1.1	0.3
0	0	0.2	0.1	1.7	<0.1	41	<0.1	<1	0.7	60	38	241	61	9	1.4	0.3
0	0	0.3	0.2	2.4	<0.1	54	0	0	0.2	54	57	310	62	15	1.9	0.5
0	0	0.2	0.1	1.6	<0.1	38	<0.1	<1	0.6	56	35	224	56	8	1.3	0.2
10	9	0.1	0.1	0.6	<0.1	16	<0.1	<1	0.5	61	42	147	32	5	0.7	0.1
0	0	0.4	0.3	3.3	<0.1	67	0	0	1.7	210	141	626	67	14	3.2	0.4
0	0	0.1	0.1	1.3	<0.1	28	0	0	0.1	23	31	175	33	8	0.9	0.3
1	4	0.7	0.5	6.6	<0.1	41	<0.1	<1	0.1	14	90	7	98	22	3.8	0.8

ERA, EatRight Analysis CD-ROM; **AMT,** amount; **WT,** weight; **WTR,** water; **CAL,** calories; **PROT,** protein; **CARB**, carbohydrate; **FIBR,** fiber; **FAT,** fat; **SATF,** saturated fat; **MONO,** monounsaturated fat; **POLY,** polyunsaturated fat

ERA CODE	FOOD DESCRIPTION	AMT	UNIT	WT (g)	WTR (g)	CAL (kcal)	PROT (g)	CARB (g)	FIBR (g)	FAT (g)	SATF (g)	MONO (g)	POLY (g)
Grains and Grain Products (continued)													
Breads and Rolls (continued)													
42047	Mixed grain bread, slice	1	pce	26	10	65	3	12	2	1	0.2	0.4	0.2
42097	Multigrain bread, low cal	1	pce	23	10	46	2	10	3	1	0.1	0.1	0.3
42190	Pannetone, Italian sweetbread	1	pce	27	8	87	2	15	1	2	1.2	0.7	0.2
42007	Pita pocket bread, white	1	ea	60	19	165	5	33	1	1	0.1	0.1	0.3
42080	Pita pocket bread, whole wheat	1	ea	64	20	170	6	35	5	2	0.3	0.2	0.7
42454	Pretzel, soft	1	ea	138		390	12	84	3	1	0		
42456	Pretzel, soft, whole wheat	1	ea	140		390	13	82	8	2	0		
42006	Pumpernickel bread, slice	1	pce	26	10	65	2	12	2	1	0.1	0.2	0.3
42051	Raisin bread	1	pce	26	9	71	2	14	1	1	0.3	0.6	0.2
42005	Rye bread	1	pce	32	12	83	3	15	2	1	0.2	0.4	0.3
42045	Sourdough bead, med slice	1	pce	25	9	68	2	13	1	1	0.2	0.3	0.2
42034	Submarine roll/hoagie	1	ea	135	46	386	11	68	4	7	1.6	3.4	1.2
42013	Wheat berry bread	1	pce	25	9	65	2	12	1	1	0.2	0.4	0.2
42136	Wheat bran bread	1	pce	36	14	89	3	17	1	1	0.3	0.6	0.2
42012	Wheat bread	1	pce	25	9	65	2	12	1	1	0.2	0.4	0.2
42095	Wheat bread, low cal	1	pce	23	10	46	2	10	3	1	0.1	0.1	0.2
42216	White bread	1	pce	30	11	80	2	15	1	1	0.2	0.2	0.6
42084	White bread, low cal	1	pce	23	10	48	2	10	2	1	0.1	0.2	0.1
42014	Whole wheat bread	1	pce	28	11	69	3	13	2	1	0.3	0.5	0.3
42057	Whole wheat roll	1	ea	28.35	9	75	2	14	2	1	0.2	0.3	0.6
Bread Crumbs, Croutons, Stuffing													
42004	Bread crumbs, dry, grated	1	cup	108	7	427	14	78	3	6	1.3	2.6	1.2
42144	Bread crumbs, seasoned, dry	1	cup	120	7	440	17	84	5	3	0.9	1.2	0.8
42016	Croutons	1	cup	30	2	122	4	22	2	2	0.5	0.9	0.4
42148	Croutons, seasoned	1	cup	40	1	186	4	25	2	7	2.1	3.8	0.9
42037	Stuffing mix, bread, prep	0.5	cup	100		178	3	22	3	9	1.7	3.8	2.6
42147	Stuffing mix, cornbread, prep	0.5	cup	100		179	3	22	3	9	1.8	3.9	2.7
Crackers													
43562	100% StoneWheat crackers	3	ea	12	<1	53	1	8	1	2	0.4	1.1	0.3
43555	Better Chedd crackers, low sod	3	ea	3.9	<1	20	<1	2	<1	1	0.4	0.4	0.2
139	Butter crackers (Club)	2	ea	8	<1	40	1	5	<1	2	0.3	0.9	0.8
43500	Cheese crackers, Cheez-its	10	ea	10	<1	50	1	6	<1	3	0.9	1.2	0.2
43501	Cheese crackers, pnut butter filled	6	ea	42	2	202	5	24	1	10	2.3	4.9	2
43527	Graham cracker, chocolate	1	ea	14	<1	68	1	9	<1	3	1.9	1.1	0.1
43502	Graham cracker, plain	2	ea	14	1	59	1	11	<1	1	0.2	0.6	0.5
43534	Matzoh crackers, plain	1	ea	28.35	1	112	3	24	1	<1	0.1	<0.1	0.2
43509	Melba toast, plain	1	pce	5	<1	20	1	4	<1	<1	<0.1	<0.1	0.1
43507	Oyster crackers	1	ea	1	<1	4	<1	1	<1	<1	<0.1	0.1	<0.1
43505	Oyster crackers, crushed	1	cup	70	3	304	6	50	2	8	2.1	4.5	1.2
43543	Round crackers (Ritz)	10	ea	30	1	151	2	18	<1	8	1.1	3.2	2.9
43541	Rye crackers, cheese filled	6	ea	42	2	202	4	26	2	9	2.5	5.1	1.2
43532	Rye crispbread	1	ea	10	1	37	1	8	2	<1	<0.1	<0.1	0.1
43506	Saltine crackers	4	ea	12	<1	52	1	9	<1	1	0.4	0.8	0.2
43586	Saltine crackers, unsalted tops	2	ea	6		25	1	4	0	<1	0	0	0

< = Trace amount present   Blank = Not available

CHOL, cholesterol; **V,** vitamin; **THI,** thiamin; **RIB,** riboflavin; **NIA,** niacin; **FOL,** folate;
CALC, calcium; **PHOS,** phosphate; **SOD,** sodium; **POT,** potassium; **MAG,** magnesium

CHOL (mg)	V-A (RE)	THI (mg)	RIB (mg)	NIA (mg)	V-B6 (mg)	FOL (μg)	V-B12 (μg)	V-C (mg)	V-E (mg)	CALC (mg)	PHOS (mg)	SOD (mg)	POT (mg)	MAG (mg)	IRON (mg)	ZINC (mg)
0	0	0.1	0.1	1.1	0.1	21	<0.1	<1	0.3	24	46	127	53	14	0.9	0.3
2	0	0.1	0.1	0.9	<0.1	14	0	0	<0.1	18	57	117	40	20	0.6	0.5
19	23	0.1	0.1	1	<0.1	19	0.1	<1	0.1	16	40	28	54	5	0.8	0.2
0	0	0.4	0.2	2.8	<0.1	57	0	0	0.4	52	58	322	72	16	1.6	0.5
0	0	0.2	0.1	1.8	0.2	22	0	0	0.6	10	115	340	109	44	2	1
0	0									40		1100			2.7	
0	0									40		1290			2.7	
0	0	0.1	0.1	0.8	<0.1	21	0	0	0.1	18	46	174	54	14	0.7	0.4
0	0	0.1	0.1	0.9	<0.1	23	0	<1	0.2	17	28	101	59	7	0.8	0.2
0	<1	0.1	0.1	1.2	<0.1	28	0	<1	0.2	23	40	211	53	13	0.9	0.4
0	0	0.1	0.1	1.2	<0.1	24	0	0	0.1	19	26	152	28	7	0.6	0.2
0	0	0.7	0.4	5.3	0.1	36	<0.1	0	0.6	188	119	756	190	27	4.3	0.8
0	0	0.1	0.1	1	<0.1	19	0	0	0.1	26	38	132	50	12	0.8	0.3
0	0	0.1	0.1	1.6	0.1	25	0	0	0.2	27	67	175	82	29	1.1	0.5
0	0	0.1	0.1	1	<0.1	19	0	0	0.1	26	38	132	50	12	0.8	0.3
0	0	0.1	0.1	0.9	<0.1	16	0	<1	<0.1	18	23	118	28	9	0.7	0.3
<1	0	0.1	0.1	1.2	<0.1	28	<0.1	0	0.1	32	28	161	36	7	0.9	0.2
0	<1	0.1	0.1	0.8	<0.1	22	0.1	<1	<0.1	22	28	104	17	5	0.7	0.3
0	0	0.1	0.1	1.1	0.1	14	<0.1	0	0.3	20	64	148	71	24	0.9	0.5
0	0	0.1	<0.1	1	0.1	9	0	0	0.4	30	64	136	77	24	0.7	0.6
0	<1	0.8	0.5	7.4	0.1	118	<0.1	0	1	245	159	931	239	50	6.6	1.3
1	2	0.2	0.2	3.3	0.2	131	<0.1	<1	0.2	119	160	3180	324	46	3.8	1.1
0	0	0.2	0.1	1.6	<0.1	40	0	0	0.2	23	34	209	37	9	1.2	0.3
3	4	0.2	0.2	1.9	<0.1	35	0.1	0	0.9	38	56	495	72	17	1.1	0.4
0	81	0.1	0.1	1.5	<0.1	101	<0.1	0	1.4	32	42	543	74	12	1.1	0.3
0	85	0.1	0.1	1.2	<0.1	97	<0.1	1	1.4	26	34	455	62	13	0.9	0.2
0	0	<0.1	<0.1	0.5	<0.1	3	0	0	0.5	6	35	79	36	12	0.4	0.3
1	1	<0.1	<0.1	0.2	<0.1	1	<0.1	0	<0.1	6	9	18	4	1	0.2	<0.1
0	0	<0.1	<0.1	0.3	<0.1	6	0	0	0.4	10	18	68	11	2	0.3	0.1
1	3	0.1	<0.1	0.5	0.1	8	<0.1	0	0.3	15	22	100	14	4	0.5	0.1
2	14	0.2	0.1	2.7	0.6	37	<0.1	<1	1.9	33	136	417	103	24	1.2	0.5
0	<1	<0.1	<0.1	0.3	<0.1	2	0	0	0.2	8	19	41	29	8	0.5	0.1
0	0	<0.1	<0.1	0.6	<0.1	8	0	0	0.3	3	15	85	19	4	0.5	0.1
0	0	0.1	0.1	1.1	<0.1	33	0	0	0.1	4	25	1	32	7	0.9	0.2
0	0	<0.1	<0.1	0.2	<0.1	6	0	0	<0.1	5	10	41	10	3	0.2	0.1
0	0	<0.1	<0.1	0.1	0	1	0	0	<0.1	1	1	13	1	<1	0.1	<0.1
0	0	0.4	0.3	3.7	<0.1	87	0	0	1.2	83	74	911	90	19	3.8	0.5
0	0	0.1	0.1	1.2	<0.1	23	0	0	1.4	36	68	254	40	8	1.1	0.2
4	16	0.3	0.2	1.5	<0.1	34	0.1	<1	0.8	93	142	438	144	16	1	0.3
0	0	<0.1	<0.1	0.1	<0.1	5	0	0	0.1	3	27	26	32	8	0.2	0.2
0	0	0.1	0.1	0.6	<0.1	15	0	0	0.2	14	13	156	15	3	0.6	0.1
0									0.1			50	5		0.4	

ERA, EatRight Analysis CD-ROM; **AMT,** amount; **WT,** weight; **WTR,** water; **CAL,** calories; **PROT,** protein; **CARB**, carbohydrate; **FIBR,** fiber; **FAT,** fat; **SATF,** saturated fat; **MONO,** monounsaturated fat; **POLY,** polyunsaturated fat

ERA CODE	FOOD DESCRIPTION	AMT	UNIT	WT (g)	WTR (g)	CAL (kcal)	PROT (g)	CARB (g)	FIBR (g)	FAT (g)	SATF (g)	MONO (g)	POLY (g)
Grains and Grain Products (continued)													
Crackers (continued)													
43561	Saltines, whole wheat	3	ea	9	<1	39	1	6	1	1	0.3	0.7	0.2
43593	SnackWell fat-free wheat crckr	7	ea	15	<1	60	2	12	1	<1	0.1	0.1	0.1
43595	SnackWell low-fat golden crackr	1	ea	14	<1	58	1	11	<1	1	0.2	0.3	0.1
43508	Triscuits whole wheat cracker	2	ea	8	<1	35	1	5	1	1	0.3	0.5	0.5
43547	Wheat crackers	5	ea	10	<1	47	1	6	<1	2	0.5	1.1	0.3
43548	Wheat crackers, cheese filled	6	ea	42	1	209	4	24	1	10	1.7	4.3	3.8
43564	Wheat crackers, thin	4	ea	8	<1	38	1	5	<1	2	0.3	0.9	0.2
43549	Wheat crackers, pnut btr filled	1	ea	7	<1	35	1	4	<1	2	0.3	0.8	0.6
43554	WheatThin crackers, low sod	5	ea	10	<1	46	1	7	<1	2	0.6	0.7	0.4
Flours, Cooked Grains													
38030	All purpose white flour, enrich	1	cup	125	15	455	13	95	3	1	0.2	0.1	0.5
38003	Barley, pearled, cooked	1	cup	157	108	193	4	44	6	1	0.1	0.1	0.3
38001	Barley, whole, cooked	1	cup	200	130	270	7	59	14	2	0.4	0.3	1.2
38171	Bread flour, enriched	0.25	cup	31		100	4	22	1	0	0	0	0
38028	Bulgur wheat, cooked	1	cup	182	142	151	6	34	8	<1	0.1	0.1	0.2
38039	Cake flour, baked value	1	cup	109	14	394	9	85	2	1	0.1	0.1	0.4
38041	Cornmeal, enrich, baked value	1	cup	138	16	505	12	107	10	2	0.3	0.6	1
30000	Cornstarch	1	Tbs	8	1	30	<1	7	<1	<1	0	<0.1	<0.1
38076	Couscous, cooked	1	cup	157	114	176	6	36	2	<1	<0.1	<0.1	0.1
38044	Light rye flour, baked value	1	cup	102	9	374	9	82	15	1	0.1	0.2	0.6
38052	Millet, cooked	0.5	cup	120	86	143	4	28	2	1	0.2	0.2	0.6
38078	Oat bran, cooked	1	cup	219	184	88	7	25	6	2	0.4	0.6	0.7
38064	Oat bran, dry	1	cup	94	6	231	16	62	14	7	1.2	2.2	2.6
38043	Rolled oats, baked value	1	cup	80	7	307	13	54	8	5	0.9	1.6	1.8
38008	Rolled oats, dry	1	cup	81	7	311	13	54	9	5	0.9	1.6	1.9
38024	Wheat bran, crude	0.5	cup	29	3	63	5	19	12	1	0.2	0.2	0.6
38055	Wheat germ, honey crunch	1	cup	113	4	420	30	66	12	9	1.5	1.2	5.5
38026	Wheat germ, toasted	1	cup	113	6	432	33	56	15	12	2.1	1.7	7.5
38318	Wheat flour, unbleach, all purpose	1	cup	125	15	455	13	95	3	1	0.2	0.1	0.5
38037	White flour, enr, baked	1	cup	125	15	455	13	95	4	1	0.2	0.1	0.5
38032	Whole wheat flour	1	cup	120	12	407	16	87	15	2	0.4	0.3	0.9
38040	Whole wheat flour, baked	1	cup	120	12	407	16	87	15	2	0.4	0.3	0.9
Granola and Cereal Bars, Diet and Energy Bars													
62729	Balance bar, banana coconut	1	ea	50		190	14	21	1	6	3		
53227	Cereal bar, Nutrigrain, mix berry	100	g	100		370	4	73	2	8	1.5	5	1.1
23100	Granola bar, almond, hard	1	ea	23.6	1	117	2	15	1	6	3	1.8	0.9
23105	Granola bar, choc chip, soft	1	ea	42.5	2	178	3	29	2	7	4.3	1.5	0.8
23108	Granola bar, peanut butter, soft	1	ea	23.6	2	100	2	15	1	4	0.9	1.6	1
23059	Granola bar, plain, hard	1	ea	24.5	1	115	2	16	1	5	0.6	1.1	3
23097	Granola bar, raisin, soft	1	ea	42.5	3	190	3	28	2	8	4.1	1.2	1.4
23104	Granola bar, soft	1	ea	28.35	2	126	2	19	1	5	2.1	1.1	1.5
23065	Kudos bar, nutty fudge	1	ea	28.35		120	1	20	1	4	2		
62206	Power bar	1	ea	65		230	10	45	3	2			
62640	SlimFast NutriBar, Dutch choc	1	ea	34	3	140	5	20	2	5	2	1.5	1

< = Trace amount present

Blank = Not available

CHOL, cholesterol; **V,** vitamin; **THI,** thiamin; **RIB,** riboflavin; **NIA,** niacin; **FOL,** folate;
CALC, calcium; **PHOS,** phosphate; **SOD,** sodium; **POT,** potassium; **MAG,** magnesium

CHOL (mg)	V-A (RE)	THI (mg)	RIB (mg)	NIA (mg)	V-B6 (mg)	FOL (μg)	V-B12 (μg)	V-C (mg)	V-E (mg)	CALC (mg)	PHOS (mg)	SOD (mg)	POT (mg)	MAG (mg)	IRON (mg)	ZINC (mg)
0	0	<0.1	<0.1	0.5	<0.1	2	0	0	0.2	2	17	93	19	6	0.4	0.1
<1	<1	<0.1	0.1	0.7	<0.1		<0.1	0		28	61	169	43	7	0.6	0.2
<1	<1	0.1	0.1	0.7	<0.1		<0.1	<1		28	51	144	15	3	0.6	0.1
0	0	<0.1	<0.1	0.4	<0.1	2	0	0	0.3	4	24	53	24	8	0.2	0.2
0	0	0.1	<0.1	0.5	<0.1	4	0	0	0.4	5	22	80	18	6	0.4	0.2
3	4	0.2	0.2	1.3	0.1	27	0.1	1	0.3	86	160	383	128	23	1.1	0.4
0	0	<0.1	<0.1	0.4	<0.1	1	0	0	0.3	4	18	64	15	5	0.4	0.1
0	0	<0.1	<0.1	0.4	<0.1	5	0	0	<0.1	12	24	56	21	3	0.2	0.1
0	2	<0.1	<0.1	0.5	<0.1	3	0	0	0.1	3	19	25	22	5	0.4	0.1
0	0	1	0.6	7.4	0.1	192	0	0	1.7	19	135	2	134	28	5.8	0.9
0	2	0.1	0.1	3.2	0.2	25	0	0	0.3	17	85	5	146	35	2.1	1.3
0	0	0.2	0.1	2.8	0.2	16	0	0	3.1	26	230	1	230	44	2.1	1.6
0	0	0.2	0.1	1.6		40		0		0		0			1.4	
0	0	0.1	0.1	1.8	0.2	33	0	0	0.5	18	73	9	124	58	1.7	1
0	0	0.8	0.4	6.7	<0.1	118	0	0	0.2	15	93	2	114	17	8	0.7
0	57	0.8	0.5	6.3	0.3	181	0	0	3	7	116	4	224	55	5.7	1
0	0	0	0	0	0	0	0	0	0	<1	1	1	<1	<1	<0.1	<0.1
0	0	0.1	<0.1	1.5	0.1	24	0	0	<0.1	13	35	8	91	13	0.6	0.4
0	0	0.3	0.1	0.7	0.2	16	0	0	0.9	21	198	2	238	71	1.8	1.8
0	0	0.1	0.1	1.6	0.1	23	0	0	0.7	4	120	2	74	53	0.8	1.1
0	0	0.3	0.1	0.3	0.1	13	0	0	0.5	22	261	2	201	88	1.9	1.2
0	0	1.1	0.2	0.9	0.2	49	0	0	2	55	690	4	532	221	5.1	2.9
0	8	0.5	0.1	0.6	0.1	18	0	0	0.9	42	379	3	280	118	3.4	2.5
0	8	0.6	0.1	0.6	0.1	26	0	0	0.6	42	384	3	284	120	3.4	2.5
0	0	0.2	0.2	3.9	0.4	23	0	0	2.6	21	294	1	343	177	3.1	2.1
0	11	1.5	0.8	5.3	0.6	376	0	0	31	56	1142	12	1089	307	9.1	15.7
0	0	1.9	0.9	6.3	1.1	398	0	7	33.6	51	1294	5	1070	362	10.3	18.8
0	0	1	0.6	7.4	0.1	192	0	0	1.7	19	135	2	134	28	5.8	0.9
0	0	0.8	0.6	6.6	0.1	135	0	0	1.7	19	135	2	134	28	5.8	0.9
0	0	0.5	0.3	7.6	0.4	53	0	0	2.8	41	415	6	486	166	4.7	3.5
0	0	0.4	0.2	6.9	0.4	37	0	0	2.8	41	415	6	486	166	4.7	3.5
5	500	0.5	0.6	4	0.6	80	1.8	60	42	200	200	150	105	16	3.6	5.2
0	405	1	1.1	13.5	1.4	108	0	0	0	39	98	297	188	26	4.9	4.1
0	1	0.1	<0.1	0.1	<0.1	3	0	0	0.4	8	54	60	64	19	0.6	0.4
<1	2	0.1	0.1	0.4	<0.1	9	0.1	0	0.4	40	98	116	144	33	1.1	0.6
<1	<1	0.1	<0.1	0.7	<0.1	8	<0.1	0	0.3	21	59	97	69	20	0.5	0.4
0	4	0.1	<0.1	0.4	<0.1	6	0	<1	0.3	15	68	72	82	24	0.7	0.5
<1	0	0.1	0.1	0.5	<0.1	9	0.1	0	0.5	43	94	120	154	31	1	0.6
<1	0	0.1	<0.1	0.1	<0.1	7	0.1	0	0.3	30	65	79	92	21	0.7	0.4
0	20							1		200		75		8	0.4	
0		1.5	1.7	20	2	400	6	60		300	350	110	150	140	5.4	5.2
	375	0.4	0.4	5	0.4	40	1.5	15	5	40	40	80	150	16	4.5	3.7

ERA, EatRight Analysis CD-ROM; **AMT,** amount; **WT,** weight; **WTR,** water; **CAL,** calories; **PROT,** protein; **CARB**, carbohydrate; **FIBR,** fiber; **FAT,** fat; **SATF,** saturated fat; **MONO,** monounsaturated fat; **POLY,** polyunsaturated fat

ERA CODE	FOOD DESCRIPTION	AMT	UNIT	WT (g)	WTR (g)	CAL (kcal)	PROT (g)	CARB (g)	FIBR (g)	FAT (g)	SATF (g)	MONO (g)	POLY (g)
Grains and Grain Products (continued)													
Granola and Cereal Bars, Diet and Energy Bars (continued)													
62205	Tiger sport bar	1	ea	65.2		230	11	40	4	2			
62643	UltrSlmFst bar, chwy carml crnch	1	ea	28.35	2	110	0	20	2	3	2.5		
62641	UltrSlmFst bar, pnt carml crnch	1	ea	28.35	2	120	1	22	1	3	1.7	0.9	0.4
Muffins													
44520	Blueberry muffin, made w/2% milk	1	ea	57	23	162	4	23	1	6	1.2	1.5	3.1
44528	Bran muffin, made w/2% milk	1	ea	57	20	161	4	24	2	7	1.3	1.7	3.6
44530	Chocolate chip muffin	1	ea	58	19	188	4	27	1	7	2.4	2.9	1.6
44524	Corn muffin, made w/2% milk	1	ea	57	19	180	4	25	2	7	1.3	1.7	3.5
42059	English muffin	1	ea	57	24	134	4	26	2	1	0.1	0.2	0.5
42082	English muffin, 100% wheat	1	ea	66	30	134	6	27	4	1	0.2	0.3	0.6
42214	English muffin, cheese	1	ea	63	26	153	5	28	2	2	0.8	0.5	0.6
42060	English muffin, sourdough	1	ea	56	24	132	4	26	2	1	0.1	0.2	0.5
44515	Muffin, plain, made w/2% milk	1	ea	57	21	169	4	24	2	6	1.2	1.6	3.3
44514	Oat bran muffin	1	ea	57	20	154	4	28	3	4	0.6	1	2.4
42017	Popover, recipe, whole milk	1	ea	40	22	90	3	11	<1	3	1.1	1	1
44522	Toasted muffin, corn	1	ea	33	8	114	2	19	1	4	0.6	0.9	2.1
44518	Toaster muffin, blueberry	1	ea	33	10	103	2	18	1	3	0.5	0.7	1.8
44531	Whole wheat muffin	1	ea	47	16	140	4	20	2	6	1.3	2.3	1.6
44536	Zucchini muffin w/nuts	1	ea	58	16	219	3	27	1	11	1.5	3.4	5.3
Pancakes, French Toast, and Waffles													
45006	Crepe, pancake, no filling	1	ea	102	58	230	9	22	1	11	3.2	4.6	2.6
42156	French toast, rec w/2% milk	1	pce	65	36	149	5	16	1	7	1.8	2.9	1.7
45023	Pancake, blueberry, recipe	1	ea	38	20	84	2	11	<1	3	0.8	0.9	1.6
45025	Pancake, buttermilk, recipe	1	ea	38	20	86	3	11	<1	4	0.7	0.9	1.7
45044	Pancake, Chinese	1	ea	28	14	58	1	13	<1	<1	<0.1	<0.1	<0.1
45067	Pancake, frozen, heated, 6 in	1	ea	73	33	167	4	32	1	2	0.6	0.9	0.7
45002	Pancake, mix, prepared	1	ea	38	20	74	2	14	<1	1	0.2	0.3	0.3
45001	Pancake, plain, recipe	1	ea	38	20	86	2	11	1	4	0.8	0.9	1.7
45008	Pancake, whole wheat	1	ea	44	23	92	4	13	1	3	0.8	0.8	1.1
45036	Rye pancakes, 4 inch	1	ea	21	7	63	1	10	1	2	0.5	0.9	0.6
45035	Sourdough pancakes, 4 inch	1	ea	21	11	46	1	7	<1	1	0.3	0.4	0.6
45038	Waffle, blueberry, round	1	ea	75	35	178	4	28	2	5	0.9	2.1	1.8
45093	Waffle, buttermilk, Eggo	1	ea	39		110	2	15	0	4	0.8		
45005	Waffle, frozen, toasted	1	ea	33	14	87	2	13	1	3	0.5	1.1	0.9
45003	Waffles, from recipe	1	ea	75	32	218	6	25	1	11	2.1	2.6	5.1
45017	Waffle, whole grain, frozen	1	ea	39	17	105	4	13	1	4	1.2	1.8	1.1
Pasta													
38048	Chow mein noodles, dry	1	cup	45	<1	237	4	26	2	14	2	3.5	7.8
38047	Egg noodles, enr, cooked	1	cup	160	110	213	8	40	2	2	0.5	0.7	0.7
38103	Lasagna, noodles, cooked	2	ea	110	73	155	5	31	1	1	0.1	0.1	0.3
38119	Linguini noodles, cooked	1	cup	140	92	197	7	40	2	1	0.1	0.1	0.4
38102	Macaroni, enriched, cooked	1	cup	140	92	197	7	40	2	1	0.1	0.1	0.4
38150	Noodle Roni, prepared	1	cup	165	111	247	8	40	2	6	1.2	2.5	1.7

< = Trace amount present   Blank = Not available

CHOL, cholesterol; **V,** vitamin; **THI,** thiamin; **RIB,** riboflavin; **NIA,** niacin; **FOL,** folate;
CALC, calcium; **PHOS,** phosphate; **SOD,** sodium; **POT,** potassium; **MAG,** magnesium

CHOL (mg)	V-A (RE)	THI (mg)	RIB (mg)	NIA (mg)	V-B6 (mg)	FOL (μg)	V-B12 (μg)	V-C (mg)	V-E (mg)	CALC (mg)	PHOS (mg)	SOD (mg)	POT (mg)	MAG (mg)	IRON (mg)	ZINC (mg)
	50	1.5	1.7	20	2	400	6	60	20	350	400	100	280	140	4.5	
5	225	<0.1	0.3	3	0.3	60	0.9	60	20.1	250	150	45			2.7	0.6
5	15	0.2	0.3	3	0.3	60	0.9	6	3	150	150	35			2.7	0.6
21	22	0.2	0.2	1.3	<0.1	27	0.1	1	1	108	83	251	70	9	1.3	0.3
19	142	0.2	0.3	2.3	0.2	30	0.1	4	1.3	106	162	335	181	44	2.4	1.6
23	21	0.2	0.2	1.4	<0.1	7	0.1	<1	0.7	91	87	117	92	16	1.5	0.4
24	29	0.2	0.2	1.4	0.1	35	0.1	<1	1	148	101	333	83	13	1.5	0.3
0	0	0.3	0.2	2.2	<0.1	46	<0.1	0	0.8	99	76	264	75	12	1.4	0.4
0	0	0.2	0.1	2.2	0.1	32	0	0	0.5	175	186	420	139	47	1.6	1.1
3	9	0.3	0.2	2.3	<0.1	23	<0.1	<1	0.1	127	96	297	82	13	1.5	0.5
0	0	0.2	0.2	2.2	<0.1	45	<0.1	0	0.8	97	74	260	73	12	1.4	0.4
22	23	0.2	0.2	1.3	<0.1	29	0.1	<1	1	114	87	266	69	10	1.4	0.3
0	0	0.1	0.1	0.2	0.1	30	<0.1	0	1.2	36	214	224	289	89	2.4	1
47	28	0.1	0.1	0.7	<0.1	7	0.1	<1	0.2	37	56	82	64	7	0.8	0.3
4	7	0.1	0.1	0.8	<0.1	19	<0.1	0	0.5	6	50	142	30	5	0.5	0.1
2	22	0.1	0.1	0.7	<0.1	18	<0.1	0	0.6	4	19	158	27	4	0.2	0.1
20	18	0.1	0.1	1.2	0.1	9	0.1	<1	0.9	102	122	140	119	31	1	0.7
38	22	0.1	0.1	1	<0.1	9	0.1	1	2	39	48	113	66	8	1.2	0.3
161	99	0.2	0.4	1.3	0.1	19	0.5	<1	1.3	94	148	77	162	17	1.6	0.8
75	86	0.1	0.2	1.1	<0.1	28	0.2	<1	0.7	65	76	311	87	11	1.1	0.4
21	19	0.1	0.1	0.6	<0.1	14	0.1	1	0.4	78	57	156	52	6	0.7	0.2
22	11	0.1	0.1	0.6	<0.1	14	0.1	<1	0.5	60	53	198	55	6	0.6	0.2
0	0	<0.1	<0.1	0.3	<0.1	1	0	0	<0.1	5	18	1	18	4	0.1	0.2
7	21	0.3	0.3	2.9	0.1	36	0.1	<1	0.5	45	272	372	53	10	2.5	0.5
5	3	0.1	0.1	0.6	<0.1	14	0.1	<1	0.4	48	127	239	66	8	0.6	0.1
22	21	0.1	0.1	0.6	<0.1	14	0.1	<1	0.4	83	60	167	50	6	0.7	0.2
27	28	0.1	0.2	1	<0.1	13	0.1	<1	1.3	110	164	252	123	20	1.4	0.5
8	4	<0.1	<0.1	0.3	<0.1	2	<0.1	<1	0.3	22	25	58	97	15	0.5	0.2
8	4	0.1	0.1	0.6	<0.1	7	<0.1	0	0.3	3	16	53	17	3	0.5	0.1
15	235	0.3	0.3	2.9	0.6	23	1.6	2	0.7	150	271	506	96	15	2.9	0.4
12	150	0.2	0.2	2	0.2	40	0.6	0		20		240	32		1.8	
8	120	0.1	0.2	1.5	0.3	15	0.8	0	0.3	77	139	260	42	7	1.5	0.2
52	49	0.2	0.3	1.6	<0.1	34	0.2	<1	2.2	191	142	383	119	14	1.7	0.5
37	30	0.1	0.1	0.8	<0.1	7	0.2	<1	0.6	102	95	132	90	16	0.8	0.4
0	4	0.3	0.2	2.7	<0.1	40	0	0	9	9	72	198	54	23	2.1	0.6
53	10	0.3	0.1	2.4	0.1	102	0.1	0	0.1	19	110	11	45	30	2.5	1
0	0	0.2	0.1	1.8	<0.1	77	0	0	<0.1	8	59	1	34	20	1.5	0.6
0	0	0.3	0.1	2.3	<0.1	98	0	0	0.1	10	76	1	43	25	2	0.7
0	0	0.3	0.1	2.3	<0.1	98	0	0	<0.1	10	76	1	43	25	2	0.7
53	47	0.3	0.1	2.4	0.1	11	0.1	<1	0.6	21	112	56	47	31	2.5	1

ERA, EatRight Analysis CD-ROM; **AMT,** amount; **WT,** weight; **WTR,** water; **CAL,** calories; **PROT,** protein; **CARB**, carbohydrate; **FIBR,** fiber; **FAT,** fat; **SATF,** saturated fat; **MONO,** monounsaturated fat; **POLY,** polyunsaturated fat

ERA CODE	FOOD DESCRIPTION	AMT	UNIT	WT (g)	WTR (g)	CAL (kcal)	PROT (g)	CARB (g)	FIBR (g)	FAT (g)	SATF (g)	MONO (g)	POLY (g)
Grains and Grain Products (continued)													
Pasta (continued)													
57319	Noodles & sce, romanoff (Lipton)	0.66	cup	65		260	9	41	2	7	3.5		
57323	Pasta & sce, cream brocc (Lipton)	0.66	cup	69		260	8	45	1	6	2.5		
38092	Pasta/noodles, fresh, cooked	2	oz	57	39	75	3	14	1	1	0.1	0.1	0.2
38067	Ramen noodles, cooked	1	cup	227	195	154	3	20	1	7	1.7	1.2	3.3
38147	Rice noodles, cooked	1	cup	160	127	135	<1	33	<1	<1	<0.1	<0.1	<0.1
38104	Rotini noodles, cooked	1	cup	140	92	197	7	40	2	1	0.1	0.1	0.4
38109	Shells pasta, jumbo, cooked	2	ea	46	30	65	2	13	1	<1	<0.1	<0.1	0.1
38105	Shells pasta, small, cooked	1	cup	115	76	162	5	33	1	1	0.1	0.1	0.3
38113	Shells pasta, whl wheat, cooked	1	cup	140	94	174	7	37	4	1	0.1	0.1	0.3
38118	Spaghetti noodles, enr, cooked	1	cup	140	92	197	7	40	2	1	0.1	0.1	0.4
38121	Spag noodles, enr, ckd+salt	1	cup	140	92	197	7	40	2	1	0.1	0.1	0.4
38066	Spag noodles, spinach, cooked	1	cup	140	95	182	6	37	5	1	0.1	0.1	0.4
38060	Spag noodles, whl wheat, cooked	1	cup	140	94	174	7	37	6	1	0.1	0.1	0.3
56129	Spinach tortellini	1	cup	122	75	232	12	25	1	9	3.3	3.4	1.3
Rice													
38010	Brown rice, long grain, cooked	1	cup	195	142	216	5	45	4	2	0.4	0.6	0.6
38082	Brown rice, med grain, cooked	0.5	cup	97.5	71	109	2	23	2	1	0.2	0.3	0.3
38145	Fried rice, meatless	1	cup	166	112	271	5	34	1	12	1.8	3.2	6.7
38083	Glutinous sticky rice, ckd	1	cup	174	133	169	4	37	2	<1	0.1	0.1	0.1
56316	Rice pilaf	1	cup	206	149	261	4	45	1	7	1.3	3.2	1.9
57360	Rice & sauce, Oriental (Lipton)	0.5	cup	59		230	6	46	1	1	0		
57337	Rice & sauce, original (Lipton)	0.5	cup	63		250	7	51	2	1	0		
57355	Rice, saute, herb butr (Lipton)	0.5	cup	60		240	6	42	1	5	2		
57341	Rice, saute, Oriental (Lipton)	0.5	cup	61		240	6	43	1	4	1.5		
56131	Spanish rice	1	cup	243	190	216	5	42	3	4	0.6	1.5	1.4
38013	White rice, long grain, cooked	1	cup	158	108	205	4	44	1	<1	0.1	0.1	0.1
38019	White rice, long grain, inst, ckd	1	cup	165	126	162	3	35	1	<1	0.1	0.1	0.1
38097	White rice, med grain, cooked	1	cup	186	128	242	4	53	1	<1	0.1	0.1	0.1
38021	Wild rice, cooked	1	cup	164	121	166	7	35	3	1	0.1	0.1	0.3
Tortillas and Taco/Tostada Shells													
42027	Taco shell, corn	1	ea	13.6	1	64	1	8	1	3	0.5	1.3	1.2
42023	Tortilla, corn, enr, reg, 6 inch	1	ea	26	11	58	1	12	1	1	0.1	0.2	0.3
42011	Edible bowl, corn, 6.25 inch	1	ea	44		165	5	25	0	5	3		
42025	Tortilla, flour, 8 inch	1	ea	72	19	234	6	40	2	5	1.3	2.7	0.8
42079	Tortilla, whole wheat	1	ea	35	11	73	3	20	2	<1	0.1	0.1	0.2
Infant Foods													
60616	Baby fd cereal, rice+mix fruit	1	Tbs	15	12	12	<1	3	<1	<1	<0.1	<0.1	<0.1
60491	Beef stew, toddler	1	Tbs	16	14	8	1	1	<1	<1	0.1	0.1	<0.1
60660	Baby fd vegetable+beef	1	Tbs	16	14	10	<1	1	<1	<1	0.1	0.1	<0.1
60638	Baby fd turkey meat sticks	10	ea	100		182	14	1	<1	14	4.1	4.7	3.6
60500	Baby fd carrots	1	Tbs	14	13	4	<1	1	<1	<1	<0.1	<0.1	<0.1
60632	Baby fd sweet potatoes	1	Tbs	14	12	8	<1	2	<1	<1	<0.1	0	<0.1
60309	Similac infant formula	0.46	cup	114		100	3	10		5			

< = Trace amount present

Blank = Not available

CHOL, cholesterol; **V,** vitamin; **THI,** thiamin; **RIB,** riboflavin; **NIA,** niacin; **FOL,** folate;
CALC, calcium; **PHOS,** phosphate; **SOD,** sodium; **POT,** potassium; **MAG,** magnesium

CHOL (mg)	V-A (RE)	THI (mg)	RIB (mg)	NIA (mg)	V-B6 (mg)	FOL (μg)	V-B12 (μg)	V-C (mg)	V-E (mg)	CALC (mg)	PHOS (mg)	SOD (mg)	POT (mg)	MAG (mg)	IRON (mg)	ZINC (mg)
70	20							0		60		920			2.7	
10	20							0		40		840			2.7	
19	3	0.1	0.1	0.6	<0.1	36	0.1	0	0.1	3	36	3	14	10	0.6	0.3
<1	2	<0.1	<0.1	0.3	<0.1	3	<0.1	<1	2.3	13	24	802	49	10	0.4	0.2
0	0	<0.1	0	0.1	<0.1	<1	0	0	<0.1	11	11	7	3	2	0.7	0.2
0	0	0.3	0.1	2.3	<0.1	98	0	0	<0.1	10	76	1	43	25	2	0.7
0	0	0.1	<0.1	0.8	<0.1	32	0	0	<0.1	3	25	<1	14	8	0.6	0.2
0	0	0.2	0.1	1.9	<0.1	80	0	0	<0.1	8	62	1	36	21	1.6	0.6
0	0	0.2	0.1	1	0.1	7	0	0	0.1	21	125	4	62	42	1.5	1.1
0	0	0.3	0.1	2.3	<0.1	98	0	0	0.1	10	76	1	43	25	2	0.7
0	0	0.3	0.1	2.3	<0.1	98	0	0	0.4	10	76	140	43	25	2	0.7
0	21	0.1	0.1	2.1	0.1	17	0	0	0.1	42	151	20	81	87	1.5	1.5
0	0	0.2	0.1	1	0.1	7	0	0	1.2	21	125	4	62	42	1.5	1.1
158	183	0.2	0.4	1.8	0.1	35	0.5	1	0.9	143	168	252	138	24	2.4	1
0	0	0.2	<0.1	3	0.3	8	0	0	1.4	20	162	10	84	84	0.8	1.2
0	0	0.1	<0.1	1.3	0.1	4	0	0	0.6	10	75	1	77	43	0.5	0.6
43	21	0.2	0.1	2.2	0.1	22	0.1	4	2.5	28	89	261	128	23	1.9	0.9
0	0	<0.1	<0.1	0.5	<0.1	2	0	0	0.2	3	14	9	17	9	0.2	0.7
0	64	0.3	<0.1	2.5	0.1	8	<0.1	1	1.1	25	76	151	111	19	2.3	0.8
2	0							0		0		750			1.8	
0	0							1		20		890			1.8	
2	0							0		0		870			1.1	
0	0							1		0		910			1.1	
0	115	0.2	0.1	3	0.3	20	0	37	1.4	77	90	295	537	39	2.4	0.9
0	0	0.3	<0.1	2.3	0.1	92	0	0	0.3	16	68	2	55	19	1.9	0.8
0	0	0.1	0.1	1.5	<0.1	68	0	0	0.2	13	23	5	7	8	1	0.4
0	0	0.3	<0.1	3.4	0.1	108	0	0	0.3	6	69	0	54	24	2.8	0.8
0	0	0.1	0.1	2.1	0.2	43	0	0	0.5	5	134	5	166	52	1	2.2
0	5	<0.1	<0.1	0.2	0.1	1	0	0	0.4	22	34	50	24	14	0.3	0.2
0	0	<0.1	<0.1	0.4	0.1	30	0	0	0.3	46	82	42	40	17	0.4	0.2
0	0	0.2	0.1			114			0				52			
0	0	0.4	0.2	2.6	<0.1	89	0	0	1.3	90	89	344	94	19	2.4	0.5
0	0	0.1	<0.1	0.9	0.1	8	0	0	0.4	10	82	171	82	26	0.7	0.5
0	<1	<0.1	<0.1	0.3	<0.1	<1	<0.1	1	<0.1	2	3	2	8	1	0.4	<0.1
2	40	<0.1	<0.1	0.2	<0.1	1	0.1	<1	<0.1	1	7	55	23	2	0.1	0.1
1	41	<0.1	<0.1	0.1	<0.1	1	<0.1	<1	<0.1	2	6	12	20	2	0.1	0.1
65	6	<0.1	0.2	1.8	0.1	11	1	2	0.4	72	103	483	91	16	1.2	1.8
0	165	<0.1	<0.1	0.1	<0.1	2	0	1	0.1	3	3	7	28	2	0.1	<0.1
0	93	<0.1	<0.1	0.1	<0.1	1	0	1	0.1	2	3	3	34	2	0.1	<0.1
	90	0.1	0.2	1	0.1	15	0.2	9	2	90	70	34	132	7	0.2	0.8

ERA, EatRight Analysis CD-ROM; **AMT,** amount; **WT,** weight; **WTR,** water; **CAL,** calories; **PROT,** protein; **CARB**, carbohydrate; **FIBR,** fiber; **FAT,** fat; **SATF,** saturated fat; **MONO,** monounsaturated fat; **POLY,** polyunsaturated fat

ERA CODE	FOOD DESCRIPTION	AMT	UNIT	WT (g)	WTR (g)	CAL (kcal)	PROT (g)	CARB (g)	FIBR (g)	FAT (g)	SATF (g)	MONO (g)	POLY (g)
Juices: Fruit, Vegetable, Blends													
3008	Apple juice, canned/bottled	1	cup	248	218	116	<1	29	<1	<1	<0.1	<0.1	0.1
3010	Apple juice, frzn conc+water	1	cup	239	210	112	<1	28	<1	<1	<0.1	<0.1	0.1
3015	Apricot nectar, canned	1	cup	251	213	140	1	36	2	<1	<0.1	0.1	<0.1
5226	Carrot juice, canned	1	cup	236	210	94	2	22	2	<1	0.1	<0.1	0.2
20042	Clam and tomato juice	1	cup	242	211	116	1	26	<1	3	0.1	<0.1	<0.1
3042	Cranberry juice cocktail	1	cup	253	216	144	0	36	<1	<1	<0.1	<0.1	0.1
3276	Cranberry jce cocktail, low cal	1	cup	237	226	45	0	11	0	0	0	0	0
3062	Grape juice, canned/bottled	1	cup	253	213	154	1	38	<1	<1	0.1	<0.1	0.1
3064	Grape juice, frzn conc+water	1	cup	250	217	128	<1	32	<1	<1	0.1	<0.1	0.1
3052	Grapefruit juice, canned	1	cup	247	222	94	1	22	<1	<1	<0.1	<0.1	0.1
3053	Grapefruit juice, frzn conc+water	1	cup	247	220	101	1	24	<1	<1	<0.1	<0.1	0.1
3304	Guava nectar	1	cup	250	211	149	<1	38	2	<1	0.1	<0.1	0.1
3069	Lemon juice, bottled	1	cup	244	226	51	1	16	1	1	0.1	<0.1	0.2
3073	Lime juice, bottled	1	cup	246	228	52	1	16	1	1	0.1	0.1	0.2
3303	Mango nectar	1	cup	250	211	146	1	38	2	<1	0.1	0.1	0.1
3046	Orange juice+calcium	1	cup	247.2		110	2	26	0	0	0	0	0
3092	Orange juice, chilled	1	cup	249	220	110	2	25	<1	1	0.1	0.1	0.2
3090	Orange juice, fresh	1	cup	248	219	112	2	26	<1	<1	0.1	0.1	0.1
3091	Orange juice, frzn conc+water	1	cup	249	219	112	2	27	<1	<1	<0.1	<0.1	<0.1
3226	Orange strawberry banana juice	1	cup	247.2		110	1	27	0	0	0	0	0
3095	Papaya nectar, canned	1	cup	250	212	142	<1	36	2	<1	0.1	0.1	0.1
3120	Pineapple juice, canned, unswt	1	cup	250	214	140	1	34	<1	<1	<0.1	<0.1	0.1
3128	Prune juice, bottled	1	cup	256	208	182	2	45	3	<1	<0.1	0.1	<0.1
3102	Tangerine orange juice	1	cup	247.2		110	2	25	0	0	0	0	0
5397	Tomato juice, canned, low sod	1	cup	243	228	41	2	10	2	<1	<0.1	<0.1	0.1
5188	Tomato juice, canned, regular	1	cup	243	228	41	2	10	1	<1	<0.1	<0.1	0.1
20080	V-8 juice, low sodium	1	cup	242	226	46	2	11	2	<1	<0.1	<0.1	0.1
Meals, Entrees, and Mixed Dishes													
Canned Meals, Entrees, and Dishes													
7040	Baked beans w/pork, canned	1	cup	253	181	268	13	51	14	4	1.5	1.7	0.5
7037	Baked beans, homemade	1	cup	253	165	382	14	54	14	13	4.9	5.4	1.9
7038	Baked beans, vegetarian, cnd	0.5	cup	127	92	118	6	26	6	1	0.1	<0.1	0.2
56092	Chicken chow mein, canned	1	cup	250	222	95	6	18	2	1	0	0.1	0.8
7004	Pork & beans+tomato sc, can	1	cup	253	184	248	13	49	12	3	1	1.1	0.3
56096	Spaghetti+sauce+cheese, can	1	cup	250	200	190	6	38	2	2	0	0.4	0.5
Frozen Meals, Entrees, and Dishes													
16234	Beef pot pie, Banquet	1	ea	198		330	9	38	3	15	7		
70734	Beef pot pie, Swansons	1	ea	198		415	11	41	2	23	9		
11094	Beef pot roast, Lean Cuisine	1	ea	255		206	17	22	4	5	1.3	2.3	0.8
11118	Beef pot roast din, Healthy Choice	1	ea	312		300	20	41	8	6	2		
56737	Cheese cannelloni, Lean Cuisine	1	ea	259		270	21	28	3	8	3.5	1.5	0.5
56901	Cheese ravioli, Lean Cuisine	1	ea	241		250	12	32	4	8	3	2	1
15964	Chicken chow mein+rice, Ln Cuis	1	ea	255		210	13	28	2	5	1	2	1
15967	Chicken parmesan, Lean Cuisine	1	ea	308		220	22	22	5	5	1.5	1.5	1

< = Trace amount present   Blank = Not available

CHOL, cholesterol; **V,** vitamin; **THI,** thiamin; **RIB,** riboflavin; **NIA,** niacin; **FOL,** folate;
CALC, calcium; **PHOS,** phosphate; **SOD,** sodium; **POT,** potassium; **MAG,** magnesium

CHOL (mg)	V-A (RE)	THI (mg)	RIB (mg)	NIA (mg)	V-B6 (mg)	FOL (μg)	V-B12 (μg)	V-C (mg)	V-E (mg)	CALC (mg)	PHOS (mg)	SOD (mg)	POT (mg)	MAG (mg)	IRON (mg)	ZINC (mg)
0	<1	0.1	<0.1	0.2	0.1	<1	0	2	<0.1	17	17	7	295	7	0.9	0.1
0	0	<0.1	<0.1	0.1	0.1	1	0	1	<0.1	14	17	17	301	12	0.6	0.1
0	331	<0.1	<0.1	0.7	0.1	3	0	2	0.7	18	23	8	286	13	1	0.2
0	2584	0.2	0.1	0.9	0.5	9	0	20	1	57	99	68	689	33	1.1	0.4
0	53	0.1	0.1	0.5	0.2	38	73.9	10	1.2	29	188	874	217	53	1.4	2.6
0	1	<0.1	<0.1	0.1	<0.1	1	0	90	0	8	5	5	46	5	0.4	0.2
0	1	<0.1	<0.1	0.1	<0.1	<1	0	76	0	21	2	7	52	5	0.1	<0.1
0	3	0.1	0.1	0.7	0.2	7	0	<1	0	23	28	8	334	25	0.6	0.1
0	2	<0.1	0.1	0.3	0.1	3	0	60	0.1	10	10	5	52	10	0.2	0.1
0	2	0.1	<0.1	0.6	<0.1	26	0	72	0.4	17	27	2	378	25	0.5	0.2
0	2	0.1	0.1	0.5	0.1	9	0	83	0.4	20	35	2	336	27	0.3	0.1
0	21	<0.1	<0.1	0.4	<0.1	3	0	47	0.4	11	10	7	93	5	0.2	0.1
0	5	0.1	<0.1	0.5	0.1	25	0	61	0.5	27	22	51	249	20	0.3	0.1
0	5	0.1	<0.1	0.4	0.1	19	0	16	0.2	30	25	39	184	17	0.6	0.1
0	292	<0.1	0.1	0.5	0.1	7	0	19	1.1	12	11	6	141	10	0.2	0.1
0	0	0.2		0.8	0.1	60		108	0	350		0	450		0	
0	20	0.3	0.1	0.7	0.1	45	0	82	0.5	25	27	2	473	27	0.4	0.1
0	50	0.2	0.1	1	0.1	75	0	124	0.5	27	42	2	496	27	0.5	0.1
0	20	0.2	<0.1	0.5	0.1	109	0	97	0.5	22	40	2	473	25	0.2	0.1
0	0	0		0	0	0		6	0	20		5	380		0	
0	28	<0.1	<0.1	0.4	<0.1	5	0	8	0.1	25	0	12	78	8	0.9	0.4
0	1	0.1	0.1	0.6	0.2	58	0	27	0.1	42	20	2	335	32	0.6	0.3
0	1	<0.1	0.2	2	0.6	1	0	10	0.4	31	64	10	706	36	3	0.5
0	0	0.2		0.8	0.1	60		27	0	20		0	450		0	
0	136	0.1	0.1	1.6	0.3	48	0	44	2.2	22	46	24	535	27	1.4	0.3
0	136	0.1	0.1	1.6	0.3	48	0	44	2.2	22	46	877	535	27	1.4	0.3
0	283	0.1	0.1	1.8	0.3	51	0	67	0.8	27	41	653	467	27	1	0.5
18	46	0.1	0.1	1.1	0.2	92	0	5	1	134	273	1047	782	86	4.3	3.7
13	0	0.3	0.1	1	0.2	122	0	3	1.3	154	276	1067	906	109	5	1.8
0	22	0.2	0.1	0.5	0.2	30	0	4	0.7	64	132	504	376	41	0.4	1.8
8	28	0.1	0.1	1	0.1	12	0.1	12	0.9	45	85	725	418	14	1.2	1.3
18	30	0.1	0.1	1.3	0.2	57	0	8	1.5	142	296	1113	759	89	8.3	14.8
8	120	0.3	0.3	4.5	0.1	6	0	10	2.1	40	88	955	302	21	2.8	1.1
25	150							0		20		1000			1.1	
25	150							0		20		740			1.8	
38	195											495				
40	250							18		20		600			1.8	
30	60	0.1	0.3	1.6	0.1	<1	0	12		350		500	400	36	1.1	1.6
55	150	0.1	0.3	1.2	0.2	48	0.3	6		200	168	500	400	42	1.1	1.5
35	20	0.2	0.2	5				6		20		510	300	30	0.4	1.1
50	150	0.2	0.3	7				6		100		530	820	59	1.4	1.3

ERA, EatRight Analysis CD-ROM; **AMT,** amount; **WT,** weight; **WTR,** water; **CAL,** calories; **PROT,** protein; **CARB**, carbohydrate; **FIBR,** fiber; **FAT,** fat; **SATF,** saturated fat; **MONO,** monounsaturated fat; **POLY,** polyunsaturated fat

Meals, Entrees, and Mixed Dishes (continued)

Frozen Meals, Entrees, and Dishes (continued)

ERA CODE	FOOD DESCRIPTION	AMT	UNIT	WT (g)	WTR (g)	CAL (kcal)	PROT (g)	CARB (g)	FIBR (g)	FAT (g)	SATF (g)	MONO (g)	POLY (g)
16260	Chicken broc alfredo, Healthy Chce	1	ea	326		300	25	34	2	7	3		
82034	Chicken enchilada din, Hlthy Chce	1	ea	320		298	13	46	4	7	3.1	2.6	1
16252	Chicken fettuc alfred, Healthy Chce	1	ea	241		280	25	30	4	7	2.5		
83000	Egg roll, chicken, ChunKing	6	pce	106		210	6	30	3	7	1.5		
83001	Egg roll, shrimp, ChunKing	6	pce	106		190	5	29	3	6	1		
56740	Lasagna w/meat sauce, Ln Cuisine	1	ea	291		270	19	34	5	6	2.5	1.5	0.5
56731	Lasagna, zucchini, Lean Cuisine	1	ea	312		240	17	33	4	4	1.5	2	0.5
18825	Lemon pepper fish din, Hlthy Chc	1	ea	303		320	14	50	5	7	2		
66047	Macaroni & cheese, Healthy Chce	1	ea	255		240	12	36	3	5	2.5		
81080	Manicotti, 3 cheese, Healthy Chce	1	ea	312		300	15	40	5	9	3		
11093	Meatloaf, Lean Cuisine	1	ea	266		270	21	24	4	10	4	2.5	0.5
70767	Mexican-style dinner, HungryMan	1	ea	567		690	26	87	13	27	9		
56739	Rigatoni, Lean Cuisine	1	ea	255		180	10	25	4	4	1.5	0.5	0.5
11063	Salisbury steak dinner, Swansons	1	ea	312		340	16	35	6	15	6		
56732	Spaghetti w/meatballs, Ln Cuisine	1	ea	269	201	298	18	40	5	8	2.1	2.7	1.3
56076	Spinach souffle	1	cup	136	100	219	11	3	3	18	7.1	6.8	3.1
56738	Stuffed cabbage, Lean Cuisine	1	ea	269		199	12	26	6	6	1.7	2.4	0.7
16928	Turkey Pot Pie, Banquet	1	ea	198		370	10	38	3	20	8		

Homemade and Generic Meals, Entrees, and Dishes

ERA CODE	FOOD DESCRIPTION	AMT	UNIT	WT (g)	WTR (g)	CAL (kcal)	PROT (g)	CARB (g)	FIBR (g)	FAT (g)	SATF (g)	MONO (g)	POLY (g)
15907	Almond chicken	1	cup	242	186	280	22	16	3	15	1.9	6.1	5.6
10081	Beef cube steak, flour fried	1	ea	165	79	460	44	18	1	22	6.2	8.2	5.8
11008	Beef stroganoff	1	cup	256	183	408	26	16	1	27	10.6	7.9	6.3
66025	Burrito, bean	2	ea	217	114	447	14	71	8	13	6.9	4.7	1.2
56629	Burrito, bean+cheese	2	ea	186	100	378	15	55		12	6.8	2.5	1.8
66024	Burrito, beef	2	ea	220	109	524	27	59	2	21	10.4	7.4	0.9
15930	Cashew chicken	1	cup	162	88	431	29	11	2	31	5.2	13.9	9.7
56075	Cheese souffle, recipe	1	cup	112	79	196	12	6	<1	14	5.6	4.8	2.8
56213	Chicken Helper, chicken dumplng	1	cup	244	175	372	26	22	1	19	5.1	7.8	4.6
15927	Chicken parmigiana	1	pce	182	120	320	28	16	1	16	5.3	4.9	4
56112	Chilis rellenos	1	ea	143	84	365	17	8	1	30	12.5	9	6.7
56634	Chimichanga, beef	1	ea	174	88	424	20	43	2	20	8.5	8.1	1.1
56121	Chimichanga, beef & bean	1	ea	118	73	241	8	21	3	14	2.9	6	4.3
56243	Chop suey, beef, no noodles	1	cup	220	166	271	22	12	3	15	3.7	6.5	3.5
56248	Chop suey, pork, no noodles	1	cup	220	165	286	22	12	3	17	4.2	7.8	3.4
57618	Chow mein, pork, w/noodles	1	cup	220	136	448	22	31	4	27	4.8	7.7	12.8
57619	Chow mein, beef w/o noodles	1	cup	220	166	271	22	12	3	15	3.7	6.5	3.5
57622	Chow mein, chicken w/o noodles	1	cup	220	179	193	20	10	2	8	1.7	2.8	3
57621	Chow mein, pork w/o noodles	1	cup	220	165	286	22	12	3	17	4.2	7.8	3.4
56132	Egg foo yung patty	1	ea	86	67	113	6	3	1	8	2	3.4	2.1
57524	Egg roll, w/meat	1	ea	64	43	113	5	9	1	6	1.4	3	1.3
56060	Enchilada, chicken	1	ea	121.9		195	13	16	2	9	3.6	2.6	2.1
56124	Fajita, beef	1	ea	223	144	399	23	36	3	18	5.5	7.6	3.5
56123	Fajita, chicken	1	ea	223	145	363	20	44	5	12	2.2	5.5	3.1
56119	Flauta, beef	1	ea	113	57	354	14	13	2	28	4.8	11.8	9.4

< = Trace amount present

Blank = Not available

CHOL, cholesterol; **V,** vitamin; **THI,** thiamin; **RIB,** riboflavin; **NIA,** niacin; **FOL,** folate;
CALC, calcium; **PHOS,** phosphate; **SOD,** sodium; **POT,** potassium; **MAG,** magnesium

CHOL (mg)	V-A (RE)	THI (mg)	RIB (mg)	NIA (mg)	V-B6 (mg)	FOL (μg)	V-B12 (μg)	V-C (mg)	V-E (mg)	CALC (mg)	PHOS (mg)	SOD (mg)	POT (mg)	MAG (mg)	IRON (mg)	ZINC (mg)
50	20							12		100		530			1.8	
38	154							18		134	237	563	384		0.8	
35	0							2		100		600			1.1	
10	3	0.1	0.1	0.7				1		20	90	260	120		0.4	
10	20	0.1	<0.1	0.4				4		20	50	360	80		0.4	
25	100	0.2	0.3	3	0.3			12		150		560	620	44	1.8	2.9
15	100	0.5	0.3	2				18		200		470	570	62	1.1	2.1
30	100							30		20		480			1.1	
20	0							0		200		600			1.1	
35	150							0		250		550			1.8	
55	60							1		80		530	520		1.8	
35	300							36		300		2170			3.6	
20	200	0.2	0.3	4				6		100		560	520	44	1.4	2.9
30	1000							6		80		920			2.7	
5	0									94		465			2.4	
184	674	0.1	0.3	0.5	0.1	80	1.4	3	1.2	230	231	763	201	38	1.3	1.3
24	0							53		105		412				
45	150							0		40		850			1.1	
40	37	0.1	0.2	9.5	0.4	26	0.3	7	3.8	69	252	526	549	60	2	1.6
125	5	0.3	0.5	7	0.7	17	4.7	<1	1.7	80	380	316	652	54	6.4	8.4
85	99	0.2	0.4	4.5	0.3	20	2.6	2	2.4	92	308	677	556	40	3.6	4.9
4	33	0.6	0.6	4.1	0.3	87	1.1	2	2	113	98	985	653	87	4.5	1.5
28	238	0.2	0.7	3.6	0.2	74	0.9	2		214	180	1166	497	80	2.3	1.6
64	29	0.2	0.9	6.4	0.3	130	2	1	2.3	84	174	1491	739	81	6.1	4.7
64	58	0.2	0.1	13.2	0.6	43	0.3	8	3.9	49	263	907	428	63	2	1.5
194	167	0.1	0.4	0.3	0.1	23	0.8	<1	1.3	209	200	298	146	16	0.8	1
89	52	0.2	0.3	9.3	0.3	11	0.3	2	0.9	128	261	244	297	35	2.5	1.9
137	146	0.2	0.3	8.5	0.4	17	0.4	9	2.4	198	317	641	471	45	2.3	2.4
168	250	0.1	0.4	0.9	0.3	29	0.5	113	4.7	398	307	522	386	36	1.7	2
9	16	0.5	0.6	5.8	0.3	84	1.5	5		63	124	910	586	63	4.5	5
17	40	0.1	0.1	2.3	0.2	16	0.5	11	2.5	48	99	230	323	28	2	1.5
50	116	0.2	0.2	4.2	0.4	42	2	23	2	38	238	924	556	42	2.9	3.5
56	118	0.6	0.3	4.8	0.4	40	0.5	24	2	48	227	926	527	40	1.9	2.4
48	19	0.8	0.4	6.2	0.4	42	0.4	20	2.7	45	249	848	489	53	3.3	2.6
50	116	0.2	0.2	4.2	0.4	42	2	23	2	38	238	924	556	42	2.9	3.5
50	14	0.1	0.2	6.9	0.4	50	0.2	10	1	36	185	651	415	35	1.7	1.6
56	118	0.6	0.3	4.8	0.4	40	0.5	24	2	48	227	926	527	40	1.9	2.4
185	86	<0.1	0.3	0.4	0.1	30	0.4	5	1.2	31	93	317	117	12	1	0.7
37	16	0.2	0.1	1.3	0.1	10	0.1	2	0.8	15	57	274	124	10	0.8	0.5
36	110	0.1	0.1	3.1	0.2	15	0.2	16	2.7	162	216	312	203	34	1	1.3
45	43	0.4	0.3	5.4	0.4	23	2.1	27	1.7	84	238	316	479	38	3.8	3.5
39	65	0.4	0.3	6.1	0.4	42	0.1	37	1.7	101	188	343	534	48	3.3	1.6
37	21	0.1	0.1	1.9	0.2	10	1.2	19	4.7	51	179	68	313	28	1.9	3.4

ERA, EatRight Analysis CD-ROM; **AMT,** amount; **WT,** weight; **WTR,** water; **CAL,** calories; **PROT,** protein; **CARB**, carbohydrate; **FIBR**, fiber; **FAT,** fat; **SATF,** saturated fat; **MONO,** monounsaturated fat; **POLY,** polyunsaturated fat

ERA CODE	FOOD DESCRIPTION	AMT	UNIT	WT (g)	WTR (g)	CAL (kcal)	PROT (g)	CARB (g)	FIBR (g)	FAT (g)	SATF (g)	MONO (g)	POLY (g)
Meals, Entrees, and Mixed Dishes (continued)													
Homemade and Generic Meals, Entrees, and Dishes (continued)													
56120	Flauta, chicken	1	ea	113	62	330	13	12	2	26	4.2	10.7	9.3
56232	Greek meat pie, 8 inch	1	ea	417	247	947	34	73	5	57	13.5	25.6	14.2
56242	Gumbo w/Rice	1	cup	244	203	193	14	17	2	8	1.6	2.6	2.7
56153	Hamburger Helper, beef+tom	1	cup	249	185	275	29	24	2	7	2.3	2.9	0.6
56310	Hamburger Helper, mac+cheese	1	cup	243	173	340	28	22	1	15	7.7	5.1	0.7
56150	Hash, roast beef	1	cup	190	131	312	21	21	2	16	4.9	5.7	3.3
56239	Jambalaya, shrimp	1	cup	243	176	310	27	28	1	9	1.8	3.8	2.8
56296	Knish, meat	1	ea	50	19	175	7	13	1	11	2.6	4.9	2.3
56294	Knish, potato	1	ea	61	22	215	5	21	1	12	2.6	5.8	3.3
13900	Lamb curry	1	cup	236	188	256	28	3	1	14	3.9	4.9	3.4
56108	Lasagna w/meat, recipe	1	pce	245	164	392	23	40	3	16	8	5.2	0.8
18800	Lobster Newburg	1	cup	244	150	611	30	11	<1	50	29.6	14.7	2.3
56082	Macaroni+cheese, recipe	1	cup	200	116	430	17	40	1	22	8.9	8.8	3.6
56250	Moo goo gai pan	1	cup	216	168	272	15	12	3	19	3.8	6.7	7
56080	Moussaka, lamb/eggplant	1	cup	250	204	237	16	13	4	13	4.6	5.4	1.9
19403	Oysters Rockefeller	1	cup	224	165	301	16	21	3	17	7.7	5.7	2.4
56234	Pork chop suey+noodles	1	cup	220	136	448	22	31	4	27	4.8	7.7	12.8
56292	Pork dumpling, fried	1	ea	100		341	13	25	1	21	4.8	9.1	5.7
56288	Pork egg foo yung, patty	1	ea	86	65	124	8	4	1	8	2.1	3	2.3
56122	Quesadilla	1	ea	54	19	183	6	18	1	10	3.5	3.4	2.2
56098	Quiche Lorraine, 1/8 pie	1	pce	176	93	526	15	25	1	41	18.9	14.3	5.2
56128	Ravioli, cheese+tom sce, svg	1	ea	250	180	341	15	38	2	15	6.4	5	1.9
56303	Ravioli, meat w/tomato sauce	2	ea	70	48	110	6	10	1	5	1.7	2.1	0.5
57517	Shrimp Creole w/rice	1	cup	243	176	310	27	28	1	9	1.8	3.8	2.8
57523	Spring roll, fresh	1	ea	64	43	113	5	9	1	6	1.4	3	1.3
56291	Spring roll, meat	1	ea	64	43	113	5	9	1	6	1.4	3	1.3
56236	Stuffed grape leaves, lamb	1	ea	21	12	56	2	2	1	4	1.1	2.5	0.5
56074	Stuffed green pepper	1	ea	172		229	11	20	2	11	5	4.9	0.5
56244	Sukiyaki	1	cup	162	126	172	19	7	1	8	2.9	3.1	0.7
56315	Sushi+egg, seaweed rolled	1	cup	166	124	202	9	22	<1	8	2.2	3.2	1.6
56313	Sushi+fish+vegetables	1	cup	166	109	232	9	47	2	1	0.2	0.2	0.2
56314	Sushi+veg, seaweed rolled	1	cup	166	118	194	4	43	1	<1	0.1	0.1	0.1
56312	Sushi, no fish+vegetables	1	cup	166	106	240	5	53	2	<1	0.1	0.1	0.1
56311	Sushi, no fish, no veges	1	cup	145	82	256	5	57	1	<1	0.1	0.1	0.1
56235	Sweet & sour pork+rice	1	cup	244	182	270	13	40	1	6	1.6	2.4	1.7
56061	Taco, chicken	1	ea	77.3		173	15	9	1	8	3.2	3.1	1.4
56113	Tamale, meat	1	ea	70	45	134	6	11	1	7	2.6	3.1	1
56130	Tortellini, meat	1	cup	190	115	373	24	33	1	15	5.4	5.7	2.1
56645	Tostada, beef+cheese	1	ea	163	101	314	19	23		16	10.4	3.3	1
56089	Tuna noodle casserole	1	cup	202	151	237	17	25	1	7	1.9	1.5	3.2
11902	Veal scallopini	1	pce	96	57	238	18	1	<1	17	4.8	7.4	3.2
Pizza													
56996	Cheese sausage, Bagel Bites	4	pce	88		200	10	24	3	7	2.5		
57166	Deluxe pizza, Kraft, piece	1	pce	125	65	298	14	27	2	15	6.5		

< = Trace amount present

Blank = Not available

CHOL, cholesterol; **V,** vitamin; **THI,** thiamin; **RIB,** riboflavin; **NIA,** niacin; **FOL,** folate;
CALC, calcium; **PHOS,** phosphate; **SOD,** sodium; **POT,** potassium; **MAG,** magnesium

CHOL (mg)	V-A (RE)	THI (mg)	RIB (mg)	NIA (mg)	V-B6 (mg)	FOL (μg)	V-B12 (μg)	V-C (mg)	V-E (mg)	CALC (mg)	PHOS (mg)	SOD (mg)	POT (mg)	MAG (mg)	IRON (mg)	ZINC (mg)
35	26	0.1	0.1	3.1	0.2	8	0.1	18	4.4	50	140	71	268	27	0.9	1.1
66	829	0.7	0.6	8.8	0.5	42	2.4	15	6.5	45	355	1032	751	62	6.5	4.7
40	63	0.2	0.2	4.5	0.2	46	2.4	14	1.4	71	152	542	446	40	2.6	15.2
86	98	0.3	0.3	5.6	0.5	19	2.7	13	1.6	26	289	666	740	55	4	4.5
92	70	0.2	0.3	4	0.3	16	2	0	0.3	188	335	736	348	36	3.4	4.6
57	<1	0.2	0.2	3.7	0.5	16	1.8	7	1.2	19	204	470	587	36	2.5	5
181	133	0.3	0.1	4.8	0.2	12	1.2	17	2.3	104	300	370	439	64	4.4	1.7
52	89	0.1	0.2	1.5	<0.1	8	0.3	<1	1.2	12	61	107	88	8	1.2	1
59	130	0.2	0.2	1.5	0.1	10	0.1	1	1.7	16	60	140	96	10	1.3	0.4
89	2	0.1	0.3	8.1	0.2	28	2.9	1	1.2	36	284	323	496	40	3	6.6
58	158	0.2	0.3	4.2	0.2	20	1	14	1.2	270	299	391	460	50	3.1	3.3
369	523	0.1	0.4	1.6	0.2	32	4	1	2	241	398	647	607	55	1.2	4.1
42	234	0.2	0.4	1.8	0.1	10	0.3	1	3.5	362	322	1086	240	37	1.8	1.2
35	142	0.2	0.3	4.4	0.3	42	0.3	34	3.7	130	199	304	488	34	1.7	1.6
97	105	0.2	0.3	4.1	0.2	45	1.4	6	0.9	68	179	432	557	40	1.8	2.6
87	805	0.4	0.4	4	0.3	122	21	27	2.2	195	254	708	583	115	10.3	97.9
48	19	0.8	0.4	6.2	0.4	42	0.4	20	2.7	45	249	848	489	53	3.3	2.6
27	11	0.5	0.3	3.6	0.2	9	0.3	<1	2.3	33	131	86	198	18	1.8	1.1
167	86	0.1	0.2	0.8	0.1	22	0.4	3	1.1	27	105	131	157	12	0.8	0.9
13	41	0.1	0.1	1.1	<0.1	6	0.1	15	1	132	107	230	77	13	1.2	0.6
221	279	0.3	0.5	2	0.1	19	0.6	1	2	231	261	221	239	24	1.9	1.5
162	236	0.3	0.4	2.9	0.2	30	0.4	9	2.1	172	220	574	405	33	3.1	1.5
48	49	0.1	0.1	1.7	0.1	8	0.5	2	0.7	20	62	50	148	11	1.2	1
181	133	0.3	0.1	4.8	0.2	12	1.2	17	2.3	104	300	370	439	64	4.4	1.7
37	16	0.2	0.1	1.3	0.1	10	0.1	2	0.8	15	57	274	124	10	0.8	0.5
37	16	0.2	0.1	1.3	0.1	10	0.1	2	0.8	15	57	274	124	10	0.8	0.5
5	145	<0.1	<0.1	0.6	<0.1	6	0.1	2	0.5	22	19	14	41	8	0.4	0.3
34	44	0.1	0.1	2.7	0.3	17	0.7	55	0.7	16	85	201	232	20	1.8	2.3
148	256	0.1	0.4	3.1	0.4	61	1.5	5	0.7	62	204	675	463	47	3.2	3.6
224	145	0.1	0.3	1.4	0.1	30	0.5	2	0.9	45	140	562	136	19	1.7	1
11	136	0.3	0.1	3	0.2	15	0.3	4	0.6	25	109	93	218	27	2.3	0.8
0	66	0.2	<0.1	2	0.1	11	0	3	0.1	22	64	5	106	21	1.6	0.7
0	152	0.3	0.1	2.6	0.1	16	0	4	0.2	25	84	88	169	24	2.6	0.9
0	0	0.3	<0.1	2.7	0.1	4	0	0	0.1	20	71	6	78	18	2.7	0.7
28	23	0.5	0.2	3.8	0.4	10	0.3	14	0.8	28	142	618	311	35	2	1.5
45	39	0.1	0.1	4.2	0.2	16	0.2	1	0.8	94	153	106	166	28	1	1.3
19	14	0.2	0.1	2.5	0.1	4	0.2	1	0.3	24	67	84	140	21	1.4	0.9
240	134	0.5	0.6	4.5	0.2	29	0.9	<1	1.1	178	290	437	231	28	3.1	2.2
41	96	0.1	0.6	3.1	0.2	75	1.2	3		217	179	896	572	64	2.9	3.7
41	13	0.2	0.1	7.8	0.2	10	1.5	1	1.2	34	155	772	182	31	2.3	1.2
65	101	<0.1	0.2	5.1	0.2	12	0.9	1	1.7	54	172	278	253	19	1	2.8
15	80							12		100		500	140		0.7	
28	93							8		233		597			1.3	

ERA, EatRight Analysis CD-ROM; **AMT,** amount; **WT,** weight; **WTR,** water; **CAL,** calories; **PROT,** protein; **CARB**, carbohydrate; **FIBR,** fiber; **FAT,** fat; **SATF,** saturated fat; **MONO,** monounsaturated fat; **POLY,** polyunsaturated fat

Meals, Entrees, and Mixed Dishes (continued)

Pizza (continued)

ERA CODE	FOOD DESCRIPTION	AMT	UNIT	WT (g)	WTR (g)	CAL (kcal)	PROT (g)	CARB (g)	FIBR (g)	FAT (g)	SATF (g)	MONO (g)	POLY (g)
56733	Fr bread cheese pizza, Ln Cuisine	1	ea	145	73	298	19	41	3	7	3.4	1.3	0.4
56736	Fr bread deluxe pizza, Ln Cuisine	1	ea	174		330	23	45	5	6	2.5	2	1
56735	Fr bread pepperoni pizza, Ln Cuisine	1	ea	149		330	20	46	4	7	3	2.5	1
57215	Supreme pizza, light, Kraft	1	ea	640		1252	116	139	9	42	16.2		

Meats

Beef

ERA CODE	FOOD DESCRIPTION	AMT	UNIT	WT (g)	WTR (g)	CAL (kcal)	PROT (g)	CARB (g)	FIBR (g)	FAT (g)	SATF (g)	MONO (g)	POLY (g)
10051	Beef jerky, large piece	1	ea	19.8	5	81	7	2	<1	5	2.1	2.2	0.2
10008	Corned beef, canned	1	cup	140	81	350	38	0	0	21	8.7	8.3	0.9
10036	Corned beef, cooked, lean	1	pce	42	25	105	8	<1	0	8	2.7	3.9	0.3
10060	Filet mignon steak, broiled, lean	1	ea	156	94	329	44	0	0	16	5.8	5.9	0.6
10724	Ground beef, lean, broiled	3	oz	85	45	238	24	0	0	15	5.9	6.6	0.6
10463	Ground beef, reg, broiled	3	oz	85	44	248	23	0	0	17	6.5	7.2	0.6
10722	Ground beef, X lean, broiled	3	oz	85	46	225	24	0	0	13	5.3	5.9	0.5
10021	London broil, broiled, lean	3	oz	85	52	176	23	0	0	9	3.7	3.5	0.3
11018	Meat loaf, beef only	1	pce	108	67	231	18	7	<1	14	4.9	6.1	0.7
10028	Porterhouse steak, broiled, ln	1	ea	170	102	366	44	0	0	20	6.9	8.9	0.6
10024	Rib eye steak, broiled, lean	3	oz	85	50	191	24	0	0	10	4	4.2	0.3
10016	Round, pot roasted, lean+fat	1	pce	42	22	116	12	0	0	7	2.7	3.1	0.3
40067	Salisbury steak, flame brld	1	ea	72	42	160	16	3	1	10	3.9	4.2	0.4
10624	Short ribs, braised	3	oz	85	30	400	18	0	0	36	15.1	16	1.3
10005	Sirloin steak, broiled, lean	1	ea	156	96	315	47	0	0	12	4.9	5.3	0.5
10050	Stew meat, cooked, lean only	1	cup	140	79	330	44	0	0	16	6	6.9	0.5
10064	Strip steak, broiled, lean	1	ea	241	144	499	69	0	0	23	8.7	9.1	0.7
10007	T-bone steak, broiled, lean	1	ea	184	113	377	49	0	0	18	6.6	8.3	0.6

Game Meats

ERA CODE	FOOD DESCRIPTION	AMT	UNIT	WT (g)	WTR (g)	CAL (kcal)	PROT (g)	CARB (g)	FIBR (g)	FAT (g)	SATF (g)	MONO (g)	POLY (g)
14008	Beefalo meat, roasted	3	oz	85	52	160	26	0	0	5	2.3	2.3	0.2
14009	Bison/buffalo meat, roasted	3	oz	85	57	122	24	0	0	2	0.8	0.8	0.2
14013	Deer/venison, roasted	3	oz	85	55	134	26	0	0	3	1.1	0.7	0.5
14014	Elk meat, roasted	3	oz	85	56	124	26	0	0	2	0.6	0.4	0.3
14029	Frog legs, steamed	2	ea	100		106	24	0	0	<1	0.1	0.1	0.1
14004	Rabbit, roasted	3.5	oz	100		197	29	0	0	8	2.4	2.2	1.6
14030	Turtle meat, cooked	1	cup	140	96	220	33	<1	0	9	1.8	4.1	2.6
14032	Venison steak, fried	1	ea	85	53	147	28	0	0	3	1.2	0.9	0.6

Goat

ERA CODE	FOOD DESCRIPTION	AMT	UNIT	WT (g)	WTR (g)	CAL (kcal)	PROT (g)	CARB (g)	FIBR (g)	FAT (g)	SATF (g)	MONO (g)	POLY (g)
13530	Goat meat, boiled	1	oz	28.35	19	41	8	0	0	1	0.3	0.4	0.1
14016	Goat ribs, cooked	1	ea	46	31	66	12	0	0	1	0.4	0.6	0.1

Lamb

ERA CODE	FOOD DESCRIPTION	AMT	UNIT	WT (g)	WTR (g)	CAL (kcal)	PROT (g)	CARB (g)	FIBR (g)	FAT (g)	SATF (g)	MONO (g)	POLY (g)
13524	Ground lamb, broiled	3	oz	85	47	240	21	0	0	17	6.9	7.1	1.2
13522	Kabob meat, broiled lean	2	oz	56.7	36	105	16	0	0	4	1.5	1.7	0.4
13513	Loin chop, broiled, lean	1	ea	46	28	99	14	0	0	4	1.6	2	0.3
13523	Stew meat, braised, lean	3	oz	85	48	190	29	0	0	7	2.7	3	0.7
13501	Leg of lamb, roasted, lean	3	oz	85	54	162	24	0	0	7	2.3	2.9	0.4

< = Trace amount present   Blank = Not available

CHOL, cholesterol; **V,** vitamin; **THI,** thiamin; **RIB,** riboflavin; **NIA,** niacin; **FOL,** folate; **CALC,** calcium; **PHOS,** phosphate; **SOD,** sodium; **POT,** potassium; **MAG,** magnesium

CHOL (mg)	V-A (RE)	THI (mg)	RIB (mg)	NIA (mg)	V-B6 (mg)	FOL (μg)	V-B12 (μg)	V-C (mg)	V-E (mg)	CALC (mg)	PHOS (mg)	SOD (mg)	POT (mg)	MAG (mg)	IRON (mg)	ZINC (mg)
17	51							5		384		341	315		3.1	
30	100							6		250		560	380		3.6	
25	100							6		250		590	350		3.6	
93	928							28		1855		3292			8.3	
10	0	<0.1	<0.1	0.3	<0.1	27	0.2	0	0.1	4	81	438	118	10	1.1	1.6
120	0	<0.1	0.2	3.4	0.2	13	2.3	0	1.1	17	155	1408	190	20	2.9	5
41	0	<0.1	0.1	1.3	0.1	3	0.7	0	0.1	3	52	476	61	5	0.8	1.9
131	0	0.2	0.5	6.1	0.7	11	4	0	0.2	11	371	98	654	47	5.6	8.7
86	0	0.1	0.2	5.1	0.3	9	2.3	0	0.2	10	155	76	297	20	2.1	5.3
86	0	<0.1	0.2	5.5	0.3	8	2.8	0	0.2	10	162	79	278	19	2.3	4.9
84	0	0.1	0.3	5	0.3	9	2.2	0	0.2	8	162	70	314	21	2.4	5.5
57	0	0.1	0.2	4.3	0.3	7	2.8	0	0.1	6	201	71	352	20	2.2	4.1
90	20	0.1	0.3	4	0.1	12	1.7	1	0.1	43	161	133	295	22	2	3.7
117	0	0.2	0.4	7.9	0.7	14	3.9	0	0.2	12	359	117	624	46	5.3	9
68	0	0.1	0.2	4.1	0.3	7	2.8	0	0.1	11	177	59	335	23	2.2	5.9
40	0	<0.1	0.1	1.6	0.1	4	1	0	0.2	3	103	21	118	9	1.3	2.1
42	18	0.1	0.1	2.6	0.3	6	1.6	2	0.1	29	232	500	259	26	2	4.5
80	0	<0.1	0.1	2.1	0.2	4	2.2	0	0.2	10	138	42	190	13	2	4.1
139	0	0.2	0.5	6.7	0.7	16	4.4	0	0.6	17	381	103	629	50	5.2	10.2
143	0	0.1	0.4	4.5	0.4	11	3.7	0	0.2	14	346	94	388	33	5	12.3
183	0	0.2	0.5	12.9	1	19	4.8	0	0.3	19	525	164	954	65	6	12.6
108	0	0.2	0.5	8.5	0.7	15	4.2	0	0.5	11	396	131	696	52	5.8	9.8
49	0	<0.1	0.1	4.2	0.3	15	2.2	8	0.2	20	212	70	390	<1	2.6	5.4
70	0	0.1	0.2	3.2	0.3	7	2.4	0	0.1	7	178	48	307	22	2.9	3.1
95	0	0.2	0.5	5.7	0.3	4	2.7	0	0.2	6	192	46	285	20	3.8	2.3
62	0	0.2	0.7	4.9	0.2	3	5.5	0	<0.1	4	153	52	279	20	3.1	2.7
72	20	0.2	0.3	1.6	0.2	16	0.5	0	1.4	26	160	84	372	29	2	1.4
82	0	0.1	0.2	8.4	0.5	11	8.3	0	0.9	19	263	47	383	21	2.3	2.3
82	126	0.2	0.2	1.7	0.2	21	1.5	<1	2.1	197	299	209	383	33	2.3	1.6
103	0	0.1	0.6	5.8	0.2	5	5.3	0	0.2	5	207	52	307	24	4.1	2.5
21	0	<0.1	0.2	1.1	0	1	0.3	0	<0.1	5	57	24	115	0	1.1	1.5
34	0	<0.1	0.3	1.8	0	2	0.5	0	<0.1	8	92	40	186	0	1.7	2.4
82	0	0.1	0.2	5.7	0.1	16	2.2	0	0.2	19	171	69	288	20	1.5	4
51	0	0.1	0.2	3.7	0.1	13	1.7	0	0.1	7	127	43	190	18	1.3	3.3
44	0	0.1	0.1	3.2	0.1	11	1.2	0	0.1	9	104	39	173	13	0.9	1.9
92	0	0.1	0.2	5.1	0.1	18	2.3	0	0.2	13	174	60	221	24	2.4	5.6
76	0	0.1	0.2	5.4	0.1	20	2.2	0	0.2	7	175	58	287	22	1.8	4.2

ERA, EatRight Analysis CD-ROM; **AMT,** amount; **WT,** weight; **WTR,** water; **CAL,** calories; **PROT,** protein; **CARB**, carbohydrate; **FIBR,** fiber; **FAT,** fat; **SATF,** saturated fat; **MONO,** monounsaturated fat; **POLY,** polyunsaturated fat

ERA CODE	FOOD DESCRIPTION	AMT	UNIT	WT (g)	WTR (g)	CAL (kcal)	PROT (g)	CARB (g)	FIBR (g)	FAT (g)	SATF (g)	MONO (g)	POLY (g)
Meats (continued)													
Lunchmeats and Sausages													
13006	Bologna, beef & pork	1	pce	28.4	15	90	3	1	0	8	3	3.8	0.7
13007	Bologna, turkey	1	pce	28.4	18	57	4	<1	0	4	1.4	1.4	1.2
13079	Bratwurst sausage link, cooked	1	ea	85	48	256	12	2	0	22	7.9	10.4	2.3
13066	Braunschweiger sausage	2	pce	57	27	205	8	2	0	18	6.2	8.5	2.1
13052	Breakfast sausage, turkey	1	pce	28.4	17	65	6	0	0	5	1.6	1.8	1.2
13070	Chorizo sausage, link	1	ea	60	19	273	14	1	0	23	8.6	11	2.1
56668	Corndog (hot dog+coating)	1	ea	175	82	460	17	56		19	5.2	9.1	3.5
13034	Ham salad spread	1	Tbs	15	9	32	1	2	0	2	0.8	1.1	0.4
13250	Hot dog, beef, fat free	1	ea	50		39	7	3	0	<1	0.1	0.1	<0.1
13009	Hot dog, beef & pork	1	ea	57	31	182	6	1	0	17	6.1	7.8	1.6
13008	Hot dog, beef, 2 oz	1	ea	57	31	180	7	1	0	16	6.9	7.8	0.8
13012	Hot dog, turkey	1	ea	45	28	102	6	1	0	8	2.7	2.5	2.2
13015	Italian pork sausage link, ckd	1	ea	67	33	216	13	1	0	17	6.1	8	2.2
13043	Kielbasa sausage	1	pce	26	14	81	3	1	0	7	2.6	3.4	0.8
13019	Liverwurst, pork	1	pce	18	9	59	3	<1	0	5	1.9	2.4	0.5
13020	Pastrami, turkey	2	pce	57	40	80	10	1	0	4	1	1.2	0.9
13021	Pepperoni sausage	4	pce	22	6	109	5	1	0	10	3.5	4.6	1
13051	Pickle & pimento loaf	2	pce	57	33	149	7	3	0	12	4.5	5.5	1.5
13022	Polish sausage, pork	1	ea	227	121	740	32	4	0	65	23.4	30.7	7
13023	Salami, beef, cooked	1	pce	23	13	60	3	1	0	5	2.1	2.2	0.2
13026	Salami, dry, beef & pork	2	pce	20	7	84	5	1	0	7	2.4	3.4	0.6
10035	Sizzlean formed bacon, cooked	3	pce	34	9	153	11	<1	0	12	4.9	5.7	0.5
13105	Spam, canned	1	pce	28.35	14	95	4	1	<1	9			
13328	Turkey lunchmeat, roasted	1	oz	28.35	21	28	5	1	0	1	0.1	0.2	0.1
13112	Turkey breast, smkd, fat free	1	pce	28		23	4	1	0	<1	0.1	0.1	<0.1
Pork and Ham													
12000	Bacon, regular, cooked	3	pce	19	2	109	6	<1	0	9	3.3	4.5	1.1
12002	Canadian bacon, grilled	2	pce	46.5	29	86	11	1	0	4	1.3	1.9	0.4
12225	Ham, canned, unheated, X lean	1	cup	140	100	202	25	0	0	10	3.4	5	1.1
12006	Ham, whole, rstd, lean only	1	cup	140	92	220	35	0	0	8	2.6	3.5	0.9
12082	Pork chop, breaded, baked	1	ea	80	44	184	21	5	<1	8	2.9	3.7	0.9
12086	Pork chop, smoked, lean	1	ea	67	43	114	17	0	0	5	1.6	2.2	0.5
12236	Pork country rib, lean, rstd	3	oz	85	49	210	23	0	0	13	4.5	5.5	0.9
12035	Pork loin chop, broiled, lean	1	ea	79	48	166	23	0	0	8	2.9	3.5	0.6
12031	Pork loin, roasted slice	1	ea	89	51	221	24	0	0	13	4.8	5.8	1.1
12098	Spareribs, braised, lean	3	oz	85	51	199	22	0	0	12	4.2	5	0.9
Veal													
11900	Breaded veal patty, fried	1	ea	79	41	212	16	7	<1	13	4.4	5.9	1.2
11530	Ground veal, broiled	3	oz	85	57	146	21	0	0	6	2.6	2.4	0.5
11514	Veal chop, med, fried, lean	1	ea	85	52	156	28	0	0	4	1.1	1.4	0.3
11527	Veal sirloin, roasted	3	oz	85	53	172	21	0	0	9	3.8	3.5	0.6
11517	Veal loin cutlet, brsd, lean+fat	1	ea	80	42	227	24	0	0	14	5.4	5.4	0.9
11519	Veal rib, roasted, lean+fat	3	oz	85	51	194	20	0	0	12	4.6	4.6	0.8

< = Trace amount present

Blank = Not available

CHOL, cholesterol; **V,** vitamin; **THI,** thiamin; **RIB,** riboflavin; **NIA,** niacin; **FOL,** folate;
CALC, calcium; **PHOS,** phosphate; **SOD,** sodium; **POT,** potassium; **MAG,** magnesium

CHOL (mg)	V-A (RE)	THI (mg)	RIB (mg)	NIA (mg)	V-B6 (mg)	FOL (μg)	V-B12 (μg)	V-C (mg)	V-E (mg)	CALC (mg)	PHOS (mg)	SOD (mg)	POT (mg)	MAG (mg)	IRON (mg)	ZINC (mg)
16	0	<0.1	<0.1	0.7	0.1	1	0.4	0	0.1	3	26	289	51	3	0.4	0.6
28	0	<0.1	<0.1	1	0.1	2	0.1	0	0.2	24	37	249	57	4	0.4	0.5
51	0	0.4	0.2	2.7	0.2	2	0.8	1	0.2	37	127	473	180	13	1.1	2
89	2405	0.1	0.9	4.8	0.2	25	11.4	0	0.2	5	96	652	113	6	5.3	1.6
23	0	<0.1	0.1	1.4	0.1	1	0.5	0	0.2	5	52	191	76	6	0.5	1
53	0	0.4	0.2	3.1	0.3	1	1.2	0	0.1	5	90	741	239	11	1	2
79	37	0.3	0.7	4.2	0.1	103	0.4	0	0.7	102	166	973	262	18	6.2	1.3
6	0	0.1	<0.1	0.3	<0.1	<1	0.1	0	0.7	1	18	137	22	2	0.1	0.2
15	0							0		10	64	464	234	10	1	1.2
28	0	0.1	0.1	1.5	0.1	2	0.7	0	0.2	6	49	638	95	6	0.7	1
35	0	<0.1	0.1	1.4	0.1	2	0.9	0	0.2	11	50	585	95	2	0.8	1.2
48	0	<0.1	0.1	1.9	0.1	4	0.1	0	0.3	48	60	642	81	6	0.8	1.4
52	0	0.4	0.2	2.8	0.2	3	0.9	1	0.2	16	114	618	204	12	1	1.6
17	0	0.1	0.1	0.7	<0.1	1	0.4	0	0.1	11	38	280	70	4	0.4	0.5
28	1494	<0.1	0.2	0.8	<0.1	5	2.4	0	0.1	5	41	155	31	2	1.2	0.4
31	0	<0.1	0.1	2	0.2	3	0.1	0	0.4	5	114	596	148	8	0.9	1.2
17	0	0.1	0.1	1.1	0.1	1	0.6	0	0.1	2	26	449	76	4	0.3	0.6
21	4	0.2	0.1	1.2	0.1	3	0.7	0	0.1	54	80	792	194	10	0.6	0.8
159	0	1.1	0.3	7.8	0.4	5	2.2	2	0.6	27	309	1988	538	32	3.3	4.4
15	0	<0.1	<0.1	0.7	<0.1	<1	0.7	0	0.2	2	26	270	52	3	0.5	0.5
16	0	0.1	0.1	1	0.1	<1	0.4	0	0.1	2	28	372	76	3	0.3	0.6
40	0	<0.1	0.1	2.2	0.1	3	1.2	0	0.1	3	80	766	140	9	1.1	2.2
16	5	<0.1	0.1	0.9						2		445	54	3	0.4	0.7
11	0							0		2	71	313	63	6	0.3	0.3
10	0							0		3	69	300	61	8	0.2	0.2
16	0	0.1	0.1	1.4	0.1	1	0.3	0	0.1	2	64	303	92	5	0.3	0.6
27	0	0.4	0.1	3.2	0.2	2	0.4	0	0.2	5	138	719	181	10	0.4	0.8
53	0	1.2	0.3	6.4	0.6	8	1.1	0	0.7	8	290	1786	468	22	1.3	2.6
77	0	1	0.4	7	0.7	6	1	0	0.4	10	318	1857	442	31	1.3	3.6
57	1	0.7	0.3	3.9	0.4	5	0.5	1	0.4	17	197	333	331	22	0.8	1.8
32	0	0.5	0.2	3.2	0.2	3	0.7	0	0.2	7	163	825	196	11	0.7	2
79	2	0.5	0.3	4	0.4	4	0.7	<1	0.4	25	188	25	297	20	1.1	3.2
62	2	0.7	0.3	4.1	0.4	5	0.6	1	0.3	13	200	51	346	23	0.7	2
73	3	0.9	0.3	5	0.5	5	0.6	1	0.3	17	215	53	363	23	0.9	2.1
73	2	0.5	0.2	3.5	0.3	3	0.6	1	0.4	21	143	54	293	15	1.2	3.4
80	8	0.1	0.2	5.9	0.3	11	0.7	0	1	35	153	142	227	20	1.1	2
88	0	0.1	0.2	6.8	0.3	9	1.1	0	0.2	14	184	71	286	20	0.8	3.3
91	0	0.1	0.3	10.7	0.4	14	1.3	0	0.4	6	246	65	376	27	0.7	2.9
87	0	0.1	0.3	7.5	0.3	13	1.2	0	0.4	11	190	71	298	22	0.8	2.8
94	0	<0.1	0.2	7.2	0.2	11	1	0	0.9	22	176	64	224	19	0.9	2.9
94	0	<0.1	0.2	5.9	0.2	11	1.2	0	0.8	9	167	78	251	19	0.8	3.5

ERA, EatRight Analysis CD-ROM; **AMT,** amount; **WT,** weight; **WTR,** water; **CAL,** calories; **PROT,** protein; **CARB**, carbohydrate; **FIBR,** fiber; **FAT,** fat; **SATF,** saturated fat; **MONO,** monounsaturated fat; **POLY,** polyunsaturated fat

ERA CODE	FOOD DESCRIPTION	AMT	UNIT	WT (g)	WTR (g)	CAL (kcal)	PROT (g)	CARB (g)	FIBR (g)	FAT (g)	SATF (g)	MONO (g)	POLY (g)
Meats (continued)													
Variety Meats and Byproducts													
10015	Beef heart, simmered	3	oz	85	54	149	24	<1	0	5	1.4	1.1	1.2
10010	Beef liver, fried	3	oz	85	47	184	23	7	0	7	2.3	1.4	1.5
10019	Beef tripe, pickled	1	oz	28.4	25	18	3	0	0	<1	0.1	0.1	<0.1
15025	Chicken gizzards, simmered	1	cup	145	98	222	39	2	0	5	1.5	1.3	1.5
15005	Chicken livers, simmered	7	ea	140	96	220	34	1	0	8	2.6	1.9	1.3
16048	Smoked goose liver pate, cnd	1	Tbs	13	5	60	1	1	0	6	1.9	3.3	0.1
Meat Substitutes, Tofu, Vegetarian Foods													
Generic													
7518	Firm tofu, raw	1	cup	252	211	194	20	7	1	11	1.6	2.5	6.3
7503	Miso (soybean)	1	cup	275	114	566	32	77	15	17	2.4	3.7	9.4
7508	Natto, soybean, fermented	1	cup	175	96	371	31	25	9	19	2.8	4.3	10.9
7718	Soy burger, black bean & salsa	1	ea	142		200	19	20	3	4	1.5		
7564	Tempeh	1	cup	166	99	320	31	16	9	18	3.7	5	6.4
8835	Tofu franks/wiener, each	1	ea	38		45	9	5	2	0	0	0	0
7520	Tofu, fried	1	pce	13	7	35	2	1	1	3	0.4	0.6	1.5
7500	Tofu, regular	1	cup	248	216	151	16	4	<1	9	1.3	2	5.2
7511	Vegetarian breakfast links	1	ea	25	13	64	5	2	1	5	0.7	1.1	2.3
7512	Vegetarian breakfast patty	1	ea	38	19	97	7	4	1	7	1.1	1.7	3.5
7548	Vegetarian chicken, bread fried	1	pce	57	40	97	6	3	3	7	1	1.6	3.9
7549	Vegetarian fish sticks	2	ea	57	26	165	13	5	3	10	1.6	2.5	5.3
7550	Vegetarian frankfurter	1	ea	51	30	102	10	4	2	5	0.8	1.2	2.6
7551	Vegetarian luncheon meat	1	pce	67	31	188	17	6	3	11	1.7	2.6	5.6
7561	Vegetarian meat patties	1	ea	71	41	142	15	6	3	6	1	1.6	3.3
7552	Vegetarian meatballs	7	ea	70	41	140	15	6	3	6	1	1.5	3.3
7554	Vegetarian soyburger	1	ea	71	41	142	15	6	3	6	1	1.6	3.3
Green Giant													
7673	Harvest Burger, Italian, frozen	1	ea	90		140	17	8	5	4	1.5	0.5	0.5
7674	Harvest Burger, original, frozen	1	ea	90	58	137	18	7	6	4	1	2.1	0.3
Lightlife Foods													
8169	Vegetarian baloney, pce	1	pce	14.33	10	20	3	1	0	1	0.3		
8173	Vegetarian ham, country, piece	1	pce	14.33	10	17	3	1	0	0	0	0	0
8159	Vegetarian Italian sausage, lean	1	ea	40		60	5	5	0	2	1		
8166	Vegetarian sausage, lean, bfast	1	ea	35		60	4	4	0	3	1		
Loma Linda													
7727	Vege chicken nugget, frozen	5	pce	85	40	244	12	13	5	16	2.5	4	8.8
7666	Vege sandwich spread, canned	1	ea	55	38	85	4	7	3	4	0.9	2.1	1.4
Morningstar Farms													
7726	Black bean burger	1	ea	78	47	115	12	15	5	1	0.2	0.2	0.4
7752	Breakfast strip, frozen	2	pce	16	7	56	2	2	1	4	0.7	1.1	2.6
7724	Deli franks	1	ea	45	23	112	10	4	3	6	0.9	2	3.3
7665	Vege chicken patties, frozen	1	ea	71		177	7	15	2	10	1.3	2.6	5.9

< = Trace amount present   Blank = Not available

CHOL, cholesterol; **V,** vitamin; **THI,** thiamin; **RIB,** riboflavin; **NIA,** niacin; **FOL,** folate;
CALC, calcium; **PHOS,** phosphate; **SOD,** sodium; **POT,** potassium; **MAG,** magnesium

CHOL (mg)	V-A (RE)	THI (mg)	RIB (mg)	NIA (mg)	V-B6 (mg)	FOL (μg)	V-B12 (μg)	V-C (mg)	V-E (mg)	CALC (mg)	PHOS (mg)	SOD (mg)	POT (mg)	MAG (mg)	IRON (mg)	ZINC (mg)
164	0	0.1	1.3	3.5	0.2	2	12.1	1	0.6	5	212	54	198	21	6.4	2.7
410	9119	0.2	3.5	12.3	1.2	187	95	20	1.4	9	392	90	309	20	5.3	4.6
19	0	0	<0.1	0.5	<0.1	<1	0.3	0	<0.1	36	24	13	5	2	0.5	0.5
281	81	<0.1	0.4	5.8	0.2	77	2.8	2	2.3	14	225	97	260	29	6	6.4
883	6878	0.2	2.4	6.2	0.8	1078	27.1	22	2.4	20	437	71	196	29	11.9	6.1
20	130	<0.1	<0.1	0.3	<0.1	8	1.2	<1	0.2	9	26	91	18	2	0.7	0.1
0	2	0.2	0.3	<0.1	0.2	83	0	1	0.1	408	370	20	444	116	3.7	2.5
0	25	0.3	0.7	2.4	0.6	91	0	0	<0.1	182	421	10029	451	116	7.5	9.1
0	0	0.3	0.3	0	0.2	14	0	23	<0.1	380	304	12	1275	201	15.1	5.3
0												660				
0	0	0.1	0.6	4.4	0.4	40	0.1	0	<0.1	184	442	15	684	134	4.5	1.9
0	0	0.2					0.6	0		20		240	90		1.1	
0	0	<0.1	<0.1	<0.1	<0.1	3	0	0	<0.1	48	37	2	19	8	0.6	0.3
0	2	0.1	0.1	1.3	0.1	109	0	<1	8.4	275	228	20	298	67	2.8	1.6
0	16	0.6	0.1	2.8	0.2	6	0	0	0.5	16	56	222	58	9	0.9	0.4
0	24	0.9	0.2	4.3	0.3	10	0	0	0.8	24	86	337	88	14	1.4	0.6
0	0	0.4	0.3	2.7	0.3	32	1.2	0	1.1	13	140	228	171	7	1	0.4
0	0	0.6	0.5	6.8	0.9	58	2.4	0	2.3	54	256	279	342	13	1.1	0.8
0	0	0.6	0.6	8.2	0.5	40	1.2	0	1	17	175	219	76	9	0.9	0.6
0	0	0.6	0.4	7.4	0.7	67	1.7	0	2	27	296	576	188	15	1.5	1.1
0	0	0.6	0.4	7.1	0.9	55	1.7	0	1.2	21	244	390	128	13	1.5	1.3
0	0	0.6	0.4	7	0.8	55	1.7	0	1.2	20	241	385	126	13	1.5	1.3
0	0	0.6	0.4	7.1	0.9	55	1.7	0	1.2	21	244	390	128	13	1.5	1.3
0	0	0.3	0.1	4	0.3		1.5	0		80		370			2.7	6.8
0	0	0.3	0.2	6.3	0.4	22	0	0	1.6	102	225	411	432	70	3.9	8.1
0	0							1		7		80			0.2	
0	0							<1		0		100			1.8	
0	0							2		20		160			1.1	
0	0							2		20		130			0.9	
2	0	0.7	0.3	2.9	0.4		4.5	0		40	172	709	153		1.4	0.4
1	10	0.3	0.3	1.8	0.5		3.6	0		20	73	255	139		1.3	0.4
1	14	8.1	0.1	0	0.2		0.1	0	0.4	56	150	499	269	44	1.8	0.9
<1	0	0.8	<0.1	0.6	0.1		0.4	0		7	48	220	15		0.3	0.1
<1	0	0.1	<0.1	0	<0.1		<0.1	0	1.3	17	42	431	50	4	0.6	0.4
1	0	2.2	0.2	1.5	0.1		0.9	0		11	106	536	163		1	0.3

ERA, EatRight Analysis CD-ROM; **AMT,** amount; **WT,** weight; **WTR,** water; **CAL,** calories; **PROT,** protein; **CARB**, carbohydrate; **FIBR,** fiber; **FAT,** fat; **SATF,** saturated fat; **MONO,** monounsaturated fat; **POLY,** polyunsaturated fat

ERA CODE	FOOD DESCRIPTION	AMT	UNIT	WT (g)	WTR (g)	CAL (kcal)	PROT (g)	CARB (g)	FIBR (g)	FAT (g)	SATF (g)	MONO (g)	POLY (g)
Meat Substitutes, Tofu, Vegetarian Foods (continued)													
Morningstar Farms (continued)													
7722	Vege patties	1	ea	67	40	119	11	10	4	4	0.5	1.1	2.2
7746	Vegetarian grillers	1	ea	64	35	139	14	5	3	7	1.7	2.2	3
Natural Touch													
7792	Black bean burger	1	ea	78	46	123	13	15	5	1	0.2	0.3	0.5
7758	Lentil rice loaf	1	pce	90	57	166	8	14	4	9	2.6	1.7	4.3
7669	Nine bean loaf	1	ea	85	55	147	8	13	6	7	1.2	2.4	3.4
7670	Vegan burger	1	ea	85	61	91	14	8	4	1	0.1	0.3	0.2
Worthington Foods													
8127	Vegetarian frank/wiener, jumbo	1	ea	76		80	16	4	1	0	0	0	0
7634	Vegetarian beef, frozen	3	pce	55	32	113	9	4	3	7	1.2	2.7	2.6
7732	Vegetarian burger	0.25	cup	55	39	60	9	2	1	2	0.3	0.5	1.1
7636	Vegetarian chicken, frozen	2	pce	57	39	86	10	1	1	5	0.8	1.2	2.6
7610	Vegetarian choplets, canned	2	pce	92	66	93	17	3	2	2	0.9	0.3	0.3
7607	Vegetarian country stew, frozen	1	cup	240	195	208	13	20	5	9	1.6	2.3	4.8
7639	Vegetarian cutlets, canned	1	pce	61	43	66	11	3	2	1	0.5	0.4	0.2
7632	Vegetarian egg rolls, frozen	1	ea	85		181	6	20	2	8	1.7	4.5	2.3
7642	Vegetarian fillets, frozen	2	pce	85	48	183	16	8	4	10	1.9	3.5	4.3
7734	Vegetarian leanies, frozen	1	pce	40	22	106	7	2	1	8	1.3	2.9	3.5
7618	Vegetarian salami, frozen	3	pce	57	32	130	12	2	2	8	0.9	1.4	5.8
7624	Vegetarian tuno, frozen	1	ea	55	39	83	6	2	1	5	0.9	1.3	3.2
7626	Vegetarian veelets, frozen	1	ea	85		171	15	10	5	8	1.5	2.5	3.9
Nuts, Seeds, and Products													
4548	Almonds, blanched, sliced	1	cup	105	5	610	23	21	11	53	4.1	33.9	12.6
4503	Almonds, slivered, pkd measure	1	cup	108	6	624	23	21	13	55	4.2	34.7	13.2
4566	Almonds, toasted, whole	1	oz	28.35	1	167	6	6	3	14	1.4	9.4	3
4525	Black walnuts, chopped	1	cup	125	5	759	30	15	6	71	4.5	15.9	46.9
4519	Cashews, dry roasted+salt	1	cup	137	2	786	21	45	4	63	12.5	37.4	10.7
4621	Cashews, dry roast, no salt	1	cup	137	2	786	21	45	4	63	12.5	37.4	10.7
4596	Cashews, oil roasted	1	cup	130	5	749	21	37	5	63	12.4	36.9	10.6
4622	Cashews, oil roast, no salt	1	cup	130	5	749	21	37	5	63	12.4	36.9	10.6
4538	Chestnuts, roasted	1	cup	143	58	350	5	76	7	3	0.6	1.1	1.2
4649	Coconut cream, canned	1	cup	296	211	568	8	25	7	52	46.5	2.2	0.6
4528	Coconut milk, raw	1	cup	240	162	552	5	13	5	57	50.7	2.4	0.6
4511	Coconut, dried, sweet, shred	1	cup	93	12	466	3	44	4	33	29.3	1.4	0.4
4510	Coconut, dried, unsweet	1	cup	78	2	515	5	19	13	50	44.6	2.1	0.6
4508	Coconut, raw piece, 2.5x2 in	1	pce	45	21	159	1	7	4	15	13.4	0.6	0.2
4556	English walnuts, chopped	1	cup	120	5	785	18	16	8	78	7.4	10.7	56.6
4557	English walnuts, halves	1	cup	100		654	15	14	7	65	6.1	8.9	47.2
4514	Filberts/hazelnuts, chopped	1	cup	115	6	722	17	19	11	70	5.1	52.5	9.1
4513	Filberts/hazelnuts, whole	1	cup	135	7	848	20	23	13	82	6	61.7	10.7
4587	Macadamia nuts, oil roasted	1	cup	134	2	962	10	17	12	102	15.4	80.9	1.8
4533	Mixed nuts+pnuts, oil roast	1	cup	142	3	876	24	30	14	80	12.4	45	18.9

< = Trace amount present   Blank = Not available

CHOL, cholesterol; **V,** vitamin; **THI,** thiamin; **RIB,** riboflavin; **NIA,** niacin; **FOL,** folate;
CALC, calcium; **PHOS,** phosphate; **SOD,** sodium; **POT,** potassium; **MAG,** magnesium

CHOL (mg)	V-A (RE)	THI (mg)	RIB (mg)	NIA (mg)	V-B6 (mg)	FOL (μg)	V-B12 (μg)	V-C (mg)	V-E (mg)	CALC (mg)	PHOS (mg)	SOD (mg)	POT (mg)	MAG (mg)	IRON (mg)	ZINC (mg)
1	77	6.5	0.1	0	0	29	0	0	1	48	124	382	180	29	1.2	0.6
2	0	11.7	0.2	3	0.4		4.9	0		43	111	256	127		1.2	0.5
1	15							0		76	156	323	228		1.9	1
2	78	0.1	0.1	0	<0.1		0.1	0		21	202	366	161		1.2	1
2	151	0.1	0.1	0				1		27	180	319	187		0.6	0.9
0	0	0.3	0.6	4.1	0.2	246	0	0	<0.1	87	181	382	434	16	2.9	0.7
0	0							1		40		590			0.7	
0	0	0.9	0.3	6.5	0.6		4	0		4	92	624	44		2.6	0.2
0	0	0.1	0.1	2	0.2		1.1	0		4	56	269	25		1.7	0.4
1	0	0.3	0.1	1.2	0.2		0.9	0		12	113	374	276		2.1	0.3
0	0	<0.1	0.1	0	0.1		0	0		6	75	500	40		0.4	0.7
2	216	1.8	0.3	4.2	0.9		3.7	0		51	187	826	270		5.1	1
0	0	<0.1	<0.1	0	<0.1		0	0		4	50	340	29		0.2	0.4
1	0	1.2	0.2	0	<0.1		0.1	0		15	93	384	96		0.6	0.3
2	0	0.7	0.1	1	0.4		2.7	0		15	183	749	132		2.1	0.9
1	0	0.2	0.1	1	0.2		0.8	0		25	93	425	43		0.9	0.2
2	0	0.8	0.1	1.1	0.3		0.6	0		26	67	930	93		1.4	0.3
<1	0	0.1	<0.1	1.2	0.3		2	0		20	88	287	34		1.2	0.4
1	0	1.8	0.2	1.6	0.3		3	0		36		388	121		0.5	0.6
0	1	0.2	0.6	3.8	0.1	32	0	0	26.2	227	504	29	721	289	3.9	3.3
0	1	0.3	0.9	4.2	0.1	31	0	0	28.3	268	512	1	786	297	4.6	3.6
0	0	<0.1	0.2	0.8	<0.1	18	0	<1	6.7	80	156	3	219	86	1.4	1.4
0	38	0.3	0.1	0.9	0.7	82	0	4	3.3	72	580	1	655	252	3.8	4.3
0	0	0.3	0.3	1.9	0.3	95	0	0	15.1	62	671	877	774	356	8.2	7.7
0	0	0.3	0.3	1.9	0.3	95	0	0	10.2	62	671	22	774	356	8.2	7.7
0	0	0.6	0.2	2.3	0.3	88	0	0	14.3	53	554	814	689	332	5.3	6.2
0	0	0.6	0.2	2.3	0.3	88	0	0	10.4	53	554	22	689	332	5.3	6.2
0	3	0.3	0.2	1.9	0.7	100	0	37	1.7	41	153	3	846	47	1.3	0.8
0	0	0.1	0.1	0.1	0.1	42	0	5	2.2	3	65	148	299	50	1.5	1.8
0	0	0.1	0	1.8	0.1	39	0	7	1.8	38	240	36	631	89	3.9	1.6
0	0	<0.1	<0.1	0.4	0.3	8	0	1	1.3	14	100	244	313	46	1.8	1.7
0	0	<0.1	0.1	0.5	0.2	7	0	1	1.1	20	161	29	424	70	2.6	1.6
0	0	<0.1	<0.1	0.2	<0.1	12	0	1	0.3	6	51	9	160	14	1.1	0.5
0	5	0.4	0.2	2.3	0.6	118	0	2	3.5	125	415	2	529	190	3.5	3.7
0	4	0.3	0.2	1.9	0.5	98	0	1	2.9	104	346	2	441	158	2.9	3.1
0	5	0.7	0.1	2.1	0.6	130	0	7	17.5	131	334	0	782	187	5.4	2.8
0	5	0.9	0.2	2.4	0.8	152	0	8	20.5	154	392	0	918	220	6.3	3.3
0	1	0.3	0.1	2.7	0.3	21	0	0	19	60	268	348	441	157	2.4	1.5
0	3	0.7	0.3	7.2	0.3	118	0	1	17	153	659	16	825	334	4.6	7.2

ERA, EatRight Analysis CD-ROM; **AMT,** amount; **WT,** weight; **WTR,** water; **CAL,** calories; **PROT,** protein; **CARB**, carbohydrate; **FIBR,** fiber; **FAT,** fat; **SATF,** saturated fat; **MONO,** monounsaturated fat; **POLY,** polyunsaturated fat

Nuts, Seeds, and Products (continued)

ERA CODE	FOOD DESCRIPTION	AMT	UNIT	WT (g)	WTR (g)	CAL (kcal)	PROT (g)	CARB (g)	FIBR (g)	FAT (g)	SATF (g)	MONO (g)	POLY (g)
4594	Mixed nuts, no pnts, oil roast	1	cup	144	5	886	22	32	8	81	13.1	47.7	16.5
4668	Peanut butter, natural	2	Tbs	32	<1	187	8	7	2	16	2.2	7.9	5
4626	Peanut butter, smooth, salted	2	Tbs	32	<1	188	8	7	2	16	3.1	7.5	4.5
4576	Peanut butter, chunky, no salt	2	Tbs	32	<1	188	8	7	2	16	3.1	7.5	4.5
4590	Peanuts, dry roasted w/salt	1	oz	28.35	<1	166	7	6	2	14	2	7	4.4
4542	Peanuts, oil roasted, unsalted	1	cup	133	3	773	35	25	9	66	9.1	32.5	20.7
4578	Pecans, dried halves	1	cup	108	4	746	10	15	10	78	6.7	44	23.3
4577	Pecans, dried, chopped	1	cup	119	4	822	11	16	11	86	7.3	48.5	25.7
4554	Pine nuts/pinon, dried	10	ea	1	<1	6	<1	<1	<1	1	0.1	0.2	0.3
4520	Pistachio nuts, dried	1	cup	128	5	705	26	37	13	55	6.8	29	16.7
4564	Pumpkin seeds, roasted+salt	1	cup	64	3	285	12	34	3	12	2.3	3.9	5.7
4523	Sesame seeds, whole, dried	1	cup	144	7	825	26	34	17	72	10	27	31.4
4545	Sunflower seeds, dry	1	cup	144	8	821	33	27	15	71	7.5	13.6	47.1
4552	Sunflower seeds, oil roasted	1	cup	135	4	830	29	20	9	78	8.1	14.8	51.2
4532	Tahini (sesame butter)	1	Tbs	15	<1	91	3	3	1	8	1.2	3.2	3.7

Poultry

Chicken

ERA CODE	FOOD DESCRIPTION	AMT	UNIT	WT (g)	WTR (g)	CAL (kcal)	PROT (g)	CARB (g)	FIBR (g)	FAT (g)	SATF (g)	MONO (g)	POLY (g)
15016	Boned chicken+broth, canned	1	ea	142	97	234	31	0	0	11	3.1	4.5	2.5
15003	Chicken breast+skin, flour fried	1	ea	196	111	435	62	3	<1	17	4.8	6.9	3.8
15001	Chicken breast+skin, roastd	1	ea	196	122	386	58	0	0	15	4.3	5.9	3.3
15057	Chicken breast, no skin, fried	1	ea	172	104	322	58	1	0	8	2.2	3	1.8
15004	Chicken breast, no skin, roasted	1	ea	172	112	284	53	0	0	6	1.7	2.1	1.3
15042	Chicken drumstick, fried	1	ea	42	26	82	12	0	0	3	0.9	1.2	0.8
15008	Chicken drumstick, roasted	1	ea	52	33	112	14	0	0	6	1.6	2.2	1.3
15035	Chicken drumstk, no skin, roast	1	ea	44	29	76	12	0	0	2	0.7	0.8	0.6
15028	Chicken meat, all, fried	1	cup	140	81	307	43	2	<1	13	3.4	4.7	3
15000	Chicken meat, all, roasted	1	cup	140	89	266	40	0	0	10	2.9	3.7	2.4
15006	Chicken meat, all, stewed	1	cup	140	94	248	38	0	0	9	2.6	3.3	2.2
15902	Chicken patty, breaded, cooked	1	ea	75	37	213	12	11	<1	13	4.1	6.4	1.7
15009	Chicken thigh+skin, flour fried	1	ea	62	34	162	17	2	<1	9	2.5	3.6	2.1
15010	Chicken thigh+skin, roasted	1	ea	62	37	153	16	0	0	10	2.7	3.8	2.1
15011	Chicken thigh, no skin, fried	1	ea	52	31	113	15	1	0	5	1.4	2	1.3
15012	Chicken thigh, no skin, roast	1	ea	52	33	109	13	0	0	6	1.6	2.2	1.3
15002	Chicken wing+skin, roasted	1	ea	34	19	99	9	0	0	7	1.9	2.6	1.4
15029	Chicken wing, flour fried	1	ea	32	16	103	8	1	<1	7	1.9	2.8	1.6
15027	Chicken, dark meat, roasted	1	cup	140	88	287	38	0	0	14	3.7	5	3.2
15032	Chicken, light meat, roasted	1	cup	140	91	242	43	0	0	6	1.8	2.2	1.4
15903	Chicken wings, buffalo/spicy	1	pce	16	9	49	4	<1	<1	3	0.9	1.3	0.9

Turkey

ERA CODE	FOOD DESCRIPTION	AMT	UNIT	WT (g)	WTR (g)	CAL (kcal)	PROT (g)	CARB (g)	FIBR (g)	FAT (g)	SATF (g)	MONO (g)	POLY (g)
16003	Ground turkey, patty, cooked	1	ea	82	49	193	22	0	0	11	2.8	4	2.6
16040	Tom turkey, no skin, roasted	1	cup	140	91	235	41	0	0	7	2.2	1.4	1.9
16002	Turkey dark meat, roasted	1	cup	140	88	262	40	0	0	10	3.4	2.3	3
16000	Turkey meat, all, roasted	1	cup	140	91	238	41	0	0	7	2.3	1.4	2
16001	Turkey white meat, roasted	1	cup	140	96	196	42	0	0	2	0.5	0.3	0.4

< = Trace amount present   Blank = Not available

CHOL, cholesterol; **V,** vitamin; **THI,** thiamin; **RIB,** riboflavin; **NIA,** niacin; **FOL,** folate;
CALC, calcium; **PHOS,** phosphate; **SOD,** sodium; **POT,** potassium; **MAG,** magnesium

CHOL (mg)	V-A (RE)	THI (mg)	RIB (mg)	NIA (mg)	V-B6 (mg)	FOL (μg)	V-B12 (μg)	V-C (mg)	V-E (mg)	CALC (mg)	PHOS (mg)	SOD (mg)	POT (mg)	MAG (mg)	IRON (mg)	ZINC (mg)
0	3	0.7	0.7	2.8	0.3	81	0	1	17.3	153	646	16	783	361	3.7	6.7
0	0	0.1	<0.1	4.3	0.1	46	0	0	2.4	17	114	2	210	56	0.7	1.1
0	0	<0.1	<0.1	4.4	0.1	29	0	0	2.4	13	101	156	239	51	0.6	0.9
0	0	<0.1	<0.1	4.4	0.1	29	0	0	3.2	13	101	5	239	51	0.6	0.9
0	0	0.1	<0.1	3.8	0.1	41	0	0	2.8	15	101	230	186	50	0.6	0.9
0	0	0.3	0.1	19	0.3	167	0	0	9.9	117	688	8	907	246	2.4	8.8
0	8	0.7	0.1	1.3	0.2	24	0	1	4	76	299	0	443	131	2.7	4.9
0	9	0.8	0.2	1.4	0.2	26	0	1	4.4	83	330	0	488	144	3	5.4
0	<1	<0.1	<0.1	<0.1	<0.1	1	0	<1	0.1	<1	<1	1	6	2	<0.1	<0.1
0	71	1.1	0.2	1.7	2.2	65	0	6	5.9	137	627	1	1250	155	5.5	2.8
0	4	<0.1	<0.1	0.2	<0.1	6	0	<1	2.5	35	59	368	588	168	2.1	6.6
0	1	1.1	0.4	6.5	1.1	139	0	0	3.3	1404	906	16	674	505	21	11.2
0	7	3.3	0.4	6.5	1.1	327	0	2	72.4	167	1015	4	992	510	9.7	7.3
0	7	0.4	0.4	5.6	1.1	316	0	2	67.9	76	1537	814	652	171	9	7
0	1	0.2	<0.1	0.8	<0.1	15	0	0	0.3	21	118	<1	69	53	1	1.6
88	48	<0.1	0.2	9	0.5	6	0.4	3	0.6	20	158	714	196	17	2.2	2
174	29	0.2	0.3	26.9	1.1	12	0.7	0	1.4	31	457	149	508	59	2.3	2.2
165	53	0.1	0.2	24.9	1.1	8	0.6	0	1.1	27	419	139	480	53	2.1	2
156	12	0.1	0.2	25.4	1.1	7	0.6	0	0.7	28	423	136	475	53	2	1.9
146	10	0.1	0.2	23.6	1	7	0.6	0	0.7	26	392	127	440	50	1.8	1.7
39	8	<0.1	0.1	2.6	0.2	4	0.1	0	0.2	5	78	40	104	10	0.6	1.4
47	16	<0.1	0.1	3.1	0.2	4	0.2	0	0.3	6	91	47	119	12	0.7	1.5
41	8	<0.1	0.1	2.7	0.2	4	0.1	0	0.3	5	81	42	108	11	0.6	1.4
132	25	0.1	0.3	13.5	0.7	10	0.5	0	0.6	24	287	127	360	38	1.9	3.1
125	22	0.1	0.2	12.8	0.7	8	0.5	0	0.8	21	273	120	340	35	1.7	2.9
116	21	0.1	0.2	8.6	0.4	8	0.3	0	0.7	20	210	98	252	29	1.6	2.8
45	22	0.1	0.1	5	0.2	8	0.2	<1	1.5	12	150	399	184	15	0.9	0.8
60	18	0.1	0.2	4.3	0.2	7	0.2	0	0.7	9	116	55	147	16	0.9	1.6
58	30	<0.1	0.1	3.9	0.2	4	0.2	0	0.7	7	108	52	138	14	0.8	1.5
53	11	<0.1	0.1	3.7	0.2	5	0.2	0	0.4	7	103	49	135	14	0.8	1.5
49	10	<0.1	0.1	3.4	0.2	4	0.2	0	0.4	6	95	46	124	12	0.7	1.3
29	16	<0.1	<0.1	2.3	0.1	1	0.1	0	0.5	5	51	28	63	6	0.4	0.6
26	12	<0.1	<0.1	2.1	0.1	2	0.1	0	0.5	5	48	25	57	6	0.4	0.6
130	31	0.1	0.3	9.2	0.5	11	0.4	0	1	21	251	130	336	32	1.9	3.9
119	13	0.1	0.2	17.4	0.8	6	0.5	0	0.5	21	302	108	346	38	1.5	1.7
13	9	<0.1	<0.1	1	0.1	<1	<0.1	<1	0.1	2	24	13	29	3	0.2	0.3
84	0	<0.1	0.1	4	0.3	6	0.3	0	0.3	20	161	88	221	20	1.6	2.3
108	0	0.1	0.3	7.4	0.7	11	0.5	0	0.6	35	300	104	421	36	2.5	4.4
119	0	0.1	0.3	5.1	0.5	13	0.5	0	1.2	45	286	111	406	34	3.3	6.2
106	0	0.1	0.3	7.6	0.6	10	0.5	0	0.6	35	298	98	417	36	2.5	4.3
120	0	0.1	0.2	9.7	0.8	8	0.5	0	0.1	21	302	78	388	39	2.2	2.9

ERA, EatRight Analysis CD-ROM; **AMT,** amount; **WT,** weight; **WTR,** water; **CAL,** calories; **PROT,** protein; **CARB,** carbohydrate; **FIBR,** fiber; **FAT,** fat; **SATF,** saturated fat; **MONO,** monounsaturated fat; **POLY,** polyunsaturated fat

ERA CODE	FOOD DESCRIPTION	AMT	UNIT	WT (g)	WTR (g)	CAL (kcal)	PROT (g)	CARB (g)	FIBR (g)	FAT (g)	SATF (g)	MONO (g)	POLY (g)
Poultry (continued)													
Turkey (continued)													
16276	Turkey chunk white, cnd, water	0.25	cup	62		90	16	4	1	2	0.5		
Duck, Emu, Ostrich, and Other													
15069	Cornish game hen, roasted	1	ea	306	180	796	68	0	0	56	15.4	24.5	11
14001	Duck+skin, domestic, roasted	1	cup	140	73	472	27	0	0	40	13.5	18.1	5.1
14000	Duck, meat only, roasted	1	ea	442	284	888	104	0	0	50	18.4	16.4	6.3
16289	Emu thigh, raw	3	oz	85		79	17			1			
14002	Goose meat, no skin, roasted	1	ea	1182	676	2813	342	0	0	150	53.9	51.3	18.2
14003	Goose+skin, domestic, roast	0.5	ea	774	402	2360	195	0	0	170	53.2	79.3	19.5
16332	Ostrich, tenderloin, ckd	1	oz	28.35	19	38	7	0	0	1	0.3	0.4	0.3
Salad Dressings, Dips, and Mayonnaise													
Dips													
7083	Jalapeno pepper bean dip	1	cup	262	180	376	16	49	18	14	1.9	3.4	8.2
8136	Sour cream dip, cup meas	1	cup	243	160	536	9	20	2	48	29.5	14.2	1.9
Mayonnaise													
8046	Mayonnaise	1	Tbs	13.8	2	99	<1	<1	0	11	1.6	3.1	5.7
8069	Mayonnaise, fat free	1	Tbs	16	13	11	<1	2	<1	<1	0.1		
8032	Mayonnaise, imitation	1	Tbs	15	9	35	<1	2	0	3	0.5	0.7	1.6
8033	Mayonnaise, low cal	1	Tbs	15	9	35	<1	2	0	3	0.5	0.7	1.6
8148	Mayonnaise, low cal, low sod	1	Tbs	14	9	32	<1	2	0	3	0.5	0.6	1.5
8021	Miracle Whip	1	Tbs	14.7	6	57	<1	4	0	5	0.7	1.3	2.6
8122	Miracle Whip, light	1	Tbs	14	8	36	<1	3	0	3	0.4	0.6	1.5
Salad Dressings, Lower Calorie/Fat/Sodium/Cholesterol													
8023	1000 Island dressing, low cal	1	Tbs	15.31	11	24	<1	2	<1	2	0.2	0.4	0.9
286	Benecol French dressing	1	Tbs	15		65	0	3	0	6	1		
287	Benecol ranch dressing	1	Tbs	14.5		65	0	2	0	6	1		
8498	Catalina dressing, fat free	1	Tbs	17.5		22	0	6	<1	0	0	0	0
8017	Dijon vinaigrette, lite	1	Tbs	15	12	16	<1	1	<1	1	0.2	0.3	0.9
8499	French dressing, fat free	1	Tbs	17.5		20	0	6	<1	0	0	0	0
8014	French dressing, low cal	1	Tbs	16.25	11	22	<1	4	0	8	0.1	0.2	0.6
8504	Honey dijon dressing, fat free	1	Tbs	17.5		25	<1	6	<1	0	0	0	0
8491	Italian dressing, fat free	1	Tbs	16.5	13	10	<1	2	<1	<1	0.1		
8016	Italian dressing, low cal	1	Tbs	15	12	16	<1	1	<1	1	0.2	0.3	0.9
8493	Ranch dressing, fat free	1	Tbs	17.5	11	24	<1	5	<1	<1	<0.1		
Salad Dressings, Regular													
8024	1000 Island dressing	1	Tbs	15.625	7	59	<1	2	0	6	0.9	1.3	3.1
8013	Blue cheese dressing	1	Tbs	15.31	5	77	1	1	0	8	1.5	1.9	4.3
8066	Caesar salad dressing	1	Tbs	11.5	4	53	1	<1	<1	5	0.9	3.6	0.5
8015	French dressing	1	Tbs	15.6	6	67	<1	3	0	6	1.5	1.2	3.4
8124	Honey mustard dressing	1	Tbs	15.6	5	51	<1	7	<1	3	0.3	0.9	1.4
8020	Italian dressing	1	Tbs	14.7	6	69	<1	1	0	7	1	1.6	4.1
8035	Oil & vinegar dressing	1	Tbs	16	8	72	0	<1	0	8	1.5	2.4	3.9

< = Trace amount present   Blank = Not available

CHOL, cholesterol; **V,** vitamin; **THI,** thiamin; **RIB,** riboflavin; **NIA,** niacin; **FOL,** folate;
CALC, calcium; **PHOS,** phosphate; **SOD,** sodium; **POT,** potassium; **MAG,** magnesium

CHOL (mg)	V-A (RE)	THI (mg)	RIB (mg)	NIA (mg)	V-B6 (mg)	FOL (μg)	V-B12 (μg)	V-C (mg)	V-E (mg)	CALC (mg)	PHOS (mg)	SOD (mg)	POT (mg)	MAG (mg)	IRON (mg)	ZINC (mg)
35	0							0		0		220			0	
401	98	0.2	0.6	18	0.9	6	0.9	2	0.8	40	447	196	750	55	2.8	4.6
118	88	0.2	0.4	6.8	0.3	8	0.4	0	1.8	15	218	83	286	22	3.8	2.6
393	102	1.1	2.1	22.5	1.1	44	1.8	0	7.7	53	897	287	1113	88	11.9	11.5
42															4.2	
1134	142	1.1	4.6	48.2	5.6	142	5.8	0	33	165	3652	898	4586	296	33.9	37.5
704	162	0.6	2.5	32.3	2.9	15	3.2	0	20	101	2089	542	2546	170	21.9	20.3
27												20			0.8	
0	78	0.3	0.1	0.9	0.3	188	0	37	3.1	86	283	12	793	101	3.9	1.8
100	437	0.1	0.4	1.1	0.1	27	0.7	2	1.5	288	252	1820	449	37	0.4	0.7
8	12	0	0	0	0.1	1	<0.1	0	8	2	4	78	5	<1	0.1	<0.1
2	3							0	0.5	1	4	120	8		<0.1	
4	0	0	0	0	0	0	0	0	2.7	<1	<1	75	2	<1	0	<0.1
4	0	0	0	0	0	0	0	0	2.7	<1	<1	75	2	<1	0	<0.1
3	1	0	<0.1	0	0	<1	<0.1	0	0.5	0	0	15	1	0	0	<0.1
4	12	<0.1	<0.1	<0.1	<0.1	1	<0.1	0	4.4	2	4	104	1	<1	<0.1	<0.1
4	9	<0.1	<0.1	0	<0.1	1	<0.1	0	0.6	2	4	99	1	<1	<0.1	<0.1
2	15	<0.1	<0.1	<0.1	<0.1	1	<0.1	0	0.2	2	3	153	17	<1	0.1	<0.1
0	0							0		0		85			0	
0	0							0		0		125			0	
0	75							0		0		180	30		0	
1	0	0	0	0	0	0	0	0	1.4	<1	1	118	2	0	<0.1	<0.1
0	75							0		0		150	20		0	
0	21	0	0	0	0	0	0	0	0.8	2	2	128	13	0	0.1	<0.1
0	0							0		0		165	25		0.2	
<1	5							<1		7	34	215	19		<0.1	
1	0	0	0	0	0	0	0	0	1.4	<1	1	118	2	0	<0.1	<0.1
<1	<1							<1		5	14	177	15		<0.1	
4	15	<0.1	<0.1	<0.1	<0.1	1	<0.1	0	0.2	2	2	109	18	<1	0.1	<0.1
3	10	<0.1	<0.1	<0.1	<0.1	1	0.4	<1	7.5	12	11	168	6	0	<0.1	<0.1
12	6	<0.1	<0.1	0.5	<0.1	2	0.1	1	0.7	22	19	198	20	3	0.2	0.1
0	20	<0.1	<0.1	0	<0.1	1	<0.1	0	5.9	2	2	214	12	0	0.1	<0.1
0	0	<0.1	<0.1	<0.1	<0.1	<1	0	<1	0.6	3	3	37	10	2	0.1	0.1
0	4	<0.1	<0.1	0	<0.1	1	<0.1	0	1.5	1	1	116	2	<1	<0.1	<0.1
0	0	0	0	0	0	0	0	0	8.3	0	0	<1	1	0	0	0

ERA, EatRight Analysis CD-ROM; **AMT,** amount; **WT,** weight; **WTR,** water; **CAL,** calories; **PROT,** protein; **CARB**, carbohydrate; **FIBR,** fiber; **FAT,** fat; **SATF,** saturated fat; **MONO,** monounsaturated fat; **POLY,** polyunsaturated fat

ERA CODE	FOOD DESCRIPTION	AMT	UNIT	WT (g)	WTR (g)	CAL (kcal)	PROT (g)	CARB (g)	FIBR (g)	FAT (g)	SATF (g)	MONO (g)	POLY (g)
Salad Dressings, Dips, and Mayonnaise (continued)													
Salad Dressings, Regular (continued)													
8022	Russian dressing	1	Tbs	15.31	5	76	<1	2	0	8	1.1	1.8	4.5
8019	Vinaigrette dressing	1	Tbs	14.7	6	69	<1	1	0	7	1	1.6	4.1
8123	Yogurt dressing	1	Tbs	15.4	13	11	<1	1	<1	1	0.3	0.2	0.1
Salads													
56109	Carrot raisin salad	1	cup	175	101	405	3	42	4	28	4	7.8	14.5
56628	Chef-style salad	1.5	cup	326	269	267	26	5		16	8.2	5.2	1.4
56002	Chicken salad w/celery	0.5	cup	78	41	268	11	1	<1	25	3.1	4.5	15.8
56253	Crab salad	1	cup	208	153	282	27	11	1	14	2	3.5	7.1
5638	Cucumber salad w/vinegar	1	cup	159	145	48	1	12	1	<1	<0.1	<0.1	0.1
56003	Egg salad	1	cup	183	105	584	17	3	0	56	10.5	17.4	23.9
5637	Mixed salad greens/lettuce	1	cup	55	52	9	1	2	1	<1	<0.1	<0.1	0.1
56005	Potato salad+mayo+eggs	1	cup	250	190	358	7	28	3	20	3.6	6.2	9.3
56257	Seafood salad	1	cup	208	152	328	26	5	1	23	3.2	16	2.4
56256	Shrimp salad	1	cup	182	131	282	27	6	1	17	2.6	4.5	8.4
5537	Spinach salad, no dressing	1	cup	74	51	108	5	11	2	5	1.4	2.2	0.7
56916	Tabbouleh/tabbuli	1	cup	160	124	199	3	16	4	15	2	10.8	1.4
56643	Taco salad	1.5	cup	198	143	279	13	24		15	6.8	5.2	1.7
56118	Three-bean salad	1	cup	150	121	140	4	15	5	8	1.1	1.7	4.4
5677	Tossed green salad	0.75	cup	104	98	19	1	4	1	<1	<0.1	<0.1	0.1
56007	Tuna salad	1	cup	205	129	383	33	19	0	19	3.2	5.9	8.4
56006	Waldorf salad	1	cup	137	79	408	4	13	2	40	4.2	7.3	27
Sandwiches													
10047	Beef sand steak, Steak Ums	1	ea	41	24	104	10	0	0	7	2.6	2.9	0.2
56008	BLT sandwich, firm white	1	ea	133		336	11	32	2	18	4.5	6.1	6.1
56281	Bologna sandwich	1	ea	83	34	256	7	26	1	13	4.1	6.3	2.1
56016	Chicken salad san, firm white	1	ea	118.8		397	12	35	2	23	3.7	6	12
57519	Chicken fajita w/cheese on pita	1	ea	207	142	311	22	28	2	12	4.5	3.4	3.3
56020	Corned beef+swiss on rye	1	ea	156		420	28	22	<1	26	9.4	7.4	6.3
56024	Egg salad sandwich on white	1	ea	125.6		409	11	35	2	25	4.4	6.8	12
66011	Fish sandwich+cheese+tartar sc	1	ea	183	83	523	21	48	<1	29	8.1	8.9	9.4
56268	French dip sandwich au jus	1	ea	193	118	363	25	34	2	13	4.7	5.8	0.9
69017	Grilled chicken sandwich	1	ea	113		210	18	24	2	5	2		
56012	Grilled cheese sandw on white	1	ea	127.8		428	19	34	1	24	13.1	7.5	2
56272	Gyro sandwich	1	ea	105	67	170	12	21	1	4	1.5	1.4	0.4
56033	Ham & swiss on rye sandwich	1	ea	149.5		338	22	22	<1	19	6.5	5.1	6
56066	Ham salad sandwich on wheat	1	ea	130.6		356	11	35	3	20	4.5	6.8	7.4
56031	Ham sandwich on wheat	1	ea	156.3		329	22	28	3	14	2.7	4.4	6
56267	Pastrami sandwich	1	ea	134	71	331	14	27	2	18	6.2	8.7	1
56038	Patty melt sandwich on rye	1	ea	181.9		561	37	22	3	37	13.2	11.7	8.4
56040	Peanut butter & jelly on white	1	ea	101		351	12	47	3	15	3.1	6.7	3.9
56266	Reuben sandwich, grilled	1	ea	181	97	464	21	30	3	29	9.9	9.7	6.7
56046	Roast beef sandwich on wheat	1	ea	155.8		397	29	32	3	17	3.2	4.3	8.3
56671	Submarine sandwich w/coldcuts	1	ea	228	132	456	22	51	2	19	6.8	8.2	2.3

< = Trace amount present   Blank = Not available

CHOL, cholesterol; **V,** vitamin; **THI,** thiamin; **RIB,** riboflavin; **NIA,** niacin; **FOL,** folate;
CALC, calcium; **PHOS,** phosphate; **SOD,** sodium; **POT,** potassium; **MAG,** magnesium

CHOL (mg)	V-A (RE)	THI (mg)	RIB (mg)	NIA (mg)	V-B6 (mg)	FOL (μg)	V-B12 (μg)	V-C (mg)	V-E (mg)	CALC (mg)	PHOS (mg)	SOD (mg)	POT (mg)	MAG (mg)	IRON (mg)	ZINC (mg)
3	32	<0.1	<0.1	0.1	<0.1	2	<0.1	1	7.3	3	6	133	24	<1	0.1	0.1
0	4	<0.1	<0.1	0	<0.1	1	<0.1	0	1.5	1	1	116	2	<1	<0.1	<0.1
2	4	<0.1	<0.1	<0.1	<0.1	1	<0.1	<1	<0.1	15	12	6	22	2	<0.1	0.1
20	2889	0.2	0.1	1.3	0.4	18	0.1	11	20.5	53	92	235	630	28	1.5	0.4
140	137	0.4	0.4	6	0.4	101	0.8	16		235	401	743	401	49	2	3.1
48	31	<0.1	0.1	3.3	0.3	8	0.2	1	6.3	16	80	200	138	11	0.6	0.8
142	37	0.2	0.1	4.5	0.3	79	9.8	7	2.8	157	292	700	536	49	1.5	5.7
0	20	<0.1	<0.1	0.2	0.1	16	0	6	0.1	19	29	3	206	21	0.5	0.2
581	262	0.1	0.7	0.1	0.5	61	1.6	0	7.7	74	238	464	181	13	1.8	1.4
0	150	<0.1	0.1	0.2	<0.1	64	0	9	0.4	30	18	14	174	13	0.7	0.2
170	82	0.2	0.2	2.2	0.4	17	0	25	19	48	130	1322	635	38	1.6	0.8
132	51	0.1	0.1	2.4	0.2	31	1.8	12	4	92	283	352	503	54	2	3.3
206	42	0.1	0.1	3.3	0.3	15	1.3	6	3.4	87	280	392	366	52	3.4	1.5
77	176	0.1	0.3	1.7	0.1	60	0.2	7	0.9	46	83	227	242	27	1.5	0.6
0	69	0.1	0.1	1.1	0.1	31	0	28	2.2	29	64	799	246	36	1.2	0.5
44	77	0.1	0.4	2.5	0.2	83	0.6	4		192	142	762	416	51	2.3	2.7
0	20	0.1	0.1	0.4	<0.1	56	<0.1	4	1.7	35	76	520	246	27	1.5	0.6
0	209	0.1	<0.1	0.4	0.1	36	0	11	0.4	14	24	11	201	11	0.5	0.2
27	55	0.1	0.1	13.7	0.2	16	2.5	5	21.9	35	365	824	365	39	2	1.1
21	39	0.1	<0.1	0.4	0.4	27	0.1	6	27.6	43	84	236	270	39	0.9	0.6
33	0	<0.1	0.1	1.9	0.1	4	0.8	0	0.1	3	66	29	128	9	1	2.2
22	31	0.4	0.2	3.5	0.1	37	0.3	12	6.1	67	133	630	252	22	2.2	1
16	37	0.3	0.2	2.7	0.1	19	0.4	<1	0.8	60	74	598	112	15	2	0.9
33	24	0.3	0.2	4	0.2	29	0.1	1	14.8	76	114	498	158	20	2.3	0.9
51	102	0.3	0.3	5.1	0.3	35	0.4	33	1.5	187	221	784	372	37	2.1	2
82	81	0.2	0.3	2.7	0.2	19	1.7	1	7.3	268	272	1392	225	28	3.1	3.6
157	76	0.3	0.3	2.3	0.2	41	0.4	0	10.8	87	134	566	133	18	2.4	0.8
68	97	0.5	0.4	4.2	0.1	92	1.1	3	1.8	185	311	939	353	37	3.5	1.2
54	0	0.4	0.4	5.9	0.2	25	2	0	0.4	104	212	616	380	32	4.2	5.1
20	0							0		60		420	220		1.4	
56	212	0.3	0.4	2.2	0.1	28	0.4	<1	2.5	414	491	1182	174	27	2.1	2.1
34	11	0.2	0.2	3.1	0.1	18	0.9	4	0.3	46	116	272	209	21	1.9	2.3
57	79	0.7	0.4	4.1	0.3	16	1.2	15	6.8	257	327	1597	343	29	2.2	2.6
29	8	0.5	0.2	3.7	0.2	25	0.5	4	9.2	69	166	933	215	33	2.4	1.3
45	8	1	0.3	6.5	0.5	27	0.7	22	6.5	72	277	1634	422	43	2.7	2.3
51	3	0.3	0.3	4.8	0.1	21	1	2	0.3	68	135	1334	243	23	2.6	2.7
113	123	0.3	0.5	6.1	0.3	25	2.4	<1	10.4	221	327	701	391	36	4.2	7.1
2	<1	0.3	0.2	5.3	0.1	40	0	<1	1.1	60	141	293	245	56	2.3	1.1
82	94	0.2	0.4	3.4	0.2	37	1.3	4	0.8	299	291	1348	261	39	2.9	4
43	12	0.3	0.3	6.8	0.4	34	2.2	12	9.1	72	232	1605	484	42	4.3	4
36	80	1	0.8	5.5	0.1	87	1.1	12		189	287	1650	394	68	2.5	2.6

ERA, EatRight Analysis CD-ROM; **AMT,** amount; **WT,** weight; **WTR,** water; **CAL,** calories; **PROT,** protein; **CARB,** carbohydrate; **FIBR,** fiber; **FAT,** fat; **SATF,** saturated fat; **MONO,** monounsaturated fat; **POLY,** polyunsaturated fat

ERA CODE	FOOD DESCRIPTION	AMT	UNIT	WT (g)	WTR (g)	CAL (kcal)	PROT (g)	CARB (g)	FIBR (g)	FAT (g)	SATF (g)	MONO (g)	POLY (g)
Sandwiches (continued)													
56047	Tuna salad sandwich on white	1	ea	131		356	15	40	2	15	2.4	3.8	7.9
56053	Turkey sandwich, whole wheat	1	ea	168.8		364	26	33	4	15	2.3	3.5	8.4
56103	Turkey ham sandwich on rye	1	ea	149.5		280	21	20	<1	14	2.5	2.8	6.9
56059	Turkey ham+cheese on wheat	1	ea	156.3		396	23	28	3	22	8.2	5.3	6.8
Snack Foods: Chips, Pretzels, Popcorn													
44061	Bagel chips	5	pce	70	2	298	6	52	4	7	1.3	2.1	3.4
44029	Bugles corn chips, plain	2	oz	56.7	1	289	3	36	1	15	12.9	1	0.4
44001	Cheetos cheese puffs	1	cup	20	<1	111	2	11	<1	7	1.3	4.1	1
44032	Chex party mix	1	cup	42.5	1	181	5	28	2	7	2.3	3.9	1.1
44033	Combos pretzels w/cheese	10	pce	30	1	139	3	20		5			
44002	Corn chips (Fritos)	1	cup	26	<1	140	2	15	1	9	1.2	2.5	4.3
44031	Cornnuts, toasted corn nuggets	10	pce	18	<1	79	2	13	1	3	0.5	1.3	0.6
44037	Cracker Jacks snack	1	cup	42.5	1	170	3	34	2	3	0.4	1.2	1.4
44004	Dorito chips, nacho flavor	1	cup	26	<1	129	2	16	1	7	1.3	3.9	0.9
44012	Popcorn, air popped, plain	1	cup	8	<1	31	1	6	1	<1	<0.1	0.1	0.2
44014	Popcorn, caramel corn	1	cup	35.2	1	152	1	28	2	5	1.3	1	1.6
44038	Popcorn, cheese	1	cup	11	<1	58	1	6	1	4	0.7	1.1	1.7
44013	Popcorn, cooked in oil+salt	1	cup	11	<1	55	1	6	1	3	0.5	0.9	1.5
44006	Potato chips	10	pce	20	<1	107	1	11	1	7	2.2	2	2.4
44040	Potato chips, BBQ	20	pce	26	<1	128	2	14	1	8	2.1	1.7	4.3
44043	Potato chips, light	20	pce	40	<1	188	3	27	2	8	1.7	1.9	4.4
44015	Pretzels, Dutch twist	10	pce	60	2	229	5	48	2	2	0.4	0.8	0.7
44017	Rice cake, carmel corn, mini	1	ea	3.2	<1	13	<1	3	<1	<1	0.1	<0.1	<0.1
44016	Rice cake, plain, regular size	1	ea	9		35	1	7	<1	<1	0.1	0.1	0.1
44064	Rice cake, unsalted	2	ea	18	1	70	1	15	1	1	0.1	0.2	0.2
44266	Tortilla chips, low fat	13	pce	28		110	2	24	2	1	0	0.3	0.7
44267	Tortilla chips, no salt	13	pce	28		110	3	24	2	1	0		
44054	Tortilla chips, nacho, low fat	10	ea	16	<1	71	1	11	1	2	0.5	1.4	0.3
44058	Trail mix, regular	1	cup	150	14	693	21	67	8	44	8.3	18.8	14.5
44085	Trail mix, regular, unsalted	1	cup	150	14	693	21	67	8	44	8.3	18.8	14.5
44060	Trail mix, tropical	1	cup	140	13	570	9	92	9	24	11.9	3.5	7.2
Soups, Stews, and Chilis													
50000	Bean+bacon soup w/water	1	cup	253	213	172	8	23	9	6	1.5	2.2	1.8
50001	Beef broth/bouillon, prepared	1	cup	240	234	17	3	<1	0	1	0.3	0.2	<0.1
50183	Beef broth, canned, low sodium	1	cup	240	230	38	5	1	0	1	0.4	0.7	0.3
50033	Beef broth, cube+water	1	cup	241	236	7	1	1	0	<1	0.1	0.1	0
50003	Beef noodle soup+water	1	cup	244	224	83	5	9	1	3	1.1	1.2	0.5
50066	Beef soup, chunky, prepared	1	cup	240	200	170	12	20	1	5	2.5	2.1	0.2
50060	Black bean soup+water	1	cup	247	216	116	6	20	4	2	0.4	0.5	0.5
50204	Bouillabaise soup/chowder	1	cup	227	177	241	34	5	1	9	2	3.9	1.5
50071	Cheese soup+milk	1	cup	251	207	231	9	16	1	15	9.1	4.1	0.5
50004	Chicken broth, can+water	1	cup	244	234	39	5	1	0	1	0.4	0.6	0.3
50035	Chicken broth, cube+water	1	cup	243	237	12	1	2	0	<1	0.1	0.1	0.1
50005	Chicken noodle soup+water	1	cup	241	222	75	4	9	1	2	0.6	1.1	0.6

< = Trace amount present   Blank = Not available

CHOL, cholesterol; **V,** vitamin; **THI,** thiamin; **RIB,** riboflavin; **NIA,** niacin; **FOL,** folate;
CALC, calcium; **PHOS,** phosphate; **SOD,** sodium; **POT,** potassium; **MAG,** magnesium

CHOL (mg)	V-A (RE)	THI (mg)	RIB (mg)	NIA (mg)	V-B6 (mg)	FOL (μg)	V-B12 (μg)	V-C (mg)	V-E (mg)	CALC (mg)	PHOS (mg)	SOD (mg)	POT (mg)	MAG (mg)	IRON (mg)	ZINC (mg)
15	22	0.3	0.2	5.8	0.1	29	0.7	1	11.9	76	167	605	180	25	2.5	0.7
43	12	0.3	0.2	9.8	0.5	39	1.8	0	9.7	59	359	1664	418	77	2.7	2.3
55	8	0.2	0.3	4.3	0.3	17	0.3	<1	7	51	213	1182	341	25	4.1	3
64	90	0.3	0.4	4.4	0.3	30	0.4	0	6.6	246	411	1389	354	44	3.7	3.2
0	0	0.1	0.1	1.6	0.2	46	0	<1	1.7	9	145	419	167	39	1.4	0.9
0	18	0.2	0.1	0.8	<0.1	2	0	0	1.1	2	25	579	46	6	1.4	0.1
1	7	0.1	0.1	0.6	<0.1	24	<0.1	<1	1	12	22	210	33	4	0.5	0.1
0	6	0.7	0.2	7.2	0.7	0	5.3	20	0.1	15	79	432	114	27	10.5	0.9
2	2	0.1	0.2	1	<0.1	2	<0.1	0	0.1	59	43	335	39	7	0.3	0.2
0	2	<0.1	<0.1	0.3	0.1	5	0	0	1.6	33	48	164	37	20	0.3	0.3
0	0	<0.1	<0.1	0.3	<0.1	0	0	0	0.2	2	50	99	50	20	0.3	0.3
0	3	<0.1	0.1	0.8	0.1	7	0	0	0.6	28	54	125	151	34	1.7	0.5
1	11	<0.1	<0.1	0.4	0.1	4	<0.1	<1	1	38	63	184	56	21	0.4	0.3
0	2	<0.1	<0.1	0.2	<0.1	2	0	0	<0.1	1	24	<1	24	10	0.2	0.3
2	4	<0.1	<0.1	0.8	<0.1	1	<0.1	0	0.4	15	29	73	38	12	0.6	0.2
1	5	<0.1	<0.1	0.2	<0.1	1	0.1	<1	<0.1	12	40	98	29	10	0.2	0.2
0	2	<0.1	<0.1	0.2	<0.1	2	0	<1	<0.1	1	28	97	25	12	0.3	0.3
0	0	<0.1	<0.1	0.8	0.1	9	0	6	1.3	5	33	119	255	13	0.3	0.2
0	6	0.1	0.1	1.2	0.2	22	0	9	1.3	13	48	195	328	20	0.5	0.2
0	0	0.1	0.1	2.8	0.3	11	0	10	1.2	8	77	197	698	36	0.5	<0.1
0	0	0.3	0.4	3.2	0.1	103	0	0	0.5	22	68	1029	88	21	2.6	0.5
<1	1	<0.1	<0.1	0.1	<0.1	1	0	<1	<0.1	1	6	14	6	3	<0.1	<0.1
0	0	<0.1	<0.1	0.6	0.1	2	0	0	<0.1	1	33	14	25	14	0.1	2
0	1	<0.1	<0.1	1.4	<0.1	4	0	0	<0.1	2	65	5	52	24	0.3	0.5
0 0	0	<0.1	<0.1	0.4				0		37	80	200 0	85		0.4	0
<1	7	<0.1	<0.1	0.1	<0.1	4	0	<1	0.1	25	51	160	44	16	0.3	
0	3	0.7	0.3	7.1	0.4	106	0	2	5.3	117	518	344	1027	237	4.6	4.8
0	3	0.7	0.3	7.1	0.4	106	0	2	5.3	117	518	15	1027	237	4.6	4.8
0	7	0.6	0.2	2.1	0.5	59	0	11	3.1	80	260	14	993	134	3.7	1.6
3	89	0.1	<0.1	0.6	<0.1	32	0.1	2	0.1	81	132	951	402	46	2	1
0	0	<0.1	0.1	1.9	<0.1	5	0.2	0	0	14	31	782	130	5	0.4	0
0	0	0	0.1	3.3	<0.1	5	0.2	0	<0.1	10	72	72	206	2	0.5	0.2
0	1	<0.1	<0.1	0.2	0	2	0	0	<0.1	2	12	1156	19	2	0.1	<0.1
5	63	0.1	0.1	1.1	<0.1	20	0.2	<1	<0.1	15	46	952	100	5	1.1	1.5
14	262	0.1	0.2	2.7	0.1	13	0.6	7	0.2	31	120	866	336	5	2.3	2.6
0	49	0.1	0.1	0.5	0.1	25	<0.1	1	0.1	44	106	1197	274	42	2.1	1.4
90	89	0.2	0.2	5	0.4	28	10.4	12	2	83	340	416	732	74	3.9	1.9
48	148	0.1	0.3	0.5	0.1	10	0.4	1	0.3	289	251	1019	341	20	0.8	0.7
0	0	<0.1	0.1	3.3	<0.1	5	0.2	0	<0.1	10	73	776	210	2	0.5	0.2
0	5	<0.1	<0.1	0.2	0	2	<0.1	0	<0.1	12	12	792	24	2	0.1	<0.1
7	72	0.1	0.1	1.4	<0.1	22	0.1	<1	0.1	17	36	1106	55	5	0.8	0.4

ERA, EatRight Analysis CD-ROM; **AMT,** amount; **WT,** weight; **WTR,** water; **CAL,** calories; **PROT,** protein; **CARB**, carbohydrate; **FIBR,** fiber; **FAT,** fat; **SATF,** saturated fat; **MONO,** monounsaturated fat; **POLY,** polyunsaturated fat

ERA CODE	FOOD DESCRIPTION	AMT	UNIT	WT (g)	WTR (g)	CAL (kcal)	PROT (g)	CARB (g)	FIBR (g)	FAT (g)	SATF (g)	MONO (g)	POLY (g)
Soups, Stews, and Chilis (continued)													
50037	Chicken noodle soup, dry+water	1	cup	252	237	58	2	9	<1	1	0.3	0.5	0.4
50020	Chicken rice soup+water	1	cup	241	226	60	4	7	1	2	0.5	0.9	0.4
56001	Chili+beans, canned	1	cup	256	193	287	15	30	11	14	6	6	0.9
50007	Chili beef soup+water	1	cup	250	212	170	7	21	10	7	3.3	2.8	0.3
7557	Chili, vegetarian	1	cup	214	138	282	38	30	10	4	0.6	1.3	1.8
50008	Clam chowder, New Eng+milk	1	cup	248	211	164	9	17	1	7	3	2.3	1.1
50093	Clam chowder, Manhattan, prep	1	cup	240	206	134	7	19	3	3	2.1	1	0.1
50098	Consommé+gelatin+water	1	cup	241	232	29	5	2	0	0	0	0	0
50213	Crab bisque soup	1	cup	248	202	236	20	12	<1	12	3.4	4.7	2.7
50011	Cream mushroom soup+milk	1	cup	248	210	203	6	15	<1	14	5.1	3	4.6
50049	Cream mushroom soup+water	1	cup	244	220	129	2	9	<1	9	2.4	1.7	4.2
50189	Cream of broccoli soup	1	cup	237	197	206	9	17	2	12	4	5.1	2.5
50006	Cream of chicken soup+milk	1	cup	248	210	191	7	15	<1	11	4.6	4.5	1.6
50018	Cream of chicken soup+water	1	cup	244	221	117	3	9	<1	7	2.1	3.3	1.5
50026	Cream potato soup+milk	1	cup	248	215	149	6	17	<1	6	3.8	1.7	0.6
50190	Egg drop soup	1	cup	244	229	73	8	1	0	4	1.1	1.5	0.6
50103	Gazpacho soup, prepared	1	cup	244	229	46	7	4	<1	<1	<0.1	<0.1	0.1
50182	Hot & sour soup	1	cup	244	211	162	15	5	1	8	2.7	3.4	1.2
50105	Lentil & ham soup, prepared	1	cup	248	213	139	9	20	2	3	1.1	1.3	0.3
50214	Lobster bisque soup	1	cup	248	199	252	20	13	<1	13	4.2	5.5	2.7
50009	Minestrone soup+water	1	cup	241	220	82	4	11	1	3	0.6	0.7	1.1
50040	Onion soup, dry mix+water	1	cup	246	237	27	1	5	1	1	0.1	0.3	0.1
50024	Oyster stew+milk	1	cup	245	218	135	6	10	0	8	5	2.1	0.3
50025	Split pea+ham soup+water	1	cup	253	207	190	10	28	2	4	1.8	1.8	0.6
50209	Sweet & sour soup	1	cup	244	222	72	3	14	2	1	0.3	0.3	0.1
50012	Tomato soup+milk	1	cup	248	210	161	6	22	3	6	2.9	1.6	1.1
50028	Tomato soup+water	1	cup	244	220	85	2	17	<1	2	0.4	0.4	1
50186	Vege soup, low sod+water	1	cup	241	220	78	3	15	3	1	0.2	0.2	0.5
50144	Vegetable soup, chunky, prep	1	cup	240	210	122	4	19	1	4	0.6	1.6	1.4
50013	Vegetarian vege soup+water	1	cup	241	222	72	2	12	<1	2	0.3	0.8	0.7
50027	Vichyssoise soup	1	cup	248	215	149	6	17	<1	6	3.8	1.7	0.6
50181	Wonton soup	1	cup	241	203	182	14	14	1	7	2.3	3	1
Spices, Flavors, and Seasonings and Miscellaneous Baking Products													
23010	Baking chocolate, square	1	ea	28.4	<1	148	3	8	4	16	9.2	5.2	0.5
28004	Baking powder	1	tsp	4.6	<1	2	0	1	<1	0	0	0	0
28003	Baking soda	1	tsp	4.6	<1	0	0	0	0	0	0	0	0
26001	Basil, dried	1	Tbs	4.5	<1	11	1	3	2	<1	<0.1	<0.1	0.1
26040	Celery seed	1	Tbs	6.5	<1	25	1	3	1	2	0.1	1	0.2
26002	Chili powder	1	Tbs	7.5	1	24	1	4	3	1	0.2	0.3	0.6
23012	Chocolate chips, semisweet	1	cup	168	1	805	7	106	10	50	29.8	16.7	1.6
26003	Cinnamon	1	Tbs	6.8	1	18	<1	5	4	<1	<0.1	<0.1	<0.1
28200	Cocoa powder	1	cup	86	3	197	17	47	29	12	6.9	3.9	0.4
26038	Coriander/cilantro, fresh	0.25	cup	4	4	1	<1	<1	<1	<1	0	<0.1	<0.1
26004	Curry powder	1	Tbs	6.3	1	20	1	4	2	1	0.1	0.3	0.2
26021	Dill weed, dried	1	Tbs	3.1	<1	8	1	2	<1	<1	<0.1	0.1	<0.1

< = Trace amount present   Blank = Not available

CHOL, cholesterol; **V,** vitamin; **THI,** thiamin; **RIB,** riboflavin; **NIA,** niacin; **FOL,** folate;
CALC, calcium; **PHOS,** phosphate; **SOD,** sodium; **POT,** potassium; **MAG,** magnesium

CHOL (mg)	V-A (RE)	THI (mg)	RIB (mg)	NIA (mg)	V-B6 (mg)	FOL (μg)	V-B12 (μg)	V-C (mg)	V-E (mg)	CALC (mg)	PHOS (mg)	SOD (mg)	POT (mg)	MAG (mg)	IRON (mg)	ZINC (mg)
10	5	0.2	0.1	1.1	<0.1	18	0.1	0	0.1	5	30	577	33	8	0.5	0.2
7	65	<0.1	<0.1	1.1	<0.1	1	0.1	<1	0.1	17	22	814	101	0	0.7	0.3
44	87	0.1	0.3	0.9	0.3	58	0	4	1.9	120	394	1336	934	115	8.8	5.1
12	150	0.1	0.1	1.1	0.2	18	0.3	4	1.4	42	148	1035	525	30	2.1	1.4
0	148	0.2	0.1	2.4	0.3	164	0	11	2.5	107	435	709	730	71	8.8	2.5
22	40	0.1	0.2	1	0.1	10	10.2	3	0.1	186	156	992	300	22	1.5	0.8
14	329	0.1	0.1	1.8	0.3	9	7.9	12	0.1	67	84	1000	384	19	2.6	1.7
0	0	<0.1	<0.1	0.7	<0.1	3	0	1	<0.1	10	31	636	154	0	0.5	0.4
85	145	0.2	0.3	2.9	0.2	47	5.8	5	2	253	299	584	490	46	1	3.7
20	37	0.1	0.3	0.9	0.1	10	0.5	2	1.3	178	156	918	270	20	0.6	0.6
2	0	<0.1	0.1	0.7	<0.1	5	<0.1	1	1.2	46	49	881	100	5	0.5	0.6
15	258	0.1	0.4	0.8	0.2	40	0.4	48	2.4	256	222	204	481	41	0.9	1
27	94	0.1	0.3	0.9	0.1	8	0.5	1	0.2	181	151	1046	273	17	0.7	0.7
10	56	<0.1	0.1	0.8	<0.1	2	0.1	<1	0.2	34	37	986	88	2	0.6	0.6
22	67	0.1	0.2	0.6	0.1	9	0.5	1	0.1	166	161	1061	322	17	0.5	0.7
103	41	<0.1	0.2	3	0.1	15	0.5	0	0.3	21	108	728	220	5	0.8	0.5
0	261	<0.1	<0.1	0.9	0.1	10	0	7	0.5	24	37	739	224	7	1	0.2
34	2	0.3	0.3	5	0.2	13	0.4	1	0.1	29	188	1010	384	29	1.9	1.5
7	35	0.2	0.1	1.4	0.2	50	0.3	4	0.2	42	184	1319	357	22	2.7	0.7
63	196	0.1	0.4	1	0.1	17	2.6	2	2.1	275	310	450	548	50	0.5	2.7
2	234	0.1	<0.1	0.9	0.1	36	0	1	0.1	34	55	911	313	7	0.9	0.7
0	0	<0.1	0.1	0.5	0	1	0	<1	0.1	12	30	849	64	5	0.1	0.1
32	44	0.1	0.2	0.3	0.1	10	2.6	4	0.5	167	162	1041	235	20	1.1	10.3
8	46	0.1	0.1	1.5	0.1	3	0.3	2	0.2	23	212	1006	400	48	2.3	1.3
5	31	0.1	0.1	0.9	0.1	16	<0.1	17	0.5	27	43	1291	227	15	0.6	0.3
17	109	0.1	0.2	1.5	0.2	21	0.4	68	2.6	159	149	744	449	22	1.8	0.3
0	68	0.1	0.1	1.4	0.1	15	0	66	2.5	12	34	695	264	7	1.8	0.2
0	301	0.1	0.1	1.9	0.2	17	0	1	1.9	27	54	468	522	31	0.8	0.5
0	588	0.1	0.1	1.2	0.2	17	0	6	0.6	55	72	1010	396	7	1.6	3.1
0	301	0.1	<0.1	0.9	0.1	11	0	1	0.8	22	34	822	210	7	1.1	0.5
22	67	0.1	0.2	0.6	0.1	9	0.5	1	0.1	166	161	1061	322	17	0.5	0.7
53	99	0.4	0.3	4.6	0.2	19	0.4	3	0.4	31	152	543	316	21	1.8	1.1
0	3	<0.1	<0.1	0.3	<0.1	2	0	0	1.7	21	118	4	236	88	1.8	1.1
0	0	0	0	0	0	0	0	0	0	270	101	488	1	1	0.5	0
0	0	0	0	0	0	0	0	0	0	0	0	1258	0	0	0	0
0	42	<0.1	<0.1	0.3	0.1	12	0	3	0.1	95	22	2	154	19	1.9	0.3
0	<1	<0.1	<0.1	0.2	<0.1	1	0	1	0.1	115	36	10	91	29	2.9	0.4
0	262	<0.1	0.1	0.6	0.1	8	0	5	0.1	21	23	76	144	13	1.1	0.2
0	4	0.1	0.2	0.7	0.1	5	0	0	10.1	54	222	18	613	193	5.3	2.7
0	2	<0.1	<0.1	0.1	<0.1	2	0	2	0	84	4	2	34	4	2.6	0.1
0	2	0.1	0.2	1.9	0.1	28	0	0	1.9	110	631	18	1310	429	11.9	5.9
0	11	<0.1	<0.1	<0.1	<0.1	<1	0	<1	0.1	4	1	1	22	1	0.1	<0.1
0	6	<0.1	<0.1	0.2	<0.1	10	0	1	<0.1	30	22	3	97	16	1.9	0.3
0	18	<0.1	<0.1	0.1	<0.1		0	2		55	17	6	102	14	1.5	0.1

ERA, EatRight Analysis CD-ROM; **AMT,** amount; **WT,** weight; **WTR,** water; **CAL,** calories; **PROT,** protein; **CARB,** carbohydrate; **FIBR,** fiber; **FAT,** fat; **SATF,** saturated fat; **MONO,** monounsaturated fat; **POLY,** polyunsaturated fat

ERA CODE	FOOD DESCRIPTION	AMT	UNIT	WT (g)	WTR (g)	CAL (kcal)	PROT (g)	CARB (g)	FIBR (g)	FAT (g)	SATF (g)	MONO (g)	POLY (g)
Spices, Flavors, and Seasonings and Miscellaneous Baking Products (continued)													
26007	Garlic powder	1	Tbs	8.4	1	28	1	6	1	<1	<0.1	<0.1	<0.1
26023	Ginger, ground	1	Tbs	5.4	1	19	<1	4	1	<1	0.1	0.1	0.1
26008	Onion powder	1	Tbs	6.5	<1	23	1	5	<1	<1	<0.1	<0.1	<0.1
26009	Oregano, ground	1	Tbs	4.5	<1	14	<1	3	2	<1	0.1	<0.1	0.2
26010	Paprika	1	Tbs	6.9	1	20	1	4	1	1	0.1	0.1	0.6
26016	Pepper, black	1	Tbs	6.4	1	16	1	4	2	<1	0.1	0.1	0.1
26037	Pepper, white	1	Tbs	7.1	1	21	1	5	2	<1	<0.1	0.1	<0.1
26031	Sage, ground	1	Tbs	2	<1	6	<1	1	1	<1	0.1	<0.1	<0.1
26014	Salt	1	Tbs	18	<1	0	0	0	0	0	0	0	0
26091	Salt substitute (Morton)	0.25	tsp	1.1	<1	1	<1	<1		<1			
26048	Salt, light (Morton)	0.25	tsp	1.4	0	<1	0	<1		0	0	0	0
28002	Yeast, brewer's	1	Tbs	8	<1	23	3	3	3	<1	<0.1	<0.1	0
28000	Yeast, dry, active, baker's	1	tsp	4	<1	12	2	2	1	<1	<0.1	0.1	0
Sweets, Sugars, Candy													
Candies and Confections, Gum													
23049	Almond Joy candy bar	1	ea	49	5	229	2	29	2	13	8.5	3.2	0.7
23110	Baby Ruth candy bar	1	ea	60	3	289	4	39	2	13	7.1	3.7	1.9
23226	Breathsaver mints, spearmint	1	pce	2		10	0	0	0	0	0	0	0
23066	Butterfinger candy bar	1	ea	61	1	293	8	40	1	11	6.3	3.4	1.7
23015	Caramel, plain/chocolate	1	pce	10.1	1	39	<1	8	<1	1	0.7	0.1	<0.1
23082	Chewing gum	1	pce	3	<1	10	0	3	0	<1	<0.1	<0.1	<0.1
23083	Chewing gum, sugarless	1	pce	4	<1	11	0	4	0	<1	<0.1	<0.1	<0.1
23063	Chocolate candy kisses	6	pce	28.4	<1	145	2	17	1	9	5.2	2.8	0.3
23021	Chocolate-coated peanuts	1	cup	149	3	773	20	74	7	50	21.8	19.2	6.5
23022	Chocolate-covered raisins	1	cup	190	21	741	8	130	8	28	16.7	9	1
23053	Divinity candy, homemade	1	pce	11	1	38	<1	10	0	0	0	0	0
23036	English toffee candy bar	1	ea	39	1	217	2	23	1	13	8.5	4.3	0.5
23024	Fondant candy	1	pce	16	1	57	0	15	0	0	0	0	0
23025	Fudge, chocolate	1	pce	17	2	65	<1	14	<1	1	0.9	0.4	0.1
23026	Fudge, chocolate, nuts	1	pce	19	1	81	1	14	<1	3	1.1	0.8	1
23029	Gumdrops candy, small	10	pce	36	<1	139	0	36	0	0	0	0	0
23030	Gummy Bears candy	10	pce	22	<1	85	0	22	0	0	0	0	0
23031	Hard candy, all flavors	1	pce	6	<1	24	0	6	0	<1	0	0	0
23033	Jelly beans candy	10	pce	11	1	40	0	10	0	<1	<0.1	<0.1	<0.1
23048	M&M's peanut choc candy	10	pce	20	<1	103	2	12	1	5	2.1	2.2	0.8
23046	M&M's plain choc candy	10	pce	7	<1	34	<1	5	<1	1	0.9	0.5	<0.1
23064	Marshmallow creme	2	Tbs	12		40	0	10	0	0	0	0	0
23007	Marshmallows	1	ea	7.2	1	23	<1	6	<1	<1	<0.1	<0.1	<0.1
23018	Milk choc bar+almonds	1	ea	41	1	216	4	22	3	14	7	5.5	0.9
23019	Milk choc bar+peanuts	1	ea	28.4		157	5	11	2	12	3.4	5.1	2.6
23058	Milk choc bar+rice cereal	1	ea	40	1	198	3	25	1	11	6.4	3.5	0.3
23016	Milk chocolate candy bar	1	ea	44	1	226	3	26	1	14	8.1	4.4	0.5
23038	Milky Way candy bar	1	ea	60	4	254	3	43	1	10	4.7	3.6	0.4
23081	Peanut brittle, homemade	1	cup	147	3	666	11	102	3	28	7.4	12.5	6.9
23138	Praline candy, homemade	1	pce	39	4	177	1	24	1	9	0.7	5.9	2.4

< = Trace amount present   Blank = Not available

CHOL, cholesterol; **V,** vitamin; **THI,** thiamin; **RIB,** riboflavin; **NIA,** niacin; **FOL,** folate;
CALC, calcium; **PHOS,** phosphate; **SOD,** sodium; **POT,** potassium; **MAG,** magnesium

CHOL (mg)	V-A (RE)	THI (mg)	RIB (mg)	NIA (mg)	V-B6 (mg)	FOL (μg)	V-B12 (μg)	V-C (mg)	V-E (mg)	CALC (mg)	PHOS (mg)	SOD (mg)	POT (mg)	MAG (mg)	IRON (mg)	ZINC (mg)
0	0	<0.1	<0.1	0.1	0.2	<1	0	2	<0.1	7	35	2	92	5	0.2	0.2
0	1	<0.1	<0.1	0.3	0.1	2	0	<1	<0.1	6	8	2	72	10	0.6	0.3
0	0	<0.1	<0.1	<0.1	0.1	11	0	1	<0.1	24	22	3	61	8	0.2	0.2
0	31	<0.1	<0.1	0.3	0.1	12	0	2	0.1	71	9	1	75	12	2	0.2
0	418	<0.1	0.1	1.1	0.1	7	0	5	0.6	12	24	2	162	13	1.6	0.3
0	1	<0.1	<0.1	0.1	<0.1	1	0	1	0.1	28	11	3	81	12	1.8	0.1
0	0	<0.1	<0.1	<0.1	<0.1	1	0	1	0.2	19	12	<1	5	6	1	0.1
0	12	<0.1	<0.1	0.1	<0.1	5	0	1	<0.1	33	2	<1	21	9	0.6	0.1
0	0	0	0	0	0	0	0	0	0	4	0	6976	1	<1	0.1	<0.1
							0					<1	476			
							0			1		273	364	1		
0	0	1.2	0.3	3	0.4	313	<0.1	0		17	140	10	151	18	1.4	0.6
0	<1	0.1	0.2	1.6	0.1	94	0	<1	0.2	3	52	2	80	4	0.7	0.3
2	2	<0.1	0.1	0.2	<0.1		0.1	<1	1.2	30	69	72	120	32	0.7	0.4
2	0	0.1	0.1	1.7	<0.1	19	<0.1	0	1.1	25	91	136	238	48	0.1	0.8
0												0	0			
1	0	0.1	<0.1	1.5	<0.1	16	<0.1	0	1	16	80	121	232	48	0.5	0.7
1	1	<0.1	<0.1	<0.1	<0.1	1	0	<1	<0.1	14	12	25	22	2	<0.1	<0.1
0	0	0	0	0	0	0	0	0	0	0	0	<1	<1	0	0	0
0	0	0	0	0	0	0	0	0	0	1	0	<1	0	0	0	0
6	16	<0.1	0.1	0.1	<0.1	2	0.1	<1	0.4	54	61	23	109	17	0.4	0.4
13	0	0.2	0.3	6.3	0.3	12	0.4	0	14.5	155	316	61	748	140	2	2.9
6	13	0.2	0.3	0.8	0.2	10	0.3	<1	4	163	272	68	977	86	3.2	1.5
0	<1	0	<0.1	<0.1	0	0	<0.1	0		<1	<1	5	2	<1	<0.1	<0.1
20	27	<0.1	0.1	<0.1	<0.1		0.1	<1	3.7	51	58	108	93	13	0.2	0.3
0	<1	0	<0.1	0	0	0	0	0	0	<1	<1	6	3	<1	<0.1	<0.1
2	8	<0.1	<0.1	<0.1	<0.1	<1	<0.1	<1	<0.1	7	10	11	18	4	0.1	0.1
3	9	<0.1	<0.1	<0.1	<0.1	2	<0.1	<1	0.5	10	18	11	30	9	0.1	0.1
0	0	0	0	0	0	0	0	0	0	1	<1	16	2	<1	0.1	0
0	0	0	0	0	0	0	0	0	0	1	<1	10	1	<1	0.1	0
0	0	0	0	0	0	0	0	0	0	<1	<1	2	<1	<1	<0.1	0
0	0	0	0	0	0	0	0	0	0	<1	<1	3	4	<1	0.1	<0.1
2	5	<0.1	<0.1	0.7	<0.1	7	<0.1	<1	1	20	46	10	69	15	0.2	0.5
1	4	<0.1	<0.1	<0.1	<0.1	<1	<0.1	<1	0.2	7	10	4	19	3	0.1	0.1
0	0							0	0	0		10	0		0	
0	<1	0	0	<0.1	0	<1	0	0	0	<1	1	3	<1	<1	<0.1	<0.1
8	6	<0.1	0.2	0.3	<0.1	5	0.1	<1	3.7	92	108	30	182	37	0.7	0.5
3	6	0.1	0.1	2.1	<0.1	24	<0.1	0	2.2	33	83	11	152	35	0.5	0.7
8	4	<0.1	0.1	0.2	<0.1	4	0.1	<1	1.6	68	77	58	137	20	0.3	0.4
10	24	<0.1	0.1	0.1	<0.1	4	0.2	<1	2.2	84	95	36	169	26	0.6	0.6
8	19	<0.1	0.1	0.2	<0.1	6	0.2	1	1	78	86	144	145	20	0.5	0.4
19	69	0.3	0.1	5.1	0.2	103	<0.1	0	2.4	44	163	664	306	74	2	1.4
0	2	0.1	<0.1	0.1	<0.1	5	0	<1	0.6	12	43	24	82	20	0.5	0.8

ERA, EatRight Analysis CD-ROM; **AMT,** amount; **WT,** weight; **WTR,** water; **CAL,** calories; **PROT,** protein; **CARB**, carbohydrate; **FIBR,** fiber; **FAT,** fat; **SATF,** saturated fat; **MONO,** monounsaturated fat; **POLY,** polyunsaturated fat

ERA CODE	FOOD DESCRIPTION	AMT	UNIT	WT (g)	WTR (g)	CAL (kcal)	PROT (g)	CARB (g)	FIBR (g)	FAT (g)	SATF (g)	MONO (g)	POLY (g)
Sweets, Sugars, Candy (continued)													
Candies and Confections, Gum (continued)													
23043	Reese's peanut butter cup	1	ea	50	1	270	5	27	2	16	5.6	6.6	2.8
23143	Skittles bite size candy	10	pce	10.7	<1	43	<1	10	0	<1	0.1	0.3	<0.1
23040	Snickers candy bar	1	ea	57	3	273	5	34	1	14	5.1	6	2.8
23144	Starburst fruit candy	1	pce	5	<1	20	<1	4	0	<1	0.1	0.2	0.2
23147	Taffy candy, homemade	1	pce	15	1	56	<1	14	0	<1	0.3	0.1	<0.1
23075	Three Musketeers candy bar	1	ea	60	3	250	2	46	1	8	3.9	2.6	0.3
23173	Toffee candy, homemade	1	pce	12	<1	65	<1	8	0	4	2.4	1.1	0.1
23117	Tootsie Roll candy, bite size	7	ea	35	3	126	1	31	<1	1	0.2	0.4	0.3
23154	Twizzlers, small pkg	1	ea	71	12	237	2	55	1	1	0.3		
23089	Yogurt-covered raisins	1	cup	191	19	750	8	139	5	22	19.5	0.4	0.6
23152	York peppermint patty, large	1	ea	42	4	165	1	34	1	3	1.8	1	0.1
Jams and Jellies													
23000	Apple butter	1	Tbs	18	10	31	<1	8	<1	0	0	0	0
23054	Jam/preserves	1	Tbs	20	6	56	<1	14	<1	<1	<0.1	<0.1	0
23003	Jelly	1	Tbs	19	6	54	<1	13	<1	<1	<0.1	<0.1	<0.1
23278	Fruit spread, low cal, strawberry	1	Tbs	20		20	0	5	0	0	0	0	0
23005	Marmalade, orange	1	Tbs	20	7	49	<1	13	<1	0	0	0	0
23165	Jelly, reduced sugar	1	Tbs	18.8	10	34	<1	9	<1	<1	<0.1	0	<0.1
Sugars and Syrups													
25010	Corn syrup, dark	1	cup	328	75	925	0	251	0	0	0	0	0
25000	Corn syrup, light	1	cup	328	75	925	0	251	0	0	0	0	0
25001	Honey, strained/extracted	1	cup	339	58	1030	1	279	1	0	0	0	0
25002	Maple syrup	1	Tbs	20	6	52	0	13	0	<1	<0.1	<0.1	<0.1
25004	Molasses, blackstrap cane	1	cup	328	94	771	0	199	0	0	0	0	0
23042	Pancake syrup	1	Tbs	20	5	57	0	15	0	0	0	0	0
23091	Pancake syrup, lite	1	Tbs	18	10	29	0	8	0	0	0	0	0
23172	Pancake syrup, reduced cal	1	Tbs	15	8	25	0	7	0	0	0	0	0
25005	Sugar, brown	1	cup	220	4	827	0	214	0	0	0	0	0
25071	Sugar, raw	1	cup	195	3	733	0	190	0	0	0	0	0
25006	Sugar, white, granulated	1	cup	200	0	774	0	200	0	0	0	0	0
25009	Sugar, white, powdered	1	cup	120	<1	467	0	119	0	<1	<0.1	<0.1	0.1
Vegetables and Legumes													
5314	Acorn squash, baked	1	cup	205	170	115	2	30	9	<1	0.1	<0.1	0.1
5010	Alfalfa sprouts	0.5	cup	16.5	15	5	1	1	<1	<1	<0.1	<0.1	0.1
5191	Artichoke hearts, marinated, cnd	2	pce	28		25	1	3	1	2	0		
5000	Artichoke, globe, cooked	1	ea	120	101	60	4	13	6	<1	<0.1	<0.1	0.1
6033	Arugula, chopped, raw	0.5	cup	10	9	2	<1	<1	<1	<1	<0.1	<0.1	<0.1
5842	Asparagus, canned+liq, low sod	0.5	cup	122	115	18	2	3	1	<1	0.1	<0.1	0.1
5007	Asparagus, spears, canned	1	pce	18	17	3	<1	<1	<1	<1	<0.1	<0.1	0.1
5004	Asparagus, spears, cooked	4	ea	60	55	14	2	3	1	<1	<0.1	<0.1	0.1
5401	Bamboo shoots, canned slices	1	cup	131	124	25	2	4	2	1	0.1	<0.1	0.2
5249	Bamboo shoots, cooked slices	1	cup	120	115	14	2	2	1	<1	0.1	<0.1	0.1
5250	Bamboo shoots, whole, boiled	1	ea	144	138	17	2	3	1	<1	0.1	<0.1	0.1

< = Trace amount present   Blank = Not available

CHOL, cholesterol; **V,** vitamin; **THI,** thiamin; **RIB,** riboflavin; **NIA,** niacin; **FOL,** folate; **CALC,** calcium; **PHOS,** phosphate; **SOD,** sodium; **POT,** potassium; **MAG,** magnesium

CHOL (mg)	V-A (RE)	THI (mg)	RIB (mg)	NIA (mg)	V-B6 (mg)	FOL (μg)	V-B12 (μg)	V-C (mg)	V-E (mg)	CALC (mg)	PHOS (mg)	SOD (mg)	POT (mg)	MAG (mg)	IRON (mg)	ZINC (mg)
2	10	0.1	0.1	2.3	0.1	28	0.1	<1	3.9	39	102	158	176	44	0.6	0.9
0	0	0	<0.1	<0.1	0	0	0	7	<0.1	0	<1	2	1	<1	<0.1	<0.1
7	22	0.1	0.1	2.4	0.1	23	0.1	<1	2.3	54	126	152	185	41	0.4	1.3
0	0	0	0	0	0	0	0	3	0.1	<1	<1	3	<1	<1	<0.1	0
1	5	0	<0.1	<0.1	0	0	<0.1	0	0.1	<1	<1	13	1	<1	<0.1	<0.1
7	14	<0.1	0.1	0.1	<0.1	0	0.1	<1	0.4	50	55	116	80	17	0.4	0.3
13	38	<0.1	<0.1	<0.1	<0.1	<1	<0.1	<1	0.2	4	4	22	6	<1	<0.1	<0.1
0	1	<0.1	<0.1	<0.1	<0.1	<1	<0.1	<1	0.1	9	14	28	36	11	0.1	0.2
0	0	<0.1	<0.1	0.1	<0.1		0	0		5	220	175	45	4	0.2	0.1
1	2	0.2	0.3	1.5	0.3	17	0.6	4	2.6	214	249	85	1061	46	2.5	0.9
<1	<1	<0.1	<0.1	0.4	<0.1		<0.1	0	0.1	6	40	10	54	26	0.4	0.3
0	2	<0.1	<0.1	<0.1	<0.1	<1	0	<1	<0.1	3	2	1	16	1	0.1	<0.1
0	<1	0	<0.1	<0.1	<0.1	7	0	2	0	4	2	6	15	1	0.1	<0.1
0	<1	0	<0.1	<0.1	<0.1	<1	0	<1	0	2	1	5	12	1	<0.1	<0.1
0	0							0		0		20	25		0	
0	1	<0.1	<0.1	<0.1	<0.1	7	0	1	0	8	1	11	7	<1	<0.1	<0.1
0	<1	<0.1	<0.1	<0.1	<0.1	<1	0	0	<0.1	1	1	<1	13	1	<0.1	<0.1
0	0	<0.1	<0.1	0.1	<0.1	0	0	0	0	59	36	508	144	26	1.2	0.1
0	0	<0.1	<0.1	0.1	<0.1	0	0	0	0	10	7	397	13	7	0.2	0.1
0	0	0	0.1	0.4	0.1	7	0	2	0	20	14	14	176	7	1.4	0.7
0	0	<0.1	<0.1	<0.1	0	0	0	0	0	13	<1	2	41	3	0.2	0.8
0	0	0.1	0.2	3.5	2.3	3	0	0	0	2820	131	180	8173	705	57.4	3.3
0	0	<0.1	<0.1	<0.1	0	0	0	0	0	<1	2	17	<1	<1	<0.1	<0.1
0	0	<0.1	<0.1	<0.1	0	0	0	0	0	2	1	37	6	1	0.3	<0.1
0	0	<0.1	<0.1	<0.1	0	0	0	0	0	<1	6	30	<1	0	<0.1	<0.1
0	0	<0.1	<0.1	0.2	0.1	2	0	0	0	187	48	86	761	64	4.2	0.4
0	0	<0.1	<0.1	0.2	0.1	2	0	0	0	166	43	76	675	57	3.7	0.4
0	0	0	<0.1	0	0	0	0	0	0	2	4	2	4	0	0.1	0.1
0	0	0	0	0	0	0	0	0	0	1	2	1	2	0	0.1	<0.1
0	88	0.3	<0.1	1.8	0.4	38	0	22	1.4	90	92	8	896	88	1.9	0.3
0	3	<0.1	<0.1	0.1	<0.1	6	0	1	<0.1	5	12	1	13	4	0.2	0.2
0	0							10		0		105			0	
0	22	0.1	0.1	1.2	0.1	61	0	12	0.2	54	103	114	425	72	1.5	0.6
0	24	<0.1	<0.1	<0.1	<0.1	10	0	2	<0.1	16	5	3	37	5	0.1	<0.1
0	65	0.1	0.1	1	0.1	104	0	20	0.2	18	46	32	210	11	0.7	0.6
0	10	<0.1	<0.1	0.2	<0.1	17	0	3	0.2	3	8	52	31	2	0.3	0.1
0	32	0.1	0.1	0.6	0.1	88	0	6	0.6	12	32	7	96	6	0.4	0.3
0	1	<0.1	<0.1	0.2	0.2	4	0	1	0.5	10	33	9	105	5	0.4	0.9
0	0	<0.1	0.1	0.4	0.1	3	0	0	0.8	14	24	5	640	4	0.3	0.6
0	0	<0.1	0.1	0.4	0.1	3	0	0	1	17	29	6	768	4	0.3	0.7

ERA, EatRight Analysis CD-ROM; **AMT,** amount; **WT,** weight; **WTR,** water; **CAL,** calories; **PROT,** protein; **CARB**, carbohydrate; **FIBR,** fiber; **FAT,** fat; **SATF,** saturated fat; **MONO,** monounsaturated fat; **POLY,** polyunsaturated fat

ERA CODE	FOOD DESCRIPTION	AMT	UNIT	WT (g)	WTR (g)	CAL (kcal)	PROT (g)	CARB (g)	FIBR (g)	FAT (g)	SATF (g)	MONO (g)	POLY (g)
Vegetables and Legumes (continued)													
7084	Bean cake	1	ea	32	7	130	2	16	1	7	1	2.9	2.6
5319	Beans, baby Limas, boiled	0.5	cup	85	57	104	6	20	5	<1	0.1	<0.1	0.1
7058	Beans, baby Limas, dry, boiled	0.5	cup	91	61	115	7	21	7	<1	0.1	<0.1	0.2
7012	Beans, black, dry, cooked	1	cup	172	113	227	15	41	15	1	0.2	0.1	0.4
7021	Beans, great Northern, boiled	1	cup	177	122	209	15	37	12	1	0.2	<0.1	0.3
5231	Beans, green, cannd+liq, low sod	1	cup	240	227	36	2	8	4	<1	0.1	<0.1	0.1
5015	Beans, green, canned, drained	1	cup	135	126	27	2	6	3	<1	<0.1	<0.1	0.1
5011	Beans, green, fresh, boiled	0.5	cup	62.5	56	22	1	5	2	<1	<0.1	<0.1	0.1
5013	Beans, green, frozen, boiled	1	cup	135	123	38	2	9	4	<1	0.1	<0.1	0.1
7087	Beans, kidney, canned+liquid	0.5	cup	128	100	104	7	19	4	<1	0.1	<0.1	0.2
7022	Beans, navy, dry, cooked	1	cup	182	115	258	16	48	12	1	0.3	0.1	0.4
7051	Beans, pinto, canned+liquid	0.5	cup	120	93	103	6	18	6	1	0.2	0.2	0.3
7013	Beans, pinto, dry, cooked	1	cup	171	110	234	14	44	15	1	0.2	0.2	0.3
7047	Beans, red kidney, boiled	1	cup	177	118	225	15	40	13	1	0.1	0.1	0.5
7135	Beans, red kidney, canned, drain	1	cup	256	176	302	19	55	23	1			
5022	Beets, fresh, diced, cooked	0.5	cup	85	74	37	1	8	2	<1	<0.1	<0.1	0.1
5310	Beets, pickled, slices	1	cup	227	186	148	2	37	6	<1	<0.1	<0.1	0.1
5311	Beets, whole, pickled	1	ea	50	41	32	<1	8	1	<1	<0.1	<0.1	<0.1
5679	Broccoflower, cooked	1	cup	156	140	50	5	10	5	<1	0.1	<0.1	0.2
5678	Broccoflower, raw	1	cup	100		32	3	6	3	<1	<0.1	<0.1	0.1
5653	Broccoli pieces, steamed	1	cup	156	141	44	5	8	5	1	0.1	<0.1	0.3
5029	Broccoli spear, cooked	1	ea	180	163	50	5	9	5	1	0.1	<0.1	0.3
5028	Broccoli, pieces, boiled	0.5	cup	78	71	22	2	4	2	<1	<0.1	<0.1	0.1
5030	Broccoli, pieces, frozen, cooked	1	cup	184	167	52	6	10	6	<1	<0.1	<0.1	0.1
5026	Broccoli, raw, chopped	1	cup	88	80	25	3	5	3	<1	<0.1	<0.1	0.1
5033	Brussels sprouts, cooked	1	cup	156	136	61	4	14	4	1	0.2	0.1	0.4
5035	Brussels sprouts, frozen, cooked	1	cup	155	134	65	6	13	6	1	0.1	<0.1	0.3
5237	Cabbage, bok choy, boiled	1	cup	170	162	20	3	3	3	<1	<0.1	<0.1	0.1
5041	Cabbage, bok choy, raw	1	cup	70	67	9	1	2	1	<1	<0.1	<0.1	0.1
5671	Cabbage, Chinese, steamed	1	cup	170	162	22	3	4	2	<1	<0.1	<0.1	0.2
5038	Cabbage, cooked	1	cup	150	140	33	2	7	3	1	0.1	<0.1	0.3
5040	Cabbage, pe tsai, raw, pieces	1	cup	76	72	12	1	2	2	<1	<0.1	<0.1	0.1
5235	Cabbage, pe tsai, boiled	1	cup	119	113	17	2	3	3	<1	<0.1	<0.1	0.1
5036	Cabbage, raw, shredded	1	cup	70	64	18	1	4	2	<1	<0.1	<0.1	0.1
5042	Cabbage, red, raw	1	cup	70	64	19	1	4	1	<1	<0.1	<0.1	0.1
5046	Carrot, raw, grated	0.5	cup	55	48	24	1	6	2	<1	<0.1	<0.1	<0.1
5045	Carrot, raw, whole	1	ea	72	63	31	1	7	2	<1	<0.1	<0.1	0.1
5439	Carrots, baby, raw, 2.75 inch	1	ea	10	9	4	<1	1	<1	<1	<0.1	<0.1	<0.1
5047	Carrots, cooked	0.5	cup	78	68	35	1	8	3	<1	<0.1	<0.1	0.1
5358	Carrots, frozen, cooked	0.5	cup	73	66	26	1	6	3	<1	<0.1	<0.1	<0.1
5625	Cassava/yuca blanca, cooked	1	cup	137	81	221	2	53	2	<1	0.1	0.1	0.1
5052	Cauliflower flowerets, boiled	3	ea	54	50	12	1	2	1	<1	<0.1	<0.1	0.1
5053	Cauliflower, frozen, cooked	1	cup	180	169	34	3	7	5	<1	0.1	<0.1	0.2
5049	Cauliflower, raw, cup	0.5	cup	50	46	12	1	3	1	<1	<0.1	<0.1	<0.1
5054	Celery, raw, chopped	0.5	cup	60	57	10	<1	2	1	<1	<0.1	<0.1	<0.1
5055	Celery, raw, large outer stalk	1	ea	40	38	6	<1	1	1	<1	<0.1	<0.1	<0.1

< = Trace amount present

Blank = Not available

CHOL, cholesterol; **V,** vitamin; **THI,** thiamin; **RIB,** riboflavin; **NIA,** niacin; **FOL,** folate;
CALC, calcium; **PHOS,** phosphate; **SOD,** sodium; **POT,** potassium; **MAG,** magnesium

CHOL (mg)	V-A (RE)	THI (mg)	RIB (mg)	NIA (mg)	V-B6 (mg)	FOL (μg)	V-B12 (μg)	V-C (mg)	V-E (mg)	CALC (mg)	PHOS (mg)	SOD (mg)	POT (mg)	MAG (mg)	IRON (mg)	ZINC (mg)
0	0	0.1	<0.1	0.5	<0.1	9	0	0	1.2	3	21	1	58	6	0.7	0.2
0	31	0.1	0.1	0.9	0.2	22	0	9	1.4	27	110	14	484	63	2.1	0.7
0	0	0.1	0.1	0.6	0.1	136	0	0	0.2	26	116	3	365	48	2.2	0.9
0	2	0.4	0.1	0.9	0.1	256	0	0	1	46	241	2	611	120	3.6	1.9
0	<1	0.3	0.1	1.2	0.2	181	0	2	1.9	120	292	4	692	88	3.8	1.6
0	77	0.1	0.1	0.5	0.1	44	0	8	0.3	58	46	34	221	31	2.2	0.5
0	47	<0.1	0.1	0.3	<0.1	43	0	6	0.2	35	26	354	147	18	1.2	0.4
0	42	<0.1	0.1	0.4	<0.1	21	0	6	0.1	29	24	2	187	16	0.8	0.2
0	54	<0.1	0.1	0.5	0.1	31	0	6	0.2	66	42	12	170	32	1.2	0.6
0	0	0.1	0.1	0.6	0.1	63	0	2	0.3	35	134	444	329	40	1.6	0.7
0	<1	0.4	0.1	1	0.3	255	0	2	2.1	127	286	2	670	107	4.5	1.9
0	3	0.1	0.1	0.3	0.1	72	0	1	1.1	52	110	353	292	32	1.8	0.8
0	<1	0.3	0.2	0.7	0.3	294	0	4	1.6	82	274	3	800	94	4.5	1.8
0	0	0.3	0.1	1	0.2	229	0	2	0.1	50	251	4	713	80	5.2	1.9
0	1	0.4	0.3	1.6	0.1	179	0				333			99		2
0	3	<0.1	<0.1	0.3	0.1	68	0	3	0.3	14	32	65	259	20	0.7	0.3
0	2	<0.1	0.1	0.6	0.1	60	0	5	0.3	25	39	599	336	34	0.9	0.6
0	<1	<0.1	<0.1	0.1	<0.1	13	0	1	0.1	6	8	132	74	8	0.2	0.1
0	11	0.1	0.1	1.2	0.3	76	0	98	0.5	50	100	36	502	31	1.1	0.8
0	7	0.1	0.1	0.8	0.2	57	0	74	0.3	32	64	23	322	20	0.1	0.5
0	228	0.1	0.2	0.9	0.2	94	0	123	0.7	75	103	42	505	39	1.4	0.6
0	250	0.1	0.2	1	0.3	90	0	134	3	83	106	47	526	43	1.5	0.7
0	108	<0.1	0.1	0.4	0.1	39	0	58	1.3	36	46	20	228	19	0.7	0.3
0	348	0.1	0.1	0.8	0.2	104	0	74	3	94	101	44	331	37	1.1	0.6
0	136	0.1	0.1	0.6	0.1	62	0	82	1.5	42	58	24	286	22	0.8	0.4
0	112	0.2	0.1	0.9	0.3	94	0	97	1.3	56	87	33	494	31	1.9	0.5
0	91	0.2	0.2	0.8	0.4	157	0	71	1.3	37	84	36	504	37	1.1	0.6
0	437	0.1	0.1	0.7	0.3	69	0	44	0.2	158	49	58	631	19	1.8	0.3
0	210	<0.1	<0.1	0.3	0.1	46	0	32	0.1	74	26	46	176	13	0.6	0.1
0	15	0.1	0.1	0.8	0.3	95	0	5	0.2	178	63	110	427	32	1.4	0.3
0	20	0.1	0.1	0.4	0.2	30	0	30	2.5	46	22	12	146	12	0.3	0.1
0	91	<0.1	<0.1	0.3	0.2	60	0	21	0.1	59	22	7	181	10	0.2	0.2
0	115	0.1	0.1	0.6	0.2	64	0	19	0.2	38	46	11	268	12	0.4	0.2
0	9	<0.1	<0.1	0.2	0.1	30	0	23	1.2	33	16	13	172	10	0.4	0.1
0	3	<0.1	<0.1	0.2	0.1	14	0	40	1.2	36	29	8	144	10	0.3	0.1
0	1547	0.1	<0.1	0.5	0.1	8	0	5	0.3	15	24	19	178	8	0.3	0.1
0	2025	0.1	<0.1	0.7	0.1	10	0	7	0.4	19	32	25	232	11	0.4	0.1
0	150	<0.1	<0.1	0.1	<0.1	3	0	1	<0.1	2	4	4	28	1	0.1	<0.1
0	1914	<0.1	<0.1	0.4	0.2	11	0	2	0.4	24	23	51	177	10	0.5	0.2
0	1292	<0.1	<0.1	0.3	0.1	8	0	2	0.7	20	19	43	115	7	0.3	0.2
0	2	0.1	0.1	1.1	0.1	24	0	19	0.3	21	34	18	338	28	0.4	0.4
0	1	<0.1	<0.1	0.2	0.1	24	0	24	<0.1	9	17	8	77	5	0.2	0.1
0	4	0.1	0.1	0.6	0.2	74	0	56	0.1	31	43	32	250	16	0.7	0.2
0	1	<0.1	<0.1	0.3	0.1	28	0	23	<0.1	11	22	15	152	8	0.2	0.1
0	8	<0.1	<0.1	0.2	0.1	17	0	4	0.4	24	15	52	172	7	0.2	0.1
0	5	<0.1	<0.1	0.1	<0.1	11	0	3	0.3	16	10	35	115	4	0.2	0.1

ERA, EatRight Analysis CD-ROM; **AMT,** amount; **WT,** weight; **WTR,** water; **CAL,** calories; **PROT,** protein; **CARB,** carbohydrate; **FIBR,** fiber; **FAT,** fat; **SATF,** saturated fat; **MONO,** monounsaturated fat; **POLY,** polyunsaturated fat

ERA CODE	FOOD DESCRIPTION	AMT	UNIT	WT (g)	WTR (g)	CAL (kcal)	PROT (g)	CARB (g)	FIBR (g)	FAT (g)	SATF (g)	MONO (g)	POLY (g)
Vegetables and Legumes (continued)													
5399	Chili peppers, hot, green, raw	0.5	cup	75	66	30	2	7	1	<1	<0.1	<0.1	0.1
5288	Chili peppers, red, raw, pieces	0.5	cup	75	66	30	2	7	1	<1	<0.1	<0.1	0.1
5061	Collard greens, boiled	1	cup	190	174	49	4	9	5	1	0.1	<0.1	0.3
5062	Collard greens, frozen, boiled	1	cup	170	150	61	5	12	5	1	0.1	<0.1	0.4
5515	Corn w/red pepper, Mexican	1	cup	227	176	170	5	41	5	1	0.2	0.4	0.6
5201	Corn, canned+liquid	0.5	cup	128	104	82	2	20	2	1	0.1	0.2	0.3
5066	Corn, canned, drained	0.5	cup	82	63	66	2	15	2	1	0.1	0.2	0.4
5364	Corn on cob, small, frozen, ckd	1	ea	63	46	59	2	14	2	<1	0.1	0.1	0.2
5380	Corn on cob, yellow, med, boiled	1	ea	77	54	83	3	19	2	1	0.2	0.3	0.5
5560	Corn, white, boiled	1	ea	77	54	83	3	19	2	1	0.2	0.3	0.5
5562	Corn, white, canned+liquid	0.5	cup	128	104	82	2	20	1	1	0.1	0.2	0.3
5563	Corn, white, canned, drained	0.5	cup	82	63	66	2	15	2	1	0.1	0.2	0.4
5393	Corn, white, frozen, cooked	0.5	cup	82	63	66	2	16	2	<1	0.1	0.1	0.2
5379	Corn, yellow, boiled	0.5	cup	82	57	89	3	21	2	1	0.2	0.3	0.5
5065	Corn, yellow, frozen, boiled	0.5	cup	82	63	66	2	16	2	<1	0.1	0.1	0.2
5068	Creamed corn, canned	0.5	cup	128	101	92	2	23	2	1	0.1	0.2	0.3
5071	Cucumber, raw, pieces w/peel	0.5	cup	52	50	7	<1	1	<1	<1	<0.1	<0.1	<0.1
5070	Cucumber, whole, 8 inch	1	ea	301	289	39	2	8	2	<1	0.1	<0.1	0.2
5673	Eggplant pieces, steamed	1	cup	96	88	25	1	6	2	<1	<0.1	<0.1	<0.1
5674	Eggplant pieces, stir fried	1	cup	96	88	25	1	6	2	<1	<0.1	<0.1	<0.1
5202	Escarole/curly endive	1	cup	50	47	8	1	2	2	<1	<0.1	<0.1	<0.1
7055	Fava/broadbeans, canned+liq	0.5	cup	128	103	91	7	16	5	<1	<0.1	0.1	0.1
7027	Fava/broadbeans, dry, cooked	1	cup	170	122	187	13	33	9	1	0.1	0.1	0.3
5139	French fries, frozen, heated	10	pce	50	18	166	2	20	2	9	3	5.7	0.7
5460	French fries, veg oil, serving	1	ea	115	41	393	5	46	4	21	4.4	12.2	3.6
5536	Fried green tomatoes	1	ea	144	97	284	5	19	1	22	4.6	9.4	6.4
56638	Frijoles+cheese	1	cup	167	115	225	11	29		8	4.1	2.6	0.7
7088	Garbanzo beans/chickpeas+liq	0.5	cup	120	84	143	6	27	5	1	0.1	0.3	0.6
7001	Garbanzo beans/chickpeas, ckd	1	cup	164	99	269	15	45	12	4	0.4	1	1.9
26005	Garlic cloves, fresh	4	ea	12	7	18	1	4	<1	<1	<0.1	<0.1	<0.1
5140	Hash brown potatoes, frzn, ckd	1	cup	156	88	340	5	44	3	18	7	8	2.1
5141	Hash browns, frozen, fried patty	1	ea	29	16	63	1	8	1	3	1.3	1.5	0.4
5640	Hominy, cooked	1	cup	165	136	119	2	24	4	1	0.2	0.4	0.7
38077	Hominy, white, canned	1	cup	165	136	119	2	24	4	1	0.2	0.4	0.7
5470	Hominy, yellow, canned	1	cup	160	132	115	2	23	4	1	0.2	0.4	0.6
7081	Hummous/hummus	1	cup	246	160	421	12	50	13	21	3.1	8.7	7.8
5293	Jalapeno peppers, chop, can	0.5	cup	68	60	18	1	3	2	1	0.1	<0.1	0.3
6099	Jalapeno peppers, raw	1	ea	45	40	11	<1	2		<1			
6208	Japanese stir fry veg (Birdseye)	0.5	cup	116	106	35	2	7	2	<1	<0.1		
5224	Jicama	1	cup	120	108	46	1	11	6	<1	<0.1	<0.1	0.1
5075	Kale, cooked	1	cup	130	118	36	2	7	3	1	0.1	<0.1	0.2
5206	Leeks, raw	1	ea	89	74	54	1	13	2	<1	<0.1	<0.1	0.1
7086	Lentil loaf, 3/4 in slice	1	pce	47	29	83	4	10	3	4	0.4	0.9	2.1
7006	Lentils, cooked	1	cup	198	138	230	18	40	16	1	0.1	0.1	0.3
5080	Lettuce, butterhead, chopped	1	cup	56	54	7	1	1	1	<1	<0.1	<0.1	0.1
5083	Lettuce, iceberg, chopped	1	cup	55	53	7	1	1	1	<1	<0.1	<0.1	0.1

< = Trace amount present   Blank = Not available

CHOL, cholesterol; **V,** vitamin; **THI,** thiamin; **RIB,** riboflavin; **NIA,** niacin; **FOL,** folate;
CALC, calcium; **PHOS,** phosphate; **SOD,** sodium; **POT,** potassium; **MAG,** magnesium

CHOL (mg)	V-A (RE)	THI (mg)	RIB (mg)	NIA (mg)	V-B6 (mg)	FOL (μg)	V-B12 (μg)	V-C (mg)	V-E (mg)	CALC (mg)	PHOS (mg)	SOD (mg)	POT (mg)	MAG (mg)	IRON (mg)	ZINC (mg)
0	58	0.1	0.1	0.7	0.2	18	0	182	0.5	14	34	5	255	19	0.9	0.2
0	806	0.1	0.1	0.7	0.2	18	0	182	0.5	14	34	5	255	19	0.9	0.2
0	595	0.1	0.2	1.1	0.2	177	0	35	1.7	226	49	17	494	32	0.9	0.8
0	1016	0.1	0.2	1.1	0.2	129	0	45	0.9	357	46	85	427	51	1.9	0.5
0	52	<0.1	0.2	2.2	0.2	77	0	20	2.5	11	141	788	347	57	1.8	0.8
0	19	<0.1	0.1	1.2	<0.1	49	0	7	0.2	5	65	273	210	20	0.5	0.5
0	13	<0.1	0.1	1	<0.1	40	0	7	0.1	4	53	175	160	16	0.7	0.3
0	13	0.1	<0.1	1	0.1	19	0	3	0.2	2	47	3	158	18	0.4	0.4
0	17	0.2	0.1	1.2	<0.1	36	0	5	0.4	2	79	13	192	25	0.5	0.4
0	0	0.2	0.1	1.2	<0.1	36	0	5	0.1	2	79	13	192	25	0.5	0.4
0	0	<0.1	0.1	1.2	<0.1	49	0	7	0.4	5	65	15	210	20	0.5	0.5
0	0	<0.1	0.1	1	<0.1	40	0	7	0.1	4	53	265	160	16	0.7	0.3
0	0	0.1	0.1	1.1	0.1	25	0	3	0.1	3	47	4	120	16	0.3	0.3
0	18	0.2	0.1	1.3	<0.1	38	0	5	0.4	2	84	14	204	26	0.5	0.4
0	18	0.1	0.1	1.1	0.1	25	0	3	0.1	3	47	4	120	16	0.3	0.3
0	13	<0.1	0.1	1.2	0.1	57	0	6	0.4	4	65	365	172	22	0.5	0.7
0	11	<0.1	<0.1	0.1	<0.1	7	0	3	0.1	7	10	1	75	6	0.1	0.1
0	63	0.1	0.1	0.7	0.1	39	0	16	0.8	42	60	6	433	33	0.8	0.6
0	6	0.1	<0.1	0.5	0.1	18	0	1	0.1	7	21	3	208	11	0.3	0.1
0	6	0.1	<0.1	0.5	0.1	18	0	1	0.1	7	21	3	208	11	0.3	0.1
0	102	<0.1	<0.1	0.2	<0.1	71	0	3	0.2	26	14	11	157	8	0.4	0.4
0	1	<0.1	0.1	1.2	0.1	42	0	2	0.1	33	101	580	310	41	1.3	0.8
0	3	0.2	0.2	1.2	0.1	177	0	1	0.2	61	212	8	456	73	2.5	1.7
0	0	<0.1	<0.1	1.3	0.1	11	0	3	0.3	6	48	306	270	12	0.8	0.2
0	0	0.1	<0.1	3.3	0.4	44	0	13	1.4	16	148	228	792	45	0.9	0.5
41	82	0.2	0.2	1.4	0.1	13	0.1	21	3	101	102	134	254	17	1.5	0.4
37	70	0.1	0.3	1.5	0.2	112	0.7	2		189	175	882	604	85	2.2	1.7
0	2	<0.1	<0.1	0.2	0.6	80	0	5	0.2	38	108	359	206	35	1.6	1.3
0	5	0.2	0.1	0.9	0.2	282	0	2	1.9	80	276	11	477	79	4.7	2.5
0	0	<0.1	<0.1	0.1	0.1	<1	0	4	<0.1	22	18	2	48	3	0.2	0.1
0	0	0.2	<0.1	3.8	0.2	10	0	10	0.3	23	112	53	680	27	2.4	0.5
0	0	<0.1	<0.1	0.7	<0.1	2	0	2	0.1	4	21	10	126	5	0.4	0.1
0	0	<0.1	<0.1	0.1	<0.1	2	0	0	0.1	16	58	346	15	26	1	1.7
0	0	<0.1	<0.1	0.1	<0.1	2	0	0	0.1	16	58	346	15	26	1	1.7
0	18	<0.1	<0.1	0.1	<0.1	2	0	0	0.2	16	56	336	14	26	1	1.7
0	5	0.2	0.1	1	1	146	0	19	2.5	123	276	600	428	71	3.9	2.7
0	116	<0.1	<0.1	0.3	0.1	10	0	7	0.5	16	12	1136	131	10	1.3	0.2
	30						0	53	0.4			2	2			
0	74	0.1	0.1	0.9	0.1	35	0	32		31	42	439	191	15	0.7	
0	2	<0.1	<0.1	0.2	0.1	14	0	24	0.5	14	22	5	180	14	0.7	0.2
0	962	0.1	0.1	0.6	0.2	17	0	53	1.1	94	36	30	296	23	1.2	0.3
0	9	0.1	<0.1	0.4	0.2	57	0	11	0.8	53	31	18	160	25	1.9	0.1
0	<1	0.1	<0.1	0.7	0.1	61	0	1	2.2	18	88	44	156	27	1.5	0.6
0	2	0.3	0.1	2.1	0.4	358	0	3	1.2	38	356	4	731	71	6.6	2.5
0	54	<0.1	<0.1	0.2	<0.1	41	0	4	0.4	18	13	3	144	7	0.2	0.1
0	18	<0.1	<0.1	0.1	<0.1	31	0	2	0.4	10	11	5	87	5	0.3	0.1

ERA, EatRight Analysis CD-ROM; **AMT,** amount; **WT,** weight; **WTR,** water; **CAL,** calories; **PROT,** protein; **CARB**, carbohydrate; **FIBR,** fiber; **FAT,** fat; **SATF,** saturated fat; **MONO,** monounsaturated fat; **POLY,** polyunsaturated fat

ERA CODE	FOOD DESCRIPTION	AMT	UNIT	WT (g)	WTR (g)	CAL (kcal)	PROT (g)	CARB (g)	FIBR (g)	FAT (g)	SATF (g)	MONO (g)	POLY (g)
Vegetables and Legumes (continued)													
5084	Lettuce, iceberg, leaf	1	pce	15	14	2	<1	<1	<1	<1	<0.1	<0.1	<0.1
5086	Lettuce, looseleaf, chopped	1	cup	56	53	10	1	2	1	<1	<0.1	<0.1	0.1
5087	Lettuce, looseleaf, leaf	1	pce	10	9	2	<1	<1	<1	<1	<0.1	<0.1	<0.1
5305	Mixed vegetable, canned, drain	1	cup	163	142	77	4	15	5	<1	0.1	<0.1	0.2
5516	Mixed vegetables, cnd, low sod	1	cup	182	164	66	3	13	6	<1	0.1	<0.1	0.2
5187	Mixed vegetables, frzn, cooked	1	cup	182	151	107	5	24	8	<1	0.1	<0.1	0.1
5021	Mung bean sprouts, boiled	1	cup	124	116	26	3	5	1	<1	<0.1	<0.1	<0.1
5197	Mung bean sprouts, canned	1	cup	125	120	15	2	3	1	<1	<0.1	<0.1	<0.1
5092	Mushroom pieces, boiled	0.5	cup	78	71	21	2	4	2	<1	<0.1	<0.1	0.1
5094	Mushroom pieces, canned	0.5	cup	78	71	19	1	4	2	<1	<0.1	<0.1	0.1
5090	Mushroom slices, raw	0.5	cup	35	32	9	1	1	<1	<1	<0.1	<0.1	<0.1
5514	Mushroom, batter fried	5	ea	70	44	156	2	11	1	12	1.5	3.6	6
5091	Mushroom, raw, whole	1	ea	23	21	6	1	1	<1	<1	<0.1	<0.1	<0.1
5096	Mustard greens, boiled	1	cup	140	132	21	3	3	3	<1	<0.1	0.2	0.1
5098	Okra pods, boiled	8	ea	85	76	27	2	6	2	<1	<0.1	<0.1	<0.1
5100	Okra pods, frozen, boiled	0.5	cup	92	84	26	2	5	3	<1	0.1	<0.1	0.1
5099	Okra slices, boiled	0.5	cup	80	72	26	1	6	2	<1	<0.1	<0.1	<0.1
5644	Okra, batter fried	1	cup	92	62	175	2	14	2	12	1.7	3.1	7.1
5190	Onion rings, frozen, heated	2	ea	20	6	81	1	8	<1	5	1.7	2.2	1
5106	Onion slices, raw	1	pce	38	34	14	<1	3	1	<1	<0.1	<0.1	<0.1
5104	Onion, raw, medium, whole	1	ea	110	99	42	1	9	2	<1	<0.1	<0.1	0.1
5108	Onions, boiled	0.5	cup	105	92	46	1	11	1	<1	<0.1	<0.1	0.1
5101	Onions, chopped, raw	1	cup	160	143	61	2	14	3	<1	<0.1	<0.1	0.1
26012	Parsley, fresh, chopped	0.5	cup	30	26	11	1	2	1	<1	<0.1	0.1	<0.1
5212	Parsnips, boiled	1	cup	156	121	126	2	30	6	<1	0.1	0.2	0.1
5281	Peas+carrots, canned+liquid	1	cup	255	225	97	6	22	5	1	0.1	0.1	0.3
5123	Peas+carrots, frozen, boiled	0.5	cup	80	69	38	2	8	2	<1	0.1	<0.1	0.2
7016	Peas, cowpea/blackeye, canned	1	cup	240	191	185	11	33	8	1	0.3	0.1	0.6
7018	Peas, cowpea/blackeye, dry, boil	1	cup	172	120	200	13	36	11	1	0.2	0.1	0.4
5117	Peas, green, boiled	1	cup	160	124	134	9	25	9	<1	0.1	<0.1	0.2
5214	Peas, green, canned+liquid	0.5	cup	124	106	66	4	12	4	<1	0.1	<0.1	0.2
5267	Peas, green, low sod, cnd+liq	0.5	cup	124	106	66	4	12	4	<1	0.1	<0.1	0.2
5118	Peas, greens, frozen, boiled	0.5	cup	80	64	62	4	11	4	<1	<0.1	<0.1	0.1
5124	Pepper, sweet green, fresh	1	cup	149	137	40	1	10	3	<1	<0.1	<0.1	0.2
5126	Pepper, sweet green, cooked	0.5	cup	68	62	19	1	5	1	<1	<0.1	<0.1	0.1
5125	Pepper, sweet green, whole	1	ea	74	68	20	1	5	1	<1	<0.1	<0.1	0.1
5128	Pepper, sweet red, raw, chpd	1	cup	149	137	40	1	10	3	<1	<0.1	<0.1	0.2
5441	Pepper, sweet yellow, large	1	ea	186	171	50	2	12	2	<1	0.1	<0.1	0.2
5622	Pickled vegetables	1	cup	163	149	44	2	10	3	<1	<0.1	<0.1	0.1
5227	Pimento, canned	1	Tbs	12	11	3	<1	1	<1	<1	<0.1	<0.1	<0.1
5228	Pimento slices, canned	20	pce	20	19	5	<1	1	<1	<1	<0.1	<0.1	<0.1
5352	Potato pieces, canned	0.5	cup	90	76	54	1	12	2	<1	<0.1	<0.1	0.1
5339	Potato skin, oven baked	1	ea	58	27	115	2	27	5	<1	<0.1	<0.1	<0.1
5130	Potato, baked, flesh, medium	0.5	cup	61	46	57	1	13	1	<1	<0.1	<0.1	<0.1
5947	Potato, baked, salted w/skin	1	ea	202	144	220	5	51	5	<1	0.1	<0.1	0.1
5276	Potatoes, au gratin from mix	1	cup	245	194	228	6	31	2	10	6.3	2.9	0.3

< = Trace amount present   Blank = Not available

CHOL, cholesterol; **V,** vitamin; **THI,** thiamin; **RIB,** riboflavin; **NIA,** niacin; **FOL,** folate; **CALC,** calcium; **PHOS,** phosphate; **SOD,** sodium; **POT,** potassium; **MAG,** magnesium

CHOL (mg)	V-A (RE)	THI (mg)	RIB (mg)	NIA (mg)	V-B6 (mg)	FOL (μg)	V-B12 (μg)	V-C (mg)	V-E (mg)	CALC (mg)	PHOS (mg)	SOD (mg)	POT (mg)	MAG (mg)	IRON (mg)	ZINC (mg)
0	5	<0.1	<0.1	<0.1	<0.1	8	0	1	0.1	3	3	1	24	1	0.1	<0.1
0	106	<0.1	<0.1	0.2	<0.1	28	0	10	0.6	38	14	5	148	6	0.8	0.2
0	19	<0.1	<0.1	<0.1	<0.1	5	0	2	0.1	7	2	1	26	1	0.1	<0.1
0	1898	0.1	0.1	0.9	0.1	38	0	8	1	44	68	243	474	26	1.7	0.7
0	924	0.1	0.1	0.9	0.1	33	0	7	0.4	38	67	47	251	27	1.2	0.9
0	779	0.1	0.2	1.5	0.1	35	0	6	0.8	46	93	64	308	40	1.5	0.9
0	1	0.1	0.1	1	0.1	36	0	14	0.1	15	35	12	125	17	0.8	0.6
0	2	<0.1	0.1	0.3	<0.1	12	0	<1	0.1	18	40	175	34	11	0.5	0.3
0	0	0.1	0.2	3.5	0.1	14	0	3	0.2	5	68	2	278	9	1.4	0.7
0	0	0.1	<0.1	1.2	<0.1	10	0	0	0.2	9	51	332	101	12	0.6	0.6
0	0	<0.1	0.1	1.4	<0.1	4	<0.1	1	0.1	2	36	1	130	4	0.4	0.3
2	6	0.1	0.3	2.3	<0.1	8	<0.1	1	2.3	15	119	112	154	7	1.2	0.4
0	0	<0.1	0.1	0.9	<0.1	3	<0.1	1	0.1	1	24	1	85	2	0.2	0.2
0	424	0.1	0.1	0.6	0.1	103	0	35	3	104	57	22	283	21	1	0.2
0	49	0.1	<0.1	0.7	0.2	39	0	14	0.6	54	48	4	274	48	0.4	0.5
0	47	0.1	0.1	0.7	<0.1	134	0	11	0.6	88	42	3	215	47	0.6	0.6
0	46	0.1	<0.1	0.7	0.1	37	0	13	0.6	50	45	4	258	46	0.4	0.4
2	39	0.2	0.1	1.4	0.1	38	<0.1	10	3	61	122	122	190	36	1.3	0.5
0	5	0.1	<0.1	0.7	<0.1	13	0	<1	1.3	6	16	75	26	4	0.3	0.1
0	0	<0.1	<0.1	0.1	<0.1	7	0	2	0.1	8	13	1	60	4	0.1	0.1
0	0	<0.1	<0.1	0.2	0.1	21	0	7	0.3	22	36	3	173	11	0.2	0.2
0	0	<0.1	<0.1	0.2	0.1	16	0	5	0.4	23	37	3	174	12	0.3	0.2
0	0	0.1	<0.1	0.2	0.2	30	0	10	0.5	32	53	5	251	16	0.4	0.3
0	156	<0.1	<0.1	0.4	<0.1	46	0	40	0.5	41	17	17	166	15	1.9	0.3
0	0	0.1	0.1	1.1	0.1	91	0	20	1.6	58	108	16	572	45	0.9	0.4
0	1471	0.2	0.1	1.5	0.2	47	0	17	1.4	59	117	663	255	36	1.9	1.5
0	621	0.2	0.1	0.9	0.1	21	0	6	0.9	18	39	54	126	13	0.8	0.4
0	2	0.2	0.2	0.8	0.1	123	0	6	0.2	48	168	718	413	67	2.3	1.7
0	3	0.3	0.1	0.9	0.2	358	0	1	0.5	41	268	7	478	91	4.3	2.2
0	96	0.4	0.2	3.2	0.3	101	0	23	0.8	43	187	5	434	62	2.5	1.9
0	47	0.1	0.1	1	0.1	35	0	12	0.3	22	66	310	124	21	1.3	0.9
0	47	0.1	0.1	1	0.1	35	0	12	0.8	22	66	11	124	21	1.3	0.9
0	54	0.2	0.1	1.2	0.1	47	0	8	0.4	19	72	70	134	23	1.3	0.8
0	94	0.1	<0.1	0.8	0.4	33	0	133	1	13	28	3	264	15	0.7	0.2
0	40	<0.1	<0.1	0.3	0.2	11	0	51	0.5	6	12	1	113	7	0.3	0.1
0	47	<0.1	<0.1	0.4	0.2	16	0	66	0.5	7	14	1	131	7	0.3	0.1
0	849	0.1	<0.1	0.8	0.4	33	0	283	1.1	13	28	3	264	15	0.7	0.2
0	45	0.1	<0.1	1.7	0.3	48	0	341	1.3	20	45	4	394	22	0.9	0.3
0	1128	0.1	0.1	0.8	0.2	27	0	56	0.5	32	45	332	348	19	0.7	0.3
0	32	<0.1	<0.1	0.1	<0.1	1	0	10	0.1	1	2	2	19	1	0.2	<0.1
0	53	<0.1	<0.1	0.1	<0.1	1	0	17	0.1	1	3	3	32	1	0.3	<0.1
0	0	0.1	<0.1	0.8	0.2	6	0	5	0.1	4	25	197	206	13	1.1	0.3
0	0	0.1	0.1	1.8	0.4	13	0	8	<0.1	20	59	12	332	25	4.1	0.3
0	0	0.1	<0.1	0.9	0.2	6	0	8	<0.1	3	30	3	238	15	0.2	0.2
0	0	0.2	0.1	3.3	0.7	22	0	26	0.1	20	115	493	844	55	2.7	0.6
37	76	<0.1	0.2	2.3	0.1	16	0	8	2.9	203	233	1075	536	37	0.8	0.6

ERA, EatRight Analysis CD-ROM; **AMT,** amount; **WT,** weight; **WTR,** water; **CAL,** calories; **PROT,** protein; **CARB**, carbohydrate; **FIBR,** fiber; **FAT,** fat; **SATF,** saturated fat; **MONO,** monounsaturated fat; **POLY,** polyunsaturated fat

ERA CODE	FOOD DESCRIPTION	AMT	UNIT	WT (g)	WTR (g)	CAL (kcal)	PROT (g)	CARB (g)	FIBR (g)	FAT (g)	SATF (g)	MONO (g)	POLY (g)
Vegetables and Legumes (continued)													
5569	Potatoes, mashed w/milk+butter	1	cup	210	160	223	4	35	4	9	5.8	2.5	0.3
5464	Potatoes, mashed, flakes, prep	1	cup	210	160	237	4	32	5	12	7.2	3.3	0.5
5269	Potatoes, O'Brien, frozen, cooked	1	cup	194	120	396	4	42	3	26	6.4	11.3	6.7
5270	Potatoes, scalloped recipe	1	cup	245	198	211	7	26	5	9	3.4	3.3	1.8
5271	Potatoes, scalloped from mix	1	cup	245	194	228	5	31	3	11	6.4	3	0.5
5136	Potato, peeled, boiled, pieces	0.5	cup	78	60	67	1	16	1	<1	<0.1	<0.1	<0.1
5451	Radicchio, raw, shredded	0.5	cup	20	19	5	<1	1	<1	<1	<0.1	<0.1	<0.1
5144	Radish, red, slices	0.5	cup	58	55	12	<1	2	1	<1	<0.1	<0.1	<0.1
5143	Radish, red, whole	10	ea	45	43	9	<1	2	1	<1	<0.1	<0.1	<0.1
5238	Red cabbage, boiled	0.5	cup	75	70	16	1	3	2	<1	<0.1	<0.1	0.1
7024	Refried beans/frijoles, canned	1	cup	252	191	237	14	39	13	3	1.2	1.4	0.4
5088	Romaine lettuce, chopped	1	cup	56	53	8	1	1	1	<1	<0.1	<0.1	0.1
5969	Rutabaga, mashed w/salt	0.5	cup	120	107	47	2	10	2	<1	<0.1	<0.1	0.1
5145	Sauerkraut, canned+liquid	1	cup	236	218	45	2	10	6	<1	0.1	<0.1	0.1
5531	Sauerkraut, canned, low sod	1	cup	142	131	27	1	6	4	<1	<0.1	<0.1	0.1
5427	Shallots, raw, chopped	1	Tbs	10	8	7	<1	2	<1	<1	<0.1	<0.1	<0.1
5385	Shiitake mushrooms, boiled, pieces	1	cup	145	121	80	2	21	3	<1	0.1	0.1	<0.1
5122	Snow pea pods, boiled	1	cup	160	142	67	5	11	4	<1	0.1	<0.1	0.2
5296	Snow pea pods, frozen, boiled	0.5	cup	80	69	42	3	7	2	<1	0.1	<0.1	0.1
7015	Soybeans, dry, cooked	1	cup	172	108	298	29	17	10	15	2.2	3.4	8.7
5147	Spinach, boiled	1	cup	180	164	41	5	7	4	<1	0.1	<0.1	0.2
5146	Spinach, raw, chopped	1	cup	30	27	7	1	1	1	<1	<0.1	<0.1	<0.1
7020	Split peas, cooked	1	cup	196	136	231	16	41	16	1	0.1	0.2	0.3
5114	Spring/green onion, pieces	0.5	cup	50	45	16	1	4	1	<1	<0.1	<0.1	<0.1
5317	Squash, butternut, baked	1	cup	205	180	82	2	22	6	<1	<0.1	<0.1	0.1
5453	Squash, Hubbard, baked	1	cup	240	204	120	6	26	6	1	0.3	0.1	0.6
5455	Squash, spaghetti, boiled	1	cup	155	143	42	1	10	2	<1	0.1	<0.1	0.2
5152	Squash, summer, boiled	1	cup	180	169	36	2	8	3	1	0.1	<0.1	0.2
5303	Squash, winter, baked	1	cup	205	182	80	2	18	6	1	0.3	0.1	0.5
5251	Succotash, boiled	1	cup	192	131	221	10	47	9	2	0.3	0.3	0.7
5154	Succotash, frozen, boiled	1	cup	170	126	158	7	34	7	2	0.3	0.3	0.7
5601	Succotash, whole corn, canned	1	cup	255	209	161	7	36	7	1	0.2	0.2	0.6
5155	Sweet potato, baked+skin	1	ea	114	83	117	2	28	3	<1	<0.1	<0.1	0.1
5166	Sweet potatoes, candied	1	pce	105	70	144	1	29	3	3	1.4	0.7	0.2
5059	Swiss chard, boiled	1	cup	175	162	35	3	7	4	<1	<0.1	<0.1	<0.1
5302	Taro slices, cooked	1	cup	132	84	187	1	46	7	<1	<0.1	<0.1	0.1
5266	Tater Tots, frozen, heated	10	ea	79	42	175	3	24	3	8	4	3.4	0.6
5476	Tomato puree, canned	1	cup	250	219	100	4	24	5	<1	0.1	0.1	0.2
5178	Tomatoes, boiled, cup measure	1	cup	240	221	65	3	14	2	1	0.1	0.2	0.4
5179	Tomatoes, canned	1	cup	240	225	46	2	10	2	<1	<0.1	<0.1	0.1
5171	Tomatoes, cherry	1	ea	17	16	4	<1	1	<1	<1	<0.1	<0.1	<0.1
5170	Tomatoes, fresh, chopped	1	cup	180	169	38	2	8	2	1	0.1	0.1	0.2
5474	Tomatoes, stewed, cnd, low sod	1	cup	255	232	71	2	17	3	<1	<0.1	0.1	0.1
5446	Tomatoes, sun dried	1	cup	54	8	139	8	30	7	2	0.2	0.3	0.6
5169	Tomato, fresh, medium	1	ea	123	115	26	1	6	1	<1	0.1	0.1	0.2
5173	Tomato, fresh, slices	2	pce	40	38	8	<1	2	<1	<1	<0.1	<0.1	0.1

< = Trace amount present Blank = Not available

CHOL, cholesterol; **V,** vitamin; **THI,** thiamin; **RIB,** riboflavin; **NIA,** niacin; **FOL,** folate;
CALC, calcium; **PHOS,** phosphate; **SOD,** sodium; **POT,** potassium; **MAG,** magnesium

CHOL (mg)	V-A (RE)	THI (mg)	RIB (mg)	NIA (mg)	V-B6 (mg)	FOL (μg)	V-B12 (μg)	V-C (mg)	V-E (mg)	CALC (mg)	PHOS (mg)	SOD (mg)	POT (mg)	MAG (mg)	IRON (mg)	ZINC (mg)
25	42	0.2	0.1	2.3	0.5	17	0	13	0.6	55	97	620	607	38	0.5	0.6
29	44	0.2	0.1	1.4	<0.1	16	0.2	20	1.5	103	118	697	489	38	0.5	0.4
0	37	0.1	0.3	2.8	0.7	24	0	20	0.4	39	180	83	918	66	1.9	1.1
15	47	0.2	0.2	2.6	0.4	27	0	26	0.8	140	154	821	926	47	1.4	1
27	51	<0.1	0.1	2.5	0.1	23	0	8	0.4	88	137	835	497	34	0.9	0.6
0	0	0.1	<0.1	1	0.2	7	0	6	<0.1	6	31	4	256	16	0.2	0.2
0	1	<0.1	<0.1	0.1	<0.1	12	0	2	0.5	4	8	4	60	3	0.1	0.1
0	1	<0.1	<0.1	0.2	<0.1	16	0	13	0	12	10	14	134	5	0.2	0.2
0	<1	<0.1	<0.1	0.1	<0.1	12	0	10	0	9	8	11	104	4	0.1	0.1
0	2	<0.1	<0.1	0.2	0.1	9	0	26	0.1	28	22	6	105	8	0.3	0.1
20	0	0.1	<0.1	0.8	0.4	28	0	15	0	88	217	753	673	83	4.2	2.9
0	146	0.1	0.1	0.3	<0.1	76	0	13	0.4	20	25	4	162	3	0.6	0.1
0	67	0.1	<0.1	0.9	0.1	18	0	23	0.2	58	67	305	391	28	0.6	0.4
0	5	<0.1	0.1	0.3	0.3	56	0	35	4	71	47	1559	401	31	3.5	0.4
0	3	<0.1	<0.1	0.2	0.1	34	0	21	0.1	43	28	437	241	18	2.1	0.3
0	12	<0.1	<0.1	<0.1	<0.1	3	0	1	<0.1	4	6	1	33	2	0.1	<0.1
0	0	0.1	0.2	2.2	0.2	30	0	<1	0.2	4	42	6	170	20	0.6	1.9
0	21	0.2	0.1	0.9	0.2	47	0	77	4.7	67	88	6	384	42	3.2	0.6
0	14	0.1	0.1	0.4	0.1	28	0	18	2.3	47	46	4	174	22	1.9	0.4
0	2	0.3	0.5	0.7	0.4	93	0	3	3.4	175	421	2	886	148	8.8	2
0	1474	0.2	0.4	0.9	0.4	262	0	18	3.6	245	101	126	839	157	6.4	1.4
0	202	<0.1	0.1	0.2	0.1	58	0	8	0.8	30	15	24	167	24	0.8	0.2
0	2	0.4	0.1	1.7	0.1	127	0	1	1.5	27	194	4	710	71	2.5	2
0	20	<0.1	<0.1	0.3	<0.1	32	0	9	0.2	36	18	8	138	10	0.7	0.2
0	1435	0.1	<0.1	2	0.3	39	0	31	1.4	84	55	8	582	59	1.2	0.3
0	1449	0.2	0.1	1.3	0.4	39	0	23	0.3	41	55	19	859	53	1.1	0.4
0	17	0.1	<0.1	1.3	0.2	12	0	5	0.2	33	22	28	181	17	0.5	0.3
0	52	0.1	0.1	0.9	0.1	36	0	10	0.3	49	70	2	346	43	0.6	0.7
0	730	0.2	<0.1	1.4	0.1	57	0	20	0.2	29	41	2	896	16	0.7	0.5
0	56	0.3	0.2	2.5	0.2	63	0	16	2.2	33	225	33	787	102	2.9	1.2
0	39	0.1	0.1	2.2	0.2	56	0	10	1.7	26	119	76	450	39	1.5	0.8
0	38	0.1	0.1	1.6	0.1	81	0	12	2.4	28	140	564	416	48	1.4	1.3
0	2487	0.1	0.1	0.7	0.3	26	0	28	0.3	32	63	11	397	23	0.5	0.3
8	440	<0.1	<0.1	0.4	<0.1	12	0	7	4	27	27	74	198	12	1.2	0.2
0	550	0.1	0.2	0.6	0.1	15	0	32	3.3	102	58	313	961	150	4	0.6
0	0	0.1	<0.1	0.7	0.4	25	0	7	0.6	24	100	20	639	40	0.9	0.4
0	2	0.2	0.1	1.7	0.2	13	0	5	0.1	24	38	589	300	15	1.2	0.2
0	320	0.2	0.1	4.3	0.4	28	0	26	6.3	42	100	998	1065	60	3.1	0.6
0	178	0.2	0.1	1.8	0.2	31	0	55	2.8	14	74	26	670	34	1.3	0.3
0	144	0.1	0.1	1.8	0.2	19	0	34	1.6	72	46	355	530	29	1.3	0.4
0	11	<0.1	<0.1	0.1	<0.1	3	0	3	0.2	1	4	2	38	2	0.1	<0.1
0	112	0.1	0.1	1.1	0.1	27	0	34	1.7	9	43	16	400	20	0.8	0.2
0	138	0.1	0.1	1.8	<0.1	14	0	29	1	84	51	564	607	31	1.9	0.4
0	47	0.3	0.3	4.9	0.2	37	0	21	<0.1	59	192	1131	1850	105	4.9	1.1
0	76	0.1	0.1	0.8	0.1	18	0	23	1.1	6	30	11	273	14	0.6	0.1
0	25	<0.1	<0.1	0.3	<0.1	6	0	8	0.4	2	10	4	89	4	0.2	<0.1

ERA, EatRight Analysis CD-ROM; **AMT,** amount; **WT,** weight; **WTR,** water; **CAL,** calories; **PROT,** protein; **CARB**, carbohydrate; **FIBR,** fiber; **FAT,** fat; **SATF,** saturated fat; **MONO,** monounsaturated fat; **POLY,** polyunsaturated fat

ERA CODE	FOOD DESCRIPTION	AMT	UNIT	WT (g)	WTR (g)	CAL (kcal)	PROT (g)	CARB (g)	FIBR (g)	FAT (g)	SATF (g)	MONO (g)	POLY (g)
Vegetables and Legumes (continued)													
5174	Tomato, fresh, wedge	1	pce	31	29	7	<1	1	<1	<1	<0.1	<0.1	<0.1
5172	Tomato, Italian/plum, fresh	1	ea	62	58	13	1	3	1	<1	<0.1	<0.1	0.1
5183	Turnip cubes, boiled	0.5	cup	78	73	16	1	4	2	<1	<0.1	<0.1	<0.1
5185	Turnip greens, boiled	1	cup	144	134	29	2	6	5	<1	0.1	<0.1	0.1
5186	Turnip greens, frozen, boiled	0.5	cup	82	74	25	3	4	3	<1	0.1	<0.1	0.1
7490	Wasabi radish, cooked	1	cup	147	140	25	1	5	2	<1	0.1	0.1	0.2
5387	Water chestnuts, canned, slices	0.5	cup	70	60	35	1	9	2	<1	<0.1	0	<0.1
5223	Watercress sprigs, fresh	10	ea	25	24	3	1	<1	<1	<1	<0.1	<0.1	<0.1
5222	Watercress, fresh	0.5	cup	17	16	2	<1	<1	<1	<1	<0.1	<0.1	<0.1
7053	White beans, boiled	1	cup	179	113	249	17	45	11	1	0.2	0.1	0.3
5553	Yams, orange+syrup, canned	1	cup	228	176	203	2	48	6	<1	0.1	<0.1	0.2
5160	Yams, orange, peeled, boiled	1	cup	328	239	344	5	80	6	1	0.2	<0.1	0.4
5667	Zucchini slices, steamed	1	cup	180	172	25	2	5	2	<1	0.1	<0.1	0.1
5327	Zucchini squash, boiled	1	cup	180	170	29	1	7	3	<1	<0.1	<0.1	<0.1
5326	Zucchini squash, raw	1	cup	130	124	18	2	4	2	<1	<0.1	<0.1	0.1

CHOL, cholesterol; **V,** vitamin; **THI,** thiamin; **RIB,** riboflavin; **NIA,** niacin; **FOL,** folate;
CALC, calcium; **PHOS,** phosphate; **SOD,** sodium; **POT,** potassium; **MAG,** magnesium

CHOL (mg)	V-A (RE)	THI (mg)	RIB (mg)	NIA (mg)	V-B6 (mg)	FOL (μg)	V-B12 (μg)	V-C (mg)	V-E (mg)	CALC (mg)	PHOS (mg)	SOD (mg)	POT (mg)	MAG (mg)	IRON (mg)	ZINC (mg)
0	19	<0.1	<0.1	0.2	<0.1	5	0	6	0.3	2	7	3	69	3	0.1	<0.1
0	38	<0.1	<0.1	0.4	<0.1	9	0	12	0.6	3	15	6	138	7	0.3	0.1
0	0	<0.1	<0.1	0.2	0.1	7	0	9	<0.1	17	15	39	105	6	0.2	0.2
0	792	0.1	0.1	0.6	0.3	170	0	39	2.5	197	42	42	292	32	1.2	0.2
0	654	<0.1	0.1	0.4	0.1	32	0	18	2.4	125	28	12	184	21	1.6	0.3
0	0	0	<0.1	0.2	0.1	26	0	22	0	25	35	19	419	13	0.2	0.2
0	0	<0.1	<0.1	0.3	0.1	4	0	1	0.3	3	13	6	83	4	0.6	0.3
0	118	<0.1	<0.1	0.1	<0.1	2	0	11	0.2	30	15	10	82	5	0.1	<0.1
0	80	<0.1	<0.1	<0.1	<0.1	2	0	7	0.2	20	10	7	56	4	<0.1	<0.1
0	0	0.2	0.1	0.2	0.2	144	0	0	0.4	161	202	11	1004	113	6.6	2.5
0	1304	0.1	0.1	1	0.1	15	0	24	0.5	34	62	100	422	30	1.8	0.4
0	5592	0.2	0.5	2.1	0.8	36	0	56	0.9	69	89	43	604	33	1.8	0.9
0	58	0.1	0.1	0.7	0.1	34	0	14	0.2	27	58	5	446	40	0.8	0.4
0	43	0.1	0.1	0.8	0.1	30	0	8	0.3	23	72	5	455	40	0.6	0.3
0	44	0.1	<0.1	0.5	0.1	29	0	12	0.5	20	42	4	322	29	0.5	0.3

APPENDIX B Exchange Lists for Meal Planning

Starch List

Cereals, grains, pasta, breads, crackers, snacks, starchy vegetables, and cooked dried beans, peas, and lentils are starches. In general, one starch is:

- ½ cup of cereal, grain, pasta, or starchy vegetable
- 1 ounce of a bread product, such as 1 slice of bread
- ¾ to 1 ounce of most snack foods (some snack foods may also have added fat)

One starch exchange equals

15 grams carbohydrate,

3 grams protein,

0–1 gram fat,

and 80 calories.

Bread

Bagel	½ (1 oz)
Bread, reduced-calorie	2 slices (1½ oz)
Bread, white, whole-wheat, pumpernickel, rye	1 slice (1 oz)
Bread sticks, crisp, 4 in. long x ½ in.	2 (⅔ oz)
English muffin	½
Hot dog or hamburger bun	½ (1 oz)
Pita, 6 in. across	½
Roll, plain, small	1 (1 oz)
Raisin bread, unfrosted	1 slice (1 oz)
Tortilla, corn, 6 in. across	1
Tortilla, flour, 6 in. across	1
Waffle, 4½ in. square, reduced-fat	1

Cereals and Grains

Bran cereals	½ cup
Bulgur	½ cup
Cereals	½ cup
Cereals, unsweetened, ready-to-eat	¾ cup
Cornmeal (dry)	3 Tbsp
Couscous	⅓ cup
Flour (dry)	3 Tbsp
Granola, low-fat	¼ cup
Grape-Nuts	¼ cup
Grits	½ cup
Kasha	½ cup
Millet	¼ cup
Muesli	¼ cup
Oats	½ cup
Pasta	½ cup
Puffed cereal	1½ cups
Rice milk	½ cup
Rice, white or brown	⅓ cup
Shredded Wheat	½ cup
Sugar-frosted cereal	½ cup
Wheat germ	3 Tbsp

Starchy Vegetables

Baked beans	⅓ cup
Corn	½ cup
Corn on cob, medium	1 (5 oz)
Mixed vegetables with corn, peas, or pasta	1 cup
Peas, green	½ cup
Plantain	½ cup
Potato, baked or boiled	1 small (3 oz)
Potato, mashed	½ cup
Squash, winter (acorn, butternut, pumpkin)	1 cup
Yam, sweet potato, plain	½ cup

Crackers and Snacks

Animal crackers	8
Graham crackers, 2½ in. square	3
Matzoh	¾ oz
Melba toast	4 slices
Oyster crackers	24
Popcorn (popped, no fat added, or low-fat microwave)	3 cups
Pretzels	¾ oz
Rice cakes, 4 in. across	2
Saltine-type crackers	6
Snack chips, fat-free (tortilla, potato)	15–20 (¾ oz)
Whole-wheat crackers, no fat added	2–5 (¾ oz)

Dried Beans, Peas, and Lentils

(Count as 1 starch exchange, plus 1 very lean meat exchange.)

Beans and peas (garbanzo, pinto, kidney, white, split, black-eyed)	½ cup
Lima beans	⅔ cup
Lentils	½ cup
Miso	3 Tbsp

Starchy Foods Prepared with Fat

(Count as 1 starch exchange, plus 1 fat exchange.)

Biscuit, 2½ in. across	1
Chow mein noodles	½ cup
Cornbread, 2 in. cube	1 (2 oz)
Crackers, round butter type	6
Croutons	1 cup
French-fried potatoes	16–25 (3 oz)
Granola	¼ cup

= 400 mg or more of sodium per serving.

Muffin, small . . . . . . 1 (1½ oz)
Pancake, 4 in. across 2
Popcorn, microwave . . . . . . 3 cups
Sandwich crackers, cheese or peanut butter filling 3
Stuffing, bread (prepared) . . . . . . ⅓ cup
Taco shell, 6 in. across 2
Waffle, 4½ in. square 1
Whole-wheat crackers, fat added . . . . . . 4–6 (1 oz)

Fruit List

Fresh, frozen, canned, and dried fruits and fruit juices are on this list. In general, one fruit exchange is:

- 1 small to medium fresh fruit
- ½ cup of canned or fresh fruit or fruit juice
- ¼ cup of dried fruit

One fruit exchange equals

15 grams carbohydrate and

60 calories.

The weight includes skin, core, seeds, and rind.

Fruit

Apple, unpeeled, small . . . . . . 1 (4 oz)
Applesauce, unsweetened . . . . . . ½ cup
Apples, dried . . . . . . 4 rings
Apricots, fresh . . . . . . 4 whole (5½ oz)
Apricots, dried . . . . . . 8 halves
Apricots, canned . . . . . . ½ cup
Banana, small . . . . . . 1 (4 oz)
Blackberries . . . . . . ¾ cup
Blueberries . . . . . . ¾ cup
Cantaloupe, small . . . . . . ⅓ melon (11 oz) or 1 cup cubes
Cherries, sweet, fresh . . . . . . 12 (3 oz)
Cherries, sweet, canned . . . . . . ½ cup
Dates 3
Figs, fresh . . . . . . 1½ large or 2 medium (3½ oz)
Figs, dried 1½
Fruit cocktail . . . . . . ½ cup
Grapefruit, large . . . . . . ½ (11 oz)
Grapefruit sections, canned . . . . . . ¾ cup
Grapes, small . . . . . . 17 (3 oz)
Honeydew melon . . . . . . 1 slice (10 oz) or 1 cup cubes
Kiwi . . . . . . 1 (3½ oz)
Mandarin oranges, canned . . . . . . ¾ cup
Mango, small . . . . . . ½ fruit (5½ oz) or ½ cup
Nectarine, small . . . . . . 1 (5 oz)
Orange, small . . . . . . 1 (6½ oz)
Papaya . . . . . . ½ fruit (8 oz) or 1 cup cubes
Peach, medium, fresh . . . . . . 1 (6 oz)
Peaches, canned . . . . . . ½ cup
Pear, large, fresh . . . . . . ½ (4 oz)
Pears, canned . . . . . . ½ cup
Pineapple, fresh . . . . . . ¾ cup
Pineapple, canned . . . . . . ½ cup
Plums, small . . . . . . 2 (5 oz)
Plums, canned . . . . . . ½ cup
Prunes, dried 3
Raisins . . . . . . 2 Tbsp
Raspberries . . . . . . 1 cup
Strawberries . . . . . . 1¼ cup whole berries
Tangerines, small . . . . . . 2 (8 oz)
Watermelon . . . . . . 1 slice (13½ oz) or 1¼ cup cubes

Fruit Juice

Apple juice/cider . . . . . . ½ cup
Cranberry juice cocktail . . . . . . ⅓ cup
Cranberry juice cocktail, reduced-calorie . . . . . . 1 cup
Fruit juice blends, 100% juice . . . . . . ⅓ cup
Grape juice . . . . . . ⅓ cup
Grapefruit juice . . . . . . ½ cup
Orange juice . . . . . . ½ cup
Pineapple juice . . . . . . ½ cup
Prune juice . . . . . . ⅓ cup

Milk List

Different types of milk and milk products are on this list. Cheeses are on the Meat list, and cream and other dairy fats are on the Fat list. Based on the amount of fat they contain, milks are divided into fat-free/low-fat milk, reduced-fat milk, and whole milk. One choice of these includes the following.

	Carbohydrate (grams)	Protein (grams)	Fat (grams)	Calories
Fat-free/ low-fat	12	8	0–3	90
Reduced-fat	12	8	5	120
Whole	12	8	8	150

One milk exchange equals

12 grams carbohydrate and

8 grams protein.

Fat-Free and Low-Fat Milk

(0–3 grams fat per serving)

Fat-free milk . . . . . . 1 cup
½% milk . . . . . . 1 cup
1% milk . . . . . . 1 cup
Fat-free or low-fat buttermilk . . . . . . 1 cup
Evaporated fat-free milk . . . . . . ½ cup
Fat-free dry milk . . . . . . ⅓ cup dry
Plain nonfat yogurt . . . . . . ¾ cup
Nonfat or low-fat fruit-flavored yogurt sweetened with aspartame or with a non-nutritive sweetener . . . . . . 1 cup

Reduced-Fat

(5 grams fat per serving)

2% milk	1 cup
Plain low-fat yogurt	¾ cup
Sweet acidophilus milk	1 cup

Whole Milk

(8 grams fat per serving)

Whole milk	1 cup
Evaporated whole milk	½ cup
Goat's milk	1 cup
Kefir	1 cup

Other Carbohydrates List

Substitute food choices from this list for a starch, fruit, or milk choice on your meal plan. Some choices will also count as one or more fat choices.

One exchange equals

15 grams carbohydrate,
or 1 starch,
or 1 fruit,
or 1 milk.

Food	Serving Size	Exchanges per Serving
Angel food cake, unfrosted	1/12th cake	2 carbohydrates
Brownie, small, unfrosted	2 in. square	1 carbohydrate, 1 fat
Cake, unfrosted	2 in. square	1 carbohydrate, 1 fat
Cake, frosted	2 in. square	2 carbohydrates, 1 fat
Cookie, fat-free	2 small	1 carbohydrate
Cookie or sandwich cookie with creme filling	2 small	1 carbohydrate, 1 fat
Cranberry sauce, jellied	¼ cup	1½ carbohydrates
Cupcake, frosted	1 small	2 carbohydrates, 1 fat
Doughnut, plain cake	1 medium (1½ oz)	1½ carbohydrates, 2 fats
Doughnut, glazed	3¾ in. across (2 oz)	2 carbohydrates, 2 fats
Fruit juice bars, frozen, 100% juice	1 bar (3 oz)	1 carbohydrate
Fruit snacks, chewy (pureed fruit concentrate)	1 roll (¾ oz)	1 carbohydrate
Fruit spreads, 100% fruit	1 Tbsp	1 carbohydrate
Gelatin, regular	½ cup	1 carbohydrate
Gingersnaps	3	1 carbohydrate
Granola bar	1 bar	1 carbohydrate, 1 fat
Granola bar, fat-free	1 bar	2 carbohydrates
Honey	1 Tbsp	1 carbohydrate
Hummus	⅓ cup	1 carbohydrate, 1 fat
Ice cream	½ cup	1 carbohydrate, 2 fats
Ice cream, light	½ cup	1 carbohydrate, 1 fat
Ice cream, fat-free, no sugar added	½ cup	1 carbohydrate
Jam or jelly, regular	1 Tbsp	1 carbohydrate
Milk, chocolate, whole	1 cup	2 carbohydrates, 1 fat
Pie, fruit, 2 crusts	1/6 pie	3 carbohydrates, 2 fats
Pie, pumpkin or custard	1/8 pie	2 carbohydrates, 2 fats
Potato chips	12–18 (1 oz)	1 carbohydrate, 2 fats
Pudding, regular (made with low-fat milk)	½ cup	2 carbohydrates
Pudding, sugar-free (made with low-fat milk)	½ cup	1 carbohydrate
Salad dressing, fat-free ✎	¼ cup	1 carbohydrate
Sherbet, sorbet	½ cup	2 carbohydrates
Spaghetti or pasta sauce, canned ✎	½ cup	1 carbohydrate, 1 fat
Sugar	1 Tbsp	1 carbohydrate
Sweet roll or Danish	1 (2½ oz)	2½ carbohydrates, 2 fats

✎ = *400 mg or more of sodium per serving.*

Syrup, light	2 Tbsp	1 carbohydrate
Syrup, regular	1 Tbsp	1 carbohydrate
Syrup, regular	¼ cup	4 carboydrates
Tortilla chips	6–12 (1 oz)	1 carbohydrate, 2 fats
Vanilla wafers	5	1 carbohydrate, 1 fat
Yogurt, frozen, low-fat, fat-free	⅓ cup	1 carbohydrate, 0–1 fat
Yogurt, frozen, fat-free, no sugar added	½ cup	1 carbohydrate
Yogurt, low-fat with fruit	1 cup	3 carbohydrates, 0–1 fat

Vegetable List

Vegetables that contain small amounts of carbohydrates and calories are on this list. In general, one vegetable exchange is:

- ½ cup of cooked vegetables or vegetable juice
- 1 cup of raw vegetables

One vegetable exchange equals

5 grams carbohydrate,

2 grams protein,

0 grams fat, and

25 calories.

Artichoke
Artichoke hearts
Asparagus
Beans (green, wax, Italian)
Bean sprouts
Beets
Broccoli
Brussels sprouts
Cabbage
Carrots
Cauliflower
Celery
Cucumber
Eggplant
Green onions or scallions
Greens (collard, kale, mustard, turnip)
Kohlrabi
Leeks
Mixed vegetables (without corn, peas, or pasta)
Mushrooms
Okra
Onions
Pea pods
Peppers (all varieties)
Radishes
Salad greens (endive, escarole, lettuce, romaine, spinach)
Sauerkraut
Spinach
Summer squash
Tomato
Tomatoes, canned
Tomato sauce
Tomato/vegetable juice
Turnips
Water chestnuts
Watercress
Zucchini

Meat and Meat Substitutes List

Meat and meat substitutes that contain both protein and fat are on this list. In general, one meat exchange is:

- 1 oz meat, fish, poultry, or cheese
- ½ cup dried beans

Based on the amount of fat they contain, meats are divided into very lean, lean, medium-fat, and high-fat lists. One ounce (one exchange) of each of these includes the following.

	Carbohydrate (grams)	Protein (grams)	Fat (grams)	Calories
Very lean	0	7	0–1	35
Lean	0	7	3	55
Medium-fat	0	7	5	75
High-fat	0	7	8	100

Very Lean Meat and Substitutes List

One exchange equals

0 grams carbohydrate,

7 grams protein,

0–1 gram fat,

and 35 calories.

One very lean meat exchange is equal to any one of the following items.

Poultry: Chicken or turkey (white meat, no skin), Cornish hen (no skin) . . . . . 1 oz

Fish: Fresh or frozen cod, flounder, haddock, halibut, trout; tuna, fresh or canned in water . . . 1 oz
Shellfish: Clams, crab, lobster, scallops, shrimp, imitation shellfish . . . 1 oz
Game: Duck or pheasant (no skin), venison, buffalo, ostrich . . . 1 oz
Cheese with 1 gram or less fat per ounce:
Nonfat or low-fat cottage cheese . . . ¼ cup
Fat-free cheese . . . 1 oz
Other: Processed sandwich meats with 1 gram or less fat per ounce, such as deli thin, shaved meats, chipped beef, turkey ham . . . 1 oz
Egg whites . . . 2
Egg substitutes, plain . . . ¼ cup
Hot dogs with 1 gram or less fat per ounce . . . 1 oz
Kidney (high in cholesterol) . . . 1 oz
Sausage with 1 gram or less fat per ounce . . . 1 oz
Count as one very lean meat and one starch exchange:
Dried beans, peas, lentils (cooked) . . . ½ cup

Lean Meat and Substitutes List

One exchange equals

0 grams carbohydrate,

7 grams protein,

3 grams fat,

and 55 calories.

One lean meat exchange is equal to any one of the following items.

Beef: USDA Select or Choice grades of lean beef trimmed of fat, such as round, sirloin, and flank steak; tenderloin; roast (rib, chuck, rump); steak (T-bone, porterhouse, cubed), ground round . . . 1 oz
Pork: Lean pork, such as fresh ham; canned, cured, or boiled ham; Canadian bacon; tenderloin, center loin chop . . . 1 oz
Lamb: Roast, chop, leg . . . 1 oz
Veal: Lean chop, roast . . . 1 oz
Poultry: Chicken, turkey (dark meat, no skin), chicken (white meat with skin), domestic duck or goose (well drained of fat, no skin) . . . 1 oz
Fish:
Herring (uncreamed or smoked) . . . 1 oz
Oysters . . . 6 medium
Salmon (fresh or canned), catfish . . . 1 oz
Sardines (canned) . . . 2 medium
Tuna (canned in oil, drained) . . . 1 oz
Game: Goose (no skin), rabbit . . . 1 oz
Cheese:
4.5%-fat cottage cheese . . . ¼ cup
Grated Parmesan . . . 2 Tbsp
Cheeses with 3 grams or less fat per ounce . . . 1 oz
Other:
Hot dogs with 3 grams or less fat per ounce . . . 1½ oz
Processed sandwich meat with 3 grams or less fat per ounce, such as turkey pastrami or kielbasa . . . 1 oz
Liver, heart (high in cholesterol) . . . 1 oz

Medium-Fat Meat and Substitutes List

One exchange equals

0 grams carbohydrate,

7 grams protein,

5 grams fat,

and 75 calories.

One medium-fat meat exchange is equal to any one of the following items.

Beef: Most beef products fall into this category (ground beef, meatloaf, corned beef, short ribs, Prime grades of meat trimmed of fat, such as prime rib) . . . 1 oz
Pork: Top loin, chop, Boston butt, cutlet . . . 1 oz
Lamb: Rib roast, ground . . . 1 oz
Veal: Cutlet (ground or cubed, unbreaded) . . . 1 oz
Poultry: Chicken dark meat (with skin), ground turkey or ground chicken, fried chicken (with skin) . . . 1 oz
Fish: Any fried fish product . . . 1 oz
Cheese: With 5 grams or less fat per ounce
Feta . . . 1 oz
Mozzarella . . . 1 oz
Ricotta . . . ¼ cup (2 oz)
Other:
Egg (high in cholesterol, limit to 3 per week) . . . 1
Sausage with 5 grams or less fat per ounce . . . 1 oz
Soy milk . . . 1 cup
Tempeh . . . ¼ cup
Tofu . . . 4 oz or ½ cup

High-Fat Meat and Substitutes List

One exchange equals

0 grams carbohydrate,

7 grams protein,

8 grams fat,

and 100 calories.

One high-fat meat exchange is equal to any one of the following items.

Pork: Spareribs, ground pork, pork sausage . . . 1 oz
Cheese: All regular cheeses, such as American, cheddar, Monterey Jack, Swiss . . . 1 oz
Other: Processed sandwich meats with 8 grams or less fat per ounce, such as bologna, pimento loaf, salami . . . 1 oz
Sausage, such as bratwurst, Italian, knockwurst, Polish, smoked . . . 1 oz

= 400 mg or more of sodium per serving.

Hot dog (turkey or chicken)	1 (10/lb)
Bacon	3 slices (20 slices/lb)

Count as one high-fat meat plus one fat exchange:

Hot dog (beef, pork, or combination)	1 (10/lb)

Count as one high-fat meat plus two fat exchanges:

Peanut butter (contains unsaturated fat)	2 Tbsp

Fat List

Fats are divided into three groups, based on the main type of fat they contain: monounsaturated, polyunsaturated, and saturated. Small amounts of monounsaturated and polyunsaturated fats in the foods we eat are linked with good health benefits. Saturated fats are linked with heart disease and cancer. In general, one fat exchange is:

- 1 teaspoon of regular margarine or vegetable oil
- 1 tablespoon of regular salad dressings

Monounsaturated Fats List

One fat exchange equals

5 grams fat and

45 calories.

Avocado, medium	⅛ (1 oz)
Oil (canola, olive, peanut)	1 tsp
Olives: ripe (black)	8 large
green, stuffed	10 large
Nuts	
almonds, cashews	6 nuts
mixed (50% peanuts)	6 nuts
peanuts	10 nuts
pecans	4 halves
Peanut butter, smooth or crunchy	2 tsp
Sesame seeds	1 Tbsp
Tahini paste	2 tsp

Polyunsaturated Fats List

One fat exchange equals

5 grams fat and

45 calories.

Margarine: stick, tub, or squeeze	1 tsp
lower-fat (30% to 50% vegetable oil)	1 Tbsp
Mayonnaise: regular	1 tsp
reduced-fat	1 Tbsp
Nuts, walnuts, English	4 halves
Oil (corn, safflower, soybean)	1 tsp
Salad dressing: regular	1 Tbsp
reduced-fat	2 Tbsp
Miracle Whip Salad Dressing: regular	2 tsp
reduced-fat	1 Tbsp
Seeds: pumpkin, sunflower	1 Tbsp

Saturated Fats List*

One fat exchange equals

5 grams of fat

and 45 calories.

Bacon, cooked	1 slice (20 slices/lb)
Bacon, grease	1 tsp
Butter: stick	1 tsp
whipped	2 tsp
reduced-fat	1 Tbsp
Chitterlings, boiled	2 Tbsp (½ oz)
Coconut, sweetened, shredded	2 Tbsp
Cream, half and half	2 Tbsp
Cream cheese: regular	1 Tbsp (½ oz)
reduced-fat	2 Tbsp (1 oz)
Fatback or salt pork, see below†	
Shortening or lard	1 tsp
Sour cream: regular	2 Tbsp
reduced-fat	3 Tbsp

**Saturated fats can raise blood cholesterol levels.*

†Use a piece 1 in. × 1 in. × ¼ in. if you plan to eat the fatback cooked with vegetables. Use a piece 2 in. × 1 in. × ½ in. when eating only the vegetables with the fatback removed.

Free Foods List

A *free food* is any food or drink that contains less than 20 calories or less than 5 grams of carbohydrate per serving. Foods with a serving size listed should be limited to three servings per day. Foods listed without a serving size can be eaten as often as you like.

Fat-free or Reduced-Fat Foods

Cream cheese, fat-free	1 Tbsp
Creamers, nondairy, liquid	1 Tbsp
Creamers, nondairy, powdered	2 tsp
Mayonnaise, fat-free	1 Tbsp
Mayonnaise, reduced-fat	1 tsp
Margarine, fat-free	4 Tbsp
Margarine, reduced-fat	1 tsp
Miracle Whip, nonfat	1 Tbsp
Miracle Whip, reduced-fat	1 tsp
Nonstick cooking spray	
Salad dressing, fat-free	1 Tbsp
Salad dressing, fat-free, Italian	2 Tbsp
Salsa	¼ cup
Sour cream, fat-free, reduced-fat	1 Tbsp
Whipped topping, regular or light	2 Tbsp

Sugar-Free or Low-Sugar Foods

Candy, hard, sugar-free . . . . 1 candy
Gelatin dessert, sugar-free
Gelatin, unflavored
Gum, sugar-free
Jam or jelly, low-sugar or light . . . . 2 tsp
Sugar substitutes†
Syrup, sugar-free . . . . 2 Tbsp

†Sugar substitutes, alternatives, or replacements that are approved by the Food and Drug Administration (FDA) are safe to use. Common brand names include:

Equal (aspartame)
Sprinkle Sweet (saccharin)
Sweet One (acesulfame K)
Sweet-10 (saccharin)
Sugar Twin (saccharin)
Sweet 'n Low (saccharin)

Drinks

Bouillon, broth, consommé 🧂
Bouillon or broth, low-sodium
Carbonated or mineral water
Club soda
Cocoa powder, unsweetened . . . . 1 Tbsp
Coffee
Diet soft drinks, sugar-free
Drink mixes, sugar-free
Tea
Tonic water, sugar-free

Condiments

Ketchup . . . . 1 Tbsp
Horseradish
Lemon juice
Lime juice
Mustard
Pickles, dill 🧂 . . . . 1½ large
Soy sauce, regular or light 🧂
Taco sauce . . . . 1 Tbsp
Vinegar

Seasonings

Be careful with seasonings that contain sodium or are salts, such as garlic or celery salt, and lemon pepper.

Flavoring extracts
Garlic
Herbs, fresh or dried
Pimento
Spices
Tabasco or hot pepper sauce
Wine, used in cooking
Worcestershire sauce

Combination Foods List

Many of the foods we eat are mixed together in various combinations. These combination foods do not fit into any one exchange list. This is a list of exchanges for some typical combination foods.

Food Entrees	Serving Size	Exchanges per Serving
Tuna noodle casserole, lasagna, spaghetti with meatballs, chili with beans, macaroni and cheese 🧂	1 cup (8 oz)	2 carbohydrates, 2 medium-fat meats
Chow mein (without noodles or rice)	2 cups (16 oz)	1 carbohydrate, 2 lean meats
Pizza, cheese, thin crust 🧂	¼ of 10 in. (5 oz)	2 carbohydrates, 2 medium-fat meats, 1 fat
Pizza, meat topping, thin crust 🧂	¼ of 10 in. (5 oz)	2 carbohydrates, 2 medium-fat meats, 2 fats
Pot pie 🧂	1 (7 oz)	2 carbohydrates, 1 medium-fat meat, 4 fats
Frozen Entrees		
Salisbury steak with gravy, mashed potato 🧂	1 (11 oz)	2 carbohydrates, 3 medium-fat meats, 3–4 fats
Turkey with gravy, mashed potato, dressing 🧂	1 (11 oz)	2 carbohydrates, 2 medium-fat meats, 2 fats
Entree with less than 300 calories 🧂	1 (8 oz)	2 carbohydrates, 3 lean meats
Soups		
Bean 🧂	1 cup	1 carbohydrate, 1 very lean meat
Cream (made with water) 🧂	1 cup (8 oz)	1 carbohydrate, 1 fat
Split pea (made with water) 🧂	½ cup (4 oz)	1 carbohydrate
Tomato (made with water) 🧂	1 cup (8 oz)	1 carbohydrate
Vegetable beef, chicken noodle, or other broth-type 🧂	1 cup (8 oz)	1 carbohydrate

🧂 *= 400 mg or more of sodium per serving.*

Fast Foods*

Food	Serving Size	Exchanges per Serving
Burritos with beef	2	4 carbohydrates, 2 medium-fat meats, 2 fats
Chicken nuggets	6	1 carbohydrate, 2 medium-fat meats, 1 fat
Chicken breast and wing, breaded and fried	1 each	1 carbohydrate, 4 medium-fat meats, 2 fats
Fish sandwich/tartar sauce	1	3 carbohydrates, 1 medium-fat meat, 3 fats
French fries, thin	20–25	2 carbohydrates, 2 fats
Hamburger, regular	1	2 carbohydrates, 2 medium-fat meats
Hamburger, large	1	2 carbohydrates, 3 medium-fat meats, 1 fat
Hot dog with bun	1	1 carbohydrate, 1 high-fat meat, 1 fat
Individual pan pizza	1	5 carbohydrates, 3 medium-fat meats, 3 fats
Soft-serve cone	1 medium	2 carbohydrates, 1 fat
Submarine sandwich	1 sub (6 in.)	3 carbohydrates, 1 vegetable, 2 medium-fat meats, 1 fat
Taco, hard shell	1 (6 oz)	2 carbohydrates, 2 medium-fat meats, 2 fats
Taco, soft shell	1 (3 oz)	1 carbohydrate, 1 medium-fat meat, 1 fat

**Ask at your fast-food restaurant for nutrition information about your favorite fast foods.*

***Source:** Exchange Lists for Meal Planning. The American Diabetes Association, Alexandria, VA, and The American Dietetic Association, Chicago, IL. 1995.*

APPENDIX C Nutrition and Health for Canadians

- Guidelines for Nutrition
- *Canada's Food Guide to Healthy Eating*
- *Canada's Physical Activity Guide to Healthy Active Living*
- Nutrient Intake Recommendations for Canadians
- Nutrition Labeling for Canadians
- Food Choice System

Canadian Guidelines for Nutrition

For the past 60 years, the government has worked to promote healthy and nutritious eating habits in Canadians. In 1987, Health and Welfare Canada began a major review of the system for guiding Canadians on their food choices. To perform the review, the government appointed two advisory committees—the Scientific Review Committee and the Communications and Implementation Committee.

After examining research evidence available on nutrition and public health, the Scientific Review Committee issued a report in 1990 called *Nutrition Recommendations.* The report included both updated Recommended Nutrient Intakes (RNI) and a scientific description of a healthy dietary pattern that would deliver adequate nutrients for health and reduce the risk of nutrition-related chronic diseases.

Meanwhile, the Communications and Implementation Committee translated these scientific findings into understandable guidelines and outlined implementation strategies in a report called *Action Towards Healthy Eating: Technical Report* (1990). This report suggested that Canada develop a "total diet approach" towards healthy eating. A total diet approach would give consumers a better idea of eating patterns associated with reducing the risk of developing chronic diseases.

In 1990, the government issued *Nutrition Recommendations: A Call for Action,* a summary report produced jointly by the Scientific Review Committee and the Communications and Implementation Committee.

A Revised Food Guide

In accordance with the recommendations of its two advisory groups, the Health Department undertook to revise *Canada's Food Guide.* In 1992, the agency launched *Canada's Food Guide to Healthy Eating* and an explanatory document called *Using the Food Guide.* This promotes dietary diversity, reducing total fat intake, and an active lifestyle. It also offers consumers a pattern for establishing healthy eating habits in their daily selection of foods.

Moreover, the guide introduced a number of new concepts. A range of servings from the four food groups accommodates the wide range of energy needs for different ages, body sizes, activity levels, genders and conditions such as pregnancy and nursing. The wide range of servings in grain products, vegetables, and fruits is designed to give consumers a better idea of the type of diet that would help reduce the risk of developing nutrition-related chronic diseases.

The guide also introduced a category of "other" foods such as sweets, fats such as butter, and drinks like coffee, that, though part of the diets of many Canadians, would traditionally not have been mentioned in a food guide. The guide recommends moderation in the consumption of these foods and acknowledges their role, along with the wide range of servings in grains, vegetables, and fruits, as a "total diet approach" to healthy eating.

A Work in Progress

Some groups and organizations challenged specific aspects of the government's *Nutrition Recommendations.* In a typically Canadian twist, the government responded to challengers by including them in the development process. When the Canadian Pediatric Society, for example, queried the dietary recommendations on fat consumption in children, the Society was invited to join Health Canada in researching the issue. The result was *Nutrition Recommendations Update: Dietary Fat and Children* (1993), which adjusted the recommendation of appropriate levels of dietary fat for growing children. In 1995, Health Canada issued *Canada's Food Guide to Healthy Eating: Focus on Preschoolers* as a background paper for educators and communicators.

Health Canada also has positioned nutrition in a broader health context, which includes physical activity and a positive outlook on life. One result of this comprehensive approach was the *Vitality Leaders Kit* (1994), intended to help community leaders promote healthy eating, active living, and positive self- and body-image in an integrated way.

Looking Ahead

The job of keeping Canada's nutrition policy and consumer guidelines up-to-date is an ongoing task. New scientific research on nutrition and health continually uncovers new relationships and connections between them. Consumer tastes in foods vary in response to prevailing fashions and shifting demographics. Global trade also influences the food choices that appear on the Canadian dinner table.

The science underlying nutrition recommendations knows no borders. An increasingly complex knowledge base on nutrients, food and health, global trade, and international agreements requires international efforts. Scientists from Canada and the United States are working with the National Academy of Sciences to achieve a set of harmonized dietary reference intakes for both countries.

Information about Canadian standards is integrated throughout the main body of this text, especially in the chapters on nutrition guidelines, sports nutrition, and nutrition throughout the life cycle. In Chapter 2, "Nutrition Guidelines," for example, you can find more information on *Canada's Food Guide to Healthy Eating*, DRIs, and RNIs, and the concept of vitality. To keep abreast of the latest developments in Canada's nutrition policies, visit the Food and Nutrition area of the Health Canada Web site at: http://www.hc-sc.gc.ca/english/lifestyles/food_nutr.html or http://www.hc-sc.gc.ca/francais/vie_saine/nutrition.html.

Canada's Food Guide to Healthy Eating

Scientists have known for some time that adequate nutrition is essential for proper growth and development. More recently, healthy eating has been accepted as a significant factor in reducing the risk of developing nutrition-related problems, including heart disease, cancer, obesity, hypertension (high blood pressure), osteoporosis, anemia, dental decay, and some bowel disorders.

What "Reducing Risk" Means

Reducing risk means lowering the chances of developing a disease. It does not guarantee the prevention of a disease. Since the development of disease involves several factors, risk reduction usually involves several different strategies or approaches. Healthy eating is just one positive action that may help to avoid a potential problem.

Healthy Eating in Canada

The Food Guide is based on nutrition and food science. A key reference is *Nutrition Recommendations: The Report of the Scientific Review Committee*, published in 1990 by Health Canada. This report contains a review of nutrition research conducted by a committee of scientists and provides recommendations describing the desired characteristics of the Canadian diet. The Nutrition Recommendations, which are reviewed regularly, act as the foundation for all nutrition and healthy eating programs in the country.

Canada's Guidelines for Healthy Eating

A committee of experts in communications and program planning worked with the committee of scientists and prepared the report *Action Towards Healthy Eating*. They adapted the Nutrition Recommendations into a more user-friendly set of statements called *Canada's Guidelines for Healthy Eating*. These Guidelines promote healthy eating in a general way:

- Enjoy a *variety* of foods.
- Emphasize cereals, breads, other grain products, vegetables, and fruits.
- Choose lower-fat dairy products, leaner meats, and foods prepared with little or no fat.
- Achieve and maintain a healthy body weight by enjoying regular physical activity and healthy eating.
- Limit salt, alcohol, and caffeine.

Canada's Food Guide to Healthy Eating

Canada's Food Guide to Healthy Eating takes *Canada's Guidelines for Healthy Eating* one step further and provides consumers with more detailed information for establishing healthy eating habits through the daily selection of food. The Food Guide is a basic nutrition education tool used:

- to help plan healthy meals for individuals or groups; and
- to evaluate a person's eating habits in a general way but not to assess nutritional status.

The Food Guide meets the nutritional needs of all Canadians four years of age and over and has been designed specifically for the general public with a reading level of grade seven. It is not appropriate for those under the age of four because the number of servings and the serving sizes are too large for toddlers and preschoolers.

Food Guide Materials

- *Canada's Food Guide to Healthy Eating*: a tear sheet for consumers.
- *Using the Food Guide*: a booklet for consumers that explains the basic concepts of the tear sheet more fully.
- *Food Guide Facts: Background for Educators and Communicators*: fact sheets that provide background information for nutrition professionals, health educators, home economists, fitness leaders, and others involved in promoting healthy eating.
- *Canada's Food Guide to Healthy Eating*: tear sheet, consumer booklet and the fact sheets for educators and communicators are available from provincial or local health departments or from: Publications, Health Canada, Ottawa, Ontario K1A 0K9, tel. (613) 954-5995.

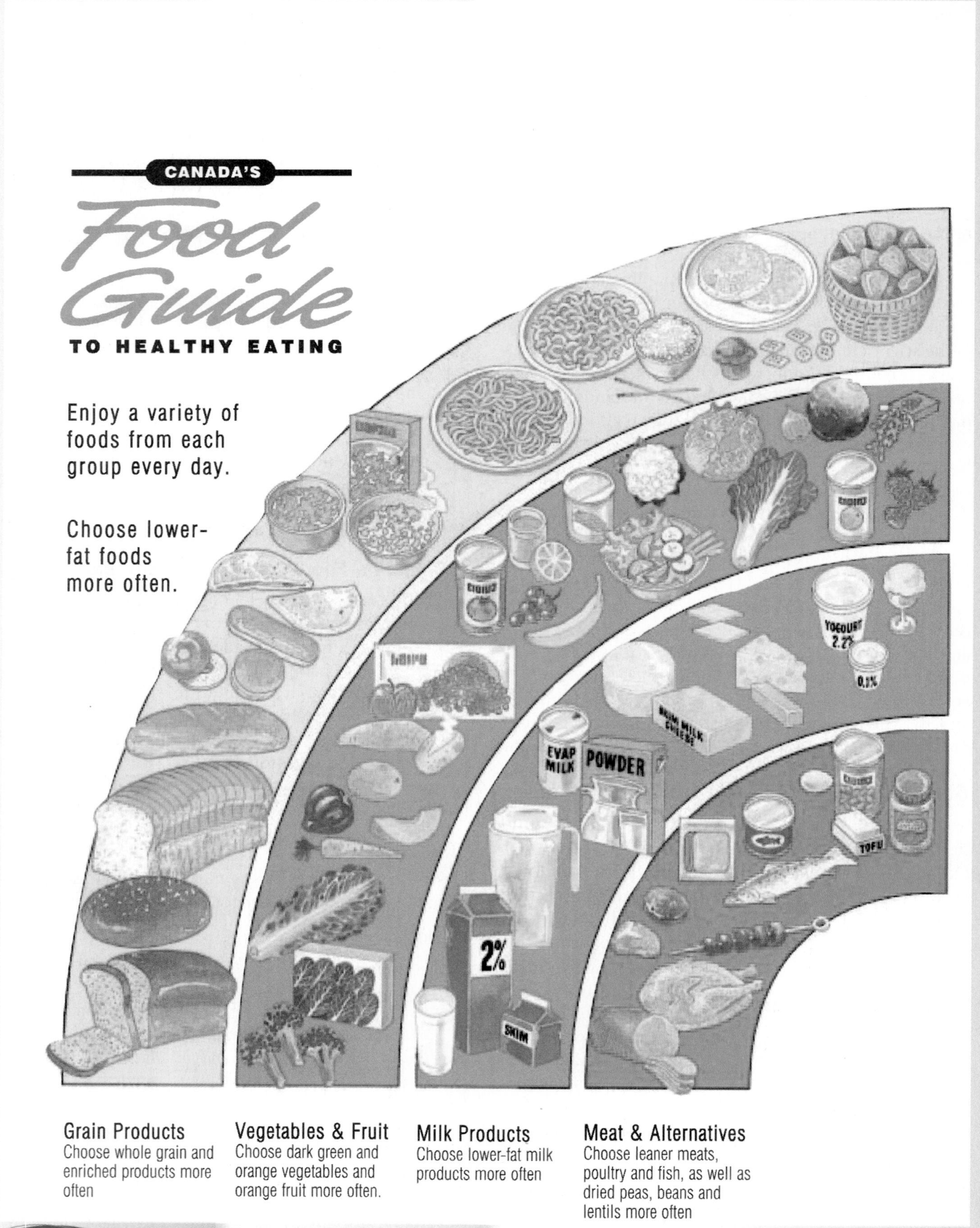
CANADA'S
Food Guide
TO HEALTHY EATING
Enjoy a variety of foods from each group every day.
Choose lower-fat foods more often.
EVAP MILK
POWDER
2%
SKIM
YOGOURT 2.2%
0.1%
TOFU
Grain Products
Choose whole grain and enriched products more often
Vegetables & Fruit
Choose dark green and orange vegetables and orange fruit more often.
Milk Products
Choose lower-fat milk products more often
Meat & Alternatives
Choose leaner meats, poultry and fish, as well as dried peas, beans and lentils more often

Figure C.1 The Canadian Food Guide. **Source:** © Minister of Public Works and Government Services Canada, 1997.

CANADA'S
Food Guide
TO HEALTHY EATING
FOR PEOPLE FOUR YEARS AND OVER

Different People Need Different Amounts of Food

The amount of food you need every day from the 4 groups and other foods depends on your age, body size, activity level, whether you are male or female and if you are pregnant or breast-feeding. That's why the Food Guide gives a lower and higher number of servings for each food group. For example, young children can choose the number of servings, while male teenagers can go to the higher number. Most other people can choose servings somewhere in between.

Grain Products
5 – 12
SERVINGS PER DAY

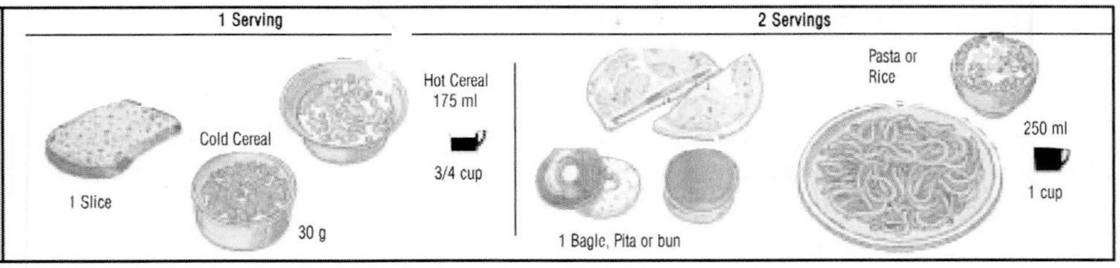

Vegetables and Fruit
5 – 10
SERVINGS PER DAY

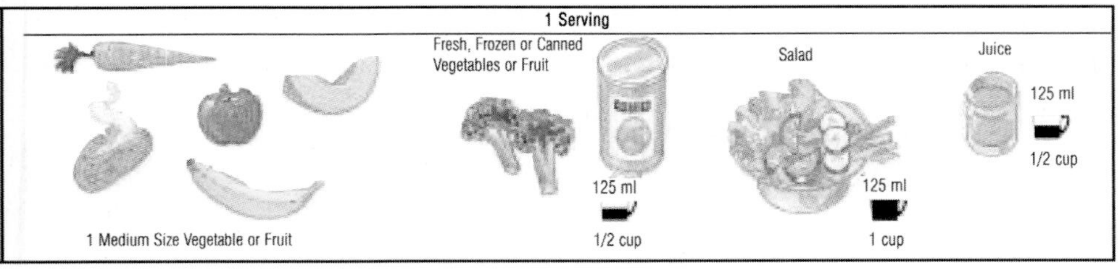

Milk Products
SERVINGS PER DAY
Children 4–9 years: 2–3
Youth 10–16 years: 3–4
Adults: 2–4
Pregnant and Breast-feeding Women 3–4

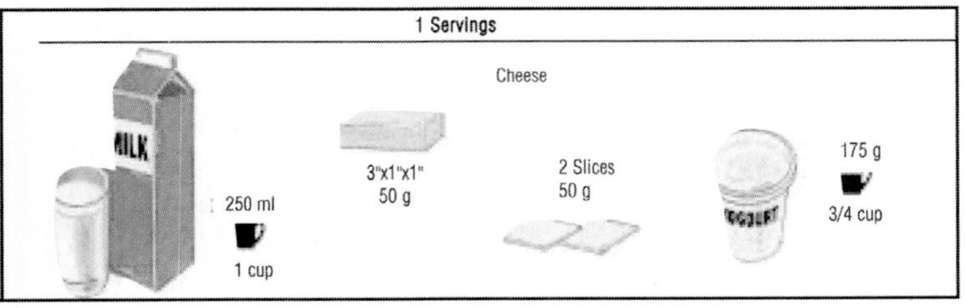

Meat and Alternatives
2–3
SERVINGS PER DAY

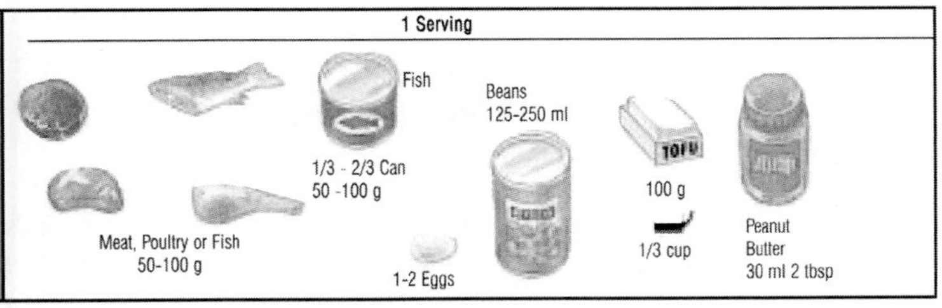

Other Foods

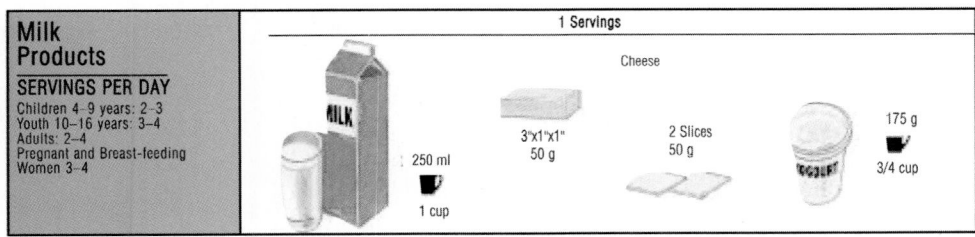

Taste and enjoyment can also come from other foods and beverages that are not part of the 4 food groups. Some of these foods are higher in fat or calories, so use these foods in moderation.

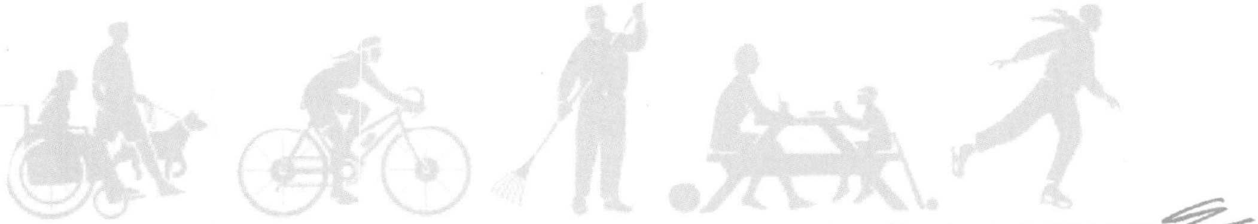

Enjoy eating well, being active and feeling good about yourself. That's VITALITÉ

ISBN 0-662-19648-1

Canada's Physical Activity Guide to Healthy Active Living

High levels of physical inactivity are a serious threat to public health in Canada. Nearly two-thirds of Canadians are not active enough to achieve optimal health benefits. These Canadians are at risk for heart disease, obesity, high blood pressure, adult-onset diabetes, osteoporosis, stroke, depression, and colon cancer. Although physical activity levels increased during the 1980s and early 1990s, the progress has stalled. Health Canada estimates that physical inactivity results in at least 21,000 premature deaths annually.

Canada's Physical Activity Guide to Healthy Active Living, produced by a joint effort of Health Canada and the Canadian Society for Exercise Physiology, provides the first set of Canadian guidelines for physical activity. It provides information to help Canadians understand how to achieve health benefits by being physically active. The guide complements the popular *Canada's Food Guide to Healthy Eating* and provides concrete examples of how to incorporate physical activity into daily life.

Designed for adults, the guide recommends 60 minutes of physical activity every day to stay healthy or improve your health. As a person progresses to more intense activity, they can cut down to 30 minutes, four days a week. The guide also suggests Canadians can add up their activities in periods of at least 10 minutes each, starting slowly and building up.

Federal, provincial, and territorial governments are working to reduce the number of inactive Canadians. *Canada's Physical Activity Guide to Healthy Active Living* is a major step toward building the knowledge and awareness necessary for all Canadians to become more active. The healthy active living series now also includes *Physical Activity Guide to Healthy Active Living for Older Adults, Physical Activity Guide for Youth, Physical Activity Guide for Children,* and *Active Living at Work.*

Nutrient Intake Recommendations for Canadians

Health Canada has reviewed and made recommendations on nutrient requirements on a periodic basis since 1938. The last update on nutrient requirements, which were termed Recommended Nutrient Intakes, was published in 1990 as part of *Nutrition Recommendations: The Report of the Scientific Review Committee.* Since that time, there have been advances in science and by 1994, it was clear that it was time to initiate another review of the scientific data.

At the same time, the Food and Nutrition Board of the National Academy of Sciences was beginning a consultation process on the review of the Recommended Dietary Allowances. Health Canada considered that participating in

Table C-1 Protein: Recommended Nutrient Intakes for Canadians, 1990

Age	Sex	Weight (kg)	Protein (g/day)[a]
Infants (months)			
0–4	Both	6	12[b]
5–12	Both	9	12
Children (years)			
1	Both	11	13
2–3	Both	14	16
4–6	Both	18	19
7–9	M	25	26
	F	25	26
10–12	M	34	34
	F	36	36
13–15	M	50	49
	F	48	46
16–18	M	62	58
	F	53	47
Adults (years)			
19–24	M	71	61
	F	58	50
25–49	M	74	64
	F	59	51
50–74	M	73	63
	F	63	54
75+	M	69	59
	F	64	55
Pregnancy (additional amount needed)			
1st trimester			5
2nd trimester			20
3rd trimester			24
Lactation (additional amount needed)			20

NOTE: Recommended intakes during periods of growth are taken as appropriate for individuals representative of the midpoint in each age group. All recommended intakes are designed to cover individual variations in essentially all of a healthy population subsisting upon a variety of common foods available in Canada.

Source: Health and Welfare Canada, *Nutrition Recommendations: The Report of the Scientific Review Committee* (Ottawa: Canadian Government Publishing Centre, 1990), Table 20, p. 204.

[a]The primary units are expressed per kilogram of body weight. The figures shown here are examples.

[b]The assumption is made that the protein is from breast milk or has the same biological value as breast milk and that, between 3 and 9 months, adjustment for the quality of the protein is made.

the U.S. review would offer several advantages to Canada. These were as follows:

- The science underlying nutrient requirements knows no borders and scientists everywhere are utilizing the same knowledge produced from studies conducted all over the world.
- The knowledge base on nutrients, foods, and health is increasing rapidly in scope and complexity. This increases the need for specialized expertise. Participating in the U.S. review permits Canada to expand the base of scientific expertise that could be utilized.
- International trade considerations, including NAFTA, suggest that the harmonization of the science base underlying nutrition policy will facilitate harmonization of such trade-related matters as nutrition labeling and food composition.

Canadian and American scientists are establishing Dietary Reference Intakes (DRIs) through a review process overseen by the Food and Nutrition Board of the Institute of Medicine, National Academy of Sciences. DRIs are replacing the 1990 Recommended Nutrient Intakes (RNIs).

The National Academy of Sciences is an American private non-profit society of distinguished scholars engaged in scientific and engineering research, dedicated to the advancement of science and technology and to their use for the general welfare. The Academy has a mandate that requires it to advise the U.S. federal government on scientific and technical matters. The National Research Council is the operating agency of the National Academy of Sciences.

The Food and Nutrition Board (FNB) is a unit of the Institute of Medicine, part of the National Academy of

Table C-2 Average Energy Requirements for Canadians

		Average Height	Average Weight	Requirements[a]					
Age	**Sex**	**(cm)**	**(kg)**	**(kcal/kg)[b]**	**(MJ/kg)[b]**	**(kcal/day)**	**(MJ/day)**	**(kcal/cm)**	**(MJ/cm)**
Infants (months)									
0–2	Both	55	4.5	120–100	0.50–0.42	500	2.0	9	0.04
3–5	Both	63	7.0	100–95	0.42–0.40	700	2.8	11	0.05
6–8	Both	69	8.5	95–97	0.40–0.41	800	3.4	11.5	0.05
9–11	Both	73	9.5	97–99	0.41	950	3.8	12.5	0.05
Children and Adults (years)									
1	Both	82	11	101	0.42	1,100	4.8	13.5	0.06
2–3	Both	95	14	94	0.39	1,300	5.6	13.5	0.06
4–6	Both	107	18	100	0.42	1,800	7.6	17	0.07
7–9	M	126	25	88	0.37	2,200	9.2	17.5	0.07
	F	125	25	76	0.30	1,900	8.0	15	0.06
10–12	M	141	34	73	0.30	2,500	10.4	17.5	0.07
	F	143	36	61	0.25	2,200	9.2	15.5	0.06
13–15	M	159	50	57	0.24	2,800	12.0	17.5	0.07
	F	157	48	46	0.19	2,200	9.2	14	0.06
16–18	M	172	62	51	0.21	3,200	13.2	18.5	0.08
	F	160	53	40	0.17	2,100	8.8	13	0.05
19–24	M	175	71	42	0.18	3,000	12.6		
	F	160	58	36	0.15	2,100	8.8		
25–49	M	172	74	36	0.15	2,700	11.3		
	F	160	59	32	0.13	1,900	8.0		
50–74	M	170	73	31	0.13	2,300	9.7		
	F	158	63	29	0.12	1,800	7.6		
75+	M	168	69	29	0.12	2,000	8.4		
	F	155	64	23	0.10	1,500	6.3		

[a]Requirements can be expected to vary within a range of ±30 percent.

[b]First and last figures are averages at the beginning and end of the three-month period.

Source: Health and Welfare Canada, *Nutrition Recommendations: The Report of the Scientific Review Committee* (Ottawa: Canadian Government Publishing Centre, 1990), Tables 5 and 6, pp. 25, 27.

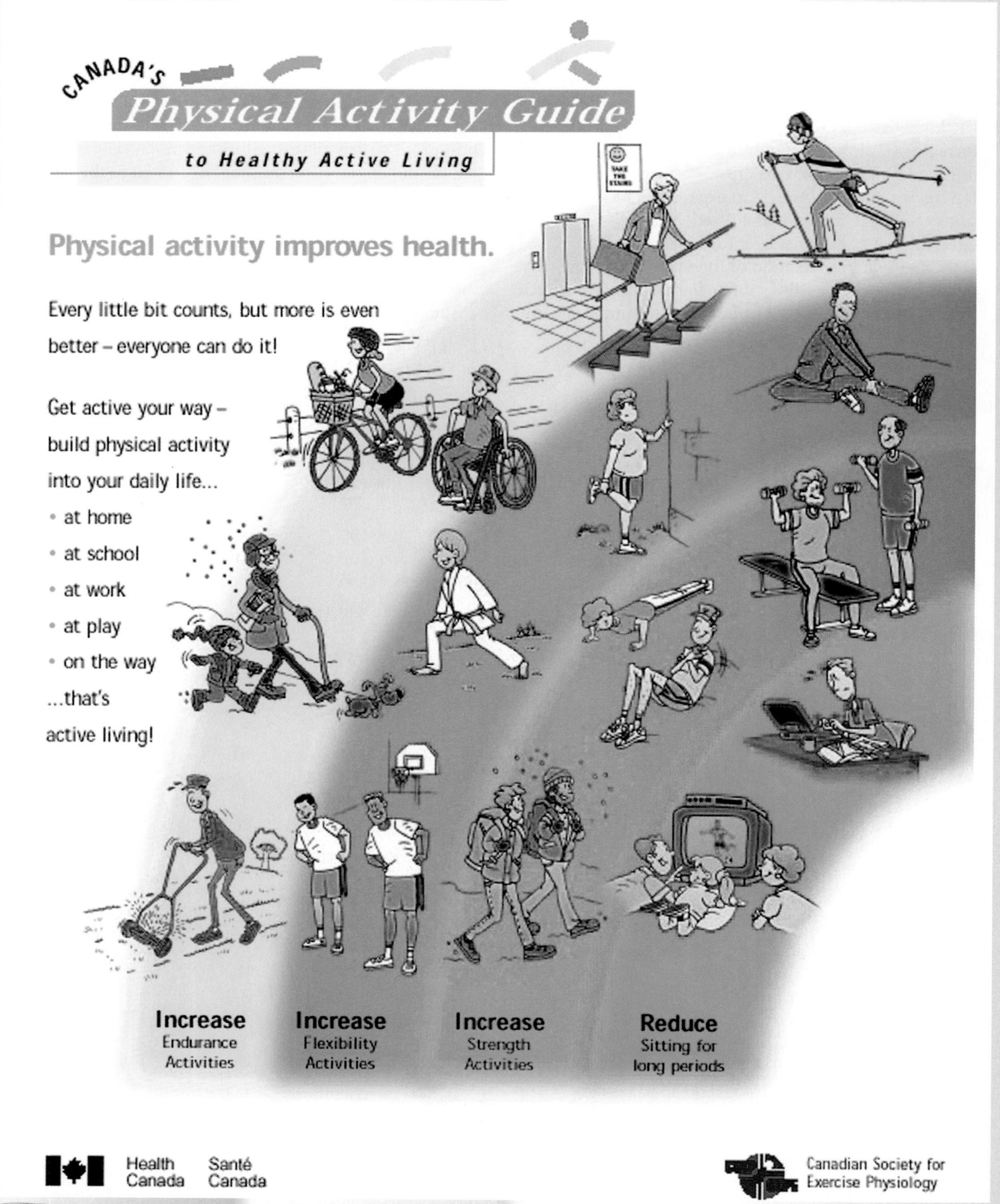

CANADA'S
Physical Activity Guide
to Healthy Active Living
Physical activity improves health.
Every little bit counts, but more is even better – everyone can do it!
Get active your way – build physical activity into your daily life...
• at home
• at school
• at work
• at play
• on the way
...that's active living!
Increase Endurance Activities
Increase Flexibility Activities
Increase Strength Activities
Reduce Sitting for long periods
Health Canada
Santé Canada
Canadian Society for Exercise Physiology

Figure C.2 Canada's Physical Activity Guide. **Source:** © Minister of Public Works and Government Services Canada, 1997.

Choose a variety of activities from these three groups:

Endurance

4-7 days a week
Continuous activities for your heart, lungs and circulatory system.

Flexibility

4-7 days a week
Gentle reaching, bending and stretching activities to keep your muscles relaxed and joints mobile.

Strength

2-4 days a week
Activities against resistance to strengthen muscles and bones and improve posture.

Starting slowly is very safe for most people. Not sure? Consult your health professional.

For a copy of the *Guide Handbook* and more information: **1-888-334-9769**, or **www.paguide.com**

Eating well is also important. Follow *Canada's Food Guide to Healthy Eating* to make wise food choices.

Get Active Your Way, Every Day—For Life!

Scientists say accumulate 60 minutes of physical activity every day to stay healthy or improve your health. As you progress to moderate activities you can cut down to 30 minutes, 4 days a week. Add-up your activities in periods of at least 10 minutes each. Start slowly... and build up.

Time needed depends on effort

Very Light Effort	Light Effort *60 minutes*	Moderate Effort *30-60 minutes*	Vigorous Effort *20-30 minutes*	Maximum Effort
• Strolling • Dusting	• Light walking • Volleyball • Easy gardening • Stretching	• Brisk walking • Biking • Raking leaves • Swimming • Dancing • Water aerobics	• Aerobics • Jogging • Hockey • Basketball • Fast swimming • Fast dancing	• Sprinting • Racing

Range needed to stay healthy

You Can Do It – Getting started is easier than you think

Physical activity doesn't have to be very hard. Build physical activities into your daily routine.

- Walk whenever you can – get off the bus early, use the stairs instead of the elevator.
- Reduce inactivity for long periods, like watching TV.
- Get up from the couch and stretch and bend for a few minutes every hour.
- Play actively with your kids.
- Choose to walk, wheel or cycle for short trips.
- Start with a 10 minute walk – gradually increase the time.
- Find out about walking and cycling paths nearby and use them.
- Observe a physical activity class to see if you want to try it.
- Try one class to start – you don't have to make a long-term commitment.
- Do the activities you are doing now, more often.

Benefits of regular activity:	Health risks of inactivity:
• better health • improved fitness • better posture and balance • better self-esteem • weight control • stronger muscles and bones • feeling more energetic • relaxation and reduced stress • continued independent living in later life	• premature death • heart disease • obesity • high blood pressure • adult-onset diabetes • osteoporosis • stroke • depression • colon cancer

Active Living — Physical Activity Guide

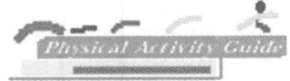

Sciences. The Board is a multidisciplinary group of biomedical scientists with expertise in various aspects of nutrition, food sciences, biochemistry, medicine, public health, epidemiology, food toxicology, and food safety. The major focus of the FNB is to evaluate emerging knowledge of nutrient requirements and relationships between diet and the reduction of risk of common chronic diseases and to relate this knowledge to strategies for promoting health and preventing disease.

Nutrition Labeling for Canadians

The nutrition label is one of the most useful tools in selecting foods for healthy eating. The Food Guide outlines a pattern of healthy eating; the nutrition label supports the Food Guide by helping consumers to choose foods according to healthy eating messages.

Consumers can use labels to compare products and make choices on the basis of nutrient content. For example, consumers can choose a lower-fat product based on the fat content given on the labels.

Consumers also can use label information to evaluate products in relation to healthy eating. For instance, the Nutrition Recommendations advise Canadians to get 30 percent or less of their day's energy (kilocalories/kilojoules) from fat. This translates into a range of fat, in grams, that can be used as a benchmark against which individual foods and meals can be evaluated. The Food Guide covers a range of energy needs from 1,800 to 3,200 kilocalories (7,500 to 13,400 kilojoules) per day. A fat intake of 30 percent or less of a day's calories means a fat intake between 60 and 105 grams of fat.

Label Claims

A claim on a food label highlights a nutritional feature of a product. It is known to influence consumer's buying habits. Manufacturers often position label claims in a bold, banner-format on the front panel of a package or on the side panel along with the nutrition label. Since a label claim must be backed up by detailed facts relating to the claim, the consumer should look for the nutrition label for more information.

Nutrient Content Claims

A nutrient content claim describes the amount of a nutrient in a food. A food whose label carries the claim *high fiber* must contain 4 grams or more fiber per reference amount and serving of stated size. A "sodium-free" food must contain less than 5 mg of sodium per reference amount and serving of stated size.

Diet-Related Health Claims

Optional health claims highlight the characteristics of a diet that reduces the chance of developing a disease such as cancer or heart disease. They also tell how the food fits into the diet.

Characteristic of the Diet:	Reduced Risk of:
Low in sodium and high in potassium	High blood pressure
Adequate in calcium and vitamin D	Osteoporosis
Low in saturates and *trans* fats	Heart disease
Rich in fruit and vegetables	Some types of cancer
Sugar alcohols (such as sorbitol)	Tooth decay

The Nutrition Facts Box

The Nutrition Facts box allows consumers to make informed choices.

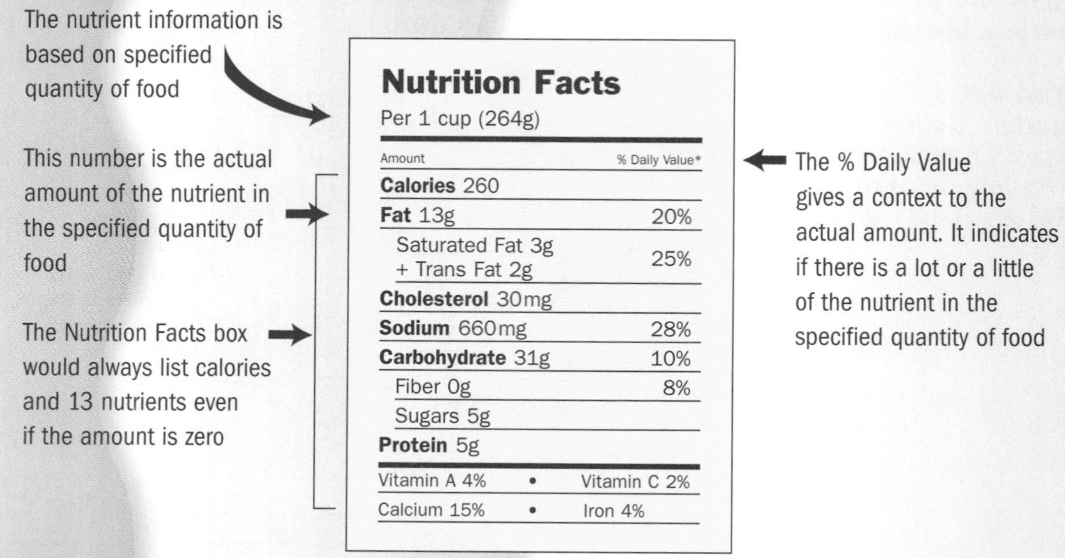

The nutrient information is based on specified quantity of food
This number is the actual amount of the nutrient in the specified quantity of food
The Nutrition Facts box would always list calories and 13 nutrients even if the amount is zero
The % Daily Value gives a context to the actual amount. It indicates if there is a lot or a little of the nutrient in the specified quantity of food
Nutrition Facts
Per 1 cup (264g)
Amount
% Daily Value*
Calories 260
Fat 13g 20%
Saturated Fat 3g
+ Trans Fat 2g 25%
Cholesterol 30mg
Sodium 660mg 28%
Carbohydrate 31g 10%
Fiber 0g 8%
Sugars 5g
Protein 5g
Vitamin A 4% • Vitamin C 2%
Calcium 15% • Iron 4%

Figure C.3 How to read a food label.

INGREDIENTS: Fructose Syrup (from Grapes, Corn and Pears), Oat Bran, Maltodextrin (Complex Carbohydrate), Modified Milk Ingredients (Milk Protein with Lactose removed), Brown Rice, Almond Butter, Natural Berry Flavours, Carmine, Citric Acid, **VITAMINS AND MINERALS:** Dicalcium phosphate, Potassium bicarbonate, Ascorbic acid, Magnesium carbonate, Alpha tocopherol (vit. E), Zinc gluconate, Ferrous fumarate, Salt, Potassium iodide, Beta carotene (vit. A), Copper gluconate, Manganese sulfate, Calcium pantothenate, Pyridoxine hydrochloride (vit. B_6), Riboflavin (vit B_2), Niacin, Thiamin hydrochloride (vit. B_1), Cholecalciferol (vit. D), Folic acid, Biotin, Cyanocobalamin (vit. B_{12}).

INGRÉDIENTS: Sirop de fructose (de Raisin, de Maïs et de Poire), Son d'avione, Maltodextrine (glucide complexe), Substances latières modifées (protéines du lait, lactose enlevé), Riz brun, Beurre d'amande, Arômes naturels de baie, Carmin, Acide citrique, **VITAMINES ET MINERAUX:** Phosphate bicalcique, Bicarbonate de potassium, Acide ascorbique, Carbonate de magnésium, Alpha tocophérol (vit. E), Gluconate de zinc Fumarate ferreux, Sel, Iodure de potassium, Bêta-carotène (vit. A), Gluconate de cuivre, Sulfate de manganèse, Pantothénate de calcium, Chlorhydrate de pyridoxine (vit. B_6) Riboflavine (vit. B_2), Niacine, Chlorhydrate de thiamine (vit. B_1) Cholécalciférol (vit. D), Acide folique, Biotine, Cyanocobalamine (vit. B_{12}).

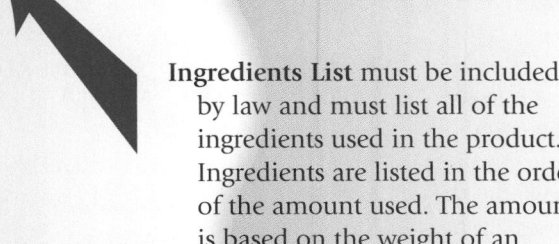

Ingredients List must be included by law and must list all of the ingredients used in the product. Ingredients are listed in the order of the amount used. The amount is based on the weight of an ingredient rather than its volume.

Figure C.4 Ingredients list.

Health Canada is finalizing the nutrition labeling standards. For the latest information, visit the Nutrition Labeling area of the Health Canada Web site at: http:// www.hc-sc.gc.ca/hppb/nutrition/labels/index.html.

Food Choice System

The CDA Food Choice System is a method of meal planning created by the Canadian Diabetes Association to make it easier for people with diabetes to eat the right amount of food for their insulin supply. This system is based on two concepts: Most foods are eaten by people with diabetes in measured amounts, and foods within each of the system's seven food groups can be interchanged.

The CDA Food Choice System started with the nutritional principles in *Canada's Food Guide to Healthy Eating* and modified them to meet the special needs of people with diabetes. People with diabetes must eat a certain amount of carbohydrate, protein, and fat at each meal in order to control the amount of glucose (sugar) that enters the blood after a meal. The CDA Food Choice System helps them select the proper type and amount of food to manage their diabetes.

The Food Choice System classifies foods into seven food groups according to the food's carbohydrate, protein, and fat content. The Food Choice Values tell a person with diabetes what group a food belongs to and how much of that food is interchangeable with another food in the same food group. The Food Choice Values, therefore, help someone with diabetes eat a balance of foods in the right amounts.

In the Food Choice System, the seven food groups and their symbols are:

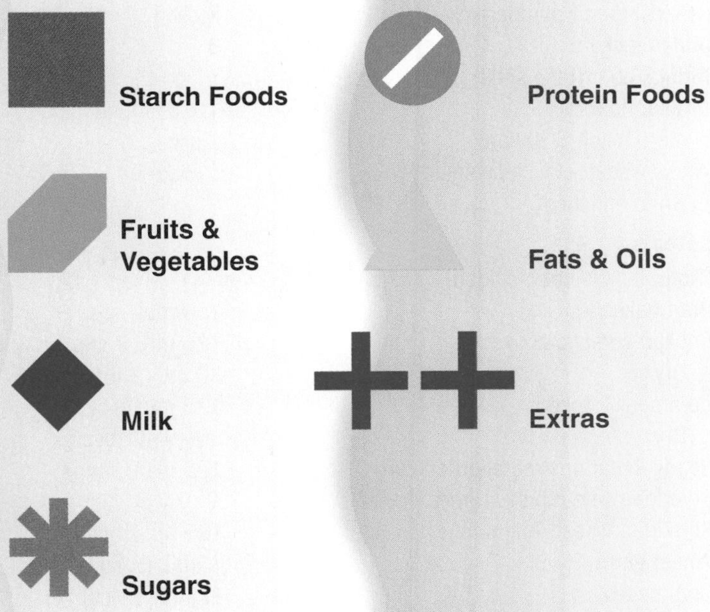

Because food groups in CDA's Food Choice System may be confused with the food groups in *Canada's Food Guide to Healthy Eating*, the government does not permit them to be listed by name on food labels. The Federal government regulation states that only the assigned quantity, the Food Choice "Symbol" and the word "Choice" can be published on a label.

Table C-3 CDA Food Choice System: Starch Foods

Note: 1 Starch choice contains about 15 g of carbohydrate, 2 g of protein, 290 kJ (68 Calories) of energy.

FOOD	MEASURE	MASS (WEIGHT)
Breads		
Bagel	½	30 g
Bread crumbs	50 mL (¼ cup)	30 g
Bread cubes	250 mL (1 cup)	30 g
Bread sticks	2	20 g
Brewis, cooked	50 mL (¼ cup)	45 g
Chapati	1	20 g
Cookies, plain	2	20 g
English muffin, crumpet	½	30 g
Flour	40 mL (2½ tbsp.)	20 g
Hamburger bun	½	30 g
Hot dog bun	½	30 g
Kaiser roll	½	30 g
Matzo, 15 cm	1	20 g
Melba toast, rectangular	4	15 g
Melba toast, rounds	7	15 g
Pita, 20 cm (8") diameter	¼	30 g
Pita, 15 cm (6") diameter	½	30 g
Plain roll	1 small	30 g
Pretzels	7	20 g
Raisin bread	1 slice	30 g
Rice cakes	2	30 g
Roti	1	20 g
Rusks	2	20 g
Rye, coarse or pumpernickel	½ slice	30 g
Soda crackers	6	20 g
Tortilla, corn (taco shell)	1	30 g
Tortilla, flour	1 – 9" round	30 g
White (French & Italian)	1 slice	25 g
Whole-wheat, cracked-wheat, rye, white enriched	1 slice	30 g
Cereals		
(Note: Milk is not included)		
Bran flakes	150 mL	18 g
Cooked cereals, cooked	125 mL (½ cup)	125 g
Dry	30 mL (2 tbsp.)	20 g
Cornmeal, cooked	125 mL (½ cup)	125 g
Dry	30 mL (2 tbsp.)	20 g
Ready-to-eat unsweetened cereal	125 mL (½ cup)	20 g
Shredded wheat biscuit, rectangular or round	1	20 g
Shredded wheat, bite size	125 mL (½ cup)	20 g
Wheat germ	75 mL (⅓ cup)	30 g
Corn flakes	175 mL (⅔ cup)	17 g
Rice krispies	150 mL	18 g
Muffets	1 muffet	21 g
Puffed rice	300 mL (1¼ cup)	15 g
Puffed wheat	425 mL (1⅔ cup)	20 g
Grains		
Barley, cooked	125 mL (½ cup)	120 g
dry	30 mL (2 tbsp.)	20 g

Source: *The Good Health Eating Guide Resource,* © Canadian Diabetes Association, 2002. Reprinted with permission.

FOOD	MEASURE	MASS (WEIGHT)
Grains (Continued)		
Bulgar, kasha,		
Cooked moist	125 mL (½ cup)	70 g
Cooked crumbly	75 mL (⅓ cup)	40 g
Dry	30 mL (2 tbsp.)	20 g
Rice, brown & white, cooked	75 mL (⅓ cup)	60 g
Rice, short & long grain, dry	15 mL (1 tbsp.)	20 g
Rice, wild, cooked	75 mL (⅓ cup)	60 g
Tapioca, pearl and granulated		
quick-cooking, dry	30 mL (2 tbsp.)	15 g
Couscous, cooked moist	125 mL (½ cup)	70 g
Dry	30 mL (2 tbsp.)	20 g
Quinoa, cooked moist	125 mL (½ cup)	70 g
Dry	30 mL (2 tbsp.)	20 g
Pasta		
Macaroni, cooked	125 mL (½ cup)	70 g
Noodles, cooked	125 mL (½ cup)	80 g
Spaghetti, cooked	125 mL (½ cup)	70 g
Starch Vegetables		
Breadfruit	1 slice	75 g
Corn, canned whole kernel	125 mL (½ cup)	85 g
Corn-on-the-cob	½ medium cob	70 g
Cornstarch	30 mL (2 tbsp.)	15 g
Plantain	⅓ small	50 g
Popcorn, air-popped, unbuttered	750 mL (3 cups)	20 g
Potatoes, with skin	½ potato	95 g
Without skin	½ potato	75 g
Yam, sweet potatoes, with skin	½ potato	95 g
Without skin	½ potato	75 g

Note: Each of the following measured foods equals more than 1 Starch choice:

FOOD	MEASURE	FOOD CHOICES	MASS (WEIGHT)
Bran flakes	250 mL (1 cup)	1½ starch	30 g
100% Bran	125 mL (½ cup)	½ starch + ½ sugar + ½ fat	30 g
Croissant, small	1 small	1 starch + 1½ fat	35 g
Large	½ large	1 starch + 1½ sugar	30 g
Corn, canned creamed	125 mL (½ cup)	1 starch + ½ sugar	120 g
Potato chips	15 chips	1 starch + 2 fat	30 g
Tortilla chips (nachos)	13 chips	1 starch + 1½ fat	30 g
Corn chips	30 chips	1 starch + 2 fat	30 g
Cheese twists	30 chips	1 starch + 1½ fat	30 g
Cheese puffs	27 chips	1 starch + 2 fat	30 g
Tea biscuit	1	1 starch + 2 fat	30 g
Pancake, homemade using 50 mL (¼ cup) batter (6" diameter)	1 medium	1 starch + 1 fat	50 g
Potatoes, French fried (homemade or frozen)	10 regular size	1 starch + 1 fat	35 g
Soup, canned[a] (prepared with equal volume of water)	250 mL (1 cup)	1 starch	260 g
Waffle, packaged	1	1 starch + 1 fat	35 g

[a]Soup can vary according to brand and type. Check the label for CDA Food Choice Values and Symbols or the core nutrient listing.

Table C-4 CDA Food Choice System: Fruits and Vegetables

Note: 1 Fruits & Vegetables choice contains about 10 g of carbohydrate, 1 g of protein, 190 kJ (44 Calories) of energy.

FOOD	MEASURE	MASS (WEIGHT)
Fruits *(fresh, frozen, without sugar, canned in water)*		
Apple, raw (with or without skin)	½ medium	75 g
Sauce unsweetened	125 mL (½ cup)	120 g
Apple butter	20 mL (4 tsp.)	20 g
Apricot, raw	2 medium	115 g
Canned in water	4 halves plus 30 mL (2 tbsp.) liquid	110 g
Bake-apple (cloudberries), raw	125 mL (½ cup)	120 g
Banana, with peel	½ small	75 g
Peeled	½ small	50 g
Berries	250 mL (1 cup)	150 g
Blackberries, boysenberries, raspberries		
Blueberries, loganberries, huckleberries	125 mL (½ cup)	70 g
Cantaloupe, wedge with rind (no seeds)	¼ of cantaloupe	160 g
Cubed or diced	175 mL (⅔ cup)	135 g
Cherries, raw with pits	10	75 g
Raw without pits	10	70 g
Canned in water, with pits	75 mL (⅓ cup), includes 30 mL (2 tbsp.) liquid	90 g
Canned in water, without pits	75 mL (⅓ cup), includes 30 mL (2 tbsp.) liquid	85 g
Crabapple, raw	1 small	55 g
Cranberries, raw	250 mL (1 cup)	100 g
Figs, raw	1 medium	50 g
Canned in water	3 medium plus 30 mL (2 tbsp.) liquid	100 g
Foxberries, raw	250 mL (1 cup)	100 g
Fruit cocktail, canned in water	125 mL (½ cup), includes 30 mL (2 tbsp.) liquid	120 g
Fruit, mixed cut-up	125 mL (½ cup)	120 g
Gooseberries, raw	250 mL (1 cup)	150 g
Canned in water	250 mL (1 cup), includes 30 mL (2 tbsp.) liquid	230 g
Grapefruit, raw with rind	½ small	185 g
Raw sectioned	125 mL (½ cup)	100 g
Canned in water	125 mL (½ cup), includes 30 mL (2 tbsp.) liquid	120 g
Grapes, raw slip skin	125 mL (½ cup)	75 g
Raw seedless	125 mL (½ cup)	75 g
Canned in water	75 mL (⅓ cup), includes 30 mL (2 tbsp.) liquid	115 g
Honeydew melon, raw with rind	⅒ wedge	130 g
Cubed or diced	175 mL (⅔ cup)	115 g
Guava, raw	½	50 g
Kiwi, raw with skin	1 medium	76 g
Kumquats, raw	3	60 g
Loquats, raw	8	130 g
Lychee fruit, raw	8	120 g
Mandarin orange, raw with rind	1	135 g
Raw sectioned	125 mL (½ cup)	100 g
Canned in water	125 mL (½ cup), includes 30 mL (2 tbsp.) liquid	100 g

FOOD	MEASURE	MASS (WEIGHT)
Fruits (Continued)		
Mango, raw without skin and seeds, diced	75 mL (⅓ cup)	65 g
Nectarine	½ medium	75 g
Orange, raw with rind	1 small	130 g
Raw sectioned	125 mL (½ cup)	95 g
Papaya, raw with skin and seeds	¼ medium	150 g
Raw without skin and seeds	¼ medium	100 g
Cubed or diced	125 mL (½ cup)	100 g
Peaches, raw with pit and skin	1 large	100 g
Raw sliced or diced	125 mL (½ cup)	85 g
Canned in water, halves or slices	125 mL (½ cup), includes 30 mL (2 tbsp.) liquid	120 g
Pear, raw with skin and core	½	90 g
Raw without skin and core	½	85 g
Halves canned in water	½ plus 30 mL (2 tbsp.) liquid	90 g
Persimmons, raw native	1	30 g
Raw Japanese	¼	50 g
Pineapple, raw	1 slice	75 g
Raw diced	125 mL (½ cup)	75 g
Sliced canned in water	2 slices plus 15 mL (1 tbsp.) liquid	100 g
Diced canned in water	125 mL (½ cup), includes 30 mL (2 tbsp.) liquid	100 g
Sliced canned in juice	1 slice plus 15 mL (1 tbsp.) liquid	55 g
Diced canned in juice	75 mL (⅓ cup), includes 15 mL (1 tbsp.) liquid	55 g
Plum, raw	2 small	60 g
Damson	6	65 g
Japanese	1	70 g
Canned in water	3 plus 30 mL (2 tbsp.) liquid	100 g
Canned in apple juice	2 plus 30 mL (2 tbsp.) liquid	70 g
Pomegranate, raw	½	140 g
Strawberries, raw	250 mL (1 cup)	150 g
Frozen/canned in water	250 mL (1 cup), includes 30 mL (2 tbsp.) liquid	240 g
Tangelo, raw	1	205 g
Tangerine, raw	1 medium	115 g
Raw, sectioned	125 mL (½ cup)	100 g
Watermelon, raw with rind	1 wedge	310 g
Cubed or diced	250 mL (1 cup)	160 g
Dried Fruit		
Apple	5 pieces	15 g
Apricot	4 halves	15 g
Banana flakes	30 mL (2 tbsp.)	15 g
Currants	30 mL (2 tbsp.)	15 g
Dates, without pits	2	15 g
Peach	½	15 g
Pear	½	15 g
Prunes, raw with pits	2	15 g
Raw without pits	2	10 g
Stewed no liquid	2	20 g
Stewed with liquid	2 plus 15 mL (1 tbsp.) liquid	35 g
Raisins	30 mL (2 tbsp.)	15 g

(table continues on next page)

Table C-4 CDA Food Choice System: Fruits and Vegetables *(Continued)*

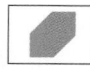

Note: 1 Fruits & Vegetables choice contains about: 10 g of carbohydrate, 1 g of protein, 190 kJ (44 Calories) of energy.

FOOD	MEASURE	MASS (WEIGHT)
Juices *(no sugar added or unsweetened)*		
Apricot, grape, guava, mango, prune	50 mL (¼ cup)	55 g
Apple, carrot, papaya, pear, pineapple, pomegranate	75 mL (⅓ cup)	80 g
Cranberry	*see Sugars section*	
Clamato	*see Sugars section*	
Grapefruit, loganberry, orange, raspberry, tangelo, tangerine	125 mL (½ cup)	130 g
Tomato, tomato-based mixed vegetables	250 mL (1 cup)	255 g
Vegetables *(fresh, frozen or canned)*		
Artichokes, French, globe	2 small	50 g
Beets, diced or sliced	125 mL (½ cup)	85 g
Carrots, diced, cooked or uncooked	125 mL (½ cup)	75 g
Chestnuts, fresh	5	20 g
Parsnips, mashed	125 mL (½ cup)	80 g
Peas, fresh or frozen	125 mL (½ cup)	80 g
Canned	75 mL (⅓ cup)	55 g
Pumpkin, mashed	125 mL (½ cup)	45 g
Rutabagas, mashed	125 mL (½ cup)	85 g
Sauerkraut	250 mL (1 cup)	235 g
Snow peas	250 mL (1 cup)	135 g
Squash, yellow or winter, mashed	125 mL (½ cup)	115 g
Succotash	75 mL (⅓ cup)	55 g
Tomatoes, canned	250 mL (1 cup)	240 g
Tomato paste	50 mL (¼ cup)	55 g
Tomato sauce*	75 mL (⅓ cup)	100 g
Turnip, mashed	125 mL (½ cup)	115 g
Vegetables, mixed	125 mL (½ cup)	90 g
Water chestnuts	8 medium	50 g

Table C-5 CDA Food Choice System: Milk

TYPE OF MILK	CARBOHYDRATE	PROTEIN	FAT	ENERGY
Skim (0%)	6 g	4 g	0 g	170 kJ (40 Cal)
1%	6 g	4 g	1 g	206 kJ (49 Cal)
2%	6 g	4 g	2 g	244 kJ (58 Cal)
Homo (4%)	6 g	4 g	4 g	319 kJ (76 Cal)

(table continues on next page)

*Tomato sauce varies according to brand name. Check the label or discuss with your dietitian.

FOOD	MEASURE	MASS (WEIGHT)
Milk	125 mL (½ cup)	125 g
Buttermilk (higher in salt)	125 mL (½ cup)	125 g
Evaporated milk	50 mL (¼ cup)	50 g
Powdered milk, regular	30 mL (2 tbsp.)	15 g
Instant	50 mL (¼ cup)	15 g
Plain yogurt	125 mL (½ cup)	125 g

Note: Each of the following measured foods equals more than 1 Milk choice:

FOOD	FOOD CHOICES	MEASURE	MASS (WEIGHT)
Milkshake	1 milk + 3 sugars + ½ protein	250 mL (1 cup)	300 g
Chocolate milk, 2%	2 milk 2% + 1 sugar	250 mL (1 cup)	300 g
Frozen yogurt	1 milk + 1 sugar	125 mL (½ cup)	125 g

Table C-6 CDA Food Choice System: Sugars

FOOD	MEASURE	MASS (WEIGHT)
Beverages		
Condensed milk	15 mL (1 tbsp.)	
Cranberry cocktail	75 mL (⅓ cup)	
Cranberry cocktail, light	350 mL (1⅓ cup)	
[a]Flavoured fruit crystals	75 mL (⅓ cup)	
[a]Iced tea mixes	75 mL (⅓ cup)	
Regular soft drinks	125 mL (½ cup)	
[a]Sweet drink mixes	75 mL (⅓ cup)	
Tonic water	125 mL (½ cup)	
Miscellaneous		
Bubble gum (large square)	1 piece	10 g
Cranberry sauce	30 mL (2 tbsp.)	
Hard candy	2	10 g
Honey, molasses, corn & cane syrup	10 mL (2 tsp.)	15 g
Jelly beans	4	10 g
Licorice	1 short stick	10 g
Marshmallows	2 large	15 g
Popsicle	½ popsicle (1 stick)	
Powdered gelatin mix (Jello®) reconstituted	50 mL (¼ cup)	
Regular jam, jelly, marmalade	15 mL (1 tbsp.)	
Sugar, white, brown, icing, maple	10 mL (2 tsp.)	10 g
Sweet pickles	2 small	100 g
Sweet relish	30 mL (2 tbsp.)	

Note: Each of the following measured foods equals more than 1 Sugars choice:

FOOD	FOOD CHOICES	MEASURE	MASS (WEIGHT)
Brownie	1 sugar + 1 fat	1	20 g
Clamato juice	1½ sugars	175 mL (⅔ cup)	
Fruit salad, light syrup	1 sugar + 1 starch	125 mL (½ cup)	130 g
Aero® bar	2½ sugars + 2½ fats	1 bar	43 g
Smarties®	4½ sugars + 2 fats	1 box	60 g
Sherbet	3 sugars + ½ fat	125 mL (½ cup)	95 g

See Combined Food Choices for more foods containing Sugars.

[a]These have been made with water.

Table C-7 CDA Food Choice System: Protein Foods

Note: 1 choice from the Protein Foods group contains about 7 g protein, 3 g fat, 230 kJ (55 Calories) of energy.
Note: All of the weights and measures in this section are for **cooked** meats, fish, and poultry, unless it is otherwise stated.

FOOD	MEASURE	MASS (WEIGHT)
Cheese		
Low-fat cheese about 7% milk fat (M.F.)	1 slice	30 g
Cottage cheese, 2% M.F. or less	50 mL (¼ cup)	55 g
Ricotta cheese, about 7% M.F.	50 mL (¼ cup)	60 g
Fish		
Anchovy (see Extras)		
Canned, drained, e.g., tuna packed in water, mackerel, salmon	50 mL (¼ cup) (⅓ of 6.5 oz. can)	30 g
Cod tongues, cheeks	75 mL (⅓ cup)	50 g
Fillet or steak, e.g., Boston blue, cod, flounder, haddock, halibut, mackerel, orange roughy, perch, pickerel, pike, salmon, shad, snapper, sole, swordfish, trout, tuna, whitefish	1 piece	30 g
Herring	⅓ fish	30 g
Sardines, smelts	2 medium or 3 small	30 g
Squid, octopus	50 mL (¼ cup)	40 g
Shellfish		
Clams, mussels, oysters, scallops, snails	3 medium	30 g
Crab, lobster, flaked	50 mL (¼ cup)	30 g
Shrimp: fresh	5 large	30 g
Frozen	10 medium	30 g
Canned	18 small	30 g
Dry pack	50 mL (¼ cup)	30 g
Meat and Poultry ***(e.g., beef, chicken, goat, ham, lamb, pork, turkey, veal, wild game)***		
Back, peameal bacon	3 thin slices	30 g
Chop	½ chop, with bone	40 g
Minced or ground, lean or extra-lean	30 mL (2 tbsp.)	30 g
Sliced, lean	1 slice	30 g
Steak, lean	1 piece	30 g
Organ Meats		
Heart, liver	1 slice	30 g
Kidney, sweetbreads, chopped	50 mL (¼ cup)	30 g
Tongue	1 slice	30 g
Tripe	5 pieces	60 g
Soyabean		
Bean curd or tofu	½ block	70 g
Eggs		
Egg in shell, raw or cooked	1 medium	50 g
Egg without shell, cooked or poached in water	1 medium	45 g
Egg, scrambled	50 mL (¼ cup)	55 g

(table continues on next page)

Note: Each of the following measured foods equals a higher fat protein choice:

FOOD	CHOICES	MEASURES	MASS (WEIGHT)
Cheese	1 protein + 1 fat	1 piece	25 g
Cheese, coarsely grated, e.g., cheddar	1 protein + 1 fat	50 mL (¼ cup)	25 g
Cheese, dry, finely grated, e.g., parmesan	1 protein + 1 fat	45 mL	15 g
Cheese, ricotta, high fat	1 protein + 1 fat	50 mL (¼ cup)	55 g
Eel	1 protein + 1 fat	1 slice	50 g
Bologna	1 protein + 1 fat	1 slice	20 g
Canned luncheon meat	1 protein + 1 fat	1 slice	20 g
Corned beef, fresh	1 protein + 1 fat	1 slice	25 g
Corned beef, canned	1 protein + 1 fat	1 slice	25 g
Ground beef, medium fat	1 protein + 1 fat	30 mL (2 tbsp.)	25 g
Meat spreads, canned	1 protein + 1 fat	45 mL	35 g
Mutton chop	1 protein + 1 fat	½ chop (with bone)	35 g
Paté (see Fats & Oils group)			
Sausage, pork link	1 protein + 1 fat	1 link	25 g
Sausage, garlic Polish or knockwurst	1 protein + 1 fat	1 slice	50 g
Summer sausage or salami	1 protein + 1 fat	1 slice	40 g
Spareribs or short ribs, with bone	1 protein + 1 fat	1 large	65 g
Stewing beef	1 protein + 1 fat	1 cube	25 g
Weiner, hot dog	½ protein + 1½ fats	1 wiener	38 g
Blood pudding	1 protein + 1 fat	1 slice	25 g
Peanut butter	1 protein + 1 fat	15 mL (1 tbsp.)	15 g

Table C-8 CDA Food Choice System: Fats and Oils

FOOD	MEASURE	MASS (WEIGHT)
Avocado	⅛	30 g
Bacon, side, crisp[a]	1 slice	5 g
Butter[a]	5 mL (1 tsp.)	5 g
Cheese spread[a]	15 mL (1 tbsp.)	15 g
Coconut, fresh[a]	45 mL (3 tbsp.)	15 g
Dried[a]	15 mL (1 tbsp.)	10 g
Cream, half-and-half (cereal) 10%[a]	30 mL (2 tbsp.)	30 g
Coffee 20%[a]	15 mL (1 tbsp.)	15 g
Whipping 32-37%[a]	15 mL (1 tbsp.)	15 g
Cream cheese[a]	15 mL (1 tbsp.)	15 g
Gravy[a]	30 mL (2 tbsp.)	30 g
Lard[a]	5 mL (1 tsp.)	5 g
Margarine, brick[a]	5 mL (1 tsp.)	5 g
Soft tub	5 mL (1 tsp.)	5 g
Nuts, shelled		
Almonds	8 nuts	5 g
Brazil Nuts	2 nuts	10 g
Cashews	5 nuts	10 g
Filberts, Hazelnuts	5 nuts	10 g
Macadamia	3 nuts	5 g
Peanuts	10 nuts	10 g
Pecans	5 halves	5 g
Pignolias, Pine nuts	25 mL (5 tsp.)	10 g
Pistachios, shelled	20 nuts	10 g
in shell	20 nuts	20 g
Pumpkin and Squash Seeds	20 mL (4 tsp.)	10 g
Sesame Seeds	15 mL (1 tbsp.)	10 g
Sunflower Seeds, shelled	15 mL (1 tbsp.)	10 g
in shell	45 mL (3 tbsp.)	15 g
Walnuts	4 halves	10 g
Oil, cooking and salad	5 mL (1 tsp.)	5 g
Olives, green	10	45 g
black (ripe)	7	57 g
Paté, liverwurst, meat spreads[a]	15 mL (1 tbsp.)	15 g
Salad dressing		
Blue cheese, French, Italian, mayonnaise,	10 mL (2 tsp.)	10 g
Thousand Island	5 mL (1 tsp.)	5 g
Salad dressing, low-calorie	30 mL (2 tbsp.)	30 g
Salt pork, raw or cooked[a]	5 mL (1 tsp.)	5 g
Sesame oil	5 mL (1 tsp.)	5 g
Sour cream, 12% M.F.[a]	30 mL (2 tbsp.)	30 g
7% M.F.[a]	60 mL (4 tbsp.)	60 g
Shortening[a]	5 mL (1 tsp.)	

[a]These items contain higher amounts of saturated fats.

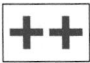

Table C-9 CDA Food Choice System: Extras ++

Note: Use less than 125 mL (½ cup) for all vegetables listed, larger quantities may need to be counted as Fruits and Vegetables choice.

Extra Vegetables

Artichokes	Cucumber	Peppers, green, red, yellow
Asparagus	Eggplant	Radish
Bamboo shoots	Endive	Rapini
Beans, string, green or yellow	Fiddleheads	Rhubarb
Bean sprouts, mung or soya	Greens, beet, dandelion, etc.	Sauerkraut
Bitter melon (balsam pear)	Kale	Shallots
Bok choy	Kohlrabi	Spinach
Broccoli	Leeks	Sprouts, alfalfa, radish, etc.
Brussel sprouts	Lettuce	Tomato wedges
Cabbage	Mushroom	Watercress
Cauliflower	Okra	Zucchini
Celery	Onions, green, mature	
Chard	Parsley	

Note: Use the amount listed. Your dietitian may limit use of these items to no more than two per day.

FOOD	MEASURE	FOOD	MEASURE	FOOD	MEASURE
Condiments					
Anchovy	2 fillets	Cranberry sauce, unsweetened	15 mL (1 tbsp.)	Pickles, unsweetened (cont.) Sour mixed	11
Barbecue sauce	15 mL (1 tbsp.)	Dietetic fruit spreads	5 mL (1 tsp.)	Sour cream, Fat-free	15 mL (1 tbsp.)
Bran, natural	30 mL (2 tbsp.)	Ketchup	5 mL (1 tsp.)	Sugar substitutes, granular	5 mL (1 tsp.) (3 to 4 packets)
Brewers yeast	5 mL (1 tsp.)	Maraschino cherry	1	Whipped topping	15 mL (1 tbsp.)
Carob powder	5 mL (1 tsp.)	Nuts, chopped pieces	5 mL (1 tsp.)		
Chili sauce	5 mL (1 tsp.)	Non-Dairy Coffee Whitener	5 mL (1 tsp.)		
Cocoa powder	5 mL (1 tsp.)	Pickles, unsweetened dill	2		

(table continues on next page)

Table C-9 CDA Food Choice System: Extras *(Continued)* ++

Note: These items do not need to be measured.

Free Foods

Artificial sweetener, such as cyclamate or aspartame	Garlic	Pimentos
Baking powder, soda	Gelatin, unsweetened	Soda water, club soda
Bouillon or clear broth	Ginger root	Soya sauce
Bouillon from cube, powder or liquid	Herbal teas, unsweetened	Sugar-free jelly powder
Chow Chow, unsweetened	Horseradish, uncreamed	Sugar-free soft drink
Coffee, clear	Lemon juice/lemon wedge	Sugar-free crystal drink
Consomme	Lime juice/lime wedge	Tea, clear
Dulse	Marjoram, cinnamon, etc.	Vinegar
Flavouring and extracts	Mineral water	Water
	Mustard	Worcestershire sauce
	Parsley	Salt, pepper, thyme

ATP Produced from Macronutrients APPENDIX D

Pathway	ATP formed by pathway	ATP formed by electron transport chain
Glycolysis (1 Glucose)		
Net 2 ATP (4 produced – 2 used)	2	
2 NADH*		3 to 5
Pyruvate to Acetyl CoA (2 Pyruvate)		
First pyruvate → Acetyl CoA		
1 NADH		2.5
Second pyruvate → Acetyl CoA		
1 NADH		2.5
Citric Acid Cycle (twice)		
First acetyl CoA → Citric acid cycle		
1 GTP (ATP)	1	
1 $FADH_2$		1.5
3 NADH		7.5
Second acetyl CoA → Citric acid cycle		
1 GTP (ATP)	1	
1 $FADH_2$		1.5
3 NADH		7.5
Subtotal	4	26 to 28
		Total = 30 to 32

*Each NADH molecule formed in the cytosol by glycolysis will produce either 2.5 or 1.5 ATP molecules in the electron transport chain. NADH formed by the citric acid cycle will produce 2.5 ATP molecules in the electron transport chain.

Figure D.1 **The complete breakdown of glucose.** These metabolic pathways and molecules move energy from glucose to ATP. Complete breakdown of one glucose molecule yields 30 to 32 ATP molecules.

Pathway	ATP yield
Beta oxidation (stearic acid C18:0)	
8 NADH	20
8 $FADH_2$	12
Citric Acid Cycle (9 acetyl CoA)	
1 GTP x 9 = 9 GTP	9
1 $FADH_2$ x 9 = 9 $FADH_2$	13.5
3 NADH x 9 = 27 NADH	67.5
Subtotal	122
ATP needed to start beta-oxidation	–2
Net yield	**120**

The grand total:
120 ATP molecules from one molecule of stearic acid

Figure D.2 **The complete breakdown of stearic acid.** The complete breakdown of one 18-carbon fatty acid yields about four times as much ATP as the complete breakdown of one glucose molecule.

Pathway	ATP yield
Alanine to Pyruvate	0
Pyruvate to Acetyl CoA	
1 NADH	2.5
Citric Acid Cycle	
1 GTP (ATP)	1
1 $FADH_2$	1.5
3 NADH	7.5
Total	**12.5**

Figure D.3 **The complete breakdown of alanine.** The complete breakdown of the amino acid alanine yields about one-third the ATP of the complete breakdown of one glucose molecule.

Pathway	ATP yield
Methionine to Succinyl CoA*	0
Citric Acid Cycle (partial)	
1 GTP (ATP)	1
1 $FADH_2$	1.5
1 NADH	2.5
Total	**5**

*Succinyl CoA is an intermediate of the citric acid cycle.

Figure D.4 **The complete breakdown of methionine.** The complete breakdown of the amino acid methionine yields about one-sixth the ATP of the complete breakdown of one glucose molecule.

APPENDIX E Vitamin and Mineral Summary Tables

Fat-Soluble Vitamins

NAME	MAIN ROLES	RECOMMENDED INTAKE (ADULT)
Vitamin A (retinol, retinal, and retinoic acid) **Provitamin A carotenoids**	Regulates cell growth and cell death. Growth/maintenance of bones/teeth; skin, mucous membranes, and other epithelial cells. Required for reproduction, immune function, vision/night vision, wound healing.	**RDA** Men: 900 μg RAE Women: 700 μg RAE RAE is Retinol Activity Equivalent 1 RAE = 1 μg retinol = 12 μg beta-carotene = 24 μg alpha-carotene, beta-cryptoxanthin, other provitamin A carotenoids. = 2 μg beta-carotene in oil base/supplements
Vitamin D (cholecalciferol and calcitriol; ergocalciferol is D_2, cholecalciferol is D_3)	Regulates calcium and phosphorus levels by regulating their intestinal absorption, retention by the kidneys, deposition into bone, and absorption from bone when calcium and phosphorus blood levels dip. Required for bone/teeth growth and maintenance.	**AI** Ages 19–50 yr: 5 μg 51–70 yr: 10 μg >70 yr: 15 μg
Vitamin E (alpha-tocopherol) (Includes natural alpha-tocopherol and several, but not all, synthetic variations.)	As a fat-soluble antioxidant, it protects unsaturated fats, phospholipids, and other fat-soluble substances; discourages oxidation of blood lipids and their subsequent deposition in arteries; helps prevent oxygen damage in the lungs, skin, eyes, liver, and other organs. Helps maintain red blood cell integrity, nervous system function.	**RDA** Adults: 15 mg
Vitamin K (phylloquinone and menaquinone)	Required in production of thrombin for blood clotting. Involved in bone formation and maintenance.	**RDA** Men: 120 μg Women: 90 μg

RDA, Recommended Dietary Allowance; UL, Tolerable Upper Intake Level; AI, Adequate Intake.

DEFICIENCY	GOOD FOOD SOURCES	TOXICITY
Eyes: Night blindness, Bitot's spots (foamy deposits on cornea), keratomalacia (corneal dryness, itching), progressing to xerophthalmia (corneal scarring and degeneration, blindness). Skin, mucous membranes: Hyperkeratosis (bumpy dry skin from clogged hair follicles); compromised linings of respiratory, digestive, and reproductive systems. Impaired immunity, growth, and reproduction.	Vitamin A (animal sources): Liver, egg yolk, butterfat, cream, cheese, whole milk, fortified low-fat milks, fortified margarine. Provitamin A (vegetable sources): Spinach, collards, and other dark-green vegetables; pumpkin, sweet potato, carrots, apricots, peaches, cantaloupe, mango, and other orange or dark yellow fruits and vegetables (the carotenoid in oranges/tangerines is not converted to vitamin A).	**UL:** 3,000 μg Teratogenic (birth defects from excessive use during pregnancy). Dry itchy skin. Hair loss. Bone/joint pain. Bone abnormalities. Loss of appetite. Liver abnormalities/damage. (UL does not apply to provitamin carotenoids.)
Growth retardation. Rickets (bowed legs, knocked knees, other skeletal deformities) develop in childhood. Adults develop osteomalacia (excessive loss of calcium from bones) with risk of bone fracture. Severe deficiency due to illness or metabolic error causes twitching and muscle spasms.	Synthesis by the body when skin is exposed to sunlight is the most important source of vitamin D. Vitamin D-fortified milk. Fish liver oils. Salmon, mackerel, and other fatty fish; egg yolk; butter; and liver. (Vitamin D levels in foods vary widely.)	**UL:** 50 μg Impairs kidney function; excessive urination and thirst. Kidney stones and calcium deposition in other soft tissues—heart, blood vessels, and membranes in bone joints. Joint pain. Bone loss. Growth retardation.
Hemolysis (breaking) of red blood cells and hemolytic anemia, especially in premature babies. Retinopathy of prematurity. Neurological problems.	Wheat germ. Nuts and seeds such as pumpkin, sunflower, sesame. Vegetable oils, margarine, salad dressings.	**UL:** 1,000 μg Interferes with blood clotting. (UL applies only to vitamin E in supplements or fortified foods; includes natural-form alpha-tocopherol and all synthetic versions.)
Hemorrhage. Possible decrease in bone density.	Synthesis by intestinal bacteria. Vegetable source (phylloquinone): Dark green leafy vegetables, vegetables in cabbage family. Animal source (menaquinone): Egg yolk, butterfat, liver.	Possible interference with anti-coagulation medication. No UL has been set.

Water-Soluble Vitamins and Choline

NAME	MAIN ROLES	RECOMMENDED INTAKE (ADULT)
Thiamin (vitamin B_1)	As part of coenzyme TPP (thiamin pyrophosphate), it functions in several energy-producing pathways, is required for RNA and DNA synthesis, and is involved in nervous system function.	**RDA** Men: 1.2 mg Women: 1.1 mg
Riboflavin (vitamin B_2)	As part of coenzymes FMN (flavin mononucleotide) and FAD (flavin adenine dinucleotide), it functions in energy production and metabolism of amino acids. Involved in oxidation/reduction reactions. Required for vision.	**RDA** Men: 1.3 mg Women: 1.1 mg
Niacin (vitamin B_3, niacinamide, nicotinic acid, nicotinamide)	As part of coenzymes NAD and NADP (nicotinamide adenine dinucleotide/phosphate), it functions in energy metabolism and synthesis of fatty acids, steroid hormones, DNA, and amino acids.	**RDA** Men: 16 mg NE Women: 14 mg NE NE is niacin equivalent 1 NE = 1 mg niacin = 60 mg tryptophan
Pantothenic acid	As part of coenzyme A, it has many metabolic activities, including energy production and synthesis of lipids, steroid hormones, and proteins.	**AI** Adults: 5 mg
Biotin	As part of several coenzymes, it has many metabolic activities, including DNA and lipid synthesis, and energy production from carbohydrates, proteins, and fats.	**AI** Adults: 30 μg

DEFICIENCY	GOOD FOOD SOURCES	TOXICITY
Beriberi deficiency disease: Painful leg muscles, overall muscle weakness and wasting, loss of reflexes, and ultimately paralysis; edema, enlarged heart and heart failure; loss of appetite; depression, mental confusion; death. When complicated by alcoholism, Wernicke/Korsakoff syndrome with mental/emotional symptoms, involuntary eye movements or eye paralysis.	Pork. Organ meats. Enriched or fortified bread, pasta, rice, breakfast cereals; whole grain products. Nuts, seeds, legumes. (Widely distributed in small amounts in most fruits, vegetables, animal products, and dairy foods.)	Not determined. No UL has been set.
Ariboflavinosis deficiency disease: Glossitis and stomatitis (inflamed tongue and mouth), cheilosis (fissures at corners of mouth), seborrheic dermatitis (inflammation of skin's oil-producing glands). Sensitivity to light. Ariboflavinosis usually coexists with other vitamin deficiencies.	Milk, other dairy products. Liver, other organ meats. Enriched or fortified grain products; whole-grain products. Dark-green vegetables.	Not determined. No UL has been set.
Pellagra deficiency disease: The 4 Ds—dementia, diarrhea, dermatitis, death. Rough, darkened skin rash where exposed to sun. Inflamed mouth and tongue. Neuritis, confusion, anxiety.	Eggs, organ meats, meats, poultry, fish. Peas, peanuts, soybeans. Enriched or fortified grain products; whole-grain products. Milk, cheese, yogurt. (Tryptophan can be converted to niacin; 60 mg tryptophan provides 1 NE.)	**UL:** 35 mg >35 mg may cause flushing. >250 mg may cause itching, rash, headache, nausea; glucose intolerance; blurred vision. Extremely high doses (over 3 g/d) are associated with liver damage. (UL applies only to niacin in supplements and fortified foods.)
Irritability, fatigue, apathy, nausea, vomiting, tingling, muscle cramps. (Deficiency symptoms seen only in experimental settings.)	Widely distributed in most foods. Eggs, milk, yogurt. Fish, shellfish, meat, poultry. Peas, potatoes, winter squash.	Not determined. No UL has been set.
Hair loss, rash, convulsions, impaired growth. (Deficiency symptoms seen in infants with rare genetic error of biotin metabolism.)	Cauliflower, liver, nuts, peanuts, cheese, egg yolks (raw egg whites interfere with biotin absorption). Little information is available on food sources.	Not determined. No UL has been set.

(table continues on next page)

Water-Soluble Vitamins and Choline (Continued)

NAME	MAIN ROLES	RECOMMENDED INTAKE (ADULT)
Vitamin B_6 (pyridoxine, pyridoxal, pyridoxamine)	As part of PLP (pyridoxal phosphate) and other coenzymes, it functions in amino acid, carbohydrate, and fatty acid metabolism; red and white blood cell synthesis; conversion of tryptophan to niacin; synthesis of several neurotransmitters.	**RDA** Ages 19–50 yrs: 1.3 mg Men >51 yrs: 1.7 mg Women >51 yrs: 1.5 mg
Folate (folic acid, folacin)	As the coenzyme THFA (tetrahydrofolic acid), involved in DNA and RNA synthesis, red blood cell maturation, synthesis of neurotransmitters, and metabolism of homocysteine and other amino acids. Important for reproduction.	**RDA** Adults: 400 μg DFE DFE is dietary folate equivalent 1 μg DFE = 1 μg food folate = 0.5 μg supplemental folic acid on empty stomach = 0.6 μg supplemental folic acid taken with food or folic acid from fortified food
Vitamin B_{12} (cobalamin)	As part of cobalamin coenzymes, involved in cell synthesis, red blood cell maturation. Regeneration of folate. Maintenance of protective sheath around nerve fibers. Involved in fatty acid metabolism.	**RDA** Adults: 2.4 μg
Vitamin C (ascorbic acid)	An antioxidant. Needed for collagen synthesis: wound healing, blood vessel integrity, maintenance of gums, bone growth and maintenance. Aids iron absorption. Involved in thyroxin metabolism; synthesis of neurotransmitters, carnitine, and amino acids.	**RDA** Men: 90 mg Women: 75 mg Smokers: add 35 mg to above
Choline	A methyl donor. A component of bile, and of the neurotransmitter acetylcholine. As part of the phospholipid lecithin, it is an emulsifier and functions in cell membranes.	**AI** Men: 550 mg Women: 425 mg

AI, Adequate Intake; RDA, Recommended Dietary Allowance; UL, Tolerable Upper Intake Level.

DEFICIENCY	GOOD FOOD SOURCES	TOXICITY
Anemia. Depression, confusion, headache, convulsions. Seborrheic dermatitis. Possible relation to cardiovascular disease from homocysteine buildup.	Fortified breakfast cereals. Liver, other meat, poultry, seafood, fish. Bananas, avocados, green and leafy vegetables, legumes, potatoes.	**UL:** 100 mg Nerve damage causing weakness, numbness, inability to walk. At high doses, damage may be irreversible.
Anemia. Impaired immunity. Diarrhea. Neuropathy, depression, confusion, fatigue. Sore, inflamed mouth and tongue. Possible relation to cardiovascular disease from homocysteine buildup. Inadequate folate early in pregnancy related to neural tube birth defects such as spina bifida.	Fortified breakfast cereals, wheat germ. Leafy green vegetables, asparagus, broccoli, cauliflower. Oranges. Peanuts, legumes, seeds such as pumpkin or sunflower. Liver.	**UL:** 1,000 μg Masks vitamin B_{12} deficiency. Allergic reactions possible. May interfere with antiseizure medications. (UL applies only to folic acid in supplements and fortified foods.)
Pernicious anemia. Impaired immunity. Diarrhea. Neuropathy, which becomes irreversible. Possible relation to cardiovascular disease from homocysteine buildup.	Liver and other meats, poultry, fish, and seafood. Milk, cheese, eggs. Only vegetable sources are fortified foods and Cyanobacteria (blue-green algae). (For adults > 51 yr, B_{12} supplements or fortified foods are recommended.)	Not determined. No UL has been set.
Scurvy deficiency disease: Broken blood vessels with tiny hemorrhages; easily bruised; bleeding gums and loose or missing teeth; pain in joints, bones, muscles; nonhealing wounds, bedsores; delayed bone growth, bone fragility; anemia. Severe scurvy can be fatal.	Citrus fruits, kiwi, strawberries, peppers, cabbage-family vegetables, dark leafy greens, potatoes, melon, papaya.	**UL:** 2,000 mg May cause diarrhea. Tooth erosion. Excessive iron absorption. Buildup of oxalates and uric acid may cause kidney stones. Interference with diagnostic testing and with some medications.
Fatty liver and liver damage.	Egg yolk, liver, milk and dairy products, soybeans, peanuts.	**UL:** 3,500 mg Fishy body odor, vomiting, excess sweating and salivation, liver damage, digestive disturbance, low blood pressure.

Major Minerals

NAME	MAIN ROLES	RECOMMENDED INTAKE (ADULT)
Sodium	Major cation in extracellular fluid. Involved in regulating body water distribution, blood pressure, acid–base balance, and nerve and muscle function.	**DV** Adults: 2,400 mg American Heart Association recommends limiting daily intake to this amount.
Potassium	Major intracellular cation. Involved in transmitting nerve impulses, regulating blood pressure, and controlling muscle contractility.	**DV** Adults: 3,500 mg
Chloride	Major anion in extracellular fluid. Involved in maintaining fluid and electrolyte balance. Component of gastric juice.	**DV** Adults: 3,400 mg
Calcium	Structural material for bones and teeth. Involved in regulating nerve conduction, blood clotting, membrane permeability, nerve irritability, and muscle contraction.	**AI** 19–50 yrs: 1,000 mg >51 yrs: 1,200 mg
Phosphorus	Structural material for bones and teeth. Component of nucleic acids, of phospholipids, of numerous enzymes, and of high-energy compounds such as ATP.	**RDA** Adults: 700 mg
Magnesium	Participates in hundreds of enzyme reactions. Regulates muscle contractility. Involved in nerve function and blood clotting, release of energy from ATP.	**RDA** 19–30 yrs / >30 yrs Men: 400 mg / 420 mg Women: 310 mg / 320 mg
Sulfur	Component of some amino acids, biotin, thiamin, other important compounds. Helps regulate acid–base balance. Drug detoxification.	Not established

AI, Adequate Intake; DV, Daily Value; RDA, Recommended Dietary Allowance; UL, Tolerable Upper Intake Level.

DEFICIENCY	GOOD FOOD SOURCES	TOXICITY
Muscle cramps, fatigue.	Table salt, salty snacks and condiments, processed meats, pickles, sauerkraut, salty cheeses, soy sauce, flavoring salts.	Excess sodium is associated with excessive fluid retention, high blood pressure and its consequences. No UL has been set.
Muscle cramps, heartbeat irregularities, loss of appetite, weakness, drowsiness.	Bananas, potatoes, avocados, oranges, other fruits and vegetables; meats, fish, seafood, poultry; milk and dairy products.	Excess unlikely in healthy people. No more than 18,000 mg is advised. Acute hyperkalemia from excess intake can cause cardiac arrest. No UL has been set.
Hypochloremic metabolic alkalosis, confusion, stupor.	Occurs along with sodium.	Not determined. No UL has been set.
Slow, stunted growth; osteoporosis (bone loss) with dowager's hump, bone fractures, bone pain. Tooth loss. Muscle cramping.	Milk, cheese, yogurt, ice cream; canned fishes with bones; tofu made with calcium carbonate; fortified fruit juices; broccoli, kale, almonds.	**UL:** 2,500 mg May interfere with absorption of iron, zinc, magnesium, and other minerals. May cause kidney stones; may be constipating. Very high blood calcium levels cause coma and cardiac arrest.
Weakness, muscle loss, bone loss and pain, anorexia. (Rare. Most likely in people taking phosphorus-binding drugs.)	Protein-rich foods. Cereal grains. Soft drinks. Present in most foods.	**UL:** 4,000 mg Contributor to osteoporosis. Lowers blood calcium levels. Severe calcium depletion causes convulsions, muscle spasms.
Weakness, confusion. Constipation. Disturbed heart rhythm.	Whole grain products; green vegetables; nuts; legumes; bananas; seafood; molasses; cocoa and chocolate.	**UL:** 350 mg Nausea, vomiting, low blood pressure, diarrhea. Severe hypermagnesemia (from magnesium-containing drugs) depresses breathing, causes coma, cardiac arrest. (UL applies only to magnesium in supplements and drugs.)
None reported.	All protein-rich foods.	Not determined. No UL has been set.

Trace and Ultra-Trace Minerals

NAME	MAIN ROLES	RECOMMENDED INTAKE (ADULT)
Iron	Component of hemoglobin, which transports oxygen in blood; component of myoglobin, which holds oxygen for muscle use. Required for energy utilization, immune function.	**RDA** Men: 8 mg Women: 19–50 yr: 18 mg >50 yr: 8 mg
Zinc	As a cofactor in many enzymes, it is involved with gene expression, protein metabolism, sexual maturation, sperm production, fetal development, and bone health. It is needed for vitamin A metabolism, wound healing, and taste perception.	**RDA** Men: 11 mg Women: 8 mg
Selenium	Component of the antioxidant enzyme glutathione peroxidase. Works synergistically with vitamin E. Involved in immune function and thyroid metabolism.	**RDA** Adults: 55 µg
Iodine	As a component of thyroid hormones, it is involved with regulating body temperature, metabolic rate, reproduction, and growth.	**RDA** Adults: 150 µg
Copper	Functions of copper-containing enzymes include antioxidant activity; participation in electron transport, synthesis of connective tissue, synthesis of melanin; myelination of nerve tissue. It is involved with immune function and heart health. The copper-containing enzyme ceruloplasmin catalyzes oxidation of ferrous to ferric iron.	**RDA** Adults: 900 µg
Manganese	As a cofactor for many enzymes, it assists in energy metabolism, urea synthesis, growth, and reproduction.	**AI** Men: 2.3 mg Women: 1.8 mg

DEFICIENCY	GOOD FOOD SOURCES	TOXICITY
Anemia with weakness, fatigue, reduced learning ability, impaired reactivity and coordination, pale skin or pallor, intolerance of cold. Slowed wound healing. Lowered resistance to infection.	Liver, gizzards, red meat, seafood and fish; enriched grain products; dark green leafy vegetables; nuts, legumes, dried fruits.	**UL:** 45 mg Gastric distress. Accidental iron poisoning in children can cause death. People with hemochromatosis are at risk of toxicity: fatigue; joint pain; liver, kidney, and heart damage; increased oxidation of blood lipids.
Growth retardation, delayed puberty, hypogonadism; loss of taste sensations, anorexia, weight loss, diarrhea; hair loss; delayed wound healing; night blindness; impaired immunity.	Protein-rich foods, especially oysters, red meat, other seafood; whole-grain products.	**UL:** 40 mg Impaired immunity, impaired copper absorption. Acute toxicity (2,000–4,000 mg zinc intake) causes nausea, vomiting, cramping.
Impaired immunity. Susceptibility to Keshan disease (a heart disorder).	Brazil nuts; tuna fish, seafood, meats and poultry, other fish; whole-grain products.	**UL:** 400 μg. Fatigue, "garlic body odor," irritability, abnormal fingernails, hair loss, skin lesions.
Simple goiter is deficiency disease: enlargement of the thyroid gland, cold intolerance, weight gain, sluggishness, decreased body temperature. Cretinism is deficiency disease caused by inadequate iodine intake during pregnancy: mental retardation, stunted growth, deafness.	Iodized salt; ocean fish and seafood; seaweed; foods produced on iodine-rich soils (usually near an ocean); bread made with dough conditioners; dairy products (if iodine-containing disinfectants are used to clean processing areas).	**UL:** 1,100 μg Toxicity produces goiter.
Anemia, bone abnormalities, immune impairment. Menkes' syndrome is a rare, usually fatal genetic disorder causing copper deficiency.	Liver, seafood, nuts, whole grain products, seeds, legumes.	**UL:** 10 mg Wilson's disease is a genetic disorder of copper retention; untreated it causes nerve and liver problems.
None identified in humans.	Whole-grain and cereal products; tea, coffee; cloves; fruits, dried fruits, and vegetables.	**UL:** 11 mg Toxicity is likely to occur from breathing manganese-containing dust, not from diet. Impaired coordination and memory.

(table continues on next page)

Trace and Ultra-Trace Minerals (Continued)

NAME	MAIN ROLES	RECOMMENDED INTAKE (ADULT)
Fluoride	A component of bones and teeth; promotes bone and tooth formation; discourages tooth decay; may reduce risk of osteoporosis.	**AI** Men: 4 mg Women: 3 mg
Chromium	Assists in glucose metabolism.	**AI** 19–50 yr / >50 yr Men: 35 μg / 25 μg Women: 30 μg / 20 μg
Molybdenum	Enzyme cofactor.	**RDA** Adults: 45 μg
Arsenic	Function unclear.	None set.
Boron	Appears to be involved in bone metabolism.	Probable need of ~1 mg.
Nickel	Enzyme cofactor.	Probable need of ~100–300 μg
Silicon	Appears to be involved in bone metabolism.	None set.
Vanadium	Function unclear.	None set.

AI, Adequate Intake; RDA, Recommended Dietary Allowance; UL, Tolerable Upper Intake Level.

DEFICIENCY	GOOD FOOD SOURCES	TOXICITY
Increased tooth decay; possibly increased risk of bone fractures from osteoporosis.	Water, fluoridated or with naturally occurring fluoride. Beverages and foods made with fluoride-containing water.	**UL:** 10 mg Chronic excessive consumption causes fluorosis: discoloration of the teeth, kidney problems, possible muscle or nerve problems. Chronic intake of 2–8 mg daily can mottle children's teeth. Acute fluoride toxicity causes headaches, nausea, abnormal heart rhythm.
Neurological disorders from long-term chromium-free total parenteral nutrition.	Nuts, chocolate, whole grains, mushrooms, asparagus.	Airborne chromium is toxic, but toxicity of dietary sources is unclear.
Weakness, confusion from long-term molybdenum-free total parenteral nutrition.	Peas, beans, organ meats, cereals.	**UL:** 2 mg Possible reproductive problems.
None reported.		Not determined. Excess is clearly toxic. No UL has been set.
None reported.		**UL:** 20 mg Poor appetite, nausea.
None reported.		**UL:** 1 mg Possible delayed growth. Airborne nickel is toxic.
None reported.		Not determined. Airborne silicon causes lung disease. No UL has been set.
None reported.		**UL:** 1.8 mg Possible kidney problems.

APPENDIX F Calculations and Conversions

- Energy from Food
- Recommended Protein Intake for Adults
- Niacin Equivalents (NE)
- Dietary Folate Equivalents (DFE)
- Retinol Activity Equivalents (RAE)
- Vitamin D
- Vitamin E
- Estimating Energy Expenditure
- Body Mass Index (BMI)
- Metric Prefixes
- Length: Metric and U.S. Equivalents
- Capacities or Volumes
- Food Measurement Equivalents
- Food Measurement Conversions: U.S. to Metric
- Food Measurement Conversions: Metric to U.S.
- Conversion Factors
- Fahrenheit and Celsius (Centigrade) Scales

Energy from Food

grams carbohydrate × 4 kcal/g
grams protein × 4 kcal/g
grams fat × 9 kcal/g
grams alcohol × 7 kcal/g
total = energy from food

Example:

Carbohydrate	275 g × 4 kcal/g =	1,100 kcal
Protein	64 g × 4 kcal/g =	256 kcal
Fat	60 g × 9 kcal/g =	540 kcal
Alcohol	15 g × 7 kcal/g =	105 kcal
	TOTAL ENERGY	2,001 kcal

Calculating the percentage of calories for each:

Carbohydrate	(1,100 kcal ÷ 2,001 kcal) × 100 = 54.97% (55%)
Protein	(256 kcal ÷ 2,001 kcal) × 100 = 12.79% (13%)
Fat	(540 kcal ÷ 2,001 kcal) × 100 = 26.99% (27%)
Alcohol	(105 kcal ÷ 2,001 kcal) × 100 = 5.25% (5%)

1 kilocalorie = 4.184 kilojoules
1 kilojoule = 0.239 kilocalories

Recommended Protein Intake for Adults

grams of recommended protein = weight in kilograms × 0.8 g/kg

Example:
A 70-kg (154-lb) person
grams of recommended protein = 70 kg × 0.8 g/kg = 56 grams protein, or
grams of recommended protein = (154 lb ÷ 2.2) × 0.8 g/kg = 56 grams protein

Note: Endurance athletes involved in heavy training require 1.2 to 1.4 grams of protein per kilogram of body weight per day.

Niacin Equivalents (NE)

Determining the amount of niacin from tryptophan:

NE = milligrams niacin
NE from tryptophan = grams excess protein ÷ 6
NE from tryptophan = (grams dietary protein − protein RDA) ÷ 6

Example: Assume dietary protein = 86 g and protein RDA = 56 g
NE from tryptophan = (86 g − 56 g) ÷ 6
NE from tryptophan = 5

Dietary Folate Equivalents (DFE)

Dietary folate equivalents account for differences in the absorption of food folate, synthetic folic acid in dietary supplements, and folic acid added to fortified foods. Food in the stomach also affects bioavailability. Folic acid taken as a supplement when fasting is two times more bioavailable than food folate. Folic acid taken with food and folic acid in fortified foods are 1.7 times more bioavailable than food folate.

1 μg DFE = 1 microgram of food folate
= 0.5 μg of folic acid supplement taken on an empty stomach
= 0.6 μg of folic acid supplement consumed with meals
= 0.6 μg of folic acid in fortified foods

1 μg folic acid as a fortificant = 1.7 μg DFE
1 μg folic acid as a supplement, fasting = 2.0 μg DFE

Example:

Food folate in cooked spinach	100 μg = 100 μg DFE
Ready-to-eat cereal fortified with folic acid	100 μg = 170 μg DFE
Supplemental folic acid taken without food	100 μg = 200 μg DFE

Estimating DFE from Daily Value:
DFE = %DV × DV × bioavailability factor

Example:
Assume that a serving of fortified breakfast cereal contains 10% of the Daily Value for folate
Daily Value = 400 μg folic acid

DFE = %DV × DV × bioavailability factor
DFE = 0.10 × 400 μg × 1.7
DFE = 68 μg, which can be rounded to 70 μg DFE

Retinol Activity Equivalents (RAE)

Retinol activity equivalents are a standardized measure of vitamin A activity that account for differences in the bioavailability of different sources of vitamin A. Of the provitamin A carotenoids, beta-carotene produces the most vitamin A.

1 RAE = 1 μg retinol
= 12 μg beta-carotene
= 24 μg of other vitamin A precursors

Although outdated, many vitamin supplements still report vitamin A content as International Units (IU).

1 IU = 0.3 μg retinol
= 3.6 μg beta-carotene

Vitamin D

Although outdated, many vitamin supplements still report vitamin D content as International Units (IU).

1 IU = 0.025 μg cholecalciferol
μg cholecalciferol = IU ÷ 40

Example:
A vitamin supplement contains 100 IU vitamin D
μg cholecalciferol = 100 ÷ 40 = 2.5

Vitamin E

Although outdated, many vitamin supplements still report vitamin E content as International Units (IU) rather than as milligrams of α-tocopherol. Two conversion factors are used to convert IU to milligrams of α-tocopherol. If the form of the supplement is "natural" or RRR-α-tocopherol (historically labeled as *d*-alpha-tocopherol), the conversion factor is 0.67 mg/IU. If the form of the supplement is *all rac-α-*tocopherol (historically labeled *dl-α*-tocopherol), the conversion factor is 0.45 mg/IU.

Examples:
A multivitamin supplement contains 30 IU of *d*-α-tocopherol
30 IU × 0.67 = 20 mg α-tocopherol
A multivitamin supplement contains 30 IU of *dl*-α-tocopherol
30 IU × 0.45 = 13.5 mg α-tocopherol

Estimating Energy Expenditure

Resting Energy Expenditure (REE)

Harris-Benedict Equations

Adult men **REE = 66 + 13.7*W* + 5.0*H* − 6.8*A***

Adult women **REE = 655 + 9.6*W* + 1.8*H* − 4.7*A***

(*W* = weight in kilograms, *H* = height in centimeters, *A* = age)

Note: Harris-Benedict equations can overestimate resting energy expenditure, especially for obese people.

Quick Estimate

Adult men **REE = weight (kg) × 1.0 kcal/kg × 24 hours**
REE = weight (kg) × 1.0 × 24

Adult women **REE = weight (kg) × 0.9 kcal/kg × 24 hours**
REE = weight (kg) × 0.9 × 24

Equation Table for Estimating REE (Most accurate method)

Age (years)	REE Males	REE Females
0–3	(60.9 × wt) − 54	(61.0 × wt) − 51
3–10	(22.7 × wt) + 495	(22.5 × wt) + 499
10–18	(17.5 × wt) + 651	(12.2 × wt) + 746
18–30	(15.3 × wt) + 679	(14.7 × wt) + 496
30–60	(11.6 × wt) + 879	(8.7 × wt) + 829
>60	(13.5 × wt) + 487	(10.5 × wt) + 596

Body weight is in kg, and REE is kcal/day.

Total Energy Expenditure (TEE)

Activity Factor* Men	Women	Activity Level	Description
1.3	1.3	Sedentary	Mostly resting, with little or no activity
1.6	1.5	Light	Occasional unplanned activity (e.g., going for a stroll)
1.7	1.6	Moderate	Daily planned activity, such as brisk walks
2.1	1.9	Heavy	Daily workout routine requiring several hours of continuous exercise
2.4	2.2	Exceptional	Daily vigorous workouts for extended hours; training for competition

*The activity factor accounts for the thermic effect of food.

Source: Adapted from Recommended Dietary Allowances, 10th ed. Washington, DC: National Academy Press; 1989.

Total energy expenditure (TEE) = REE × activtiy factor

Example: A 120-pound (54.5-kilogram), 19-year-old woman engages in moderate activity

REE = (14.7 × wt) + 496
= (14.7 × 54.5) + 496
= 1,297 kcal/day
TEE = 1,297 kcal/day × 1.6

Body Mass Index (BMI)

U.S. Formula

BMI = [weight in pounds ÷ (height in inches)^2] × 703

Example: **A 154-pound man is 5 ft 8 inches (68 inches) tall**
BMI = [154 ÷ (68 in × 68 in)] × 703
BMI = (154 ÷ 4,624) × 703
BMI = 23.41

Metric Formula

BMI = weight in kilograms ÷ [height in meters]^2
or
BMI = [weight in kilograms ÷ (height in cm)^2] × 10,000

Example: **A 70-kg man is 1.75 meters tall**
BMI = 70 kg ÷ (1.75 m × 1.75 m)
BMI = 70 ÷ 3.0625
BMI = 22.86

Metric Prefixes

giga-	G	1,000,000,000
mega-	M	1,000,000
kilo-	k	1,000
hecto-	h	100
deka-	da	10
deci-	d	0.1
centi-	c	0.01
milli-	m	0.001
micro-	μ	0.000001
nano-	n	0.000000001

Length: Metric and U.S. Equivalents

1 centimeter	0.3937 inch
1 decimeter	3.937 inches
1 foot	0.3048 meter
1 inch	2.54 centimeters
1 meter	39.37 inches
	1.094 yards
1 micron	0.001 millimeter
	0.00003937 inch
1 millimeter	0.03937 inch
1 yard	0.9144 meter

Capacities or Volumes

1 cup, measuring	8 fluid ounces
	1/2 liquid pint
1 gallon (U.S.)	231 cubic inches
	3.785 liters
	0.833 British gallon
	128 U.S. fluid ounces
1 gallon (British Imperial)	277.42 cubic inches
	1.201 U.S. gallons
	4.546 liters
	160 British fluid ounces

1 liter	1.057 liquid quarts
	0.908 dry quart
	61.024 cubic inches
1 milliliter	0.061 cubic inches
1 ounce, fluid or liquid (U.S.)	1.805 cubic inches
	29.574 milliliters
	1.041 British fluid ounces
1 pint, dry	33.600 cubic inches
	0.551 liter
1 pint, liquid	28.875 cubic inches
	0.473 liter
1 quart, dry (U.S.)	67.201 cubic inches
	1.101 liters
	0.969 British quart
1 quart, liquid (U.S.)	57.75 cubic inches
	0.946 liter
	0.833 British quart
1 quart (British)	69.354 cubic inches
	1.032 U.S. dry quarts
	1.201 U.S. liquid quarts
1 tablespoon, measuring	3 teaspoons
	1/2 fluid ounce
1 teaspoon, measuring	1/3 tablespoon
	1/6 fluid ounce
1 kilogram	2.205 pounds
1 microgram (μg)	0.000001 gram

Food Measurement Equivalents

16 tablespoons = 1 cup
12 tablespoons = 3/4 cup
10 tablespoons + 2 teaspoons = 2/3 cup
8 tablespoons = 1/2 cup
6 tablespoons = 3/8 cup
5 tablespoons + 1 teaspoon = 1/3 cup
4 tablespoons = 1/4 cup
2 tablespoons = 1/8 cup
2 tablespoons + 2 teaspoons = 1/6 cup
1 tablespoon = 1/16 cup
2 cups = 1 pint
2 pints = 1 quart
3 teaspoons = 1 tablespoon
48 teaspoons = 1 cup

Food Measurement Conversions: U.S. to Metric

Capacity

1/5 teaspoon	1 milliliters
1 teaspoon	5 milliliters
1 tablespoon	15 milliliters
1 fluid ounce	30 milliliters
1/5 cup	47 milliliters
1 cup	237 milliliters
2 cups (1 pint)	473 milliliters
4 cups (1 quart)	0.95 liter
4 quarts (1 gal.)	3.8 liters

Weight

1 ounce	28 grams
1 pound	454 grams

Food Measurement Conversions: Metric to U.S.

Capacity

1 milliliter	1/5 teaspoon
5 milliliters	1 teaspoon
15 milliliters	1 tablespoon
100 milliliters	3.4 fluid oz
240 milliliters	1 cup
1 liter	34 fluid oz
	4.2 cups
	2.1 pints
	1.06 quarts
	0.26 gallon

Weight

1 gram	0.035 ounce
100 grams	3.5 ounces
500 grams	1.10 pounds
1 kilogram	2.205 pounds
	35 ounces

Conversion Factors

To change	To	Multiply by
centimeters	inches	0.3937
centimeters	feet	0.03281
cubic feet	cubic meters	0.0283
cubic meters	cubic feet	35.3145
cubic meters	cubic yards	1.3079
cubic yards	cubic meters	0.7646
feet	meters	0.3048
gallons (U.S.)	liters	3.7853
grams	ounces avdp	0.0353
grams	pounds	0.002205
inches	millimeters	25.4000
inches	centimeters	2.5400
inches	meters	0.0254
kilograms	pounds	2.2046
liters	gallons (U.S.)	0.2642
liters	pints (dry)	1.8162
liters	pints (liquid)	2.1134
liters	quarts (dry)	0.9081
liters	quarts (liquid)	1.0567
meters	feet	3.2808
meters	yards	1.0936
millimeters	inches	0.0394
ounces avdp	grams	28.3495
ounces	pounds	0.0625
pints (dry)	liters	0.5506
pints (liquid)	liters	0.4732
pounds	kilograms	0.4536
pounds	ounces	16
quarts (dry)	liters	1.1012
quarts (liquid)	liters	0.9463

Fahrenheit and Celsius (Centigrade) Scales

°Celsius	°Fahrenheit
−273.15	−459.67
−250	−418
−200	−328
−150	−238
−100	−148
−50	−58
−40	−40
−30	−22
−20	−4
−10	14
0	32
5	41
10	50
15	59
20	68
25	77
30	86
35	95
40	104
45	113
50	122
55	131
60	140
65	149
70	158
75	167
80	176
85	185
90	194
95	203
100	212

Zero on the Fahrenheit scale represents the temperature produced by the mixing of equal weights of snow and common salt.

	°Fahrenheit	°Celsius
Boiling point of water	212°	100°
Freezing point of water	32°	0°
Normal body temperature	98.6°	37°
Comfortable room temperature	68–77°	20–25°
Absolute zero	−459.6°	−273.1°

Absolute zero is theoretically the lowest possible temperature, the point at which all molecular motion would cease.

To Convert Temperature Scales

To convert Fahrenheit to Celsius (Centigrade), subtract 32 and multiply by $\frac{5}{9}$.

$$°C = \frac{5}{9}(°F - 32)$$

To convert Celsius (Centigrade) to Fahrenheit, multiply by $\frac{9}{5}$ and add 32.

$$°F = \left(\frac{9}{5} \times °C\right) + 32$$

Nutrition Assessment: Determining Nutritional Health

In a nutritional sense, what does it mean to be healthy? Nutritional health is quite simply obtaining all the nutrients in amounts needed to support body processes. We can measure nutritional health in a number of ways. Taken together, such measurements can give you much insight into your current and long-term well-being. The process of measuring nutritional health is usually termed **nutrition assessment**.

Nutrition assessment serves a variety of purposes. It may help evaluate nutrition-related risks that may jeopardize a person's current or future health. Nutrition assessment is a routine part of the nutritional care of hospitalized patients. In this setting, nutrition assessment not only identifies risks, but also measures the effectiveness of treatment. In public health, nutrition assessment helps identify people in need of nutrition-related interventions and monitors the effectiveness of intervention programs. Sometimes, assessments determine the nutritional health of an entire population—identifying health risks common in a population group so specific policy measures can be developed to combat them.

nutrition assessment Measurement of the nutritional health of the body. It can include anthropometric measurements, biochemical tests, clinical observations, and dietary intake, as well as medical histories and socioeconomic factors.

ABCDs of nutrition assessment Nutrition assessment components: Anthropometric measurements, Biochemical tests, Clinical observations, and Dietary intake.

Nutrition Assessment of Individuals

In health care settings, a registered dietitian or physician may do an individual nutrition assessment of a patient or client. Depending on the purpose of the nutrition assessment, the measures may be very comprehensive and detailed. A dietitian can then use this information to plan individualized nutrition counseling. Nutrition assessment measures often are repeated in order to assess the effectiveness of nutrition counseling or a change in diet.

Nutrition Assessment of Populations

Population-based nutrition assessment is done in conjunction with programs to monitor the status of nutrition in the United States or Canada or as part of large-scale epidemiological studies. Typically, nutrition assessment of populations is not as comprehensive as an assessment of an individual. One of the largest ongoing nationwide surveys of dietary intake and health status is the National Health and Nutrition Examination Survey (NHANES). To date, four of these surveys have been completed, and they have told us a great deal about the nutritional status of our population. Another tool for monitoring the dietary intake of Americans is the Continuing Survey of Food Intake by Individuals (CSFII).

Nutrition Assessment Methods

Just as there is not one measure of physical fitness, there is not just one indicator of nutritional health. Nutrients play many roles in the body, so measures of nutritional status must look at many factors. Often these factors are termed the **ABCDs of nutrition assessment:** Anthropometric measurements, Biochemical tests, Clinical observations, and Dietary intake (see **Table G.1**).

Table G.1 **The ABCDs of Nutrition Assessment**

Assessment Method	*Why It's Done*
Anthropometric measures	Measure growth in children; show changes in weight that can reflect diseases (e.g., cancer or thyroid problems); monitor progress in fat loss
Biochemical tests	Measure blood, urine, and feces for nutrients or metabolites that indicate infection or disease
Clinical observations	Assess change in skin color and health, hair texture, fingernail shape, etc.
Dietary intake	Evaluate diet for nutrient (e.g., fat, calcium, protein) or food (e.g., number of fruits and vegetables) intake

Anthropometric Measurements

Anthropometric measurements are physical measurements of the body, such as height and weight, head circumference, girth measurement, or skinfold measurements.

Height and Weight

To provide useful information, height and weight must be measured accurately. For infants and very young children, measurement of height is really measurement of recumbent length (that is, when they are lying down). Careful measurement of length at each checkup gives a clear indication of a child's growth rate. Standard growth charts show how the child's growth compares with that of others of the same age and gender. For children 2 to 20 years old, charts illustrating growth are based on standing height, or stature. (See Appendix H.)

The standing height of older children and adults can be determined with a tape measure fixed to a wall and a sliding right-angle headboard for reading the measurement. Aging adults lose some height due to bone loss and curvature, so it is important to measure height and not simply rely on remembered values. Because many calculations/standards use metric measures, it's important to be familiar with standard conversion factors.

To convert inches to centimeters, multiply the number of inches by 2.54

inches × 2.54 = centimeters

To convert pounds to kilograms, divide the number of pounds by 2.2

pounds ÷ 2.2 = kilograms

Weight is a critical measure in nutrition assessment. It is used to assess children's growth, predict energy expenditure and protein needs, and determine body composition. Weight should be measured using a calibrated scale. For assessments that need a high degree of precision, subtract the weight of the clothing.

For the anthropometric assessment of infants and young children, a third measurement is common: head circumference. This is measured using a flexible tape measure, put snugly around the head. Head circumference measures are another useful indicator of normal growth and development, especially during rapid growth from birth to age 3.

anthropometric measurements Measurements of the physical characteristics of the body, such as height, weight, head circumference, girth, and skinfold measurements. Anthropometric measurements are particularly useful in evaluating the growth of infants, children, and adolescents and in determining body composition.

skinfold measurements A method to estimate body fat by measuring with calipers the thickness of a fold of skin and subcutaneous fat.

Skinfolds

Skinfold measurements serve a variety of purposes. Because a significant amount of the body's fat stores are right beneath the skin (subcutaneous fat), the sizes of skinfolds at various sites around the body can give a good indication of body fatness. This information may be used to evaluate the physical fitness of an athlete or predict the risk of obesity-related disorders. Skinfold measurements are also useful in cases of illness; the maintenance of fat stores in a patient's body may be a valuable indicator of dietary adequacy. Skinfold measurements are done with special calipers (see **Figure G.1**). For reliable measurements, training in the use of calipers is essential. Skinfold measurements can be used to estimate the percentage of body fat, or can be compared with percentile tables for specific gender and age categories.

Biochemical Tests

Because of their relation to growth and body composition, anthropometric measurements give a broad picture of nutritional health—whether the diet contains enough calories and protein to maintain normal patterns of growth, normal body composition, and normal levels of lean body mass. However, anthropometric measures do not give specific information about *nutrients.* For that information, a variety of biochemical tests are useful.

Biochemical assessment measures a nutrient or metabolite (a related compound) in one or more body fluids such as blood and urine, or in feces. For example, the concentration of albumin (an important transport protein) in the blood can be an indicator of the body's protein status. If little protein is eaten, the body produces smaller amounts of body proteins such as albumin.

biochemical assessment Assessment by measuring a nutrient or its metabolite in one or more body fluids such as blood and urine, and in feces. Also called laboratory assessment.

Biochemical assessment may include measurements of a nutrient metabolite, a storage or transport compound, an enzyme that depends on a vitamin or mineral, or another indicator of the body's functioning in relation to a particular nutrient. These measures usually are a better indicator of nutritional status than directly measuring blood levels of nutrients such as vitamin A or calcium. The levels of nutrients excreted in the urine or feces also provide valuable information.

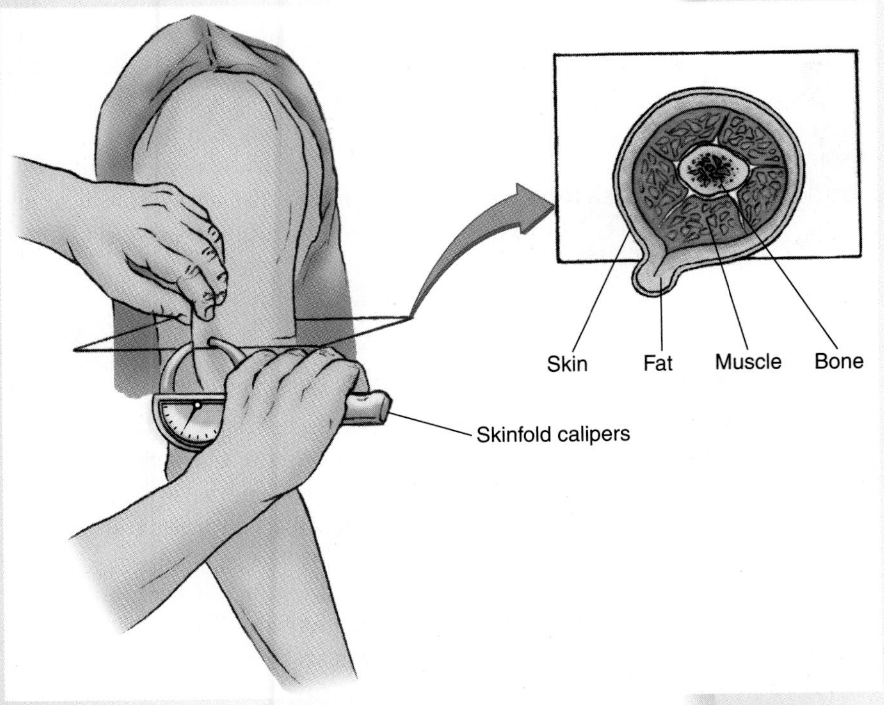

Figure G.1 **Skinfold measurements.** A significant amount of the body's fat stores lie just beneath the skin, so when done correctly skinfold measurements can provide an indication of body fatness. An inexperienced or careless measurer, however, can easily make large errors. Skinfold measurements usually work better for monitoring malnutrition than for identifying overweight and obesity. They also are widely used in large population studies.

Clinical Observations

Clinical observations—the characteristics of health that can be seen during a physical exam—help complete the picture of nutritional health. While often nonspecific, clinical signs are clues to nutrient deficiency or excess that can be confirmed or ruled out by further testing. In a clinical nutrition examination, a clinician observes the hair, nails, skin, eyes, lips, mouth, bones, muscles, and joints. Specific findings, such as cracking at the corners of the mouth (suggestive of riboflavin, vitamin B_6, or niacin deficiency) or petechiae (small, pinpoint hemorrhages on the skin indicative of vitamin C deficiency) need to be followed by other assessments.

Dietary Intake

A picture of nutritional health would not be complete without information about dietary intake. Dietary information may confirm the lack or excess of a dietary component suggested by anthropometric, biochemical, or clinical evaluations.

There are a number of ways to collect dietary intake data. Each has strengths and weaknesses. It is important to match the method to the type and quantity of data needed. Remember, too, that the quality of information obtained about people's diets often relies heavily on people's memories, as well as their honesty in sharing those recollections. How well do you remember *everything* you ate yesterday?

clinical observations Assessment by evaluating the characteristics of well-being that can be seen in a physical exam. Nonspecific, clinical observations can provide clues to nutrient deficiency or excess that can be confirmed or ruled out by biochemical testing.

diet history Record of food intake and eating behaviors that includes recent and long-term habits of food consumption. Done by a skilled interviewer, the diet history is the most comprehensive form of dietary intake data collection.

food records Detailed information about day-to-day eating habits; typically includes all foods and beverages consumed for a defined period, usually three to seven consecutive days.

weighed food records Detailed food records obtained by weighing foods before eating, and then weighing leftovers to determine the exact amount consumed.

food frequency questionnaire (FFQ) A questionnaire for nutrition assessment that asks how often the subject consumes specific foods or groups of foods, rather than what specific foods the subject consumes daily. Also called food frequency checklist.

Diet History

The most comprehensive form of dietary intake data collection is the **diet history.** In this method, a skilled interviewer finds out not only what the client has been eating in the recent past but also the client's long-term food consumption habits. The interviewer's questions also may address other risk factors for nutrition-related problems, such as economic issues.

Food Record

Food records, or diaries, provide detailed information about day-to-day eating habits. Typically, a person records all foods and beverages consumed during a defined period, usually three to seven consecutive days. Because food records are recorded concurrently with intake, they are less prone to inaccuracy from lapses in memory. Because the data are completely self-reported, however, food records will not be accurate if the person fails to record all items. To make food records more precise, the items in a meal can be weighed before consumption. Remaining portions are weighed at the end of the meal to determine exactly how much was eaten. **Weighed food records** are much more time consuming to complete.

Food Frequency Questionnaire

A **food frequency questionnaire (FFQ)** asks how often the subject consumes specific foods or groups of foods, rather than what specific foods the subject consumes daily. A food frequency questionnaire may ask, for example, "How often do you drink a cup of milk?" with response options of daily, weekly, monthly, and so on (see **Figure G.2**). This information is used to estimate that person's average daily intake.

Although food frequency questionnaires do not require a trained interviewer and can be completed relatively quickly, there are disadvantages to this method of data collection. One problem is that it is often difficult to translate a person's response to how often they drink milk, or how many

Food Item	Average Use during Past Year					
	<1 serving per month	1–3 servings per month	1–4 servings per week	5–7 servings per week	2–4 servings per day	5+ servings per day
Coffee					√	
Dark bread	√					
Ice cream				√		

Food Item	Medium Serving	Your Serving Size			How Often?				
		S	M	L	Day	Week	Month	Year	Never
Coffee	(1 cup)			√	2				
Dark bread	(1 slice)								√
Ice cream	(1/2 cup)		√			3			

Figure G.2 **Examples of food frequency questionnaire formats.**
Source: Adapted from Lee RD, Nieman DC. *Nutritional Assessment.* 2nd ed. St. Louis: Mosby; 1996.

cups of milk they drink per week, into specific nutrient values without more detailed information. More importantly, food frequency questionnaires require a person to average, over a long period, foods that may be consumed erratically in portions that are sometimes large and sometimes small.

Twenty-Four-Hour Dietary Recall

The **twenty-four-hour dietary recall** is the simplest form of dietary intake data collection. In a twenty-four-hour recall, the interviewer takes the client through a recent 24-hour period (usually midnight to midnight) to determine what foods and beverages the client consumed. To get a complete, accurate picture of the subject's diet, the interviewer must ask probing questions like, "Did you put anything on your toast?" but not leading questions like, "Did you put butter and jelly on your toast?" Comprehensive population surveys frequently use twenty-four-hour recalls as the main method of data collection. While a single twenty-four-hour recall is not very useful for describing the nutrient content of an individual's overall diet (there's too much day-to-day variation), in large-scale studies it gives a reasonably accurate picture of the average nutrient intake of a population. Multiple diet recalls also are useful for estimating nutrient intake of individuals.

twenty-four-hour dietary recall A form of dietary intake data collection. The interviewer takes the client through a recent 24-hour period (usually midnight to midnight) to determine what foods and beverages the client consumed.

Methods of Evaluating Dietary Intake Data

Once the data are collected, the next step is to determine the nutrient content of the diet and evaluate that information in terms of dietary standards or other reference points. This is commonly done using nutrient analysis software. Computer programs remove the tedium of looking up foods in tables of nutrient composition; large databases allow for simple access to food composition, and the computer does the math automatically.

Comparison to Dietary Standards

It is possible to compare a person's nutrient intake to dietary standards such as the RDA or AI values. Although this will give a qualitative idea of dietary adequacy, it cannot be considered a definitive evaluation of a person's diet because we don't know that individual's specific nutrient requirements. Comparisons of individual diets to RDA or AI values should be interpreted with caution.

Comparison to Food Guide Pyramid

Another type of dietary analysis compares a person's food intake to the Food Guide Pyramid. This involves categorizing foods into the various groups and determining the number of servings the subject has eaten. Evaluators often have trouble making these comparisons because many common foods (e.g., pizza, sandwiches, casseroles) contain servings or partial servings from multiple food groups.

Comparison to Dietary Guidelines for Americans

For a general picture of the subject's dietary habits, the evaluator can compare the person's diet to the *Dietary Guidelines for Americans.* While these evaluations usually are not specific, they give a general idea of whether the subject's diet is high or low in saturated fat, or whether the subject is eating enough fruits and vegetables.

Outcomes of Nutrition Assessment

When taken together, anthropometric measures, biochemical tests, clinical exams, and dietary evaluation, along with the individual's family history, socioeconomic situation, and other factors give a complete picture of nutritional health. A client's assessment may lead to a recommendation for a diet change to reduce weight or blood cholesterol, the addition of a vitamin or mineral supplement to treat a deficiency, the identification of abnormal growth due to inadequate infant feeding, or simply the affirmation that dietary intake is adequate for current nutrition needs.

2 to 20 years: Boys
Stature-for-Age and Weight-for-Age Percentiles

NAME ______________________

RECORD # ______________

Mother's Stature ____________ Father's Stature ____________

Date	Age	Weight	Stature	BMI*

***To Calculate BMI**: Weight (kg) ÷ Stature (cm) ÷ Stature (cm) x 10,000
or Weight (lb) ÷ Stature (in) ÷ Stature (in) x 703

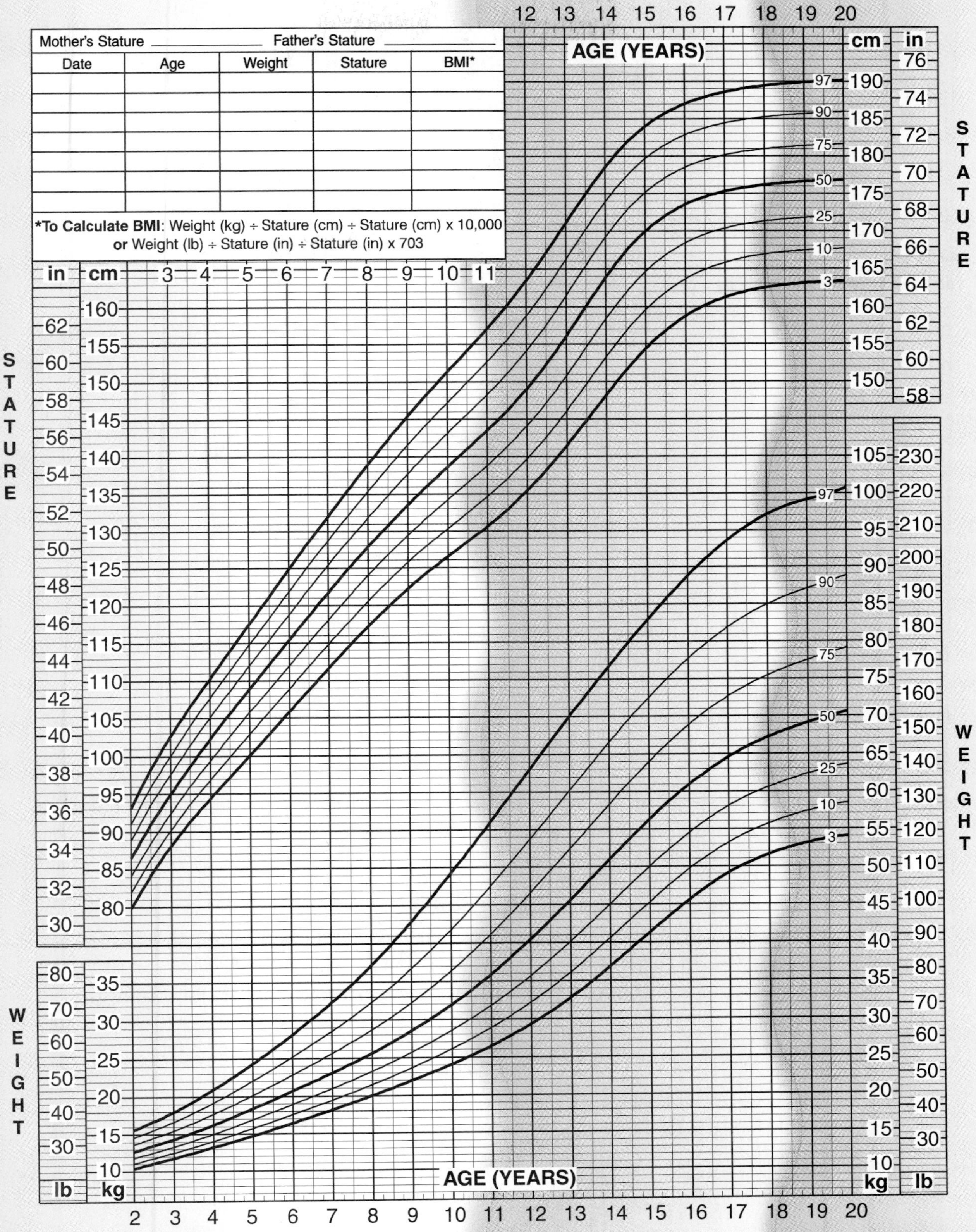

SOURCE: Developed by the National Center for Health Statistics in collaboration with the National Center for Chronic Disease Prevention and Health Promotion (2000).
http://www.cdc.gov/growthcharts

CDC

APPENDIX I Food Safety Tables

- Minimum Internal Cooking Temperatures
- Cold Storage Chart

Minimum Internal Cooking Temperatures

Fresh ground beef, veal, lamb, pork	160°F
Beef, veal, lamb roasts, steaks, chops	
Medium	160°F
Well done	170°F
Fresh pork roasts, steaks, chops	
Medium	160°F
Well done	170°F
Ham	
Cook before eating	160°F
Fully cooked, to reheat	140°F
Poultry	
Ground chicken, turkey	165°F
Whole chicken, turkey	180°F
Breasts, roasts	170°F
Thighs and wings	Cook until juices run clear
Egg dishes, casseroles	160°F
Leftovers	165°F

Source: USDA Food Safety and Inspection Service

Cold Storage Chart

Since product dates aren't a guide for safe use of a product, consult this chart and follow these tips. These short but safe time limits will help keep refrigerated food (40°F) from spoiling or becoming dangerous.

- Purchase the product before "sell-by" or expiration dates.
- Follow handling recommendations on product.
- Keep meat and poultry in its package until just before using.
- If freezing meat and poultry in its original package longer than two months, overwrap these packages with airtight heavy-duty foil, plastic wrap, or freezer paper, or place the package inside a plastic bag.

Because freezing (0°F) keeps food safe indefinitely, recommended freezer storage times are for quality only.

Product	Refrigerator	Freezer
Eggs		
Fresh, in shell	3 weeks	Don't freeze
Raw yolks, whites	2 to 4 days	1 year
Hard cooked	1 week.	Doesn't freeze well
Liquid pasteurized eggs or egg substitutes		
Opened	3 days	Don't freeze
Unopened	10 days	1 year
Cooked egg dishes	3 to 4 days	Doesn't freeze well

Product	Refrigerator	Freezer
Dairy Products		
Swiss, brick, processed cheese	3 to 4 weeks	Can be frozen, but freezing affects texture and taste
Mayonnaise, Commercial		
Refrigerate after opening	2 months	Don't freeze
TV Dinners, Frozen Casseroles		
Keep frozen until ready to heat	Keep frozen	3 to 4 months
Deli and Vacuum-Packed Products		
Store-prepared (or homemade) egg, chicken, tuna, ham, macaroni salads	3 to 5 days	Doesn't freeze well
Pre-stuffed pork and lamb chops, chicken breasts stuffed with dressing	1 day	Doesn't freeze well
Store-cooked convenience meals	3 to 4 days	Doesn't freeze well
Commercial brand vacuum-packed dinners with USDA seal, unopened	2 weeks	Doesn't freeze well
Raw Hamburger, Ground and Stew Meat		
Hamburger and stew meats	1 to 2 days	3 to 4 months
Ground turkey, veal, pork, lamb, and mixtures of them	1 to 2 days	3 to 4 months
Ham, Corned Beef		
Corned beef in pouch with pickling juices	5 to 7 days	Drained, 1 month
Ham, canned, labeled "Keep Refrigerated"		
Opened	3 to 5 days	1 to 2 months
Unopened	6 to 9 months	Don't freeze
Ham, fully cooked, whole	7 days	1 to 2 months
Ham, fully cooked, half	3 to 5 days	1 to 2 months
Ham, fully cooked, slices	3 to 4 days	1 to 2 months
Hot Dogs and Lunch Meats (in freezer wrap)		
Hot dogs		
Opened package	1 week	1 to 2 months
Unopened package	2 weeks	1 to 2 months
Lunch meats		
Opened package	3 to 5 days	1 to 2 months
Unopened package	2 weeks	1 to 2 months
Soups and Stews		
Vegetable or meat-added	3 to 4 days	2 to 3 months
Bacon and Sausage		
Bacon	7 days	1 month
Sausage, raw from pork, beef, chicken, or turkey	1 to 2 days	1 to 2 months
Smoked breakfast links, patties	7 days	1 to 2 months
Summer sausage labeled "Keep Refrigerated"		
Opened	3 weeks	1 to 2 months
Unopened	3 months	1 to 2 months
Fresh Meat (Beef, Veal, Lamb, and Pork)		
Steaks	3 to 5 days	6 to 12 months
Chops	3 to 5 days	4 to 6 months
Roasts	3 to 5 days	4 to 12 months
Variety meats (tongue, kidneys, liver, heart, chitterlings)	1 to 2 days	3 to 4 months

Product	Refrigerator	Freezer
Meat Leftovers		
Cooked meat and meat dishes	3 to 4 days	2 to 3 months
Gravy and meat broth	1 to 2 days	2 to 3 months
Fresh Poultry		
Chicken or turkey, whole	1 to 2 days	1 year
Chicken or turkey, parts	1 to 2 days	9 months
Giblets	1 to 2 days	3 to 4 months
Cooked Poultry, Leftover		
Fried chicken	3 to 4 days	4 months
Cooked poultry dishes	3 to 4 days	4 to 6 months
Pieces, plain	3 to 4 days	4 months
Pieces covered with broth, gravy	1 to 2 days	6 months
Chicken nuggets, patties	1 to 2 days	1 to 3 months
Fish		
Lean (such as cod)	1 to 2 days	up to 6 months
Fatty (such as blue, perch, salmon)	1 to 2 days	2 to 3 months

Sources: Food Marketing Institute for fish and dairy products, USDA Food Safety and Inspection Service for all other foods.

Academic

www.mayoclinic.com/findinformation/healthylivingcenter/index.cfm
Mayo Clinic nutrition information

www.navigator.tufts.edu
Tufts University Nutrition Navigator

Aging

www.aoa.gov
Administration on Aging
330 Independence Avenue SW
Washington, DC 20201
(202) 619-7501

www.aarp.org
American Association of Retired Persons (AARP)
601 E Street NW
Washington, DC 20049
(800) 424-3410

www.americangeriatrics.org
American Geriatrics Society
The Empire State Building
350 Fifth Avenue, Suite 801
New York, NY 10118
(212) 308-1414

www.aoa.gov/naic
National Aging Information Center
330 Independence Avenue SW
Washington, DC 20201
(202) 619-7501

www.ncoa.org
National Council on the Aging
1828 L Street NW
Washington, DC 20036

www.nia.nih.gov
National Institute on Aging
Building 31, Room 5C27
31 Center Drive, MSC 2292
Bethesda, MD 20892
(301) 496-1752

www.nof.org
National Osteoporosis Foundation
1232 22nd Street NW
Washington, DC 20037-1292
(202) 223-2226

Alcohol and Drug Abuse

www.al-anon.alateen.org
Al-Anon/Alateen
1600 Corporate Landing Parkway
Virginia Beach, VA 23154-5617
(888) 425-2666, (757) 563-1600

www.aa.org
Alcoholics Anonymous (AA)
General Service Office
Grand Central Station
P.O. Box 459
New York, NY 10163
(212) 870-3400

www.covesoft.com/csap.html
Center for Substance Abuse Prevention
1010 Wayne Avenue, Suite 850
Silver Spring, MD 20910
(301) 459-1591 ext. 244; fax: (301) 495-2919

www.wsoinc.com
Narcotics Anonymous (NA)
P.O. Box 9999
Van Nuys, CA 91409
(818) 773-9999; fax: (818) 700-0700

www.health.org
National Clearinghouse for Alcohol and Drug Information (NCADI)
P.O. Box 2345
Rockville, MD 20847-2345
(800) 729-6686

www.ncadd.org
National Council on Alcoholism and Drug Dependence (NCADD)
20 Exchange Place
Suite 2902
New York, NY 10005
(800) 622-2255; (212) 269-7797; fax: (212) 269-7510

Canadian Government: Federal

www.agr.gc.ca
Agriculture and Agri-Food Canada
Public Information Request Services
Sir John Carling Building
930 Carling Avenue
Ottawa, Ontario K1A 0C5
(613) 759-1000; fax: (613) 759-6726

www.hc-sc.gc.ca/food-aliment/ns-sc/e_nutrition.html
Bureau of Nutritional Sciences
Nutrition Research Division
Sir Fredrick G. Banting Research Center
Tunney's Pasture (2203C)
Ottawa, Ontario K1A 0L2
(613) 957-0919; fax: (613) 941-6182

Canadian Government: Federal (continued)

www.hc-sc.gc.ca/food-aliment/ns-sc/e_nutrition.html
Bureau of Nutritional Sciences
Nutrition Evaluation Division
Sir Fredrick G. Banting Research Center
Tunney's Pasture (2203A)
Ottawa, Ontario K1A 0L2
(613) 957-0352; fax: (613) 941-6636

www.inspection.gc.ca
Canadian Food Inspection Agency
59 Camelot Drive
Ottowa, Ontario K1A 0Y9
(800) 442-2342, (613) 225-2342; fax: (613) 228-6653

www.cihi.ca
Canadian Institute for Health Information
377 Dalhousie Street
Suite 200
Ottawa, Ontario K1N 9N8
(613) 241-7860; fax: (613) 241-8120

www.cpha.ca
Canadian Public Health Association
400-1565 Carling Avenue
Ottawa, Ontario K1Z 8R1
(613) 725-3769; fax: (613) 725-9826

www.agr.ca/food/nff/enutrace.html
Functional Foods and Nutraceuticals
Food Bureau
597-930 Carling Avenue
Ottawa, ON K1A 0C5

www.hc-sc.gc.ca
Health Canada

www.nin.ca
National Institute of Nutrition
265 Carling Avenue, Suite 302
Ottawa, Ontario K1S 2E1
(613) 235-3355; fax: (613) 235-7032

Canadian Government: Provincial and Territorial

Consultant, Nutrition
Health and Wellness Promotion, Population Health, Department of Health and Social Services, Government of the Northwest Territories
Center Square Tower, 6th Floor
P.O. Box 1320
Yellowknife, NT X1A 2L9

Coordinator, Health Information Resource Center
Department of Health and Social Services
1 Rochford Street, Box 2000
Charlottetown, PEI C1A 7N8

Director, Health Promotion
Department of Health, Government of Newfoundland and Labrador
P.O. Box 8700
Confederation Building, West Block
St. John's, NF A1B 4J6

Director, Nutrition Services
Yukon Hospital Corporation
#5 Hospital Road
Whitehorse, YT Y1A 3H7

Executive Director
Health Programs
2nd Floor 800 Portage Avenue
Winnipeg, MB R3G 0P4

Health Promotion Unit
Population Health Branch
Saskatchewan Health
3475 Albert Street
Regina, SK S4S 6X6

Nutritionist
Preventive Services Branch
Ministry of Health
1520 Blanshard Street
Victoria, BC V8W 3C8

Population Health Strategies Branch
Alberta Health
23rd Floor, TELUS Plaza, North Tower
10025 Jasper Avenue
Edmonton, AB T5J 2N3

Project Manager, Public Health Management Services
Health and Community Services
P.O. Box 5100
520 King Street
Fredericton, NB E3B 5G8

Public Health Nutritionist
Central Health Region
201 Brownlow Avenue, Unit 4
Dartmouth, NS B3B 1W2

Responsables de la santé cardiovasculaire et de la nutrition
Ministère de la Santé et des Services sociaux, Service de la Prévention en Santé
3e étage, 1075, chemin Sainte-Foy
Quèbec, (Quèbec) G1S 2M1

Senior Consultant, Nutrition
Public Health Branch
Ministry of Health, 8th Floor
5700 Yonge St.
New York, Ontario M2M 4K5

Complementary and Alternative Nutrition

http://nccam.nih.gov/
National Center for Complementary and Alternative Medicine, NIH

www.hc-sc.gc.ca/hpb/onhp/
Office of Natural Health Products
171 Slater Street
9th Floor
Ottawa, ON K1P 5H7
(613) 946-1615

Consumer Organizations

www.diabetes.ca
Canadian Diabetes Association
15 Toronto Street
Suite 800
Toronto, ON M5C 2E3
(800) 226-8464; (416) 363-3373

www.cspinet.org
Center for Science in the Public Interest (CSPI)
1875 Connecticut Ave NW, Suite 300
Washington, DC 20009-5728
(202) 332-9110; fax: (202) 265-4954

www.consumersunion.org
Consumers Union
101 Truman Avenue
Yonkers, NY 10703-1057
(914) 378-2000

www.pueblo.gsa.gov
Federal Consumer Information Center
Pueblo, CO 81009
(800) 688-9889; (888) 878-3256

www.ncahf.org
National Council Against Health Fraud, Inc. (NCAHF)
119 Foster Street
Peabody, MA 01960
(978) 532-9383

www.partnershipforcaring.org/HomePage
Partnership for Caring
1620 I Street NW, Suite 202
Washington, DC 20006
(202) 296-8071; fax: (202) 296-8352

www.quackwatch.com
Stephen Barrett, MD
P.O. Box 1747
Allentown, PA 18105
(610) 437-1795

Eating Disorders

www.anred.com
Anorexia Nervosa and Related Eating Disorders (ANRED)
P.O. Box 5102
Eugene, OR 97405
(541) 344-1144

www.anad.org
National Association of Anorexia Nervosa and Associated Disorders, Inc. (ANAD)
P.O. Box 7
Highland Park, IL 60035
(847) 831-3438; fax: (847) 433-4632

www.nedic.ca
National Eating Disorder Information Centre
200 Elizabeth Street, CW 1-211
Toronto, Ontario M5G 2C4
(866) 633-4220, (416) 340-4156; fax: (416) 340-4736

www.nationaleatingdisorders.org
National Eating Disorders Association
603 Stewart Street, Suite 803
Seattle, WA 98101
(206) 382-3587

Food Safety

www.foodsafetyalliance.org
Alliance for Food & Farming
Food Safety Hotline
(800) 266-0200

www.cfsan.fda.gov
FDA Center for Food Safety and Applied Nutrition
5100 Paint Branch Parkway
College Park, MD 20740
(888) 723-3366

www.epa.gov/opptintr/lead/nlic.htm
National Lead Information Center
(800) 424-5323

www.npic.orst.edu/index.html
National Pesticide Information Center
Oregon State University
333 Weniger Hall
Corvallis, OR 97331-6502
(800) 858-7378

Seafood Safety Hotline
(800) 332-4010; (202) 205-4314

U.S. EPA Safe Drinking Water Hotline
(800) 426-4791

www.fsis.usda.gov
USDA Food Safety and Inspection Service
Food Safety Education Office
Room 1180-S
Washington, DC 20250
(202) 720-3333

USDA Meat and Poultry Hotline
(800) 535-4555

Infancy, Childhood, and Adolescence

www.aap.org
American Academy of Pediatrics
141 Northwest Point Boulevard
Elk Grove Village, IL 60007-1098
(847) 434-4000; fax: (847) 434-8000

www.birthdefects.org
Birth Defect Research for Children, Inc.
930 Woodcock Road
Suite 225
Orlando, FL 32803
(407) 895-0802

www.cps.ca
Canadian Paediatric Society
100-2204 Walkley Road
Ottawa, ON K1G 4G8
(613) 526-9397; fax: (613) 526-3332

Infancy, Childhood, and Adolescence (continued)

www.childrensfoundation.net
Children's Foundation
725 Fifteenth Street NW
Suite 505
Washington, DC 20005-2109
(202) 347-3300; fax: (202) 347-3382

www.KidsHealth.org
KidsHealth
The Nemours Foundation

www.ncemch.org
National Center for Education in Maternal & Child Health
2000 15th Street North
Suite 701
Arlington, VA 22201-2617
(703) 524-7802

International Agencies

www.fao.org
Food and Agriculture Organization of the United Nations (FAO)
Liaison Office for North America
2175 K Street, Suite 300
Washington, DC 20437
(202) 653-2400

www.ific.org
International Food Information Council Foundation
1100 Connecticut Avenue NW
Suite 430
Washington, DC 20036
(202) 296-6540

www.unicef.org
UNICEF
3 United Nations Plaza
New York, NY 10017
(212) 326-7000; fax: (212) 887-7465

www.who.int/home-page
World Health Organization (WHO)
Regional Office
525 23rd Street NW
Washington, DC 20037
(202) 974-3000; fax: (202) 974-3663

Pregnancy and Lactation

www.acog.org
American College of Obstetricians and Gynecologists
Resource Center
409 12th Street SW
Washington, DC 20024-2188
(202) 638-5577

www.lalecheleague.org
La Leche League International, Inc.
1400 N. Meacham Road
Schaumburg, IL 60173-4048
(847) 519-7730

www.modimes.org
March of Dimes Birth Defects Foundation
1275 Mamaroneck Avenue
White Plains, NY 10605
(888) 663-4637

Professional Nutrition Organizations

ADA, The Nutrition Line
(800) 366-1655

www.eatright.org
American Dietetic Association (ADA)
216 West Jackson Boulevard
Suite 800
Chicago, IL 60606-6995
(800) 877-1600, (312) 899-0040

www.faseb.org/ascn
American Society for Clinical Nutrition
9650 Rockville Pike
Bethesda, MD 20814-3998
(301) 530-7110; fax: (301) 571-1863

www.faseb.org/asns
American Society for Nutritional Sciences
9650 Rockville Pike
Suite 4500
Bethesda, MD 20814
(301) 530-7050; fax: (301) 571-1892

Canadian Dietetic Association
480 University Avenue
Suite 601
Toronto, ON M5G 1V2

Canadian Society for Nutritional Sciences
Department of Food and Nutrition
University of Manitoba
Winnipeg, Manitoba R3T 2N2

www.dietitians.ca
Dietitians of Canada
480 University Avenue, Suite 604
Toronto, Ontario M5G 1V2
(416) 596-0857; fax: (416) 596-0603

http://hni.ilsi.org
ILSI Human Nutrition Institute (HNI)
One Thomas Circle
Washington, DC 20005
(202) 659-0524; fax: (202) 659-3617

www.ift.org
Institute of Food Technologists
525 West Van Buren
Suite 1000
Chicago, IL 60607
(312) 782-8424; fax: (312) 782-8348

www.nationalacademies.org/nrc
National Academy of Sciences/National Research Council (NAS/NRC)
2101 Constitution Avenue NW
Washington, DC 20418
(202) 234-2000

www.stfx.ca/academic/human-nutrition/organization/one.html
Organization for Nutrition Education
Woodlawn Postal Outlet
P.O. Box 25
Guelph, ON N1H 8H6

www.sne.org
Society for Nutrition Education
9202 North Meridian
Suite 200
Indianapolis, IN 46260
(800) 235-6690

Sports Nutrition

www.acsm.org
American College of Sports Medicine (ACSM)
401 W. Michigan Street
Indianapolis, IN 46202-3233
(317) 637-9200; fax: (317) 634-7817

www.acefitness.org
American Council on Exercise (ACE)
4851 Paramount Drive
San Diego, CA 92123
(800) 825-3636

www.cahperd.ca
Canadian Association for Health, Physical Education, Recreation, and Dance
403-2197 Riverside Drive
Ottawa, ON K1H 7X3
(613) 523-1348

www.csep.ca
Canadian Society for Exercise Physiology
185 Somerset St. West
Suite 202
Ottawa, ON K2P 0J2
(613) 234-3755; fax: (613) 234-3565

www.fitness.gov
President's Council on Physical Fitness and Sports
Humphrey Building, Room 738
200 Independence Avenue SW
Washington, DC 20201
(202) 690-9000; fax: (202) 690-5211

www.runnersworld.com
Runners World
Rodale, Inc.
Emmaus, PA 18098
(610) 967-8809

Sports Medicine and Science Council of Canada
1600 James Naismith Drive
Suite 306
Gloucester, Ontario K1B 5N4
(613) 748-5671; fax: (613) 748-5729

Sports Safety Board of Quebec
100 Laviolette
Bureau 306
Trois-Riveres, Quebec G9A 5S9
(819) 371-6033

www.nutrifit.org
Sports, Cardiovascular and Wellness Nutritionists (SCAN)
P.O. Box 4995
Buena Vista, CO 81211
(719) 395-9271

www.ideafit.com
The International Association for Fitness Professionals (IDEA)
6190 Cornerstone Court East # 204
San Diego, CA 92121-3773
(800) 999-4332 ext 7; fax: (858) 535-8234

www.veggie.org/
Veggie Sports Association

Supplements

http://dietary-supplements.info.nih.gov/databases/ibids.html
International Bibliographic Information on Dietary Supplements (IBIDS)

http://dietary-supplements.info.nih.gov
Office of Dietary Supplements
National Institutes of Health
Building 31, Room 1B29
31 Center Drive, MSC 2086
Bethesda, MD 20892-2086
(301) 435-2590; fax: (301) 480-1845

Trade and Industry Organizations

www.aibonline.org
American Institute of Baking
1213 Bakers Way
P.O. Box 3999
Manhattan, KS 66505-3999
(800) 633-5137, (785) 537-4750; fax: (785) 537-1493

www.meatami.org
American Meat Institute
1700 North Moore Street
Suite 1600
Arlington, VA 22209
(703) 841-2400; fax: (703) 527-0938

www.beechnut.com
Beech-Nut Nutrition Corporation
100 S. 4th Street
St. Louis, MO 63102
(800) 233-2468

Trade and Industry Organizations (continued)

www.gssiweb.com
Gatorade Sports Science Institute
617 West Main Street
Barrington, IL 60010
(800) 616-4774

www.GeneralMills.com/corporate
General Mills, Inc.
Number One General Mills Boulevard
Minneapolis, MN 55426
(800) 328-6787

www.gerber.com
Gerber Products Co.
445 State Street
Fremont, MI 49413-0001
(800) 443-7237

www.heinz.com
H.J. Heinz Company
World Headquarters
P.O. Box 57
Pittsburgh, PA 15230-0057
(412) 456-5700

www.kelloggs.com
Kellogg Company
P.O. Box 3599
Battle Creek, MI 49016-3599
(616) 961-2000

www.kraftfoods.com
Kraft Foods
Consumer Response and Information Center
One Kraft Court
Glenview, IL 60025
(800) 323-0768

www.nationaldairycouncil.org
National Dairy Council
10255 West Higgins Road
Suite 900
Rosemont, IL 60018-5616
(847) 803-2000

www.pillsbury.com
Pillsbury Company
2866 Pillsbury Center
Minneapolis, MN 55402
(800) 775-4777

www.pg.com
Procter & Gamble Company
One Procter and Gamble Plaza
Cincinnati, OH 45202
(513) 983-1100

www.sunkist.com
Sunkist Growers
Consumer Affairs, Fresh Fruit Division
14130 Riverside Drive
Sherman Oaks, CA 91423
(800) 248-7875

www.dannon.com
The Dannon Company
120 White Plains Road
Tarrytown, NY 10591-5536
(877) 326-6668

www.nutrasweet.com
The NutraSweet Company
P.O. Box 2986
Chicago, IL 60654-0986
(800) 323-5316

www.uffva.org
United Fresh Fruit and Vegetable Association
727 North Washington Street
Alexandria, VA 22314
(703) 836-3410

www.usarice.com
USA Rice Federation
4301 North Fairfax Drive
Suite 305
Arlington, VA 22203
(703) 351-8161

http://63.81.122.102/cognis/verisonline/default.asp
VERIS Research Information Service
5325 S. 9th Avenue
LaGrange, IL 60525
(800) 554-1708; (612) 927-7104; fax: (612) 927-6406

Weight Management

http://nutrition.uvm.edu/bodycomp/
Body Composition Analysis Tutorials

www.overeatersanonymous.org
Overeaters Anonymous (OA)
World Service Office
6075 Zenith Court NE
Rio Rancho, NM 87124
(505) 891-2664; fax: (505) 891-4320

www.shapeup.org
Shape Up America!
6707 Democracy Boulevard
Suite 306
Bethesda, MD 20817
(301) 493-5368

www.tops.org
TOPS (Take Off Pounds Sensibly)
4575 South Fifth Street
P.O. Box 07360
Milwaukee, WI 53207-0360
(800) 932-8677; (414) 482-4620

www.niddk.nih.gov/health/nutrit/win.htm
Weight-control Information Network
1 WIN Way
Bethesda, MD 20892-3665
(877) 946-4627, (202) 828-1025; fax: (202) 828-1028

www.weightwatchers.com
Weight Watchers International
Consumer Affairs Department/IN
175 Crossways Park West
Woodbury, NY 11797
(516) 390-1400; fax: (516) 390-1632

World Hunger

www.bread.org
Bread for the World
50 F Street, NW
Suite 500
Washington, DC 20001
(800) 822-7323, (202) 639-9400

http://hunger.tufts.edu
Center on Hunger, Poverty and Nutrition Policy
Tufts University School of Medicine
11 Curtis Avenue
Medford, MA 02155
(617) 627-6223; fax: (617) 627-3688

www.freefromhunger.org
Freedom from Hunger
1644 DaVinci Court
Davis, CA 95616
(800) 708-2555; fax: (530) 758-6241

www.oxfamamerica.org
Oxfam America
26 West Street
Boston, MA 02111-1206
(800) 776-9326; fax: (617) 728-2594

www.worldwatch.org
Worldwatch Institute
1776 Massachusetts Avenue NW
Suite 800
Washington, DC 20036
(202) 452-1999

U.S. Government

www.nutrition.gov
Online federal government information on nutrition

www.cdc.gov
Centers for Disease Control and Prevention
1600 Clifton Road
Atlanta, GA 30333
(800) 311-3435, (404) 639-3534

FDA Consumer Information Line
(301) 827-4420

FDA Office of Nutritional Products, Labeling and Dietary Supplements
HFS-800
200 C Street SW
Washington, DC 20204
(202) 205-4561; fax: (202) 205-4594

FDA Office of Plant and Dairy Foods and Beverages
HFS-300
200 C Street SW
Washington, DC 20204
(202) 205-4064; fax: (202) 205-4422

www.ftc.gov
Federal Trade Commission (FTC)
CRC-240
Washington, DC 20580
(877) 382-4357

www.fda.gov
Food and Drug Administration (FDA)
Office of Consumer Affairs, HFE 1
Room 16-85
5600 Fishers Lane
Rockville, MD 20857
(888) 463-6332, (301) 443-1544

www.nal.usda.gov/fnic
Food and Nutrition Information Center
National Agricultural Library, Room 105
10301 Baltimore Avenue
Beltsville, MD 20705-2351
(301) 504-5719; fax: (301) 504-6409

www.frac.org
Food Research and Action Center (FRAC)
1875 Connecticut Avenue NW
Suite 540
Washington, DC 20009
(202) 986-2200; fax: (202) 986-2525

www.healthfinder.gov
Gateway for health and nutrition information
www.nidr.nih.gov
National Institute of Dental and Cranofacial Research (NIDCR)
National Institutes of Health
Bethesda, MD 20892-2190
(301) 496-4261

www.niddk.nih.gov
National Institute of Diabetes & Digestive & Kidney Diseases
Office of Communications and Public Liaison
NIDDK, NIH
Building 31, Room 9A04 Center Drive, MSC 2560
Bethesda, MD 20892-2560

www.nih.gov/health
National Institutes of Health search engine and free access to MEDLINE and PubMed databases

www.usda.gov
U.S. Department of Agriculture (USDA)
14th Street SW and Independence Avenue
Washington, DC 20250
(202) 720-2791

U.S. Government (continued)

www.dhhs.gov
U.S. Department of Health and Human Services
200 Independence Avenue SW
Washington, DC 20201
(877) 696-6775, (202) 619-0257

www.epa.gov
U.S. Environmental Protection Agency (EPA)
1200 Pennsylvania Avenue NW
Washington, DC 20460
(202) 260-2090

www.pueblo.gsa.gov
U.S. General Services Administration
Federal Communication Information Center
Pueblo, CO 81009

www.access.gpo.gov/su_docs
U.S. Government Printing Office
Superintendent of Documents
Washington, DC 20402
(202) 512-1071

www.hhs.gov/phs/
U.S. Public Health Service
200 Independence Avenue SW
Washington, DC 20201
(877) 696-6775, (202) 619-0257

www.usda.gov/cnpp
USDA Center for Nutrition Policy and Promotion
3101 Park Center Drive
Room 1034
Alexandria, VA 22302-1594
(703) 305-7600; fax: (703) 305-3400

Index/Glossary

Key terms in the text appear here in **bold** followed by the definition.

ABC model of behavior A behavioral model that includes the external and internal events that precede and follow the behavior. The "A" stands for antecedents, the events that precede the behavior ("B"), which is followed by consequences ("C") that positively or negatively reinforce the behavior, 286

ABCDs of nutrition assessment Nutrition assessment components: Anthr.opometric measurements, Biochemical tests, Clinical observations, and Dietary intake, G1–G6

Absorption The movement of substances into or across tissues; in particular, the passage of nutrients and other substances into the walls of the gastrointestinal tract and then into the bloodstream, 94, 97–106
- of alcohol, 356, 361
- of calcium, 316–317, 393–395
- of carbohydrates, 133–134
- of carotenoids, 315
- of chromium, 416
- of copper, 412
- factors, 12, 112–113
- of iron, 400–401, 404
- of lipids, 174–176
- of medications, 545
- of minerals, 384
- of niacin, 330
- of olestra, 181–183
- of phosphorus, 396
- and pregnancy, 493
- of proteins, 206
- of sterols, 176
- of vitamins, 302–303, 334, 336
- of zinc, 406–409

Acesulfame K [ay-see-SUL-fame] An artificial sweetener that is 200 times sweeter than common table sugar (sucrose). Because it is not digested and absorbed by the body, acesulfame contributes no calories to the diet and yields no energy when consumed, 147

Acetaldehyde A toxic intermediate compound formed by the action of alcohol dehydrogenase enzyme during the metabolism of alcohol, 356–357

Acetaminophen, 545

Acetylcholine, 341

Acetyl CoA A key intermediate product in the metabolic breakdown of carbohydrates, fatty acids, and amino acids. It consists of a two-carbon acetate group linked to coenzyme A, which is derived from pantothenic acid, 238–240, 243, 244–245, D1
- and cholesterol, 251
- and pantothenic acid, 337

Acid-base balance, 203, 390–391

Acidosis An abnormally low blood pH (below about 7.35) due to increased acidity, 203

Acne An inflammatory skin eruption that usually occurs in or near the sebaceous glands of the face, neck, shoulders, and upper back, 534

Acquired Immune Deficiency Syndrome (AIDS), 500, 600–601, 602

Acrolein A pungent decomposition product of fats, generated from dehydrating the glycerol component of fats; responsible for the coughing attacks caused by the fumes released by burning fat. This toxic water-soluble liquid vaporizes easily and is highly flammable, 112

Active transport The movement of substances into or out of cells against a concentration gradient. Active transport requires energy (ATP) and involves carrier (transport) proteins in the cell membrane, 99

Added fiber The isolated nondigestible carbohydrates added to foods, which have beneficial physiological effects in humans, 130, 143

Additives Substances added to food to perform various functions, such as adding color or flavor, replacing sugar or fat, improving nutritional content, or improving texture or shelf life, 65–68, 214

Adenosine triphosphate. *See* ATP

Adequate Intake (AI) The nutrient intake that appears to sustain a defined nutritional state or some other indicator of health (e.g., growth rate of normal circulating nutrient values) in a specific population or subgroup. AI is used when there is insufficient scientific evidence to establish an EAR, 45, G6

Adipocytes Fat cells, 164, 175

Adipose tissue Body fat tissue, 164, 249, 251–252

Adolescence The period between onset of puberty an adulthood, 531–536
- and alcohol, 534, 535
- athletes, 443, 447–448
- and minerals, 395, 443, 531
- pregnant, 501
- and substance (ab)use, 534, 535
- *See also* Eating disorders

ADP (adenosine diphosphate) [ah-DEN-oh-seen di-FOS-fate] A molecule composed of adenosine and two phosphate groups, 236

Adrenaline. *See* Epinephrine

Advertising
- and children, 525–526
- of dietary supplements, 78
- as influential factor, 7
- regulation, 572

Aerobic [air-ROW-bic] Referring to the presence of or need for oxygen. The complete breakdown of glucose, fatty acids, and amino acids to carbon dioxide and water occurs only via aerobic metabolism. The citric acid cycle and electron transport chain are aerobic pathways, 237, 431

Aerobic endurance The ability of skeletal muscle to obtain a sufficient supply of oxygen from the heart and lungs to maintain muscular activity for a prolonged time, 435

Aflatoxins Carcinogenic and toxic factors produced by food molds, 569

Africa, 126, 603

African Americans, 529

Age factors
- and exercise, 448
- and fiber, 151
- and magnesium, 397
- and obesity, 276
- and perspiration, 448
- and protein intake, 210–211
- and starvation, 254
- and sugar, 148
- *See also* Adolescence; Babies; Childhood; Elderly; Infancy

Agriculture, 604–605

AIDS, 500, 600–601, 602

Air, swallowing, 117

Alanine, 253, D1

Albumin A protein that circulates in the blood and helps transport many minerals and some drugs, 412

Alcohol
- and central nervous system, 361–362

Alcohol Common name for ethanol or ethyl alcohol. As a general term, it refers to any organic compound with one or more hydroxyl (–OH) groups.
- absorption, 356
- abuse, 371
- and adolescents, 534, 535
- and athletes, 446

Photo Credits

Chapter openers created by Studio Montage.

All incidental and background photos and art © PhotoDisc, Corbis Digital Images, Hemera Photo Objects.

4 Mickey Pfleger/PictureQuest; 5 PhotoDisc; 6 (A) Karl Weatherly/PhotoDisc; (B) Owen Franken/Corbis; (C) Suza Scalora/PhotoDisc; 7 Courtesy of The National Dairy Council; 8 Ryan McVay/PhotoDisc; 9 (T) PhotoDisc; 9 (B) Peter Menzel/Stock, Boston Inc./PictureQuest; 24 Courtesy of the FDA; 30 NovaStock/Photo Researchers, Inc.,; 43 Hisham F. Ibrahim/PhotoDisc ; 44 Hisham F. Ibrahim/PhotoDisc; 46 Jones and Bartlett; 48 Jones and Bartlett; 50 (A) Jones and Bartlett; 50 (B) Jones and Bartlett; 60 PhotoDisc; 61 PhotoDisc; 68 Jones and Bartlett; 69 David Young-Wolff/PhotoEdit; 74 Bonnie Kamin/PhotoEdit; 92 Prof P. Motta/Dept. of Anatomy/University "La Sapienza", Rome/Science Photo Library; 112 (A) EyeWire; (B) Chris Shorten/Cole Group/PhotoDisc; (C) PhotoLink/PhotoDisc; (D) USDA/Science Source/Photo Researchers, Inc.; 119 (T) © A.B. Dowsett/SPL/Photo Researchers, Inc.; 119 (B) Dr. E. Walker/Science Photo Library; 120 PhotoDisc; 126 (A) Sylvan Wittwer/Visuals Unlimited; (B) David Nance/ARS Photo Library/USDA; (D) USDA; 131 J.D. Litvay/Visuals Unlimited; 139 Barros & Barros/ImageBank; 140 (T) Digital Vision; 140 (B) PhotoDisc; 142 Don Tremain/PhotoDisc; 143 PhotoDisc (top); © Health Canada (top middle); USDA photo (bottom middle); USDA photo (bottom); 148 Digital Stock; 163 Steve Mason/PhotoDisc; 164 Veronica Burmeister/Visuals Unlimited; 165 PhotoDisc; 166 Jones and Bartlett; 183 PhotoDisc; 209 (L) EyeWire; 209 (M) Keith Brofsky/PhotoDisc; 209 (R) EyeWire; 210 © Health Canada (top); USDA photo (middle); USDA photo (bottom); 211 Don Smetzer/Tony Stone; 212 PhotoDisc; 214 Jones and Bartlett; 216 PhotoDisc; 221 (A) Charles Cecil/Visuals Unlimited; (B) Seamus Murphy/SABA; 230 Quest/Science Photo Library; 252 Bob Montesciaros/Cole Group/PhotoDisc; 260 PhotoDisc; 267 Jones and Bartlett ; 271 Jones and Bartlett; 271 Courtesy of Life Measurement Instruments; 279 (T) The Bridgeman Art Library; 279 (M) Pix/FPG; 279 (B) AP Photo/Doug Mills; 281 Michael Philip Manheim/Photo Network/PictureQuest; 283 Karl Weatherly/PhotoDisc; 290 Jones and Bartlett Publishers; 323 CNRI/Science Photo Library/Photo Researchers, Inc.; 327 L. V. Bergman/The Bergman Collection; 328 Richard Pasley/Stock, Boston/PictureQuest; 330 Peter Essick/PictureQuest; 353 (A) Jack Star/PhotoLink/PhotoDisc; (B) Mitch Hrdlicka/PhotoDisc; (C) Yoav Levy/PictureQuest; 354 David M. Phillips/Visuals Unlimited; 356 (A–C) PhotoDisc; 359 PhotoDisc; 361 PhotoDisc; 362 Tomi/PhotoLink/PhotoDisc; 366 OJ Staats/Custom Medical Stock Photography; 384 Scott Bauer/ARS Photo Library/USDA; 386 Dr. Michael Klein/Peter Arnold, Inc.; 391 CNRI/Science Photo Library/Photo Researchers, Inc.; 411 Martin Rotker/Phototake; 415 NIH/Custom Medical Stock Photograpy; 430 PhotoDisc; 431 PhotoDisc; 432 PhotoDisc; 441 AP Photo/Nils Meilvang; 449 Jones and Bartlett; 454 AP Photo/Kamran Jebrili; 464 PhotoDisc; 466 (T) Hulton-Deutch Collection/CORBIS; 466 (B) Linda DeBruyn; 469 Tony Latham/Tony Stone; 472 Jack Star/PhotoLink; 474 Jack Star/PhotoLink; 477 Jack Star/PhotoLink/PhotoDisc; 478 AP Photo/AP World Wide; 480 Gerard Loucel/Tony Stone Images; 488 PhotoDisc; 490 Mel Curtis/PhotoDisc; 492 Lennart Nilsson/A Child Is Born; 494 Ian O'Leary/Tony Stone Images; 498 David H. Wells/CORBIS; 506 (T) David R. Austen/Stock Boston/PictureQuest; 506 (M) Lynne Siler/Focus Group/PictureQuest; 506 (B) Michael Newman/PhotoEdit/PictureQuest; 509 PhotoDisc; 511 Jones and Bartlett; 512 Myrleen Ferguson Cate/Photo Network/PictureQuest; 514 Gill/Custom Medical Stock Photography; 533 Rubber Ball Productions/EyeWire; 534 SW Productions/PhotoDisc; 539 (T) PhotoLink/PhotoDisc; 539 (B) PhotoLink/PhotoDisc; 546 Susan Lerner/Design Conceptions/Joel Gordon; 548 Bill Aron/PhotoEdit; 566 (A) PhotoDisc; (B) Scott Camazine/Photo Researchers, Inc.; 571 (TL) PhotoDisc; 571 (BL) PhotoLink/PhotoDisc; 571 (TR) C Squared Studios/PhotoDisc; 571 (BR) Siede Preis/PhotoDisc; 576 Illustration courtesy of Partnership for Food Safety Education; 595 (T) PhotoDisc; 595 (TM) Skip Nall/PhotoDisc; 595 (BM) Jack Star/PhotoLink/PhotoDisc; 595 (B) PhotoDisc; 598 (T) AP Photo/Danny Johnston; 598 (B) Bob Daemmrich/Stock, Boston/PictureQuest;

Tolerable Upper Intake Levels (UL[1])

Life stage group	Vitamin A[2] (µg/d)	Vitamin D (µg/d)	Vitamin E[3,4] (mg/d)	Niacin[4] (mg/d)	Vitamin B_6 (mg/d)	Folate[4] (µg/d)	Vitamin C (mg/d)	Choline (g/d)	Calcium (g/d)	Phosphorus (g/d)	Magnesium[5] (mg/d)
Infants											
0-6 mo	600	25	ND[7]	ND	ND	ND	ND	ND	ND	ND	ND
7-12 mo	600	25	ND	ND	ND	ND	ND	ND	ND	ND	ND
Children											
1-3 y	600	50	200	10	30	300	400	1.0	2.5	3	65
4-8 y	900	50	300	15	40	400	650	1.0	2.5	3	110
Males, females											
9-13 y	1,700	50	600	20	60	600	1,200	2.0	2.5	4	350
14-18 y	2,800	50	800	30	80	800	1,800	3.0	2.5	4	350
19-70 y	3,000	50	1,000	35	100	1,000	2,000	3.5	2.5	4	350
>70 y	3,000	50	1,000	35	100	1,000	2,000	3.5	2.5	3	350
Pregnancy											
≤18 y	2,800	50	800	30	80	800	1,800	3.0	2.5	3.5	350
19-50 y	3,000	50	1,000	35	100	1,000	2,000	3.5	2.5	3.5	350
Lactation											
≤18 y	2,800	50	800	30	80	800	1,800	3.0	2.5	4	350
19-50 y	3,000	50	1,000	35	100	1,000	2,000	3.5	2.5	4	350

Life stage group	Iron (mg/d)	Zinc (mg/d)	Selenium (µg/d)	Iodine (µg/d)	Copper (µg/d)	Manganese (mg/d)	Fluoride (mg/d)	Molybdenum (µg/d)	Boron (mg/d)	Nickel (mg/d)	Vanadium[6] (mg/d)
Infants											
0-6 mo	40	4	45	ND	ND	ND	0.7	ND	ND	ND	ND
7-12 mo	40	5	60	ND	ND	ND	0.9	ND	ND	ND	ND
Children											
1-3 y	40	7	90	200	1,000	2	1.3	300	3	0.2	ND
4-8 y	40	12	150	300	3,000	3	2.2	600	6	0.3	ND
Males, females											
9-13 y	40	23	280	600	5,000	6	10	1,100	11	0.6	ND
14-18 y	45	34	400	900	8,000	9	10	1,700	17	1.0	ND
19-70 y	45	40	400	1,100	10,000	11	10	2,000	20	1.0	1.8
>70 y	45	40	400	1,100	10,000	11	10	2,000	20	1.0	1.8
Pregnancy											
≤18 y	45	34	400	900	8,000	9	10	1,700	17	1.0	ND
19-50 y	45	40	400	1,100	10,000	11	10	2,000	20	1.0	ND
Lactation											
≤18 y	45	34	400	900	8,000	9	10	1,700	17	1.0	ND
19-50 y	45	40	400	1,100	10,000	11	10	2,000	20	1.0	ND

[1]UL = The maximum level of daily nutrient intake that is likely to pose no risk of adverse effects. Unless otherwise specified, the UL represents total intake from food, water, and supplements. Due to lack of suitable data, ULs could not be established for vitamin K, thiamin, riboflavin, vitamin B_{12}, pantothenic acid, biotin, carotenoids, arsenic, chromium, or silicon. In the absence of ULs, extra caution may be warranted in consuming levels above recommended intakes.
[2]As preformed vitamin A (retinol) only.
[3]As α-tocopherol; applies to any form of supplemental α-tocopherol.
[4]The ULs for vitamin E, niacin, and folate apply to synthetic forms obtained from supplements, fortified foods, or a combination of the two.
[5]The ULs for magnesium represent intake from a pharmacological agent only and do not include intake from food and water.
[6]Although vanadium in food has not been shown to cause adverse effects in humans, there is no justification for adding vanadium to food and vanadium supplements should be used with caution. The UL is based on adverse effects in laboratory animals and these data could be used to set a UL for adults but not children or adolescents.
[7]ND = Not determinable due to lack of data on adverse effects in this age group and concern with regard to lack of ability to handle excess amounts. Source of intake should be from food only to prevent high levels of intake.

Sources: Data compiled from *Dietary Reference Intakes for Calcium, Phosphorus, Magnesium, Vitamin D, and Fluoride.* Washington, DC: National Academy Press; 1997. *Dietary Reference Intakes for Thiamin, Riboflavin, Niacin, Vitamin B_6, Folate, Vitamin B_{12}, Pantothenic Acid, Biotin, and Choline.* Washington, DC: National Academy Press; 1998. *Dietary Reference Intakes for Vitamin C, Vitamin E, Selenium, and Carotenoids.* Washington, DC: National Academy Press; 2000. *Dietary Reference Intakes for Vitamin A, Vitamin K, Arsenic, Boron, Chromium, Copper, Iron, Manganese, Molybdenum, Nickel, Silicon, Vanadium, and Zinc.* Washington, DC: National Academy Press; 2001. These reports may be accessed via http://nap.edu.